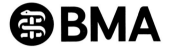 BRITISH MEDICAL ASSOCIATION

COMPLETE HOME
MEDICAL
GUIDE

BMA Consulting Medical Editor

Dr Michael Peters

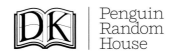

DK London
Consulting Editor Martyn Page
Senior Editor Janet Mohun
Senior Art Editor Ina Stradins
Managing Editor Angeles Gavira
Managing Art Editor Michael Duffy
Jacket Designer Mark Cavanagh
Jacket Editor Claire Gell
Jacket Designer Development Manager Sophia MTT
Preproduction Producer Luca Frassinetti
Producer Mary Slater
Publisher Liz Wheeler
Publishing Director Jonathan Metcalf

DK India
Head of Publishing Operations Aparna Sharma
Managing Editor Rohan Sinha
Design Manager Sudakshina Basu
Designer Konica Juneja
Assistant Editors Shramana Purkayastha, Sneha Sunder Benjamin
DTP Manager Balwant Singh
DTP Designer Anita Yadav

First published in Great Britain in 2000 by Dorling Kindersley Limited
80 Strand, London WC2R ORL

First UK edition, 2000
Second UK edition, 2005
Third UK edition, 2010
Fourth UK edition, 2016

Copyright © 2000, 2005, 2010, 2016 Dorling Kindersley Limited, London
A Penguin Random House Company

2 4 6 8 10 9 7 5 3 1

001 – 283259 – June/2016

A CIP catalogue record for this book is available from the British Library

ISBN 978-0-2412-2594-3

British Medical Association

Chair of Council Dr Mark Porter
Treasurer Dr Andrew Dearden
Chair of Representative Body Dr Ian Wilson
BMA Consulting Medical Editor Dr Michael Peters MB BS

Medical Editors and Reviewers

Dr Jeremy Beider MB BS MSc MRCPsych
Les Bernhardt FRCOG FRCS
Dr Jocelyn A.S. Brooks MB BS FRCR FRCP
Mr Rudy Crawford MBE BSc (Hons) MB ChB FRCS (Glasg) FRCEM
Miss Clare Davey BSc MB BS FRCS FRCOphth
Dr Sue Davidson MB BS FRCP MRCGP
Dr Tamara Everington MB BS MRCP FRCPath PhD
Prof Julian Halcox MA MD FRCP
Dr Lara Hawkes MB BCh MRCP
Lauren Limb MSc
Dr Alasdair D. Mace DLO FRCS (ORL-HNS)
Dr Janice Main MB ChB FRCP
Dr Tanya Malkiel BDS
Dr Hadi Manji MA MD FRCP

Dr Steven Mann MB ChB FRCP
Dr Stephen Motto BM DipSportsMed DM-SMed FFSEM(UK)
Dr Neal Navani MA MSc PhD FRCP
Dr Dean Noimark BSc MRCP
Dr Lee Noimark MRCPCH
Mr Mark Ornstein FRCS
Mr Adam Rodin BSc MB BS FRCOG
Dr Kevin M. O'Shaughnessy MA BM BCh DPhil FRCP
Dr Richard Smith BSc MSc MB BS FRCP PGDip
Mr Peter Whelan MS FRCS
Dr Frances Williams MA MB BChir MRCP DTM&H MRCPCH
Dr Stuart Wolfman MB ChB MRCP

Previous Editions

Medical Editors

BMA Consulting Medical Editor Dr Michael Peters MB BS
Medical Editor Tony Smith MA BM BCh
Deputy Medical Editor Sue Davidson MB BS MRCP MRCGP DRCOG
Assistant Medical Editors Naomi Craft BSc MB BS MRCGP, Gabrielle Murphy BA BSc MB ChB, Fiona Payne MB BS, Penny Preston MB ChB MRCGP, Amanda Rouse BSC MB BS MRCP MRCGP, Frances Williams MA MB BChir MRCP DTM&H MRCPCH
Medical Editor-in-Chief (US) David Goldman MD FACP
Associate Medical Editor (US) David A. Horowitz MD

Medical Reviewers and Contributors

Michael Adler MD FRCP FFPHM
Robert N. Allan MD FRCP
Samir Alvi BSc MB BS PhD DFFP DRCOG
Ursula Arens
Helen Barnett BPharm
Jeffrey L. Barron MB ChB MSc MMed FRCPath
Sir Peter Beale KBE FRCP FFCM FFOM DTM&H
Ian R. Beider BDS (U.Lond.)
Jacky Bernett BSc RD
Huw Beynon BSc MD FRCP
A. Graham Bird FRCP FRCPath

Robin L. Blair MB FRCS (Ed.) FRCS (C.) FACS
Fiona Boag MB BS FRCP
Sue Bosanko
Charles G. D. Brook MA MD FRCP FRCPCH
Jocelyn A. S. Brookes MB BS MRCP FRCR
Jane de Burgh RGN
Helen Byrt PhD
Frank Chinegwundoh MB BS MS FRCS (Eng & Ed) FRCS (Urol) FEBU
Clare Davey BSc MB BS FRCS FRCOphth
Christopher Davidson MA (Cantab.) MB FRCP FESC

Dorling Kindersley London

Dorling Kindersley India

Contents

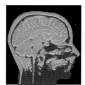

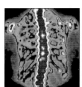

Treating disease 566–624

taking control of your health

GOOD HEALTH IS SOMETHING most of us take for granted. When it fails, it is often for reasons that could have been avoided. Protecting your health is mainly a matter of understanding what causes disease and other problems so that you can take appropriate steps to avoid them. Modern techniques of immunization and screening offer protection against a wide range of illnesses. By taking advantage of these and maintaining a healthy lifestyle, you can safeguard your health not only for the present but for the future as well.

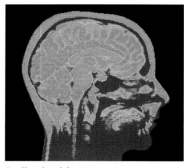

Feeling healthy
Certain psychological factors, such as how well you sleep and cope with stress, affect your general wellbeing, which in turn can influence your physical health.

Feeling healthy involves more than simply being free from disease; it also involves a general sense of wellbeing. Your health and wellbeing depend in part on factors that are often beyond your control, such as the amount of pollution in your environment and the security of your employment. However, there are many aspects of your lifestyle that you can change or adapt to improve your physical and mental health, which will reduce your chance of becoming ill. This part of the book explores a number of strategies that can help you to take control of your own health. It also includes information about screening programmes that help to identify potential health problems at an early stage.

What determines health?

Your health is partly determined by your genes, but it is also inextricably linked with your environment and lifestyle. Your chance of developing many diseases is determined

The moment of conception
Your susceptibility to many diseases is programmed at conception when the sperm and egg cells fuse, bringing together half a set of genes from each parent.

at the moment of conception by the mix of genetic material that you inherit from your parents. Sometimes, you inherit a specific faulty gene, such as the gene that causes cystic fibrosis, that will inevitably lead to the development of a disease. However, it is more common for a person's genetic inheritance merely to predispose him or her to a disease or disorder that may develop later in life, such as diabetes mellitus.

Even if you are genetically susceptible to a disease, your chance of developing it can be influenced by a number of other factors, many of which are related to the way you live. For example, lifestyle factors such as diet, exercise, smoking, and alcohol consumption are important determinants of health. If you adopt a healthy lifestyle and have appropriate screening tests, you may be able to reduce your risk of developing the diseases that are common in your family.

The environment you live in can have an influence on both your general health and your susceptibility to particular diseases.

For example, high levels of pollution in the atmosphere, such as airborne particles of soot and smoke, may exacerbate the symptoms of respiratory diseases such as asthma. Many environmental effects are more pronounced in children, as their bodies are still developing.

Other determining factors of health include age, gender, ethnicity, and occupation. For example, the risk of developing heart disease increases with age and is more common in men, Asian people, and people who have sedentary jobs.

Assessing your health

To understand your inheritance and reduce your risk of disease, you need to know about conditions that run in your family. There may be certain disorders, especially types of cancer or heart disease, that have occurred in several family members under the age of 50. You can create a family medical tree of disorders and discuss them with your doctor. He or she will check your state of health and advise you about lifestyle changes, such as changing to a healthier diet or taking exercise, that could reduce your risk of developing these diseases.

At certain times in your life, particularly as you get older, you will be offered screening tests for early signs of diseases, such as breast or bowel cancer. Depending on your family medical history, your doctor may suggest extra, or earlier, screening to pick up on any signs of disorders that run in your family at the earliest stage possible.

Choosing a healthy lifestyle

In recent years, there has been clear evidence that people can reduce their susceptibility to disease by targeting unhealthy aspects of their lifestyle. The fall in the numbers of deaths before the age of 65 from stroke, coronary

Exercise
Cardiovascular exercise, like cycling, can lower blood pressure, reduce body fat, and alleviate stress, which all helps to prevent heart disease.

artery disease, and certain types of cancer in the past 25 years has been largely attributed to a fall in the number of smokers and a better understanding of what makes a healthy diet. By contrast, the strains of modern living, such as the break-up of relationships, long working hours in stressful jobs, and loss of contact with family and friends, can affect mental and physical wellbeing.

Nearly everyone is aware of the features that make up a healthy lifestyle, but too few people manage to act on this information. By adopting a healthy diet, taking regular exercise, not smoking, and limiting your alcohol consumption, you can bring about an almost instant improvement in your general health. In the longer term, you will benefit from a reduced risk of developing diseases in the future.

Unhealthy habits can be hard to break, especially if they do not seem to cause immediate damage to your health. Committing yourself to long-term changes such as giving up smoking or losing weight takes considerable willpower; you may find it easier if you seek support from family and friends.

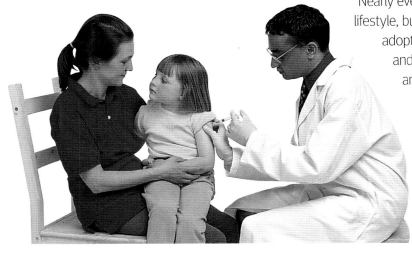

Immunization
Making sure your children are immunized at the recommended times will help to protect them from many infectious diseases.

Inheritance and health

Your physical characteristics are inherited from your parents and so are many genes that influence your health. Your genes partly determine how your body ages and whether you are predisposed to certain diseases. You cannot alter your genes, but medical intervention may help to prevent diseases to which you are prone. Genetic diagnosis and expert counselling may enable you to control your risk of disease by adapting your lifestyle.

THE GENES THAT you inherit from your parents form the basis of your physical and mental characteristics. Half of your genes come from your mother and the other half from your father, via the egg and sperm cells respectively. Each child receives a different mix of the genes provided by each parent. These different gene combinations account for the marked differences in appearance, health, and personality among most siblings. The genes you inherit determine many aspects of your appearance, such as the colour of your eyes and hair. They direct the striking bodily changes that are brought about by growth and aging, noticeably during infancy and puberty. Genes also affect your body chemistry, which may influence your risk of disease.

Your inheritance

At conception, the fertilized egg, or zygote, is a single cell that contains all the information necessary to make a new human being. This information is unique to each individual and is carried in genes, which are sections of tightly coiled DNA strands. DNA is found in the nuclei of cells and contains the instructions that control the physical characteristics, growth, development, and functioning of an individual. As the fertilized egg divides, the information is duplicated so that a copy exists in every cell of the growing baby's body.

Humans have about 20,000–25,000 pairs of genes but only certain ones are active in cells, depending on the cell's specialized function; for example, different sets of genes are active in brain and liver cells. The genes direct the activity of cells, usually by controlling the production of specific proteins. Many of these proteins are involved in the formation of body structures or in regulating the body's activities. For example, some genes are responsible for the production of proteins that cause cells to form tissues, such as skin, hair, and muscle; others give rise to proteins that control processes in the body, such as enzymes that regulate particular chemical reactions, or immunoglobulins, which fight infectious organisms.

Some genes, called control genes, produce proteins that influence certain other genes by switching those genes "on" or "off". Control genes regulate the processes of growth and development, such as the limits of cell growth. They also determine the specialization of cells. However, if control genes malfunction, the cells multiply out of control. This is one of the mechanisms

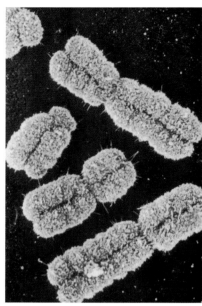

Chromosomes
All body cells (except red blood cells, eggs, and sperm) contain 23 pairs of chromosomes. These carry the genetic material inherited from your parents.

by which cancers develop. In cell division, during the copying of the genetic material, a fault occasionally occurs, leading to a mutation or change in the gene. This altered gene is then passed on to the new cells each time the cell divides. Disorders that result from such mutated genes are known as genetic disorders.

Altered genes may cause an organ to develop or function abnormally, and particular genes are known to cause rare genetic diseases. If a genetic disease runs in your family, you may decide to have tests to find out if you have inherited the altered gene. More common disorders, such as heart disease, have also been shown to have a genetic component. Screening tests to detect these diseases early on are particularly important if your family history suggests that you are at risk.

Changing health needs

As you age and pass through distinct life stages, your body's needs and your health concerns change accordingly. For example, infants need high-energy diets to promote rapid growth, whereas elderly people require less energy and eat proportionately less.

Young adults are most at risk from accidents, but later in life people are increasingly susceptible to degenerative disease as the functioning of their body organs and major body systems gradually declines. Natural healing processes also tend to become less efficient as the immune system's resistance to disease is reduced with age. The body's systems tend to age at different rates and are affected by genetic and lifestyle factors that vary from one person to the next.

Although life expectancy has risen dramatically in the UK over the past century, due to improved nutrition, health care, and sanitation, your personal good health throughout life and during old age is inevitably the result of the genes you have inherited and the way you live your life.

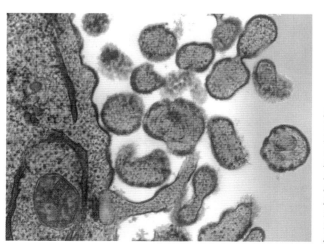

Measles virus
This highly magnified image shows measles virus particles budding from an infected cell. Measles can be prevented by immunization with the combined MMR (measles, mumps, rubella) vaccine.

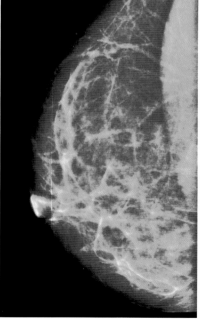

Mammogram
This mammogram shows healthy breast tissue. Mammography is used to screen for breast cancer so that it can be detected and treated at an early stage.

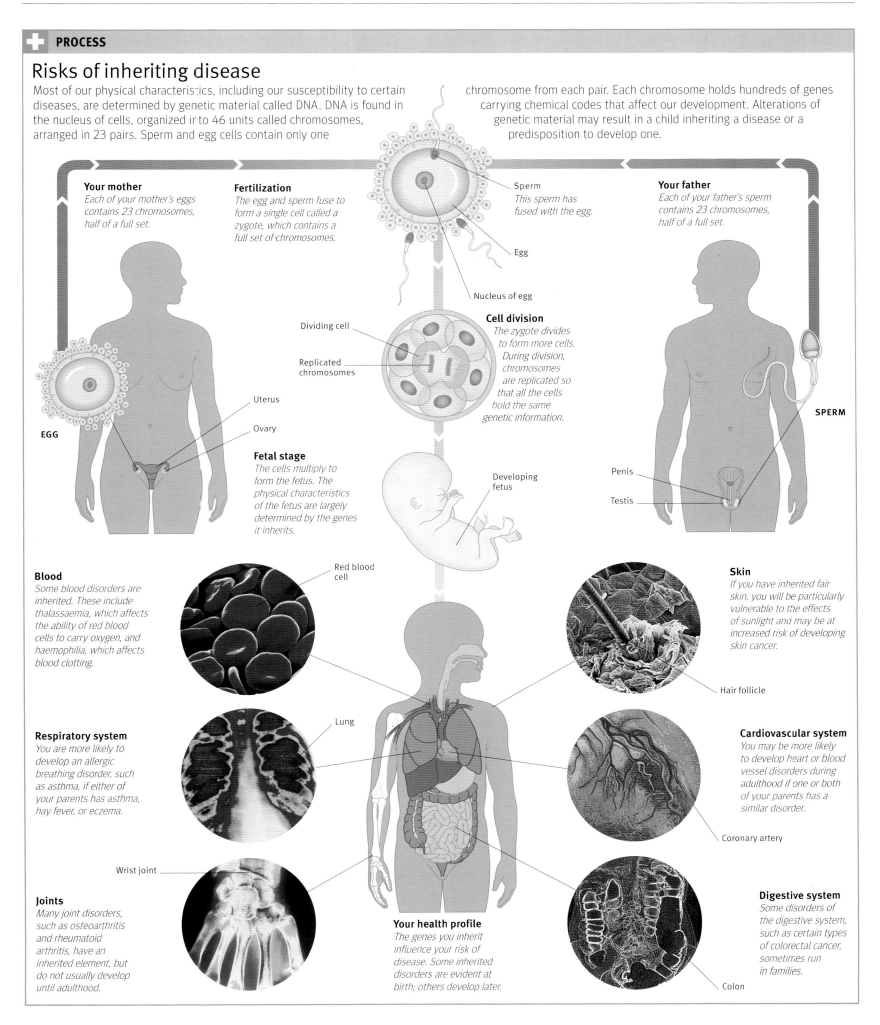

✚ **PROCESS**

Risks of inheriting disease

Most of our physical characteristics, including our susceptibility to certain diseases, are determined by genetic material called DNA. DNA is found in the nucleus of cells, organized into 46 units called chromosomes, arranged in 23 pairs. Sperm and egg cells contain only one chromosome from each pair. Each chromosome holds hundreds of genes carrying chemical codes that affect our development. Alterations of genetic material may result in a child inheriting a disease or a predisposition to develop one.

Your mother
Each of your mother's eggs contains 23 chromosomes, half of a full set.

Fertilization
The egg and sperm fuse to form a single cell called a zygote, which contains a full set of chromosomes.

Sperm
This sperm has fused with the egg.

Egg

Your father
Each of your father's sperm contains 23 chromosomes, half of a full set.

Nucleus of egg

Cell division
The zygote divides to form more cells. During division, chromosomes are replicated so that all the cells hold the same genetic information.

Dividing cell

Replicated chromosomes

Uterus

Ovary

EGG

SPERM

Fetal stage
The cells multiply to form the fetus. The physical characteristics of the fetus are largely determined by the genes it inherits.

Developing fetus

Penis

Testis

Blood
Some blood disorders are inherited. These include thalassaemia, which affects the ability of red blood cells to carry oxygen, and haemophilia, which affects blood clotting.

Red blood cell

Skin
If you have inherited fair skin, you will be particularly vulnerable to the effects of sunlight and may be at increased risk of developing skin cancer.

Hair follicle

Respiratory system
You are more likely to develop an allergic breathing disorder, such as asthma, if either of your parents has asthma, hay fever, or eczema.

Lung

Cardiovascular system
You may be more likely to develop heart or blood vessel disorders during adulthood if one or both of your parents has a similar disorder.

Coronary artery

Wrist joint

Joints
Many joint disorders, such as osteoarthritis and rheumatoid arthritis, have an inherited element, but do not usually develop until adulthood.

Your health profile
The genes you inherit influence your risk of disease. Some inherited disorders are evident at birth; others develop later.

Digestive system
Some disorders of the digestive system, such as certain types of colorectal cancer, sometimes run in families.

Colon

Understanding inheritance

In recent years, evidence has emerged showing the influence of inherited factors on our risk of developing a wide range of diseases. We take for granted the fact that children resemble their parents and other relatives and that families typically share physical and behavioural characteristics. It is this shared biological inheritance that also accounts for certain diseases "running in families".

Many of our physical and behavioural characteristics are determined by our genes. An explanation of the structure and function of genes and how they are inherited is given elsewhere (*see* **Genes and inheritance**, pp.144–149).

Genetic factors, along with lifestyle factors, contribute to many common diseases. The genes that you inherit from your parents help to explain why susceptibility to certain diseases varies from one family to the next, although only relatively few disorders are directly caused by altered genes.

By collecting information on your family's medical history, you may be able to identify diseases that appear to be particularly common in your family. This type of information can provide a valuable early indication of genetic tendencies to particular diseases.

The range of genetic tests used to determine whether either partner in a couple has inherited specific altered genes is increasing all the time. Genetic sts can assess the risk of

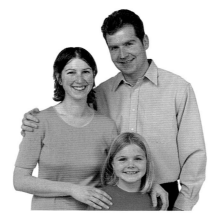

Family similarities
Children resemble their parents not only in appearance and personality but also in susceptibility to certain diseases.

the couple's children inheriting the altered genes and give advice on the likely effects on their health. In some cases, this allows the symptoms of a genetic disorder to be treated early or relieved effectively.

You and your inheritance

Understanding how the genes you inherit may influence your health

The genes you inherit from your parents programme your development from a single fertilized cell at the moment of conception to adulthood. Humans have about 20,000–25,000 pairs of genes arranged on 23 pairs of chromosomes. One chromosome from each pair is inherited from your mother, the other from your father. The mix of genes is slightly different in each sibling.

Genes control the metabolism, growth, repair, and reproduction of cells. They are responsible for the development of the embryo, first into a baby, then a child, and eventually an adult. Throughout your life, genes control cell functions and the repair and replacement of dead or damaged cells.

Blood relatives have many genes in common, and these genes help to determine family physical characteristics and other traits. Many of these traits, such as the shape of the nose, have no significance for your health. Other traits, such as being unusually tall or short

or having a tendency to be overweight, can be associated with an increased risk of certain diseases.

Some diseases, such as haemophilia (p.274) and cystic fibrosis (p.535), are directly caused by a fault or mutation in a single gene or pair of genes. These rare diseases follow a predictable pattern of inheritance, and this means that families in which the altered gene is present can usually be given clear, reliable information regarding the probability of the disease affecting future generations.

More common than these genetic disorders are those in which genes, along with other factors, contribute to a family's susceptibility to certain diseases. For example, some disorders, such as coronary artery disease (p.243), tend to run in families, but lifestyle factors such as an unhealthy diet, smoking, and lack of exercise also play a part in determining whether these diseases develop.

In some diseases that have a genetic component, including asthma (p.295), environmental factors, such as living in a polluted area, also play a crucial role.

The complex interplay between genetic susceptibility and environment makes it difficult to predict the risks in adult life for children who are born into families affected by disorders of this kind.

Your family medical history

Assessing your chance of developing a genetic disorder or passing one on to your children

You may have noticed that some diseases seem to "run in your family". These disorders may have a genetic basis or be due to lifestyle factors or a combination of the two. You can create a record of the disorders that have affected your family by making a medical family tree (opposite page), which may help you to assess your own risk of disease.

Gathering information

Information on your parents, brothers, and sisters is the most important, but you can provide a fuller picture by finding out about as many generations as possible, including your uncles, aunts, and grandparents. It is also helpful to know something about your relatives' lifestyles to help you and your doctor to assess whether any diseases were largely due to behaviour or inheritance.

You may want to find out about your medical family tree out of curiosity, but you will find this information useful whenever a doctor needs to ask questions about illnesses in your family. You are likely to be asked about your family medical history when you first see a new doctor; you are expecting a baby; if you are admitted to hospital; and if you develop symptoms of a disorder with a genetic component, such as asthma.

Assessing the information

You may be able to come to some conclusions about your risk of disease by looking at your medical family tree. If your investigation suggests that a particular disease has affected more than one member of your family, you should consult your doctor. In some cases, you may be referred for genetic counselling to assess your chance of developing a disorder or passing it on to your children.

Drawing your own conclusions Longevity runs in families, and, if many of your relatives lived beyond the age of 80, you have a good chance of doing the same, especially if you adopt a healthy lifestyle. If many of your relatives died young, you should try to find out the causes of death. You may be susceptible to disorders that have occurred more than once in your family.

You should suspect an inherited disorder if more than one child in your family was stillborn or died in childhood; if more than one adult died from heart disease at an early age; if more than two people in the family had a long-term disorder, such as arthritis (p.220); if several family members developed cancer at an early age; or if more than one family member had the same disabling or fatal disease. Deaths before the age of 60 are especially rele-

vant, unless they were caused by accidents or by an infection that occurred before effective treatment was available.

Professional interpretation Genetic counsellors are trained to interpret genetic family histories, to assess your risk of genetic disease, and to determine whether you are a carrier of an altered gene that causes a genetic disorder. Carriers do not show signs of the disorder because the altered gene is masked by a normal gene, but children of carriers can inherit the altered gene. The counsellor will try to find out whether a high frequency of a disease in your family is due more to genetics or to environmental factors, such as lifestyle. For example, in some families where there are several people with colorectal cancer (p.421), this could be due more to environmental factors, such as diet, whereas in other families there may be an inherited predisposition to the disease.

Considering the options Your family medical history may suggest that you have a higher than average probability of having an inherited disorder. In this case, the counsellor will tell you whether a specific gene alteration for the disorder has been identified and whether there is a test to see if you have the altered gene. If a test is available, the counsellor can provide information that will help you decide whether or not to have the test.

Some people decide not to proceed with genetic tests for a variety of reasons. Prospective parents may feel there is no point in worrying about a disorder that would not necessarily affect them or their child, or they may choose to carry on with a pregnancy even if there is an increased probability of their child being affected by a genetic disease. They may also be concerned by the stigma associated with "labelling" someone as having or being a carrier of a disorder. Other people want to know the results of a test even if they would not act on them. Bear in mind that the test result for one family member may have implications for other family members who may not want to know the outcome.

Members of some groups of the population are susceptible to particular genetic disorders, and individuals may be offered a screening test based on this fact. For example, about 1 in 10 people of African or Caribbean descent carries the gene for sickle-cell disease (p.272), a disorder of red blood cells. If you are Jewish, a genetic counsellor may recommend that you consider a screening test for the metabolic disorder Tay–Sachs disease (p.562) because 1 in 25 Ashkenazi Jews, compared with only 1 in 250 of the general population, carries the altered gene that causes the disease.

What you can do

If tests show that you have an altered gene, your course of action will depend on whether you already have the symptoms of a genetic disorder or whether you are at high risk of developing the disorder. If you carry an altered gene and you are planning a family, there are several options to consider.

▶ **ASSESSMENT**

Making a medical family tree

To make your medical family tree, you need key pieces of information about your relatives. You should research at least as far back as your grandparents because a genetic predisposition to a certain disease may be masked in one generation but nevertheless passed on to succeeding generations. Key facts include date of birth and, if the person is deceased, cause of death and the age at which it occurred. If possible, you should find out about lifestyle factors, such as smoking, body weight, alcohol consumption, and exercise.

Your paternal grandfather (1926–1988)

Medical history
Angina

Lifestyle factors
Smoker

Cause of death
Heart attack at the age of 62

Your paternal grandmother (1929–1985)

Medical history
None

Lifestyle factors
Nonsmoker

Cause of death
Colorectal cancer at the age of 56

Your maternal grandfather (1932–)

Medical history
None

Lifestyle factors
Active, nonsmoker

Health status
In good health

Your maternal grandmother (1935–2005)

Medical history
Diabetes mellitus

Lifestyle factors
Smoker

Cause of death
Stroke at the age of 70

Your paternal uncle (1952–)

Medical history
None

Lifestyle factors
Active, nonsmoker

Health status
In good health

Your paternal uncle (1949–)

Medical history
Coronary artery disease

Lifestyle factors
Sedentary, smoker

Health status
In poor health

Your father (1948–)

Medical history
Treated for polyps in the colon

Lifestyle factors
Active, nonsmoker

Health status
In good health

Your mother (1956–)

Medical history
Diabetes mellitus

Lifestyle factors
Nonsmoker

Health status
Overweight

Your maternal uncle (1958–1965)

Medical history
None

Lifestyle factors
Was active

Cause of death
Measles at the age of 7

Your maternal uncle (1960–)

Medical history
None

Lifestyle factors
Nonsmoker

Health status
In good health

Sister (1984–)

Medical history
None

Lifestyle factors
Active, smoker

Health status
Overweight

Sister (1986–)

Medical history
Kidney failure, aged 12 years. Kidney transplant at 14

Lifestyle factors
Smoker

Health status
In good health

Brother (1988–)

Medical history
None

Lifestyle factors
Nonsmoker

Health status
In good health

You (female) (1990–)

Medical history
None

Lifestyle factors
Nonsmoker

Health status
In good health

Partner
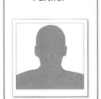

Example of a family tree
A family tree enables you to detect disease trends, but you will need your doctor's help to interpret your risk of disease. This example assumes that you are female and were born in 1990. From this record, the doctor would conclude that you and your siblings are at risk of polyps in the colon, which may lead to colorectal cancer, and diabetes mellitus. If you are planning to have a child, you should look at both your own and your partner's family trees to assess possible health risks for the child.

People with a genetic disorder Certain genetic disorders can be treated. For example, a person who has inherited a tendency to high levels of cholesterol in the blood (*see* **Inherited hyperlipidaemias**, p.440) may be treated with a low-fat diet and lipid-lowering drugs (p.603). Children with the genetic disorder haemophilia (p.274) may be given regular transfusions of Factor VIII, a protein that helps the blood to clot.

People at risk If you find that you have an altered gene that predisposes you to a particular disorder, such as breast cancer (p.486), you may be offered regular screening to detect signs of the disorder at an early stage. You may also be able to make lifestyle changes to help to reduce the likelihood of developing a disease. For example, if your family history suggests that you are at increased risk of develop-

ing diabetes mellitus (p.437), you should keep your weight within the normal range.
Carriers If you and your partner are carriers of an altered gene for the same condition, you may decide not to have children or may consider various family planning options, such as adoption or artificial insemination (p.497). You may be able to take advantage of advances in assisted conception (p.498) such as preimplanation

genetic diagnosis, in which embryos resulting from in vitro fertilization are tested for certain altered genes, and then only healthy embryos are transferred to the uterus. If you are already expecting a baby, you will be offered antenatal genetic testing (p.509). If you discover that your baby is affected by a genetic disorder, options you may want to consider include terminating the pregnancy (p.510).

Health care throughout life

Until the mid-20th century, people consulted a doctor only when they were ill, injured, or pregnant. Although for many people this is still the case, the intervening period has seen an explosion in public knowledge about health and disease and a growing emphasis on health care that prevents as well as treats disease.

The main point of contact with health services for most people is with their GPs or other primary health-care professionals, such as practice nurses, dentists, and opticians. The first article offers advice on choosing a practice and getting the best from consultations with your doctor.

The next subject is immunization. In developed countries, programmes of immunization from birth onwards have dramatically reduced many of the infections that used to be common in childhood. Immunization also protects people from serious illness in later life.

As well as treating disorders, primary health-care providers are responsible for two important elements in preventive health care: checkups carried out during childhood and

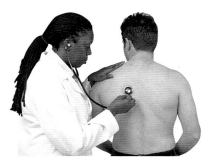

Having your health checked
Checkups are a chance to discuss ways of improving your health while your doctor examines you for early signs of disease.

later in life, and screening tests to identify risk factors and early signs of disease. These topics are covered in the last two articles.

You and your doctor

Choosing a practice and finding the right doctor for your primary care

Good health care should be a partnership between you and your GP. You should feel comfortable discussing any aspect of your health with your doctor and be confident that you are getting proper care from the practice with which you are registered.

Most GPs work in group practices but a minority of GPs still work single-handedly. Most practices provide a range of family health services. These typically include examination and treatment; antenatal care; immunizations; minor surgery; clinics for people with diabetes and asthma; health education advice; and referrals to other health services and social services. Some large practices also have other health-care practitioners, such as nurses, midwives, health visitors, physiotherapists, and dentists.

Finding a practice
Before you can consult a GP, you need to register with him or her. You can get a list of GPs over the Internet or from your library. However, before you register with a particular GP, find out about the various options. Take a look around a few practices and ask for their practice leaflet to see what it offers. This way you can check whether the opening hours suit you and if the practice offers the kind of services you need (for example, baby clinics) before you register.

Once you have registered, you will probably be asked by your GP to have a health check, which will usually be carried out by a nurse. You will also be asked to fill in a questionnaire about your health and lifestyle.

Consulting your doctor
When you need to see a doctor or other health professional (such as a nurse), you will usually have to make an appointment. You can ask to see a male or female doctor or nurse, although it may not always be possible to grant your request. You will need to make a separate appointment for each member of the family. It is important to keep your appointment, or to notify the surgery if you have to cancel or change it.

If you think you need to see the doctor urgently, tell the receptionist when you make the appointment and you will be seen that day, if appropriate. If the doctor thinks you are too ill to come to the surgery, he or she may make arrangements for you to be visited at home.

If you need to see a doctor out of normal surgery hours for an urgent medical problem that cannot wait, all doctors have an out-of-hours service. You will be given contact details about this service when you register with your GP. Alternatively, you can phone the NHS 111 service (dial 111). This service, which is available 24 hours a day, every day of the year, provides medical advice and details of local services that can provide care. For minor injuries or illnesses, you can also go to an NHS walk-in centre. For emergency medical help for serious health problems, you can dial 999 (or 112) and ask for an ambulance or go directly to the Accident and Emergency Department of a hospital.

Making the most of a visit
The key to a successful appointment with your GP is good communication. You should try to provide accurate information about your symptoms, past history, and lifestyle. Your GP should offer medical and health advice in a way that is easy to understand and encourage you to be involved in maintaining your health and in any treatment (*see* **Visiting your doctor**, pp.126–128). You should not feel anxious about asking questions about your treatment or raising issues that are important to you.

Consultations with your doctor vary between surgeries but generally average 7–12 minutes. If you feel that you may need substantially longer than this, ask for a double appointment. If possible, try to plan what you want to discuss before you arrive at the surgery. This will help your doctor to focus on your most important concerns and given them priority. It is also useful if you wear clothes or dress your child in clothes that can be easily removed in case a physical examination is necessary.

Your health records
Before your first visit, you will have been asked to complete a questionnaire about your medical history and lifestyle. Your doctor will use this as a starting point for asking further questions during the visit. Topics will probably include the amount of alcohol you drink, the exercise you take, and whether or not you smoke. Your doctor will also check that you are up to date with immunizations (right) and screening tests (*see* **Screening**, opposite page).

During subsequent visits your doctor will make notes that become part of your medical records. People have the right to see their medical records, and they also have the right to read letters and notes if they are referred for secondary care. Your complete health records, including letters to and from consultants, hospital admissions, and summaries of any treatment, are transferred with you if you change your GP.

Confidentiality
Doctors are governed by the rules of confidentiality and cannot divulge a patient's medical history, even to their closest family members, without permission. If your doctor is asked to report on your medical history and state of health for life insurance purposes, welfare benefits, for a new employer, or for evidence in court, he or she must have your written consent before passing on this information. However, doctors must disclose information about patients when required to do so by law, or when they are faced with injuries or disorders that indicate a serious crime. Doctors are also required to notify the appropriate authority about patients with specified infectious diseases.

Treatment of young children is usually discussed with the parents, but an older child's request for confidentiality is generally respected if the doctor feels he or she is competent enough to understand the issues involved.

Immunization

A method of producing artificial immunity to infectious diseases, usually involving a course of injections

Immunization is a way of boosting the body's defences against infectious diseases. Most immunizations use a vaccine containing a tiny amount of a weakened or inactivated form of a disease-causing organism (*see* **Vaccines and immunoglobulins**, p.571). When the vaccine is introduced into your body, it stimulates your immune system to produce antibodies against the disease so that you are protected if you are exposed to the actual organism at some time in the future. Most vaccines are given by injection. For most immunizations, several injections of the vaccine are given over a period of months or years to build up adequate protection.

Timing of immunizations
Most routine immunizations (opposite page) are given during infancy and childhood according to an immunization schedule. In addition, certain immunizations, such as influenza, are routinely offered to certain groups of adults. There are also immunizations that are not routinely available for everybody but are available for special at-risk groups (*see* **Special circumstances**, below), such as pregnant women, those with certain long-term health problems, and health-care workers. You should keep records of all your immunizations and those of your children in case a doctor other than your GP needs to know about your immune status.

Babies and children Most immunizations are given to babies during their first year, when infectious diseases are most likely to be serious. A baby has some natural protection from antibodies that pass through the placenta during pregnancy, but this immunity wears off by about 6 months after birth. Premature babies are immunized routinely because they are at high risk of serious illness if they develop an infection.

By the time children start school, they will have completed most of their routine immunizations, although some immunizations are given during the school years. If a child starts the schedule late, the timings of vaccinations can usually be adjusted so that he or she receives the full complement.

Special circumstances Adults sometimes need a booster dose in special circumstances. For example, you may need an extra injection against tetanus (p.173) if you sustain a deep or dirty cut. Certain at-risk groups, such as pregnant women, people with certain long-term health problems, and health-care workers, may also be offered vaccines that are not part of the routine

Routine immunizations

Immunizations help to protect against various infectious diseases and most are scheduled during childhood. Serious reactions to immunizations are rare; consult your doctor if you are concerned.

Routine schedule
The timing of immunizations can usually be adjusted if some doses are missed.

Age	Diseases immunized against
2 months	Diphtheria/tetanus/pertussis/poliomyelitis/*Haemophilus influenzae* B (Hib)* Pneumococcus Rotavirus Meningitis B
3 months	Diphtheria/tetanus/pertussis/poliomyelitis/*Haemophilus influenzae* B (Hib)* Rotavirus Meningitis C
4 months	Diphtheria/tetanus/pertussis/poliomyelitis/*Haemophilus influenzae* B (Hib)* Pneumococcus Meningitis B
12 to 13 months	*Haemophilus influenzae* B (Hib)/meningitis C* Measles/mumps/rubella* Pneumococcus Meningitis B
2, 3, and 4 years, plus school years 1 and 2	Childhood influenza (every year)
3 years 4 months, or soon after	Diphtheria/tetanus/pertussis/poliomyelitis* Measles/mumps/rubella*
12 to 13 years (girls only)	Human papillomavirus (helps to protect against cervical cancer)
13 to 18 years	Diphtheria/tetanus/polio* Meningitis A, C, W, and Y*
19 to 25 years (first time students only)	Meningitis A, C, W, and Y*
65 years and older	Influenza (every year) Pneumococcus
70 years (and 78 and 79 years, as a catch-up)	Shingles

* Given as a single injection

immunization schedule, notably vaccines against hepatitis B (p.408), tuberculosis (p.300), and chickenpox (p.165). Extra immunizations may also be recommended if you plan to travel to a country that has a high incidence of infectious diseases, such as hepatitis or yellow fever (*see* **Travel immunizations**, p.35).

Risks of immunization

Immunizations have few side effects, although there may be some inflammation around the injection site or a mild fever. If you or your child have any reactions to initial doses, tell your doctor so that he or she can advise you about subsequent doses. Serious side effects are extremely rare, and research has shown that, in general, the risks from immunizations are substantially lower than the risks associated with the diseases that they protect against.

Homeopathic types of vaccine have been shown to be ineffective. If you rely on them, you could be putting yourself or your children at risk.

Health checkups

Visits to the doctor or a health clinic to check on your state of health, or to monitor a child's growth and development

Health checkups are an opportunity to talk about your or your child's general health with a primary health-care specialist, such as a doctor or health visitor. In babies and infants, health checks tend to focus on healthy growth and development. In adults, checks are usually done to monitor disorders and their treatment or to screen for specific conditions. Pregnant women have regular health checks with their doctor or midwife as part of their antenatal care (*see* **Routine antenatal care**, p.506). You may also be offered a health check when you register with a new GP or may be required to have checkups for insurance purposes of when you begin a new job.

Some employers and private health-care providers offer regular health checks as part of their general provisions. However, no health checkup can check for every possible illness or condition and it is therefore important to consult your doctor if you have any concerns about your health, even if you have recently had a health checkup.

Checkups in childhood All newborn babies have a complete physical examination within 72 hours of their birth to identify potential problems. This examination includes listening to the baby's heart for problems such as a heart murmur (*see* **Congenital heart disease**, p.542) and checking the eyes for abnormalities such as cataracts (p.357). Newborn babies are also given a blood spot screening test (p.561) to check for certain congenital disorders, and a hearing test (*see* **Hearing tests in children**, p.557).

Until a child reaches school age, subsequent checkups are carried out at regular intervals by your doctor or a health visitor. These checks include monitoring physical growth by measuring weight, length, and head circumference. These measurements are recorded in a Personal Child Health Record book (known as "the red book"), which every mother is given shortly before or after her baby is born. This enables her to keep track of her child's health and progress and is a useful source of information if her child needs medical care.

The purpose of preschool health checks is to ensure that the child's physical, social, and intellectal development are progressing satisfactorily. Although the exact age at which children reach developmental milestones varies (*see* **Gaining skills during the first five years**, p.528), the doctor or health visitor will check that the child has gained certain skills within predicted age ranges. These include gross motor skills, such as the ability to sit up; fine motor skills, such as picking up a small object; and social skills, such as using language. Your child will also have regular hearing and vision tests.

On starting school, your child will be offered a school entry health check, which includes measuring height and weight and checking your child's vision and hearing. Your child's height and weight will be measured again at age 10 to 11. Your child will also have other checkups during his or her school years if he or she has a problem that needs monitoring.

Checkups in adults Health checks in adults mainly rely on a few basic tests, such as measurement of blood pressure; on various screening tests (p.14) to detect any early signs of certain diseases, such as breast cancer; and on questionnaires about lifestyle and health. Your doctor may also measure your height and weight and use those measurements to calculate your body mass index to check whether you are within a healthy weight range (*see* **Are you a healthy weight?**, p.19). Some GP practices run "well person clinics",

where, in addition to height, weight, and blood pressure checks, you may also be offered blood cholesterol checks, and urine tests to check for diabetes and kidney disease. As well as health checks provided by your doctor, there are also specialist sexual health clinics, where you can go to get checked (and treated) for sexually transmitted infections.

Acting on your checkup

Using the results of your checkup, your doctor will suggest ways in which you can maintain your health and promote your own or your child's health. You can also discuss any health concerns you may have. You may need further tests if there are factors that increase your risk of disease, such as your lifestyle, family history, occupation, or travel abroad.

Screening

Detecting disease or risk factors for a disease before symptoms develop

Screening is an important element of preventive medicine. Most screening tests are used to detect risk factors associated with disease or to make an early diagnosis of a treatable condition. Less commonly, if there is a rare inherited disease in your family history, screening may be carried out to find out if you have an abnormal gene that could cause a disorder in you or your children.

You may be offered screening tests at different stages of your life. A few tests are offered as part of national screening programmes, while others are available on request or might be recommended if there are risk factors that predispose you to a particular disease.

Before accepting a test, you should ask your doctor what it involves, if it carries risks, and how reliable it is. You should also consider the possible implications of the test results. No test is completely accurate, and sometimes a test can miss disease or suggest disease when it is not present. An abnormal result may lead to further tests for which you might not be prepared.

Why people are screened

It is not possible or even worthwhile to screen for every risk factor or disease. Tests are useful only if they detect a disease or risk factor that can be treated effectively, and which benefits from early treatment. For example, women are screened for cervical abnormalities such as cervical intraepithelial neoplasia (p.480) that can be treated before cancer of the cervix (p.481) develops.

Some screening tests are offered to adults at stages of life when the risk of certain diseases increases (*see* **Common screening tests**, p.14). You may be offered other tests if you have a higher than normal risk of a disorder due to lifestyle factors such as smoking, your age, family history of disease, or a pre-existing illness.

▶ **ASSESSMENT**

Common screening tests

In the UK, various screening tests are offered nationwide. The more common ones are outlined in the table below. Your doctor may also recommend other tests on the basis of your age, occupation, family or personal medical history, and lifestyle factors. Some tests may be performed by your GP while others may be carried out in hospital clinics or special centres.

Screening for glaucoma is carried out by your optometrist during routine eye tests. Screening in pregnancy is performed as part of routine antenatal care (p.506)

Screening test	Disease/disorder	When recommended	Comments
Abdominal aortic aneurysm screening test	Aneurysm of the aorta (a potentially dangerous swelling in the aorta, p.259)	In the 65th year	The test consists of an ultrasound scan of the abdomen. It is offered to men only. Men over 65 can request the test
Blood spot screening tests (p.561)	Phenylketonuria (p.562), hypothyroidism (p.432), cystic fibrosis (p.535), sickle cell disease (p.272), MCADD (p.562), and sometimes also other conditions	Soon after birth, ideally at 5 days	Blood sample is taken for analysis from the heel of all newborn babies
Blood pressure measurement (p.242)	Hypertension (p.242)	All adults should have their blood pressure checked at least every 5 years, or more frequently for those with conditions such as diabetes and/or raised blood pressure	Blood pressure is often checked during visits to the doctor. High blood pressure is a risk factor for heart disease and stroke
Bowel scope screening	Colorectal cancer (p.421)	A single test at age 55	The test consists of examining the inside of the bowel with a flexible endoscope (viewing instrument). Subsequently, faecal occult blood testing resumes at age 60. Bowel scope screening is only offered in certain areas of the UK
Cervical screening test (p.480)	Cervical intraepithelial neoplasia (p.480), cancer of the cervix (p.481)	Every 3 years from age 25 to 49, then every 5 years from age 50 to 64	The test is not necessary for women who have had a total hysterectomy (removal of the uterus and cervix)
Diabetic eye screening	Diabetic retinopathy (p.361)	Every year from the age of 12	The test consists of taking photographs of the retina to check for any damage
Eye pressure measurement (see Tonometry, p.358)	Glaucoma (p.358)	Every 2 years from age 40, or more frequently and from a younger age if there is a family history of glaucoma	Eye tests by an optometrist are free for people over 60 or for those at high risk of glaucoma
Faecal occult blood test	Colorectal cancer (p.421)	Every 2 years from age 50 or 60 to age 69 or 74	The age at which this test is offered varies in different parts of the UK
Mammography (p.487)	Breast cancer (p.486)	Every 3 years from age 50 to 70	Women aged over 70 may have mammography on request

Stage of life Your risk of developing certain disorders depends on your age. For this reason, the type and frequency of screening tests that your doctor may recommend will change as you grow older. Women are offered a specific programme of tests during pregnancy (see **Routine antenatal care**, p.506), in which they are tested regularly for conditions such as pre-eclampsia (p.513) or diabetes mellitus (p.437) that can be harmful to the mother or the baby or both. The fetus may also be screened by ultrasound (see **Ultrasound scanning in pregnancy**, p.512) for abnormalities that may require treatment after birth. Shortly after birth, all babies are screened with a blood spot screening test (p.561) for a range of metabolic diseases.

Adult screening Screening for early signs of breast cancer (p.486) and cervical cancer is offered on the NHS to women in specific age groups. Cervical cancer screening is offered to women every 3–5 years from the age of 25 until the age of 64. Mammography to screen for breast cancer is offered to women every 3 years from age 50 to age 70. The faecal occult blood test to screen for colorectal cancer (p.421) is offered to men and women every 2 years from the age of 50 or 60 to the age of 69 or 74 (the start and end ages vary according to where you live). In some areas, a once-only bowel scope screening test for colorectal cancer is also offered at the age of 55. Men in their 65th year are offered screening with ultrasound scanning for abdominal aortic aneurysm; this test is not offered to women or younger men because the condition is rare in these groups. One of the most common screening tests carried out is blood pressure measurement, because high blood pressure (see **Hypertension**, p.242) itself is symptomless but is a major risk factor for heart disease and stroke. Blood pressure is usually measured in the doctor's surgery, often when you see the doctor for another health problem.

Inherited disorders A number of disorders, including abnormally high levels of cholesterol and other lipids in the blood (see **Inherited hyperlipidaemias**, p.440), colorectal cancer, and breast cancer, tend to run in families. If any members of your family have been affected by one of these disorders, your doctor may suggest screening tests to look for early disease. For example you may be offered regular faecal occult blood tests earlier than normal if you have a family history of colorectal cancer. A woman with a family history of breast cancer, may be offered mammography (p.487) earlier or more often than is usual. Particular forms of breast cancer are caused by inherited faulty genes. There are tests that can identify specific abnormal genes.

Chronic conditions If you have a long-term disorder, you may be offered regular screening to detect early signs of complications. For example, people with diabetes mellitus are screened routinely for kidney disease, cardiovascular disorders, nerve damage, and damage to the blood vessels of the eye.

Hazardous occupations In some occupations, workers are exposed to substances that can increase the risk of some diseases. If your occupation carries known health risks, take appropriate safety measures (see **Safety and health at work**, p.34) and participate in any screening offered by your employer.

Who carries out screening?

Most screening is carried out at your doctor's surgery or at special clinics. Your doctor may refer you to a specialist for certain tests, such as colonoscopy (p.418). Testing for glaucoma is carried out by an optometrist as part of a routine eye test.

There are several simple health checks that you can regularly perform yourself to help detect early indications of disease. They include breast awareness (p.484), examining the testes (p.460), and inspecting the skin for signs of skin cancer (p.200). If you discover any abnormal signs, discuss them with your doctor as soon as possible. Although you can now buy screening test kits for some disorders over the counter, such kits do not always produce accurate results. Furthermore, the significance of the results in your individual case may need expert interpretation and you are therefore advised to always consult your doctor if you are concerned about a health risk.

Your test results

Some tests, such as those for metabolic disorders in children (see **Blood spot screening tests**, p.561), produce a clear positive or negative result that does not usually require further investigation. The results of other tests may not be as easy to interpret.

If your test results are negative, no further action may be needed until the next screening test. No screening test is 100 per cent accurate, and, rarely, a disorder may be present even though test results were negative. When this happens, the result is called a false-negative.

Sometimes a disease develops soon after a test: if symptoms become apparent, consult your doctor even if your test result was negative. You will be advised if further action is needed. In most cases, regular screening tests pick up diseases before symptoms develop.

If your result is positive, your doctor may repeat the test or arrange for further investigations to confirm the result and perhaps provide more information. For example, if a mammogram reveals an abnormality, a test in which a sample of cells is collected (see **Fine-needle aspiration of a breast lump**, p.484) may be needed to find out the cause.

Lifestyle and health

Your health is influenced by two major factors: your genetic make-up, which determines your predisposition to disease, and your lifestyle. You cannot change inherited factors, but you can adapt your behaviour to control your risk of disease or injury. You have some control over what you eat and drink and whether you smoke, exercise, or practise safe sex. Your lifestyle choices affect your present and future health.

IN THE DEVELOPED world, life expectancy has risen greatly over the last century due to improvements in public health. However, in England and Wales in 2014, more than 79,000 people died before the age of 65, often from long-term diseases such as cancer or heart disease. You can reduce your risk of developing some of these diseases by adopting a healthy lifestyle. All aspects of life, including work, travel, home, and leisure, carry risks and benefits to health. You need to balance these risks and benefits by lifestyle choices that enable you to enjoy your life while staying healthy.

Understanding the risks

It is important to be aware of the lifestyle factors associated with certain diseases so that you can make informed choices. For example, tobacco smoking is a critical factor in more than a quarter of all cancer deaths. Several lifestyle factors, including an unhealthy diet, are known to contribute to the development of heart disease and cancer. Many people enjoy drinking alcohol as part of social activity. However, regularly drinking to excess can severely damage your liver, brain, and heart, and drinking in pregnancy may harm your developing baby.

In order to make informed decisions about your health priorities, you need to take into account your individual circumstances. Your doctor can help you to do this. Your age is one of the most important factors and greatly influences the lifestyle decisions that you need to make. For example, young adults are statistically more likely to experience illness or injury associated with risk-taking behaviour, such as sexually transmitted infections or reactions to recreational drugs, than to suffer from ill health due to long-term disease. Another consideration is work: if you have a dangerous occupation, such as construction work, paying close attention to safety could be the most important factor in protecting your health in the short term. Nevertheless, it is important to recognize that some lifestyle choices, such as tobacco smoking, do not carry an immediate and obvious threat but have a cumulative effect and can ultimately cause serious damage to your health.

Making lifestyle choices

Activities that take place in the home, such as eating, sleeping, and being with your family, have a major influence on physical and mental health. A balanced diet is vital for good health. Age, sex, activity levels, and pregnancy all affect the amount and type of food you need to include in your daily diet. Sleep helps you to stay healthy and improves mental skills. Regular exercise improves fitness and builds muscle, but you should tailor programmes to your own needs. You should also consider the benefits and risks of different leisure activities.

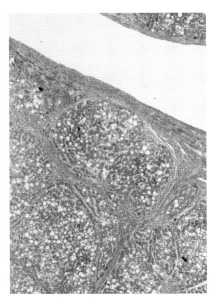

Liver cirrhosis
This light micrograph of liver tissue shows that scar tissue (green) has developed around the liver lobules and fat deposits (yellow-white) have built up as a result of heavy alcohol use.

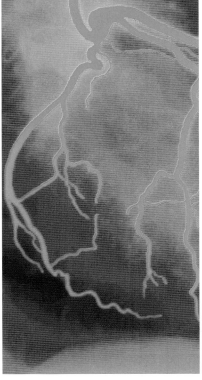

Healthy heart
Lifestyle factors such as diet can affect the coronary arteries and thus the health of your heart.

Sports, hobbies, and social activities can all benefit your physical and mental health, although some, such as sunbathing or listening to loud music, may carry a risk of injury or harm.

Making lifestyle changes

Most health habits, such as food choices and taking exercise, are formed in our families when we are children. Giving children a healthy lifestyle from birth maximizes their chances of growing into healthy adults and establishes habits that they may find easier to maintain in later life. Some families may find it difficult to make healthy lifestyle choices. For example, they may not be able to afford good food or housing. However, everyone can do something to improve health.

The first step towards a healthier lifestyle is to identify activities that pose significant risks to your health. It is easier to change these activities if you can see immediate benefits. Some activities, such as hang-gliding, are clearly dangerous and carry a significant risk every time you do them. For other types of behaviour, the risks to health may not be as obvious but tend to be cumulative; they are likely to damage your health only if carried out repeatedly over a period of time. Eating one unhealthy meal does not damage your health, but consistently eating an unhealthy diet may increase your risk of developing heart disease over time. Long-term changes, such as giving up smoking, increasing the amount of exercise that you take, or changing your diet, are often more difficult to make and maintain, especially if they involve overcoming social pressure. You may need to seek support from family, friends, and health professionals.

Diet and health

By far the most common problem with the British diet is excess. People in the UK tend to consume too much food, especially too much saturated fat, salt, and sugar. Overconsumption of these nutrients has been linked to some of the main causes of death in the UK: heart disease, cancer, and stroke. Making informed choices about your diet could improve your chance of avoiding these diseases.

The huge growth in the availability and popularity of fast food has led to a corresponding rise in poor eating habits because packaged snacks and meals often contain large amounts of ingredients that can be harmful. The first article in this section provides easy-to-follow guidelines on how to assess and improve your diet, explains how food energy is measured, and describes how each of the major food groups (carbohydrate, protein, and fat) contributes to your nutritional needs. Many people in the UK have a diet that provides more energy than they need, and, as a result, a significant percentage of the population is obese and suffers from health problems associated with being overweight. The second article explains how to determine your ideal weight and explores various methods of losing or gaining weight.

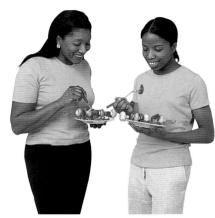

Eating well
Food is essential for good health but is also an important aspect of social life for most people. Cooking and sharing healthy food can be an enjoyable part of daily life.

A healthy diet

A diet that contains the right balance of foods for optimum health

Variation in diet among people living in different countries is closely associated with national patterns of disease. For example, the high-calorie, high-saturated-fat diet common in the UK is linked to the high national rates of obesity (p.400), heart disease (see **Coronary artery disease**, p.243), cancer (pp.152–159), and stroke (p.329). In contrast, the traditional Mediterranean diet, which includes plenty of fresh vegetables, olive oil, and fish and is therefore low in saturated fat, seems to be related to the low incidence of heart disease in Mediterranean countries. In Japan, the typical diet is high in fibre, and the incidence of colorectal cancer (p.421) is low. In many countries, an excessive amount of salt in the diet has been associated with people having high blood pressure (see **Hypertension**, p.242).

Just as an excess of certain elements in the diet can lead to health problems, deficiencies in essential nutrients can result in poor health (see **Nutritional deficiencies**, p.399). Such deficiencies, however, are rare in developed countries such as the UK.

The knowledge gained by nutritionists from studying the effects of diet on health in countries around the world has led to the development of guidelines to ensure a healthy, balanced diet that can reduce the risk of ill health.

Balancing your diet
There are five essential components of food: carbohydrates, protein, fats, vitamins, and minerals. Each one of these elements makes an important contribution to health, but it is important that they are consumed in the correct proportions, with carbohydrates forming the bulk of the diet and fats only a small proportion (see **Healthy eating**, opposite page). By eating plenty of fruit and vegetables, you can ensure you are getting enough vitamins and minerals. You should also include plenty of water in your diet. Drinks that contain sugar, caffeine, or alcohol (see **Alcohol and health**, p.24) should be consumed in moderation. Sugar is known to contribute to tooth decay. Carbonated drinks, even those that are low in sugar, can damage the teeth because they are acidic. Excess caffeine from drinks such as coffee and cola can cause palpitations (a feeling that the heart is beating rapidly) and insomnia, and caffeine may worsen symptoms of anxiety.

Other important health factors are the amount of salt you have in your diet and the types of fat you eat.

Carbohydrates These should be the body's main energy source. However, if you eat more carbohydrate than your body needs, the excess will be stored as fat. There are two main types of carbohydrate in food: simple and complex.

Simple carbohydrates are made up of sugars. They provide your body with a quick energy boost but can be harmful to the teeth. Foods such as biscuits, cakes, and sweets contain large quantities of simple carbohydrates.

Complex carbohydrates have a more complicated structure than simple carbohydrates and are made up of starches and dietary fibre. Starches are digested slowly and therefore provide sustained energy. Pasta, bread, vegetables such as potatoes, and rice contain high levels of starch. Dietary fibre consists of the fibrous parts of plants that are not completely broken down during digestion. Fibre can be divided into two kinds: soluble fibre and insoluble fibre.

Insoluble fibre adds bulk to faeces, aiding the passage of material through the intestines. People who have plenty of this type of fibre in their diet seem to have a reduced risk of colorectal cancer. Major sources of insoluble fibre include unrefined carbohydrate foods such as wholemeal bread, cereals, brown pasta, brown rice, fruits, pulses, vegetables, seeds, and whole grains.

Soluble fibre may lower blood cholesterol levels and has been associated with a reduced risk of heart disease and stroke. Good sources of soluble fibre include fruits, oats, beans and pulses, and vegetables.

Complex carbohydrates should form the major part of your daily diet. Simple carbohydrates should be kept to a minimum because, although they provide energy, they are low in vitamins and minerals and contain little fibre.

Protein Protein is essential for building and repairing cells in the body. Insufficient protein in the diet causes serious health problems, but such deficiency is largely restricted to developing countries where the availability of food is limited. A more common problem in the UK is too much protein in the diet, particularly animal protein. Excess protein is converted into fat in the body. Many protein-rich foods are also high in calories and saturated fat. A high-protein diet may therefore lead to obesity. Foods that are high in protein include meat, fish, cheese, and nuts. For a healthy diet, about a sixth of your total calorie intake should ideally be obtained from protein.

Fats Fats are a source of energy and are essential for the absorption of certain vitamins. The amount and type of fat in your diet are important in determining your general health and also affect your risk of developing coronary artery disease or of having a stroke. The link is cholesterol, a fat-like substance that is essential for normal body functioning but can be a risk to health in excess. There are two types of cholesterol in the body: high density lipoprotein (HDL) cholesterol and low density lipoprotein

▶ **HEALTH ACTION**

Healthy eating

A healthy diet combines a variety of foods in different proportions. Foods are divided into five groups, shown here in the relative proportions in which they should be eaten to form a balanced, healthy diet. Enjoy your food and vary your diet to ensure that you get all of the nutrients your body needs. Eat the correct amount to maintain a healthy weight. Fresh fruit and vegetables and carbohydrate-rich foods such as potatoes should form the bulk of your diet, with meat, fish, and dairy products forming a smaller part of your daily intake.

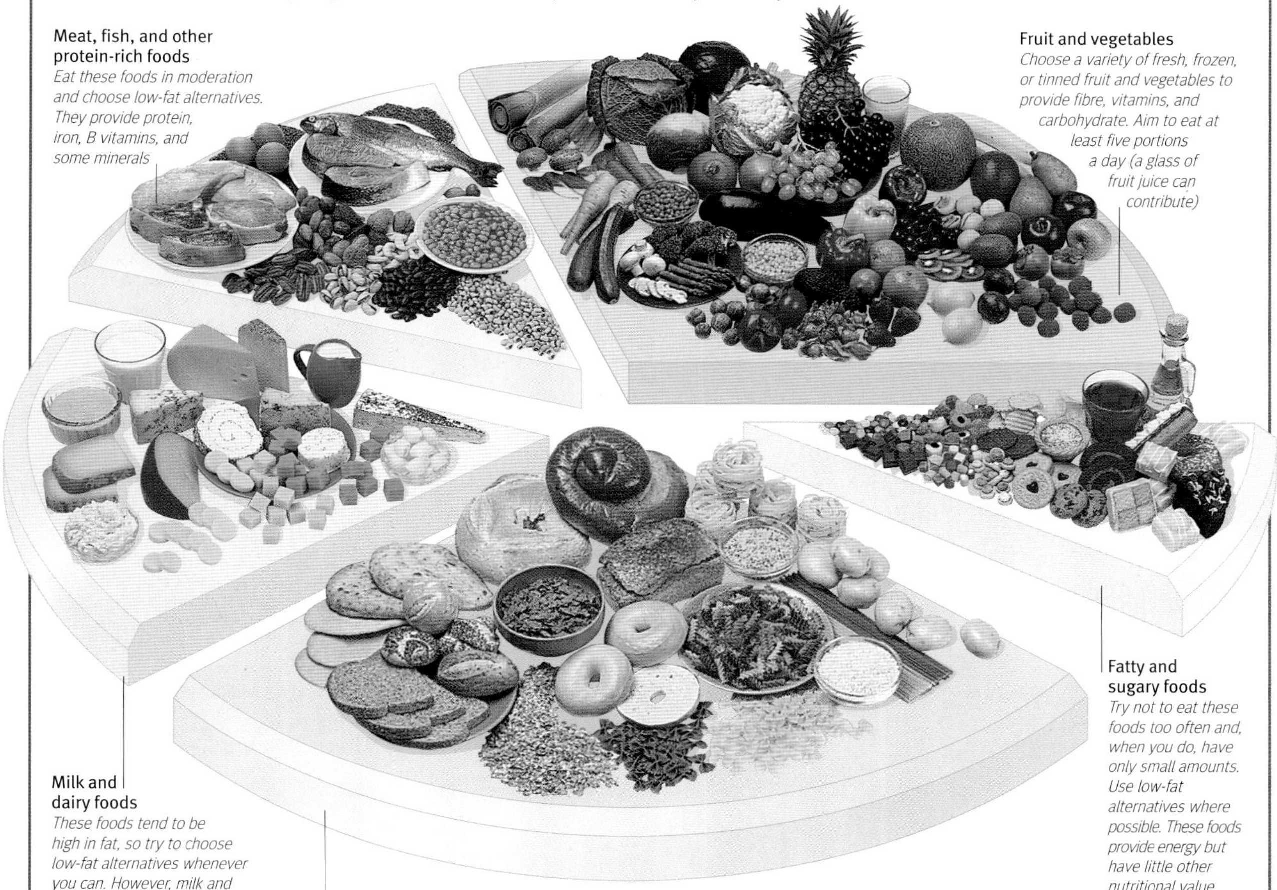

Meat, fish, and other protein-rich foods
Eat these foods in moderation and choose low-fat alternatives. They provide protein, iron, B vitamins, and some minerals

Fruit and vegetables
Choose a variety of fresh, frozen, or tinned fruit and vegetables to provide fibre, vitamins, and carbohydrate. Aim to eat at least five portions a day (a glass of fruit juice can contribute)

Fatty and sugary foods
Try not to eat these foods too often and, when you do, have only small amounts. Use low-fat alternatives where possible. These foods provide energy but have little other nutritional value

Milk and dairy foods
These foods tend to be high in fat, so try to choose low-fat alternatives whenever you can. However, milk and dairy products provide protein and are a good source of calcium and certain vitamins, such as B₁₂, A, and D

Bread, potatoes, pasta, and other complex carbohydrates
These foods provide plenty of dietary fibre; complex carbohydrate; some minerals, particularly calcium and iron; and vitamins in the B group

Food groups
You should aim to eat foods from each of the five main food groups in the proportions represented here by slices of a plate. Foods in the larger slices should form a greater part of your diet than foods in the smaller slices. The total amount of food you need to eat depends on your body size, age, and activity levels.

(LDL) cholesterol. High levels of LDL cholesterol in the blood increase the risk of developing atherosclerosis (p.241), narrowing of the arteries that may eventually lead to cardiovascular disease, which is why LDL cholesterol is commonly known as "bad" cholesterol. Conversely, HDL cholesterol helps to lower the blood level of LDL cholesterol, and so HDL cholesterol is often called "good" cholesterol.

An individual's level of blood cholesterol depends partly on genetic factors, but in many cases the main influence is the amount and type of fat in the diet. Fats can be either saturated or unsaturated, depending on their chemical structure; it is the saturated fats found in dairy products and meat that mainly contribute to raised LDL cholesterol levels in the body. It is also advisable to avoid hydrogenated fats, sometimes known as transfats, which are artificially produced and have properties that are similar to satu-

rated fats. Hydrogenated fats are often found in butter substitutes and manufactured food items such as biscuits and cakes. In contrast, unsaturated fats seem to provide some protection against cardiovascular disease by reducing LDL cholesterol levels, with polyunsaturates having a greater effect than monounsaturates.

For a healthier diet, the average man should eat no more than 30g of saturated fat a day, and the average woman no more than 20g a day. You should also choose foods that contain unsaturated rather than saturated fats.

Vitamins and minerals Vitamins and minerals play vital roles in growth and metabolism (*see* **Good sources of vitamins and minerals**, p.18). Apart from vitamin K, which is formed by intestinal bacteria, and vitamin D, which is produced in the skin by the action of sunlight, all vitamins and minerals must be obtained from your diet.

The majority of people in the UK obtain adequate amounts of vitamins and minerals from their diet. Some vitamins, including vitamins A, D, E, and K, are harmful if consumed in excess. However, some people may need to take vitamin and mineral supplements (pp.598–600). For example, women who regularly lose iron through heavy menstrual bleeding may be advised to take iron supplements. Women are advised to take supplementary folic acid before pregnancy and for the first 12 weeks of pregnancy. During pregnancy, women are also advised to take supplementary vitamin D. Children who are reluctant to eat a normal range of foods may be given vitamins A, C, and D. Elderly people who have a low or restricted intake of food may also need supplements. Older women should make sure they have adequate calcium in their diet to help prevent osteoporosis (p.217). People who eat a vegetarian diet usually

have an adequate intake of vitamins and minerals, but vegans, who eat no animal products, are at risk of vitamin B₁₂ deficiency and should also ensure that they get enough calcium in their diet.

Fluids Water is essential for life, and makes up almost four-fifths of the body. Water is lost by sweating and passing urine and must be replaced. Inadequate water intake may lead to kidney problems, such as kidney stones (p.447), and constipation (p.398). Some water is obtained from solid foods, but you should also drink plenty of fluids. Try to drink at least 8 glasses (2 litres/3½ pints) of nonalcoholic fluid a day. In hot weather or during exercise, you may need more. The need for water is also increased by diarrhoea, vomiting, diuretics (drugs that increase urine output), and caffeine.

Your energy requirements
The body needs a constant reserve of energy to function properly. Energy from food is measured in units called kilojoules (kJ) or kilocalories (kcal), which are usually referred to simply as calories.

The number of calories you need to obtain from your diet depends on how much energy your body uses. This depends partly on how efficiently your body cells use energy, which is genetically determined, and partly on your level of physical activity. The rate at which your body uses energy simply to maintain basic processes such as breathing and digestion is called your basal metabolic rate (BMR). Extra calories are needed for all your day-to-day activities. Energetic activities, such as sports, increase the calorie requirement. Most of these extra calories should come from complex carbohydrates, such as bread. However, people who have physically demanding jobs also require extra fat and sugar, both of which are rich sources of energy.

Your stage of life also has an influence on your energy requirements. For example, a growing, active teenager usually needs more calories than an adult. Calorie requirements tend to decrease as you get older because BMR declines with age and activity may be reduced. A pregnant woman needs more calories than a nonpregnant woman.

Choosing nutritious food
Fresh foods tend to be healthy, but they often have a short shelf life. Processing techniques are used to increase shelf life. Many processed foods have as many vitamins and minerals as fresh food. Food preservatives prevent the growth of microorganisms, which could cause food poisoning (p.398). However, processed and refined foods may contain high levels of fats, sugar, or salt, so it is important to check the food labels (*see* **Understanding food labels**, opposite page). In addition to listing food ingredients and nutritional information, many food labels provide extra information so that people who restrict their diet in some way can make decisions about which foods to select.

▶ **HEALTH ACTION**

Good sources of vitamins and minerals

Vitamins and minerals are essential for growth and health, and certain vitamins play a key role in preventing disease. Requirements for some of these elements depend on gender, stage of life, and age. For example, women planning a pregnancy or in the first 12 weeks of pregnancy are advised to take folic acid at the recommended dose to help prevent neural tube defects in the fetus. Most vitamins and all minerals have to come from food or supplements because they are not produced in the body. Some vitamins are toxic if consumed in excess. For example, pregnant women should avoid foods that contain high levels of vitamin A because of potential harmful effects on the fetus.

Eating for health

The body needs vitamins and minerals to stay healthy, although the exact daily requirements for the various vitamins and minerals may differ according to factors such as stage of life and gender.

Vitamins and minerals	Good sources	Effects
Vitamin A	Calves' liver, eggs, carrots, melon	■ Important for healthy eyes, hair, skin, and bones ■ Can be toxic in excess
Vitamin B₁ (Thiamine)	Meat, whole grains, peas, fortified cereals and breads	■ Helps in energy production ■ Essential for the proper functioning of the nervous system
Vitamin B₂ (Riboflavin)	Eggs, meat, milk products, leafy vegetables	■ Involved in the release of proteins from nutrients ■ Helps to maintain the nervous system and muscles
Vitamin B₃ (Niacin)	Fish, whole grains, peanuts, peas	■ Essential for the utilization of energy from food ■ Helps to maintain healthy skin
Vitamin B₆	Meat, fish, whole grains, bananas	■ Necessary for blood formation ■ Helps to regulate the cells in the nervous system
Vitamin B₁₂	Milk, fish, meat, eggs, yeast extract	■ Vital for the growth of blood cells in the bone marrow ■ Essential for a healthy nervous system
Vitamin C	Many fruits and vegetables	■ Helps maintain healthy tissues ■ Helps the body to use iron
Vitamin D	Dairy products, oily fish, also formed in the skin by sunlight	■ Enhances calcium absorption for strong teeth and bones ■ Can be toxic in excess
Vitamin E	Vegetables, eggs, fish, margarine	■ Protects tissues and organs against degenerative disease ■ Can be toxic in excess
Vitamin K	Leafy green vegetables, pigs' liver, also formed by intestinal bacteria	■ Essential for proper blood clotting ■ Necessary for bone formation ■ Can be toxic in excess
Folic acid	Leafy green vegetables, organ meats, whole grains, fortified bread, nuts	■ Helps to prevent neural tube defects (p.547) in fetuses ■ Contributes to healthy cells and blood
Calcium	Tofu, sardines, milk, cheese, yoghurt, sesame seeds	■ Necessary for healthy bones, teeth, and muscles ■ Helps with conduction of nerve impulses
Iron	Eggs, meat, leafy green vegetables, pulses, fortified cereals	■ Aids formation of red blood cells and certain proteins ■ Maintains healthy muscles

There is continuing debate about the health benefits of organic food and the possibility of health risks from genetically modified (GM) food. However, there is no unequivocal scientific evidence that organic food offers health benefits over non-organic food nor that the GM foods currently produced pose a risk to human health. So-called superfoods – foods that are purported to have health benefits – are another area of debate. In most cases, the health claims are not supported by scientific evidence. An exception is oily fish, for which there is evidence that it can reduce blood cholesterol levels and reduce the risk of cardiovascular disease. There is also limited evidence that oily fish may reduce the risk of age-related macular degeneration (p.362). It is therefore recommended that oily fish should be eaten as part of a healthy diet.

Fad diets

Diets that promise rapid weight loss but may have only short-term effects

People who are overweight often look for a quick way to lose weight and many are keen to try any new diet that appears on the market. There are new diets coming out all the time, each with its own unique formula, promising easy and rapid weight loss. A fad diet is a weight loss plan that gives this type of quick fix. However, most of these diets do not provide a long-term solution to the problem of excess weight. Furthermore, some fad diets may make you feel unwell and may even damage your health.

What are the types?

Fad diets that promise quick weight loss often recommend only a particular food or type of food. They are popular because many of them work for a short time. They ensure that a person following the diet takes in fewer calories than usual because he or she stops eating certain types of food or eats combinations of specific foods. However, much of the weight lost is not from body fat, but from water and lean muscle.

High protein–low carbohydrate diets People following these diets often lose weight very rapidly. However, the weight loss is not sustained once the diets are discontinued. A high fat intake may increase the risk of heart disease. Nutritionists recommend animal proteins such as lean chicken and fish, and plant proteins such as nuts and beans, but advise against cutting

out whole groups of foods, such as starchy carbohydrates, or limiting the consumption of fruit and vegetables.

Food-combining diets These diets are based on the belief that different food types are digested in different ways and should not be eaten together in the same meal. For example, carbohydrates and proteins should not be combined in a meal. However, these diets can be unbalanced and unhealthy. Each of the five components in a balanced diet – carbohydrates, fats, proteins, vitamins, and minerals – contributes to health and should be consumed in correct proportions (*see* **A healthy diet**, p.16).

Liquid meal replacement diets These very low-calorie diets result in rapid weight loss. They can be effective and nutritionally balanced, and may help to motivate people to change their diet and lifestyle. However, they should be followed only for short periods. People on meal-replacement diets may find it difficult to maintain a lower weight if they return to their previous eating habits. If you are pregnant or breast-feeding, have health problems, or wish to lose a lot of weight, consult your doctor before starting.

Intermittent-fasting diets These are based on fasting for a number of days per week and eating normally for the rest of the week. Although strict calorie counting is not usually necessary during the normal-eating days, you should still make healthy food choices and keep physically active. As a method of weight-loss, the evidence for the effectiveness of these diets is limited. Fasting may also cause effects such as dizziness, headaches, irritability, and difficulty concentrating, and it is not suitable for certain groups of people, such as pregnant women or those with diabetes or some other health problems.

What are the risks?

Fad diets often involve theories that lack adequate scientific support, such as the belief that carbohydrates are fattening. In fact, a balanced diet with less fat, adequate carbohydrate, and a limited calorie intake will help people to lose weight in a more controlled way, especially when combined with plenty of exercise.

A high-fat diet is more likely to result in overconsumption of calories than a high-carbohydrate diet. This is because fat contains about twice the amount of calories as carbohydrates. For example, 1 g of fat has 9 calories while 1 g of carbohydrate contains 4 calories.

Repeated episodes of rapid weight loss while on a fad diet are often followed by weight gain (the "yo-yo" effect). This can cause people to gain even more excess weight than they had originally.

Health risks include wasting of body muscle, including the heart muscle. Fad diets can also cause nutritional deficiencies. For example, iron deficiency may cause anaemia (p.271) and calcium deficiency may aggravate osteoporosis (p.217). In addition, a lack of vitamins in the diet may lead to deficiency diseases.

It is important to assess the diet you choose to follow. People who need to take special care are children, adolescents, women who are pregnant or breast-feeding, the elderly, those with conditions such as diabetes mellitus or those who have heart, kidney, or musculoskeletal problems.

What might be done?

The only effective way to lose weight is to plan a weight-loss programme that involves a gradual and long-term change in eating habits and exercise. If you wish to lose weight, you should consult your doctor. He or she can help you to plan your weight loss in a safe and effective way. You should eat a variety of foods, such as whole grains, pulses, vegetables, and fruit, but in limited quantities. You should never skip a meal, but limit your intake of saturated fats and sugar. You should also be more physically active, and make a concerted effort to exercise regularly (*see* **Exercise and health**, pp.20–23). Losing weight means taking in fewer calories relative to energy expenditure in a sustained way. There are no quick and easy solutions.

Controlling your weight

Maintaining your weight within a healthy range for your height

An essential part of a healthy lifestyle is maintaining your body weight within the range considered normal for your height. In recent decades, the number of overweight and obese people (including children) in many developed countries has increased significantly. In the UK, an estimated 1 in 4 adults (*see* **Obesity in adults**, p.400) and 1 in 5 children (*see* **Obesity in children**, p.552) are obese.

Obesity is a major threat to health. Disorders associated with being obese, such as coronary artery disease (p.243), high blood pressure (*see* **Hypertension**, p.242), cancer (pp.152–159), and stroke (p.329), rank among the leading causes of illness and death in developed countries such as the UK. Being underweight can also cause health problems, including an increased risk of infertility (pp.497–499) and the bone disorder osteoporosis (p.217).

Causes of weight problems

In the UK, the main factor contributing to the general weight gain of the population is lack of exercise combined with overeating. Children's pastimes are far more sedentary than those of former generations, and many adults do not exercise at all. In addition, an increasing number of people rely on convenience foods, which tend to be high in saturated fat and simple carbohydrates, both of which are high in calories.

There are various reasons why someone may be underweight. Some people are naturally thin and find it difficult to gain weight.

Others start within the normal weight range but then develop an eating disorder, such as anorexia nervosa (p.348) or bulimia (p.349), and lose a great deal of weight, eventually becoming abnormally thin. Weight loss can also result from loss of appetite due to long-term illness such as depression (p.343), tuberculosis (p.300), or rheumatoid arthritis (p.222).

Finding your ideal weight

Height and weight charts offer an easy way to find out whether you are within the recommended weight range for your height. Your ideal body weight depends on your height and on the amount of muscle tissue you have. For example, an athlete should weigh more than a healthy but relatively sedentary person of the same height. This is because exercise increases muscle, which is heavier than other types of body tissue. For this reason, the charts provide ranges and not precise measurements.

Research indicates that the distribution of fat around the body is an important determinant of health. Excess fat around the abdomen is more closely linked to cardiovascular diseases than fat elsewhere. To find out whether you are a healthy weight, you should both check if your weight falls within the recommended range for your height and measure your waist size (*see* below).

Doctors and dietitians use weight and height measurements to calculate body mass index (BMI). This is a widely accepted and more precise method of checking if you are underweight, a healthy weight, or overweight by providing an indication of the degree of fatness, although it is not a direct measure of body fat. The BMI is calculated by dividing a person's weight (in kilograms) by his or her height (in metres) squared. A BMI of 18.4 or less is classed as underweight; 18.5–24.9 is classed as a healthy weight; 25–29.9 is classed as overweight; and a BMI over 30 is classed as obese. These figures are general ones that apply to most healthy adults. They are not applicable to children; those with chronic health problems; women who are pregnant or breast-feeding; or athletes, weight-trainers, or similar groups of people with a high proportion of body muscle.

Body mass index is also used to check whether children are a healthy weight or not, although the BMI value is used in a slightly way from how it is used in adults. A child's BMI is plotted on a chart and compared with how it relates to the BMI values of children of the same age.

Losing weight

If the height/weight chart confirms that you are overweight, you can lose weight by following a slimming diet and taking exercise. Rarely, a doctor may advise drug treatment or surgery as well as a slimming diet to aid weight loss in a very obese person.

Before you attempt to lose weight, you should try to identify why you may be overweight. The most likely cause is a combination of overeating and lack of exercise, but you may find it helpful to look at your reasons for overeating. For example, do you tend to eat when you feel unhappy or is overeating a habit that has become established in your family?

The best way to lose weight is to combine calorie reduction with regular exercise. Plan what you need to do to succeed. For example, if you need more exercise, arrange a time each day to take a brisk walk. If you are tempted by the wrong foods, make a list of healthy foods before going shopping.

Success in dieting also depends on being realistic about how much weight you can lose. Set yourself a practical, short-term target, revising it as you go along. About 2–4 kg (4.5–9 lb) a month is sensible. If you want to lose more than this or have any health problems, consult your doctor before you start.

You also need to consider what you hope to achieve by losing excess weight. You should recognize that weight loss may not solve all your problems. It may make you feel more self-confident and will certainly improve some aspects of your health, but it is unlikely to help a failing relationship. However, the health benefits alone are worth the effort.

Slimming diets If your diet does not provide enough calories for all your energy needs, your body will start to use up excess fat for energy. Therefore, you should begin to lose weight if you eat fewer calories. Publications that list the calorie content of foods are widely available, and this information can also be found on the labels of most packaged food (*see* **Understanding food labels**, p.16). A good starting point for most people is to try to reduce their daily calorie intake by about 500 calories. This can be achieved by cutting down on high-fat foods, such as cakes, pastries, cheese, and fried dishes, and replacing them with healthy, low-calorie foods, such as fruit, vegetables, and grilled dishes.

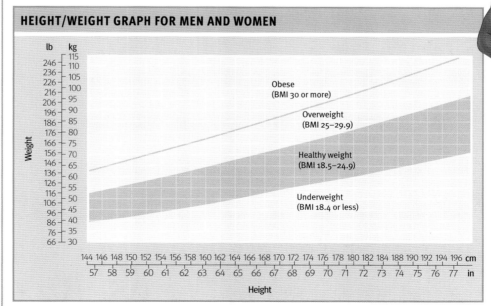

▶ **ASSESSMENT**

Are you a healthy weight?

You can check whether you are a healthy weight by using the height/weight graph below. Height and weight measurements can be used to calculate your body mass index (BMI), an indicator of body fat. Even if the graph indicates that you are a healthy weight, you are still at increased risk of cardiovascular disease if your waist measurement is greater than 89 cm (35 in) for women and 102 cm (40 in) for men.

HEIGHT/WEIGHT GRAPH FOR MEN AND WOMEN

Obese (BMI 30 or more)

Overweight (BMI 25–29.9)

Healthy weight (BMI 18.5–24.9)

Underweight (BMI 18.4 or less)

Weight

Height

Measuring your waist
Your waist measurement indicates whether you have excess abdominal fat.

Using the graph
Find your height and weight on the axes. Trace a vertical line from your height and a horizontal line from your weight. The point at which the lines cross on the graph indicates whether or not you are within a healthy range.

If your normal diet already consists mainly of low-calorie foods, you simply need to cut down on the quantity of food you eat. The best type of slimming diet is one that is low in calories but balanced so that you stay well nourished (*see* **Healthy eating**, p.17).

Alcohol contains no healthy nutrients and is high in calories. It is therefore advisable to reduce your alcohol consumption as much as possible when you are trying to lose weight.

Rapid weight-loss plans (*see* **Fad diets**, p.18) and fasting to lose weight should be avoided. They can damage your health by depriving your body of the range of nutrients it needs to function well. Such plans do not produce sustainable weight loss or encourage sensible, healthy eating habits.

Exercise Exercising to lose weight need not be strenuous, but it does have to be regular. Sustained regular exercise raises your basal metabolic rate (BMR), the rate at which your body uses energy to maintain basic processes such as breathing, digestion, and the heartbeat. If your BMR rises, you use up more calories (*see* **Exercise and health**, pp.20–23) and will lose weight if you also follow a calorie-controlled diet. Exercise tones and builds muscles, which weigh more than fat. Therefore, as you become fitter, you may find that the scales initially register a few more kilograms, although you will not actually be any fatter. Exercise can also stimulate your appetite; you must resist eating more than your new diet allows. As you become older, your metabolism slows down, and therefore your body uses up fewer calories. It is important to remain as active as possible to prevent the gradual weight gain that is common among older people.

Drugs and surgery Anti-obesity drugs are usually recommended only for people who are obese and for whom exercise and diet alone has not helped, especially if they also have other risk factors to health, such as diabetes mellitus and/or high blood pressure. Anti-obesity drugs are always used in conjunction with diet and exercise and should not be taken long term.

Certain drugs for weight loss are available over the counter, such as bulking agents and orlistat (Xenical). Bulking agents, such as methyl cellulose, make you feel full but may cause bloating and flatulence. Orlistat inhibits the absorption of fat in the intestine; possible side effects include headaches, flatulence, an urgent need to defecate, an oily discharge from the rectum, and liquid or oily faeces.

Weight-loss surgery (*see* **Obesity in adults**, p.400) carries the risk of potentially serious complications and so is generally considered only for people who are severely obese and for whom other weight-loss measures have been unsuccessful.

Gaining weight

Many people think that being underweight is not a health risk. It can be just as unhealthy as being overweight and requires careful treatment. If your BMI is 18.4 or less and if you have other symptoms, such as excessive tiredness and an inability to keep warm, you should see your doctor to exclude an underlying condition that requires treatment.

It is important to gain weight sensibly to build up muscle and bone and achieve a healthy level of body fat. Although fatty and fast foods are high in calories, you should avoid eating large quantities to gain weight because of their unhealthy effects, such as causing high blood pressure and increasing risk of heart disease. Put on weight slowly by eating a healthy, balanced diet. Several small, nutritious meals each day provide a better supply of energy than one or two large meals.

Regular exercise helps to build muscles, increases strength, and may also improve your appetite. You should start slowly, especially if you tire easily, and build up the amount you do gradually.

Exercise and health

Exercise is an essential part of any healthy lifestyle. This idea is not a new one; the fact that physical activity is linked to good health can be traced back to the Greeks in the fifth century BC. Since then, research has proven that exercise prolongs life, protects health, and can reduce the risk of disease. Taking part in team sports also provides the opportunity for social contact.

Many people in developed countries lead a sedentary lifestyle, and too few people exercise regularly. By making a concerted effort to incorporate physical activity into your daily life, you can become significantly healthier.

The first article in this section outlines the overwhelming physical and psychological benefits of being active. Exercise also has an effect on other aspects of your lifestyle. For example, people who exercise tend to smoke less than those who do not. Developing a habit of regular physical activity may encourage you to give up smoking.

The second article provides practical guidelines for assessing how fit you are and improving your level of fitness.

The last article explores safe habits and routines to adopt when exercising to minimize the risk of injury.

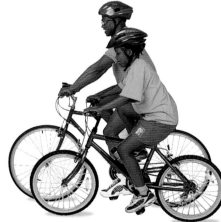

Exercise for life
Exercising on a regular basis can improve the quality of your life by improving your strength, stamina, and psychological health and by providing you with the opportunity to socialize.

developing type 2 diabetes mellitus (p.437) or, if you have the condition, can help to control your blood sugar level. When you make exercise a part of your daily routine, you will probably find it a lot easier to perform ordinary tasks, such as shopping, gardening, doing housework, and climbing stairs. In addition to the more obvious physical benefits, exercising regularly can improve your psychological wellbeing. Developing a habit of exercising with other people can also help you to make new friends.

Cardiovascular health

Research has shown that people who do little or no exercise are at increased risk of coronary artery disease (p.243), heart attack (*see* **Myocardial infarction**, p.245), and stroke (p.329). However, for exercise to give you effective protection against heart disease, it has to be regular and sustained over your lifetime. Exercising only in your youth is no guarantee of benefits later in life.

When you exercise regularly, your heart becomes stronger and more efficient and can pump more blood with every heartbeat, making it able to cope with extra demands. The amount of regular exercise that you take also influences your chance of surviving a heart attack if you should ever have one; people who have exercised regularly are more likely to survive.

Regular exercise helps to reduce blood cholesterol levels and lowers blood pressure. Both of these factors reduce the risk of developing fatty plaques in your arteries (*see* **Atherosclerosis**, p.241). Research shows that people who already have coronary artery disease or lower limb ischaemia (p.261) may benefit from exercise because of the improvement that it makes to the blood supply. These benefits may be experienced within 2 months of starting regular exercise.

Respiratory health

Regular exercise improves the efficiency of your respiratory muscles and increases the usable volume of the alveoli (air sacs) in the lungs. It also increases the efficiency of the exchange of oxygen and carbon dioxide in the lungs. People who exercise regularly are able to extract more oxygen from a single breath and have a slower breathing rate. If you have a respiratory disease, such as chronic obstructive pulmonary disease (p.297), regular exercise may help to improve the amount of physical activity that you can do on a daily basis without becoming breathless.

Musculoskeletal health

Exercising improves the condition of your bones, joints, and muscles. Taking regular exercise helps you to keep yourself flexible and mobile for longer and improves your quality of life.

Maintaining strong bones Weight-bearing exercises, such as walking and running, help to improve bone strength, density, and development. This kind of exercise is particularly important for proper physical development during childhood and adolescence, when the bones are still growing.

It is also important for women of all ages to do weight-bearing exercises regularly because they help to slow down the accelerated bone loss caused by the decline in levels of the hormone oestrogen (*see* **Osteoporosis**, p.217) that occurs after the menopause.

Mobilizing and stabilizing joints Regular exercise improves the flexibility of joints and minimizes stiffness. It also helps to stabilize the joints by strengthening the muscles and ligaments surrounding them. By maintaining joint mobility, exercise can help you to remain independent and able to do more in later life. If you

The benefits of exercise

How regular exercise benefits your physical and psychological health

Most people know that exercise is part of a healthy lifestyle. In recent decades, the number of people in the UK taking regular exercise has increased, but many still do too little exercise. Exercise protects physical and mental health, and it has a particularly positive effect on the respiratory, cardiovascular, and musculoskeletal systems. By taking regular physical exercise, you can reduce your risk of developing long-term disease, increase your life expectancy, and improve your quality of life in later years. For example, regular exercise can reduce your risk of have a joint disease, such as rheumatoid arthritis (p.222), strength-building exercises may stabilize affected joints and reduce further damage.

Increasing muscle strength You should exercise your muscles regularly to keep them in good condition. Muscle size and strength can be increased with exercises that work against resistance, such as lifting moderate weights. Aerobic exercises that build stamina, such as running and cycling, make the muscles more efficient so that they can work for longer periods of time. Stronger muscles, and the increased confidence that often comes from feeling and looking fit, also improve your posture.

After about the age of 25, you lose a small amount of muscle each year as part of the normal aging process. If you keep your muscles strong and healthy, this loss of muscle bulk and strength can be kept to a minimum.

Lower back pain (p.225) is often a result of poor muscle strength and lack of flexibility. Regularly doing exercises that concentrate on strengthening particular muscle groups and improving overall flexibility can help to prevent back pain (see **Preventing back pain**, p.226) and keep you mobile.

Psychological wellbeing

When you begin a programme of regular exercise, you may experience some psychological benefits from early on. For example, many people notice a feeling of wellbeing after they have been exercising; this is commonly thought to be the result of an increase in the production by the brain of morphine-like chemical compounds known as endorphins. These chemical compounds act as natural antidepressants, and they can help you to feel more relaxed.

Mildly anxious or depressed people may notice a marked improvement in their mood after they have been exercising regularly for some time. For this reason, exercise is increasingly being incorporated into psychological therapies. You may find that exercise helps you to cope with stress (p.31). It also promotes regular, deep, and refreshing sleep (p.31).

By exercising regularly, you are likely to look and feel healthy, which can increase your self-esteem. You may also have a sense of achievement when you meet goals in your exercise routine.

Taking part in a team sport or joining a health club or gym can be a way of expanding your circle of friends. Team sports foster mutual respect, shared responsibility, and self-discipline. These benefits are widely recognized and are particularly important for children.

Research into the effects of exercise among people who work in offices has found that regular exercise generally leads to a more productive workforce.

Taking regular exercise

Taking steps to increase the amount of physical activity in your daily life

For exercise to be beneficial (see **The benefits of exercise**, opposite page), it has to be regular and consistent. The type and amount of activity you can incorporate into your lifestyle depends on the time you have available to exercise. The best form of exercise is one that you enjoy doing and can fit into your daily routine. Exercise should be tailored to your age, state of health, and lifestyle.

Recommended level of exercise

Evidence has shown that even gentle exercise has measurable positive effects on life expectancy; consequently, everyone should try to lead an active life. If your life is fairly active already, there are guidelines on the amount and the frequency of additional exercise you can take to gain the maximum benefit to your general health. Recommendations for adults are that they should do at least 30 minutes of aerobic exercise at moderate intensity on at least 5 days of the week. A brisk 30-minute walk will provide a healthy amount of exercise for the day. However, if you want to improve your muscle tone or lose excess body fat, or if you want to become even more fit, you will have to exercise harder and for a longer time.

Starting out

If your life is sedentary, begin by taking simple steps to become more active. For example, you could make a habit of climbing the stairs instead of taking the lift. If your life already includes some physical activity, think about starting a regular exercise routine, such as swimming, brisk walking, or jogging.

Make sure that your exercise routine is realistic for you, that you slowly build up the amount of exercise you take, and that you learn safe techniques (see **Exercising safely**, p.22). You may be encouraged to continue exercising on a regular basis once you begin to experience its positive effects.

Consult your doctor If you have never exercised regularly before, or if you think you may be at particular risk from exercise, you should consult your doctor before starting a regular exercise programme. You should consult your doctor if you have a chronic medical condition, such as coronary artery disease (p.243), high blood pressure (see **Hypertension**, p.242), diabetes mellitus (p.437), chronic kidney disease (p.451), or asthma (p.295). You should ask your doctor for advice if you are overweight or if you are over age 35 and have not exercised regularly for several years.

▶ HEALTH OPTION

Choices for fitness

Different exercises benefit different aspects of fitness (stamina, flexibility, or strength) to a greater or lesser extent. Some types of exercise, such as swimming, offer benefits in all of these aspects. You can choose the best activity to improve a specific aspect of fitness or review the overall fitness benefits of activities that you already do or are considering taking up.

Fitness benefits of different activities			
Activity	**Fitness benefits**		
	Stamina	Flexibility	Strength
Aerobics	★★★★	★★★	★★
Basketball	★★★★	★★★	★★
Cycling (fast)	★★★★	★★	★★★
Climbing stairs	★★★	★	★★★
Dancing (aerobic)	★★★	★★★★	★
Golf	★	★★	★
Hiking	★★★	★	★★
Jogging	★★★★	★★	★★
Swimming	★★★★	★★★★	★★★★
Tennis	★★	★★★	★★
Walking (briskly)	★★	★	★
Yoga	★	★★★★	★

Using the chart

The activities above have been graded according to their benefit to each aspect of fitness. By comparing the benefits of each activity, you can tailor an exercise programme to your own fitness needs.

KEY	
★ Small effect	★★★ Very good effect
★★ Good effect	★★★★ Excellent effect

Your doctor may recommend certain types of exercises that are appropriate for you. For example, if you are overweight and have not exercised for some years, he or she may suggest gentle exercise, such as walking or cycling, to avoid any strain on your heart and to reduce the risk of injury. If you have asthma, your doctor may suggest swimming.

Assess your fitness Overall fitness is a combination of three factors: stamina, flexibility, and strength. To improve your level of fitness, you need to do regular exercise that works your heart and lungs (builds stamina), improves your joint mobility (increases flexibility), and increases your muscle strength.

Before starting regular exercise, it is a good idea to estimate your overall fitness. Think about the activity you do in a normal day or week. You may find that you already do some exercise most days, such as walking to work.

Your resting pulse can be used as an indication of your general cardiovascular fitness. A fairly slow pulse indicates that your heart is fit. If you stop exercising regularly, you will lose the level of fitness you have attained, but can regain your fitness by restarting exercise.

Choosing the right exercise

Exercise needs vary depending on age, lifestyle, and fitness. Individual sports and activities improve different aspects of fitness (see **Choices for fitness**, above). You should choose exercises that help you to develop stamina, suppleness, and strength and that you can do all year round. Decide what your fitness goal is and then choose an activity. It is also important that you choose a type of exercise that you enjoy, because this will help you to maintain a regular exercise regime.

Getting the most from your exercise programme

If your goal from regular exercise is to achieve an optimal level of fitness, you might set yourself a target heart rate. It is a good idea to monitor and record improvements in your fitness at regular intervals, such as once a month. You can monitor your fitness level by taking your pulse while at rest and then measuring how quickly it returns to its resting rate after vigorous exercise (see **Your pulse recovery time**, p.22). As you become fitter, your pulse recovery time decreases.

▶ ASSESSMENT

Your pulse recovery time

The time it takes for your pulse to return to its resting rate after exercise can be used to monitor improvements in your fitness. As you become fitter, your pulse recovery time decreases. You should be able to notice a difference in how quickly your pulse recovers within 4 weeks of starting regular exercise that makes your heart and lungs work hard.

Neck pulse
Find your pulse on the side of the neck with your first and second fingers

Watch
Use a watch to time beats per minute

Taking your neck pulse after exercise
Count the number of beats for 10 seconds and multiply the result by 6 to calculate beats per minute. Continue taking your pulse every minute until it returns to its resting rate.

Target heart rate To calculate this, first estimate your maximum heart rate, which is normally about 220 minus your age. Your target heart rate during exercise is 60–80 percent of your maximum heart rate. You can measure your pulse to monitor your heart rate during exercise, but wearing an electronic heartrate monitor, activity tracker, or smartwatch is easier and gives a more accurate measurement.

Planning your programme When you start to increase the amount of exercise, you must build up gradually (*see* Exercising safely, below). Initially, increase the number of times each week that you exercise. When you are exercising more frequently, focus on increasing the length of time. Finally, you should increase the intensity of your exercise so that you achieve your target heart rate. For maximum benefit, you should aim to exercise every day for at least 30 minutes at your target heart rate.

Exercising safely

Taking all sensible precautions to avoid injury from exercise

Each type of exercise has its own potential hazards and may require the use of specialized equipment. Set yourself realistic goals to avoid overexertion or injury. If you are not fit or have exercised very little, begin slowly and build up gradually. Sudden strenuous exercise could result in injury (*see* Sports injuries, p.231). You may need advice from your doctor before you start exercising (*see* Taking regular exercise, p.21).

Specialized equipment and protection
Some activities, such as walking, need little or no specialized equipment, but equipment is essential for sports such as cycling. Proper footwear and clothing is important;

for example, poorly fitting shoes may aggravate hip and back problems. If you are exercising outside, it is important to protect your skin and eyes from the sun (*see* Safety in the sun, p.34). If you are using exercise equipment at home or at a gym, follow the instructions carefully.

Good exercise habits
Develop a routine of warming up and cooling down (right). If you notice signs of overexertion, you should stop at once. Serious warning symptoms include:
■ Chest pain.
■ Pain in the neck, jaw, or arms.
■ Awareness of an irregular heartbeat (palpitations).
■ Nausea.
■ Severe shortness of breath.
■ Dizziness and light-heartedness.
If you have any of these symptoms, you should discuss them with your doctor.

Dangers of overtraining
Exercising too often or too hard, which is often called overtraining, seems to undo the benefits of moderate exercise. The most common injuries due to overtraining include severe muscle stiffness, joint sprains, and stress fractures.

You may need to make small adjustments to include physical activity in your life, but take care not to become obsessive about exercise.

▶ HEALTH ACTION

Warming up and cooling down in your exercise routine

You should follow a routine to stretch your muscles, tendons, and ligaments before and after exercise to prevent cramping and stiffness and to minimize the risk of injury. Your warm-up should involve aerobic exercise followed by a series of stretches. After exercise, use a cool-down routine to slow the pace so that you are still warm while you stretch out your muscles. Repeat the stretches on both sides of the body and hold each stretch for at least 10 seconds. Some suitable warm-up and cool-down exercises are shown here.

Aerobic exercises
Aerobic activity increases the flow of blood through the soft tissues of the body. This increased blood flow raises their temperature and makes them more flexible. You should aim to do gentle aerobic exercises for between 8 and 10 minutes as part of both your warm-up and your cool-down routines.

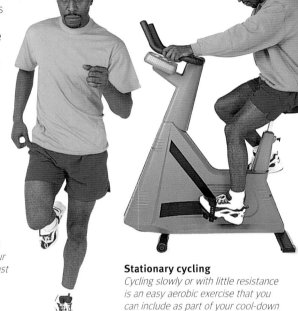

Jogging
Gentle jogging or running is a good way to warm up your muscles. You need to run fast enough to raise your heart rate and breathing rate. Moving your arms helps to raise your heart rate and create momentum.

Stationary cycling
Cycling slowly or with little resistance is an easy aerobic exercise that you can include as part of your cool-down routine. This exercise allows the heart rate to decrease gradually.

Upper body stretches
Stretching your chest and neck can help to relieve tension across the top of your back. Stretching your upper back by holding your arms out in front of you, clasping your hands, and rounding your back may also help. Upper body stretches improve your shoulder mobility.

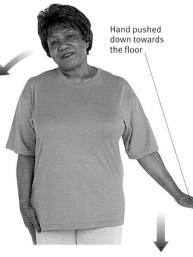

Hand pushed down towards the floor

Hands clasped behind back

Chest stretch
Clasp your hands behind you, and, while keeping your shoulders down, slowly move your arms up as far as they will go.

Neck stretch
While holding your arm out to one side, push your hand downwards. Then let your head fall to the opposite side.

Arm stretches

Like the upper body stretches, stretching your arms can help to relieve tension across the top of your back. You may find stretching easier on one side, depending on whether you are right- or left-handed. You should stretch your arms and shoulders before playing racket sports.

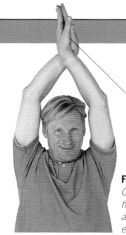

Palms of hands facing each other

Full arm stretch
Cross your arms and put your hands together. Raise your arms overhead, behind your ears, and stretch upwards.

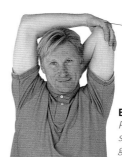

Elbow held beside head

Back of arm stretch
Put one hand between your shoulder blades and pull gently on the elbow to stretch the muscle.

Leg stretches

Many sports injuries affect the legs, so making sure that you stretch your leg muscles is especially important. You should always perform a series of leg stretches before taking part in activities that rely heavily on using your legs, such as brisk walking, running, jogging, and cycling.

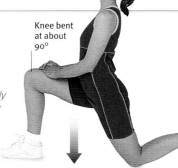

Knee bent at about 90°

Hip and thigh stretch
Kneel with one knee directly above its ankle and stretch the other leg back so that the knee touches the floor. Place your hands on your front knee for stability.

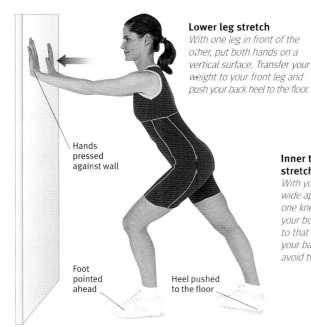

Lower leg stretch
With one leg in front of the other, put both hands on a vertical surface. Transfer your weight to your front leg and push your back heel to the floor.

Hands pressed against wall

Foot pointed ahead

Heel pushed to the floor

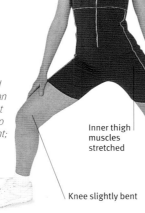

Trunk of body held upright

Inner thigh stretch
With your feet wide apart, bend one knee and lean your body weight to that side. Keep your back straight; avoid twisting.

Inner thigh muscles stretched

Knee slightly bent

Hand increases the stretch

Back of thigh stretch
In a lying position, bend both legs and bring one knee towards your chest. Grasp your toes with one hand and gently pull on the back of the thigh with the other.

Trunk stretches

Do not forget to stretch muscles in your trunk. For example, by stretching out your back and the sides of your body before and after working in the garden, you may prevent back pain.

Knee pushed back by the arm

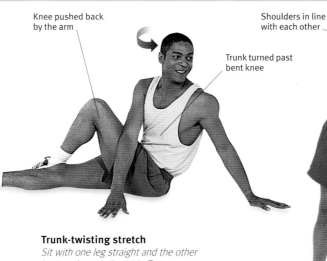

Shoulders in line with each other

Trunk turned past bent knee

Arms stretched out in front

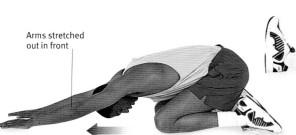

Lower back stretch
While kneeling, place your head on the floor in front of you and stretch your arms above your head, away from your body.

Trunk-twisting stretch
Sit with one leg straight and the other bent and crossed over it. Turn towards the knee that is bent, place your arm in front of the knee, and push against that leg while turning your body towards your other arm.

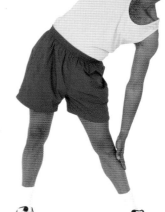

Side stretch
With your feet shoulder-width apart, stand up straight. Then put one arm over your head, lean from the waist, and reach slowly to the side with your upper hand to feel the stretch.

Alcohol, tobacco, and drugs

Many people use alcohol, tobacco, or recreational drugs for pleasure. However, all of these substances may cause severe health problems. Knowledge of their harmful effects can help you to make informed choices about whether or not to use them.

If you drink alcohol, you should do so in moderation. Having more than two drinks a day can pose short-term risks, from alcohol poisoning to traffic accidents. In the long term, excessive alcohol consumption causes serious problems, such as heart, liver, and brain disease, and can lead to alcohol dependence.

Tobacco smokers are exposed to over 4,000 chemicals, including nicotine, which is addictive, and other chemicals that increase susceptibility to cancer and to narrowing of the arteries, a cause of heart disease and stroke. The smoke may also have adverse effects on the health of people particularly children, who live around a smoker.

All recreational drugs alter your state of mind; many, such as LSD and marijuana, can impair judgment and increase the risk of

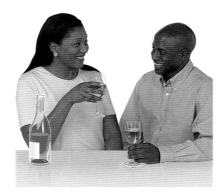

Social drinking
Alcohol consumption can be an enjoyable part of your social life, but you should keep your consumption within safe limits.

accidents. Drugs may be highly addictive and may cause death from overdose or side effects. Most recreational drugs are illegal.

Alcohol and health

How alcohol affects health and how to use alcohol responsibly

Alcohol has been used for centuries at celebrations and social occasions. It is a drug that alters a person's mental and physical state reducing tension and anxiety, and facilitating social interaction, but it may also cause loss of control over behaviour. Although moderate alcohol consumption (*see* **Safe alcohol limits**, right) promotes a feeling of relaxation, excessive use of alcohol over a long period can result in a wide range of serious physical, psychological, and social problems.

Excessive drinking severely reduces life expectancy and is a significant cause of preventable injury or death. In the UK in 2013, there were more than 8,400 deaths that were attributable to alcohol. In the same year, drink-driving accidents resulted in 8,290 casualties, including about 260 deaths (*see* **Safety on the road**, p.35).

Effects of alcohol use

When you drink alcohol, it is absorbed into the blood from the stomach and small intestine. It is carried to the liver, where it is broken down by enzymes to be used for energy or stored as fat. A small amount is eliminated unchanged in urine and in exhaled breath. Alcohol reaches its maximum concentration in the blood about 35–45 minutes after intake. The actual concentration depends on various factors, such as the weight of the

individual and whether the alcohol has been drunk with food or on an empty stomach. The rate at which alcohol is broken down (metabolized) in the liver also varies between individuals, and heavy drinkers can metabolize it more quickly. The average rate is about 1 unit per hour. On any occasion, your body cannot alter the rate at which it breaks down alcohol, so that the more you drink, the longer it will take for your blood alcohol concentration to return to normal. If you drink heavily at night, you may still be intoxicated the next morning.

Short-term effects Alcohol is a sedative, depressing the central nervous system. In particular, it affects the part of the brain that controls movement, impairing reaction times and coordination. Your inhibitions are suppressed, and, although you may feel more confident, your judgment may be impaired for several hours after drinking. Just one drink is enough to have this effect, making it dangerous to drive or operate machinery. Alcohol dilates blood vessels in the skin. Although this may make you feel warm, you are actually losing heat. Therefore, alcohol should not be given to anyone chilled from exposure to the cold.

Alcohol causes increased urine production, and you may feel dehydrated if you have several drinks in quick succession. Heavy drinking often leads to a hangover, with headache, nausea, dizziness, and a dry mouth. Hangovers are the result of adverse reactions to alcohol itself and to chemical additives, which are found particularly in dark-coloured drinks such as red wine and whisky. You can slow the absorption of alcohol by eating when you drink. Drinking very large quantities of alcohol may cause confusion and loss of memory, loss of consciousness, coma, or, in extreme cases, death.

Some Asian people have a gene that causes an immediate adverse reaction to alcohol. Affected people have reactions such as nausea and facial flushing.

▷ **HEALTH ACTION**

Safe alcohol limits

Alcohol intake is measured in units. The UK guidelines state that, in general, men and women should not regularly drink more than 14 units of alcohol a week. If you do drink as much as 14 units a week, your consumption should be spread evenly across the week. There is no established safe alcohol limit in pregnancy. However, it is known that the risk to the baby increases the more you drink. It is therefore recommended that women who

are pregnant or who are trying to conceive should not drink at all. Drinking small amounts during breast-feeding is not thought to be harmful to the baby but, if you do drink, you should wait about 2 hours before breast-feeding to ensure that there is no alcohol in your breast milk.

Units of alcohol
The number of units in a drink is calculated on the basis of the volume of the drink and the percentage of alcohol by volume (ABV).

▷ **1 UNIT OF ALCOHOL**

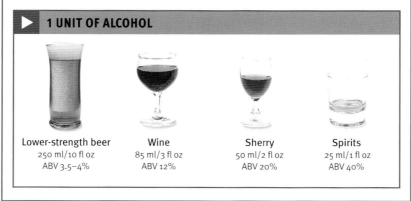

Lower-strength beer	Wine	Sherry	Spirits
250 ml/10 fl oz	85 ml/3 fl oz	50 ml/2 fl oz	25 ml/1 fl oz
ABV 3.5–4%	ABV 12%	ABV 20%	ABV 40%

Long-term effects Drinking small amounts of alcohol may protect against coronary heart disease (p.243) in women aged 55 or over. However, when safe limits are exceeded, the risks outweigh the benefits. Since alcohol has a high calorie content, regular drinkers often put on weight (*see* **Controlling your weight**, p.19). Alcohol damages most body systems and is a major cause of liver disease (*see* **Alcohol-related liver disease**, p.409). In the brain, cells that control learning and memory may be damaged (*see* **Wernicke–Korsakoff syndrome**, p.332). Drinking more than the safe alcohol limit increases the risk of cardiovascular disorders such as dilated cardiomyopathy (p.257), stroke, and high blood pressure (*see* **Hypertension**, p.242). Excessive consumption of alcohol increases the risk of several kinds of cancer, especially cancer of the nasopharynx (p.293), cancer of the larynx (p.294), mouth cancer (p.402), and cancer of the oesophagus (p.404). If you also smoke, the cancer risk is even greater. Drinking too much alcohol also causes a reduction in fertility.

Regular excessive drinking leads to alcohol dependence (p.350) and is a major cause of social problems. Regular drinking can also damage relationships and lead to stress for a drinker's family and friends.

Pregnancy and breast-feeding Drinking during pregnancy increases the risk of fetal alcohol syndrome, and also the risk of miscarriage (p.511). Babies affected by fetal alcohol syndrome are abnormally small, with small eyes and a small jaw; they may also suffer from heart defects (*see* **Congenital heart disease**, p.542) or a cleft lip and palate (p.558), may suckle poorly, sleep badly, and be irritable. It is not known whether there is a safe alcohol intake during pregnancy, but the more you drink, the greater the risk to your baby. To be safe, it is recommended that women who are pregnant or who are trying to conceive should abstain from alcohol completely.

For women who are breast-feeding, occasionally drinking small amounts of alcohol – 1 or 2 units once or twice a week – is not believed to be harmful to the baby. However, drinking more than this may reduce your milk supply and may also affect your baby's digestion, sleeping, and development. If you do choose to drink, you should wait for a couple of hours before breast-feeding so that the alcohol has had time to clear from your bloodstream and will not be in your breast milk.

Assessing your consumption

If you think you may be drinking too much, consult your doctor, who might ask you to keep a diary for several weeks to record each drink you have.

Some people drink to relieve stress or painful emotions. Stress-related consumption may lead to the development of a drinking problem. Warning signs include drinking more than you intended on any occasion, severe hangovers, and being involved in accidents or arguments after drinking.

What you can do

To enjoy alcohol safely, limit your intake. At social events, eat first, alternate alcoholic and nonalcoholic drinks, and finish each drink before refilling so that you know how many units you have had. Never drive if you intend to drink; try to go with a designated driver who will not drink. If you have children, set a good example for them. In addition, discuss the effects of alcohol with them and reinforce the message of any alcohol awareness programmes run by their school. To relieve emotional problems, try approaches such as counselling.

Tobacco and health

The effects of tobacco on health and reasons for avoiding its use

Tobacco is most commonly smoked in cigarettes but can be smoked in cigars and pipes, inhaled as snuff, or chewed. However it is used, tobacco is harmful to health. In the UK, smoking is one of the main causes of death. It accounts for about a third of all deaths from respiratory diseases, a quarter of deaths from cancer, and approximately a seventh of deaths from cardiovascular diseases. Overall, about 100,000 people a year die in the UK from smoking-related causes. Smoking also damages the health of "passive smokers", who inhale other people's smoke from the air around them. The only way to avoid the risks associated with tobacco smoking is to avoid smoking and those situations in which you come into contact with other people's smoke. In the UK, smoking is banned in workplaces and enclosed public spaces; it is also illegal to smoke in a vehicle if there is somebody under 18 present.

In the UK, the number of smokers has declined from about half the population in the early 1970s to less than 1 in 5 in 2013. The proportion of people who smoke is highest in the 25–34 age group and lowest in those aged 60 or over.

Effects of tobacco use

Tobacco smoke contains more than 7,000 different substances, many of which are toxic or irritating to the body. The substances that have been studied most extensively are tar, carbon monoxide, and nicotine. Tobacco smoke also contains carcinogenic (cancer-causing) substances that have toxic effects on the lungs and other organs.

Tar in tobacco smoke irritates and inflames the tissues of the lungs. Carbon monoxide attaches itself to red blood cells, reducing their capacity to carry oxygen. Nicotine acts as a tranquillizer, starting to take effect within 10 seconds of ingestion and producing a temporary feeling of wellbeing and relaxation. The substance is also known to increase the ability to concentrate. It stimulates the release of the hormone epinephrine (adrenaline) into the bloodstream, and this causes a rise in blood pressure. Nicotine is highly addictive, which is why most tobacco users

find it hard to give up the habit. There are many damaging long-term effects of tobacco use, some of which are exacerbated by other aspects of a person's lifestyle, such as drinking excessive amounts of alcohol.

Damage to the respiratory system Substances in cigarette smoke irritate the mucous membranes that line the air passages to the lungs, causing them to produce more mucus (sputum). These substances also paralyse the tiny hairs, called cilia, that help to expel sputum from the air passages. To clear their lungs, many smokers develop the characteristic "smoker's cough". Eventually, smoking may result in chronic obstructive pulmonary disease (p.297), which leads to severe shortness of breath.

Carcinogens in cigarette smoke cause over 8 in 10 of the deaths from lung cancer. In some countries, lung cancer has overtaken breast cancer as the leading cause of cancer-related deaths in women, a fact reflecting the large number of women who took up smoking during the second half of the 20th century. Smoking also causes cancer of the nasopharynx (p.293) and cancer of the larynx (p.294). The risk of developing cancer of the larynx is even higher for cigar or pipe smokers and for people who both smoke and drink alcohol.

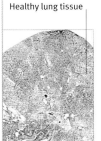 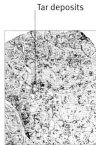

Healthy lung tissue / Tar deposits

NONSMOKER / **SMOKER**

Effects of smoking on the lungs
Over time, the tar from cigarette smoke gradually builds up in the lungs, as these sections through the lungs of a long-term smoker and a nonsmoker show.

Vascular damage Smoking is known to cause permanent damage to the cardiovascular system and has been linked to a significant number of deaths from cardiovascular disease. This damage is thought to be caused by the nicotine and carbon monoxide present in cigarette smoke, which may encourage the development of atherosclerosis (p.241), a condition in which the arteries become narrowed. Atherosclerosis in turn is known to increase the risk of stroke (p.329) and cardiovascular disorders such as coronary heart disease. In women over the age of 35, tobacco smoking increases the risk of developing disorders associated with the use of oral contraceptives (p.28), in particular deep vein thrombosis (p.263) and stroke.

Damage to other body systems Smokers are at increased risk of developing mouth cancer (p.402) and cancer of the oesophagus (p.404), particularly if they also drink alcohol. Carcinogenic chemicals from tobacco smoke that enter the bloodstream may also cause cancer in other parts of the body, such as the

bladder (*see* **Bladder tumours**, p.456) and the cervix (*see* **Cancer of the cervix**, p.481). The toxic effect of tobacco smoke may aggravate conditions such as peptic ulcers (p.406). Smoking may reduce fertility in men and women. If a pregnant woman smokes, her baby's birth weight is likely to be about 200 g (7 oz) lower than the average, and the baby is at greater risk of illness or death just after birth. The menopause may occur earlier in women who smoke. Smoking also affects the skin and accelerates skin changes, such as wrinkling, caused by aging and sunlight.

People who smoke cigars or pipes run a higher risk of developing mouth cancer and throat cancers. Snuff and chewing tobacco may also irritate the lining of the nose, mouth, and stomach.

Risks of passive smoking

Inhaling the smoke from other people's cigarettes is known as passive smoking. Secondhand smoke, also called environmental tobacco smoke (ETS), is a mixture of smoke from burning cigarettes and that exhaled by smokers.

ETS irritates the eyes, nose, and throat and may cause headaches and nausea. It may also worsen respiratory disorders such as asthma (p.295). The risk of developing lung cancer and heart disease is increased for nonsmokers who are exposed to ETS for long periods.

The children of smokers are particularly at risk from passive smoking. As babies, they are at increased risk of sudden infant death syndrome (p.532). Children of smokers are also more susceptible to asthma (*see* **Asthma in children**, p.544), and , if they have asthma, their attacks may be more severe and more frequent. They are also more prone to ear, nose, and respiratory infections, such as colds, sinusitis (p.290), acute bronchitis (p.297), and chronic secretory otitis media (p,557), a common cause of hearing impairment in children. The children of smokers are also more likely to smoke themselves when they get older, and, as adults, are at increased risk of developing chronic obstructive pulmonary disease and cancer.

What you can do

You can prevent disease by not smoking or by giving up smoking before you begin to develop any smoking-related illness. However, no matter how long you have been smoking, you can prevent further damage to your health by quitting (*see* **Health of ex-smokers**, right). As soon as you stop smoking, you begin to reduce your risk of developing lung cancer and other respiratory disorders, cardiovascular disease, and stroke. You will also be less likely to suffer from a range of conditions that are associated with smoking, such as peptic ulcer. You are never too old to benefit from this reduction in risk; even elderly people who have been smoking for most of their adult lives can improve their health and life expectancy by stopping.

Some smokers find it comparatively easy to quit but most find it difficult because they are addicted to nicotine. It is the

physiological affects of this addiction that cause the craving that gradually builds up between cigarettes and the withdrawal symptoms – such as agitation, irritability, depressed mood, increased appetite, dizziness, and difficulty sleeping – that occur after a longer period without smoking.

Various forms of help are available to help smokers quit. Your doctor, practice nurse, or pharmacist can give information and advice on stopping smoking. There are also various NHS "Stop Smoking" services, which provide advice and support for those who want to give up smoking, including an NHS helpline and a "Smokefree" website that gives information about how to quit and the various services available.

Many smokers trying to quit find nicotine replacement therapy (NRT) helpful. This is available over the counter in various forms: chewing gum, patches, tablets, lozenges, inhalators, and sprays. All of these give you a dose of nicotine, which helps reduce the tobacco craving and other withdrawal symptoms. Electronic cigarettes (e-cigarettes) are battery-powered devices that produce a vapour consisting of nicotine and water vapour. Although their long-term safety and effectiveness as an aid to stopping smoking has not yet been assessed,

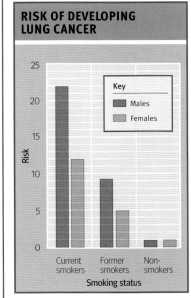

▶ **HEALTH EFFECTS**

Health of ex-smokers

The body starts to repair damage caused by smoking as soon as the habit is stopped. The risk of developing lung cancer and other disorders such as cardiovascular disease and stroke lessens the longer smoking has been stopped.

RISK OF DEVELOPING LUNG CANCER

Key: Males / Females

Risk / Current smokers / Former smokers / Non-smokers / Smoking status

Smoking and lung cancer
This graph shows the risks for smokers and former smokers relative to the risk for nonsmokers. Statistics appear to show that women have a lower risk of lung cancer than men, but this may be due to different patterns of smoking.

preliminary studies indicate that, at least in the short term, they are safer than traditional cigarettes and may be a useful aid in quitting smoking. Some people also find that complementary therapies, such as hypnotherapy and acupuncture, may be helpful in stopping smoking.

Drugs such as bupropion (Zyban) and varenicline (Champix), used in conjunction with self-help measures, may also be helpful in quitting. However, these drugs are available only on prescription and are not suitable for everybody. Bupropion should not be used by women who are pregnant or breast-feeding, by those with a history of seizures or who are at increased risk of seizures, or those who have an eating disorder. It may cause various side effects, including dry mouth, gastrointestinal disturbances, and sleep problems. Varenicline should not be used during pregnancy. Possible side effects include gastrointestinal disturbances, dry mouth, headache, drowsiness, dizziness, sleep problems, depression, and suicidal thoughts.

As well as giving up smoking yourself, it is also important to teach children about the health risks of smoking because if they can be prevented from starting, they are more likely never to smoke.

Drugs and health

Health hazards associated with the recreational use of drugs

A drug is any chemical that alters the function of an organ or a process in the body. Drugs include prescribed medicines, over-the-counter remedies, and various other substances used for nonmedical purposes. Drugs developed to improve body functions or to treat disorders are known as medicines (see **Drug treatment**, pp.568–606). Some drugs, such as temazepam (see **Sleeping drugs**, p.591), may be used as medicines and abused for recreation. Other drugs, such as ecstasy, have no medicinal value and are used only for recreational purposes.

Recreational drug use can cause serious health problems, particularly if the user takes an overdose or becomes dependent on a drug (see **Drug dependence**, p.349). Since the sale or use of most recreational drugs is illegal, a user may be arrested and even face imprisonment. Alcohol and nicotine are also drugs that can be addictive and harmful (see **Alcohol and health**, p.24, and **Tobacco and health**, p.25), as is caffeine, but they are viewed differently by society because they have been used for centuries and are sold legally.

Effects of drug use

Recreational drugs are usually used to alter mood. They can be classified according to the predominant change they cause but often have a mixture of effects. Stimulants, such as cocaine, cause increased physical and mental activity; relaxants, such as marijuana and heroin, produce a feeling of calm; intoxicants, such as solvents, make users feel giggly and

dreamy; and hallucinogens, such as LSD, alter perception and cause the user to see or hear things that do not exist.

In addition, recreational drugs can affect functions such as breathing and temperature control. These effects can be damaging in both the short and the long term and some are potentially fatal. Some of the potential health risks, such as those of dependence or of an extreme reaction, apply to many or all drugs. Drugs that are injected carry additional risks associated with the use of needles. Each drug also carries a range of specific risks to the health of users (see **Risks of specific drugs**, right). The health hazards of some recently developed recreational drugs, particularly "designer drugs", are not yet fully understood, but they could be potentially serious or even life-threatening.

Although problems arising from drug abuse are often due to the adverse effects of some drugs and drug dependence, there is also a risk of accidents during intoxication.

Extreme reactions Any recreational drug can be dangerous, even if not used regularly. One risk is an extreme reaction to a drug. The effects of any drug can vary among users, and a drug that has only mild effects on one person may severely affect another. In addition, a drug may be mixed with other substances, and the amount of active drug may vary considerably from dose to dose. Many drugs, such as cocaine and LSD, can cause delusions, leading to abnormal or hazardous behaviour. Uncertainty about the strength of a drug may lead to overdose, which can be fatal. Alcohol and certain medicinal drugs, such as aspirin, interact with recreational drugs to produce intensified or unexpected effects.

Drug dependence Regular users of recreational drugs may face the problem of physical or psychological dependence, or both.

In physical dependence, the body has adapted to the drug and begins to crave it; the user feels ill if he or she does not take the drug regularly, and may come to need that substance simply to function normally. If the drug is stopped, the user will develop withdrawal symptoms, which are relieved if the drug is taken again. Physical dependence develops more rapidly if the drug is injected.

Even if a particular drug is not physically addictive, drug users may become psychologically dependent, coming to rely on the enjoyable effects of a drug or the rituals that surround its use. They may also risk psychological disturbance and malnutrition due to self-neglect or loss of appetite. Some users may also spend a lot of time taking or obtaining drugs and withdraw from ordinary life. Since many illegal drugs are expensive, users may support their habit by crime.

Risks associated with injection Drugs that are injected take effect more rapidly than those taken by mouth because they enter the bloodstream directly. There are different routes for injection, the fastest of which is intravenous. Users who inject drugs risk causing infection and damage to blood vessels. These problems can lead to tissue death (see **Gangrene**, p.262) or septicaemia (p.171),

▶ HEALTH EFFECTS

Risks of specific drugs

People use drugs for recreation because they enjoy some of their effects, but there are also many short- and long-term effects that are unpleasant, harmful, or potentially fatal. It is important to be aware of the risks involved.

Hazardous effects
Short-term hazards may occur soon after taking a drug, possibly after only one dose. Long-term risks result from repeated use.

Drug	Short-term hazards	Long-term hazards
Stimulants		
Ecstasy	■ Nausea ■ Tense muscles ■ Panic ■ Loss of temperature control and/or fluid retention, which can cause coma and death	■ Sleep problems ■ Depression ■ Possible liver and kidney problems and brain damage
Amphetamines	■ Tension ■ Anxiety ■ Hallucinations ■ Rise in body temperature ■ Convulsions ■ Stroke	■ Heart disorders ■ Severe psychological disorders
Cocaine	■ Paranoia ■ Lethargy ■ Depression ■ Heart attack ■ Convulsions ■ Stroke	■ Damage to nose and lungs from sniffing drug ■ Anxiety ■ Paranoia ■ Heart disorders
Crack	■ Loss of self-control ■ Violent or erratic behaviour ■ Burnt mouth and throat ■ Chest pain ■ Convulsions	■ Heart disorders ■ Damage to lungs ■ Paranoia
Relaxants		
Cannabis (marijuana)	■ Decreased coordination and concentration ■ Impairment of skills, such as driving vehicles ■ Anxiety ■ Panic ■ Paranoia	■ Apathy ■ Increased risk of lung cancer and other respiratory disorders ■ High blood pressure ■ Memory problems ■ Mental illness ■ Infertility
Heroin	■ Overdose can cause coma and death ■ Infection with HIV or hepatitis if needles are shared	■ Tremor ■ Apathy ■ Blood-vessel damage from repeated injections
Intoxicants		
Solvents (eg. glue, petrol, aerosols)	■ Vomiting ■ Suffocation if inhaling from plastic bag ■ Loss of consciousness ■ Possibly fatal reaction upon inhalation	■ Cough ■ Rash around nose and mouth ■ Damage to brain, liver, kidneys, and nervous system
Hallucinogens		
Lysergic acid diethylamide (LSD)	■ Extreme anxiety ■ Loss of self-control and increased risk of accidents	■ Hallucinations that occur months or even years after use of drug
Phencyclidine, or phenocyclo-piperidine (PCP)	■ Confusion ■ Vomiting ■ Sharp rise or fall in pulse rate and blood pressure ■ Seizures ■ Heart failure ■ Overdose may be fatal	■ Loss of short-term memory and coordination ■ Paranoia ■ Speech difficulties ■ Violent behaviour ■ Depression
Anaesthetics		
Ketamine	■ Palpitations ■ Hallucinations ■ Paralysis ■ Convulsions ■ Breathing problems	■ Memory and learning problems ■ Flashbacks ■ Psychosis

both of which are potentially life-threatening. If syringes and needles are shared, users also risk infection with HIV (p.169) and hepatitis B or C (see **Acute hepatitis**, p.408).

What you can do

If you or someone close to you abuses drugs, ask your doctor about the health risks and treatment options. Controlled withdrawal programmes are available. Alternative, less harmful drugs may be given as well as treat-

ment for any withdrawal symptoms. Social service agencies and support groups may provide follow-up care. The success of treatment depends on the motivation of the affected person. Problems often recur if people return to the circumstances that originally gave rise to the drug abuse. If you have children, you should tell them about the hazards of drug use. If their school has a drug awareness programme, you should try to reinforce its messages.

Sex and health

Human beings are unique among animals in having the capacity for sexual desire even when the female is not fertile and in retaining desire into old age, long after conception has ceased to be possible. The explanation may be that sex helps to maintain partnerships. Regular sex also seems to improve cardiovascular fitness and prolong life. People who are involved in stable sexual relationships live longer than those without sexual partners.

A satisfying sexual relationship is an important part of life but not always easy to achieve, and sexual contact may be risky. In particular, casual sex and sex with multiple partners carry the risks of unwanted pregnancy and sexually transmitted infections (STIs).

The first article in the section covers the basic elements of a healthy sexual relationship. The following article, on safe sex, discusses ways in which your risk of exposure to sexually transmitted infections can be reduced. The final article provides an overview of the advantages and disadvantages of different forms of contraception. Education about sex, pregnancy, and sexually transmitted infections is particularly important for teenagers, who often fail to make use of contraceptives and ignore advice about safe sex.

Specific sexual problems and the symptoms and treatment of sexually transmitted infections are discussed in other sections of the book (see **Sexual**

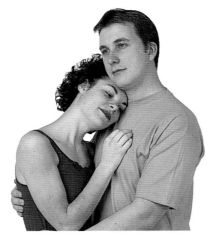

Enjoying intimacy
When two partners are establishing an intimate, sexual relationship, it is important for them to trust each other.

problems, pp.494–496, and **Sexually transmitted infections**, pp.491–493), as are possible problems in conceiving (*see* **Infertility**, pp.497–499)

Sexual relationships

The physical and emotional elements of satisfying sexual relationships

The physical maturity necessary for a sexual relationship is signalled by the onset of puberty, when the individual's body makes the transition from childhood to adulthood. The development of emotional maturity frequently takes much longer, and early sexual encounters, although sometimes exciting, may just as often be disappointing or cause anxiety. With age and experience, most people become better able to establish and fully enjoy sexual relationships.

A healthy relationship
What constitutes a healthy sexual relationship varies widely from person to person. Sexual fulfilment depends on a blend of physical and psychological factors, and what is right for one couple may not suit another. You and your partner should both be happy with the frequency of sexual activity, and you should be able to discuss which sexual activities you find pleasant and which you find unappealing.

Anyone in a sexual relationship should be aware of the risks posed by sexually transmitted infections (STIs) and know how to minimize the risk of exposure to them (*see* **Safe sex**, right). In addition, to avoid an unwanted pregnancy, you should be familiar with the options for contraception (p.28), including emergency contraception. It is important that children approaching puberty are given education about STIs, safe sex, and contraception. Most schools provide sex-education programmes.

Potential problems
It is normal to experience fluctuations in sex drive or occasional temporary loss of sexual desire, lack of sexual response, or inability to perform sexually. However, if sexual problems persist, they may be distressing and cause you anxiety, which further impairs your ability to enjoy sexual activity, and this creates a vicious circle.

Sexual problems may have a number of causes. Emotional difficulties in your current relationship will affect your sex life. External stress will also affect a relationship and may lead to problems. For example, ongoing problems at work or financial difficulties may cause anxiety, irritability, or lack of sleep, all of which may decrease your desire for sex. Past upsets of an emotional nature, such as the break-up of a

former relationship, can affect your current situation even when the problem seems to have disappeared.

Decrease in sex drive or impaired sexual function may also be the result of complications of certain long-term physical conditions, such as diabetes mellitus (p.437); disabilities that cause pain and restrict movement; convalescence from surgery or severe illness; and the use of alcohol, recreational drugs, and certain medications.

What you can do
If there are matters that are bothering you, it is important to talk about them with your partner. If the problem is persistent, discuss it with your doctor, who can refer you for appropriate help. If you have a long-term illness or a disability that impairs your sex life, you may find it helpful to get in touch with an organization that has been established to help people with the problem.

Safe sex

Sexual practices that minimize your risk of contracting sexually transmitted infections

One of the hazards of sexual contact is exposure to certain infections. These range from minor problems, such as pubic lice (p.493), to life-threatening disorders, such as HIV infection (*see* **HIV infection and AIDS**, p.169). Some disorders, such as genital herpes (p.493), genital warts (p.493), and gonorrhoea (p.491), are almost always transmitted by sexual contact and are known as sexually transmitted infections (STIs). Others, such as hepatitis B and C (*see* **Acute hepatitis**, p.408) and HIV infection, may be transmitted by other means as well as through sex. For example, people who inject drugs and share needles with others risk infection with HIV or hepatitis. Some disorders, such as scabies (p.207), are transmitted by physical contact and are common among people living in overcrowded conditions and among schoolchildren. These disorders may also be transmitted through sex.

Assessing the risks
It is important to assess your risk of exposure to STIs so that you can make informed choices about sexual activity. You need to understand how infection is spread and know which sexual activities carry the highest risks. If you think you are likely to be exposed to infection, or if you are not sure what your own risk might be, you should use a condom (*see* **Using contraceptives**, p.28) or avoid sex. You should try to ensure that you and your partner do not have unprotected sex until your relationship is well established and monogamous and both of you are known to be free of disease.

High-risk activities Diseases such as hepatitis B and C and HIV infection may be spread by contact with semen, blood, or

vaginal secretions. Other disorders, such as genital warts and genital herpes, are transmitted by contact with a wart or sore. The areas most vulnerable to infection are the skin of the genitals and mucous membranes such as the lining of the vagina, anus, mouth, and urethra.

The sexual activities that pose the highest risks are those in which the mucous membranes could be damaged, allowing infections from body fluids or body parts to enter the bloodstream. Vaginal, anal, and oral intercourse that involves penetration, and in which partners do not use a condom, are the activities carrying the highest risks. Anal penetration can be particularly hazardous because the lining of the anus and rectum is easily damaged.

Sexual history The risk of exposure to STIs increases with the more sexual partners you have and the more times that you practise unsafe sex. A monogamous relationship with someone whom you know has been screened and found free of disease carries the lowest risk. You may be more vulnerable if your partner has had sex with someone else and has not told you, particularly if you do not use a condom with that partner. You or your partner may already have an STI but have no symptoms. For example, chlamydial infections (p.492) affect both sexes but often cause no symptoms in women. In both sexes, infection with genital warts is followed by a latent period of about 9 months when you have no symptoms but are still infectious. Casual sex without using a condom carries most risk because you are unlikely to know if your partner is infected.

Some STIs are particularly prevalent in certain groups of people. For example, HIV infection is more common among people living in some parts of Africa and Asia, prostitutes, people who inject recreational drugs and share needles, and people who have unprotected anal sex. You may run a higher risk of infection if you have unsafe sex with a person from one of these groups.

Pair of bacteria

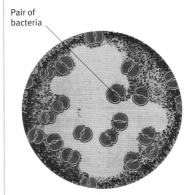

Gonorrhoea organisms
This highly magnified view shows the bacteria that cause gonorrhoea, Neisseria gonorrhoeae, *which may be found in genital, rectal, and throat secretions.*

What you can do
Condoms are able to protect you from infections that are transmitted during sexual intercourse. However, they do not protect

you from contact with sores or warts on uncovered areas of the body or from pubic lice or scabies.

If you choose not to use condoms, make sure that neither you nor your partner has an infection. Discuss your past sexual contacts honestly, particularly if either of you is in a high-risk group. If you suspect that you have been exposed to infection, arrange to have a screening test at a clinic that specializes in treating STIs. With HIV infection, there is a latent period of a few weeks between acquiring the infection and the time when the antibody to the virus can be detected in the test. For this reason, many clinics advise using condoms for the first few months of a new relationship before having an HIV test.

Once you and your partner are sure that you are free from STIs, the most effective way to protect yourselves is by remaining monogamous. If you do have sexual intercourse with other partners, make sure that you use condoms. If you are not using condoms and develop an STI, use condoms until you have been treated and are free of disease or abstain from penetrative sex. Both you and your partner should be treated at the same time to avoid the risk of reinfecting each other, and you should both be free of disease before you stop using condoms. Sexual activities that carry a relatively low risk of infection include kissing your partner's mouth (or body areas other than the genitals) and mutual masturbation by hand. The activities that have little or no risk are those that do not involve contact with your partner's genitals.

Contraception

Artificial and natural methods for controlling fertility

Contraception allows people to choose whether and when to have children. There are several types and each works differently (*see* **Using contraceptives**, right). Nearly all types, apart from the male condom and male sterilization, are designed for use by women.

Most contraceptives, apart from condoms, are supplied by your doctor, who considers your age, medical history, and sexual lifestyle. No contraceptive is entirely free from risk. Some types may not be suitable for you, while others have side effects that you must weigh against the benefits. You may need to change your contraceptive as you grow older, after having children, or if you alter your sexual lifestyle.

Barrier methods

Barrier contraceptive methods include diaphragms, condoms, and cervical caps. They act by preventing sperm from entering the uterus and reaching the egg. Male condoms cover the penis, female condoms line the vagina, and caps and diaphragms cover the cervix. Barrier contraceptives do not disrupt normal body functions or affect fertility, but they are unreliable if not used correctly and can also affect the spontaneity of sex. Some

people may be allergic to the latex from which many condoms are made; if so, latex-free condoms are available. However, when used correctly, condoms are an effective method of preventing unwanted pregnancy. Condoms may also protect women from cancer of the cervix (p.481) by reducing the risk of infection with human papillomavirus.

The male condom is the only contraceptive method that also protects users and their partners from sexually transmitted infections (*see* **Safe sex**, p.27). Condoms may also be used for protection when one partner has a longstanding infection such as HIV (*see* **HIV infections and AIDS**, p.169).

Hormonal methods

Hormonal contraceptives alter the hormone balance in a woman's body to prevent conception. They may be taken orally in the form of the combined pill or the progestogen-only pill. Hormones may also be administered as a patch; injected into a muscle; implanted in a flexible rod under the skin; administered via a hormone-containing intrauterine device (known as an intrauterine system, or IUS); or administered via a vaginal ring. These methods do not interrupt sexual activities, but they can cause side effects or health risks in some women. If you stop using them, it may take a few months for your fertility to return. Vomiting and diarrhoea may reduce the reliability of oral contraceptives. If you vomit, take another pill as soon as possible and the next pill at the usual time. If you have persistent vomiting, another method of contraception (such as a condom) should also be used. If you have severe diarrhoea, you should also continue taking the pill and should use another method of contraception as well. With either persistent vomiting or severe diarrhoea, the alternative form of contraception should be used while you are ill and for 2 days afterwards. If your vomiting or diarrhoea are long-lasting, you should consult your doctor. Certain drugs may interact with oral contraceptives so if you are taking an oral contraceptive you should tell your doctor in case it interacts with other medication. Your pharmacist should be able to advise you about possible interactions with over-the-counter medications.

Combined oral contraceptive pill This type of pill (COC), containing both oestrogen and progestogen, is highly reliable if used correctly. There may be side effects, such as changes in weight and mood, but these usually disappear after the first few months of use.

The COC pill lowers the risk of cancer of the ovary (p.477) but increases the risk of some other disorders, including a slight increase in the risk of breast cancer (p.486). It can cause a slight rise in blood pressure, so you may be advised not to use it if you have a family history of high blood pressure (*see* **Hypertension**, p.242) or of high blood lipids (*see* **Hypercholesterolaemia**, p.440). The COC pill also causes blood to clot more readily, increasing your risk of stroke (p.329), deep vein thrombosis (p.263), and heart attacks (*see* **Myocardial infarction**, p.245). The risk

▶ HEALTH OPTIONS

Using contraceptives

Contraception provides a high degree of protection against unwanted pregnancy, although the effectiveness of different methods varies. For each method described here, effectiveness is defined as the number of women per hundred per year who do not become pregnant while using it and is expressed as a percentage. For most methods, apart from the IUD, your doctor will need to explain how to use them so that they are effective. It may take some time to learn how to use a diaphragm, a cap, or natural methods, and they are not suitable for times when you need contraception immediately. A condom is usually the best method in this situation.

Barrier methods

Condoms, diaphragms, and caps form barriers between the penis and the uterus to prevent sperm from reaching the egg. Spermicide (a substance that kills sperm) should be used with diaphragms and caps but should be avoided with condoms. Barrier methods are 92–98 per cent effective, with the male condom being the most effective. Most failures are due to incorrect use.

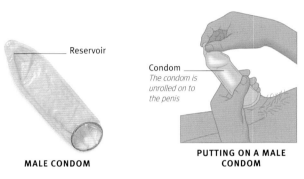

Reservoir

MALE CONDOM

Condom
The condom is unrolled on to the penis

PUTTING ON A MALE CONDOM

Male condom
Before a condom is unrolled on to the penis, the air must be squeezed out of the reservoir (end) so that the condom will not split. After intercourse, the penis must be withdrawn with the condom held on to prevent semen from leaking out.

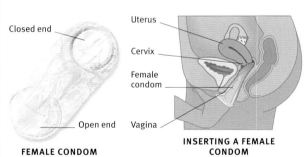

Closed end

Open end

FEMALE CONDOM

Uterus
Cervix
Female condom
Vagina

INSERTING A FEMALE CONDOM

Female condom
The closed end of the condom is pushed up to the cervix. The open end extends just beyond the vaginal opening. Make sure that the penis goes inside the condom, not between the condom and the vaginal wall.

Cervical cap
The cap is partially filled with spermicide then pushed over the cervix. If intercourse does not occur within 3 hours of inserting it, extra spermicide must be added. To be effective, the cap must be left in place for at least 6 hours after intercourse.

CERVICAL CAP

Uterus
Cervix
Cap
Vagina

IN POSITION

Diaphragm
The diaphragm is coated with spermicide on both surfaces. It is positioned so that the concave side covers the cervix. Like the cervical cap, it must be left in place for at least 6 hours after intercourse.

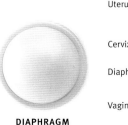

DIAPHRAGM

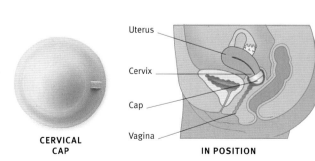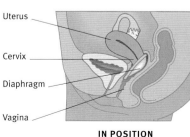

Uterus
Cervix
Diaphragm
Vagina

IN POSITION

Hormonal methods

Female hormones that prevent conception may be prescribed as pills, patches, injections, implants, the intrauterine system (IUS), or vaginal rings. Some types of hormonal contraceptive contain only progestogen. This hormone thickens the cervical mucus so that sperm cannot pass through; it also thins the lining of the uterus, which reduces the chance of a fertilized egg implanting successfully. The POP that contains desogestrel also inhibits ovulation. Hormonal contraceptives that contain oestrogen and progestogen work by suppressing ovulation. Hormonal contraceptive methods are over 99 per cent effective, but they must be used exactly as instructed.

Vaginal ring
The vaginal ring is a flexible plastic ring containing oestrogen and progestogen. It is inserted into the vagina, left in place for 3 weeks, then removed. After a ring-free interval of a week, a new ring is inserted.

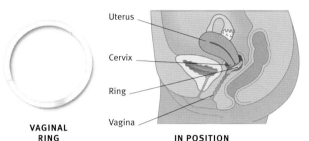

VAGINAL RING

IN POSITION

Uterus
Cervix
Ring
Vagina

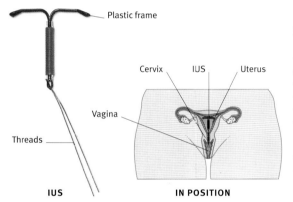

Plastic frame
Cervix   IUS   Uterus
Vagina
Threads

IUS

IN POSITION

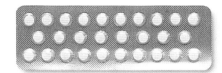

Progestogen-only pill (POP)
The traditional progestogen-only pill must be taken at about the same time each day, for every day of the menstrual cycle. Although the traditional progestogen-only pill is less effective than the combined pill, it does not have the health risks of the combined pill. There is a newer type of progestogen-only pill containing desogestrel that is more effective than the traditional type.

Intrauterine system (IUS)
The IUS resembles an IUD, consisting of a T-shaped plastic frame with threads attached to the base. Unlike an IUD, the plastic frame of the IUS is not coated with copper but contains progestogen, which is released slowly and continuously for 3 or 5 years, depending on the type. The IUS is positioned in the uterus in the same way as an IUD (see below).

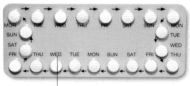

Days of week
The days of the week are marked as a guide

Combined oral contraceptive (COC)
The combined pill contains oestrogen and progestogen. There are various types. With some, you take pills for 21 days and then have 7 pill-free days. With others, you take 21 hormone pills and then 7 inactive pills. You must take the pills in the specified order.

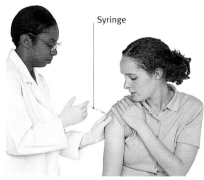

Syringe

Contraceptive injection and implant
Progestogen is injected into a muscle in your arm or buttock, and it is released into your body over 8–12 weeks. Alternatively, an implant containing progestogen can be inserted under the skin of the upper arm and will remain effective for 3 years.

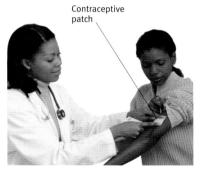

Contraceptive patch

Contraceptive patch
The contraceptive patch contains oestrogen and progestogen. It is used for 3 weeks out of every 4 of the menstrual cycle, and a new patch is used each week. A patch can be put on any part of the body that is not very hairy and is not sore.

Mechanical methods

The intrauterine device (IUD) is fitted by a doctor and is left in place for up to 10 years, depending on the type. IUDs are thought to work mainly by stopping sperm from reaching an egg; they may also prevent eggs from implanting in the wall of the uterus. IUDs are over 98 per cent effective.

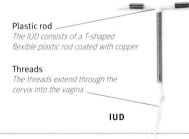

Plastic rod
The IUD consists of a T-shaped flexible plastic rod coated with copper

Threads
The threads extend through the cervix into the vagina

IUD

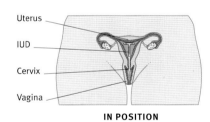

Uterus
IUD
Cervix
Vagina

IN POSITION

Intrauterine device (IUD)
An IUD has two threads that extend through the cervix. Once a month, the user should check that the threads are still there in order to make sure that the IUD has not been expelled during menstruation.

Natural methods

Natural methods of contraception are used to identify days in your menstrual cycle when you are fertile and times when you are less likely to conceive. Having identified these times, you can refrain from sex on your fertile days or use another form of contraception. The sympto-thermal method, which is only about 80 per cent effective, is the most commonly used natural method. It is based on two factors: body temperature rising just after ovulation (which occurs 12–16 days before each period) and staying high for at least 3 days; and increased amounts of mucus in the vagina around the time of ovulation. If you plan to use natural methods, seek advice from your doctor first.

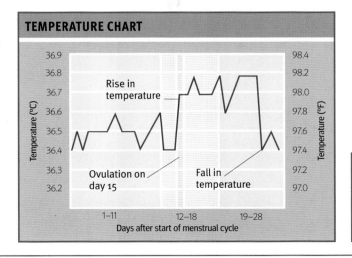

TEMPERATURE CHART

Temperature (°C): 36.9, 36.8, 36.7, 36.6, 36.5, 36.4, 36.3, 36.2
Temperature (°F): 98.4, 98.2, 98.0, 97.8, 97.6, 97.4, 97.2, 97.0

Rise in temperature

Ovulation on day 15

Fall in temperature

1–11   12–18   19–28
Days after start of menstrual cycle

Key
- Ovulation, unsafe for sex
- Fertile days, unsafe for sex
- Infertile days, safe for sex

Using a temperature chart
You can monitor your fertility by recording your temperature on a chart like the one here. Take your temperature at the same time every day, immediately after waking and before getting up. Ovulation is followed by a rise in temperature. When your temperature is higher for 3 days in a row, your fertile time is probably over. A time of infertility then follows; this lasts until the last day of your next period. Because of possible variability in the menstrual cycle and lifespan of sperm, this method does not predict the fertile period with total accuracy.

is substantially raised if you are over 35 and smoke. The COC pill may also not be advised if you are very overweight or have a parent or sibling who has had deep vein thrombosis.

Progestogen-only pill (POP) This type of contraceptive pill contains only progestogen and does not carry the health risks of the COC pill. The POP does not carry an increased risk of deep vein thrombosis, and it can be used if you are over 35 and/or smoke. The traditional POP is less effective than the COC pill and must be taken at the same time each day to be reliable. It often causes lighter periods but may also make your cycle irregular. However, its effect on menstruation does not alter its effectiveness as a contraceptive. There may be other side effects, such as acne and breast tenderness, but these should last only a few months. A newer type of POP is available that contains desogestrel, which works by inhibiting ovulation and is more effective than traditional POPs. Like traditional POPs, it may cause menstrual irregularities, acne, and breast tenderness.

Contraceptive patch This is an adhesive skin patch that contains oestrogen and progestogen (the hormones used in the COC). It delivers a constant daily dose of the hormones through the skin and works in the same way as the COC. Its reliability is similar to that of the COC. The patch is used for 3 weeks out of every 4, and a new patch needs to be applied every week. If the patch is started up to and including the 5th day of a period, it is effective immediately. If it is started at any other time, additional contraception should be used for 7 days. Because the patch contains the same hormones as the COC, the potential side effects and health risks are the same.

Injections and implants Progestogen can be given as an injection or an implant; both provide reliable long-term contraception. They are useful if you do not want to have children for some years or at all or if you forget to take pills. Initially, these may make your periods irregular or heavier. You may also gain weight. After the first period, most women stop menstruating.

Intrauterine system (IUS) The IUS is similar to an ordinary intrauterine device, or IUD (see p.29) but, unlike an IUD, it contains progestogen. The IUS consists of a T-shaped plastic frame impregnated with progestogen, which is released slowly and continuously. It prevents conception by thinning the lining of the uterus and thickening the cervical mucus. It may also suppress ovulation in some women, although most continue to ovulate.

The IUS is an extremely reliable form of contraception. It starts to work immediately if it is fitted during the first 7 days of your menstrual cycle. If it is fitted at any other time additional contraception is necessary for the first 7 days. The IUS lasts for 3 or 5 years, depending on the type. After it is removed, fertility usually returns quickly. The IUS makes periods lighter and less painful after the first three months of use. For this reason, it can be useful for women

with heavy periods or for those nearing the menopause. It may cause side effects such as irregular periods and breast tenderness but they usually wear off after a few months. The IUS shares many of the disadvantages of the IUD, such as the rare risk of being expelled from the uterus or of piercing the uterine wall and causing inflammation of the abdominal lining (*see* Peritonitis, p.421).

Vaginal ring This consists of a flexible plastic ring containing oestrogen and progestogen (the hormones used in the COC). It works in the same way as the COC and its reliability is similar. The ring is placed high inside the vagina, where it releases a constant dose of the hormones through the vaginal wall into the bloodstream. The ring is easy to insert and remove; you will be shown how to do so correctly the first time you use it, and afterwards you do it yourself. The ring is used for 3 weeks out of every 4. It is inserted on the 1st day of the menstrual cycle and left in for 3 weeks. It is then removed and left out for a week, during which time there may be withdrawal bleeding. After this ring-free interval, a new ring is inserted. When the ring is inserted on the 1st day of the menstrual cycle, it is effective immediately. If it is inserted at any other time, additional contraception is needed for the first 7 days. The ring's potential side effects and health risks are the same as those of the COC.

Mechanical methods (IUDs)

Intrauterine devices (IUDs), also known as coils, are devices that are inserted into the uterus by a doctor. They are made of plastic coated with copper, and have threads that protrude into the vagina so the user can check that her IUD is still in place.

IUDs give immediate protection and last for several years. However, they may be difficult to insert in women who have never been pregnant and may increase your susceptibility to certain infections (*see* Pelvic inflammatory disease, p.475). Rarely, an IUD may be expelled from the uterus, or may pierce the wall of the uterus and cause peritonitis. The IUD does not affect hormones or ovulation, but it may worsen heavy or painful periods (*see* Menorrhagia, p.471, and Dysmenorrhoea, p.472).

Natural methods

Natural birth control involves working out when you are fertile and avoiding intercourse at those times. It has no side effects, but can disrupt the spontaneity of sex and should not be used without training. It also requires that you have a regular menstrual cycle. There is a fertility monitoring kit available for home use. Natural birth control works best if you feel that you could accept an unplanned pregnancy.

Surgical methods

Surgical contraception, or sterilization, is an operation that makes you infertile. This surgery can be carried out on men (*see* Vasectomy, p.461) or women (*see* Female

sterilization, p.476). Since the operation is considered permanent, it is suitable only for those who are sure that they do not want children. Male sterilization is not immediately effective. The seminal vesicles (sacs that hold semen) still contain sperm after the operation, and a condom must be used until semen analysis (p.499) shows that no sperm are left. Female sterilization is immediately effective.

Emergency methods

Emergency contraception is used to prevent pregnancy if you have unprotected sex. There are two main methods: oral medications and an IUD. There are two oral medications for emergency contraception: levonorgestrel and ulipristal. The levonorgestrel pill should be taken as a single dose as soon as possible after unprotected sex, preferably within 12 hours but no later than 72 hours afterwards. The levonorgestrel pill can be obtained from your doctor, or over the counter without a prescription if you are over 16. Ulipristal should be taken as a single dose, ideally as as soon as possible after unprotected sex but no later than 5 days afterwards. It can be obtained from your doctor or over the counter without a prescription if you are over 18. An IUD is an effective alternative to oral medication for emergency contraception. One can be fitted by your doctor up to 5 days after unprotected sex.

Psychological health

Your physical and psychological health are closely linked. A long-term physical illness is likely to make you feel low, while a mental health disorder such as depression may cause physical symptoms. You can make changes in your lifestyle to improve your physical and psychological state so that you are better able to deal with the stresses and strains of daily life.

Some life events, such as a death in the family, inevitably cause stress. People's reactions to such stressful events depend in part on personality and in part on other current causes of stress, such as financial problems. The more stress you have to face, the greater your risk of developing a psychiatric disorder.

To help you to identify problems at an early stage, this section starts with a discussion of the difference between the normal range of wellbeing and a mental health disorder. The next two articles provide advice on how to develop good sleep habits and on ways to identify and minimize stress. The final article explains the process of grieving and suggests ways in which you might cope with your feelings.

Specific psychiatric disorders are covered elsewhere (*see* Mental health disorders, pp.341–350).

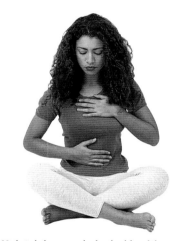

Maintaining psychological health
Learning how to relax by using techniques such as breathing exercises can be a key factor in maintaining psychological health.

Your psychological health

Your mental approach to dealing with everyday stress and life events

Growing up is a process of learning psychological responses to life events, both positive and negative. People vary in their ability to deal with these events, and everyone on occasion feels anger, frustration, sadness, mild depression, worry, loneliness, or uncertainty. However, when these feelings prevent you from functioning normally for a sustained period, you may need to see your doctor. People have different personality traits and

sometimes these can become sufficiently exaggerated to be classified as a disorder (*see* Mental health disorders, pp.341–350).

Children and adults express their concerns differently. Recognizing early signs of problems enables action to be taken before they become serious.

Recognizing problems in children

Children often cannot say if something is upsetting them, so they may express their feelings in unexpected ways, often as a change in behaviour. As a parent, it is important to be aware of warning signs. For example, your child may have a problem if he or she starts wetting the bed after a period of dryness or is unusually withdrawn, sad, or nervous. Children who are unhappy often complain of pain, typically stomach-ache. If your doctor cannot identify a physical cause, he or she may ask you about possible sources of stress.

Recognizing problems in adults

If you notice changes in your normal behaviour, such as increased moodiness, irritability, constant depression, anxiety attacks, trouble sleeping, poor concentration, or loss of appetite, you may be under emotional strain. If these feelings continue for a sustained period or grow more intense, they could signal a developing psychological problem. They may stem from a specific cause, such as the death of a relative (see **Loss and bereavement**, p.32), but may develop for no apparent reason.

Your psychological health changes with age and may reflect your physical well-being. Physical and psychological problems often coexist in older people, and if you become seriously ill or have a major operation you are more likely to suffer from psychological problems as a result (see **Mental problems due to physical illness**, p.345).

If an aspect of your behaviour or personality is making you or someone close to you unhappy and you want to change but cannot, seek advice from your doctor or a therapist (see **Psychological therapies**, pp.622–624).

Sleep

Understanding sleep and how it contributes to your health

Sleep is a fundamental human need and is an important factor in maintaining good health. When you sleep well, you wake up feeling refreshed and alert; if you regularly sleep badly, every aspect of your life can suffer as a result. Occasional lack of sleep is a very common experience. Usually, you should be able to overcome the problem by altering your lifestyle, but if you have persistent sleeping problems, you should consult your doctor (see **Insomnia**, p.343).

Why we need to sleep

Although scientists do not completely understand why people need to sleep, research shows that the body and mind

require time to rest and recover from the day's activities. While you sleep, your body undergoes a series of repair processes and conserves energy.

There are two types of sleep: rapid eye movement (REM) sleep and non-REM sleep. During REM sleep, brain activity increases and information is processed to reinforce memory and learning. Most dreaming occurs during REM sleep, although dreams also occur during non-REM sleep. Non-REM sleep consists of four stages: stage 1 is light sleep, in which you may wake spontaneously, and stage 4 is the deepest, in which you are very hard to wake. Each complete cycle of non-REM and REM sleep lasts about 90 minutes, starting with non-REM sleep. An average sleep cycle is made up of three-quarters non-REM sleep and one-quarter REM sleep.

Sleep requirements

Sleep runs on a daily cycle regulated by an internal clock. Although people tend to sleep at night and are awake during the day, the cycle adapts to individual needs. The amount of sleep needed changes over a person's lifetime and depends on the individual. Newborn babies sleep up to 16 hours a day. Most people sleep an average of 7–8 hours a night, but generally the amount of sleep you need decreases as you grow older. Many people over 60 need only about 6 hours sleep a night, although they may take a nap during the day.

Most people can cope with a couple of nights in which they have little or no sleep, without experiencing serious harmful effects on their health. At certain times, such as when you are ill or convalescing, you may find that you need more sleep than you usually have.

Promoting good sleep

The most successful approach to getting a good night's sleep is to have a healthy lifestyle and to establish a regular routine before getting into bed.

A healthy lifestyle The key lifestyle factors that will help to ensure good sleep patterns are getting sufficient exercise, moderating your alcohol and caffeine intake, and not smoking.

Exercise promotes a sense of calm and wellbeing by increasing the production of endorphins in the brain (see **The benefits of exercise**, p.20). It also helps to tire you out physically.

Caffeine and nicotine are both central nervous system stimulants and may prevent you from falling asleep. Reduce your caffeine intake during the afternoon and evening. If you smoke, giving up may improve your sleep and also your general health (see **Tobacco and health**, p.25). Alcohol is a sedative (see **Alcohol and health**, p.24), but you should not use it to help you to sleep because alcohol-induced sleep is not as refreshing as normal sleep.

Bedtime routine By adopting a consistent bedtime routine, you may find it easier to relax and sleep normally. Your routine could include listening to the radio, reading, or practising relaxation exercises (p.32). Try soaking in a warm bath 2–4 hours before going to bed or having a warm drink made with milk at bedtime. Try to avoid working late into the evening. Make sure your bed is comfortable and your bedroom is well ventilated, neither too hot nor too cold, and sheltered from outdoor light.

Dealing with sleep problems

At some time in their lives, most people experience changes in their sleep patterns. Common problems are trouble getting to sleep, waking during the night or too early in the morning, and sleepiness during the day. Snoring (p.291) is another major cause of sleep disturbance. Sleep problems are often due to stress-associated behaviour, such as drinking more alcohol than normal or working until late at night.

If you have a sleep problem, examine your lifestyle to see if a change in activity or behaviour could account for it. If you cannot sleep, get out of bed, walk around, or read until you feel sleepy. Try to establish regular times for sleep and waking up. If you have a bad night, try not to sleep during the next day, but if you feel tired a nap of up to 20 minutes may improve your alertness.

If you continue to have difficulty sleeping, you should see your doctor. Your problem may be a symptom of an illness, such as depression (p.343), or a side effect of medication.

Stress

How to identify signs of stress and find ways to manage it effectively

Stress is a physical or mental demand that provokes responses allowing us to meet challenges or escape from danger. The demand may be sudden, such as needing to avoid a speeding car, or long-term, such as pressures at work. Responses to stress

include both physical reactions, such as an increase in the heart rate and sweating, and psychological reactions, such as an intense concentration on the source of the stress.

A certain amount of stress can improve your performance in some sports and challenging physical activities, but excessive stress can be harmful to your health and interfere with your ability to cope with life. You can minimize harmful stress by identifying the types of situation that you find stressful and developing ways to avoid or limit them.

Sources of stress

Stress may result from external events or circumstances, your particular personality traits and how these affect your reaction to pressure, or a combination of both of these factors.

External events There are three main types of external circumstance that are especially likely to give rise to stress.

Long-term problems, such as an unhappy personal relationship, debilitating illness, or unemployment, are major sources of stress for many people.

Life events that require a lot of readjustment, such as marriage and moving house, can be highly stressful even if you consider the change a desirable one.

An accumulation of minor everyday occurrences, such as being late for work or getting caught in a traffic jam, can cause you to reach a breaking point if you are already under a lot of strain.

Attitudes and behaviour Some patterns of behaviour may result in stress. For example, if you suffer from low self-esteem you may doubt your ability to cope with challenges that arise in your life. You may also feel that you are not entitled to receive help from other people when you are under excessive stress. Highly competitive people may find it difficult to relax and may have a higher than usual risk of developing stress-associated disorders. People who do not express anxiety or anger even when they are under stress may suffer from accumulated tension.

Recognizing stress

You may recognize that you have been stressed only when the source of the stress is removed. However, there are early warning symptoms of excessive stress that you can learn to recognize. If you experience any of the symptoms listed below, you may need to take action to reduce your stress level.

Physical symptoms Stress may affect your general health. You may feel tired, have problems such as tension headaches (p.320), mouth ulcers (p.401), or muscle pain, or be unusually susceptible to minor infections such as colds.

Excessive stress may also lead to or aggravate a range of disorders, such as high blood pressure (see **Hypertension**, p.242), peptic ulcers (p.406), atopic

---

SLEEP CYCLES

A typical night's sleep
The cycles in a night's sleep are made up of lengthening phases of REM sleep, and four stages of non-REM sleep. In stages 1 and 2 you sleep lightly and wake easily; stages 3 and 4 are deep sleep, when you are difficult to wake.

▶ **HEALTH ACTION**

Relaxation exercises

When you are under stress, your muscles tighten, your heart beats more rapidly, and your breathing becomes fast and shallow. A good way to relax both mind and body is to learn simple relaxation routines that slow down your body's stress responses. Two simple techniques are shown here. For further information, ask your doctor about relaxation classes.

Breathing techniques

Controlled breathing, which uses the diaphragm and the abdominal muscles, is the basis of all relaxation methods. To prepare for abdominal breathing exercises, you should wear loose clothing and try to find a quiet spot away from distractions. Sit or lie in a comfortable position.

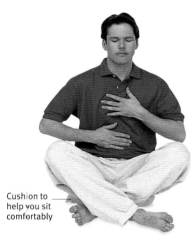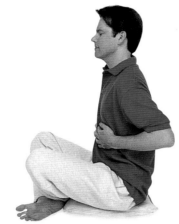

Cushion to
help you sit
comfortably

1 *Put one hand on your chest and the other hand on your abdomen. Inhale slowly, hold your breath for a moment, then exhale slowly. Try to breathe using your abdominal muscles so that the lower hand moves more than the upper hand.*

2 *Once you are breathing from your abdomen, place your hands just below your ribs. Feel your hands move as your abdomen rises and falls.*

Muscle relaxation

For muscle relaxation exercises, wear comfortable clothing and lie on a bed or on the floor. Put your arms by your sides and let your feet fall open. Tense and relax each part of your body in turn. During the exercise, keep your eyes closed. Breathe slowly using your abdominal muscles.

1 *Begin by taking one or two slow, deep breaths. Focus on your breathing. Starting with your feet, tense the muscles in each part of your body, hold for a count of three, then release the tension.*

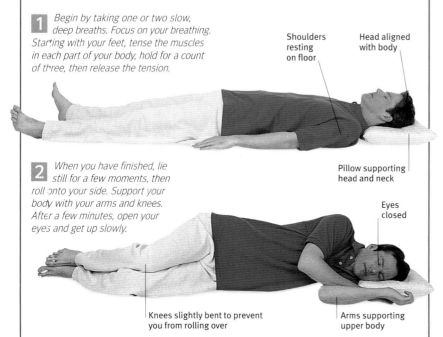

Shoulders resting on floor

Head aligned with body

2 *When you have finished, lie still for a few moments, then roll onto your side. Support your body with your arms and knees. After a few minutes, open your eyes and get up slowly.*

Pillow supporting head and neck

Eyes closed

Knees slightly bent to prevent you from rolling over

Arms supporting upper body

---

eczema (p.193), irritable bowel syndrome (p.415), psoriasis (p.192), menstrual disorders (*see* **Menstrual, menopausal, and hormonal problems**, pp.471–475), and erectile dysfunction (p.494).

Psychological symptoms If you feel very stressed, you may be anxious, tearful, or irritable. Even small problems may provoke an emotional response that is out of proportion to the cause. You may find it difficult to concentrate and be unable to make decisions. Your sleep patterns may be disrupted. You may lose your appetite and find that you have less energy than you used to have. Personal relationships may also suffer, especially if you become impatient or feel anxious when dealing with people. To distract yourself, you may begin to rely on alcohol, smoking, or drugs (*see* **Alcohol, tobacco, and drugs**, pp.24–26), which may further affect your health.

Minimizing harmful stress

To avoid excessive stress and maintain good health, you should learn to identify sources of stress and try to manage your life so that you can anticipate and prepare for problems or crises.

Maintaining good health Attempt to improve your mental health and well-being by keeping up contact with your family, maintaining friendships, and pursuing unstressful leisure activities. Exercising regularly can help to relieve physical tension (*see* **The benefits of exercise**, p.20), but you may also find it helpful to learn to relax your body consciously (*see* **Relaxation exercises**, left).

Identifying sources of stress A useful way to identify sources of stress is to keep a diary and record daily events and how you have responded to them. After a few weeks, look through your diary and identify events that you found stressful. Note whether the stress made you perform better or worse and try to identify activities that may have reduced your stress level.

Anticipating problems If you know that you will soon have to face a stressful event, prepare for it thoroughly so that you feel you have a good chance of managing it successfully. Break tasks or events down into smaller parts if they seem too big to cope with all at once. If you have several tasks to do in a limited time, list them and prioritize them. Limit the tasks that are not important or urgent in order to conserve your time and energy. If other people regularly make heavy demands on you, try to set limits.

Dealing with a crisis

Stress is a normal response to crises, and in most cases it need not be a cause for concern. However, if it leads to unmanageable symptoms, it has itself become a crisis. Seek help from your family and friends. Ask your doctor for help with the symptoms. He or she may refer you for counselling (p.624) if needed.

Loss and bereavement

Understanding and coping with the feelings, emotions, and stress that characterize the grieving process

Many types of change may result in a sense of loss, such as the break-up of a relationship, children leaving home, loss of job, or sudden disability. The loss felt after the death of a partner, relative, close friend, or a pet is called bereavement.

The grieving process

The grieving process has several elements. Throughout the process, you may find that you oscillate between focusing on your loss and distracting yourself with work or future plans.

Initial reactions At first, you may be overcome by shock or feel detached. You may even act as though nothing has happened. You are likely to experience signs of stress (p.31).

Protest After the initial shock, you may feel overcome with intense emotions, such as sadness, anger, guilt, or fear. The emotional pain may be interspersed with feelings of emptiness.

Disorganization As your mind accepts the reality of the loss, you may feel bleakness, apathy, and confusion and have no hope in the future. You may even feel suicidal.

Reorganization As time passes, you accept the loss and achieve a new normality. You may feel stronger as a result of coping. You can remember happy times and hope to be happy again.

How to cope with grief

It is important for you to acknowledge the loss, such as by viewing the dead body of a loved person and attending the funeral service if you feel you can.

There is a difference between normal and abnormal responses. The most common abnormal reactions are very intense emotions that last for a long time; inability to stop grieving, even after several years; and the inability to grieve at all. To cope with any of these reactions, it may be helpful to contact an organization for support.

Safety and health

Although most deaths and disabilities are the result of disease, a substantial number have other causes. About 1 in 40 deaths in England and Wales is caused by an accident. At home, on the road, at work, during recreational activities, and when travelling, accidents result in injuries to millions of people every year.

Accidents are the most significant single cause of death in children and young adults and are a major cause of death and disability in elderly people. They are also a major cause of serious injury in people of all ages. For example, in 2014, 1,775 people were killed, and about 22,800 were seriously injured, in traffic accidents in England and Wales alone. These injuries have substantial social and economic costs and may also have psychological effects such as post-traumatic stress disorder. The prevention of accidents has become a major concern for both medical and economic reasons. This section is designed to alert you to potentially dangerous circumstances in your everyday life, whether you are at work or at home. The first article addresses safety and health in your home and is followed by others on health and safety in the garden, in the sun, in and around water, with pets, at work, on the road, and when travelling.

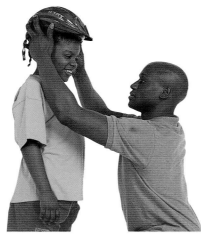

Family safety
When taking part in sports or travelling by road, make yourself aware of potential dangers and take action to minimize the risks to you and your family.

Home safety and health

How to prevent accidents and avoid health problems in the home

More accidents happen at home than anywhere else, and each year in the UK an estimated 5,000 people are killed and more than 2 million are injured due to accidents in their homes.

People over the age of 75 and children under the age of 5 have the highest rates of accidents in the home needing medical treatment.

Preventing falls
Falls are the most common accidents that occur in the home. Elderly people are especially vulnerable. To prevent falls in the home, make sure that the lighting in your house is adequate, that floor coverings are secure, that no objects are left on the stairs, and that safety rails are installed in the bathroom.

If you have a baby or a toddler, you can reduce the risk of falls by installing a stair gate, which restricts the child's access to stairways.

Avoiding poisoning
Poisoning causes a significant proportion of injuries that take place in the home. The poisons responsible include prescription and over-the-counter drugs, household cleaning materials, gases such as carbon monoxide, and lead. Since children are particularly at risk of poisoning, all drugs, cleaning materials, and other household chemicals should be kept out of their reach.

Carbon monoxide To prevent the build-up of carbon monoxide, have chimneys and flues checked, and heating systems and gas appliances inspected, yearly. For extra protection you should also fit carbon monoxide alarms, available in DIY shops.
Lead Lead pipes should be replaced with copper or plastic pipes. Any lead-based paint in your house should be removed by professional contractors. If you have any children's toys made before 1980, make sure that the toys are not coated with lead-based paint.

Preventing fires
Fire is one of the greatest hazards in the home. If you have an open fire, put a fire guard in front of it, and have both the fireplace and the chimney swept regularly. If you smoke, extinguish smoking materials carefully after use. When cooking, take care if using hot oil, and never leave frying pans or deep-fat fryers unattended. Keep a fire blanket or extinguisher in the kitchen. Teach children never to play with matches. To prevent electrical fires, take care not to overload sockets with adapters. Keep highly flammable materials locked away. In addition, have smoke detectors installed in case a fire does break out.

Monitoring air pollution in and around the home
Causes of air pollution in the home include tobacco smoke and house dust. Outside the home, sources of air pollution include industrial plants and various types of vehicle. If you are concerned about air pollution near your home, contact your local authority. Nitrogen dioxide, sulphur dioxide, and ozone from motor vehicles irritate the airways and aggravate the symptoms of respiratory diseases. The fine particles from diesel exhaust can also irritate the airways, and some have caused cancer in laboratory animals.

Other possible sources of pollution include older refrigerators and freezers that use chlorofluorocarbons (CFCs) and, in some areas of the UK, radon from granite rock, which can damage the lungs if inhaled in large amounts.

Safety in the garden

Taking precautions to keep your garden safe for all age groups

Every year, several hundred thousand people in the UK have accidents in their gardens that need medical treatment. The greatest risk is from water in ponds or pools (*see* **Safety in and around water**, p.34). Poisonous plants and chemicals, garden tools and barbecues also pose risks.

Avoiding poisonous plants
Some plants cause irritation if they come into contact with the skin. Other plants, if swallowed, may cause irritation of the mouth, throat, and stomach or nausea and vomiting. If a child swallows anything poisonous or anything you think might be poisonous, consult your doctor, or take the child to the accident and emergency department.

Using garden chemicals and tools safely
Store poisonous products in a locked shed or cabinet and follow the manufacturer's instructions. Don't leave sharp tools where

---

▶ **HEALTH ACTION**

Food hygiene

Food poisoning is usually caused by eating food contaminated by bacteria. The risk of poisoning is increased if food is left at room temperature because any bacteria present can multiply rapidly. Food is usually safe if stored in the refrigerator because the low temperature prevents bacteria from multiplying.

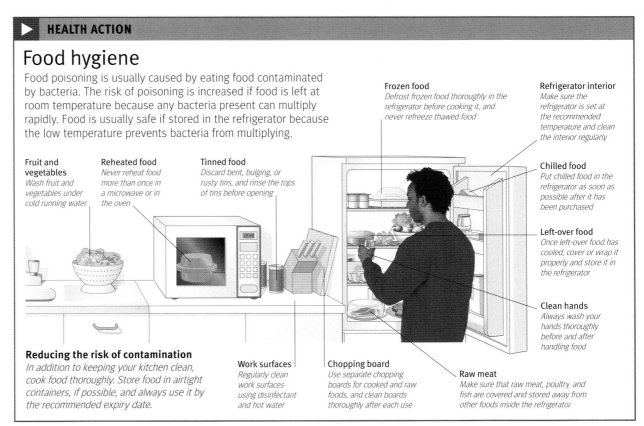

Fruit and vegetables
Wash fruit and vegetables under cold running water

Reheated food
Never reheat food more than once in a microwave or in the oven

Tinned food
Discard bent, bulging, or rusty tins, and rinse the tops of tins before opening

Frozen food
Defrost frozen food thoroughly in the refrigerator before cooking it, and never refreeze thawed food

Refrigerator interior
Make sure the refrigerator is set at the recommended temperature and clean the interior regularly

Chilled food
Put chilled food in the refrigerator as soon as possible after it has been purchased

Left-over food
Once left-over food has cooled, cover or wrap it properly and store it in the refrigerator

Clean hands
Always wash your hands thoroughly before and after handling food

Reducing the risk of contamination
In addition to keeping your kitchen clean, cook food thoroughly. Store food in airtight containers, if possible, and always use it by the recommended expiry date.

Work surfaces
Regularly clean work surfaces using disinfectant and hot water

Chopping board
Use separate chopping boards for cooked and raw foods, and clean boards thoroughly after each use

Raw meat
Make sure that raw meat, poultry, and fish are covered and stored away from other foods inside the refrigerator

children can find them. Wear goggles, ear protectors, gloves, and boots, when using tools such as chainsaws.

Using barbecues safely

Barbecues should always be supervised. Avoid lighting barbecues in a high wind, do not wear loose clothing near flames, and never pour flammable liquids onto smoking charcoal. When using a gas-fired barbecue, check for gas leaks and make sure that the flame is blue. Keep an outdoor fire extinguisher on hand.

Safety in the sun

Precautions and procedures to avoid skin damage and overexposure to heat

Overexposure to sunlight may lead to sunburn (p.207), premature aging, skin cancer (p.199), and damage to the eyes. Tanning, whether from sunlight or from sunbeds or sunlamps, is now considered to be harmful.

Damaging effects of sun

Exposure to strong sunlight without adequate protection can result in sunburn. Skin damage is caused by ultraviolet (UV) light, of which there are two main types: UVA light and UVB light. Overexposure to UVB light is known to cause skin cancer and cataracts (p.357). UVA light may also play a part in these conditions. In addition, repeated exposure to UV light can damage fibres called elastin in the skin, leading to premature aging.

Certain drugs, such as tetracycline antibiotics (p.572), may make the skin more sensitive to sunlight (see **Photosensitivity**, p.195). Oral contraceptives may cause areas of patchy skin pigmentation after exposure to the sun. Some perfumes and deodorants may cause skin discoloration in strong sunlight.

In the UK, skin cancer is the most common form of cancer, with about 115,000 new cases diagnosed in 2011. About 13,300 of these were malignant melanoma (p.201), which causes about 2,000 deaths in the UK each year. The risk of skin cancer is greater if you had severe sunburn as a child, or if you have red or blond hair and green or blue eyes. Even if you have never had severe sunburn, exposure to the sun over many years can increase your risk of skin cancer.

Protection from the sun

You can minimize the risk of sun damage by staying out of the sun between 11 am and 3 pm. If you have to be in the sun, there are three main types of protection: clothing, sunscreens, and sunglasses.

Clothing Wear a wide-brimmed hat and tightly woven clothing that covers your shoulders and neck. Protective clothing is available, such as a "legionnaire's hat" to cover the back of the neck, and swimwear that protects the body from UV light even when wet.

Sunscreens Sunscreens protect the skin by absorbing UV rays (see **Sunscreens and sunblocks**, p.577). Sunblocks block sunlight completely. Sunscreens only partially absorb UV rays, but because they are transparent, they are more acceptable for all-over use. You should choose one that protects against both UVA and UVB and with an SPF (sun protection factor) of at least 15 for adults or at least 30 for babies and children. It is preferable to choose a waterproof sunscreen because it is less likely to be washed or sweated off.

Sunscreens and sunblocks should be applied thickly before you go outside. They must be put directly onto the skin so should be applied before any insect repellent, make-up, or moisturizer. Afterwards, the sunscreen should be reapplied at least every 2 hours, or more frequently if it is rubbed, sweated, or washed off. You should use a sunscreen even on cloudy days and in the shade. Babies under 12 months old should be kept in the shade.

Sunglasses Sunglasses should give 100 per cent protection against UV light and should ideally be wrap-arounds, to stop light getting in at the sides. Never look at the sun directly, even when wearing sunglasses, or view it through a camera or binoculars, since the light can cause permanent damage to your eyes.

Sunbeds and sunlamps These typically emit concentrated UV light and so are potentially more dangerous than natural sunlight. Their use should be avoided.

Safety in and around water

Avoiding accidents and injuries in and around water

Fatalities from drowning have remained fairly consistent in recent years. In 2013, there were 381 deaths due to drowning, and it is one of the less common causes of accidental death. However, there are also other dangers associated with water, such as waterborne infections and non-fatal injury.

Preventing drowning and near-drowning

The situations that most often result in drowning or near-drowning are strong currents or very cold water and swimming or boating after drinking alcohol.

Understanding water conditions Even confident swimmers should always get information about local swimming conditions and heed advice that is given.

Avoid swimming in very cold water. Water below 5°C (41°F) stiffens muscles and may cause cardiac arrest.

Avoiding alcohol Many victims of drowning accidents have a significant amount of alcohol in their blood (see **Alcohol and health**, p.24). Never drink alcohol before swimming or boating.

Supervising children Do not leave young children alone when they are swimming or in the bath, even when the water is shallow. If you have a pond or swimming pool in your garden, fence it off or cover it.

Avoiding hazards in water

Drowning is not the only hazard associated with water. Shallow water, hidden objects, animals, and infections all present dangers.

Shallow water and hidden objects Every year, people injure their spines by diving into water that is too shallow or that contains hidden objects. Check the depth of water before diving or jumping, and check for rocks or fallen trees below the surface.

Animal life and infections On holiday, follow warnings about local dangers, such as sharks, and swim only in designated safe areas. Coral can cause cuts and abrasions.

The sea near coastal resorts may be polluted with sewage. Freshwater contaminated with rat or fox urine can cause leptospirosis (p.173). In tropical countries, avoid swimming in lakes or other bodies of fresh water (unless they are known to be safe) as there is a risk of schistosomiasis (p.179) and other waterborne parasitic infections.

Pets and health

Minimizing health risks associated with domestic pets

Diseases from pets are uncommon. However, animals can cause allergies, and infections and infestations with microorganisms, worms, or insects may spread to people. Pets that may bite should never be left alone with young children.

Check cats and dogs regularly for ticks. If your pet scratches more than usual or develops bald patches, consult your vet in case your pet has a fungal infection, such as ringworm (p.205), that could infect you.

Cat and dog faeces contain a number of dangerous organisms, such as the eggs of the toxocara worm. If ingested, these worm eggs may cause toxocariasis (p.178), a potentially serious disease that may lead to blindness. Cat faeces may also contain toxoplasma protozoa. Pregnant women in particular should avoid contact with cat faeces, because toxoplasmosis (p.176) may cause serious harm to the developing fetus. Deworm pets regularly and dispose of their faeces hygienically. Teach children to wash their hands after touching animals.

Safety and health at work

Practical steps to promote safety and health in the workplace

There are well-established connections between conditions in the workplace and certain health problems. As a result, measures have been developed to protect employees from a variety of occupational disorders, and these measures are enforced through legislation, regulation, and advisory information. In the UK in 2013/2014, there were about 1.2 million people suffering from a work-related illness. During that period, an estimated 28.2 million working days were lost due to work-related illness or injury, and there were about 142 deaths due to accidents at work. If you develop symptoms of ill-health or disease while at work and you suspect that your work environment might be the cause, you should talk to your supervisor or occupational health department, or to your doctor.

Reducing risks in the office

Your office can be a source of health hazards, particularly if you spend much of the day sitting in an awkward position at a computer.

If you work at a desk, you need to think carefully about the layout of your work area, your equipment, and your working practices. Your work area should be arranged so that everything is easy to reach and use. Make sure you have good lighting and ventilation, and that cables are not underfoot. If you are working at a computer, good posture is essential to prevent back problems. You should use an adjustable chair with a stable base and with half or no arm rests so that it can go under the desk. The seat should be flat or tipped slightly forwards and the height of the chair should be adjusted so that your feet can rest flat on the floor. The chair should have a back rest that can be adjusted to support your lower back at belt level. You should sit with shoulders relaxed, your head in a neutral position, and your chin tucked in. There should be a slight arch in your lower back, and you should sit close to the desk. The computer monitor should be an arm's length away, and the top of the monitor should be at eye level. The keyboard should be kept at elbow height, and your elbows should be kept at an angle of 90 degrees. You should take frequent short breaks from using the keyboard and monitor, and occasionally focus on a distant object to relax your eyes. Some people may also benefit from equipment that is specially modified, such as an ergonomic keyboard or a larger, more supportive mouse.

Sick building syndrome is a group of symptoms that seem to be associated with working in a building but which have no identifiable cause. It is more common in buildings where many people work together in close proximity, especially in new buildings with sealed windows. Symptoms include tiredness, headaches, dizziness, eye problems, nausea, coughing, wheezing, and nose or throat irritation. Although the cause is unknown, various causes have been suggested, including ozone from photocopiers, solvents and other chemicals, air-conditioning, and poor ventilation. Recent research has indicated that the psychological and social work environment may be a significant causative factor.

Strained relationships with your colleagues, poor job satisfaction, and difficult personal events can be causes of stress.

If this is the case, you should try to raise your concerns with your line manager or relevant supervisor. You should also seek advice on managing the symptoms of stress.

Reducing risks in the industrial workplace

Some occupations are inherently dangerous. If your work involves contact with heavy machinery, organic solvents, or other hazardous substances, loud noise, or extreme heat or cold, you should be aware of the dangers and be provided with protective equipment. Legislation, regulations, and guidelines now in place should reduce the risk of developing a work-related illness but they do need to be followed by both employers and employees.

Many substances in the workplace can cause occupational lung diseases (p.305). The most common of these conditions is asthma (p.295). More than 200 substances, ranging from latex in gloves to isocyanates used in paint spraying, are known to trigger the disorder. Your doctor can arrange for tests in order to identify asthma triggers. Several other lung disorders are associated with inhalation of specific particles. Occupations that carry particular risks include mining, farming, and any other work involving contact with asbestos or silica.

Substances such as detergents may irritate your skin and cause disorders such as eczema (p.193) or contact dermatitis (p.193). To avoid these problems, you need to wear protective clothing and use barrier creams.

If your work involves lifting heavy loads or sitting for long periods with poor back support, you are vulnerable to back pain. It is important to make sure you have any necessary training, be aware of your posture, and try to lift heavy objects safely (see **Preventing back pain**, p.226).

Taking responsibility for health at work

In many countries, including the UK, employers are required by law to meet safety standards, monitor employees' health, offer screening if needed, and compensate workers who develop permanent health problems. Employees should be aware of the health hazards associated with their occupation and of legally required safety practices. In the UK, both employers and employees are responsible for maintaining a safe working environment.

Safety on the road

Safety precautions for motorists, motorcyclists, cyclists, and pedestrians

Accidents involving motorists, motorcyclists, cyclists, and pedestrians are among the leading causes of accidental death and injury in the developed world. In the UK the number of injuries and deaths on the roads has declined in recent years but still remains

high: in England and Wales, about 22,800 people were seriously injured and 1,775 people were killed on the roads in 2014.

Most road traffic accidents in the UK are due to speeding, drink-driving, or the use of illegal drugs. Very few accidents are caused by mechanical faults. Other causes include poor eyesight, tiredness, and taking certain prescription or over-the-counter drugs.

Staying safe in cars

The most important vehicle safety device is the seat belt. Airbags have also saved many lives. Modern cars and lorries have a variety of other built-in safety features, including headrests, specially designed seats for children, and anti-lock brakes.

Staying safe on motorcycles and bicycles

Motorcyclists need helmets and special clothing to protect them from the road surface, other vehicles, and the weather.

Cyclists are particularly at risk of head injuries, so wearing a helmet is essential. Cyclists should also make sure they are easily visible, for example by wearing bright clothing and by putting reflectors on their bicycles.

Staying safe as a pedestrian

Nearly all injuries to pedestrians happen in urban areas. Children aged 5–14 years are most at risk of accidents.

If you plan to go out walking or jogging at night, wear bright clothes and reflectors. Teach children to be alert when out on busy streets.

Travel health

Staying healthy and avoiding accidents when travelling abroad

Common problems abroad include digestive upsets, injuries in traffic accidents, and sexually transmitted infections. You can minimize the risks by finding out about your destination before you travel and having recommended travel immunizations.

Staying healthy

Digestive upsets and sexually transmitted infections are common problems when travelling abroad, but hot weather and local wildlife can also present hazards.

Digestive-system problems To reduce the risk of gastroenteritis, wash your hands with soap and water before meals; avoid raw vegetables, salads, shellfish, and ice cream; and peel all fruit. Use bottled water for drinking and brushing your teeth, or purify water using tablets or a filter.

If you develop diarrhoea, rest for at least a day, eat nothing, and drink plenty of fluids (preferably special rehydration fluids). If diarrhoea persists, seek medical help.

Sexually transmitted infections The best defence against sexually transmitted infections is abstinence from sex with new partners. Also reduce the risk of infection by practising safe sex (p.27).

Hot weather Moist skin is an excellent growth medium for bacteria and fungi. Most skin and fungal infections can be prevented by frequently showering and changing, wearing loose clothing, and avoiding strong sunlight.

Bites and stings Precautions against mosquitoes will help to prevent other stings and bites (see **Avoiding bites and stings**, p.188). Keep your bed away from the wall, shake clothes and shoes before you wear them, and put on shoes whenever you get out of bed.

▶ **HEALTH ACTION**

Travel immunizations

The immunizations you will need before travelling depend on your immunization history and the area you intend to visit, although some diseases can be contracted almost anywhere. Wherever you are planning to go, make sure you have been immunized against diphtheria, tetanus, and polio (see **Routine immunizations**, p.13) and have had booster doses if necessary. Before travelling, always ask your doctor or travel clinic for up-to-date information. It is not possible to be immunized against malaria (p.175).

Immunization advice
The recommendations here are for healthy adults; you should consult your doctor about immunizations for a child, or if you are pregnant or have a health problem. Timings of the doses you receive may differ from those shown here.

Disease	Number of doses	When effective	Period of protection	Who should be immunized
Cholera (p.173)	2 oral doses 1–6 weeks apart	1 week after 2nd dose	2 years	People travelling to areas where cholera is epidemic or endemic. Immunization does not provide complete protection; travellers to these areas should pay scrupulous attention to food, water, and personal hygiene.
Hepatitis A (p.408)	2 injections 6–12 months apart	2–4 weeks after 1st dose	1st dose protects for 1 year; 2nd dose for up to 20 years	Travellers to high-risk areas outside Northern and Western Europe, North America, Australia, New Zealand, and Japan.
Hepatitis B (p.408)	3 injections 1 month between 1st and 2nd doses, 5 months between 2nd and 3rd doses	After 3rd dose	5 years	People travelling to countries in which hepatitis B is prevalent and who might need medical or dental treatment and/or likely to have unprotected sex while there.
Japanese encephalitis	2 injections 28 days apart	About 1 week after 2nd dose	1 year	People staying for an extended period in rural areas of the Indian subcontinent, China, Southeast Asia, and the Far East.
Meningitis A, C, W135, and Y	1 injection	After 2–3 weeks	5 years	People travelling to Saudi Arabia for the Hajj and Umrah pilgrimages (immunization certificate needed), and those travelling to sub-Saharan Africa.
Rabies (p.169)	3 injections; 1 week between 1st and 2nd doses, 2 or 3 weeks between 2nd and 3rd doses	After 3rd dose	2–5 years; those at continued risk need reinforcing doses from 1 year after the first course	People travelling to areas where rabies is endemic and who are at high risk (e.g. people working with animals, and those travelling into remote country).
Typhoid (p.172)	1 injection, or 3 oral doses 2 days apart	2 weeks after injection, or 7–10 days after 3rd oral dose	3 years (injection); 1 year (oral)	People travelling to areas with poor sanitation, and those at high risk of infection (e.g. laboratory workers).
Yellow fever (p.169)	1 injection	After 10 days	10 years	People travelling to parts of South America and Sub-Saharan Africa.

2 assessing your symptoms

THE BODY FUNCTIONS RELIABLY most of the time, and we are not aware of the internal processes that keep us alive and enable us to carry out everyday activities. However, sometimes we experience warning signals, or symptoms, that tell us something is wrong. Most symptoms are caused by minor illness or injury and clear up within a few days. However, it is important to be able to tell when a symptom requires medical attention, and the question-and-answer charts in this section provide guidance on how to recognize this.

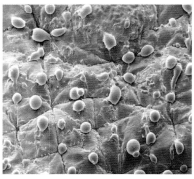

Droplets of sweat
The secretion of sweat helps to control body temperature. Excessive sweating is a common symptom of feverish illnesses.

Symptoms take many forms. Some involve a new sensation, such as pain in the chest, that only you can perceive. Others involve a change in a normal body function, such as frequent passing of urine, or a change in appearance, such as the development of a rash. Such new sensations or changes in the way we look or function alert us to the possibility of illness and may prompt us to seek medical help. However, when investigating the cause of your problem, your doctor does not rely only on a description of your symptoms. He or she will also look for signs of illness. Signs are physical evidence of a disorder or illness that the doctor can detect during a physical examination but of which you may be unaware. For example, if you have a lung condition, shortness of breath might be a symptom that you experience. When the doctor listens to your chest through a stethoscope, he or she may detect abnormal sounds with each breath; these are a sign of the disorder. The combination of symptoms and signs provides the doctor with a pattern that may suggest a diagnosis.

Understanding symptoms

Doctors learn by experience to recognize patterns of symptoms and signs, and most of us learn to do the same for a particular illness if we have had similar symptoms on several occasions. For example, a person who has recurrent attacks of migraine is usually able to recognize the symptoms at an early stage and knows the best way to bring the attacks under control. Similarly, the symptoms of many common infectious illnesses have become general knowledge. Most people recognize aching muscles, runny nose, tiredness, and fever as the usual symptoms of flu. However, dealing with unfamiliar symptoms is not as easy. In these cases, you should make a note of your symptoms so that you can describe them accurately to your doctor or other health professional. Information that may be helpful

Measuring body temperature
A temperature above 37°C (98.6°F) is a common symptom of infectious illness. Temperature can be measured using a thermometer placed in the mouth or armpit. For children, using an aural thermometer, the tip of which is gently inserted into the ear, is a safer alternative.

includes when the symptom started; which part of the body is affected; whether it came on suddenly or developed gradually; and whether it is continuous or intermittent. If you have a pain, it may also be useful for you to determine how it feels, such as whether it is dull, sharp, burning, or throbbing.

Certain symptoms can be assessed very accurately because they can be measured. Probably the most familiar example is assessing whether or not a person has a fever and, if so, how high the fever is, by measuring body temperature using a thermometer. It is especially useful to be able to measure a symptom in young children because they may not be able to understand or tell you how they are feeling.

Most people seek help for symptoms that they find troublesome, but it is not wise to assume that an apparently harmless symptom does not need treatment. For example, a rash may cause distress even though it is unlikely to have a serious cause, but a painless swelling may be the first sign of cancer and should not be ignored.

What the charts are for

The charts in this section guide you through a series of questions about your symptoms in order to suggest possible causes and the most appropriate course of action. The charts tell you whether you can safely treat your symptoms yourself or whether you need medical attention. They also say how urgently medical help should be sought if required. Some symptoms, such as loss of consciousness, are obvious emergencies. If a symptom could indicate a medical emergency in some circumstances, this is highlighted on the charts. Other symptoms, such

Checking a child's breathing rate
A rapid breathing rate in a baby or young child could be a sign of a respiratory disorder.

as a sore throat, are often due to a minor infection and should clear up whether or not they are treated. In these cases, the charts give advice on self-help measures that may relieve discomfort in the meantime. If over-the-counter remedies are appropriate, the charts will tell you. However, you should consult your doctor if you are unsure whether a remedy is suitable for you and read the manufacturer's instructions before taking medication. The charts advise on how long to keep treating yourself and when you need to see your doctor.

Self-help measures
You can treat some minor symptoms yourself at home. For example, a cold compress may help to relieve the pain of swollen joints.

Although the charts can help you to decide on the best way to deal with your symptoms, they cannot be applied across all situations. For example, even what may appear to be minor complaints should receive medical attention when they occur in people who are elderly or in those with reduced immunity, such as people undergoing chemotherapy as part of cancer treatment.

Consulting your doctor

If you do need to see your doctor, he or she will assess your condition by asking you detailed questions about the nature of your symptoms. The questions on the charts should help you to think about your symptoms so that you will be able to describe them accurately to the doctor. The doctor will probably carry out a physical examination and may also arrange tests to confirm whatever diagnosis is suggested by your symptoms and signs.

1 Tiredness

▶ For tiredness caused by poor sleep, see chart 3

It is normal to feel tired during the day if you have had difficulty sleeping or if you have been working hard or exercising. You should not be concerned unless your tiredness is persistent and severe. If you are uncertain about the cause of your tiredness, you should consult your doctor.

START

? Do you have any of the following symptoms?

Feeling faint or passing out

Shortness of breath

Paler skin than normal

None of the above

? Have you progressively lost weight without a change in eating habits or increased exercise?

No, or gained weight

Yes

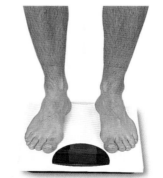

? Do you have any of the following symptoms?

Increased dryness or roughness of the skin

Feeling the cold more than you used to

Generalized hair thinning

None of the above

Possible cause

Anaemia (p.271) is a possible cause of your symptoms.

Medical help

 See your doctor within 24 hours.

? Have you been experiencing any of the following symptoms?

Increased thirst

Passing more urine than normal

Blurred vision

None of the above

Possible cause

Diabetes mellitus (p.437) may be a possibility.

Medical help

 See your doctor within 24 hours.

Go to chart 2
Loss of weight

Possible cause

Hypothyroidism (p.432) is a possible cause.

Medical help

 Make an appointment to see your doctor.

Possible cause

Regularly drinking too much alcohol can cause tiredness (*see* **Alcohol and health**, p.24).

Medical help

 Make an appointment to see your doctor for advice about reducing the amount of alcohol you drink.

Go to chart 8
Feeling depressed

? **Are you currently taking any medications, complementary remedies, or recreational drugs?**

Yes

No

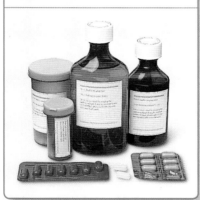

? **Do you regularly drink more than the recommended limit of alcohol (*see* Safe alcohol limits, p.24)?**

More than the limit

Within the limit

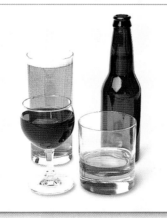

? **Do you have any of the following symptoms?**

Low self-esteem

Inability to concentrate or to make decisions

Lack of interest in sex

None of the above

? **Have you recently had a viral illness such as flu?**

Recent illness

No recent illness

Possible cause

Certain drugs and remedies may cause tiredness, for example, some drugs used to treat high blood pressure (*see* **Antihypertensive drugs**, p.580).

Medical help

 Make an appointment to see your doctor. Continue to take prescribed medication unless advised to stop by your doctor but stop taking any other medications, complementary remedies, or recreational drugs.

Possible cause

It may take several weeks to recover from an illness, particularly from some viral infections, such as **infectious mononucleosis** (p.166).

Medical help

 Make an appointment to see your doctor if you are still feeling tired 1 month after any other symptoms you had have disappeared.

If you cannot identify a possible cause for your tiredness from this chart, make an appointment to see your doctor.

2 Loss of weight

▶ For children under 12, see chart 42

Most people experience small fluctuations in their weight. However, weight loss may be a cause for concern if it occurs without a deliberate change in diet and/or increased exercise. Consult your doctor if you have been losing weight without an obvious cause.

START

? Has your weight loss been progressive?

Yes

No

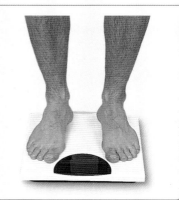

? How has your appetite been lately?

Poor

Normal or increased

? Have you been experiencing any of the following symptoms?

Recurrent fever

Profuse sweating at night

Persistent cough

Bloodstained sputum

None of the above

? Have you been experiencing any of the following symptoms?

Increased thirst

Passing more urine than usual

Blurred vision

None of the above

? Do you have any of the following symptoms?

Feeling constantly on edge

Increased sweating

Bulging eyes

None of the above

Possible cause

A small weight loss is unlikely to be a serious cause for concern unless you are below your healthy weight (*see* **Are you a healthy weight?**, p.19).

Self-help

Increase the amount of food you eat (*see* **Controlling your weight**, p.19). Make an appointment to see your doctor if you continue to lose weight or have any other symptoms.

Possible cause

Diabetes mellitus (p.437) is a possible cause.

Medical help

 See your doctor within 24 hours.

Possible causes

Hyperthyroidism (p.432) is a possibility. However, **anxiety disorders** (p.341) can cause some of these symptoms.

Medical help

 Make an appointment to see your doctor.

Possible causes

A chronic infection, such as **tuberculosis** (p.300) or an AIDS-related illness (*see* **HIV infection and AIDS**, p.169), could be the cause of your symptoms. An underlying **cancer** (pp.152–155) is also a possible cause.

Medical help

 See your doctor within 24 hours.

Possible causes

An intestinal infection, such as **giardiasis** (p.176), or a long-term bowel condition, such as **ulcerative colitis** (p.417) or **Crohn's disease** (p.417), could be the cause of your symptoms. **Colorectal cancer** (p.421) or **stomach cancer** (p.406) are also possibilities.

Medical help

 See your doctor within 24 hours.

Possible causes

Depression (p.343) could be the cause. However, **anxiety disorders** (p.341) sometimes produce similar symptoms.

Medical help

 Make an appointment to see your doctor.

Possible cause

You are probably eating less than you need to meet your energy requirements.

Medical help

 Make an appointment to see your doctor to make sure that an underlying problem is not responsible for your weight loss.

Have you noticed any of the following symptoms?

Recurrent diarrhoea

Recurrent constipation

Recurrent abdominal pain

Blood in faeces

None of the above

Do you have any of the following symptoms?

Difficulty sleeping

Low self-esteem

Lack of interest in sex

Inability to concentrate or to make decisions

Lack of energy

None of the above

Have you recently increased the amount of exercise you do?

No increase

Increased exercise

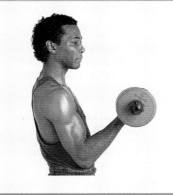

Possible cause

Your increase in energy output is the most probable cause of your weight loss.

Self-help

Increase the amount of food you eat to make up for your increased energy needs (*see* **Controlling your weight**, p.19). Make an appointment to see your doctor if you continue to lose weight or are below the healthy weight for your height (*see* **Are you a healthy weight?**, p.19)

If you cannot identify a possible cause for your weight loss from this chart, call your doctor within 24 hours.

3 Difficulty sleeping

Most people are affected by difficulty sleeping on occasion. The causes include worry, drinking too much caffeine, or insufficient exercise. If you wake feeling unrested but are not aware of difficulty sleeping, the cause may be interruption of breathing during sleep (*see* **Sleep apnoea**, p.292). Consult your doctor if you have frequent sleeping problems.

START

What kind of sleeping difficulty have you been experiencing?

Difficulty getting to sleep

Difficulty staying asleep

Are you awakened from sleep by attacks of shortness of breath?

No

Yes

Go to chart 17
Shortness of breath

Go to chart 8
Feeling depressed

Do you have any of the following symptoms?

Lack of energy

Low self-esteem

Inability to concentrate or to make decisions

Lack of interest in sex

None of the above

Do you take sleeping pills regularly or have you recently stopped taking them?

Taking sleeping pills

Recently stopped

Neither

Possible cause

The regular use of sleeping pills can lead to a gradual reduction in their effectiveness (*see* **Sleeping drugs**, p.591).

Medical help

 Make an appointment to see your doctor.

Possible cause

Withdrawal from sleeping pills can lead to difficulty sleeping as your body adapts (*see* **Sleeping drugs**, p.591).

Self-help

Follow the advice for getting a good night's sleep (*see* **Sleep**, p.31). Make an appointment to see your doctor if difficulty sleeping continues.

Possible causes

Hyperthyroidism (p.432) is a possible cause. However, **anxiety disorders** (p.341) can also cause these symptoms.

Medical help

 Make an appointment to see your doctor.

Possible cause

Consumption of any of these can lead to difficulty sleeping.

Self-help

Follow the advice for getting a good night's sleep (*see* **Sleep**, p.31). Make an appointment to see your doctor if difficulty sleeping continues.

Possible cause

Your symptoms may be a side effect of the medication, remedy, or recreational drug.

Medical help

Make an appointment to see your doctor. Continue to take prescribed medication unless advised to stop by your doctor but stop taking any other medications, complementary remedies, or recreational drugs.

Possible cause

You may need less sleep than you think. It is possible that some of the sleep that you need has been taken as naps during the day.

Self-help

Follow the advice for getting a good night's sleep (*see* **Sleep**, p.31). Make an appointment to see your doctor if difficulty sleeping continues.

? On nights that you have difficulty sleeping, have you consumed any of the following?

Large amounts of coffee, tea, or cola

Large amounts of alcohol

A late, heavy meal

None of the above

? Are you currently taking any medications, complementary remedies, or recreational drugs?

Yes

No

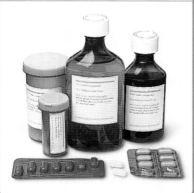

? On nights that you have difficulty sleeping, have either of the following applied?

You have taken a nap during the day

You have been awake for fewer than 18 hours

Neither

? How physically active is your usual daily routine?

Mainly sedentary

Physically active

? Do you have either of the following symptoms?

Feeling constantly on edge

Inability to concentrate

Neither

Possible cause

Insufficient physical activity in the day can lead to sleeping problems at night.

Self-help

Build more exercise into your daily routine (*see* **Taking regular exercise**, p.21). Make an appointment to see your doctor if problems with sleeping persist.

If you cannot identify a possible cause for your difficulty sleeping from this chart, make an appointment to see your doctor.

4 Fever

▶ For children under 12, see chart 45

Normal temperature varies from one person to another, but if your temperature is 38°C (100.4°F) or above, you have a fever. Most fevers are due to infection, but heat exposure or certain drugs can also raise body temperature. In all cases, follow the self-help advice for **bringing down a fever** (p.165).

❌ WARNING

High temperature

If you are feeling unwell, you should take your temperature every 4 hours. Call your doctor immediately if your temperature rises to 39°C (102°F) or above, and take steps to lower the fever without delay (*see* **Bringing down a fever**, p.165).

START

? Do you have a rash?

Rash

No rash

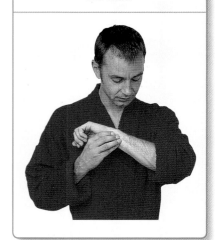

? Do you have a headache?

Severe headache

Mild headache

No headache

? Are you having problems breathing?

You are short of breath

Breathing is painful

Breathing is normal

? Do you have a cough?

Cough

No cough

Go to chart 10
Rash with fever

? Do you have any of the following symptoms?

Drowsiness or confusion

Dislike of bright light

Neck pain on bending the head forwards

None of the above

Possible cause

There is a possibility that you have **meningitis** (p.325).

Medical help

 EMERGENCY! Dial 999/112 and ask for an ambulance.

Possible causes

Cystitis (p.453) is the most likely cause of your symptoms, but **pyelonephritis** (p.446) is also possible, especially if you have back pain.

Medical help

 See your doctor within 24 hours.

Have you been coughing up sputum?

Sputum

No sputum

Possible cause

A chest infection, such as **pneumonia** (p.299), is a possible cause.

Medical help

 URGENT! Phone your doctor immediately!

Possible causes

A chest infection, such as **acute bronchitis** (p.297), may cause your symptoms. **Tuberculosis** (p.300) is also a possibility.

Medical help

See your doctor within 24 hours.

 Do you have either of the following symptoms?

Generalized aches and pains

Runny nose

Neither

Possible cause

A viral illness, such as a severe cold (see **Common cold**, p.164) or **influenza** (p.164), is the most probable cause of your symptoms.

Self-help

Follow the self-help advice for **bringing down a fever** (p.165). Consult your doctor if your symptoms worsen, if you are no better in 2 days, or if other symptoms develop.

 Have you had several bouts of fever over the past few weeks?

Recurrent fever

No other recent fever

Possible causes

A long-term infection, such as **infective endocarditis** (p.256) or an AIDS-related illness (see **HIV infection and AIDS**, p.169) may cause recurrent fever. An underlying cancer, such as **lymphoma** (p.279), or **tuberculosis** (p.300) are also possibilities.

Medical help

See your doctor within 24 hours.

 Do you have any urinary problems?

Pain on passing urine

Passing urine too frequently

Neither

 Do you have a sore throat?

Sore throat

No sore throat

Go to chart 15
Sore throat

If you cannot identify a possible cause for your fever from this chart, see your doctor within 24 hours.

5 Lumps and swellings

Lumps and swellings under the skin, particularly in the neck, under the arms, or in the groin, are often enlarged lymph nodes (glands). These glands usually become swollen due to an infection. The swelling subsides shortly after the infection clears up. If the lumps are painful or if they are persistent but painless, you should consult your doctor.

✕ WARNING

Painless lumps or swellings
Any painless lump or swelling that does not disappear within 2 weeks should be seen by a doctor.

START

? What are the characteristics of the lump or swelling?

Red and painful

Other

? Are the lumps or swellings in more than one area?

One area only

Several areas

? Do you have a rash?

Rash

No rash

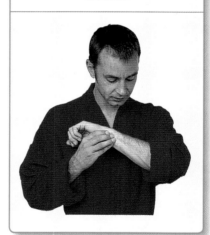

Possible cause

An abscess or a **boil** (p.204) may be the cause of a painful, inflamed swelling.

Medical help

 See your doctor within 24 hours.

? Do you have a fever – a temperature of 38°C (100.4°F) or above?

Fever

No fever

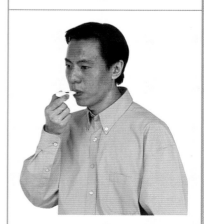

Possible causes

A viral infection is the most likely cause. There is also a possibility of a cancer of the lymphatic system (*see* **Lymphoma**, p.279) or an AIDS-related illness (*see* **HIV infection and AIDS**, p.169).

Medical help

 See your doctor within 24 hours.

Possible cause

Infectious mononucleosis (p.166) is a possible cause of swelling of the lymph nodes in several areas, especially if you feel generally unwell.

Medical help

 See your doctor within 24 hours.

Go to chart 34
Testes and scrotum problems

 What happens to the swelling if you press on it or if you lie down?

It disappears

It reduces in size

No change

Possible cause

You may have an inguinal hernia (*see* **Hernias**, p.419).

Medical help

Make an appointment to see your doctor.

 Where is the lump or swelling?

Testis

Groin

Breast

Sides or back of neck

Other

Go to chart 36
Breast problems

Possible cause

A trapped inguinal hernia (*see* **Hernias**, p.419) could be responsible for the swelling.

Medical help

URGENT! Phone your doctor immediately!

Possible causes

A number of viral illnesses can cause swollen glands and a rash. **Lyme disease** (p.174) is another possibility, particularly if you think you may have been bitten by a tick recently.

Medical help

See your doctor within 24 hours.

 Do you have a sore throat?

Sore throat

No sore throat

Go to chart 15
Sore throat

Possible causes

An injury is likely to cause some swelling as a result of damage to the tissues. An infected wound or a localized rash can also cause nearby lymph nodes to swell (*see* **Lymphadenopathy**, p.279).

Self-help

Make sure the wound is clean and protect it with an adhesive bandage or light dressing. Consult your doctor if there is any pain, redness, or pus around the wound, or if the swelling persists after the wound has healed.

If you cannot identify a possible cause for your lumps or swellings from this chart, make an appointment to see your doctor.

Do you have a recent injury near the site of the swelling?

Injury

No injury

Feeling faint and passing out

Feeling faint is a sensation of dizziness or light-headedness. It may be followed by passing out (loss of consciousness). The cause is usually lack of food or a reduction in blood flow to the brain. A brief episode of feeling faint without other symptoms is not a cause for alarm, but you should consult your doctor if such episodes recur or if you have passed out.

 WARNING

Unconsciousness

If someone remains unconscious for more than a minute or so, whatever the suspected cause, you should get emergency medical help. If you need to leave the person to call for help, first lay him or her in the recovery position. Do not move the person if you suspect spinal injury.

START

? Have you had any of the following symptoms?

- Disturbed vision
- Numbness, tingling, or weakness in any part of the body
- Confusion
- Difficulty in speaking
- None of the above

? Are any of your symptoms still present?

- Symptoms present
- Symptoms no longer present

? Have you noticed any of the following?

- Bloodstained vomit
- Red blood in the faeces
- Black, tarry faeces
- None of the above

? Did any of the following occur when you passed out?

- You twitched uncontrollably
- You bit your tongue
- You passed urine
- None of the above

Possible cause

You may have bleeding in the digestive tract, perhaps from a **peptic ulcer** (p.406).

Medical help

 EMERGENCY! Dial 999/112 and ask for an ambulance.

Possible cause

You may have had a seizure, which could be due to **epilepsy** (p.324).

Medical help

 EMERGENCY! Dial 999/112 and ask for an ambulance.

Possible cause

A **transient ischaemic attack** (p.328) is a possibility.

Medical help

 URGENT! Phone your doctor immediately!

Possible cause

It is possible that you have had a **stroke** (p.329).

Medical help

 EMERGENCY! Dial 999/112 and ask for an ambulance.

Possible causes

You may have low blood pressure (see **Hypotension**, p.248) due to worsening of a pre-existing heart condition or an irregular heartbeat (see **Arrhythmias**, p.249).

Medical help

 URGENT! Phone your doctor immediately!

Possible cause

Sudden psychological shock can result in feeling faint or passing out.

Self-help

Rest and ask someone to stay with you until you feel better. If it happens again, make an appointment to see your doctor.

Does either of the following apply?

You have diabetes

You had not eaten for several hours before passing out

Neither

Possible cause

Low blood sugar levels are a possible cause of feeling faint or passing out, often with sweating, anxiety, and nausea (*see* **Diabetes mellitus**, p.437, and **Hypoglycaemia**, p.440).

Medical help

URGENT! Phone your doctor immediately! Eat or drink something sweet.

Did you feel faint or pass out immediately after either of the following?

Getting up suddenly

Emotional shock

Neither

Do you have any of the following symptoms?

Shortness of breath

Paler skin than normal

Undue tiredness

None of the above

Possible cause

Anaemia (p.271) is a possible cause of your symptoms.

Medical help

See your doctor within 24 hours.

Possible cause

The most likely explanation is a temporary drop in blood pressure due to a change in position; it is usually not a cause for concern (*see* **Hypotension**, p.248).

Medical help

See your doctor within 24 hours if you passed out. Make an appointment to see your doctor in the next few days even if you did not pass out.

Does either of the following apply?

You have had chest pain or you have a heart condition

You have had palpitations

Neither

Possible cause

Changes in blood flow during pregnancy can cause faintness.

Medical help

Make an appointment to see your doctor.

Might you be pregnant?

Possibly pregnant

Not pregnant

If you cannot identify a possible cause for passing out from this chart, phone your doctor immediately. If you cannot identify a possible cause for feeling faint, see your doctor within 24 hours.

7 # Headache

Tension in head and neck muscles and fever are common causes of headache (*see* **Tension headaches,** p.320). Too much alcohol, caffeine, or nicotine may also cause a headache. Most headaches do not last for more than a few hours. If your headache lasts for more than 24 hours, is not improved by over-the-counter painkillers, or recurs several times in a week, consult your doctor.

✖ DANGER SIGNS

Dial 999/112 and ask for an ambulance if a headache is accompanied by any of the following symptoms:
- Flat, dark red spots that do not fade when pressed (*see* **Checking a red rash,** p.57).
- Drowsiness or confusion.
- Weakness in a limb.
- Blurred vision.
- Dislike of bright light.
- Temporary unconsciousness.

START

? **Have you hit your head within the past 24 hours?**

Head injury

No head injury

? **Do you have a fever – a temperature of 38°C (100.4°F) or above?**

Fever

No fever

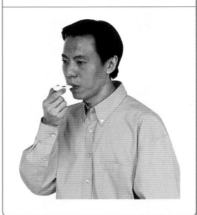

Possible causes

Many minor illnesses associated with fever are accompanied by a headache. However, a serious illness such as **meningitis** (p.325) may also be the cause. Go to **chart 4, Fever** if you are 12 or over or **chart 45, Fever in children** for a child under 12.

? **Are any of the danger signs listed in the box (above right) present, or have you vomited?**

Danger signs present

Vomited after head injury

No danger signs or vomiting

? **Have you experienced nausea and/or vomiting with your headache?**

Yes

No

Possible cause

A mild headache is common following a minor head injury (*see* **Head injuries,** p.322).

Self-help

Take a painkiller (not aspirin). If your headache lasts for more than 2 hours or if you develop other symptoms, phone your doctor immediately.

Possible cause

There may be damage to the tissues that surround the brain (*see* **Head injuries,** p.322).

Medical help

 EMERGENCY! Dial 999/112 and ask for an ambulance.

Possible cause

Sinusitis (p.290) is the likely cause of your headache.

Self-help

Try **steam inhalation** (p.291). Get medical advice if you feel no better in 2 days.

How is your vision?

Blurred vision

Disturbed in other ways

Unchanged

Possible cause

Acute glaucoma (p.358) is a possibility, particularly if the pain is around your eye.

Medical help

 URGENT! Phone your doctor immediately!

Possible cause

Your symptoms may be a side effect of the medication, remedy, or recreational drug.

Medical help

Make an appointment to see your doctor. Continue to take prescribed medication unless advised to stop by your doctor but stop taking any other medications, complementary remedies, or recreational drugs.

Possible causes

 Migraine (p.320) is the most likely cause of your headache, particularly if any visual problems occurred before the headache started. However, the possibility of another disorder, such as a **stroke** (p.329), needs to be ruled out.

Medical help

URGENT! Phone your doctor immediately if this is your first attack. Although the condition is probably not dangerous, your doctor should confirm the diagnosis.

Where is the pain?

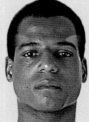

SITES OF PAIN

Over one or both temples as shown

Elsewhere

Are you currently taking any medications, complementary remedies, or recreational drugs?

Yes

No

Have you had this type of headache before?

Yes

No

Does either of the following apply?

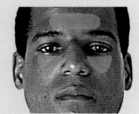

SITES OF PAIN

The pain is felt chiefly in the areas shown

You have recently had a runny or stuffy nose

Neither

Possible cause

Giant cell (temporal) arteritis (p.282) is a possibility, particularly if you are over the age of 50 and have been feeling unwell.

Medical help

URGENT! Phone your doctor immediately!

If you cannot identify a possible cause for your headache from this chart, make an appointment to see your doctor.

Possible cause

A recurrent **headache** (p.320) for which there is no obvious cause, such as drinking too much alcohol, should always be investigated by your doctor.

Medical help

Make an appointment to see your doctor.

8 Feeling depressed

Feeling depressed may include a lack of energy, sadness, and low self-esteem. It is normal to feel down from time to time, especially after disappointments. More severe feelings of depression are also natural after major upsets, such as the death of someone close. You should consult your doctor if depression is severe or if it persists for more than 2 weeks.

✖ WARNING

Having suicidal thoughts

Anyone who considers suicide is in need of urgent help. If someone close to you is suicidal, encourage the person to contact his or her doctor or seek other professional help. Alternatively, encourage him or her to contact the Samaritans, who provide advice and support and can be contacted 24 hours a day.

START

? Do you have any of the following symptoms?

- Lack of energy
- Difficulty sleeping
- Low self-esteem
- Inability to concentrate or to make decisions
- Lack of interest in sex
- None of the above

? Did your depression develop after any of the following?

- Bereavement
- Divorce
- Job loss
- Other distressing life event
- None of the above

Possible cause

Some life events can be devastating and a period of **depression** (p.343) is natural.

Medical help

 Make an appointment to see your doctor.

? Do any of the following apply?

- You have recently had a baby
- You have recently had a viral illness
- You are recuperating from major surgery or a serious illness
- None of the above

Possible cause

You are unlikely to be suffering from serious depression. Your low spirits are probably the result of a temporary stress or disappointment.

Medical help

 Make an appointment to see your doctor if your feelings of depression last for more than 2 weeks, if your depression gets worse, or if you develop other symptoms.

Possible cause

Grief and depression are normal following the loss of someone close (*see* **Loss and bereavement**, p.32).

Medical help

 Make an appointment to see your doctor, who may provide support while you come to terms with your loss.

Possible cause

Major hormonal changes after childbirth sometimes lead to depression (*see* **Depression after childbirth**, p.521).

Medical help

 Make an appointment to see your doctor.

Possible causes

A serious accident, major surgical operation, or serious illness can be followed by **depression** (p.343).

Medical help

 Make an appointment to see your doctor.

Possible cause

Viral illnesses may sometimes be followed by a period of mild **depression** (p.343).

Self-help

Follow a healthy diet and get plenty of sleep to rebuild your strength. If your depression continues longer than 2 weeks after the viral symptoms have gone, make an appointment to see your doctor.

Possible cause

Stress (p.31) is a common cause of depression.

Self-help

Try to reduce the impact of stress in your life (*see* **Stress**, p.31). Make an appointment to see your doctor if you feel unable to cope or if depression is interfering with your normal everyday activities.

Possible cause

Your symptoms may be a side effect of the medication, complementary remedy, or recreational drug.

Medical help

 Make an appointment to see your doctor. Continue to take prescribed medication unless advised to stop by your doctor but stop taking any other medications, complementary remedies, or recreational drugs.

Possible cause

Regularly drinking too much alcohol leads to depression in some people (*see* **Alcohol dependence**, p.350).

Medical help

 Make an appointment to see your doctor for advice about cutting down your alcohol intake.

Have you been suffering from particular stress at home or at work?

Yes
No

Are you currently taking any medications, complementary remedies, or recreational drugs?

Yes
No

Do you regularly drink more than the recommended limit of alcohol (*see* Safe alcohol limits, p.24)?

More than the limit
Within the limit

Are you male or female?

Male
Female

Possible cause

Your depression may be related to your monthly hormonal changes (*see* **Premenstrual syndrome**, p.472).

Medical help

 Make an appointment to see your doctor.

Do you feel depressed only in the days before your period is due?

Yes
No

If you cannot identify a possible cause for your depression from this chart, make an appointment to see your doctor.

9 General skin problems

Skin problems are often caused by localized infection, allergy, or irritation. They are not usually serious, although widespread skin problems may be distressing. You should consult your doctor if a skin problem lasts more than a month or causes severe discomfort; a new lump appears, especially if it is dark-coloured; or a sore fails to heal.

✖ WARNING

Skin changes

Consult your doctor promptly if you notice any of the following; they may be signs of skin cancer:
- An ulcer or sore that has not healed within 2–3 weeks.
- A slowly growing lump.
- A change in a longstanding mole, such as increased size or thickness; irregular edges; itching; inflammation; redness, bleeding or crusting; or a change in colour.
- The development of a new mole.

START

? What type of skin problem do you have?

Rash

Other skin problem

Go to chart 10
Rash with fever

? Is the affected skin itchy?

Itchy

Not itchy

Possible cause

Cellulitis (p.204) may be the cause of your symptoms.

Medical help

📋 **URGENT!** Phone your doctor immediately!

? Do you have a fever – a temperature of 38°C (100.4°F) or above?

Fever

No fever

Possible cause

Psoriasis (p.192) can produce this type of rash.

Medical help

📋 Make an appointment to see your doctor.

Possible cause

Skin cancer (p.199) is a possible cause.

Medical help

📋 Make an appointment to see your doctor.

? Have you noticed any of the following?

Red, tender, and hot area of skin

New mole or a change in an existing mole

An open sore that has not healed after 3 weeks

Hard, skin-coloured lump on hand or sole

None of the above

? Does your skin problem fit any of the following descriptions?

A painful, blistery rash in only one area on one side of the body

Reddened patches covered with silvery scales

Blistery, oozing rash on or around the lips

A painful red lump with a yellow centre

None of the above

Possible causes

This is likely to be a wart or verruca (*see* **Warts**, p.206), or a callus (*see* **Calluses and corns**, p.202).

Medical help

📋 Make an appointment to see your doctor if you are uncertain about the diagnosis.

Possible cause

This may be a **boil** (p.204).

Self-help

Follow the self-help measures for a **boil** (p.204). Phone your doctor if the condition has not improved in 24 hours.

? What does the affected skin look like?

Areas of inflamed skin with a scaly surface

One or more red bumps with a central dark spot

One or more red raised areas (weals) that come and go

None of the above

? What do the edges of the rash look like?

Merge into surrounding skin

Clearly defined margins

Possible causes

Seborrhoeic dermatitis (p.194) or **eczema** (p.193) may be causing your rash.

Self-help

Avoid using harsh soaps or detergents on the skin. A mild emollient cream should help to soothe the rash. Make an appointment to see your doctor if your rash does not improve within 1 week or if other symptoms develop.

Possible cause

Urticaria (p.285) is possible.

Self-help

Soothe the irritation with cold compresses or calamine lotion. Over-the-counter antihistamine tablets may help. Get medical advice at once if breathing difficulties develop.

Possible cause

Ringworm (p.205) may be the cause of your rash.

Medical help

 Make an appointment to see your doctor.

Possible cause

Insect bites may be the cause of such itchy bumps.

Self-help

Soothe the irritation with cold compresses. Get medical help at once if you are allergic to bites or stings.

Possible cause

Your symptoms may be a side effect of the medication or remedy.

Medical help

 URGENT! Phone your doctor immediately! He or she may advise you to stop taking a particular medication.

Possible cause

Shingles (*see* **Herpes zoster**, p.166) is a possible cause of this type of rash.

Medical help

 See your doctor within 24 hours.

? Does either of the following apply?

You have a rash that spreads out from a central red spot

You have been bitten by a tick

Neither

? Are you currently taking any medications or complementary remedies?

Yes

No

Possible causes

You may have **impetigo** (p.204). However, if this is a recurring problem, a **cold sore** (p.205) is more likely.

Medical help

 See your doctor within 24 hours if the diagnosis is not clear. For **cold sores** (p.205), use self-help measures.

Possible cause

There is a possibility that you have **Lyme disease** (p.174).

Medical help

 See your doctor within 24 hours.

If you cannot identify a possible cause for your skin problem from this chart, make an appointment to see your doctor.

Rash with fever

 If you have a rash without fever, see chart 9

If you or your child has a temperature of 38°C (100.4°F) or above, you should check whether a rash is also present. A rash with fever is usually caused by a viral infection. Most viral infections are not serious. However, a rash may alert you to the possibility of potentially life-threatening meningitis.

 DANGER SIGNS

Dial 999/112 and ask for an ambulance if a rash and fever are accompanied by any of the following symptoms:
- Dislike of bright light.
- Pain in the neck on bending the head forward.
- Seizures.
- Temperature of 39°C (102°F) or above.
- Noisy or difficult breathing.
- Severe headache.

START

 What are the features of the rash?

- **Widespread itchy, blistery rash**
- **A rash that spreads out from a central red spot**
- **Flat, dark red spots that do not fade when pressed**
- **Bright red rash, particularly affecting the cheeks**
- **Dull red spots or blotches that fade when pressed**
- **Light red or pink rash mainly on the trunk and/or face**
- **None of the above**

Possible cause

Chickenpox (p.165) is a possible cause of this type of rash with fever.

Medical help

See your doctor within 24 hours. Meanwhile, follow the advice for **bringing down a fever** (p.165).

Possible cause

There is a possibility that you have **Lyme disease** (p.174).

Medical help

See your doctor within 24 hours. Meanwhile, follow the advice for **bringing down a fever** (p.165).

If you cannot identify a possible cause for your rash and fever from this chart, see your doctor within 24 hours.

Possible causes

Rubella (p.168), also known as German measles, may be the cause of these symptoms. **Roseola infantum** (p.538), which mainly affects infants under 4 years, is another possibility, particularly if the rash was preceded by fever.

Medical help

 See your doctor within 24 hours to confirm the diagnosis. Meanwhile, follow the advice for **bringing down a fever** (p.165).

WARNING

Rubella and pregnancy

If you are pregnant and develop a rash, you should see your doctor as soon as possible so that the cause can be identified and any possible risk to the fetus assessed. Many viral illnesses pose no risk, but the rubella virus may cross the placenta and harm the fetus, especially in early pregnancy. Immunization in childhood against rubella may not always give permanent protection, so before trying to become pregnant you should have a blood test to check your immunity, followed by immunization if necessary.

Do you have any of the following symptoms?

Severe headache

Drowsiness or confusion

Dislike of bright light

Neck pain on bending the head forwards

Nausea or vomiting

None of the above

Possible cause

Meningitis (p.325) could be a cause of your symptoms.

Medical help

EMERGENCY! Dial 999/112 and ask for an ambulance.

Possible causes

This type of rash may be due to a severe allergic reaction, such as a reaction to penicillin (*see* **Drug allergy**, p.284). It may also be the result of a blood disorder, such as **thrombocytopenia** (p.275) or, in children, **Henoch–Schönlein purpura** (p.543).

Medical help

URGENT! Phone your doctor immediately!

▶ **SYMPTOM ASSESSMENT**

Checking a red rash

If you develop a dark red rash, check if it fades on pressure by pressing the side of a drinking glass on to it. If the rash is visible through the glass, it may be a form of **purpura** (p.196), a rash caused by bleeding from tiny blood vessels in the skin. Purpura can be caused by one of several serious disorders and needs prompt medical attention. You should call an ambulance if you have a high fever, severe headache, or any other danger sign (opposite).

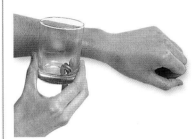

Checking a rash
In this example, the rash has faded under the glass – a sign that the rash is not purpura.

Possible cause

Fifth disease (p.168) may be the cause of such a rash and other symptoms in a young child.

Medical help

See your doctor within 24 hours. Meanwhile, follow the advice for **bringing down a fever** (p.165).

Have you noticed any of the following symptoms in the past few days?

Runny nose

Cough

Red eyes

None of the above

Possible cause

Measles (p.167) is a possible cause of your symptoms.

Medical help

See your doctor within 24 hours. Meanwhile, follow the advice for **bringing down a fever** (p.165).

Go to chart 15
Sore throat

Do you have a severe sore throat?

Yes

No

If you cannot identify a possible cause for your rash and fever from this chart, see your doctor within 24 hours.

11 Painful or irritated eye

Injury, infection, and allergy are the most common causes of discomfort or irritation of the eye and eyelids. A painless red area in the white of the eye is likely to be a burst blood vessel and should clear up without treatment. However, you should see your doctor if your eyes are sore. Consult your doctor immediately if your vision deteriorates.

START

Does either of the following apply?

You have injured your eye

You have something in your eye

Neither

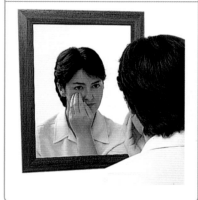

Possible cause

A foreign body in your eye is likely to cause pain and possibly redness.

Self-help

If a foreign body is floating free on the white of the eye, try to flush it out with water. If the object cannot be removed easily, seek immediate medical help in a hospital. Never try to remove an object that is embedded in the eye.

How would you describe your main symptom?

Pain in and around the eye

The eye feels gritty

Itching or irritation of the eyelid

Tender red lump on the eyelid

None of the above

Possible causes

An infected hair follicle (see **Stye**, p.363) or infected gland in the eyelid (see **Chalazion**, p.364) may be the cause of your symptoms.

Self-help

Follow the advice for **stye** (p.363) or **chalazion** (p.364). Make an appointment to see your doctor if self-help measures do not produce an improvement within 3 days.

Has your vision deteriorated since the injury?

Yes

No

Possible cause

A serious eye injury is possible.

Medical help

 URGENT! Phone your doctor immediately! Expert help may be needed to prevent permanent damage.

Possible cause

Your pain may be due to a minor eye injury.

Medical help

 URGENT! Phone your doctor immediately!

Is your vision blurred?

Blurred

Not blurred

 Is your eyelid turned inwards or outwards?

Eyelid turned inwards

Eyelid turned outwards

Appears normal

Possible cause

Entropion (p.364) may be the cause of your problem.

Medical help

Make an appointment to see your doctor.

Possible causes

Acute glaucoma (p.358) or **uveitis** (p.357) are possible causes.

Medical help

 URGENT! Phone your doctor immediately!

Possible cause

Ectropion (p.364) may be the cause of your problem.

Medical help

Make an appointment to see your doctor.

Possible cause

Cluster headaches (p.321) are a possible cause, especially if the eye is red and/or watery.

Medical help

 See your doctor within 24 hours.

Possible cause

Blepharitis (p.364) may be the cause of irritation or itching of the eyelids, especially if the skin is scaly and inflamed.

Self-help

Follow the self-help advice for **blepharitis** (p.364). Make an appointment to see your doctor if self-help measures do not help.

Possible cause

Conjunctivitis (p.355), which can occur as a result of allergy or infection, is the likely explanation.

Medical help

Make an appointment to see your doctor.

 Is there any discharge from the eye?

Watery discharge

Sticky discharge

No discharge

If you cannot identify a possible cause for your painful or irritated eye from this chart, make an appointment to see your doctor.

Possible cause

Keratoconjunctivitis sicca (p.365), in which the eye fails to produce enough tears, can lead to discomfort.

Medical help

Make an appointment to see your doctor.

12 Disturbed or impaired vision

Disturbed or impaired vision might include blurred vision or seeing double. You may also see flashing lights or floating spots. Visual disturbances may be caused by a problem in one or both eyes or by damage to the areas in the brain that process visual information. If your vision deteriorates suddenly, you should seek immediate medical help.

⊠ DANGER SIGNS

Dial 999/112 and ask for an ambulance or arrange to be taken to a hospital immediately if you experience the following:
■ Sudden loss or blurring of vision in one or both eyes.

START

Do you have pain in the affected eye?

Pain

No pain

Go to chart 11
Painful or irritated eye

Have you injured your head in the past 48 hours?

Recent head injury

No head injury

How long has your vision been disturbed or impaired?

Less than 24 hours

24 hours or longer

Do you have diabetes?

Yes

No

Possible cause

A **cataract** (p.357) can cause blurred vision in older people.

Medical help

Make an appointment to see your doctor.

Possible cause

You may have damaged the part of the brain that is responsible for vision (*see* **Head injuries**, p.322).

Medical help

EMERGENCY! Dial 999/112 and ask for an ambulance, or go to hospital immediately.

What kind of visual disturbance or impairment have you been experiencing?

Blurred vision

Increasing difficulty in focusing on nearby objects

Other disturbance

Possible causes

Diabetic retinopathy (p.361) or a high blood sugar level can lead to blurred vision.

Medical help

 See your doctor within 24 hours.

How old are you?

50 or over

Under 50

What is the nature of your disturbed or impaired vision?

Sudden loss of all or part of the vision in one or both eyes

Blurred vision

Seeing flashing lights or floating spots

Double vision

None of the above

Possible causes

Blockage of a blood vessel that supplies the brain or eye or a serious eye condition such as **retinal detachment** (p.360) are possible causes.

Medical help

 EMERGENCY! Dial 999/112 and ask for an ambulance.

Possible causes

This may be due to bleeding inside the brain (*see* **Stroke**, p.329, and **Subarachnoid haemorrhage**, p.330). It may also be due to an abnormality in the muscles moving the eyes (*see* **Double vision**, p.368).

Medical help

 EMERGENCY! Dial 999/112 and ask for an ambulance.

Possible cause

You may be developing **presbyopia** (p.367) as part of the normal aging process.

Medical help

 Make an appointment to see your optician.

Possible cause

Migraine (p.320) is a possible cause of recurrent headaches with visual disturbance, but urgent medical assessment is needed to rule out a more serious condition.

Medical help

 URGENT! Phone your doctor immediately!

If you cannot identify a possible cause for your disturbed or impaired vision from this chart, phone your doctor immediately.

 Are you currently taking any medications, complementary remedies, or recreational drugs?

Yes

No

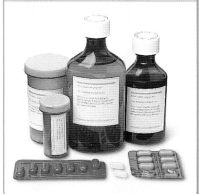

Possible cause

Your symptoms may be a side effect of the medication, remedy, or recreational drug.

Medical help

See your doctor within 24 hours. Continue to take prescribed medication unless advised to stop by your doctor but stop taking any other medications, complementary remedies, or recreational drugs.

If you cannot identify a possible cause for your disturbed or impaired vision from this chart, see your doctor within 24 hours.

13 Hearing loss

Hearing loss is a sudden or gradual reduction in the ability to hear clearly in one or both ears. Total, permanent hearing loss is rare. Wax blockage or an ear infection may cause temporary hearing loss. The normal aging process may result in partial, permanent hearing loss, which can sometimes be treated with surgery or with a hearing aid.

START

? **Do you have earache?**

Earache

No earache

Go to chart 14
Earache

? **Have you noticed any discharge from the ear?**

Discharge

No discharge

? **Do any of the following apply?**

Your ear feels blocked

You have been feeling dizzy

You have ringing in the ear

None of the above

? **Do you have either of the following symptoms?**

Runny or stuffy nose

Sore throat

Neither

Possible cause

It is likely that the tube linking your middle ear and throat has become blocked as a result of a **common cold** (p.164).

Self-help

Steam inhalation (p.291) can help. Make an appointment to see your doctor if your hearing has not returned to normal 1–2 days after the other cold symptoms have disappeared or if new symptoms develop.

Possible cause

An infection of the outer ear is a possible cause (*see* **Otitis externa**, p.374).

Medical help

 Make an appointment to see your doctor.

Possible causes

You could have **Ménière's disease** (p.380). **Acoustic neuroma** (p.380) or another problem of the nervous system are also possibilities.

Medical help

 Make an appointment to see your doctor.

Possible cause

Your symptoms may be a side effect of the medication.

Medical help

 Make an appointment to see your doctor. Continue to take prescribed medication unless advised to stop by your doctor but stop taking any other medications.

Have you recently had any of the following illnesses?

Meningitis

Encephalitis

None of the above

 Does either of the following apply?

You regularly listen to loud music

You are exposed to loud noise at work

Neither

Possible cause

Exposure to loud noise can result in damage to your hearing (*see* **Noise-induced hearing loss**, p.378).

Medical help

 Make an appointment to see your doctor.

Possible cause

These infections sometimes cause damage to hearing, which may not become obvious until later.

Medical help

Make an appointment to see your doctor.

 Have other family members suffered from increasing hearing loss that started before the age of 50?

No family history of hearing loss

Family history of hearing loss

Possible causes

Gradual loss of hearing that develops in later life may be due to **presbyacusis** (p.376). **Wax blockage** (p.374) can also cause hearing loss.

Medical help

Make an appointment to see your doctor.

 Has hearing loss developed since you started any medication?

Medication

No medication

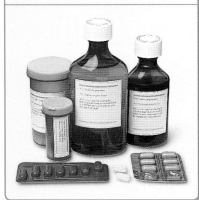

 How old are you?

50 or over

Under 50

Possible causes

Otosclerosis (p.375) or one of a group of rare inherited disorders that affect hearing are possibilities.

Medical help

Make an appointment to see your doctor.

If you cannot identify a possible cause for your hearing loss from this chart, make an appointment to see your doctor.

14 Earache

Pain in one or both ears is a distressing symptom, especially for children. Earache is usually caused by an infection in the outer or middle ear. Mild discomfort, however, may be due to wax blockage. Consult your doctor if you have earache, particularly if it is persistent. A severe or recurrent middle-ear infection may damage hearing.

START

? Does pulling the ear lobe make the pain worse?

Increases pain

Pain is no worse

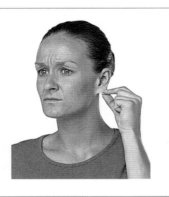

Possible causes

Your earache is probably due to an infection of the outer ear (*see* **Otitis externa**, p.374) or a **boil** (p.204) in the ear canal.

Medical help

Make an appointment to see your doctor.

Possible causes

You may have a middle-ear infection (*see* **Otitis media**, p.374) with a perforated eardrum; an outer-ear infection (*see* **Otitis externa**, p.374) is another possibility.

Medical help

See your doctor within 24 hours.

Possible cause

Barotrauma (p.375) may be the cause of your pain.

Medical help

Make an appointment to see your doctor if the discomfort persists for longer than 24 hours.

? Is there a discharge from the affected ear?

Discharge

No discharge

? Did the pain start during or immediately after an aeroplane flight?

During or immediately after an aeroplane flight

Unrelated to air travel

Possible causes

A cold (*see* **Common cold**, p.164) is often accompanied by mild earache. Persistent or severe earache is likely to be due to a middle-ear infection (*see* **Otitis media**, p.374).

Self-help

Take decongestants to relieve stuffiness and painkillers to relieve discomfort. Make an appointment to see your doctor if pain is severe or persists for longer than 2 days.

? Do you have a runny or stuffy nose?

Yes

No

If you cannot identify a possible cause for your earache from this chart, see your doctor within 24 hours.

15 Sore throat

A raw or rough feeling in the throat is a symptom that most people have from time to time. A sore throat is often the first sign of a common cold and is also a feature of other viral infections. Sore throats can usually be safely treated at home unless you otherwise do not feel well. However, if your sore throat persists or is severe, consult your doctor.

Possible cause

Infectious mononucleosis (p.166) can cause a sore throat and swollen lymph nodes.

Medical help

 Make an appointment to see your doctor.

START

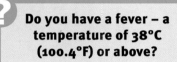 **Do you have a fever – a temperature of 38°C (100.4°F) or above?**

| Fever |
| No fever |

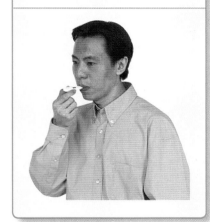

 Do you have swelling in your groin and/or armpits ?

| Yes |
| No |

Possible cause

A throat infection is a possible cause (*see* **Pharyngitis** and **tonsillitis**, p.293).

Medical help

Make an appointment to see your doctor. Follow the advice for **soothing a sore throat** (p.293) to help relieve your symptoms.

Do you have any of the following symptoms?

| Generalized aches and pains |
| Runny nose |
| Headache |
| Cough |
| None of the above |

Possible cause

A viral illness, such as a severe cold (*see* **Common cold**, p.164) or **influenza** (p.164), is the most probable cause.

Self-help

Follow the advice for **bringing down a fever** (p.165). If your symptoms worsen, change, or are no better after 2 days, consult your doctor.

Possible cause

These activities are likely to result in inflammation of the throat (*see* **Pharyngitis and tonsillitis**, p.293).

Self-help

Follow the advice for **soothing a sore throat** (p.293). If your symptoms worsen, change, or are no better in 2 days, consult your doctor.

Before the onset of your sore throat had you been doing any of the following?

| Smoking heavily or breathing smoke |
| Shouting or singing loudly |
| None of the above |

You may be developing a cold. Follow the advice for Soothing a sore throat **(p.293). Make an appointment to see your doctor if you are no better in 2 days.**

Coughing

▶ For children under 12, see chart 47

Coughing is the body's defence mechanism for clearing the airways of inhaled particles or secretions. Persistent coughing may be due to infection or inflammation in the lungs or to the effects of irritants such as tobacco smoke. Persistent coughing should be investigated by your doctor.

✖ WARNING

Coughing up blood

You should always consult your doctor if you cough up blood, although, if you otherwise feel well, a single instance of coughing up sputum that contains streaks of blood is unlikely to be serious. However, if you have more than one such episode or cough up a large amount of blood, you should see a doctor without delay.

START

 How long have you had a cough?

Less than 48 hours

Over 48 hours

Do you have a fever – a temperature of 38°C (100.4°F) or above?

Fever

No fever

Possible cause

Being in a smoky atmosphere can irritate the lungs.

Self-help

Move into a well-ventilated area. See your doctor if you become breathless or develop other symptoms.

 Are you currently taking any prescribed medication?

Medication

No medication

 Are you coughing up sputum?

Sputum

No sputum

Are you a smoker?

Smoker

Nonsmoker

Possible causes

A persistent dry cough may be due to **asthma** (p.295), **gastro-oesophageal reflux disease** (p.403), or exposure to irritants in your workplace (*see* **Occupational lung diseases**, p.305). However, the slight possibility of **primary lung cancer** (p.307) needs to be excluded.

Medical help

🗓 Make an appointment to see your doctor.

Possible cause

Your symptoms may be a side effect of the medication.

Medical help

🗓 Make an appointment to see your doctor. Continue to take the medication unless advised to stop by your doctor.

If you cannot identify a possible cause for your cough from this chart, make an appointment to see your doctor.

Are you having either of the following problems with breathing?

Breathing is painful

You are short of breath

Neither

Possible cause

Pneumonia (p.299) may be the cause of these symptoms.

Medical help

 URGENT! Phone your doctor immediately!

Possible cause

Acute bronchitis (p.297) is a possibility.

Medical help

See your doctor within 24 hours.

Possible cause

Coughing is the body's natural response to a foreign body that has lodged in the lungs.

Medical help

 Phone your doctor if coughing has not subsided within 1 hour.

Have you coughed up sputum?

Sputum

No sputum

Possible cause

A viral illness such as a severe cold (*see* **Common cold**, p.164) or **influenza** (p.164) is a likely cause of your cough.

Self-help

Follow the self-help advice for **bringing down a fever** (p.165). Consult your doctor if you are no better in 2 days or if other symptoms develop.

Have you inhaled any of the following in the last few hours?

Particle of food

Tobacco smoke

Dust, fumes, or smoke from a fire

None of the above

Possible cause

Severe inflammation of the respiratory tract can occur as a result of breathing in any of these substances.

Medical help

 URGENT! Phone your doctor immediately!

Possible cause

A cold (*see* **Common cold**, p.164) is the probable cause of your cough.

Self-help

Steam inhalation (p.291) may help. Consult your doctor if your breathing becomes painful or you start to wheeze, if you are no better in 2 days, or if other symptoms develop.

Possible causes

A persistent smoker's cough that produces sputum may be due to **chronic obstructive pulmonary disease** (p.297) or, in rare cases, to **primary lung cancer** (p.307).

Medical help

 Make an appointment to see your doctor.

Do you have either of the following symptoms?

Runny nose

Sore throat

Neither

Possible causes

A cough without any other symptoms may be caused by **asthma** (p.295). **Chronic heart failure** (p.247) is a less likely possibility.

Medical help

Make an appointment to see your doctor.

Shortness of breath

▶ For children under 12, see chart 46

Shortness of breath can be expected after strenuous exercise. Breathing should return to normal after resting. If you are short of breath at rest or after normal activities, such as getting dressed, you should consult your doctor because your symptom may be due to a serious heart or lung disorder.

❌ DANGER SIGNS

Dial 999/112 and ask for an ambulance if either you or someone you are with has one of the following:
- Severe shortness of breath.
- Blue-tinged lips.

While waiting for medical help, loosen any tight clothing and help the person to sit upright, well supported by pillows.

START

? Is breathing painful?

Painful

Not painful

Go to chart 26
Chest pain

? Do you have either of the following symptoms?

Swollen ankles

Cough with sputum on most days

Neither

? Have you been wheezing?

Wheezing

No wheezing

? How quickly did the shortness of breath start?

Gradually over a few days or longer

Suddenly within the past 48 hours

Go to chart 18
Wheezing

? Do any of the following apply?

You have recently had a surgical operation

You have recently been immobile because of injury or illness

You have had a baby within the past 2 weeks

None of the above

Possible cause

It is possible that you have a blood clot in the lung (*see* **Pulmonary embolism**, p.302).

Medical help

 EMERGENCY! Dial 999/112 and ask for an ambulance.

? Do you have any of the following symptoms?

Temperature of 38°c (100.4°F) or above

Frothy pink or white sputum

Waking at night feeling breathless

None of the above

Possible cause

A possible cause of your symptoms is **chronic heart failure** (p.247).

Medical help

 See your doctor within 24 hours.

Possible cause

Your symptoms may be the result of an **occupational lung disease** (p.305).

Medical help

 Make an appointment to see your doctor.

Possible cause

Your shortness of breath may be the result of an allergic reaction (*see* **Extrinsic allergic alveolitis**, p.307).

Medical help

 Make an appointment to see your doctor.

Possible causes

One possible cause is **chronic obstructive pulmonary disease** (p.297). However, a respiratory tract infection, such as **acute bronchitis** (p.297), can also be a cause of shortness of breath that comes on gradually.

Medical help

 See your doctor within 24 hours.

Do you have, or have you ever had, regular exposure to or contact with the following?

Dust or fumes

Grain crops, caged birds, or animals

Neither

Possible cause

Anaemia (p.271) is a possible cause of your symptoms.

Medical help

 See your doctor within 24 hours.

Possible cause

Your symptoms may be due to **pneumonia** (p.299); this is particularly likely if you also have a cough.

Medical help

 URGENT! Phone your doctor immediately!

Possible cause

You may have had a panic attack brought on by stress (*see* **Anxiety disorders,** p.341).

Medical help

 URGENT! Phone your doctor immediately if this is a first attack. Otherwise, follow the advice for **coping with a panic attack** (p.341).

Do you have any of the following symptoms?

Faintness or fainting

Paler skin than normal

Undue tiredness

None of the above

Possible cause

Your symptoms may be caused by fluid on the lungs (*see* **Acute heart failure,** p.247).

Medical help

 URGENT! Phone your doctor immediately!

Did the shortness of breath start immediately after a stressful event?

Yes

No

If you cannot identify a possible cause for your shortness of breath from this chart, see your doctor within 24 hours.

18 Wheezing

▶ For children under 12, see chart 46

Wheezing, a whistling or rasping sound on exhaling, occurs when the air passages become narrowed. Narrowing may be caused by inflammation due to infection, asthma, smoking, or inhaled dust. Rarely, it may be due to a tumour or a small foreign body in an airway.

✖ DANGER SIGNS

Dial 999/112 and ask for an ambulance if you or someone with you has one of the following:
- Severe shortness of breath.
- Blue-tinged lips.

While waiting for medical help, loosen any tight clothing and help the person to sit upright, well supported by pillows.

START

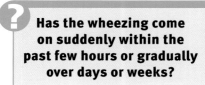

? Has the wheezing come on suddenly within the past few hours or gradually over days or weeks?

Sudden onset

Gradual onset

? Do you have either of the following symptoms?

Frothy pink or white sputum

Waking at night feeling breathless

Neither

Possible cause

You could be having an attack of **asthma** (p.295).

Medical help

 URGENT! Phone your doctor immediately!

Possible cause

There is a possibility of fluid on the lungs (*see* **Acute heart failure**, p.247).

Medical help

URGENT! Phone your doctor immediately!

? Are you short of breath?

Short of breath

Not short of breath

? Do you have a fever – a temperature of 38°C (100.4°F) or above?

Fever

No fever

Possible cause

Acute bronchitis (p.297) is a possible cause.

Medical help

 See your doctor within 24 hours.

Possible cause

A mild asthma attack (*see* **Asthma**, p.295) is the most likely cause of wheezing without shortness of breath.

Medical help

See your doctor within 24 hours.

Possible cause

Your symptoms may be caused by **chronic obstructive pulmonary disease** (p.297), especially if you are a smoker.

Medical help

 Make an appointment to see your doctor.

? Do you cough up sputum?

Most days

Seldom or never

If you cannot identify a possible cause for your wheezing from this chart, see your doctor within 24 hours.

19 Difficulty swallowing

Difficulty swallowing is most commonly the result of a sore throat due to infection. Self-treatment should ease the soreness and allow normal swallowing. However, persistent difficulty with swallowing may be due to a disorder of the stomach or oesophagus, the tube connecting the throat to the stomach, and should be investigated by your doctor.

START

Is your throat sore?

Sore

Not sore

Which of the following applies?

Food seems to stick high up in the chest

You have a feeling of something being stuck in the throat

Neither

Do you often get a burning pain in the centre of the chest in either of the following situations?

When you bend forward

When you lie down

Neither

Possible cause

Gastro-oesophageal reflux disease (p.403) is a likely cause.

Medical help

 Make an appointment to see your doctor.

Is it possible that you have swallowed something sharp, such as a fish bone?

Possible

Unlikely

Possible cause

Anxiety disorders (p.341) may be a cause of this type of difficulty with swallowing.

Medical help

 Make an appointment to see your doctor.

Go to chart 15
Sore throat

Does either of the following apply?

The swallowing difficulty is getting worse

You have lost weight

Neither

Possible cause

Something may have either scratched your throat or become lodged in it.

Medical help

 URGENT! Phone your doctor immediately!

If you cannot identify a possible cause for your difficulty swallowing from this chart, make an appointment to see your doctor.

Possible causes

These symptoms may be due to a narrowed oesophagus, which could be caused by **gastro-oesophageal reflux disease** (p.403) or rarely **cancer of the oesophagus** (p.404).

Medical help

See your doctor within 24 hours.

20 Vomiting

▶ For children under 12, see chart 43

Vomiting is most often caused by irritation or inflammation of the digestive tract. It may also be triggered by conditions affecting the brain or by an inner-ear disorder, or it can be a side effect of medication. If you have been vomiting for longer than a day, consult chart 21, **Recurrent vomiting** (p.74).

✗ DANGER SIGNS

Dial 999/112 and ask for an ambulance if your vomit contains blood, which may appear as any of the following:
- Bright red streaks.
- Black material that resembles coffee grounds.
- Blood clots.

START

Have you vomited repeatedly in the past week?

On 2 or more days

Today only

Go to chart 21
Recurrent vomiting

Do you have a headache?

Headache

No headache

Possible cause

Acute glaucoma (p.358) is a possibility, especially if your vision is also blurred.

Medical help

🖾 **URGENT!** Phone your doctor immediately!

Do you have pain in the abdomen?

Severe pain

Mild pain

No pain

Do you have pain in or around an eye?

Eye pain

No eye pain

Do you have any of the following symptoms?

Temperature of 38°C (100.4°F) or above

Diarrhoea

Dizziness

None of the above

Possible cause

You could have a serious abdominal condition, such as **appendicitis** (p.420).

Medical help

 URGENT! Phone your doctor immediately!

Possible cause

Labyrinthitis (p.380) is a possible cause of your symptoms.

Medical help

 Make an appointment to see your doctor. If symptoms are severe, you should lie down and try to remain as still as possible.

✕ WARNING

Vomiting and medications

If you are taking any oral medication, including oral contraceptives, an episode of vomiting may reduce the effectiveness of the drug because your body cannot absorb the active ingredients. If you use oral contraceptives, you will need to use an additional form of contraception (such as condoms) during the period of vomiting and for some time afterwards. You should follow the instructions given with the oral contraceptives or consult your doctor if you are not sure what to do. You should also consult your doctor if you have been taking any other prescribed oral medication and have been vomiting.

Go to chart 7
Headache

Possible cause

Your symptoms may be the result of infection (*see* **Gastroenteritis**, p.398).

Self-help

Follow the self-help advice for **preventing dehydration** (p.397). Consult your doctor if you are no better in 2 days or if other symptoms develop.

? Have you eaten or drunk any of the following?

An unusually large or rich meal

A large amount of alcohol

Food that may have been contaminated

None of the above

Possible cause

You may be suffering from **food poisoning** (p.398).

Self-help

Follow the self-help advice for **preventing dehydration** (p.397). Consult your doctor if you are no better in 2 days or if other symptoms develop.

Possible cause

Your symptoms may be a side effect of the medication, remedy, or recreational drug.

Medical help

 See your doctor within 24 hours. Continue to take prescribed medication unless advised to stop by your doctor but stop taking any other medications, complementary remedies, or recreational drugs.

Possible cause

The lining of your stomach has probably become inflamed (*see* **Gastritis**, p.405).

Self-help

Follow the self-help measures for **gastritis** (p.405). Consult your doctor if you are no better in 2 days or if other symptoms develop.

? Are you currently taking any medications, complementary remedies, or recreational drugs?

Yes

No

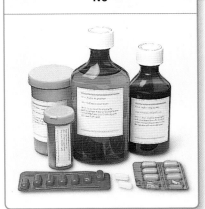

If you cannot identify a possible cause for your vomiting from this chart, see your doctor within 24 hours.

Recurrent vomiting

▶ For children under 12, see chart 43

Consult this chart if you have been vomiting repeatedly over a number of days or weeks. Recurrent vomiting may be caused by a digestive tract disorder but is also common in early pregnancy. You should consult your doctor if you have persistent or recurrent vomiting, or seek emergency medical help if your vomit contains blood (*see* **Danger signs**, right).

❌ DANGER SIGNS

Dial 999/112 and ask for an ambulance if your vomit contains blood, which may appear as any of the following:
- Bright red streaks.
- Black material that resembles coffee grounds.
- Blood clots.

START

Could you be pregnant?

Possibly pregnant

Not pregnant

Possible causes

Gastro-oesophageal reflux disease (p.403) and **nonulcer dyspepsia** (p.397) are possible causes of your symptoms.

Medical help

 Make an appointment to see your doctor.

Possible cause

Your symptoms may be due to a **peptic ulcer** (p.406).

Medical help

 Make an appointment to see your doctor.

Possible cause

Nausea and/or vomiting are often the first indicators of pregnancy (*see* **Common complaints of normal pregnancy**, p.506).

Medical help

 Make an appointment to see your doctor if vomiting is preventing you from keeping down fluids. You should see your doctor even if you are not sure whether you are pregnant.

Have you experienced any of the following kinds of recurrent pain?

Burning central chest pain if you bend or lie down

Pain in the upper right abdomen that may spread to the back

Pain in the centre of the upper abdomen that is related to eating

None of the above

Possible cause

Yellowing of the skin and the whites of the eyes, known as **jaundice** (p.407), is often accompanied by vomiting. Jaundice has many possible causes but in most cases is due to liver disease such as hepatitis (*see* **Acute hepatitis**, p.408).

Medical help

 See your doctor within 24 hours.

Possible cause

Gallstones (p.412) could be the cause of your symptoms.

Medical help

 See your doctor within 24 hours.

Have you noticed either of the following symptoms?

Yellowing of the skin

Yellowing of the whites of the eyes

Neither

Possible causes

Your symptoms may be the result of a **peptic ulcer** (p.406), but there is also a possibility of **stomach cancer** (p.406).

Medical help

 Make an appointment to see your doctor.

 Do you regularly drink more than the recommended limit of alcohol (*see* Safe alcohol limits, p.24)?

More than the limit

Within the limit

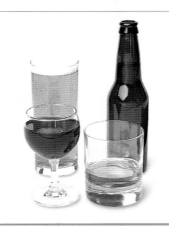

Possible cause

Excessive consumption of alcohol over a prolonged period can cause long-term inflammation of the stomach lining (*see* **Gastritis**, p.405).

Medical help

 Make an appointment to see your doctor.

 Have you had progressive unintentional weight loss or a reduced appetite?

Weight loss

Reduced appetite

Neither

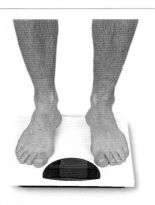

Possible cause

Your symptoms may be a side effect of the medication or remedy.

Medical help

 See your doctor within 24 hours. Continue to take any prescribed medication unless advised to stop by your doctor but stop taking any other medications or complementary remedies.

 Have you been suffering from recurrent headaches?

Headaches with vomiting but no nausea

Headaches with vomiting and nausea

No headaches

 Are you currently taking any medications or complementary remedies?

Yes

No

Possible causes

Recurrent headaches with vomiting but no nausea may, in rare cases, indicate pressure on the brain due to bleeding or a tumour (*see* **Subdural haemorrhage**, p.330, and **Brain tumours**, p.327).

Medical help

 URGENT! Phone your doctor immediately!

Possible cause

You may be suffering from **migraine** (p.320).

Medical help

 Make an appointment to see your doctor, who can review your diagnosis. He or she may recommend that you take a preventive medication in future.

If you cannot identify a possible cause for your recurrent vomiting from this chart, make an appointment to see your doctor.

Abdominal pain

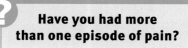 ## For children under 12, see chart 48

Mild abdominal pain is often due to a stomach or bowel upset that will clear up without treatment. However, severe or persistent abdominal pain, especially if it is accompanied by other symptoms, may indicate a more serious problem that your doctor should investigate.

DANGER SIGNS

Dial 999/112 and ask for an ambulance if you have severe abdominal pain that lasts for longer than 4 hours and is associated with any of the following additional symptoms:
- Vomiting.
- Fever.
- Swollen or tender abdomen.
- Feeling faint, drowsy, or confused.
- Blood in the urine or faeces.
- Swelling in the groin or scrotum.

START

Have you had more than one episode of pain?

Single continuous episode

Recurrent episodes

How severe is the pain?

Severe

Mild or moderate

Do you have diarrhoea?

Diarrhoea

No diarrhoea

Go to chart 23
Recurrent abdominal pain

Are any danger signs present?

Danger signs

No danger signs

Possible cause

Gallstones (p.412) are a possibility, especially if you have vomited.

Medical help

 See your doctor within 24 hours.

Possible cause

Severe abdominal pain may be an indication of a serious abdominal condition, such as **appendicitis** (p.420).

Medical help

 EMERGENCY! Dial 999/112 and ask for an ambulance.

Possible cause

Your pain may be the result of **gastroenteritis** (p.398).

Self-help

Maintain fluid intake (*see* **Preventing dehydration**, p.397). Consult your doctor if you are no better in 2 days or if other symptoms develop.

Possible cause

You may have **kidney stones** (p.447), especially if you have been vomiting.

Medical help

 URGENT! Phone your doctor immediately!

 Do any of the following apply?

Pain is related to eating

Pain is relieved by antacids

Pain comes on when lying or bending over

None of the above

Possible causes

Your abdominal pain may be caused by **nonulcer dyspepsia** (p.397) or **gastro-oesophageal reflux disease** (p.403).

Medical help

Make an appointment to see your doctor. In the meantime, follow the self-help measures for **preventing indigestion** (p.397).

Go to chart 26
Chest pain

 What kind of pain have you been experiencing?

Pain that starts in the back and may move to the groin

Pain in the centre of the upper abdomen

Pain in the upper right abdomen that may spread to the back

Pain mainly below the waist

None of the above

 Do you have either of the following symptoms?

Pain on passing urine

Passing urine more often than usual

Neither

Possible cause

You may have a urinary tract infection (*see* **Pyelonephritis**, p.446, and **Cystitis**, p.453).

Medical help

See your doctor within 24 hours.

If you cannot identify a possible cause for your abdominal pain from this chart, see your doctor within 24 hours.

 Are you female or male?

Female

Male

Go to chart 37
Lower abdominal pain in women

23 Recurrent abdominal pain

▶ For children under 12, see chart 48

Abdominal discomfort that has occurred on more than one day in the past month may be a symptom of a digestive tract disorder or, less commonly, of a urinary tract problem. It is important to consult your doctor if you experience recurrent attacks of abdominal pain even if they are short-lived.

START

Where is the pain mainly felt?

- Below the waist
- Above the waist

Possible causes

Your symptoms may be due to a **peptic ulcer** (p.406) or **nonulcer dyspepsia** (p.397). **Stomach cancer** (p.406) is also a remote possibility.

Medical help

 Make an appointment to see your doctor.

Possible cause

Gastro-oesophageal reflux disease (p.403) is the most likely cause of this type of upper abdominal pain.

Medical help

 Make an appointment to see your doctor.

What kind of pain have you been experiencing?

- Burning central chest pain when you bend or lie down
- Pain that is related to meals
- Pain in the upper right abdomen that may spread to the back
- None of the above

Possible cause

Gallstones (p.412) are a possible cause.

Medical help

 Make an appointment to see your doctor.

Is pain accompanied by bouts of diarrhoea and/or constipation?

- Diarrhoea and/or constipation
- No change in bowel habit

Do you have either of the following symptoms?

- Swelling in the groin
- Discomfort in the groin made worse by lifting or coughing
- Neither

Do you have any of these symptoms?

- Blood in the urine
- Pain on passing urine
- Passing urine more often than usual
- None of the above

Do you have any of the following symptoms?

Blood in the faeces

Progressive, unintentional weight loss

Neither

Possible causes

It is possible that you have a long-term intestinal condition such as **irritable bowel syndrome** (p.415). However, the possibility of **colorectal cancer** (p.421) also needs to be ruled out.

Medical help

 Make an appointment to see your doctor.

Possible causes

Recurrent abdominal pain in association with weight loss or blood in the faeces may be the result of a long-term intestinal condition, for example **diverticular disease** (p.420), **Crohn's disease** (p.417), or **ulcerative colitis** (p.417). However, the possibility of **colorectal cancer** (p.421) needs to be excluded.

Medical help

Make an appointment to see your doctor.

Possible cause

Such symptoms suggest the possibility of a **hernia** (p.419).

Medical help

Make an appointment to see your doctor.

Possible causes

You may have a urinary tract infection, such as **cystitis** (p.453) or **pyelonephritis** (p.446). However, there is also the slight possibility of a **bladder tumour** (p.456) or **kidney cancer** (p.450).

Medical help

See your doctor within 24 hours.

Possible cause

Your symptoms may be a side effect of the medication or remedy.

Medical help

 Make an appointment to see your doctor. Continue to take prescribed medication unless advised to stop by your doctor but stop taking any other medications or complementary remdies.

Go to chart 37
Lower abdominal pain in women

Are you currently taking any medications or complementary remedies?

Yes

No

Are you female or male?

Female

Male

If you cannot identify a possible cause for your recurrent abdominal pain from this chart, make an appointment to see your doctor.

Diarrhoea

▶ For children under 12 years, see chart 44

Diarrhoea, which is the frequent passing of abnormally loose or watery faeces, is usually a result of infection. However, persistent diarrhoea may be caused by a serious gastrointestinal disorder. Consult your doctor if diarrhoea continues for more than 2 days or if it recurs.

✖ WARNING

Dehydration
A person with severe diarrhoea can become dehydrated if fluids are not replaced quickly enough. The symptoms of dehydration include drowsiness or confusion, a dry mouth, loss of elasticity in the skin, and failure to pass urine for several hours. Seek urgent medical help if a person has symptoms of dehydration.

START

 Have you noticed blood in your faeces?

Blood

No blood

 Have you suffered from repeated bouts of diarrhoea over the past few weeks?

Recurrent diarrhoea

First attack

Possible causes

Irritable bowel syndrome (p.415) is the most likely cause of your symptoms. In rare cases, these symptoms may be an indication of **colorectal cancer** (p.421).

Medical help

📋 Make an appointment to see your doctor.

Possible causes

You may be suffering from an intestinal infection, such as **amoebiasis** (p.176), or an inflammatory condition of the intestines, such as **ulcerative colitis** (p.417). However, there is a slight possibility of **colorectal cancer** (p.421).

Medical help

🕐 See your doctor within 24 hours.

Has the diarrhoea been alternating with bouts of constipation?

Constipation and diarrhoea

Diarrhoea alone

Possible cause

Your symptoms may be due to **food poisoning** (p.398).

Self-help

Maintain your fluid intake (*see* **Preventing dehydration**, p.397). Consult your doctor if you are no better within 2 days or if any other symptoms develop.

 Have you recently consumed either of the following?

Food that may have been contaminated

Water that may have been contaminated

Neither

Do you have either of the following symptoms?

Nausea or vomiting

Temperature of 38°C (100.4°F) or above

Neither

Have the attacks of diarrhoea occurred since a visit abroad?

Foreign travel

No foreign travel

Possible causes

You may have picked up traveller's diarrhoea (*see* **Gastroenteritis**, p.398) or an intestinal infection, such as **giardiasis** (p.176), during your foreign visit.

Medical help

See your doctor within 24 hours.

Possible causes

There is a possibility that you have a **food allergy** (p.284) or **food intolerance** (p.416).

Medical help

Make an appointment to see your doctor.

 Do you have recurrent pain in the lower abdomen?

Yes

No

 Is your diarrhoea associated with either of the following?

Eating particular foods

Period of stress

Neither

Possible cause

Anxiety disorders (p.341) can be a cause of diarrhoea.

Medical help

Make an appointment to see your doctor.

Go to chart 23
Recurrent abdominal pain

Possible cause

Your symptoms may be a side effect of the medication or remedy.

Medical help

Make an appointment to see your doctor. Continue to take prescribed medication unless advised to stop by your doctor but stop taking any other medications or complementary remedies.

 Are you currently taking any medications or complementary remedies?

Yes

No

Possible causes

Gastroenteritis (p.398) or **food poisoning** (p.398) are the most likely possibilities.

Self-help

Maintain your fluid intake (*see* **Preventing dehydration,** p.397). Consult your doctor if you are no better within 2 days or if other symptoms develop.

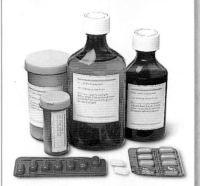

If you cannot identify a possible cause for your diarrhoea from this chart, make an appointment to see your doctor.

25 Constipation

Some people have a bowel movement once or twice a day; others do so less frequently. If you have fewer bowel movements than is usual for you or if your faeces are small and hard, you are constipated. The cause is often a lack of fluid or fibre-rich foods in the diet. If constipation occurs suddenly or persists despite a change in your diet, consult your doctor.

❌ WARNING

Blood in the faeces

Blood can appear in the faeces as red streaks or in larger amounts. It can also make the stools look black. Small amounts of blood in the faeces are usually caused by minor anal problems, such as **haemorrhoids** (p.422), but you should always consult your doctor if you notice blood in the faeces because it is vital that other causes, such as **colorectal cancer** (p.421), are ruled out.

START

 How long have you suffered from constipation?

For a few weeks or less

For several months or years

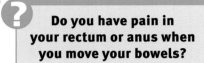 **Do you have pain in your rectum or anus when you move your bowels?**

Pain

No pain

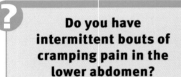 **Do you have intermittent bouts of cramping pain in the lower abdomen?**

Cramping pain

No cramping pain

Possible cause

Your bowel reflexes may have become sluggish as a result of being constantly resisted.

Self-help

Try following the advice for **preventing constipation** (p.398). Consult your doctor if your symptoms have not improved within 2 weeks.

Possible causes

Pain on defecation can cause or worsen constipation. **Haemorrhoids** (p.422) or **anal fissure** (p.423) may be the cause of your symptoms.

Medical help

📋 Make an appointment to see your doctor.

Possible causes

Your constipation could be due to a lack of fibre or fluid in your diet. Lack of exercise may also be a factor if you are not physically active (*see* **Constipation**, p.398).

Self-help

Try following the advice for **preventing constipation** (p.398). Consult your doctor if your symptoms have not improved within 2 weeks.

 Does either of the following apply?

You regularly ignore the urge to move your bowels

You regularly use stimulant laxatives

Neither

Possible cause

Regular use of stimulant **laxatives** (p.597) can seriously disrupt the normal functioning of the bowels.

Medical help

📋 Make an appointment to see your doctor.

Possible causes

Irritable bowel syndrome (p.415) is a possible cause, especially if your constipation alternates with bouts of diarrhoea. However, other causes, such as **colorectal cancer** (p.421), may need to be ruled out.

Medical help

 Make an appointment to see your doctor.

Possible cause

Hypothyroidism (p.432) is a possible cause.

Medical help

 Make an appointment to see your doctor.

Do you have any of the following symptoms?

Tiredness

Increased dryness or roughness of the skin

Feeling the cold more than you used to

Unexplained weight gain

Generalized hair thinning

None of the above

Are you currently taking any medications, complementary remedies, or recreational drugs?

Yes

No

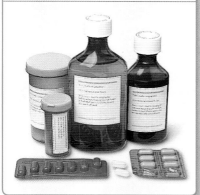

Possible cause

Constipation is common in pregnancy (*see* **Common complaints of normal pregnancy**, p.506).

Self-help

Try following the advice for **preventing constipation** (p.398). Consult your doctor if your symptoms have not improved within 2 weeks.

Possible cause

Lack of fluid in the bowel as a result of an inadequate fluid intake or excessive fluid loss can lead to constipation.

Self-help

Be sure to drink plenty of fluids, especially if the weather is hot. Consult your doctor if your symptoms have not improved within 2 weeks.

Possible cause

Your symptoms may be a side effect of the medication, remedy, or recreational drug.

Medical help

 Make an appointment to see your doctor. Continue to take prescribed medication unless advised to stop by your doctor but stop taking any other medications, complementary remedies, or recreational drugs.

Possible cause

A change in your regular diet, especially if you are travelling, can make you constipated.

Self-help

Try following the advice for **preventing constipation** (p.398). Consult your doctor if your symptoms have not improved within 2 weeks.

Do any of the following apply?

You are pregnant

You have been drinking less fluid than usual

You have changed your diet

None of the above

If you cannot identify a possible cause for your constipation from this chart, make an appointment to see your doctor.

26 Chest pain

Chest pain includes any discomfort felt in the front or back of the ribcage. Most chest pain is due to minor disorders such as muscle strain or indigestion. However, you should call an ambulance if you have a crushing pain in the centre or left side of your chest, if you are also short of breath or feel faint, or if the pain is unlike any pain you have had before.

START

What kind of pain are you experiencing?

Crushing, heavy, pressing, or tight

Spreading from the centre of the chest to the neck, arms, or jaw

Neither of the above

Does the pain subside after you rest for a few minutes?

Pain subsides

Pain persists

Possible cause
You may be having a heart attack (see **Myocardial infarction**, p.245).

Medical help
 EMERGENCY! Dial 999/112 and ask for an ambulance.

Are you short of breath?

Short of breath

Not short of breath

Possible cause
Recurrent chest pain could be an indication of **angina** (p.244), especially if pain in the chest occurs with exertion and disappears with rest.

Medical help
URGENT! Phone your doctor immediately!

Have you had this kind of pain before?

Previous episodes of this kind of pain

Never before

Do any of the following apply?

You have recently had a surgical operation

You have recently been immobile due to injury or illness

You have had a baby within the past 2 weeks

None of the above

Is pain related to breathing?

Not related to breathing

Related to breathing

Does the pain have any of the following features?

Related to eating or to particular foods

Relieved by antacids

Brought on by bending or lying down

None of the above

Possible cause

You may have a blood clot in the lung (*see* **Pulmonary embolism**, p.302).

Medical help

 EMERGENCY! Dial 999/112 and ask for an ambulance.

Possible cause

It is possible that you have a chest infection, such as **pneumonia** (p.299).

Medical help

 URGENT! Phone your doctor immediately!

Possible cause

Muscle strain and/or bruising is the most likely cause of your symptoms.

Self-help

Take a painkiller and rest for 24 hours. If the pain has not improved after this time, make an appointment to see your doctor.

? **Do you have a fever – a temperature of 38°C (100.4°F) or above?**

Fever

No fever

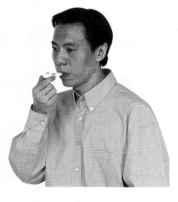

Possible cause

There is a possibility that you have a partially collapsed lung (*see* **Pneumothorax**, p.303).

Medical help

 URGENT! Phone your doctor immediately!

? **Does either of the following apply?**

You have had a chest injury

You have been exercising

Neither

? **Is the chest sore to touch?**

Sore to touch

Not sore to touch

Possible cause

You may have **pleurisy** (p.301), particularly if you have a cough and/or fever.

Medical help

 See your doctor within 24 hours.

Possible causes

This type of chest pain may be due to either **nonulcer dyspepsia** (p.397) or **gastro-oesophageal reflux disease** (p.403).

Medical help

 Make an appointment to see your doctor.

Possible cause

You may be having a heart attack (*see* **Myocardial infarction**, p.245).

Medical help

 EMERGENCY! Dial 999/112 and ask for an ambulance.

If you cannot identify a possible cause for your chest pain from this chart, make an appointment to see your doctor.

27 # Frequent urination

▶ **If passing urine is painful, see chart 28**

How often you pass urine depends largely on how much you drink and how much your bladder can hold before you feel the need to empty it. If your urine looks abnormal, the appearance may give a clue to the cause of the problem (*see* **Checking the appearance of your urine**, p.89).

? Are you female or male?

Female

Male

START

? How much urine do you pass each time you go to the toilet?

Less than usual

As much or more than usual

? Have you been experiencing either of the following?

Unexplained weight loss

Blurred vision

Neither

Possible cause

Diabetes mellitus (p.437) is a possible cause of your symptoms.

Medical help

 See your doctor within 24 hours.

Possible cause

Substances in these drinks may increase the need to pass urine.

Self-help

Reduce your consumption of such drinks. If you continue to be troubled by passing urine too frequently, consult your doctor.

? Have you been feeling more thirsty than usual?

More thirsty

No increased thirst

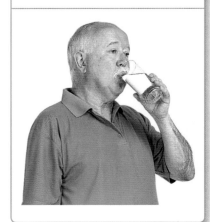

? Have you been drinking large amounts of the following?

Coffee or tea

Alcohol

Neither

Possible causes

A kidney disorder, such as **glomerulonephritis** (p.446), or a hormonal disorder, such as **diabetes insipidus** (p.431), are possible causes.

Medical help

 Make an appointment to see your doctor.

Could you be pregnant?

Not pregnant

Possibly pregnant

 Have you been experiencing either of the following ?

A strong urge to pass urine with little urine passed

Difficulty controlling urination

Neither

Possible causes

Your symptoms may be due to an irritable bladder (*see* **Urge incontinence**, p.454) or to a urinary tract infection, such as **cystitis** (p.453).

Medical help

 Make an appointment to see your doctor.

Possible cause

An increase in the frequency of passing urine is common in early, as well as later, pregnancy (*see* **Common complaints of normal pregnancy**, p.506).

Medical help

 Make an appointment to see your doctor.

 Are you currently taking any medications or complementary remedies?

Yes

No

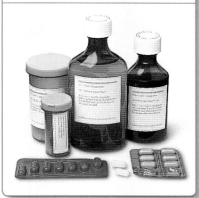

 Do you feel the need to pass urine frequently when you are anxious?

Related to anxiety

Not related to anxiety

Possible cause

Anxiety disorders (p.341) commonly cause an urge to pass urine frequently, even when the bladder is not full.

Medical help

 Make an appointment to see your doctor to discuss the causes of your anxiety.

 Do you have either of the following symptoms?

Difficulty starting to pass urine

Weak urinary system

Neither

Possible cause

Your symptoms may be a side effect of the medication or remedy.

Medical help

 Make an appointment to see your doctor. Continue to take prescribed medications unless advised to stop by your doctor but stop taking any other medications or complementary remedies.

Possible cause

You may have an **enlarged prostate gland** (p.463), especially if you are over 55.

Medical help

 Make an appointment to see your doctor.

If you cannot identify a possible cause for your frequent urination from this chart, make an appointment to see your doctor.

Painful urination

Pain or discomfort while passing urine is usually caused by inflammation of the urinary tract, often due to infection. In women, pain when passing urine may be due to vaginal infection. Discoloured urine sometimes accompanies this type of pain but can occur in the absence of disease (*see* **Checking the appearance of your urine**, opposite page).

Possible cause

A urinary tract infection, such as **cystitis** (p.453), is possible.

Medical help

 See your doctor within 24 hours. Meanwhile, follow the self-help advice for **cystitis** (p.453).

START

 Do you have either of the following symptoms?

Pain in the back just above the waist

A temperature of 38°C (100.4°F) or above

Neither

Possible cause

A kidney infection is a possible cause of your symptoms (*see* **Pyelonephritis**, p.446).

Medical help

URGENT! Phone your doctor immediately!

Are you female or male?

Female

Male

Have you felt the need to pass urine more frequently than usual?

Increased frequency

No increased frequency

 Do you have any of the following symptoms?

Lower abdominal pain

Blood in the urine

Cloudy urine

None of the above

Do you have an unusual discharge from your penis?

Discharge

No discharge

If you cannot identify a possible cause for your symptoms from this chart, make an appointment to see your doctor.

Have you noticed soreness or itching in the genital area?

Soreness

Itching

Neither

Possible cause

A urinary tract infection, such as **cystitis** (p.453), is possible.

Medical help

 See your doctor within 24 hours. Meanwhile, follow the self-help advice for **cystitis** (p.453).

Possible cause

A sexually transmitted infection, such as **gonorrhoea** (p.491) or **nongonococcal urethritis** (p.491), may be causing your symptoms.

Medical help

 See your doctor within 24 hours, or go to a clinic specializing in sexually transmitted infections.

Possible cause

A vaginal yeast infection is the most likely possibility (*see* **Vaginal thrush**, p.482).

Medical help

 Make an appointment to see your doctor if this is the first time you have had these symptoms. Otherwise, try using an over-the-counter antifungal preparation recommended by your pharmacist.

Do you have an unusual vaginal discharge?

Thick, white discharge

Yellowish-green discharge

No unusual discharge

Possible causes

The most likely cause is either a vaginal infection, such as **trichomoniasis** (p.492), or a sexually transmitted infection, such as **gonorrhoea** (p.491).

Medical help

 See your doctor within 24 hours.

▶ SYMPTOM ASSESSMENT

Checking the appearance of your urine

The appearance of urine varies considerably. For example, urine is often darker in the morning than later in the day. Some drugs and foods may also cause a temporary colour change in the urine. Beetroot, for example, may turn the urine red.

A change in your urine can indicate a disorder. Very dark urine may be a sign of liver disease (*see* **Acute hepatitis**, p.408); red or cloudy urine may be due to bleeding or infection in the kidney or bladder.

If you are not sure about the cause of a change in the appearance of your urine, consult your doctor.

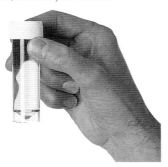

Normal appearance of urine
Normally, urine is clear, pale, and straw-coloured but may be cloudy at first in the morning.

If you cannot identify a possible cause for your symptoms from this chart, make an appointment to see your doctor.

Back pain

Mild back pain is usually caused by poor posture, sudden movements, or lifting heavy objects, all of which may strain the back. Back pain is also common in pregnancy. Persistent or severe back pain may be the result cf a more serious problem. You should consult your doctor if pain is severe cr does not start to improve after 48 hours.

> ### ✖ DANGER SIGNS
>
> Dial 999/112 and ask for an ambulance if you have back pain or have recently injured your back and you develop any of the following symptoms:
> - Difficulty in controlling your bladder or bowels.
> - Numbness, tingling, or loss of strength in a leg.
> - Numbness around your genitals, buttocks, or anus.

START

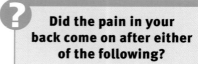

? Did the pain in your back come on after either of the following?

An injury or fall

A sudden, awkward movement

Neither

? Do you have either of the following?

Pain in the back just above the waist

A temperature of 38°C (100.4°F) or above

Neither

? Did the pain occur after any of the following?

Lifting a heavy weight

A fit of coughing

Strenuous or unaccustomed physical activity

None of the above

Possible cause

Pyelonephritis (p.446) is a likely cause of your symptoms.

Medical help

 URGENT! Phone your doctor immediately!

? Have you noticed any of the following symptoms?

Difficulty in moving a leg

Numbness or tingling in a leg

Loss of bladder or bowel control

Numbness around the genitals, buttocks, or legs

None of the above

Possible cause

Your symptoms indicate that there may be spinal damage (*see* **Spinal injuries**, p.323).

Medical help

 EMERGENCY! Dial 999/112 and ask for an ambulance.

Possible cause

Your back is probably strained and/or bruised (*see* **Muscle strains and tears**, p.234).

Self-help

Take a painkiller and try to stay as active as the pain allows. Consult your doctor if you are no better within 48 hours or if other symptoms develop.

Does either of the following apply?

Pain makes any movement difficult

Pain shoots from the back down the back of the leg

Neither

Possible causes

You may have **sciatica** (p.338), caused by a **prolapsed or herniated disc** (p.227) or by a fractured vertebra (*see* **Osteoporosis**, p.217).

Medical help

 See your doctor within 24 hours.

Possible cause

Osteoarthritis (p.221) in the back is the most likely cause of your symptoms.

Medical help

Make an appointment to see your doctor.

Possible cause

You have probably strained some of the muscles in your back or sprained some of the ligaments (*see* **Lower back pain**, p.225).

Self-help

Take a painkiller and try to stay as active as the pain allows. Consult your doctor if you are no better within 48 hours or if other symptoms develop.

How old are you?

45 or over

Under 45

Possible cause

New back pain or a worsening of existing back pain may indicate the start of labour.

Medical help

URGENT! Phone your doctor or midwife immediately if you think that you may be going into labour.

Possible cause

Ankylosing spondylitis (p.223) is a possible cause of your symptoms, especially if you are male.

Medical help

Make an appointment to see your doctor.

Have you been suffering from increasing pain and stiffness over several months or longer?

Yes

No

Possible cause

Fracture of a vertebra as a result of thinning of the bones is a possible cause (*see* **Osteoporosis**, p.217).

Medical help

See your doctor within 24 hours.

Are you in the last 3 months of pregnancy?

Pregnant

Not pregnant

Does either of the following apply?

You have recently been immobile due to illness or injury

You are over 60

Neither

If you cannot identify a possible cause for your back pain from this chart, make an appointment to see your doctor.

Neck pain or stiffness

Pain and/or stiffness in the neck is usually due to a minor problem, such as muscle strain or ligament sprain, that does not require treatment. However, if the pain occurs with fever, meningitis is a possibility. Neck pain or stiffness becomes more common as a person gets older and may then be due to a disorder of the bones and joints of the neck.

❌ DANGER SIGNS

Dial 999/112 and ask for an ambulance if you have neck pain or have recently injured your neck and you develop any of the following symptoms:
- Difficulty moving a limb.
- Pain, numbness, or tingling in a limb.
- Difficulty in controlling your bladder or bowels.

START

? How long have you had pain and/or stiffness in the neck?

Less than 24 hours

24 hours or longer

? Have you jolted or injured your neck, for example in a car accident or fall?

Neck injury

No neck injury

Possible cause

Your symptoms indicate that there may be spinal damage (*see* **Spinal injuries**, p.323).

Medical help

 EMERGENCY! Dial 999/112 and ask for an ambulance.

Possible cause

Your neck is probably strained and/or bruised (*see* **Muscle strains and tears**, p.234).

Self-help

Take a painkiller and try to stay as active as the pain allows. You may find it helpful to sleep with a supportive pillow. Consult your doctor if you are no better in 24 hours, if the pain is severe, or if other symptoms develop.

? Have you noticed any of the following symptoms?

Difficulty moving an arm or leg

Pain, numbness, or tingling in an arm or leg

Loss of bladder or bowel control

None of the above

? Which of the following describes your symptoms?

Gradually worsening pain and stiffness over many months

Neck pain with numbness or pain in the arm and/or hand

Neither

Do you have any of the following symptoms?

Temperature of 38°C (100.4°F) or above

Severe headache

Abnormal drowsiness or confusion

Dislike of bright light

Nausea or vomiting

None of the above

Possible cause

Meningitis (p.325) could be the cause of these symptoms.

Medical help

 EMERGENCY! Dial 999/112 and ask for an ambulance.

Go to chart 5
Lumps and swellings

Possible cause

The cause of your symptoms may be **cervical spondylosis** (p.222), especially if you are over the age of 45.

Medical help

 Make an appointment to see your doctor.

Does either of the following apply?

Pain is severe enough to prevent movement

Pain shoots down one arm from the neck

Neither

Possible causes

Your neck pain may be due to pressure on a nerve as a result of a **prolapsed or herniated disc** (p.227) or **cervical spondylosis** (p.222).

Medical help

 See your doctor within 24 hours.

Possible causes

You may have neck strain (*see* **Muscle strains and tears**, p.234) or **torticollis** (p.230).

Self-help

Take a painkiller and try to stay as active as the pain allows. You may find it helpful to sleep with a supportive pillow. Consult your doctor if you are no better in 24 hours, if the pain is severe, or if other symptoms develop.

Can you feel any tenderness or swelling at the sides or the back of the neck?

Yes

No

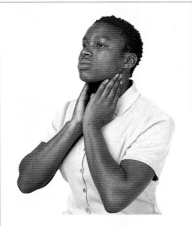

Did either of the following apply in the 24 hours before the onset of pain?

You exercised unusually strenuously

You sat or slept in an awkward position

Neither

If you cannot identify a possible cause for your neck pain or stiffness from this chart, make an appointment to see your doctor.

Painful joints

▶ **If you have a painless swollen ankle, see chart 32**

Pain in a joint may be caused by injury or strain and often gets better without a cause being found. Gout or a joint infection can cause a joint to become red, hot, and swollen. Joint pain may be due to arthritis or a reaction to an infection. Consult your doctor if pain is severe or persistent.

START

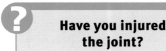
Have you injured the joint?

Injury

No injury

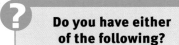
Do you have either of the following?

Hot joint(s)

Red joint(s)

Neither

How many joints are affected?

One joint

More than one

Possible causes

Septic arthritis (p.225), **gout** (p.224), or **pseudogout** (p.225), can all cause a single joint to become red, hot, and painful.

Medical help

🕐 See your doctor within 24 hours.

Does either of the following apply?

You are unable to move the joint

The joint appears misshapen or swollen

Neither

Possible causes

A severe injury is possible (*see* **Fractures**, p.232; **Muscle strains and tears**, p.234; and **Ligament injuries**, p.233).

Medical help

📞 **URGENT!** Phone your doctor immediately!

Does moving the joint affect the pain?

Considerably worsens it

Slightly worsens it or no change

Possible cause

A ligament around the joint is probably sprained.

Self-help

Put a cold compress over the joint, remove, then bandage and rest the joint. See a doctor if the joint is no better in 24 hours.

Possible cause

Osteoarthritis (p.221) is the most likely cause of pain and stiffness in the joints.

Medical help

📋 Make an appointment to see your doctor.

Did the pain come on gradually over months or years?

Yes

No

Have you recently had either of the following?

An infection with a rash

An infection without a rash

Neither

Possible causes

Certain bacterial infections of the intestines and genital tract may cause a reaction that leads to painful joints (*see* **Reactive arthritis**, p.224).

Medical help

 See your doctor within 24 hours.

Possible causes

Some viral illnesses, such as **rubella** (p.168), can cause joint pain, but **Lyme disease** (p.174) is also a possibility, particularly if you have been bitten by a tick.

Medical help

 See your doctor within 24 hours.

Possible cause

Rheumatoid arthritis (p.222) is a possible cause of your symptoms.

Medical help

 See your doctor within 24 hours.

Possible cause

A **frozen shoulder** (p.228) could be the cause.

Medical help

 Make an appointment to see your doctor.

Is the problem in a child under the age of 12 or in someone aged 12 or over?

Under 12

12 or over

Possible causes

Most childhood hip problems are not serious, but a **slipped femoral epiphysis** (p.541) or **Perthes' disease** (p.540) are rare possibilities.

Medical help

 See your doctor within 24 hours.

Which joint or joints are affected?

Hip

Shoulder

Neck

Other joint(s)

Possible causes

Your symptoms are probably a result of overuse of a joint, for example as a result of excessive exercise. A recent minor viral illness may also be the cause of such symptoms.

Medical help

 Make an appointment to see your doctor if there is no improvement in 48 hours.

Go to chart 30
Neck pain or stiffness

If you cannot identify a possible cause for your painful joints from this chart, make an appointment to see your doctor.

32 Swollen ankles

◀ If you have painful swollen ankles, see chart 31

Slight, painless swelling of the ankles is most often caused by fluid accumulating in the tissues after long periods of sitting or standing still, but it may be due to heart, liver, or kidney disorders. It is common in pregnancy. If swelling persists or if you have other symptoms, consult your doctor.

START

Are both ankles affected?

Both ankles

One ankle

Have you been suffering from increasing shortness of breath?

Shortness of breath

No shortness of breath

Possible causes

Swelling of the ankles (due to fluid retention) and shortness of breath may be a result of **chronic heart failure** (p.247). Other possible causes of these symptoms are liver problems (*see* **Cirrhosis**, p.410) or kidney problems (*see* **Nephrotic syndrome**, p.447).

Medical help

🕐 See your doctor within 24 hours.

Possible cause

You may have a blood clot in a vein in your leg (*see* **Deep vein thrombosis**, p.263).

Medical help

📞 URGENT! Phone your doctor immediately!

Possible cause

Swelling can persist or recur for several weeks following an injury. This is unlikely to be a cause for concern.

Self-help

If the injury occurred within the past 48 hours, put a cold compress on your ankle, then bandage it firmly but not tightly, and rest it. For a less recent injury, try rest alone. Make an appointment to see your doctor if swelling persists for more than 24 hours despite rest or if the ankle is painful, tender, or inflamed.

Is the calf of the affected leg either of the following?

Swollen

Tender

Neither

Have you injured your ankle within the past few weeks?

Recent injury

No recent injury

Are you pregnant?

Pregnant

Not pregnant

Possible cause

Several hours of inactivity can lead to accumulation of fluid in the ankles due to less efficient circulation. The decreased cabin pressure in a plane increases this tendency.

Self-help

Encourage the circulation by getting up and walking around at regular intervals during any long journey. When seated, keep your legs raised and take a brisk walk when you reach your destination.

Do any of the following apply?

Your face or fingers are swollen

You have gained excessive weight

You have severe headaches

You have experienced visual disturbances

None of the above

Possible cause

Retaining excessive amounts of fluid may be a sign of pre-eclampsia (*see* **Pre-eclampsia and eclampsia**, p.513).

Medical help

URGENT! Phone your doctor or midwife immediately!

Possible cause

You may have **varicose veins** (p.263), which can cause fluid to accumulate in the ankles.

Self-help

Avoid standing still for long periods. Walk as much as possible, and when sitting down try to keep your feet raised. Make an appointment to see your doctor if the swelling worsens or if other symptoms develop.

Possible cause

Fluid retention, leading to swollen ankles, is common in pregnancy (*see* **Common complaints of normal pregnancy**, p.506).

Self-help

Avoid standing still for long periods and put your feet up whenever possible to reduce swelling. Consult your doctor if your face and/or fingers become swollen or if you start to put on weight rapidly.

Possible cause

Your symptom may be a side effect of the medication or remedy.

Medical help

Make an appointment to see your doctor. Continue to take prescribed medication unless advised to stop by your doctor but stop taking any other medications or complementary remedies.

 Do you have prominent veins in the leg or legs affected by swelling?

Prominent veins

No prominent veins

Did your ankles become swollen after either of the following?

A long trip by car or train

An aeroplane flight

Neither

Are you currently taking any medications or complementary remedies?

Yes

No

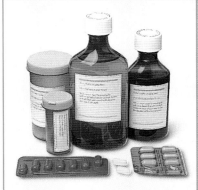

If you cannot identify a possible cause for your swollen ankles from this chart, make an appointment to see your doctor.

33 Erectile dysfunction (ED)

Erectile dysfunction (ED) is failure to have or maintain an erection. Although distressing, occasional difficulties are normal and can be caused by factors such as stress, tiredness, anxiety, or alcohol; however, there may be a physical cause in some cases. If erection problems occur frequently, you should consult your doctor. Safe and effective treatments for ED are available.

❎ WARNING

Advice for erectile dysfunction

Always consult your doctor before using a treatment for erectile dysfunction in case you have an underlying disorder that needs treating or are taking medication that may interact with drugs for erectile dysfunction. Your doctor can also advise on the most suitable treatment for you.

START

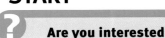

❓ Are you interested in sex?

Yes
No

❓ How often do you fail to achieve or maintain an erection?

Only occasionally
Frequently

Possible cause

Some medications, such as **antidepressant drugs** (p.592) and **antihypertensive drugs** (p.580), complementary remedies, and recreational drugs can affect sexual performance.

Medical help

 Make an appointment to see your doctor. Continue to take prescribed medication but stop taking any other medications, complementary remedies, or recreational drugs.

Possible cause

Lack of interest in sex is likely to reduce your ability to achieve an erection (see **Decreased sex drive**, p.494).

Medical help

 Make an appointment to see your doctor.

Possible causes

Most men have this experience from time to time. Occasional erection problems are most likely to be due to anxiety – for example, at the beginning of a new sexual relationship – or to factors such as tiredness or too much alcohol to drink (see **Erectile dysfunction**, p.494).

Medical help

 Make an appointment to see your doctor if you are concerned about problems with your sexual performance.

❓ Are you currently taking any medication, complementary remedies, or recreational drugs?

Yes
No

Possible cause

Anxiety about your sexual performance is the most likely reason for your problem (see **Erectile dysfunction**, p.494). A physical cause is unlikely.

Medical help

 Make an appointment to see your doctor.

❓ Do you wake with an erection or get an erection by masturbating?

Sometimes
Rarely or never

Possible causes

Various physical conditions, including **atherosclerosis** (p.241), raised blood pressure (see **Hypertension**, p.242), high blood cholesterol, **diabetes mellitus** (p.437), and **multiple sclerosis** (p.334), can cause erectile dysfunction.

Medical help

 Make an appointment to see your doctor.

34 Testes and scrotum problems

Regular self-examination (*see* **Examining your testes,** p.460) is important to detect lumps and swellings in the testes (the sperm-producing organs) and the scrotum (the sac in which the testes lie). The cause may be minor, but there is a possibility of cancer of the testis. Painful swelling in the genital area requires immediate medical attention.

START

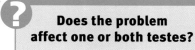
What is the nature of your symptoms?

Pain and swelling

Painless enlargement in or near testis

Generalized painless swelling of the scrotum

None of the above

Does the problem affect one or both testes?

One

Both

Possible causes

Torsion of the testis (p.459) may be the cause of pain and swelling in one testis. A less serious possible cause is **epididymo-orchitis** (p.459).

Medical help

 EMERGENCY! Dial 999/112 and ask for an ambulance.

Possible cause

Internal damage to the testes is a possibility.

Medical help

 URGENT! Phone your doctor immediately!

Possible causes

Accumulation of fluid in the scrotum (*see* **Hydrocele**, p.460), varicose veins in the scrotum (*see* **Varicocele**, p.460), or an inguinal hernia (*see* **Hernias**, p.419) are the most likely causes of your symptoms. However, there is a possibility that you may have **cancer of the testis** (p.460).

Medical help

 Make an appointment to see your doctor.

Have you had an injury in the genital area within the past 48 hours?

Injury

No injury

Possible causes

An **epididymal cyst** (p.459) is the probable cause of your symptoms. However, there is a possibility that you have **cancer of the testis** (p.460).

Medical help

 Make an appointment to see your doctor.

If you cannot identify a possible cause for your testes or scrotum problem from this chart, make an appointment to see your doctor.

Possible cause

Epididymo-orchitis (p.459), which may be due to a sexually transmitted infection or a viral infection such as mumps, may be causing your symptoms.

Medical help

 See your doctor within 24 hours.

Problems with the penis

◀ If you have erection problems, see chart 33

Pain or soreness of the penis that is not related to injury is often due to infection in the urinary tract or of the skin of the penis. Inflammation may be caused by friction during sexual intercourse. You should consult your doctor if there is any change in the appearance of the skin of the penis.

START

❌ WARNING

Blood in the semen

Blood-streaked semen is usually caused by leakage from small blood vessels in the prostate or seminal vesicles. A single episode is unlikely to be a cause for concern, but, if it recurs, you should consult your doctor. It is also important to consult your doctor if you notice a bloodstained discharge that is not related to ejaculation or if you notice blood in your urine.

? What kind of problem are you experiencing?

Painful or sore penis

Discharge from penis

Foreskin problem

Change in appearance of erect penis

None of the above

? When does the pain occur?

Only with an erection

Only when passing urine

At other times

Go to chart 28
Painful urination

? How is the foreskin affected?

Has been retracted but cannot be replaced

After childhood, cannot be fully retracted

Balloons when passing urine

None of the above

Possible cause

Inability to replace a retracted foreskin is called paraphimosis (*see* **Phimosis,** p.461).

Medical help

 EMERGENCY! Dial 999/112 and ask for an ambulance. While waiting for help, surround the affected area with an ice pack.

Possible cause

A sexually transmitted infection, such as **gonorrhoea** (p.491) or **nongonococcal urethritis** (p.491), may be the cause.

Medical help

 See your doctor within 24 hours or go to a clinic specializing in STIs.

Possible cause

Your problem may be caused by **Peyronie's disease** (p.462).

Medical help

 Make an appointment to see your doctor.

Possible cause

An abnormally tight foreskin (*see* **Phimosis,** p.461) may cause these problems.

Medical help

 Make an appointment to see your doctor.

? Has the painful erection now subsided?

Subsided

Still present

Possible cause

Priapism (p.461), in which there is an obstruction to the flow of blood leaving the penis, could be the cause of your symptoms.

Medical help

 URGENT! Phone your doctor immediately!

Possible causes

If you are not circumcised, the cause may be an abnormally tight foreskin (*see* **Phimosis**, p.461). **Peyronie's disease** (p.462) can also cause pain with erection.

Medical help

 Make an appointment to see your doctor.

? Has your penis become inflamed?

Only tip inflamed

Whole penis inflamed

Neither

Possible cause

This may be **balanitis** (p.461).

Medical help

 Make an appointment to see your doctor.

Possible cause

An allergic reaction, such as to the latex in condoms or to a contraceptive cream, may cause inflammation of this type (*see* **Eczema**, p.193, and **Contact dermatitis**, p.193).

Medical help

 Make an appointment to see your doctor.

? Do you have any of the following on the skin of your penis?

Ulcers

Sore areas

Blisters

None of the above

Possible cause

Any of these skin symptoms may be the result of a sexually transmitted infection, such as **genital herpes** (p.493).

Medical help

 Make an appointment to see your doctor or go to a clinic specializing in sexually transmitted infections.

Possible causes

This may be a chancre (*see* **Syphilis**, p.492) or **cancer of the penis** (p.462).

Medical help

 Make an appointment to see your doctor or go to a clinic for sexually transmitted infections.

Possible cause

You probably have **genital warts** (p.493).

Medical help

 Make an appointment to see your doctor or go to a clinic specializing in sexually transmitted infections.

? Have you noticed either of the following on your penis?

Flat, painless sore

Small, fleshy lumps

Neither

If you cannot identify a possible cause for your problem from this chart, make an appointment to see your doctor.

36 Breast problems

You should familiarize yourself with the normal look and feel of your breasts so that you are able to detect changes in them (*see* **Breast awareness**, p.484). Although most breast problems are not serious, consult your doctor if you notice any changes. Minor conditions clearly related to breast-feeding usually respond well to simple treatments.

START

Are you breast-feeding a baby?

Breast-feeding

Not breast-feeding

Where is the problem?

In the breast

On the nipple

Possible cause

The lump may be caused by a blocked milk duct.

Medical help

 Make an appointment to see your doctor if the lump has not disappeared within a week or if the breast becomes painful or red.

How is your nipple affected?

Tender only when feeding

Tender and painful all the time

Possible causes

Discharge from the nipple may have various causes, including a local problem in the breast or a hormonal problem (*see* **Nipple discharge**, p.486).

Medical help

 Make an appointment to see your doctor.

What is the nature of your breast problem?

Single lump in the breast

A nipple has changed in appearance

Discharge from the nipple

Breasts feel tender

Breasts feel lumpy and hard

None of the above

Possible causes

These symptoms may not have a serious cause (*see* **Breast lumps**, p.483, and **Abnormal nipples**, p.485). However, such changes must be investigated promptly to rule out the possibility of **breast cancer** (p.486).

Medical help

 Make an appointment to see your doctor.

If you cannot identify a possible cause for your breast problem from this chart, make an appointment to see your doctor.

What is the nature of your symptoms?

Small, hard lump in breast

Swollen, hard, and tender breasts

Redness of part or all of one breast

None of the above

Possible causes

This may be a breast infection (*see* **Mastitis**, p.523) or possibly a breast abscess, particularly if you are also feeling unwell.

Medical help

 See your doctor within 24 hours. In the meantime, continue to breast-feed from both of your breasts.

Possible cause

Overfull breasts are common, especially when you first start breast-feeding and your milk supply has not yet adjusted to your baby's needs (*see* **Breast engorgement**, p.522).

Self-help

Continuing to breast-feed your baby at regular intervals should solve this problem without special treatment. However, if you are concerned, consult your doctor or breast-feeding adviser.

Possible cause

This problem may be a result of your baby not latching on to your nipple properly.

Self-help

Make sure your baby takes the nipple and the surrounding area into his or her mouth (*see* **Avoiding cracked nipples**, p.523). If you are still having problems when you use the correct feeding technique, consult your doctor or breast-feeding adviser.

If you cannot identify a possible cause for your breast problem from this chart, make an appointment to see your doctor.

Possible cause

Hormonal changes associated with the menstrual cycle often lead to premenstrual breast tenderness (*see* **Premenstrual syndrome**, p.472).

Medical help

 Make an appointment to see your doctor if you are concerned.

Possible cause

Your symptoms may be due to **cracked nipples** (p.523).

Self-help

Keep your nipples dry between feeds and use moisturizing cream. If the problem persists or makes breast-feeding difficult, consult your doctor or breast-feeding adviser.

Does either of the following apply?

Menstruation is due to start within 10 days

You might be pregnant

Neither

Possible cause

Breast tenderness is common in pregnancy (*see* **Common complaints of normal pregnancy**, p.506).

Medical help

 Make an appointment to see your doctor.

If you cannot identify a possible cause for your breast problem from this chart, make an appointment to see your doctor.

Lower abdominal pain in women

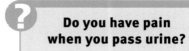 First refer to chart 22, Abdominal pain

Several disorders specific to women can cause discomfort or pain in the lower abdomen. Many of these conditions are related to the reproductive tract (ovaries, uterus, or fallopian tubes) or to pregnancy. Abdominal pain that occurs during pregnancy should always be taken seriously.

START

? Do you have pain when you pass urine?

- Yes
- No

Possible cause

You may have **cystitis** (p.453)

Medical help

 See your doctor within 24 hours. Meanwhile, drink plenty of water and take a painkiller.

? Have you had sexual intercourse in the past 3 months?

- Yes
- No

? Are you pregnant?

- More than 14 weeks pregnant
- Less than 14 weeks pregnant
- Do not think so

Possible causes

You could be having a late **miscarriage** (p.511) or the placenta may have partly separated from the wall of the uterus (*see* **Placental abruption**, p.516).

Medical help

 URGENT! Phone your doctor immediately! Rest in bed until you receive medical advice.

Possible causes

Pain at this stage of pregnancy may indicate a threatened **miscarriage** (p.511) or an **ectopic pregnancy** (p.511).

Medical help

 URGENT! Phone your doctor immediately! Rest in bed until you receive medical advice.

? Did your last period occur at the time you expected?

- On time
- Missed or late

Do you have any of the following symptoms?

Abnormal vaginal discharge

Fever

Pain during intercourse

None of the above

Possible cause

Pelvic inflammatory disease (p.475) is a possible cause of these symptoms.

Medical help

See your doctor within 24 hours.

Do you have an intrauterine contraceptive device (IUD) or intrauterine system (IUS)?

IUD or IUS

No IUD or IUS

Is the pain related to your menstrual cycle?

Occurs just before and/or during a period

Occurs briefly in midcycle

Unrelated

Possible cause

These forms of **contraception** (p.28) often cause increased period pain, particularly for the first few cycles after they have been inserted.

Medical help

Make an appointment to see your doctor.

Have you been through the menopause?

Premenopausal

Postmenopausal

Possible cause

Some women regularly have pain associated with ovulation.

Medical help

Make an appointment to see your doctor to rule out other possible causes.

Possible cause

There is a possibility of an **Ectopic pregnancy** (p.511).

Medical help

URGENT! Phone your doctor immediately!

If you cannot identify a possible cause for your lower abdominal pain from this chart, make an appointment to see your doctor.

Go to chart 41
Painful periods

Genital irritation in women

Genital irritation, which may include itching and/or soreness in the genital area, is most often caused by chemicals in toiletries or detergents. Avoiding these products should prevent irritation from occurring. Genital irritation may also be due to infection, but often the symptom has no obvious cause. If the irritation is persistent, consult your doctor.

Possible causes

You may have **eczema** (p.193), but **genital herpes** (p.493) and **cancer of the vulva** (p.483) should be ruled out.

Medical help

 Make an appointment to see your doctor.

START

 Have you noticed an unusual vaginal discharge?

Unusual discharge

Normal discharge

Have you noticed any change in the appearance of the skin in the genital area?

Skin changes

No skin changes

Have you been using a new soap, bath product, or other toiletry item, or have you switched to a new laundry detergent?

Yes

No

Go to chart 39
Abnormal vaginal discharge

Does either of the following apply?

You are over 45

Your periods are irregular or have stopped

Neither

Possible cause

You may be sensitive to one of the ingredients contained in the new product you are using (*see* **Vulvovaginitis**, p.482).

Self-help

Discontinue use of the new product and use only plain water to wash your genital area. Make an appointment to see your doctor if the irritation has not cleared up in 3–4 days.

Go to chart 27
Frequent urination

Possible causes

Pubic lice (p.493) are a possible cause. However, the symptom sometimes occurs for no obvious reason (*see* **Vulvovaginitis**, p.482).

Medical help

 Make an appointment to see your doctor.

Have you been passing urine more frequently than usual?

Increased frequency

No increased frequency

Possible cause

A change in hormone levels may be the cause of your symptoms (*see* **Menopausal problems**, p.473).

Medical help

 Make an appointment to see your doctor.

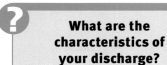 Abnormal vaginal discharge

▶ If the discharge contains blood, see chart 40

A thin, clear or whitish discharge from the vagina is normal. This discharge varies in consistency and quantity with the stage of the menstrual cycle, during sexual arousal, and during pregnancy. An abnormal discharge is usually caused by infection and should be investigated by your doctor.

START

What are the characteristics of your discharge?

- Thick and white
- Normal appearance but heavier than usual
- Greenish yellow
- None of the above

Possible cause

A vaginal yeast infection is a likely cause of your discharge, particularly if it is associated with genital irritation (*see* **Vaginal thrush**, p.482).

Medical help

 Make an appointment to see your doctor if this is the first time you have had this symptom. Otherwise, try using an over-the-counter product recommended by a pharmacist.

Possible cause

These forms of contraception may cause an increase in normal vaginal secretions.

Medical help

 Make an appointment to see your doctor if you are concerned or if you develop genital irritation.

Do any of the following apply?

- You are taking oral contraceptives
- You have an IUD
- You are pregnant
- None of the above

Possible cause

You could have an infection (*see* **Pelvic inflammatory disease**, p.475).

Medical help

 See your doctor within 24 hours.

Do you have either of the following symptoms?

- Fever
- Lower abdominal pain
- Neither

Possible cause

Increased vaginal secretion is normal in pregnancy, especially in the first trimester.

Medical help

 Make an appointment to see your doctor if you are concerned or if you develop genital irritation.

If you cannot identify a possible cause for your discharge from this chart, make an appointment to see your doctor.

Possible cause

A vaginal infection such as **trichomoniasis** (p.492) is a possible cause.

Medical help

 Make an appointment to see your doctor or go to a clinic specializing in sexually transmitted infections.

Possible cause

Cervical ectopy (p.480) may be the cause of your increased discharge.

Medical help

 Make an appointment to see your doctor.

40 Abnormal vaginal bleeding

Vaginal bleeding is considered abnormal if it occurs outside the normal menstrual cycle, during pregnancy, or after the menopause. Although there is often a simple explanation, you should always see your doctor if you have any abnormal vaginal bleeding. If you are pregnant and you are bleeding, you should consult your doctor or midwife at once.

✖ WARNING

Bleeding in pregnancy

If you have any vaginal bleeding during pregnancy, you should contact your doctor or midwife urgently. If the bleeding is heavy, call an ambulance. Although most causes of bleeding are not serious, it is important to rule out **miscarriage** (p.511) or a problem such as a low-lying placenta (*see* **Placenta praevia**, p.516) or partial separation of the placenta from the wall of the uterus (*see* **Placental abruption**, p.516).

START

 Are you pregnant?

- More than 14 weeks pregnant
- Less than 14 weeks pregnant
- Not pregnant

Possible cause

Bleeding at this stage of pregnancy could be due to a problem with the placenta (*see* **Vaginal bleeding in pregnancy**, p.511).

Medical help

 URGENT! Phone your doctor or midwife immediately! Rest in bed until you receive medical advice.

 Is the bleeding similar to that of a normal period?

- Like a period
- Different

Possible causes

You may be having a **miscarriage** (p.511) or you may have an **ectopic pregnancy** (p.511).

Medical help

 URGENT! Phone your doctor or midwife immediately! Rest in bed until you receive medical advice.

How long has it been since your last period?

- Less than 6 months
- More than 6 months

 Do you have unaccustomed pain in the lower back or abdomen?

- Lower back pain
- Abdominal pain
- Neither

Possible cause

Bleeding at this stage of pregnancy could be the first sign of a threatened **miscarriage** (p.511).

Medical help

 URGENT! Phone your doctor or midwife immediately! Rest in bed until you receive medical advice.

Possible causes

Bleeding after the menopause is most commonly from the walls of the vagina, which become dry and fragile due to lower oestrogen levels. Less commonly, bleeding may be due to **uterine polyps** (p.478) or **cancer of the uterus** (p.479).

Medical help

 URGENT! Phone your doctor immediately!

Does either of the following apply?

You have only recently started having periods

You are over 40

Neither

Possible cause

Irregular periods are fairly common in the first year or so of menstruation.

Medical help

 Make an appointment to see your doctor if you are concerned.

Possible cause

Having an occasional irregular period is unlikely to indicate that you have a serious problem if the period was normal in all other respects.

Medical help

 Make an appointment to see your doctor if you are concerned, if your pattern has not returned to normal within three menstrual cycles, or if bleeding is unusually heavy.

Possible cause

Your periods may become irregular as you approach the menopause (*see* **Irregular periods**, p.471 and **Menopausal problems**, p.473) and this is unlikely to indicate a problem if your periods are normal in all other respects.

Medical help

 Make an appointment to see your doctor so that he or she can confirm that there is no serious underlying cause.

Possible causes

You may have an abnormality of the cervix (*see* **Cervical intraepithelial neoplasia**, p.480; **Cervical ectopy**, p.480; and **Cancer of the cervix**, p.481).

Medical help

 Make an appointment to see your doctor.

Have you noticed bleeding within a few hours of intercourse?

Bleeding after intercourse

Bleeding unrelated to intercourse

Have you had sexual intercourse in the past 3 months?

Intercourse

No intercourse

If you cannot identify a possible cause for your abnormal bleeding from this chart, make an appointment to see your doctor.

Possible causes

Bleeding, especially if it is accompanied by pain in the lower abdomen, may be the first sign of an **ectopic pregnancy** (p.511) or of an impending **miscarriage** (p.511), even if you were not aware of being pregnant.

Medical help

 URGENT! Phone your doctor immediately!

Painful periods

Many women experience mild cramping pain in the lower abdomen during menstruation. This pain is considered normal unless it interferes with everyday activities; it can usually be relieved with painkillers. If you regularly have severe pain or if your periods become more painful than usual, you should consult your doctor.

Possible cause

An increase in menstrual pain is often a side effect of IUDs (*see* **Contraception**, p.28).

Medical help

 Make an appointment to see your doctor.

START

?
How does the pain you are currently experiencing compare with that of previous periods?

No worse than usual

Worse than usual

Possible cause

Some menstrual pain is quite normal; it is known as primary **dysmenorrhoea** (p.472).

Self-help

Take a painkiller. Make an appointment to see your doctor if pain interferes with normal activities.

?
Do you have an intrauterine contraceptive device (IUD)?

IUD

No IUD

?
Have you had an unusual vaginal discharge between periods?

No discharge

Discharge

?
Have you had any of the following symptoms?

Abdominal pain that persists between periods

Low back pain that persists between periods

Fever

None of the above

?
Have your periods become heavier or longer as well as more painful?

Heavier

Longer

Neither

Possible cause

You could have an infection (*see* **Pelvic inflammatory disease**, p.475).

Medical help

 See your doctor within 24 hours.

Possible causes

You may possibly have a gynaecological disorder such as **fibroids** (p.477) or **endometriosis** (p.475).

Medical help

 Make an appointment to see your doctor.

If you cannot identify a possible cause for your painful periods from this chart, make an appointment to see your doctor.

42 Weight problems in children

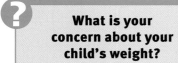 **For loss of weight in children of 12 and over, see chart 2**

Check your child is within healthy limits by regularly measuring his or her weight and height. A long-term weight problem may increase your child's risk of future health problems.

✗ WARNING

Special diets

The dietary needs of children differ from those of adults. An unbalanced diet can adversely affect growth and development. You should not put your child on a reducing diet or restrict specific food groups except on the advice of your doctor.

START

 What is your concern about your child's weight?

Overweight

Underweight

Possible cause

Your child may be eating more than is needed for the amount of exercise he or she is getting (*see* **Obesity in children**, p.552). Rarely, weight gain is due to a hormonal disorder or to prescribed drugs such as **corticosteroids** (p.600).

Medical help

Make an appointment to see your doctor.

Possible cause

Your child may be unable to absorb food properly due to a condition such as **lactose intolerance** (p.416) or **coeliac disease** (p.416).

Medical help

Make an appointment to see your doctor.

 Has your child been underweight for long?

Yes

No

Possible cause

It is likely that your child's thinness is constitutional, particularly if either parent is thin.

Medical help

Make an appointment to see your doctor to confirm that there is no additional medical cause.

Possible cause

Your child could have **diabetes mellitus** (p.437).

Medical help

URGENT! Phone your doctor immediately!

 Does your child have either of the following symptoms?

Diarrhoea

Increased thirst and need to pass urine

Neither of the above

 How is your child's appetite?

Good

Poor

If you cannot identify a possible cause for your child's loss or gain in weight, make an appointment to see your doctor.

43 Vomiting in children

For children of 12 and over, see chart 20

Children vomit as a result of many illnesses, including ear infections and urinary and digestive tract disorders. Anxiety or excitement may also cause vomiting. Rarely, vomiting may be due to an infection or injury to the brain. If vomiting is persistent, you should consult your doctor urgently.

✖ DANGER SIGNS

Dial 999/112 and ask for an ambulance if your child's vomiting is accompanied by any of the following symptoms:
- Green or bright yellow vomit.
- Abdominal pain for 4 hours.
- Flat, dark-red or purple spots that do not fade when pressed.
- Refusal to drink or feed (in babies) for over 6 hours.
- Abnormal drowsiness.
- Sunken eyes.
- Dry tongue.
- Passing no urine during the day for 3 hours (if child is under 1 year old) or 6 hours (in an older child).
- Black or bloodstained faeces.

START

? Has your child had a recent head injury?

- Head injury
- No head injury

Possible cause

Concussion (see **Head injuries**, p.322) is a possibility.

Medical help

 EMERGENCY! Dial 999/112 and ask for an ambulance. Do not allow your child to eat or drink.

? Does your child have any of the following symptoms?

- Severe headache
- Abnormal drowsiness or confusion
- Dislike of bright light
- Neck pain on bending the head forwards
- None of the above

Possible cause

Meningitis (see **Meningitis in children**, p.549) is possible.

Medical help

 EMERGENCY! Dial 999/112 and ask for an ambulance.

? How old is your child?

- Under 3 months
- 3 months or over

Possible cause

These symptoms may indicate a serious abdominal condition, such as **appendicitis** (p.420).

Medical help

 URGENT! Phone your doctor immediately!

? Does your child seem to have abdominal pain?

- Yes
- No

? Apart from the vomiting, does your baby seem generally unwell – for example, is he or she feverish or drowsy?

- Unwell
- Well

Possible causes

There may be many possible causes for these symptoms. However, any young baby who seems unwell and vomits needs prompt medical attention.

Medical help

 URGENT! Phone your doctor immediately!

What are the characteristics of the vomiting?

Frequent and effortless vomiting after feeds

Forceful vomiting after several feeds

Occasional vomiting not necessarily associated with feeding

Possible cause

This type of vomiting may be the result of a digestive tract problem, such as **pyloric stenosis in infants** (p.559).

Medical help

 URGENT! Phone your doctor immediately!

Possible causes

This type of regurgitation is rarely serious and has several possible causes (*see* **Feeding problems in babies**, p.531).

Self-help

Make sure you "burp" your baby and keep him or her upright for 30 minutes after feeding. Consult your doctor if your baby seems unwell or fails to gain weight.

Possible cause

Babies often vomit for no particular reason, and this is no cause for concern if your baby seems generally well and is gaining weight (*see* **Feeding problems in babies**, p.531).

Self-help

Be sure to "wind" your baby after each feed. Consult your doctor if your baby seems unwell or vomits frequently.

Does your child have diarrhoea?

Diarrhoea

No diarrhoea

Possible cause

This could be a digestive tract infection (*see* **Vomiting and diarrhoea**, p.559).

Medical help

 URGENT! Phone your doctor immediately if your child is under 6 months old. For older children, follow the self-help measures for **vomiting and diarrhoea** (p.559) and consult your doctor if there is no improvement in 24 hours or if other symptoms develop.

Possible causes

Your child may have **pertussis** (p.301). An infection that causes severe coughing, such as **bronchiolitis** (p.545) or **pneumonia** (p.299), can also cause vomiting.

Medical help

 URGENT! Phone your doctor immediately!

Does your child have any of the following symptoms?

Pain on passing urine

Renewed bedwetting or daytime "accidents"

Temperature of 38°C (100.4°F) or above

None of the above

Possible cause

Your child may have a **urinary tract infection** (p.564).

Medical help

See your doctor within 24 hours.

Did vomiting follow a violent bout of coughing?

Followed coughing

No coughing

If you cannot identify a possible cause for your child's vomiting from this chart, see your doctor within 24 hours.

Possible causes

Illnesses with fever, such as **acute hepatitis** (p.408), **acute otitis media** (p.557), or a **urinary tract infection** (p.564), often cause vomiting.

Medical help

 See your doctor within 24 hours.

Diarrhoea in children

 ## For children 12 and over, see chart 24

Diarrhoea is the passage of loose or watery faeces more often than normal. Breast-fed babies may pass loose faeces several times a day, and this is normal. If your child has diarrhoea, he or she should drink plenty of clear fluids to avoid dehydration. If symptoms persist, consult your doctor.

❌ DANGER SIGNS

Dial 999/112 and ask for an ambulance if your child's diarrhoea is accompanied by any of the following symptoms:
- Drowsiness or lethargy.
- Abdominal pain lasting more than 4 hours.
- No urine passed during the day for 3 hours (if under 1 year) or 6 hours (in an older child).
- Refusal to drink or feed (in babies) for over 6 hours.
- Blood in the faeces.

START

How long has your child had diarrhoea?

Less than 3 days

3 days or more

Does your child have any of the following symptoms?

Abdominal pain

Temperature of 38°C (100.4°F) or above

Vomiting

None of the above

Has your child recently taken antibiotics or is your child currently taking medications or complementary remedies?

Yes

No

Possible cause

Your child may have **gastroenteritis** (p.398).

Medical help

 URGENT! Phone your doctor immediately if your child is under 6 months old. If your child is older, follow the self-help advice for **preventing dehydration** (p.397) and consult your doctor if you are concerned, if your child has not improved in 24 hours, or if other symptoms develop.

Possible cause

Persistent constipation can lead to faeces trickling from the anus (*see* **Constipation in children**, p.560). This may be mistaken for diarrhoea.

Medical help

 See your doctor within 24 hours.

Was your child constipated before the onset of diarrhoea?

Constipated

Not constipated

What is the appearance of your child's faeces?

Uniformly runny

Contain recognizable pieces of food

Is your child gaining weight and growing normally?

Yes

No

Possible cause

Your child's symptoms may be a side effect of the drug or remedy.

Medical help

 See your doctor within 24 hours. Continue giving prescribed medications unless advised to stop by your doctor, but stop giving any other medications or complementary remedies.

Possible causes

Young children often fail to chew and digest food properly, which can lead to toddler's diarrhoea (*see* **Vomiting and diarrhoea,** p.559). Unfamiliar foods can have the same effect

Self-help

No special action is needed provided that your child is well. Consult your doctor if your child develops other symptoms.

Possible cause

Foods that are new to your baby may be the cause of digestive upsets.

Self-help

Withhold the food that seems to be causing the trouble for at least 1 week. Consult your doctor if your baby is no better in 24 hours or develops other symptoms.

? **How old is your child?**

Under 12 months

12 months – 3 years

Over 3 years

? **Is your child experiencing unusual stress, anxiety, or excitement?**

Stress or anxiety

Excitement

Neither

? **Was your baby given any of the following before the onset of diarrhoea?**

Unfamiliar foods

Sugary foods or sweetened drinks

None of the above

If you cannot identify a possible cause for your child's diarrhoea from this chart, see your doctor within 24 hours.

Possible causes

It is possible that your child has a condition affecting the digestive tract, such as **food intolerance** (p.416) or **coeliac disease** (p.416).

Medical help

 Make an appointment to see your doctor.

Possible cause

Psychological stress or unusual excitement can cause diarrhoea.

Self-help

The diarrhoea should stop as soon as the cause has disappeared. Consult your doctor if there is a long-term cause of anxiety in your child's life or if your child develops other symptoms.

Possible cause

Sugar in food and drink can cause diarrhoea in babies.

Self-help

Avoid giving your baby sweetened foods and drinks. Consult your doctor if your baby is no better in 24 hours or develops other symptoms.

45 Fever in children

◀ For children of 12 and over, see chart 4

A fever is a temperature of 38°C (100.4°F) or above. If your child is unwell, you should take his or her temperature because a high fever may need urgent treatment. If a feverish child becomes unresponsive, call an ambulance. In all cases, follow the advice for **bringing down a fever** (p.165).

✖ DANGER SIGNS

Dial 999/112 and ask for an ambulance if your child's temperature rises above 39°C (102°F) and he or she has any of the following symptoms:
- Abnormally rapid breathing (see **Checking your child's breathing rate**, p.119).
- Drowsiness.
- Severe headache.
- Dislike of bright light.
- Refusing to drink for more than 6 hours.
- A seizure.
- A rash that does not fade when pressed (see **Checking a red rash**, p.57).
- A stiff neck.

START

How old is your child?

Under 6 months

6 months or over

Possible cause

Fever in young babies is unusual unless it occurs within 48 hours of immunization; it may indicate a serious illness.

Medical help

 URGENT! Phone your doctor immediately!

Is your child reluctant to move an arm or leg?

Yes

No

Possible cause

Your child could have an infection in a bone or joint (see **Osteomyelitis**, p.219, and **Septic arthritis**, p.225).

Medical help

 URGENT! Phone your doctor immediately!

Does your child have a rash?

Rash

No rash

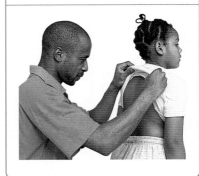

Does your child have any of the following symptoms?

Severe headache

Abnormal drowsiness, irritability, or confusion

Dislike of bright light

Neck pain on bending the head forwards

None of the above

Possible cause

Meningitis (see **Meningitis in children**, p.549) is a possible cause of these symptoms.

Medical help

 EMERGENCY! Dial 999/112 and ask for an ambulance.

Possible cause

Your child may have an infection of the middle ear (see **Acute otitis media in children**, p.557).

Medical help

 See your doctor within 24 hours.

Go to chart 10
Rash with fever

Possible cause

Your child could have a respiratory infection, such as **pneumonia** (p.299).

Medical help

 EMERGENCY! Dial 999/112 and ask for an ambulance.

 Does your child have either of the following symptoms?

Cough
Runny nose
Neither

Possible cause

A viral illness, such as a severe cold (*see* **Common cold**, p.164) or **influenza** (p.164), is the most likely cause of your child's symptoms.

Self-help

See the advice for **bringing down a fever** (p.165). Consult your doctor if your child's symptoms worsen, if your child is no better in 2 days, or if he or she develops other symptoms.

 Is your child's breathing abnormally noisy or rapid (*see* Checking your child's breathing rate, p.119)?

Abnormally rapid
Noisy
Neither

 Does your child have a sore throat?

Sore throat
No sore throat

Possible cause

Your child could be suffering from a throat infection, such as **tonsillitis** (p.546).

Self-help

See the advice for **bringing down a fever** (p.165). If your child is no better in 24 hours or if other symptoms develop, make an appointment to see your doctor.

Possible cause

This may be a severe episode of **croup** (p.545).

Medical help

 URGENT! Phone your doctor immediately!

Possible cause

A **urinary tract infection** (p.564) is a possibility.

Medical help

🕐 See your doctor within 24 hours.

 Does your child have either of the following symptoms?

Pain on passing urine
Diarrhoea with or without vomiting
Neither

Does either of the following apply?

Your child has been pulling at one ear
Your child has complained of earache
Neither

Possible cause

It is possible that your child has a digestive tract infection (*see* **Gastroenteritis**, p.398).

Medical help

URGENT! Phone your doctor immediately if your child is under 6 months old. For older children, follow the self-help measures for **vomiting and diarrhoea** (p.559), and consult your doctor if your child is no better in 24 hours or if he or she develops other symptoms.

If you cannot identify a possible cause for your child's fever from this chart, see your doctor within 24 hours.

Breathing problems in children

◀ For children of 12 and over, see charts 17 and 18

Breathing problems include noisy or rapid breathing and shortness of breath. Shortness of breath may not be obvious because a child may simply avoid exertion. A child with severe difficulty breathing needs urgent hospital treatment. Breathing problems that occur suddenly also need immediate attention.

✖ DANGER SIGNS

Dial 999/112 and ask for an ambulance if your child's breathing rate is excessively rapid (*see* **Checking your child's breathing rate**, opposite page) or if breathing problems are accompanied by any of the following symptoms:
- Bluish lips or tongue.
- Drowsiness.
- Inability to swallow, talk, or produce sounds.

START

 How long has your child had breathing problems?

Started suddenly a few minutes ago

Started more than a few minutes ago

 Is it possible that your child is choking on food or a small object?

Possible

Unlikely

Possible cause

An inhaled foreign body may be preventing your child from breathing properly.

Medical help

🏥 **EMERGENCY!** Dial 999/112 and ask for an ambulance.

 Are any of the danger signs listed in the box above present?

Danger signs present

No danger signs

Possible cause

Your child may have a serious respiratory problem.

Medical help

🏥 **EMERGENCY!** Dial 999/112 and ask for an ambulance.

Possible cause

The cause of these symptoms could be a serious lung infection such as **bronchiolitis** (p.545).

Medical help

🏥 **URGENT!** Phone your doctor immediately!

 How old is your child?

Under 6 months

6 months or over

Does your child have any of the following symptoms?

Noisy breathing

Barking cough

Shortness of breath

None of the above

Possible cause

These symptoms may be due to **croup** (p.545).

Medical help

 URGENT! Phone your doctor immediately!

Possible cause

Your child may have developed asthma (*see* **Asthma in children**, p.544).

Medical help

URGENT! Phone your doctor immediately!

Does your child suffer from repeated episodes of any of the following symptoms?

Wheezing

Coughing at night

Coughing after exercise

Coughing after going out in the cold

None of the above

If you cannot identify a possible cause for your child's breathing problems from this chart, see your doctor within 24 hours.

 Does your child have a fever – a temperature of 38°C (100.4°F) or above?

Fever

No fever

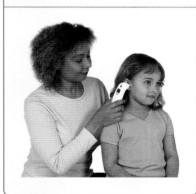

Possible cause

A lung infection, such as **pneumonia** (p.299) or **bronchiolitis** (p.545), could be the cause.

Medical help

URGENT! Phone your doctor immediately!

▶ **SYMPTOM ASSESSMENT**

Checking your child's breathing rate

A child whose breathing is unusually rapid when at rest or asleep may need medical attention. Check your child's breathing by counting the number of breaths he or she takes in one minute with your hand on his or her chest or back to feel the breaths. The normal breathing rate of a young baby is faster than that of an older child. Compare your child's breathing rate with the maximum rate for his or her age shown in the table.

Age	Breathing rate
Under 2 months	Maximum of 60 breaths a minute
2–11 months	Maximum of 50 breaths a minute
1–5 years	Maximum of 40 breaths a minute
Over 5 years	Maximum of 30 breaths a minute

Assessment of your child's breathing
Your child should be at rest and not crying when you check his or her breathing rate. Place your hand on his or her chest or back to help you to count the breaths.

Coughing in children

 For children 12 and over, see chart 16

Coughing is a normal reaction to irritation in the throat or lungs. Most coughs are caused by minor infections of the nose and/or throat, but the sudden onset of coughing may be caused by choking. Coughing is unusual in babies under 6 months old and may indicate a serious lung infection.

✖ DANGER SIGNS

Dial 999/112 and ask for an ambulance if your child is coughing and has any of the following symptoms:
- Bluish lips or tongue.
- Drowsiness.
- Inability to swallow, talk, or produce sounds.
- Excessively rapid breathing (*see* **Checking your child's breathing rate**, p.119).

START

? How long has your child been coughing?

Started suddenly a few minutes ago

Started more than a few minutes ago

? How old is your child?

6 months or over

Under 6 months

Possible cause

There is a possibility that your baby may be suffering from a serious lung infection (*see* **Bronchiolitis**, p.545), especially if he or she is also unwell.

Medical help

🏥 **URGENT!** Phone your doctor immediately!

? Is it possible that your child is choking on food or a small object?

Possible

Unlikely

? Is your child's breathing abnormally rapid (*see* Checking your child's breathing rate, p.119) or noisy?

Abnormally rapid

Noisy

Neither

? Does the cough have either of these characteristics?

Comes in fits ending with a whoop

Is followed by vomiting

Neither

Possible cause

An inhaled foreign body may be the cause of the coughing.

Medical help

 EMERGENCY! Dial 999/112 and ask for an ambulance.

Go to chart 46

Breathing problems in children

Possible cause

Pertussis (p.301) may be the cause of your child's cough.

Medical help

 See your doctor within 24 hours.

Does your child have a runny nose?

Most of the time or very often

Has developed a runny nose within the past few days

No runny nose

Possible causes

Your child may have an allergy (*see* **Allergic rhinitis**, p.283) or **enlarged adenoids** (p.546), both of which may cause these symptoms.

Medical help

Make an appointment to see your doctor.

Possible cause

A viral illness, such as a **common cold** (p.164) or **influenza** (p.164), is the most likely cause of your child's symptoms.

Self-help

See the advice for **bringing down a fever** (p.165). Consult your doctor if symptoms get worse, if your child is no better in 2 days, or if other symptoms develop.

When does the coughing occur?

Mainly at night

After exercise

When out in the cold

None of the above

Does your child have a fever – a temperature of 38°C (100.4°F) or above?

Fever

No fever

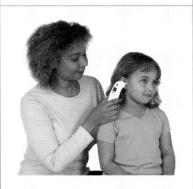

Possible cause

Your child probably has a **common cold** (p.164).

Self-help

Steam inhalation (p.291) may help relieve the cough. Consult your doctor if symptoms get worse, if your child is no better in 2 days, or if other symptoms develop.

Possible cause

Your child's cough may be a response to being in a smoky atmosphere or to smoking.

Self-help

Make sure that no one smokes in the house and avoid taking your child into a smoky atmosphere. If you suspect your child may be smoking, encourage him or her to stop.

Possible cause

There is a possibility that your child has asthma (*see* **Asthma in children**, p.544).

Medical help

 See your doctor within 24 hours.

Are there smokers in the home or might your child have been smoking?

Smokers in the home

Child might smoke

Neither

If you cannot identify a possible cause for your child's cough from this chart, see your doctor within 24 hours.

48 Abdominal pain in children

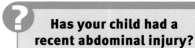 **For children 12 and over, see chart 22**

Every child suffers from abdominal pain at some time, and some children have recurrent episodes. Usually the cause is minor, and the pain subsides in a few hours without treatment. In rare cases, abdominal pain is a symptom of a serious disorder that requires prompt medical attention.

❌ DANGER SIGNS

Dial 999/112 and ask for an ambulance if your child's abdominal pain has been continuous for more than 4 hours or if the pain is associated with any of the following symptoms:
- Greenish-yellow vomit.
- Pain or swelling in the groin or scrotum.
- Blood in the faeces.

START

? Has your child had a recent abdominal injury?

Recent injury

No injury

Possible causes

A strangulated inguinal hernia (*see* **Hernias**, p.419) or **torsion of the testis** (p.459) is possible.

Medical help

 EMERGENCY! Dial 999/112 and ask for an ambulance. Do not allow your child to eat or drink.

Possible causes

Abdominal pain accompanied by blood in the faeces could indicate **intussusception** (p.560) in a young child. In older children, the cause of these symptoms may be an intestinal infection such as **food poisoning** (p.398).

Medical help

 EMERGENCY! Dial 999/112 and ask for an ambulance. Do not allow your child to eat or drink.

? Does your child have pain or swelling in either of the following places?

Groin

Scrotum

Neither

? Does your child have any of the following symptoms?

Continuous pain for more than 4 hours

Blood in the faeces

Greenish-yellow vomit

None of the above

Possible cause

An **intestinal obstruction** (p.419) is possible.

Medical help

 EMERGENCY! Dial 999/112 and ask for an ambulance. Do not allow your child to eat or drink.

Possible cause

An injury to an abdominal organ is possible.

Medical help

 URGENT! Phone your doctor immediately!

? Have your child's bowel movements (stools) been abnormal?

Hard and infrequent

Normal

Diarrhoea

Possible cause

Continuous abdominal pain for this length of time could be an indication of a serious abdominal condition, such as **appendicitis** (p.420).

Medical help

 URGENT! Phone your doctor immediately!

Possible cause

Constipation can cause abdominal pain (*see* **Constipation in children**, p.560)

Medical help

 See your doctor within 24 hours.

 Has pain been relieved by either of the following?

Vomiting

Passing wind or faeces

Neither

Possible cause

Your child could have a digestive tract infection (*see* **Gastroenteritis**, p.398).

Medical help

 URGENT! Phone your doctor immediately if your child is under 6 months old. For older children, follow the advice on **preventing dehydration** (p.397) and consult your doctor if your child is no better in 24 hours or if other symptoms develop.

 Does your child have any of the following symptoms?

Sore throat

Cough

Runny nose

None of the above

 Does your child have any of the following symptoms?

Pain on urination

Temperature of 38°C (100.4°F) or above

Renewed bedwetting or daytime "accidents"

None of the above

Possible cause

Your child may have a **urinary tract infection** (p.564).

Medical help

 See your doctor within 24 hours.

Possible cause

In young children these symptoms may be associated with an upper respiratory tract infection, such as a **common cold** (p.164).

Self-help

Encourage your child to drink and give a painkiller at the dose recommended for his or her age. If the pain is no better in 24 hours or worsens, phone your doctor.

Possible cause

Recurrent abdominal pain in children can sometimes be related to anxiety.

Medical help

 Make an appointment to see your doctor.

Has your child suffered from similar bouts of abdominal pain over the past few weeks?

Previous abdominal pain

No previous pain

If you cannot identify a possible cause for your child's abdominal pain from this chart, see your doctor within 24 hours.

looking for
disease

THE DIAGNOSTIC METHOD is the process by which a doctor identifies the disease or disorder that is causing symptoms. The doctor may use various tests to confirm or eliminate a particular diagnosis or to help to decide between several possible diagnoses. The process may include finding an underlying agent, such as a virus or bacteria. Screening tests are used to detect early signs of disease in large groups of people or are used individually to look for risk factors that predispose a person to an illness, such as cancer, in the future.

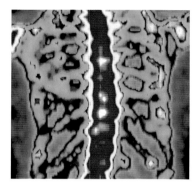

Bone scan of the chest
Radionuclide scanning may be used to detect cancer that has spread to the bones, visible here as light areas along the spine.

There are several reasons why you might visit a doctor. You may have a pain or other sensation that is causing you concern; you may have noticed a change in your body's appearance; or you may simply be anxious about your general physical or mental state. At other times, you may need to see your doctor if a medical examination is required for work-related or insurance purposes.

If you have a health problem, your doctor will base his or her diagnosis on your symptoms, medical history, a physical examination, and possibly some diagnostic tests.

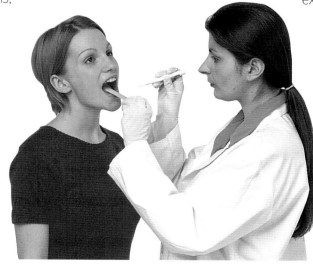

Examining the throat
The first step in the diagnostic process is often a physical examination. If you have a sore throat, the doctor will inspect it for signs of infection.

Why tests are done

Your doctor begins the diagnostic process by asking questions about your general health and any specific symptoms. The next step is to take a complete medical history by asking you questions about past illnesses, family history of disease, lifestyle, and occupation. If you have symptoms or signs of a common disease or disorder, your doctor may be able to arrive at an immediate diagnosis after examining you. If he or she is unable to arrive at a diagnosis, you may be asked to have some tests. At certain stages of your life, you may be asked to undergo screening tests. Screening uses one or more of the same tests as diagnosis but the aim of screening is to detect diseases such as cancer before symptoms develop.

Types of test

Medical tests can be simple enough to be carried out in your doctor's surgery but some require sophisticated equipment in a hospital or laboratory. Tests may be performed on body fluids, such as urine or blood, or on tissue, such as cells from the cervix. Viewing tests involve the use of instruments such as endoscopes, viewing tubes through which a doctor can look directly into the body, often through a natural opening such as the mouth or nose. Imaging tests, such as MRI, CT scanning, and ultrasound, create images of internal body structures to detect abnormalities. Certain tests, such as mammography (X-rays of the breasts), can be used for both diagnosis and screening.

You and your doctor will balance the medical value and reliability of an appropriate medical test against any health risks and discomfort.

Reliability

Some tests, such as diagnostic tests on tissue samples, are extremely accurate, but most are less reliable. There may be inaccuracies in the test equipment, the procedure, or in the interpretation of results, which, together with human errors, can lead to false results. A false positive result indicates the presence of disease in a person who is in fact healthy, causing anxiety and necessitating further tests. A false negative result indicates that a person is free of the disease when he or she actually has it. This may delay diagnosis until symptoms develop, at which stage treatment may be less effective. Since most tests are not totally reliable, all results must be carefully assessed in the context of a person's medical history and examination. Some tests may carry health risks. A risky or painful test may still be justified medically and be acceptable to the person having it if it yields information that could be lifesaving.

Screening

Screening is used to identify people who already have a disease but have not yet developed symptoms, and only if treatment is available for an early stage of the disease. For example, breast cancer screening is routine because early detection gives the best chance of a cure.

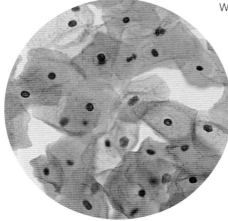

Cervical screening test result
A cervical screening test is used to detect abnormal cervical cells that might become cancerous. This common screening test enables treatment to be given at an early stage. The cells shown here are healthy.

Screening tests may also look for risk factors or a genetic predisposition to developing a disease. For example, a test might look for high blood cholesterol, associated with coronary heart disease, or for the genes associated with breast cancer. Screening may also be used to detect healthy carriers of abnormal genes, which may be passed on to children, and these tests may be offered to couples who are planning to have children. Successful, reliable, and cost-effective screening relies on careful selection of the population. Screening must be targeted at groups that are at increased risk. For example, breast cancer screening usually starts from the age of 50, because the cancer rarely occurs in younger women.

Trends in disease detection

Technological advances are making diagnosis safer and less invasive, and the use of computers is making the analysis, storage, and retrieval of test results quicker and more reliable.

Various reliable home tests, such as tests for blood sugar levels (necessary in diabetes) and blood pressure monitors, are available. Used under medical supervision, these tests can help you to monitor your long-term illnesses and the effects of treatments, enabling you to take control of your health.

Highly magnified viruses
Tiny organisms, such as viruses, can be seen only with an electron microscope. This image shows a highly magnified cluster of hepatitis A viruses.

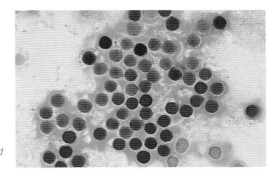

Visiting your doctor

You may need to visit your doctor for advice about symptoms or other health issues, or your doctor may ask you to come in for regular checkups or to discuss ongoing treatment. What happens during the consultation depends on its purpose, but your doctor usually assesses your health by observation, asking you questions, and carrying out a physical examination. Samples may also be collected for testing.

YOU MAY DECIDE to visit your doctor because you feel ill or because you are concerned about a physical change, such as a swelling or stiffness in a joint. You may need advice about a lifestyle change, such as losing weight or giving up smoking. If you have a long-term condition, such as diabetes mellitus, you will need regular checkups. Even if you are healthy, you may be asked to attend the surgery for screening procedures, such as cervical screening tests and blood pressure measurement.

Preparing for a visit

Whatever your reason for visiting your doctor, you may find it helpful to decide on the issues that you want to discuss before you have the appointment. For example, if you have specific symptoms, you should think about how often they occur and whether certain activities bring the symptoms on or relieve them. Your doctor also needs to know about medications or supplements that you are taking, allergies that you have to particular treatments, and any alternative therapies that you are currently using.

The consultation

There are many ways in which your doctor can assess your health. First of all, he or she will note your general appearance, such as your weight, and look for signs of anxiety or depression. Your doctor will then ask you a series of questions, known as taking your medical history, before he or she performs a physical examination. The questions that you are asked and the extent of the physical examination depend on the purpose of the consultation.

If you are visiting a doctor for the first time, he or she may take a full medical history, including details of diseases that run in your family, illnesses that you have had in the past, and lifestyle factors such as your diet. If the doctor already has your medical record, he or she may refer to it. If you have specific symptoms, the doctor will concentrate on them in order to make a diagnosis.

A full physical examination is usually given only as part of a general checkup, such as for a new insurance policy. If you have symptoms, the doctor usually checks only relevant areas of your body. Even if you are not given a full

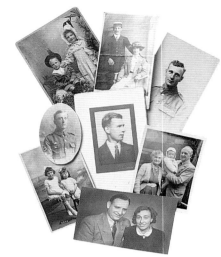

Family history
Some disorders may run in your family. Your doctor needs to know about these to help make a diagnosis.

examination, your doctor may inspect certain areas, such as your skin and nails, to assess your general health.

Your doctor may need to collect a sample, such as blood or urine. Samples are tested to confirm a diagnosis or to monitor a disease. Simple tests may be performed in the doctor's surgery, but more complex procedures are usually carried out in a laboratory. The doctor may ask you to telephone the surgery for the test results or to make another appointment to discuss the results and their implications for your health.

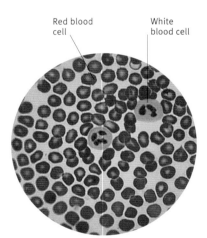

Red blood cell — White blood cell

Blood cells
Your doctor may take a blood sample, which may be sent for microscopic examination to look at the structure of the blood cells, as can be seen in this highly magnified view of normal red and white blood cells.

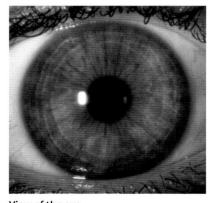

View of the eye
Your doctor may examine your eyes when you have a routine physical examination.

EQUIPMENT

The doctor's basic equipment

Your doctor may use one or more basic pieces of equipment when performing a physical examination. Each has a specific function. Some instruments enable your doctor to examine certain parts of the body more closely. Others are used to listen for abnormal sounds or to check the reflexes.

Aids to examination
An ophthalmoscope and otoscope are used to look at eyes and ears. Reflexes are tested with a hammer, and sounds, such as the heartbeat, can be heard with a stethoscope.

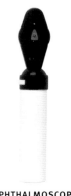

OPHTHALMOSCOPE

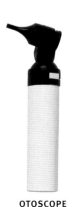

OTOSCOPE

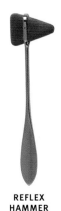

REFLEX HAMMER

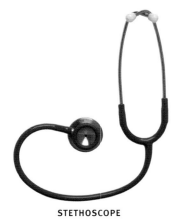

STETHOSCOPE

Medical history and examination

You may visit your doctor for a checkup or if you are feeling ill. If you have symptoms, your doctor will ask various questions and carry out an examination to take the first steps towards a diagnosis. Occasionally, this may be all that is needed for your doctor to decide what is causing your illness and what action is needed. In other cases, tests are used to gather more information.

From the moment that you walk into the surgery, your doctor starts to gather information about you from your appearance. This information may provide clues to your general health and state of mind. The doctor obtains further information about your health from a medical history and by performing a physical examination.

The first article in this section looks at the questions that your doctor may ask when taking your medical history. Such questions are an important way of gathering information about past illnesses, disorders that run in your family, and your lifestyle.

Once he or she has taken your history, your doctor may examine you to look for abnormalities or confirm a suspected diagnosis. Some common physical examination procedures are described in the second article. Your doctor may also take samples for testing.

If you need a medical examination for insurance purposes, your doctor will look for early signs of disease or for factors that may increase your risk of developing disease. Routine checkups in childhood and during pregnancy are discussed elsewhere (*see* **Health checkups**, p.13).

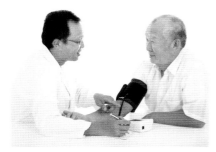

Measuring blood pressure
A physical examination may include measuring your blood pressure. High blood pressure increases the risk of stroke.

Medical history

A medical record of a person's past and present health

To diagnose a disorder or assess your risk of developing a disease, your doctor will ask questions about your current symptoms, past illnesses, medications, family medical history, or lifestyle, and then compile a medical history. If you have symptoms, your medical history will help your doctor reach a diagnosis and decide on the best course of action to take. If you are having a checkup, you may be asked about lifestyle factors that influence your health (*see* **Health checkups**, p.13).

Past medical history and medications

Information on any past disorders and operations may help your doctor decide whether a previous problem could be causing your current symptoms. The symptoms may be a side effect of or an allergic reaction to a treatment, so it is important to tell your doctor if you are taking any medications or supplements, or if you are using any alternative therapies. Your doctor needs to ensure that new medication will not react with anything that you are already taking.

Family history

If you have a family history of a particular disorder, the doctor will check whether your symptoms are due to that disorder and suggest measures that help to reduce your risk of developing the condition in the future. For example, if you have a family history of heart disease (p.243), you may be advised to restrict the amount of saturated fat in your diet and to have your blood cholesterol level tested.

Lifestyle

What you eat, what you do, and where you live are factors that can all influence your health. Your doctor may ask you about your diet, whether you exercise regularly, or drink, smoke, or use recreational drugs. He or she may ask you questions about your job, because your work may have an effect on your health. Past occupations may also be important because some work-related diseases take years to appear. For example, people who work or have worked in the mining industry may be at risk of developing certain occupational lung diseases (p.305).

Your personal relationships, living conditions, and financial circumstances can also influence your health, particularly your psychological wellbeing. If you have travelled abroad recently, you should tell your doctor as there is a possibility that your symptoms may be due to an infectious disease.

Physical examination

An examination by a doctor to check the condition or health of various body systems and organs

A physical examination is often an essential part of diagnosis or checkups. If you have symptoms, your doctor will concentrate on areas related to your symptoms or in which abnormalities can be detected. He or she may check other areas as well. For example, the doctor may examine your ankles if you have symptoms of heart failure, such as shortness of breath, because heart failure is associated with swelling of the ankles.

► TECHNIQUE

Basic examination techniques

Once your doctor has looked for obvious signs or symptoms of disease, he or she may use any of three basic techniques to examine you. An examination may include auscultation, in which a stethoscope is used to listen to your chest or other parts of your body; palpation, in which an area is felt with the hands; and percussion, which involves listening to sounds made by tapping certain areas.

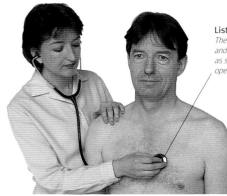

Listening to the chest
The doctor uses a stethoscope to pick up and amplify sounds within the chest, such as sounds made by heart valves as they open and close

Auscultation
A stethoscope can be used to listen not only to the chest but also to sounds made by the intestines or by blood passing through blood vessels. The doctor interprets these sounds to determine whether or not they are normal.

Feeling the abdomen
Using the flat of both hands, the doctor presses gently but firmly over the abdomen to feel for any lumps or areas of tenderness

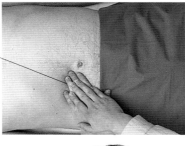

Palpation
The doctor applies pressure with one or two hands and slowly feels over the entire abdomen. This will help him or her detect enlarged or tender internal organs or abnormal swellings.

Percussing the chest
A finger of one hand is pressed on to the chest and tapped by a finger of the other hand to produce a sound

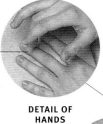

DETAIL OF HANDS

Percussion
By tapping different parts of the chest and abdomen and listening to the sounds that are produced, the doctor can distinguish solid tissue and fluids from gas-filled areas.

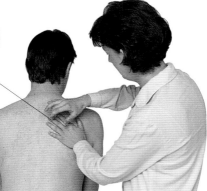

Skin, hair, and nails

Some obvious skin problems such as rashes or discoloration may be symptoms of a skin disorder, but may also indicate a more widespread problem such as systemic lupus erythematosus (p.281). Your hair and nails can also be affected by certain disorders. For example, generalized thinning of your hair may be due to a hormonal disorder, and a change in the shape or colour of your nails may indicate iron-deficiency anaemia (p.271).

Heart and circulation

Your doctor may check the strength and rate of your pulse, usually at the wrist or the side of the neck. A rapid or uneven pulse may suggest a heart problem. Pulses at other points, such as in the groin, may provide more information about your circulation. Your doctor will use a stethoscope to listen to your heart. Abnormal sounds known as heart murmurs may indicate heart valve damage. Blood pressure measurement (p.242) is a routine part of most examinations.

Lungs

If your doctor has noticed you have difficulty in breathing, he or she may listen to your chest and back with a stethoscope and tap the surface of your chest to check for fluid in the lungs. Abnormal sounds, such as wheezing, may indicate narrowed airways.

Abdomen and rectum

By feeling and tapping your abdomen, your doctor can detect abnormal swellings. Listening to the intestines with a stethoscope may help to confirm the presence of a blockage.

In a rectal examination, your doctor will insert a gloved, lubricated finger into the rectum to feel for lumps or tender areas. This is done to look for colorectal cancer (p.421), especially in people over 50. In men, the doctor may check for an enlarged prostate gland (p.463) or prostate cancer (p.464).

Reproductive organs

In men, the scrotum and testes may be examined to detect lumps. The penis is examined for signs of infection. Boys may be checked to make sure that both of their testes have descended properly. In women, internal pelvic examinations may be performed to detect disorders of the reproductive organs. A cervical screening test (p.480) should be performed every 3–5 years, depending on the woman's age, to check for early signs of cancer of the cervix (p.481). Your doctor may inspect your breasts for nipple abnormalities or puckering of the skin and also feel your breasts for any lumps or swellings.

Bones, joints, and muscles

Your doctor may examine a joint for swelling or tenderness, which could indicate a disorder such as arthritis (p.220), and test the range of pain-free movement. He or she may also check that the surrounding ligaments and muscles are working normally.

Nervous system

Your doctor may test your strength, coordination, balance, and response to sensations. By testing reflexes, such as a knee jerk, he or she will be able to assess the function of specific nerves. The doctor may also ask you questions to check mental functions such as memory.

▶ **PROCEDURE**

Having a throat swab taken

If you have a sore throat, you may need to have a throat swab taken to see if you have a bacterial infection. The doctor or nurse holds your tongue down with a depressor and uses a plastic stick with a sterile cotton end (swab) to collect a fluid sample from your throat. The swab is then sent to a laboratory. The procedure can be carried out quickly in the doctor's surgery and is not painful. However, you may gag briefly when the swab touches your throat.

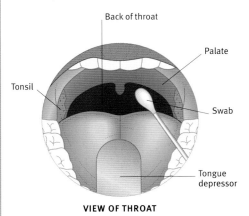

Back of throat
Palate
Tonsil
Swab
Tongue depressor

VIEW OF THROAT

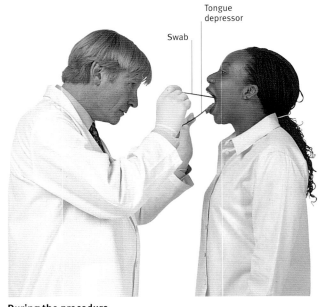

Tongue depressor
Swab

During the procedure
The doctor holds your tongue down with a depressor and wipes a swab over your tonsils and the back of your throat.

Obtaining samples

Collecting samples of body fluids, cells, or tissues for testing

As well as taking your medical history and carrying out a physical examination, your doctor may need to collect a sample, such as blood or urine, for testing, either for diagnosis or to monitor the progress of a disease or the effectiveness of treatment.

Obtaining most types of sample is straightforward and painless, and may be carried out by a doctor or nurse as part of a visit to the surgery or by yourself at home. More complex sampling procedures are performed in hospital. The samples are usually sent to a laboratory for testing, although some tests may be carried out in the doctor's surgery.

Types of sample

The sample needed and the types of tests carried out depend on the information your doctor needs. Blood and urine samples can be tested to check the function of various organs, and tests on faeces may be used to identify disorders of the digestive tract. Sputum or other body fluids, cells, or tissues may be tested to look for various diseases, such as cancer. The samples most commonly taken by your GP are described below.

Blood samples Blood tests can help the doctor assess your state of health and look for risk factors associated with certain diseases. For example, a blood sample may be taken to check your blood cholesterol level, which is an indicator of your risk for coronary heart disease. If you visit your doctor with specific symptoms, a blood test may help to diagnose the cause of your illness. Simple tests, such as for blood glucose levels, may be done in the doctor's surgery. For more complex tests, such as tests for microorganisms, tests for levels of hormones or other chemicals, and tests to look at the blood cells and functions, the sample is sent to a laboratory.

Blood tests usually require only a small sample of blood. In most cases, your doctor or nurse will take a sample from a vein using a hollow needle attached to a syringe. Occasionally, only a drop or two of capillary blood is needed, and this is obtained by using a sterile instrument called a lancet to prick the skin.

Urine samples Urine tests can provide information about the condition of the urinary tract and about changes in body chemistry associated with disorders of other systems, such as diabetes mellitus. Usually, your doctor will give you a sterile container in which to collect your urine and instructions about how to collect a suitable sample. In most cases, your doctor will carry out simple dipstick tests in the surgery to detect evidence of infection, glucose, or traces of blood or protein. If further tests are needed, the sample will be sent to a laboratory.

Faecal samples Samples of faeces may be used to help diagnose disorders of the digestive system, such as infections, and a faecal sample is used in the faecal occult blood screening test to detect early signs of colorectal cancer. If you are asked to provide a faecal sample, you will be given a special container and instructions on how to collect the sample. In most cases, the sample is sent to a laboratory for testing.

Body fluids Fluids or secretions from the skin or mucous membranes, such as those lining the throat, are usually collected on a sterile swab (see **Having a throat swab taken**, above) to look for evidence of infection. Semen may also be collected for fertility testing. You can collect some samples, such as sputum or semen yourself, and your doctor may give you a sterile container for the purpose. Techniques for collecting other body fluids are covered in the section on your body and disease. Fluid samples are usually sent to a laboratory.

Cell and tissue samples These types of samples are often used to investigate tumours and may also be used for genetic tests. Cells can sometimes be extracted from body fluids such as urine, or may be scraped from the tissue surfaces of body cavities such as the mouth, throat, or vagina, as in a cervical screening test (p.480). Removal of a larger tissue sample is known as a biopsy and is usually carried out in hospital. The various biopsy techniques are covered in the section on your body and disease. Cell and tissue samples are sent to a laboratory for analysis.

Visualizing internal organs

Modern technological advances have enabled the human body to be visualized and investigated in a wide variety of ways. Imaging creates pictures of internal structures, which may be displayed as digital images on a monitor or, more rarely, recorded on photographic film. Viewing techniques use specialized devices, including endoscopes, to look directly at internal structures of the body.

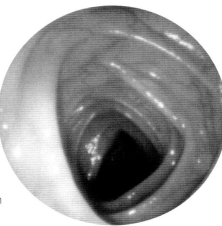

Endoscopic view of the colon
Body cavities and hollow organs such as the colon (above) can be viewed using an instrument called an endoscope.

IMAGING AND VIEWING techniques are often used to confirm a diagnosis or to make one if other tests are not conclusive. These techniques may also be used to screen for some disorders and to monitor the progress of a disease or treatment. Most imaging techniques, and some complex viewing techniques, are carried out in hospital.

Imaging techniques

Since German physicist Wilhelm Röntgen's discovery in 1895 that X-rays can be used to create "shadow pictures" of bones inside the body, X-rays have been used in medical imaging. Simple X-rays are still used today, mainly to image the skeleton although they are also used to image other parts of the body, for example, the chest in the diagnosis of diseases such as pneumonia. X-ray images may be captured by a special detector plate, which produces a signal that is converted by computer into a digital image that is displayed on a monitor, or, less commonly, may be recorded directly on photographic film.

CT (computerized tomography) scanning is a technique that uses X-rays to produce detailed images not only of hard tissues such as bones but also of soft tissues. CT scanning typically produces cross-sectional images ("slices") through the body. Liquids called contrast media can be introduced into hollow or fluid-filled body structures, such as blood vessels or the digestive tract, to enable them to be seen clearly using X-rays. Radionuclide scanning detects the radiation emitted by radioactive substances introduced into the body, allowing doctors to assess cell activity in body tissues.

Other medical imaging techniques include MRI (magnetic resonance imaging), which uses radio waves and magnets to produce clear, very detailed images, and ultrasound scanning, which uses sound waves. Neither of these techniques uses radiation.

Viewing techniques

Depending on the problem, a direct view of part of the body sometimes provides more useful information than a picture created by an imaging technique. Structures near the surface of the body, such as the eardrum, can be viewed directly using simple instruments. Endoscopes are used to look deeper inside the body.

Endoscopes are typically either rigid or flexible and are introduced into the body through a natural opening or through a small incision. They have a light to illuminate the area being viewed; a camera on the end to transmit images to a monitor, or a lens and fibre-optic system for direct visual inspection; and a channel to allow instruments to be passed along inside the endoscope. Flexible and rigid endoscopes may be used not only to examine internal structures but also to remove small samples of tissue for examination and perform various surgical operations. A newer type of endoscope, known as a wireless capsule endoscope, is a self-contained pill-sized device containing a camera, light source, and transmitter. It is swallowed and transmits images as it passes along the digestive tract but cannot be used to take samples or perform surgical procedures.

✚ COMPARISON

Viewing and imaging

The type of visualizing method that is used depends on the part of the body and the problem being investigated. Imaging creates a picture using information about the nature of a tissue, such as its density or the activity of its cells. Viewing, such as endoscopy, provides a direct view of body cavities and other internal organs and structures.

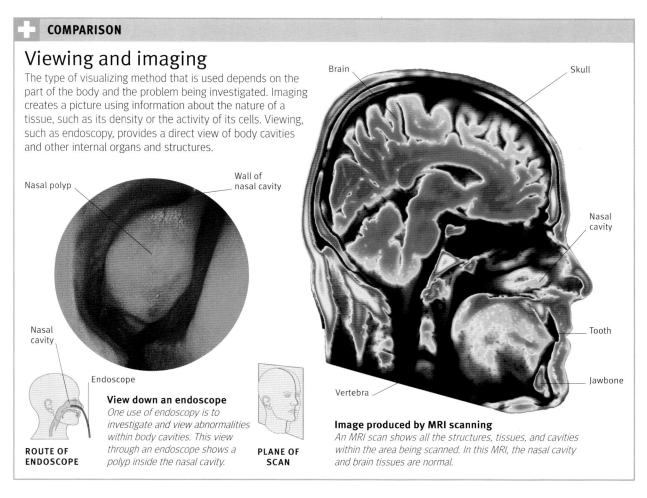

View down an endoscope
One use of endoscopy is to investigate and view abnormalities within body cavities. This view through an endoscope shows a polyp inside the nasal cavity.

Image produced by MRI scanning
An MRI scan shows all the structures, tissues, and cavities within the area being scanned. In this MRI, the nasal cavity and brain tissues are normal.

Imaging using different techniques

The imaging technique that your doctor uses depends on the part of the body being studied and the type of information needed. X-rays show dense tissue, such as bone, most clearly, whereas contrast X-rays provide a clear image of hollow or fluid-filled parts of the body. MRI and CT scanning can provide information about many types of tissue in great detail. An ultrasound scan can assess function by detecting movement, such as blood flow, and radionuclide scanning, such as SPECT and PET, gives detailed information about organ function.

MRI scan
This technique uses radio waves and a magnetic field to produce detailed images, as in this vertical section through the head.

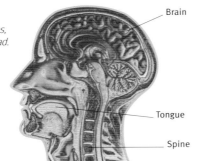

Brain

Tongue

Spine

Carotid artery

Jugular vein

Doppler ultrasound scan
In Doppler scanning, sound waves are used to create an image of blood flow, as in this scan of the blood vessels of the neck, to detect abnormal flow.

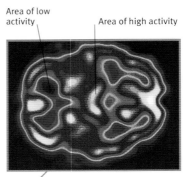

Area of low activity

Area of high activity

SPECT scan
A form of radionuclide scanning, SPECT produces images that show the function of cells. This brain scan shows the pattern of activity of brain cells.

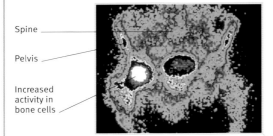

Spine

Pelvis

Increased activity in bone cells

Gas bubble

Liver

Stomach

Rib

Kidney

Spine

CT scan
In CT scanning, X-ray beams are used to create detailed cross-sectional images, as in this horizontal section of the upper abdomen.

Radionuclide scan
This technique measures levels of cell activity to detect an abnormality, such as an area of increased cell activity in this scan of the pelvis.

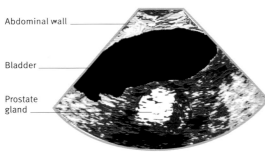

Abdominal wall

Bladder

Prostate gland

Transverse colon

Spine

Pelvis

Rectum

Ultrasound scan
This type of scan uses sound waves to produce images and is used for imaging fluid-filled structures such as the bladder.

Contrast X-ray
In contrast X-rays, an opaque substance, such as barium, is introduced into the body to visualize hollow structures such as the colon.

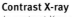

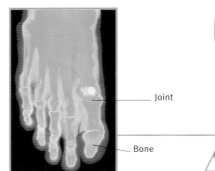

Joint

Bone

Narrowed artery

Thigh muscle

Large artery

Bone

X-ray
Ordinary X-rays produce two-dimensional images showing dense tissue, such as bone, most clearly. This view of a normal foot clearly shows the bones.

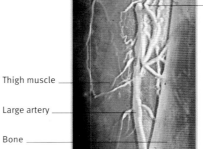

Angiogram
A special contrast X-ray, called an angiogram, can be used to detect an abnormality in a blood vessel, such as this narrowing of a large artery.

Imaging techniques

The aim of imaging is to provide detailed and reliable pictorial information about structures within the body with the minimum risk and discomfort. Most imaging is now highly computerized and has largely replaced exploratory surgery in establishing the presence and extent of disease. Recent techniques are also able to indicate how well a tissue or an organ is functioning.

The first techniques used for imaging the body were based on X-rays, a form of high-energy radiation that is able to pass through body tissues. Some X-rays require particular substances, called contrast media, to improve the visibility of certain structures.

Since then, many new techniques have been introduced, most of which involve the use of computers that control the imaging equipment and are able to create images of the body in three dimensions.

This section begins by explaining the basic imaging methods that use X-rays, which include ordinary and contrast X-rays and CT scanning. Other imaging techniques are then covered, such as MRI and ultrasound scanning, which do not involve the use of radiation, and different types of radionuclide scanning.

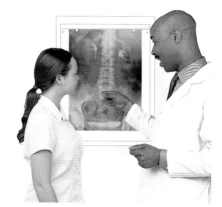

Looking at imaging results
Your doctor may show you your X-ray or scan and explain the results by pointing out the various structures that are visible along with any areas of abnormality.

X-rays

Images produced using high-energy radiation; especially suitable for looking at bone and some soft tissues

X-rays have been used in imaging since they were discovered in 1895. Ordinary X-rays, called plain X-rays, are mainly used for imaging bones and certain soft tissues, such as the breasts. Structures that are hollow or fluid-filled, such as the digestive tract or blood vessels, do not show up well on ordinary X-rays and are more successfully imaged using contrast X-rays (p.132).

Ordinary X-rays are still commonly used in imaging, despite the development of more sophisticated techniques, such as CT scanning (p.132) and MRI (p.133). This is because X-rays are inexpensive, quick, simple to perform, and often provide the doctor with sufficient information to make a diagnosis.

How do they work?
X-rays are a form of radiation similar to light waves but with a higher energy. This high energy enables X-rays to pass through body tissues. The ability of X-rays to penetrate structures depends on the tissue's density. X-rays easily penetrate soft tissues but pass less readily through dense tissue, such as bone.

X-rays blacken photographic film. If a single beam of X-rays is focused on to the body, the parts that allow X-rays through, such as air in the lungs, appear black on the film. Soft tissues, such as skin, fat, and muscle, appear as varying shades of grey. Dense substances, such as bone, are seen as white. As a result of these differences, the final image of the body created by the X-rays on the film looks like a photographic negative. Instead of photographic film, most modern X-ray machines use a special plate that detects the X-rays and converts them into a signal, which is then processed by computer into a digital image that is displayed on a monitor.

X-rays only create two-dimensional images, which means that occasionally two or more X-rays must be taken from different angles to pinpoint a condition. For example, to determine the position of a tumour in the

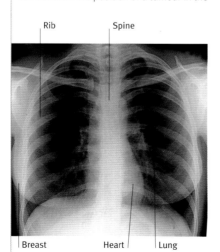

Rib · Spine

Breast · Heart · Lung

Chest X-ray
In this X-ray of a healthy woman's chest, bones appear white, soft tissue appears as shades of grey, and air appears black.

▶ **PROCEDURE**

Having an X-ray

X-rays are ideal for looking for fractures in bone and imaging certain soft tissues. You are positioned on or against a special table or surface so that the part of your body being imaged lies between the image receptor (either an X-ray detector plate or photographic film) and the X-ray source. After positioning the X-ray machine, the radiographer stands behind a screen. You are exposed to X-rays for a fraction of a second, and the whole procedure takes only a few minutes.

During the procedure
The source of the X-rays is positioned directly above the area being examined. You have to keep still so that the X-ray image is clear. In some cases, a second X-ray may be taken from a different angle to give more information.

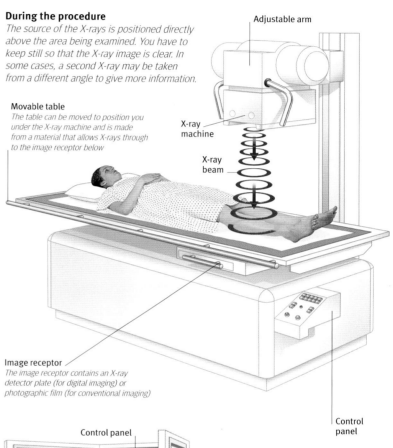

Adjustable arm

Movable table
The table can be moved to position you under the X-ray machine and is made from a material that allows X-rays through to the image receptor below

X-ray machine

X-ray beam

Image receptor
The image receptor contains an X-ray detector plate (for digital imaging) or photographic film (for conventional imaging)

Control panel

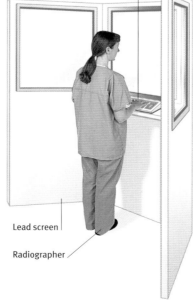

Control panel

Lead screen

Radiographer

Operating the X-ray machine
The radiographer stands behind a protective screen to minimize his or her exposure to X-rays.

RESULTS

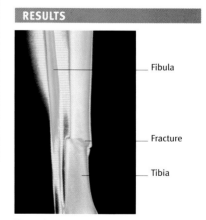

Fibula

Fracture

Tibia

X-ray image
This X-ray clearly shows the two bones of the lower leg, the tibia and the fibula. The main bone, the tibia, has an obvious fracture.

lung, X-rays would be taken of the body from the front and from the side or at a slanting angle.

What are they used for?

Ordinary X-rays produce clear images of bone and are often used to look for fractures (see Having an X-ray, p.131). Chest X-rays (p.300) may be performed to look for an enlarged heart or damaged lung tissue in a person with symptoms, such as chest pain, that may be due to heart or lung disease.

At lower doses, X-rays are useful for examining soft tissues, such as those of the breast, in detail, and they are widely used to screen for breast cancer (see Mammography, p.487). Bone densitometry (p.218) uses low-dose X-rays to measure bone density. This technique is used to screen for and diagnose osteoporosis (p.217), a common condition in postmenopausal women.

What are the risks?

There are no immediate risks from having ordinary X-rays, but there is some risk that radiation may cause damage to body cells, possibly leading to cancer later in life. This risk increases if you are repeatedly exposed to X-ray radiation. The earlier in life you are exposed to radiation, the greater the risk. Radiographers always try to use the minimum amount of radiation when taking X-rays, and modern equipment makes it possible to produce good-quality images with lower doses of radiation than in the past.

During X-ray procedures, areas that are not being imaged may be shielded. For example, when X-raying the pelvis, special care is often taken to shield the reproductive organs to avoid damage to sperm or eggs. The amount of radiation used in ordinary X-rays is not thought to pose a risk to a fetus. However, women are asked if they may be pregnant before having an X-ray and, if so, X-rays that target the uterus are not usually recommended unless they are essential; in some cases, an alternative form of imaging that does not use radiation, such as ultrasound scanning, may be possible. Radiographers are always protected by a lead apron or screen to avoid repeated exposure to radiation.

Contrast X-rays

Images produced using radiation and a substance that makes hollow or fluid-filled structures visible

Hollow or fluid-filled body structures, such as the intestines or blood vessels, do not show up well on an ordinary X-ray image (see X-rays, p.131). A substance called a contrast medium or "dye" can be introduced into these structures to make them visible. Contrast media are opaque to radiation in the same way as dense body

tissues, such as bone. X-rays cannot pass through the media, and areas containing these substances will appear white on an X-ray image.

The contrast medium is injected into the body or introduced orally or rectally, depending on the structure to be imaged. This procedure is generally straightforward, but it may cause discomfort and involve some risks, such as an adverse reaction to the dye. Contrast X-ray procedures are increasingly being replaced by other techniques, in particular CT scanning (right), MRI (opposite page), and ultrasound scanning (p.135), all of which cause less discomfort and involve fewer risks to health.

What are they used for?

Contrast X-rays can produce images of various hollow or fluid-filled structures that do not show up well on ordinary X-rays. Contrast X-rays may be used to image the blood vessels, urinary system, and digestive tract. Different types of contrast media that may be used include iodine (which is soluble in water) and barium sulphate (which is insoluble).

Blood vessels Water-soluble iodine dyes can be carried around the body in the bloodstream. For this reason, and because they show up well on X-rays, they can be used to check whether blood is flowing normally in the blood vessels. Imaging of blood vessels by using X-rays is known as angiography. In this technique, the dye is injected through a catheter that has been guided into a blood vessel until its tip is near the vessel to be studied. The dye flows into the appropriate vessels, making abnormalities, such as blockages, visible on X-rays.

Angiography is often used to look at arteries that have become narrowed or blocked due to fatty deposits in the vessel walls (see Atherosclerosis, p.241). Coronary angiography (p.245) images blood vessels that supply the heart and femoral angiography (p.260) is used to image blood vessels in the leg. Better-quality images are produced by using a computer to remove unwanted background information, a procedure called digital

Blood vessel supplying the heart

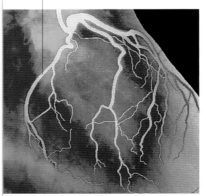

Contrast X-ray of blood vessels
These normal blood vessels supplying the heart muscle contain a water-soluble iodine dye, making them stand out on this colour-enhanced contrast X-ray image.

Large mass of barium

Junction of stomach and duodenum

Barium coating inside the stomach

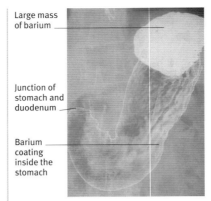

Barium contrast X-ray
A swallowed barium solution makes this normal stomach visible on an X-ray image. The barium is at the top of the stomach because the person is lying head down.

subtraction angiography. Techniques such as CT angiography, magnetic resonance angiography, and duplex ultrasound scanning (p.135) are now commonly used to obtain the same information noninvasively.

Urinary system When injected into a vein, dye circulates in the bloodstream and becomes concentrated in the kidneys before it is excreted in urine. The dye can therefore be used to image various parts of the urinary system, a technique known as intravenous urography. As the dye passes through the urinary tract, it outlines the ureter (the tube linking the kidneys and the bladder) and the bladder. If the bladder and urethra (the tube that takes urine from the bladder out of the body) alone are to be imaged by the X-rays, the contrast medium may be inserted into the bladder through a catheter that is passed up through the urethra. Intravenous urography may still be used to look for suspected kidney disease and obstructions in the urinary system, although CT urography (p.447) is now increasingly used.

Digestive tract Barium sulphate is a thick, insoluble, chalky liquid that does not allow X-rays to pass through it and shows up well on X-ray images. It moves slowly through the digestive tract and is not absorbed by the body; therefore it is a good contrast medium for examining the digestive tract. Barium X-ray examinations can also be useful for studying functions such as swallowing. However, endoscopy (p.138) is often more appropriate than barium investigations.

Barium sulphate is drunk if the upper digestive tract from the oesophagus to the duodenum (the first part of the small intestine) is to be examined. This procedure is known as a barium swallow (p.404) or a barium meal (p.404). Barium meals may be used to investigate problems of the upper digestive tract, including swallowing difficulties and indigestion (see Nonulcer dyspepsia, p.397). The progression of the barium through the digestive tract can be followed by taking X-rays at intervals or recording video images. However, barium meals are now used only rarely, having been largely superseded by a combination of endoscopy and CT scanning.

Barium sulphate may also sometimes be used to image the colon. It is given rectally as an enema after a laxative has been taken to empty the bowel. Barium enemas may be used to detect abnormal growths in the colon lining, such as polyps (see Polyps in the colon, p.418) and colorectal cancer (p.421).

In double-contrast radiography, air is introduced into the digestive tract to replace the barium, which remains only on the digestive tract lining. This technique gives a detailed image of the lining and may be used for detecting changes due to conditions such as Crohn's disease (p.417).

What are the risks?

Radiation can cause damage to body cells, which may rarely lead to cancer later in life. Contrast X-rays expose you to a relatively large quantity of radiation because they require several X-rays.

Injecting contrast media carries a minor risk of serious complications such as anaphylaxis (p.285). People who have asthma triggered by an allergy or who have a known sensitivity to iodine are advised not to have contrast X-rays or are pretreated with drugs such as antihistamines (p.585) or corticosteroids (p.600), or other contrast media may be used. Most people experience a flushing sensation as dye is injected. Barium sulphate may also cause constipation.

CT scanning

Computer-assisted imaging using a succession of X-ray beams to produce cross-sectional images through the body

Computerized tomography (CT) scanning uses X-rays (p.131) in conjunction with a computer. A series of X-rays is passed through the body at slightly different angles to produce highly detailed cross-sectional images ("slices") of the body, called tomograms. CT scanning obtains detailed information about organs painlessly and can replace exploratory surgery in many cases.

Eye **Nasal cavity**

Brain tissue

Ear

Skull **Ear cavity**

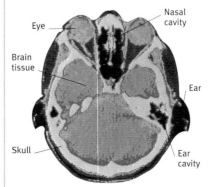

CT scan of the head
This normal CT scan of the head viewed from above clearly shows the different structures and cavities within the skull.

► **PROCEDURE**

Having a CT scan

A CT scanner uses a series of X-ray beams to build up images of the body in "slices". Several individual scans may be carried out to create detailed images of the area that is being investigated. CT scanning can detect hundreds of levels of density and is used to produce pictures of many different parts of the body. The radiographer positions you on a motorized bed and moves you into the scanner. If you feel anxious, you may be given a sedative.

RESULTS

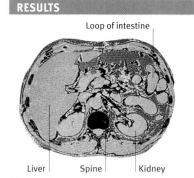

Loop of intestine

Liver | Spine | Kidney

CT scan of abdomen
Body parts of different densities are shown as different colours in this colour-enhanced CT scan of the abdomen.

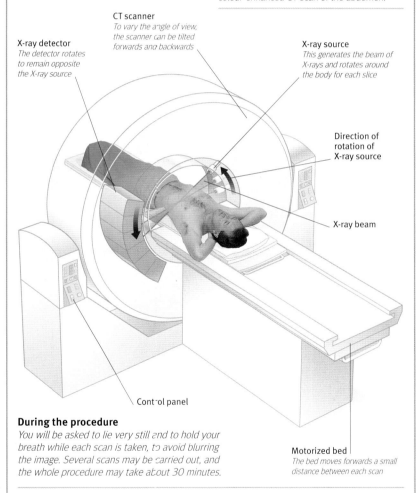

CT scanner
To vary the angle of view, the scanner can be tilted forwards and backwards

X-ray detector
The detector rotates to remain opposite the X-ray source

X-ray source
This generates the beam of X-rays and rotates around the body for each slice

Direction of rotation of X-ray source

X-ray beam

Control panel

Motorized bed
The bed moves forwards a small distance between each scan

During the procedure
You will be asked to lie very still and to hold your breath while each scan is taken, to avoid blurring the image. Several scans may be carried out, and the whole procedure may take about 30 minutes.

Operating the CT scanner
The radiographer moves to an adjacent room to operate the scanner by using a computer. A microphone allows him or her to communicate with you. Being in a separate room protects the radiographer from radiation. A doctor may oversee a scan or control the scanner.

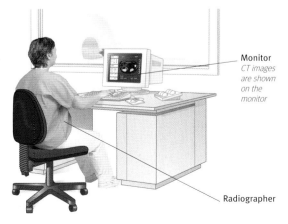

Monitor
CT images are shown on the monitor

Radiographer

How does it work?

The CT scanner consists of an X-ray source and an X-ray detector, both of which rotate during the procedure so that they remain opposite each other. CT scanning uses X-rays in a different way from an ordinary X-ray machine to give a higher-quality image. Ordinary X-rays show only a few levels of density, while the detector within a CT scanner can see hundreds of different levels of density, including fibrous tissue in solid organs such as the liver. Instead of sending one beam of radiation through your body, the X-ray source inside a CT scanner emits a succession of narrow beams as it moves through an arc. The X-ray detector then picks up the radiation after it has passed through various body tissues (*see* **Having a CT scan**, left). After each arc is completed, the bed is moved forwards a small distance.

The information from the detector is then sent to the computer, which builds up cross-sectional images of the body and displays them on a monitor. These images can be stored as computer files or printed on conventional X-ray film. More sophisticated computers can produce three-dimensional images from standard CT data.

Current CT scanners use the spiral (or helical) technique, in which the scanner rotates around you as the bed moves continuously through the scanner so that the X-ray beams follow a spiral course. This type of CT scanning produces three-dimensional images and reduces the time taken to complete the scans.

What is it used for?

The CT scans performed most often are those of the head and trunk. CT scanning of the head is commonly used to investigate the brain following a stroke (p.329) or head injury, or if a brain tumour (p.327) is suspected. Chest CT scans are used to detect lung disease and secondary tumours as well as abnormalities of the blood vessels supplying the heart and lungs. Abdominal CT scans are used to detect tumours, to investigate internal bleeding due to trauma, and to diagnose disorders in which organs are enlarged or inflamed, such as polycystic kidney disease (p.449). CT scans can also be used to guide biopsy procedures.

CT scanning is able to produce much clearer images of bone than MRI (right). Blood vessels can also be imaged. These images may be enhanced by using a contrast medium (a substance that makes a fluid-filled or hollow structure visible on the image).

What are the risks?

Imaging techniques that use radiation may damage body cells, which may increase the risk of cancer in the long term. The dose for a CT procedure depends on the number of cross sections imaged. Scanning time is reduced for spiral CT scans, but the dose is the same as in a normal CT scan. Radiation exposure during CT scans is generally quite low but nevertheless may be significant.

MRI

A radiation-free, computer-assisted imaging technique that uses a strong magnetic field and radio waves

The technique of magnetic resonance imaging (MRI) has been used since the early 1980s to provide highly detailed sectional images of internal organs and structures. These images are created by a computer using information received from a scanner. MRI does not involve potentially harmful radiation; instead, it uses magnets and radio waves.

Although MRI is a relatively expensive procedure and MRI scans tend to take longer than other techniques, it does have several advantages. Images from MRI are similar to those produced by CT scanning (opposite page), but MRI can distinguish abnormal tissue, such as a tumour, from normal tissue much more clearly. MRI scans can also be taken at a greater range of planes through the body than is possible with CT scanning and therefore can be used to image any part of the body. MRI is radiation-free and is considered to be one of the safest imaging techniques available.

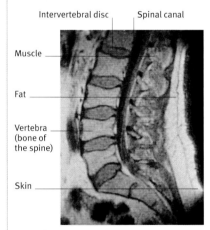

Intervertebral disc | Spinal canal

Muscle

Fat

Vertebra (bone of the spine)

Skin

MRI of the lower spine
This MRI scan of a healthy person's lower spine clearly shows the different structures, including muscle, skin, and bone.

How does it work?

During an MRI scan, you lie inside a scanner surrounded by a large, powerful magnet. A receiving magnet is then placed around the part of your body that is to be investigated. If large areas, such as the abdomen, are to be imaged, the receiving magnet is fitted inside the MRI scanner; for smaller areas, such as a joint, a magnet may be placed around the part to be scanned (*see* **Having an MRI scan**, p.134).

Your body, like everything else, is made up of atoms. When the atoms in your body are exposed to a strong magnetic field from the large magnet in the scanner, they line up parallel to each other. Short pulses of radio waves from a radiofrequency source then briefly knock the atoms out of alignment.

As they realign, the atoms emit tiny signals, which are detected by the receiving magnet. Information about these signals is then passed on to a computer, which builds up an image based on the signals' strength and location.

MRI images can be enhanced by the use of a contrast medium to highlight particular structures in the body, such as tumours and blood vessels.

What is it used for?

MRI can provide clear images of any part of the body. This type of scanning is especially useful for looking at the brain and for detecting brain tumours (p.327). MRI is also valuable for looking at the spinal cord and may be used to investigate lower back pain (p.225). Sports injuries (p.231), especially in the knee (see **Torn knee cartilage**, p.234), are increasingly being examined using MRI. MRI may also be used to examine the breasts. MRI scans show the location of tumours within the breast tissue more accurately than plain two-dimensional X-rays (see **Mammography**, p.487). In addition, because MRI does not use radiation, MRI scans can be repeated frequently, allowing doctors to monitor a condition safely.

A particular type of MRI, called magnetic resonance angiography (MRA), enables doctors to look at blood flow by comparing the signals received from stationary tissue with those received from flowing blood. Another type of MRI, called functional magnetic resonance imaging (fMRI), can reveal areas of neural activity in the brain ("brain mapping"). This technique is relatively new and is currently used mainly for research but it could potentially be used diagnostically, for example, to assess the effects on brain function of stroke, tumours, or degenerative conditions such as Alzheimer's disease (p.331).

What are the risks?

There are no known risks or side effects from MRI scanning. The scans do not use ionizing radiation and can be performed repeatedly. However, because the scanner uses a powerful magnet, it may interfere with the functioning of certain devices, such as pacemakers, cochlear implants, hearing aids, and implanted drug pumps. If you have any metal in your body, such as a surgical implant, you should tell your doctor before having MRI. You should also tell your doctor if you have an IUD fitted, because some have metal in them. During a scan, any magnetic metal items in your body will move around under the influence of the magnetic field and could cause serious damage. For this reason, your doctor may request X-rays to look for metal in your body before you have an MRI scan.

Although there is no evidence that MRI scanning poses a risk during pregnancy, doctors do not usually recommend MRI during the first three months, as a precaution.

▶ **PROCEDURE**

Having an MRI scan

MRI scanning can be used to image any part of the body but is most commonly used to investigate the brain and spinal cord, the heart and blood vessels, organs such as the liver, and bones and joints. You are positioned on a motorized bed and a receiving magnet is placed around the part of your body to be examined. You are then moved into the tunnel of the scanner.

Several individual scans will be taken during the procedure. You will have to lie within the scanner for up to about 90 minutes and therefore it is important you are as comfortable as possible. You may be given earplugs or headphones because the scanner can be noisy. Your doctor may give you a sedative if you are anxious or claustrophobic.

During the procedure
You will be asked to keep very still while an individual scan is being taken. Although complete procedures may take 15–90 minutes, each scan takes only 3–5 minutes. This knee scan would take about 30 minutes.

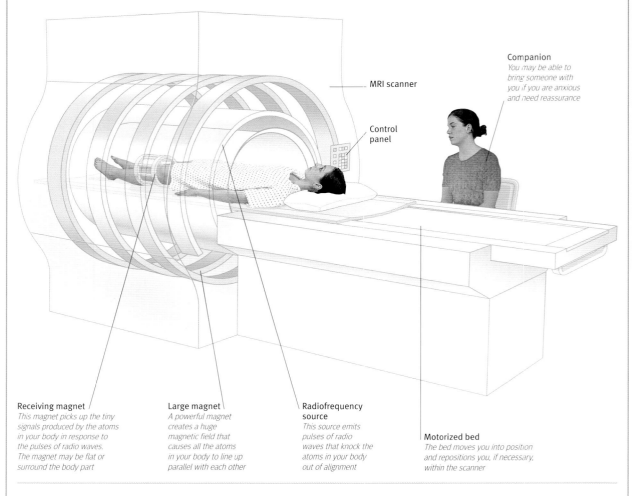

Companion
You may be able to bring someone with you if you are anxious and need reassurance

MRI scanner

Control panel

Receiving magnet
This magnet picks up the tiny signals produced by the atoms in your body in response to the pulses of radio waves. The magnet may be flat or surround the body part

Large magnet
A powerful magnet creates a huge magnetic field that causes all the atoms in your body to line up parallel with each other

Radiofrequency source
This source emits pulses of radio waves that knock the atoms in your body out of alignment

Motorized bed
The bed moves you into position and repositions you, if necessary, within the scanner

Operating the MRI scanner
The scanner is operated from an adjacent room because the computer controlling the scanner has to be protected from the powerful magnetic field created during the procedure. The radiographer may give you instructions through an intercom about when you need to keep still.

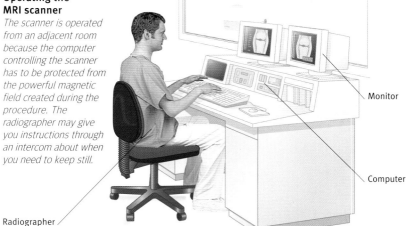

Radiographer

Monitor

Computer

RESULTS

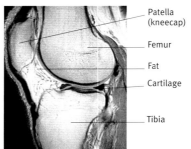

Patella (kneecap)

Femur

Fat

Cartilage

Tibia

MRI scan of a knee
An MRI scan of the knee joint gives a clear picture of its internal structure, revealing all the tissues, including bone, fat, and cartilage.

Ultrasound scanning

A technique that uses high-frequency sound waves to image internal structures or a fetus in the uterus

Ultrasound scanning uses sound waves of a very high frequency, inaudible to the human ear. The sound waves travel through the body and their echoes are processed to create images of internal structures or of a fetus in the uterus. Ultrasound scanning is a versatile technique that can show movement as well as structure, and the range of examinations using this method is constantly expanding. For example, organs situated deep within body cavities, such as those in the pelvis, which were previously difficult to image, can now be examined using ultrasound scanning. Since ultrasound does not involve ionizing radiation, it is thought to be completely safe.

How does it work?

The principle of ultrasound scanning is similar to that used in naval sonar, in which sound waves are bounced off objects deep in the ocean. In ultrasound scanning, a device called a transducer converts an electric current into high-frequency sound waves. The transducer is usually hand-held and used on the skin surface, but it is sometimes inserted on a probe into a natural opening such as the vagina or rectum. The transducer may also be incorporated into an endoscope, a viewing tube, to image deeper inside the body. Sound waves emitted by the transducer are focused in a narrow beam that passes through different parts of the body as the transducer is moved back and forth. Sound waves pass readily through soft tissue and fluid and are reflected at a point where different densities meet, such as where fluid in the bladder meets the bladder wall.

In addition to sending out the sound waves, the ultrasound transducer acts as the receiver by converting the reflected echoes back into electrical signals. These

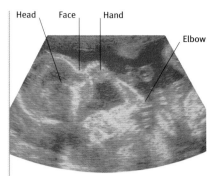

Ultrasound scan of a fetus
Imaging using ultrasound is a useful technique for looking at the movement of a fetus and monitoring fetal growth. There is no known risk to the health of the fetus.

signals are processed by a computer and displayed as a two-dimensional image on a monitor (*see* **Having an ultrasound scan**, left). The images are updated continuously, enabling scans to show movement, such as that of the fetus in the uterus (*see* **Ultrasound scanning in pregnancy**, p.512) or valves opening and closing within the heart (*see* **Echocardiography**, p.255). A specific type of ultrasound known as Doppler ultrasound scanning (p.259) uses short pulses of ultrasound to look at the direction and the speed of blood flow. Blood that is flowing away from the Doppler probe appears blue on the scan, while blood that is flowing towards it appears red. A mixture of colours indicates turbulence. The speed of blood flow is measured by a computer.

What is it used for?

Most pregnant women will have at least one ultrasound scan to examine the growing fetus. Ultrasound can also be used to image the brain of a newborn baby through the fontanelles (the soft spots in a baby's head between the bones of the skull). Using ultrasound in this way can identify bleeding into the brain from the surrounding blood vessels, a potential problem in premature babies.

Ultrasound scanning is commonly used to investigate internal organs because it produces good images of soft tissue, such as the liver, and fluid-filled structures, such as the

gallbladder. It can also be used to examine the structure of the heart and its movement. Used endoscopically through the oesophagus, ultrasound can provide more detailed information on the heart or investigate organs deep within the body, such as the stomach and pancreas. The transducer can also be inserted into the vagina on a probe to examine the female reproductive organs. Ultrasound can be used on the eye to locate foreign bodies or to investigate disorders, such as retinal detachment (p.360). It can also be used to guide tissue sampling by pinpointing an abnormal area, such as in a prostate gland biopsy (p.464).

Doppler ultrasound scans are routinely used to investigate blood vessels in which blood flow may be reduced. For example, Doppler scans are often used to detect blood clots in the veins (*see* **Deep vein thrombosis**, p.263) and to detect thickened artery walls, particularly in the arteries in the neck (*see* **Carotid doppler scanning**, p.328). Sometimes, conventional ultrasound may be combined with Doppler ultrasound (known as duplex ultrasound scanning) to investigate blood vessels and blood flow. In pregnant women with high blood pressure, Doppler ultrasound may be used to investigate the uterine artery, which carries blood to the uterus.

What are the risks?

Ultrasound scanning is not thought to cause any adverse effects and can be repeated as often as necessary. It is the only imaging technique considered safe for routine screening of a fetus.

▶ PROCEDURE

Having an ultrasound scan

In ultrasound scanning, a device called a transducer emits high-frequency sound waves and receives their echoes to produce images on a monitor. To ensure good contact between the transducer and the body, the radiographer places gel on the skin over the area to be examined before moving the transducer over it. An ultrasound scan takes 10–30 minutes and is completely painless.

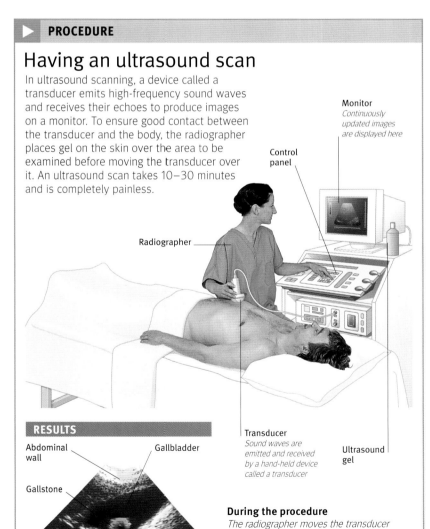

Monitor
Continuously updated images are displayed here

Control panel

Radiographer

Transducer
Sound waves are emitted and received by a hand-held device called a transducer

Ultrasound gel

RESULTS

Abdominal wall

Gallbladder

Gallstone

Ultrasound scan of gallbladder
In this ultrasound scan, the fluid-filled gallbladder and the gallstone it contains are clearly visible.

During the procedure
The radiographer moves the transducer back and forth over the area using gentle pressure. Modern scanners continually update the image on the monitor, which means the radiographer can monitor movement. He or she may use the control panel to make measurements, such as the diameter of a gallstone.

Head   Face   Hand   Elbow

Doppler ultrasound scan of an artery
The colour of the blood on a Doppler ultrasound scan indicates direction of flow. The blue in the scan above indicates blood that is flowing away from the probe.

Point where artery divides

Blood flowing away from the probe

Radionuclide scanning

A technique in which a radioactive substance is introduced into the body to assess structure and function of tissues

The technique of radionuclide scanning produces images using radiation emitted from a substance within the body. The radioactive substance called a radionuclide, is introduced into the body and taken up by the organ or tissue to be imaged. A counter positioned outside the body detects the radiation that is emitted by the radionuclide and transmits this information to a computer. The computer then converts the information into images. Radionuclide scanning is used both to image the structure of many internal organs and to provide a measure of their function. SPECT scanning (p.136) and PET scanning (p.137) are two specialized forms of radionuclide scanning.

How does it work?

Radionuclides are normally introduced into the body by a single intravenous injection and are then carried in the bloodstream to the tissues (*see* **Having a radionuclide scan**, p.136). Xenon gas, one particular type of radionuclide used during a lung scan, is inhaled (*see* **Radionuclide lung scanning**, p.302).

Different tissues take up different radionuclides. A specific radionuclide is chosen because it will accumulate in the particular tissues to be investigated; for example, iodine is taken up by the thyroid gland, and radioactive iodine is therefore injected to produce a radionuclide scan of the gland.

A radionuclide emits radiation in the form of gamma rays, which are similar to X-rays. The gamma rays are detected outside the body by a gamma camera. Within the camera are detectors that pick up the radiation and convert information about its quantity and location into a form that can be analysed by a computer. The computer then builds up an image and displays it on a monitor. The image is built up dot by dot, with each dot representing a certain amount of radiation.

Radionuclide scans show parts of the body as areas of colour of varying intensity. Areas of intense colour are called "hot spots"; these are areas where there is a high uptake of radionuclide. Areas of less intense colour, called "cold spots", are areas where the radionuclide uptake is low. The greater the amount of tissue activity, the greater the uptake.

What is it used for?
An important feature of radionuclide scanning is that it can produce a "map" of an organ based on the activity of its tissues,

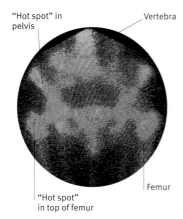

"Hot spot" in pelvis — Vertebra

Femur

"Hot spot" in top of femur

Radionuclide bone scan
This radionuclide scan of the pelvis shows "hot spots" where there is increased uptake of radioactive substance by the bone tissue. In this case, they are cancerous deposits.

therefore providing information about how that organ or tissue is functioning. This imaging technique may be used to detect abnormal levels of activity in organs such as the thyroid gland and kidneys, and it is useful for detecting some tumours of these organs. A radionuclide scan of bone will indicate areas that have increased activity, which might be due to problems such as Paget's disease of the bone (p.218) or cancer. Changes in the function of a tissue or an organ often develop

before structural changes occur, and radionuclide scanning can detect some diseases at a significantly earlier stage than most other imaging techniques. For example, a radionuclide scan of bone can detect infection of bone tissue (*see* **Osteomyelitis**, p.219) weeks before it would become apparent on an ordinary X-ray.

Radionuclide scans are particularly useful for assessing how well a treatment has worked. Scans may be done before and after a particular treatment to compare the function of an organ.

Two particular types of radionuclide scanning may be used to look at the function of the heart. Thallium scanning reveals areas of the heart muscle with a poor blood supply and is used to look at the activity of the heart muscle during exercise (*see* **Exercise testing**, p.244). MUGA (multiple-gated acquisition scanning) is a technique in which the blood flow into and out of the heart is measured to assess how efficiently the heart pumps blood.

What are the risks?
Radionuclide scanning has no immediate risks, but radiation-based imaging may damage the body cells, leading to an increased risk of cancer in later life. However, radionuclides are always administered in very small amounts, and they break down quickly in the body.

SPECT scanning

A type of radionuclide scanning that produces images of blood flow to tissues

First used in the 1970s for research, single photon emission computerized tomography (SPECT) scanning is now used for imaging. This technique is a specialized type of radionuclide scanning (p.135) and provides information on blood flow to various body tissues.

SPECT scanning is extremely sensitive and can target certain organs more easily than ordinary radionuclide scanning procedures. However, only a few centres offer SPECT scanning because expensive equipment is involved and specialist technicians are needed.

How does it work?
Before a SPECT scan, a radioactive substance (radionuclide) is intravenously injected. Radionuclides are distributed in the blood and are taken up by specific tissues. The more blood flowing through the tissues, the more radionuclide is taken up. The radionuclide emits radiation in the form of particles called photons. Photons are detected outside the body by a rotating

---

▶ **PROCEDURE**

Having a radionuclide scan

Radionuclide scanning is used both to image structures and to assess their function. In most cases, an injection of a radioactive substance (radionuclide) is given before the scan, but you may be asked to inhale radioactive gas if your lungs are being scanned (*see* **Radionuclide lung scanning**, p.302). The choice of radionuclide depends on the structure being imaged. During the scan, you lie still on a motorized bed and the radiographer moves you and a camera into position. The camera detects radiation emitted by the radionuclide, and a computer builds up an image.

RESULTS

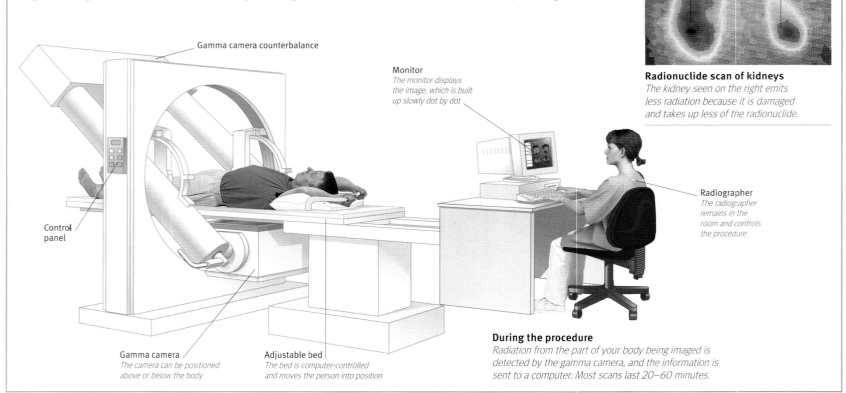

Normal kidney — Damaged kidney

Radionuclide scan of kidneys
The kidney seen on the right emits less radiation because it is damaged and takes up less of the radionuclide.

Gamma camera counterbalance

Monitor
The monitor displays the image, which is built up slowly dot by dot

Control panel

Radiographer
The radiographer remains in the room and controls the procedure

Gamma camera
The camera can be positioned above or below the body

Adjustable bed
The bed is computer-controlled and moves the person into position

During the procedure
Radiation from the part of your body being imaged is detected by the gamma camera, and the information is sent to a computer. Most scans last 20–60 minutes.

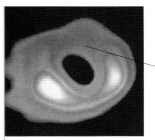

BEFORE SURGERY

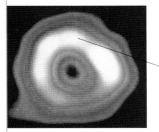

AFTER SURGERY

Area of muscle with no blood supply

Area of restored blood flow

SPECT scans of heart muscle
These SPECT scans show horizontal cross sections through the heart. Before surgery, the absence of radionuclide in part of the heart indicates there is no blood flow in that area. Surgery has restored the blood flow.

camera, which can move through 360°. A computer converts the information from the camera into cross-sectional images, on which the different tissues or organs can be coloured to assist identification. SPECT scanning can be used to produce both vertical and horizontal cross sections through the body, and the data can also be manipulated by a computer to produce three-dimensional images.

What is it used for?
SPECT scanning is mainly used to find out how well an organ is functioning by looking at the supply of blood to its tissues. SPECT scanning is particularly useful for assessing the function of the heart and brain, especially for investigating epileptic seizures (*see* **Epilepsy**, p.324).

What are the risks?
SPECT scanning presents no immediate risks to health, but it does involve radioactive substances and therefore has the potential to damage the body cells, which may increase the risk of cancer in later life. However, SPECT scanning uses only small amounts of radionuclides, which break down quickly in the body.

PET scanning

A type of radionuclide scanning that creates an image based on the function of individual cells within an organ or tissue

Positron emission tomography (PET) scanning is a special form of radionuclide scanning (p.135). The technique was originally used as a research tool in the 1970s but is now also used for medical imaging.

Unlike certain other techniques, such as CT scanning (p.132), PET does not produce good structural images; instead, it gives information about the chemical activity of tissues or organs. It can also be used to assess blood flow.

How does it work?
By measuring the uptake by a tissue or organ of certain molecules, such as glucose or oxygen, doctors can assess how well an organ is functioning. The molecules that are to be taken up by the tissue or organ are labelled with a radioactive substance (radionuclide) before being introduced into the body.

PET uses radionuclides that emit particles called positrons. The radiation that these particles generate is detected by a PET scanner. The number of positrons emitted by an area of tissue or an organ indicates how much radionuclide it has taken up and therefore how chemically active that region is. A PET scanner is a doughnut-shaped machine incorporating detectors that pick up radiation all around the patient. The technique produces cross-sectional images that can be colour coded according to the concentration of radioactivity.

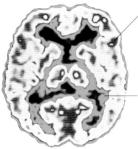

Area of high brain activity
High levels of activity are shown by red and yellow

Area of low brain activity
Low levels of activity are shown by blue and black

PET scan of brain
This normal PET scan shows high activity on the outside of the brain, the grey matter, and lower activity deeper inside.

What is it used for?
PET is mainly used to study the brain and the heart. The radionuclides used in PET can label the molecules related to blood flow as well as those involved in chemical activity. Consequently, PET can show areas of decreased blood flow while also establishing whether the cells in the area being studied are still chemically active and capable of recovery or whether they are dead. PET scanning is sometimes used to locate the origin of epileptic activity (*see* **Epilepsy**, p.324) in the brain and to investigate brain function in certain other neurological conditions, such as Alzheimer's disease (p.331). PET may also be used to detect tumours because the level of chemical activity in abnormal tissue is higher than that in healthy tissue.

What are the risks?
Like in other radiation-based imaging techniques, PET scanning carries a risk of cell damage that may lead to cancer later in life. However, radionuclides are used in small amounts and rapidly break down into harmless elements.

Viewing techniques

Viewing structures or organs in the body is often important for screening, diagnosis, or monitoring disease. Structures that are easily accessible, such as the ears, may be viewed directly using basic viewing instruments; those deeper inside the body are usually viewed indirectly, using complex optical instruments called endoscopes to transmit images on to a monitor screen.

Some viewing techniques may be used as part of a routine examination. For example, your doctor can look at your ears, eyes, and throat simply and quickly in his or her surgery. Each of the instruments used is designed to view a particular part of the body. For example, an otoscope is used to look at the ears and an ophthalmoscope to look at the eyes. The first article covers these basic viewing techniques.

To view other organs deeper within the body, your doctor may arrange for an endoscopic investigation. Endoscopy is discussed in the second article. An endoscope is a viewing device that enables body cavities or internal organs to be inspected. Most endoscopes are flexible or rigid tube-like instruments but there is also a new type (called a wireless capsule endoscope) that essentially consists of a camera in a pill-sized, self-contained capsule. Each type of endoscope is designed to view a particular part of the body.

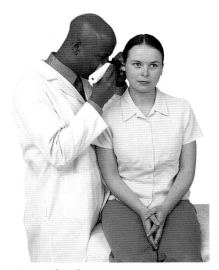

Inspecting the ear
During a routine checkup, your doctor may use a special viewing device called an otoscope to look inside the ear and examine the ear canal and eardrum.

Basic viewing techniques

The use of simple instruments to look at tissues near the surface of the body

Instruments that can be used to view body structures and organs directly have been developed and improved considerably over the past 100 years. Some of these instruments have been replaced by endoscopes (*see* **Endoscopy**, p.138). However, some basic viewing instruments are still frequently used in a doctor's surgery as part of a routine examination because they are simple to use and cause minimal discomfort.

How do they work?
In order to examine the interior of a natural opening, such as the ear canal, your doctor will usually need a source of light that can be focused on the area to be examined and some form of magnification. These two elements are often incorporated into a single viewing instrument, such as an otoscope, which is used for inspecting the ear.

For other natural openings, such as the vagina or nose, your doctor may need to use an additional instrument, called a speculum, to hold the passage open and keep other structures out of the way during viewing. In some cases, a speculum may also be used to make access easier and to enable the doctor to take samples of tissue.

The light-sensitive retina at the back of the eye can be viewed from the outside through the pupil. The instrument used to do this, called an ophthalmoscope, incorporates magnifying lenses and a source of light.

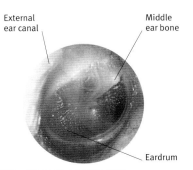

External ear canal

Middle ear bone

Eardrum

View through an otoscope
This view shows a healthy eardrum and ear canal as a doctor would see it through an otoscope. One of the bones of the middle ear is visible through the eardrum.

What are they used for?
Your doctor may perform basic viewing techniques as part of a routine physical examination to assess a particular area of the body or to investigate symptoms in that area. For example, if you have earache, your doctor may examine your ear

(*see* **Otoscopy**, p.374), and to investigate hoarseness, your doctor may look at your larynx (voice box) by using a procedure known as mirror laryngoscopy (p.294). Basic viewing techniques can also be part of screening procedures. For example, if you have a long-term disorder such as diabetes mellitus (p.437), which is associated with retinal damage, your doctor may examine your eyes by means of ophthalmoscopy (p.360) and slit-lamp examination (p.358) so that he or she can detect damage at an early stage. In addition, some types of tissue sample, such as tissue from the cervix, can be taken with the help of a viewing instrument (*see* **Colposcopy**, p.481).

In some cases, it is possible to take photographs through basic viewing instruments, such as an ophthalmoscope. Photographs taken at different times can be compared to monitor a condition.

What are the risks?

An examination using basic viewing techniques is completely safe and may be repeated as often as necessary to monitor or screen for a disorder. Most examinations cause little or no discomfort, and anaesthesia is not usually necessary. However, when viewing the larynx and throat, a local anaesthetic spray may be used to numb the throat.

Endoscopy

The use of viewing devices to look at organs or structures deep within the body

During endoscopy, a viewing device known as an endoscope is introduced deep into the body so that internal structures can be examined visually. Access into the body is usually through a natural opening, such as the mouth, anus, or urethra, although some endoscopes are introduced through small incisions made in the skin.

The first endoscopes were rigid, but various flexible instruments have since been developed. Although most endoscopes now in routine use are flexible, rigid types are preferred in certain cases, including investigations in which there is a short distance from the skin to the structure being viewed, such as in an examination of the knee joint. There is also a comparatively new type of endoscope, called a wireless capsule endoscope, which may occasionally be used to investigate certain gastrointestinal problems, such as bleeding of unknown cause. However, because this is a recently developed diagnostic tool, it is not yet widely available.

How do they work?

There are many types of endoscope, each specifically designed to investigate a particular part of the body. Flexible and rigid endoscopes differ in appearance, but they share many of the same features and operate in a similar way. For example, both forms of endoscope are tube-like instruments that use light, reflection, and magnification to show body structures clearly. Wireless capsule endoscopes essentially consist of a miniature camera, light source, and transmission circuit in a self-contained, pill-sized unit, together with an external data recorder.

Flexible endoscopes The development of flexible endoscopes has been made possible by the invention of fibre-optics. Fibre-optics use thin, flexible fibres of glass or plastic (optical fibres) that transmit light along their length by internal reflections. The main part of flexible endoscope consists of a long, thin tube containing several channels that run along its length. Some channels in the endoscope carry optical fibres to provide light or transmit the image back up to the eyepiece. Other channels contain wires to control the direction of the endoscope. Channels may also be used to pump or suck air or fluid into or out of the area being examined. Other channels may be used to pass down various instruments, such as biopsy forceps or scissors.

Most flexible endoscopes have a miniature camera built into their tip, and the view recorded by the camera is displayed on a monitor. This facility allows the doctor and his or her colleagues, and sometimes the patient, to observe an investigation together and makes it possible for a record to be kept for reference.

Rigid endoscopes These endoscopes are normally much shorter than flexible endoscopes and are usually inserted through an incision in the skin. Like flexible endoscopes, rigid endoscopes use a fibre-optic light source. However, other instruments, such as those used to hold tissues out of the way or to perform a surgical procedure, are passed through a separate incision rather than down the endoscope.

To allow the surfaces of the different organs or structures to be seen clearly, investigations using rigid endoscopes often involve expanding the organ or body cavity with gas or fluid to separate tissue

---

▶ **PROCEDURE**

Flexible endoscopy

Flexible endoscopy uses a specially designed viewing instrument to investigate organs and structures inside the body. Before you undergo an endoscopic examination, you may be given an anaesthetic or sedative. The endoscope is inserted through a natural opening, such as the mouth, or a small incision and is guided to the

appropriate area by the specialist. A tiny camera at the tip of the endoscope sends views back to the eyepiece and monitor. Very fine surgical instruments may be passed down the endoscope, allowing minor procedures, such as the removal of tissue samples, to be carried out.

During the procedure
For an investigation of the stomach and duodenum, you will be asked to lie on your side. You may be sedated or have local anaesthetic sprayed on the back of your throat. A flexible endoscope is then passed into your digestive tract through your mouth.

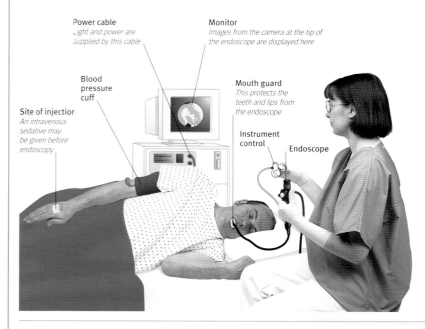

Power cable
Light and power are supplied by this cable

Monitor
Images from the camera at the tip of the endoscope are displayed here

Blood pressure cuff

Mouth guard
This protects the teeth and lips from the endoscope

Site of injection
An intravenous sedative may be given before endoscopy

Instrument control

Endoscope

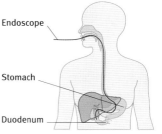

Endoscope

Stomach

Duodenum

ROUTE OF ENDOSCOPE

VIEW

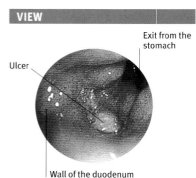

Exit from the stomach

Ulcer

Wall of the duodenum

Endoscopic view of the duodenum
This endoscopic view shows the inside of the duodenum. An ulcer is visible on the wall.

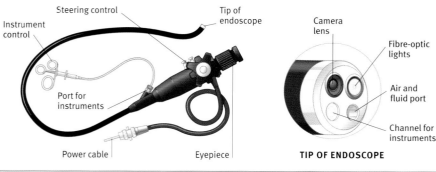

Steering control

Instrument control

Tip of endoscope

Port for instruments

Power cable

Eyepiece

Camera lens

Fibre-optic lights

Air and fluid port

Channel for instruments

TIP OF ENDOSCOPE

Flexible endoscope
A flexible endoscope contains separate channels to carry water, air, a camera lens, instruments, and optical fibres. A steering control guides the tip around bends in the structure to be viewed.

▶ **PROCEDURE**

Rigid endoscopy

Rigid endoscopes can be used to examine various internal organs and structures, especially joints and the external surfaces of organs within the abdominal cavity, such as the ovaries. The most frequently investigated joint is the knee, primarily because damage to it is common. Investigations using rigid endoscopes are often carried out under general anaesthesia. The endoscope is inserted through a small incision made in the skin. Further small incisions may be made for other instruments, such as forceps. The internal structures may be viewed on a monitor or through an eyepiece.

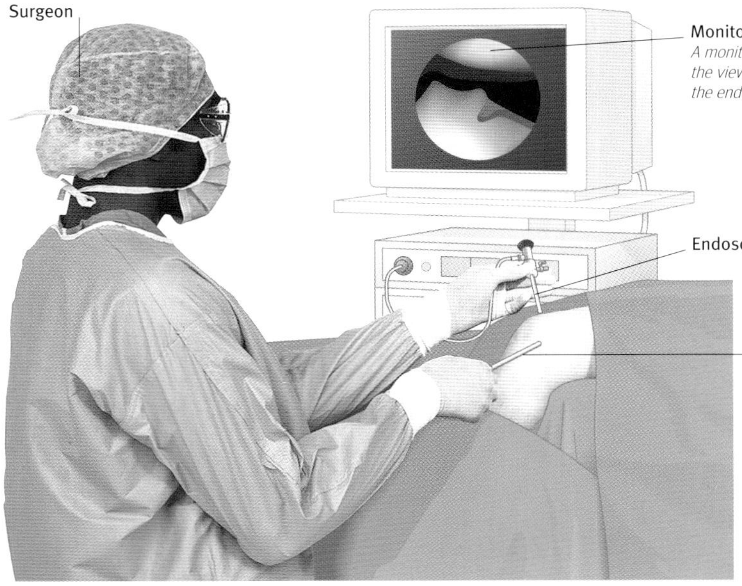

Surgeon

Monitor
A monitor shows the view down the endoscope

Endoscope

Probe

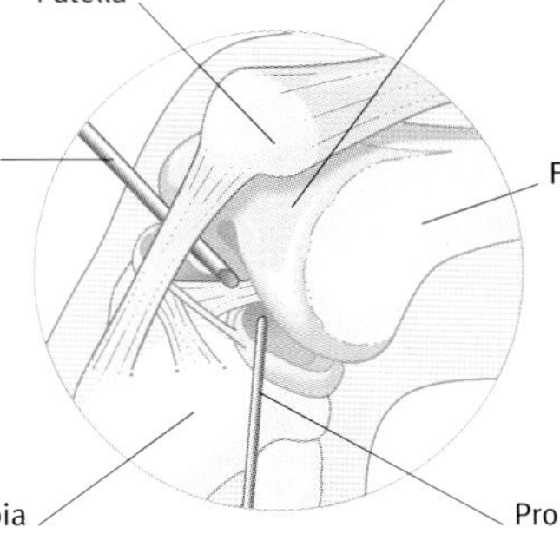

Cable for light source

Tip

Attachment for water and air

Eyepiece

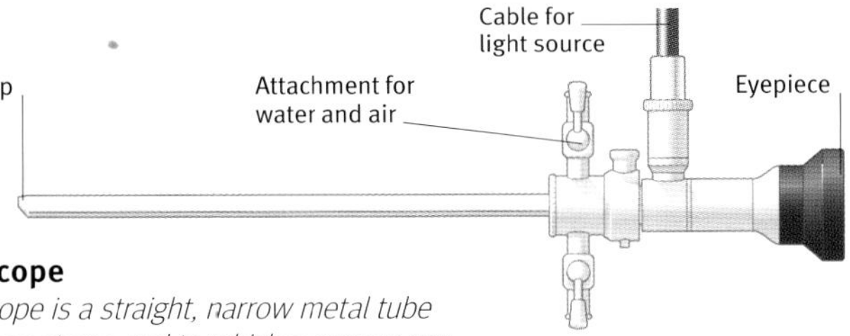

Rigid endoscope
A rigid endoscope is a straight, narrow metal tube with an eyepiece at one end to which a camera can be attached if necessary. A light source is connected to the endoscope and illuminates the structure or organ. Water and air can be pumped down the tube if necessary.

Patella

Cartilage

Endoscope

Femur

Tibia

Probe

INSIDE THE KNEE

During the procedure
For endoscopy of the knee joint, you will be given a general anaesthetic. Small incisions are made on either side of the knee through which the endoscope and other instruments are passed.

VIEW

Femur

Tibia

Damaged cartilage

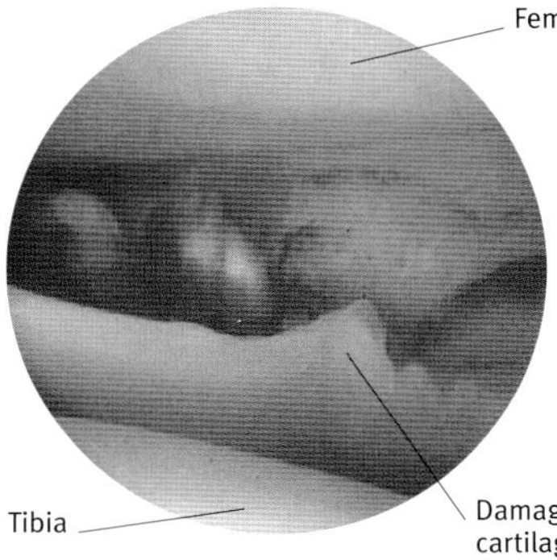

Endoscopic view of the knee joint
The cartilage in the knee joint is easily damaged. Damaged cartilage in this knee joint is seen through an endoscope.

sinuses (*see* **Endoscopy of the nose and throat**, p.291). Rigid endoscopes are used to investigate the abdominal cavity and joints (*see* **Rigid endoscopy**, left), where the structure to be viewed is near the skin surface.

If an abnormality is discovered during endoscopy, samples can be taken and, in some cases, treatment can be administered immediately. Instruments may be passed either down the channels of an endoscope or through small incisions in the skin in order to enable the doctor to carry out certain procedures such as taking tissue samples or removing foreign bodies. An endoscope can also be used to introduce a contrast medium into a particular site so that detailed images can then be produced on X-rays (*see* **ERCP**, p.414).

Some surgical procedures, such as removal of the gallbladder, that used to require a lengthy operation and a large incision can now be carried out more quickly and easily using instruments together with a rigid endoscope (*see* **Endoscopic surgery**, p.612).

Wireless capsule endoscopes are used only to examine the digestive tract, mainly to investigate bleeding when other diagnostic methods, such as flexible endoscopy, have failed to find the cause. Unlike rigid or flexible endoscopes, capsule endoscopes cannot be used to perform procedures such as taking tissue samples.

What are the risks?
Endoscopy is generally very safe, but, in rare cases, the endoscope may perforate an organ's wall. For example, if the endoscope is in the stomach, it may pierce the digestive tract. Immediate surgery will then be needed to repair the damage. If a tissue sample is taken, there may be some bleeding from the site. Wireless capsule endoscopy rarely causes serious problems, although very occasionally the capsule may not pass out of the digestive tract and may need to be surgically removed.

For some endoscopic investigations, general anaesthesia or sedation may be required (*see* **Having a general anaesthetic**, p.609), and these carry risks of their own. Your doctor will therefore make sure that you are in sufficiently good health to undergo the procedure.

---

surfaces. For example, air may be pumped into the abdomen during a laparoscopy (p.476) so that the abdominal organs can be examined.
Wireless capsule endoscopes These consist of a small capsule containing a camera, light, and transmission circuit. The capsule is swallowed by the patient and

passes through the digestive tract, eventually being passed out of the body in the faeces. As the capsule endoscope moves through the digestive tract, the images captured by its camera are transmitted wirelessly to a data recorder on a belt worn by the patient. The images are later downloaded to a computer for viewing and medical assessment.

What are they used for?
Flexible endoscopes are particularly useful for looking at the digestive and respiratory tracts, which bend in places (*see* **Flexible endoscopy**, opposite page). For example, nasendoscopes are very thin, short, flexible endoscopes that are used to inspect the nasal cavity and the surrounding

4 your body and disease

HUMAN BEINGS ARE ROBUST and adaptable, able to survive in changing environments and to endure physical and psychological stress. The body's design incorporates systems that renew and repair it continuously and others that protect it from harm. Many trivial injuries or potential illnesses heal by themselves or are controlled before we are aware of them. However, throughout a lifetime, we are exposed to a relentless stream of minor and more serious diseases and injuries with a variety of effects on the body.

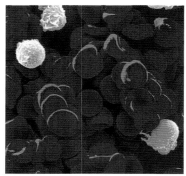

Blood cells
Two components of blood that are essential to health are white blood cells to fight disease and red blood cells to carry oxygen.

You become ill when something disrupts the normal healthy working of your body. Why you become ill is a question with multiple answers, many of which focus on your genes. Some rare diseases are caused by an inherited faulty gene, but genes are a contributing factor in many other illnesses. In particular, they predict to some extent your chance of developing major diseases of adult life, such as stroke and some types of cancer. Genes also help to determine your susceptibility to many mental health problems, such as schizophrenia and depression. As well as genes, your age, gender, lifestyle, and the environment you live in, are all factors affecting your risk of illness.

New drugs, immunizations, together with advances in hygiene and public sanitation have all contributed to a reduction in mortality from infectious diseases in the developed world, although such diseases remain a major threat to populations in the developing world. Today, major causes of death in the UK are heart disease, cancer, stroke, and accidents. These are strongly associated with lifestyle, and the risk of each can be geatly reduced by making changes in behaviour. As a result, the emphasis in medicine has changed: doctors now recognize that prevention is as important as treatment, and people are informed about how to adapt their lifestyle to stay healthy.

Understanding the body

Understanding disease is easier if you already have some appreciation of the normal structure and function of your body and the way in which its various components are organized.

The body can be divided into a number of major systems that carry out vital functions. For example, the respiratory system enables you to breathe, and the immune system protects you from infection. The bones, muscles, nerves, skin, blood, and other tissues that make up body systems are made of billions of connected cells. Each cell is a specialized, fully functioning unit, and all of its activities are controlled by the genetic code contained in the DNA (deoxyribonucleic acid), which sits within its nucleus.

In this book, diseases and disorders are mainly grouped in sections under the body system that they affect. Each section begins with a description of the normal anatomy and physiology of a body system to help you to understand the disorders that follow. When you have a problem, you may be referred to a doctor who specializes in disorders of that body system or organ. For example, you may see a dermatologist for a skin complaint and a gastroenterologist for digestive system disorders. However, diseases can also be categorized according to the mechanisms by which they damage the body.

The human body

The body consists of several integrated systems. Making up these systems are organs and tissues that work together to carry out a specific body function, such as digestion. The different types of tissue that make up organs and other body parts are specialized. For example, the stomach has muscular walls for churning food and a mucosa lining that secretes gastric juices and protective mucus. The interconnected cells that make up these tissues each contain genes that programme cell activities.

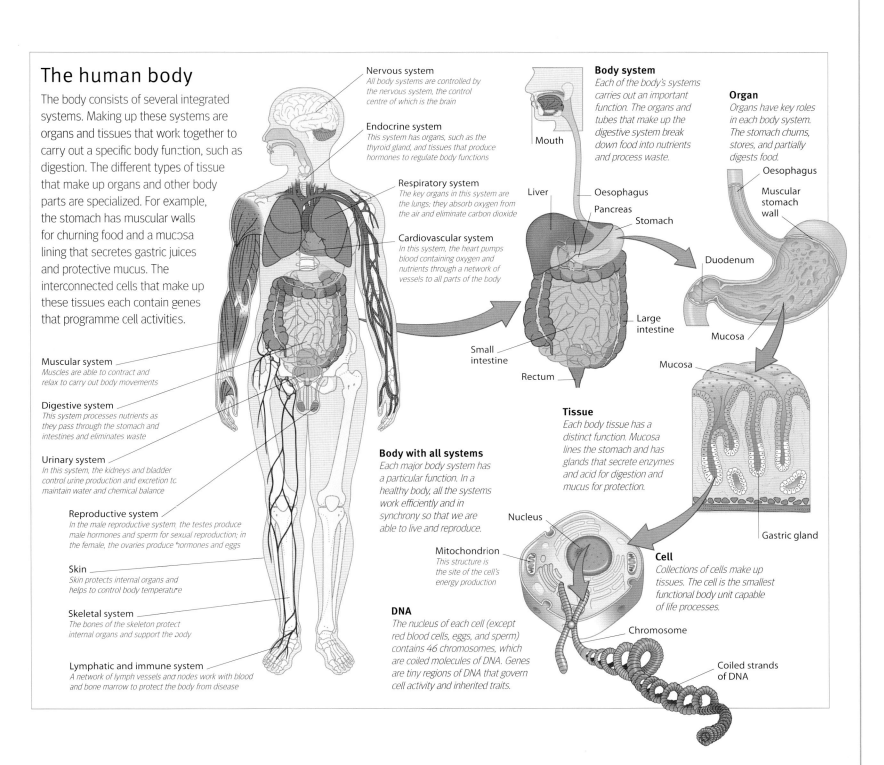

Nervous system
All body systems are controlled by the nervous system, the control centre of which is the brain

Endocrine system
This system has organs, such as the thyroid gland, and tissues that produce hormones to regulate body functions

Respiratory system
The key organs in this system are the lungs; they absorb oxygen from the air and eliminate carbon dioxide

Cardiovascular system
In this system, the heart pumps blood containing oxygen and nutrients through a network of vessels to all parts of the body

Muscular system
Muscles are able to contract and relax to carry out body movements

Digestive system
This system processes nutrients as they pass through the stomach and intestines and eliminates waste

Urinary system
In this system, the kidneys and bladder control urine production and excretion to maintain water and chemical balance

Reproductive system
In the male reproductive system, the testes produce male hormones and sperm for sexual reproduction; in the female, the ovaries produce hormones and eggs

Skin
Skin protects internal organs and helps to control body temperature

Skeletal system
The bones of the skeleton protect internal organs and support the body

Lymphatic and immune system
A network of lymph vessels and nodes work with blood and bone marrow to protect the body from disease

Body with all systems
Each major body system has a particular function. In a healthy body, all the systems work efficiently and in synchrony so that we are able to live and reproduce.

Body system
Each of the body's systems carries out an important function. The organs and tubes that make up the digestive system break down food into nutrients and process waste.

Mouth

Liver

Oesophagus

Pancreas

Stomach

Small intestine

Large intestine

Rectum

Organ
Organs have key roles in each body system. The stomach churns, stores, and partially digests food.

Oesophagus

Muscular stomach wall

Duodenum

Mucosa

Mucosa

Tissue
Each body tissue has a distinct function. Mucosa lines the stomach and has glands that secrete enzymes and acid for digestion and mucus for protection.

Gastric gland

Nucleus

Mitochondrion
This structure is the site of the cell's energy production

Cell
Collections of cells make up tissues. The cell is the smallest functional body unit capable of life processes.

Chromosome

Coiled strands of DNA

DNA
The nucleus of each cell (except red blood cells, eggs, and sperm) contains 46 chromosomes, which are coiled molecules of DNA. Genes are tiny regions of DNA that govern cell activity and inherited traits.

How disease affects the body

The different ways in which diseases damage the body are called disease processes. Several body systems may be damaged by the same process. For example, one of the major causes of death in the UK, coronary artery disease, comes under the heading of ischaemic disease. This term applies to all diseases in which there are changes in blood vessels, such as a build-up of fatty deposits, that restrict blood flow and starve organs and tissues of oxygen-carrying blood, leaving them unable to function properly.

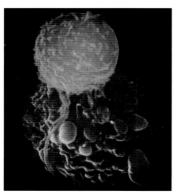

Destroying cancer cells
In this highly magnified image, a white blood cell is chemically destroying the larger cancerous cell.

Similarly cancer, a leading cause of death in the UK, is not a single disease but a group of disorders. Cancerous tumours can affect many different organs and tissues, causing different symptoms, but all cancers consist of cells that reproduce uncontrollably, invade healthy tissue, and may spread to other sites.

Infections occur when microscopic organisms, such as bacteria, invade the body, and range from minor complaints, like boils, to major infectious diseases, such as meningitis.

Metabolic disorders affect chemical processes in the body and are often caused by a failure to produce a certain enzyme or by malfunction of a hormone-producing gland. For example, in one type of diabetes mellitus, normal blood sugar levels cannot be maintained because pancreatic cells produce insufficient amounts of the hormone insulin.

A number of neurological illnesses and mental health problems are associated with disorders of brain chemistry. For example, depression and bipolar disorder are associated with imbalances in the levels of neurotransmitters, chemicals that transmit nerve signals. However, whether such neurotransmitter imbalances are a fundamental underlying cause of the disorder is not known for certain.

In autoimmune disorders, the immune system, which normally protects the body from infections and cancer, attacks the body's own tissues, disrupting the function of an organ or gland. For example, in rheumatoid arthritis, the immune system attacks and damages the linings of joints, causing pain and sometimes disability.

Although inheritance is increasingly being found to play a part in many major diseases, there is a group of several thousand rare genetic disorders caused solely by a faulty gene inherited from one or both parents. An example is cystic fibrosis, in which a faulty gene causes abnormally thick mucus to be produced in the lungs and digestive tract, resulting in the destruction of lung tissue and reduced absorption of food. In degenerative disorders, the structure and function of tissues and organs are gradually impaired by the loss of specialized cells or tissues, as in osteoarthritis, a wearing away of the smooth cartilage covering joint surfaces. Though traditionally associated with aging, a growing number of these diseases, such as cataract (loss of transparency in the lens of the eye), are also caused by exposure to strong sunlight, toxins, and prolonged use of certain drugs.

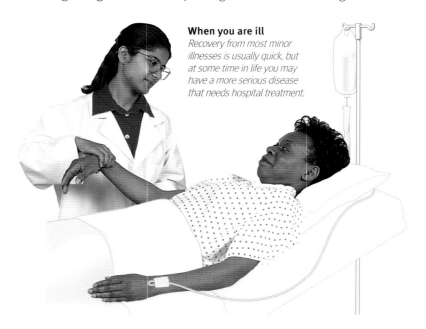

When you are ill
Recovery from most minor illnesses is usually quick, but at some time in life you may have a more serious disease that needs hospital treatment.

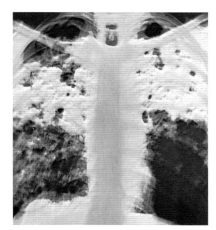

Lungs damaged by tuberculosis
This colour-enhanced chest X-ray shows areas of infected tissue at the top of the lungs due to tuberculosis.

Injury covers all types of deliberate and accidental damage to the body. Every year in the UK, there are thousands of fatal injuries; the major causes are falls, traffic accidents, intentional self-harm, and accidental poisoning.

Your susceptibility to disease

Some contributory factors for developing illness, such as your genes, gender, ethnicity, and age are largely unalterable. However, you can reduce your risk of ill health by following the guidelines for healthy living given in this book (*see* **Taking control of your health**, pp.6–35).

Many illnesses, such as psychological disorders, can occur at any age. However, particular age groups are vulnerable to certain problems. Babies are susceptible to infectious diseases because their immune system is not fully developed, and young children tend to have frequent accidents while their physical skills, coordination and balance, are still developing. People in their teens and in early adulthood are more likely to injure themselves. For example, most disability and death in young men is associated with risk-taking behaviour involving vehicles and weapons. Adolescents are prone to eating disorders, depression, and substance abuse. Young people who eat unhealthily, take too little exercise, smoke, and drink too much alcohol face a future risk of major diseases, such as heart disease, cancer, and stroke, that are increasingly common from middle age onwards. The incidence of long-term illness and disability increases with age and, for some people, poor physical health can lead to mental health problems.

Susceptibility to disease is closely linked to social factors such as poverty. For example, in the UK, rates of heart disease are higher in poor families than in those with a reasonable standard of living.

Changing patterns of disease

During the past few decades, many major infectious diseases have been brought under control in the developed world, and smallpox, one of the oldest diseases of humanity, has been eradicated globally. However, AIDS, a disease caused by HIV infection, remains a significant health concern. In addition, tuberculosis (TB) has become harder to control, because some strains have become resistant to antibiotics and due to reduced immunity in HIV-infected people.

For most of the 20th century, cardiovascular disease, cancer, and stroke were major causes of death in the developed world. They are now also becoming common in developing societies due to factors associated with affluence, such as an unhealthy diet. The high incidence of these diseases is also due in part to the increasing age of the population. As the number of people over 60 is predicted to more than double by the year 2050, these diseases are likely to continue to be major global threats to health.

Human immunodeficiency virus
This highly magnified view of a white blood cell, known as a CD4 lymphocyte, shows tiny, newly formed HIV viruses budding out from the uneven surface of the cell.

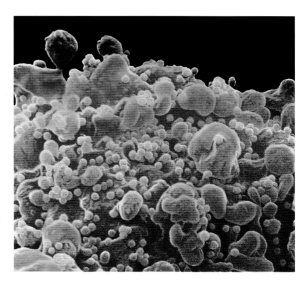

Genes and inheritance

Genes control the growth, repair, and functions of cells. Genes are made of DNA (deoxyribonucleic acid), which is found in the nucleus of cells as structures called chromosomes. DNA provides instructions for development and growth, through building proteins and making molecules that control cellular processes. Genes are the means by which physical and some mental characteristics are passed on to children.

THERE ARE ABOUT five billion cells in the adult human body, and all of them, except red blood cells, have a set of genes made of DNA. This chemical has a double helix shape and is made of two strands of molecules joined together in the centre by a series of nucleotide bases. The DNA is coiled into structures called chromosomes that are stored in the nucleus of cells.

Gene organization

Human genes are arranged on 22 pairs of matching chromosomes, plus two sex chromosomes. One chromosome in each pair is inherited from each parent. Therefore, body cells contain two copies of genes, with the genes for the same characteristic carried on the matching chromosomes in a pair. Egg and sperm cells, called sex cells, have 23 single chromosomes so that a paired set of genes is created when a sperm cell fertilizes an egg.

There are about 20,000–25,000 pairs of genes in a human body cell. These genes provide the cell with the information that enables it to make proteins. The order of nucleotide bases along the DNA provides this information. Each body cell contains the same genes, but each tissue or organ needs to make different proteins. For this reason, a system exists to turn on genes only when they are required.

Both of the genes in a matching pair can be identical. However, some matching genes occur in slightly different forms called alleles. Some genes may have two to several hundred different alleles. These different forms account for differences between individuals.

Most of the differences that occur between genes do not affect function. For example, blue eyes work as well as brown ones. However, some genetic differences have important effects and can result in inherited disorders, such as sickle-cell disease and cystic fibrosis. Genes also play a part in disorders such as coronary artery disease and some common cancers, such as colorectal and breast cancer.

Copying genes

Before a cell divides into two during growth or repair, its genes are duplicated so that each new cell has a full set. When sperm and egg cells are made, the two chromosomes of a particular pair align and exchange genetic material between each other before the cell divides. This ensures that when an egg and a sperm fuse, the new child is different both from its parents and from its siblings.

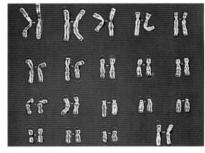

Human chromosomes
Body cells (except red blood cells) contain 46 chromosomes, organized in 23 pairs.

IN THIS SECTION

Inheritance of single gene disorders
This table lists the major single gene disorders that are covered in this book. Some disorders exist in more than one form, with different inheritance patterns. The most common pattern is indicated.

The human genome

The human genome contains about 20,000–25,000 pairs of genes. In 1990, an international research programme called the Human Genome Project was set up to identify each gene, its function, and its sequence of nucleotides (the building blocks of DNA); it was completed in 2003. The information gained from this project is being used to understand how genes are controlled and how they contribute to health and disease. Many genes for specific disorders have already been identified.

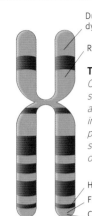

Duchenne muscular dystrophy

Retinitis pigmentosa

The X chromosome
Chromosomes can be stained, producing dark and light bands. This image shows the banding pattern and positions of some genes for disorders on the X chromosome.

Haemophilia
Fragile X syndrome
Colour blindness

SINGLE GENE DISORDERS

Autosomal dominant disorders

Achondroplasia p.540
A disorder of bone growth, resulting in short stature and abnormal proportions

Huntington's disease p.333
A brain disorder that causes abnormal movements and dementia in adulthood

Inherited hyperlipidaemias p.440
Excessive levels of lipids in the blood, of which the most common form is familial hypercholesterolaemia

Marfan's syndrome p.534
A rare disorder that mainly affects the skeleton, heart, and eyes

Neurofibromatosis p.536
A disorder in which noncancerous tumours develop along nerve fibres

Polycystic kidney disease (in adults) p.449
A disorder in which fluid-filled cysts replace normal kidney tissue

Porphyria p.441
A disorder in which chemicals called porphyrins build up in the body, causing psychological and physical symptoms

Von Willebrand disease p.275
A bleeding disorder due to a deficiency of a substance needed for blood clotting

Autosomal recessive disorders

Albinism p.563
A lack of the pigment melanin, which gives colour to the skin, hair, and eyes

Cystic fibrosis p.535
Abnormally thick secretions, leading to digestive and respiratory problems

Galactosaemia p.562
Inability to break down a form of sugar, leading to its accumulation in the blood

Haemochromatosis p.441
A condition in which too much iron is deposited in various organs

Phenylketonuria p.562
Deficiency of an enzyme needed to digest a component of protein-containing foods

Polycystic kidneys (in children) p.449
A disorder in which fluid-filled cysts replace normal kidney tissue, usually apparent at birth

Retinitis pigmentosa p.362
Progressive degeneration in the retina. It can also be inherited in an autosomal dominant and X-linked recessive manner

Sickle-cell disease p.272
A blood disorder in which red blood cells become an abnormal shape and blood flow through vessels is impeded

Tay–Sachs disease p.562
A severe disorder in which harmful substances build up in the brain

Thalassaemia p.273
A blood disorder in which production of haemoglobin, the oxygen-carrying component of red blood cells, is abnormal

X-linked disorders

Colour blindness p.369
Impaired ability to distinguish between certain colours

Fragile X syndrome p.533
A disorder that produces severe learning disabilities and a characteristic appearance

Haemophilia p.274
A disorder in which the blood does not clot normally due to a clotting factor deficiency

Duchenne muscular dystrophy p.536
A disorder causing progressive weakness and wasting of muscles

✚ STRUCTURE

Structure of genetic material

Genes are made up of DNA, which is shaped like a twisted ladder with rungs made of molecules called nucleotide bases linked in specific pairs. The arrangement of bases along the DNA provides the cell with instructions on making proteins and other molecules that control cellular processes. DNA is coiled into rod-shaped structures called chromosomes, which are stored in the nucleus of the cell. Humans have 22 pairs of chromosomes (called autosomes) plus two sex chromosomes.

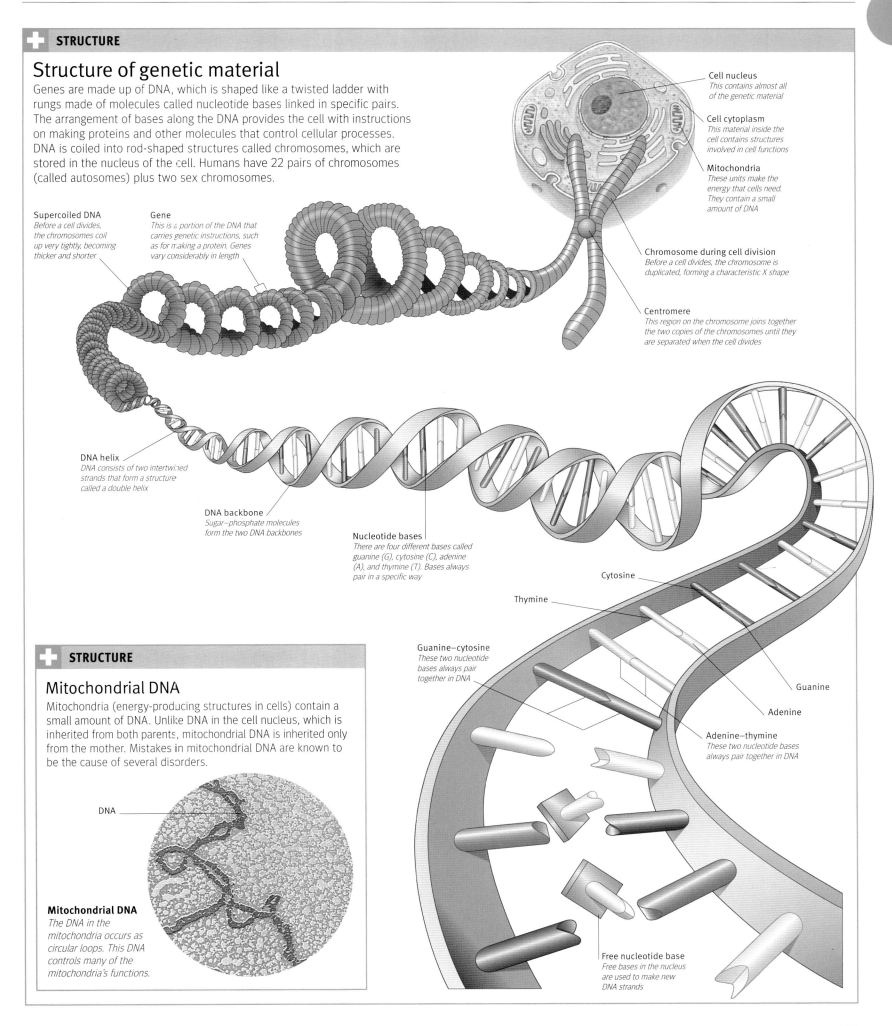

Cell nucleus
This contains almost all of the genetic material

Cell cytoplasm
This material inside the cell contains structures involved in cell functions

Mitochondria
These units make the energy that cells need. They contain a small amount of DNA

Chromosome during cell division
Before a cell divides, the chromosome is duplicated, forming a characteristic X shape

Centromere
This region on the chromosome joins together the two copies of the chromosomes until they are separated when the cell divides

Supercoiled DNA
Before a cell divides, the chromosomes coil up very tightly, becoming thicker and shorter

Gene
This is a portion of the DNA that carries genetic instructions, such as for making a protein. Genes vary considerably in length

DNA helix
DNA consists of two intertwined strands that form a structure called a double helix

DNA backbone
Sugar–phosphate molecules form the two DNA backbones

Nucleotide bases
There are four different bases called guanine (G), cytosine (C), adenine (A), and thymine (T). Bases always pair in a specific way

Cytosine

Thymine

Guanine–cytosine
These two nucleotide bases always pair together in DNA

Guanine

Adenine

Adenine–thymine
These two nucleotide bases always pair together in DNA

Free nucleotide base
Free bases in the nucleus are used to make new DNA strands

✚ STRUCTURE

Mitochondrial DNA

Mitochondria (energy-producing structures in cells) contain a small amount of DNA. Unlike DNA in the cell nucleus, which is inherited from both parents, mitochondrial DNA is inherited only from the mother. Mistakes in mitochondrial DNA are known to be the cause of several disorders.

DNA

Mitochondrial DNA
The DNA in the mitochondria occurs as circular loops. This DNA controls many of the mitochondria's functions.

Protein synthesis

Proteins have many roles in the body. Some make up body structures, such as skin and hair; others are hormones or enzymes that control cell activities. Proteins are made from amino acids, of which there are 20 types, according to instructions encoded on the DNA and relayed by messenger RNA (mRNA). An mRNA strand is a copy of a gene, which is a particular section of DNA. mRNA has four bases; three are the same as those of DNA, one is unique to mRNA.

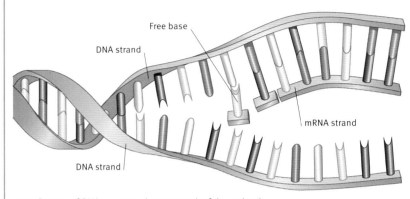

Free base

DNA strand

mRNA strand

DNA strand

1 *Strands of DNA separate along a stretch of the molecule. Free bases attach to corresponding bases on one DNA strand to make mRNA. The newly formed mRNA carries the instructions for making a protein and moves into the cytoplasm.*

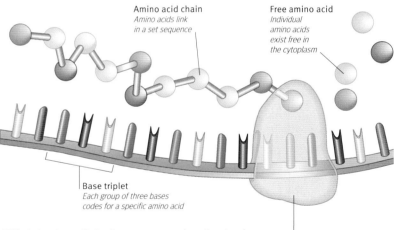

Amino acid chain
Amino acids link in a set sequence

Free amino acid
Individual amino acids exist free in the cytoplasm

Base triplet
Each group of three bases codes for a specific amino acid

Ribosome
This is the "workbench" on which amino acids are built up into proteins

2 *A structure called a ribosome moves along the strand of mRNA three bases at a time. The ribosome brings specific amino acids into place according to the sequence of bases in the mRNA triplets.*

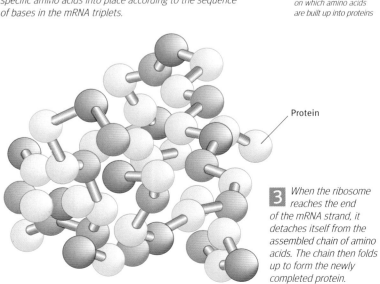

Protein

3 *When the ribosome reaches the end of the mRNA strand, it detaches itself from the assembled chain of amino acids. The chain then folds up to form the newly completed protein.*

Cell division

The process of growth requires body cells to divide and multiply constantly. Cells also divide to replace those that have become worn out. When a cell divides, its genetic material is copied. This type of cell division is called mitosis. A slightly different process of cell division, called meiosis, results in the production of egg and sperm cells. In this process, the resulting cells have only one of each pair of chromosomes and the maternal and paternal genes have been reassorted to create a new mix of genetic information.

Replication of DNA

Before a cell can divide to make new body cells or egg and sperm cells, the DNA in the cell must be copied. Each of the two strands in the original DNA acts as a template against which two new strands are built.

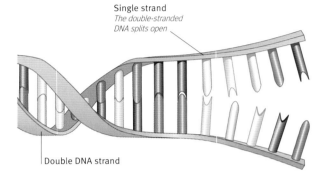

Single strand
The double-stranded DNA splits open

1 *The original DNA double helix splits open at several points along its length. This process produces areas where there are two separate single strands.*

Double DNA strand

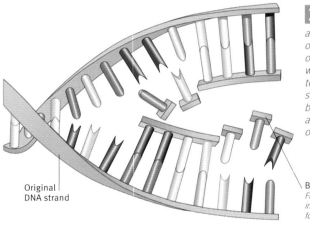

2 *New free bases (units of DNA) are attached to both of the single strands of DNA. The order in which the bases join to the single DNA strands is determined by the DNA bases that are already present on the single strand.*

Original DNA strand

Base
Free bases join to bases in the single strands to form specific pairs

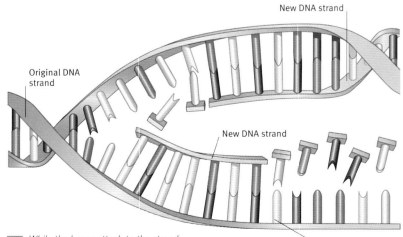

New DNA strand

Original DNA strand

New DNA strand

Base

3 *While the bases attach to the strand, each of the two newly formed double strands start to twist. The process continues along the whole length of the DNA, eventually producing two identical double DNA strands.*

Mitosis

When body cells divide, their genetic material has to be duplicated so that each new cell has a complete set of genes. This process of division is called mitosis and results in cells identical to the original cell. In the diagram below, only four chromosomes are shown for simplicity.

1 *The DNA in each chromosome is copied to form two identical copies of each chromosome joined in the centre by the centromere.*

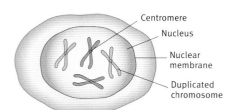

Centromere
Nucleus
Nuclear membrane
Duplicated chromosome

Centromere
Thread
Cell

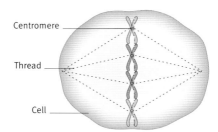

2 *The membrane around the nucleus breaks down and threads form across the cell. The chromosomes line up on the threads.*

3 *The duplicated chromosomes are pulled apart by the threads. The single chromosomes move to opposite sides of the cell.*

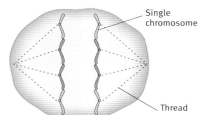

Single chromosome
Thread

Single chromosome

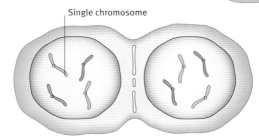

4 *A nuclear membrane forms around each set of chromosomes. The cell begins to divide into two new cells.*

Nucleus   Chromosome

5 *Two new cells form. Each cell has a central nucleus containing an identical set of chromosomes.*

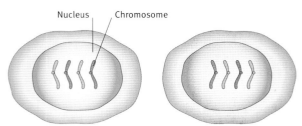

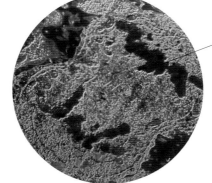

Chromosomes

Dividing cell
This highly magnified image shows a body cell dividing by mitosis. Separated chromosomes can be seen in the middle of each of the new cells.

Meiosis

Sperm cells in males and egg cells in females are produced by a form of cell division called meiosis. In this process, the amount of genetic material in the new cells is halved during two stages of cell division, so that a complete set of genes is obtained when an egg and sperm fuse. During meiosis, the two chromosomes of a particular pair exchange genetic material from one to the other. Each of the resulting egg or sperm cells then has a slightly different mixture of genes from the chromosomes of the original pair.

Sperm   Egg

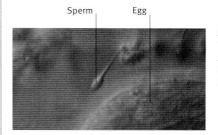

Sperm and egg
This magnified view shows an egg and sperm just before fertilization. Each of these sex cells is made by a process of division called meiosis.

1 *DNA in the chromosomes is duplicated to form X-shaped double chromosomes. Each of these is joined in the centre by a structure called a centromere.*

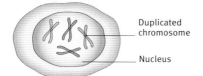

Duplicated chromosome
Nucleus

Matching pair of chromosomes
DNA may be exchanged where the chromosomes come into contact

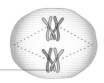

2 *The membrane around the nucleus disappears. Matching chromosomes pair and usually exchange genetic material.*

3 *Each of the duplicated chromosomes now has a mixture of genetic material. Threads form in the cell to pull the pairs of chromosomes apart.*

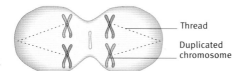

Thread
Duplicated chromosome

Duplicated chromosome

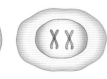

4 *The cell divides to produce two new cells. Each new cell has a full set of 23 duplicated chromosomes from the original cell.*

5 *The duplicated chromosomes line up. More threads attach to each chromosome. Each duplicated chromosome is pulled apart to form two single chromosomes.*

Single chromosome

Chromosome
Thread

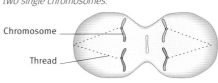

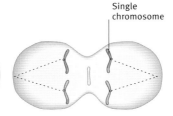

6 *The two cells divide to produce four cells from the original single cell, each with half the amount of genetic material. Each cell has a slightly different combination of the genes that were on the chromosomes that paired at the start of the process.*

Chromosome
Nucleus

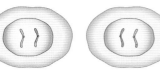

Inheritance

Physical characteristics, many disorders, and some aspects of behaviour are at least partly determined by genes passed from parents to children. Genes for each characteristic are always found at the same place on the same chromosome. At fertilization, the 23 chromosomes from the egg cell and 23 from the sperm cell come together to make the full set of 46 chromosomes containing two copies of each gene.

How genes are inherited

Half of a child's genes are inherited from its mother and half from its father. In turn, the child's parents inherited half of their genes from each of their own parents. Therefore, approximately one-quarter of a child's genes has been inherited from each of its grandparents.

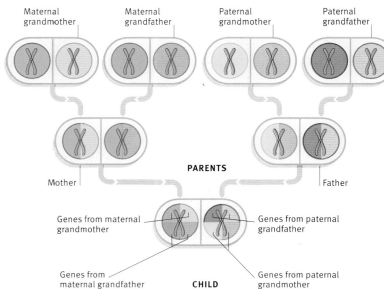

GRANDPARENTS

Maternal grandmother · Maternal grandfather · Paternal grandmother · Paternal grandfather

PARENTS

Mother · Father

Genes from maternal grandmother · Genes from paternal grandfather

Genes from maternal grandfather · **CHILD** · Genes from paternal grandmother

Child's genetic make-up
A child's genes are a mix of genes from his or her parents and grandparents. About one-quarter of each child's genes are inherited from each grandparent.

How gender is determined

There are two sex chromosomes, X and Y, that determine gender. Females have two X chromosomes and males have an X and a Y chromosome, in addition to the 22 other pairs of chromosomes. Therefore, all eggs have an X chromosome, while sperm may contain an X or a Y chromosome. The gender of a child depends on whether the sex chromosome in the sperm that fertilizes the egg is X or Y.

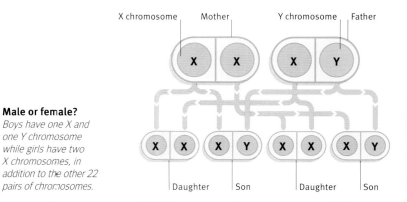

X chromosome · Mother · Y chromosome · Father

Male or female?
Boys have one X and one Y chromosome while girls have two X chromosomes, in addition to the other 22 pairs of chromosomes.

X X · X Y

X X · X Y · X X · X Y

Daughter · Son · Daughter · Son

Dominant and recessive inheritance

Many characteristics are determined by a single pair of genes. Each gene in a pair may have a dominant or recessive effect. A gene with a dominant effect (a gene for a dominant trait) overrides a gene with a recessive effect (a gene for a recessive trait), therefore a recessive trait occurs only if no genes for dominant traits are present to override the recessive trait. For example, blue eye colour is usually recessive and brown eye colour is usually dominant, as shown below.

Recessive and recessive
Each child inherits two genes for the recessive trait blue eyes, one from each parent. Since there are no genes with a dominant effect to override the effect of the recessive trait, all of the children have blue eyes.

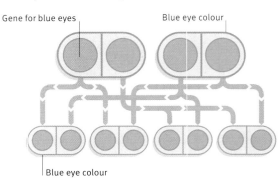

Gene for blue eyes · Blue eye colour

Blue eye colour

Gene for blue eyes · Blue eye colour · Brown eye colour · Gene for brown eyes

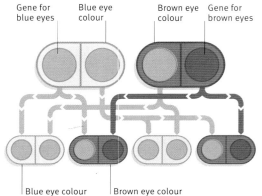

Blue eye colour · Brown eye colour

Recessive and mixed
Each child inherits a gene for the recessive trait blue eyes from one parent, and either a gene for blue eyes or for the dominant trait brown eyes from the other parent. Each child therefore has a 1 in 2 chance of having brown eyes.

Mixed and mixed
Each child has a 3 in 4 chance of inheriting at least one gene for the dominant trait brown eyes from a parent and having brown eyes. Each child has a 1 in 4 chance of inheriting two genes for the recessive trait and having blue eyes.

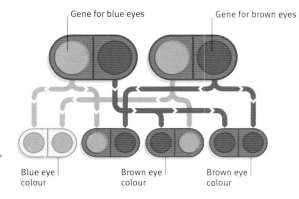

Gene for blue eyes · Gene for brown eyes

Blue eye colour · Brown eye colour · Brown eye colour

Gene for blue eyes · Gene for brown eyes

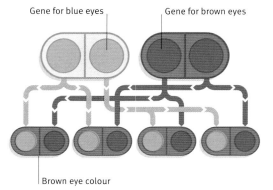

Brown eye colour

Dominant and recessive
Each child inherits a gene for the recessive trait blue eyes from one parent and a gene for the dominant trait brown eyes from the other parent. As all the children have a gene for the dominant trait, all will have brown eyes.

Sex-linked inheritance

Sex-linked traits and disorders are due to genes on the X chromosome. Males with an altered gene on the X chromosome are therefore affected as they have only one X chromosome. Females with one altered gene on one of their two X chromosomes are carriers if the genetic condition is recessive but affected if the condition is dominant. One example of an X-linked recessive trait is colour blindness. Its pattern of inheritance is illustrated in the diagram below.

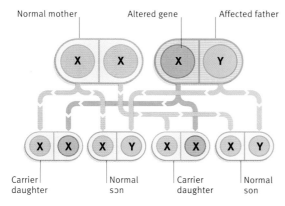

Normal mother   Altered gene   Affected father

Carrier daughter   Normal son   Carrier daughter   Normal son

Colour-blind father and normal mother
A colour-blind father passes the altered gene on his X chromosome to all his daughters. These daughters are not colour blind, although they can pass the altered gene on to the next generation. Sons inherit the X chromosome from their mother and have normal colour vision.

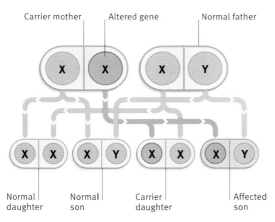

Carrier mother   Altered gene   Normal father

Normal daughter   Normal son   Carrier daughter   Affected son

Carrier mother and normal father
Each child of a carrier mother has a 1 in 2 chance of inheriting the altered gene. Sons inheriting the gene are colour blind as they have no other X chromosome. Daughters who inherit the gene are carriers.

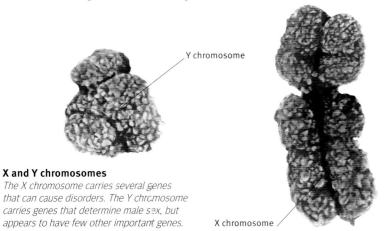

Y chromosome

X and Y chromosomes
The X chromosome carries several genes that can cause disorders. The Y chromosome carries genes that determine male sex, but appears to have few other important genes.

X chromosome

Mutations

When DNA is duplicated, errors may occur that result in a change in a gene. These changes are called mutations and they may have a dramatic effect on cell function. Mutations may occur in egg or sperm cells or in body cells but can only be passed on to a child when they are in eggs or sperm. Mutations are important for three reasons: they form the basis of evolution by providing a species with a better chance of survival if the mutation is beneficial; they account for many inherited disorders, such as haemophilia; and some mutations in body cells cause them to become cancerous.

How mutations occur

Most mutations involve a change in just one base (unit of DNA), typically substitution of an incorrect base (as shown below), deletion of a base, or addition of an extra base. Mutations may occur spontaneously as random errors in copying or may be caused by exposure to UV light, such as that present in sunlight, certain chemicals (mutagens), and radiation.

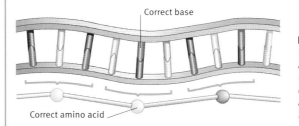

Correct base

Correct amino acid

Normal gene
The sequence of bases in a gene provides the cell with the correct sequence of amino acids that are needed to make a functioning protein.

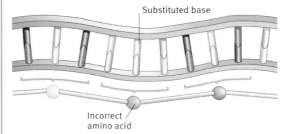

Substituted base

Incorrect amino acid

Mutated gene
If a base in a gene is incorrect, the wrong amino acid sequence may be used to make the new protein. The resulting protein may function poorly or not at all.

Mutations in eggs and sperm

A mutation in an egg or sperm cell is transmitted to a child at fertilization, and it then exists in every cell in the child's body. Some of these inherited mutations are harmless, but some may cause severe abnormalities in the child.

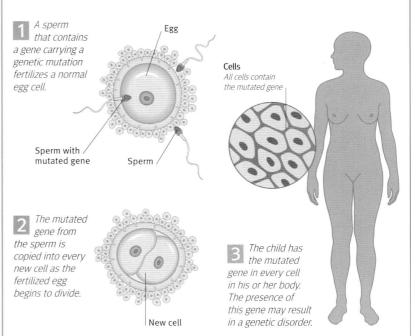

1 *A sperm that contains a gene carrying a genetic mutation fertilizes a normal egg cell.*

Egg

Cells
All cells contain the mutated gene

Sperm with mutated gene   Sperm

2 *The mutated gene from the sperm is copied into every new cell as the fertilized egg begins to divide.*

3 *The child has the mutated gene in every cell in his or her body. The presence of this gene may result in a genetic disorder.*

New cell

Genetic disorders

Genes play a part in the cause of many common diseases, such as asthma and diabetes mellitus. In these diseases, a number of genes interact with factors in the environment. However, some other rarer disorders are caused solely by altered genes or abnormal chromosomes and may be passed on from parent to child.

This section discusses the principles of chromosome and gene disorders and explains how these disorders may be inherited. The specific details of individual disorders are covered more fully in other parts of the book.

The first article discusses the way in which chromosomal abnormalities cause disease. The most common and well-known condition is Down's syndrome, which is due to an extra chromosome or extra part of a chromosome in body cells. Chromosome abnormalities often affect many systems of the body. The second article describes single gene disorders, which may be passed on through a family or may occur without a family history as the result of a gene mutation. People with a family history of a gene disorder may find genetic counselling useful.

> ### ✚ KEY ANATOMY
>
>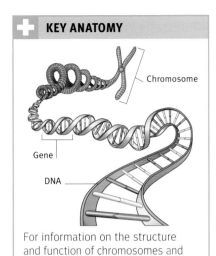
>
> For information on the structure and function of chromosomes and genes, *see* pp.144–149.

Chromosome disorders

Disorders that result from an incorrect number of or structurally altered chromosomes

 Always present at birth but effects may not become apparent until later

 Gender as a risk factor depends on the type

 Lifestyle is not a significant factor

About 1 in 150–200 babies is born with a chromosomal abnormality. Some of these do not affect health, but most may cause multiple problems, including physical abnormalities and learning difficulties. About 50–60 per cent of all miscarriages are the result of chromosome disorders.

Every cell in the body (apart from eggs, sperm, and red blood cells) has 46 chromosomes arranged in 22 pairs plus the two sex chromosomes (X and Y). One of each pair is inherited from each parent. The sex chromosomes determine an individual's gender. Females have two X chromosomes; males have one X and one Y chromosome. The other 22 pairs are known as autosomes. Humans have about 20,000–25,000 pairs of genes on these chromosomes, providing instructions for making proteins and for the growth, multiplication, and functioning of the body's cells.

Chromosomal abnormalities are usually due to an error in the division of chromosomes that occurs when eggs and sperm are formed. This process, called meiosis, involves a halving of the number of chromosomes in normal body cells. Normal meiosis results in each sex cell having only 23 chromosomes. Occasionally, a chromosomal abnormality can arise early in the division of the fertilized egg. Chromosomal abnormalities usually result in major physical and/or mental effects.

Several factors increase the likelihood of a couple having a child with a chromosomal abnormality, such as already having a child with a chromosome disorder or a maternal age of over 35 years.

What are the types?

A chromosomal abnormality involves either an incorrect number of chromosomes or a change in the structure of a chromosome. These abnormalities can affect any of the 44 autosomal chromosomes or the sex chromosomes. Disorders that are caused by autosomal chromosome abnormalities are usually more severe than those involving the sex chromosomes.

Numerical abnormalities Mistakes occasionally occur in the way chromosome pairs are divided between the new egg or sperm cells during meiosis, with one cell having too many chromosomes while the other has too few. For example, if an egg containing an extra chromosome is fertilized by a normal sperm, the embryo will have an extra chromosome in every cell in its body. If a sperm with a missing chromosome fertilizes a normal egg, the fetus will have one less chromosome in each of its cells. About two-thirds of all chromosome disorders are caused by cells that contain the wrong number of chromosomes.

Extra or missing autosomal chromosomes usually result in miscarriage of the embryo. One exception to this is having an extra chromosome 21, known as trisomy 21. Although fetuses with trisomy 21 are often miscarried, a number survive, and they have the condition known as Down's syndrome (p.533). Abnormalities in the number of sex chromosomes tend to have a less severe effect on the embryo and, in some cases, there are no obvious signs of a disorder. About 1 in 500 babies is born with an extra X or Y chromosome. An extra X chromosome in a girl or Y chromosome in a boy may have little or no physical effect. However, boys who are born with an extra X chromosome (XXY) have a disorder known as Klinefelter's syndrome (p.534), which may be associated with male secondary sexual characteristics not developing fully unless treatment with the male sex hormone testosterone is given. About 1 in 2,500 girls is born with only one X chromosome instead of the usual two, a condition known as Turner's syndrome (p.534). Girls with this condition have short stature and, if they are not treated, fail to develop normal secondary sexual characteristics at puberty.

Structural abnormalities There is a natural exchange of genetic material between two chromosomes of a particular pair during meiosis. This mixing ensures that the genetic make-up of each egg or sperm is slightly different. Occasionally, errors occur during this process, resulting in a structural chromosomal abnormality. A small section of a chromosome may be deleted, duplicated, or inserted the wrong way around (inverted). These types of structural abnormalities affecting a chromosome may result in miscarriage or birth defects, ranging from mild to extremely severe. The effect on the fetus depends on the amount of genetic material that is altered and the chromosome affected. Material may also be exchanged between two different chromosomes following breaks in each one. This process is known as translocation. If no genetic material is gained or lost during this process, it is known as a balanced translocation.

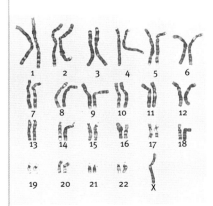

Chromosomes in Turner's syndrome
This set of chromosomes (karyotype) from a female with Turner's syndrome shows only one X chromosome rather than the two that are usual for a female.

Balanced translocations are carried by about 1 in 500 people and rarely cause health problems. However, the child of a person who carries a balanced translocation may have serious problems as a result of inheriting too much or too little chromosomal material.

Mosaicism In this condition, a person has some body cells that contain a normal set of chromosomes and other cells that contain abnormal chromosomes. Mosaicism occurs when there is an error in cell division in the embryo soon after fertilization, resulting in a population of cells with abnormal chromosomes. These cells can often, but not always, be detected by analysis of a blood sample. The effects of mosaicism depend on the proportion and distribution of cells containing abnormal chromosomes.

How are they diagnosed?

Many chromosome disorders are obvious either at birth or once symptoms appear. The diagnosis can be confirmed by a blood test.

If a fetus dies in the womb, is stillborn, or is miscarried, it may be possible to test for chromosome defects. During a pregnancy, chromosomal abnormalities can be detected by taking a sample of fetal cells and analysing the chromosomes (*see* **Antenatal genetic tests**, p.509). Antenatal genetic tests may be offered to women at increased risk of having a baby with a chromosomal abnormality due to advanced maternal age or because of previously having had a baby with such an abnormality. Certain routine tests or scans carried out in early pregnancy may also indicate an increased risk of Down's syndrome. In such cases, women may then be offered specific antenatal tests, such as amniocentesis or chorionic villus sampling, which can confirm the diagnosis of Down's syndrome in a fetus.

What is the treatment?

There is no cure for disorders caused by chromosomal abnormalities. However, surgery in infancy may rectify physical problems, such as intestinal abnormalities or heart defects, and some people with sex chromosome disorders may be treated with hormone replacement. For example, girls with Turner's syndrome can be given hormones to induce puberty and increase height.

When there is a history of chromosomal abnormality within the family or if recurrent miscarriages have occurred, prospective parents may wish to consider genetic counselling (opposite page) so that they can assess the risk of a child developing a chromosome disorder before deciding to begin a pregnancy.

Gene disorders

Disorders that result from inheriting an altered gene or genes

 Always present at birth but effects may not become apparent until later

 Gender as a risk factor depends on the type

 Lifestyle is not a significant factor for most disorders

Genes provide instructions to the cells to make enzymes and other proteins and molecules that the body needs to grow and function. A defective gene may have mild, moderate, or potentially fatal consequences or no effect at all, depending on the role of the protein or molecule for which the gene codes. The development of many common disorders, such as diabetes mellitus (p.437) and asthma (p.295), is linked with genetic factors but is also influenced by environment and lifestyle.

Several thousand disorders are the result of alterations in single genes but the majority of these conditions are extremely rare. Some of the most common single gene disorders include haemophilia (p.274), cystic fibrosis (p.535), sickle-cell disease (p.272), and thalassaemia (p.273). About 1 in 100 babies is born with a disorder that is caused by an alteration in one or both copies of a single gene.

Some communities have high frequencies of abnormal genes for certain disorders. For example, the gene that produces Tay–Sachs disease (p.562) is more common among Ashkenazi Jews, and the gene for thalassaemia is more common in people from Mediterranean countries and Asia.

Some gene disorders are obvious soon after birth or in the first few months of life. Symptoms of other disorders caused by a single altered gene, such as Huntington's disease (p.333), do not appear until adult life.

What are the causes?
In most gene disorders, an individual has an altered gene in all body cells from conception. There are two possible reasons for the presence of the altered gene. First, and most commonly, the altered gene may have been passed on from parent to child. Second, the gene may have become changed (mutated) during meiosis, the process of division by which eggs and sperm form. This is one reason why somebody with a genetic condition may be the only person in the family who is affected.

What are the types?
Genes occur in pairs; one of each pair is inherited from the mother, the other from the father. Genes are located on the 22 pairs of chromosomes known as autosomes and also on the X and Y sex chromosomes. Single gene disorders are classified by their pattern of inheritance: autosomal dominant, autosomal recessive, or X-linked. In addition, many common disorders are the result of an inter-

action between genes, the environment, and lifestyle. These are known as multifactorial (or common complex) disorders.

Autosomal dominant disorders A person with an autosomal dominant condition has one gene of a particular pair with an alteration; the other gene of the pair is the usual form. The effect of the altered gene (the dominant gene) overrides the effect of the usual gene (the recessive gene). Each child of a person with an autosomal dominant disorder has a 1 in 2 chance of inheriting the altered gene and developing the disorder. Familial hypercholesterolaemia is one of the most common conditions to follow this pattern of inheritance (see Inherited hyperlipidaemias, p.440). In this disorder, high blood levels of cholesterol lead to an increased risk of early coronary artery disease (p.243). About 1 in 500 people of European descent has this gene and is affected by the disorder.

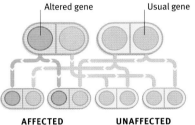

AFFECTED PARENT   UNAFFECTED PARENT
Altered gene   Usual gene

AFFECTED CHILDREN   UNAFFECTED CHILDREN

Autosomal dominant disorder
In this example, one of the parents has the altered gene and the other parent is unaffected. Each child has a 1 in 2 chance of inheriting the altered gene and therefore developing the disorder.

Autosomal recessive disorders A person with an autosomal recessive condition has two copies of an altered gene, one from each parent. If a person has one copy of the altered gene but the second copy is normal, the person is a carrier. A carrier does not usually develop the disease but may pass the altered gene on to his or her children. Most autosomal recessive disorders are rare. Cystic fibrosis, a disease that affects certain glands, is the most common autosomal recessive disorder in white Europeans. In the UK population, about 1 in 25 people is

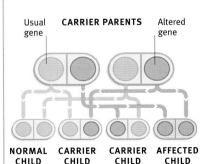

Usual gene   CARRIER PARENTS   Altered gene

NORMAL CHILD   CARRIER CHILD   CARRIER CHILD   AFFECTED CHILD

Autosomal recessive inheritance
In this example, both parents carry the altered gene but do not have the disease. Their children may be unaffected (1 in 4 chance), may be carriers of the altered gene (1 in 2), or may have the disease (1 in 4).

a carrier of the disease. The chance of two carriers meeting is therefore about 1 in 625. If two carriers have a child, there is a 1 in 4 probability of the child inheriting two altered genes and so overall, cystic fibrosis affects about 1 in 2,500 people. The most common autosomal recessive disorder among people of African or Caribbean descent is sickle-cell disease: 1 in 10 people is a carrier and about 1 in 400 has the disorder.

X-linked recessive disorders In a disorder of this type, such as haemophilia, the altered gene is on the X chromosome. Women who have one altered gene are usually unaffected carriers because the usual gene on the second X chromosome counterbalances the effects of the altered gene. However, they may pass on the altered gene to their children. Since each child inherits one X chromosome from the mother, each child of a carrier has a 1 in 2 chance of inheriting the altered gene. If a boy inherits the altered gene, he will develop the disorder because he has a Y chromosome and not a second X chromosome. Girls are carriers because the normal gene on the X chromosome inherited from their father masks the effects of the altered gene. A man with an X-linked autosomal recessive condition will pass on the altered gene to all his daughters (who will be carriers) but not to his sons.

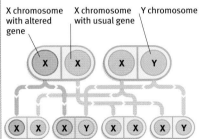

CARRIER MOTHER   UNAFFECTED FATHER

X chromosome with altered gene   X chromosome with usual gene   Y chromosome

X | X   X | Y

X | X | X | Y   X | X | X | Y

CARRIER DAUGHTER   AFFECTED SON   UNAFFECTED DAUGHTER AND SON

X-linked recessive inheritance
In this example, a mother carries the altered gene on the X chromosome but is unaffected. Each son has a 1 in 2 chance of inheriting the disease; each daughter has a 1 in 2 chance of being a carrier but is unlikely to have symptoms of the disease.

Multifactorial disorders There are many common disorders, including asthma, that run in families but for which no single gene appears to be responsible. In these disorders, it is likely that several different genes interact with lifestyle and environmental factors to cause the disease. Certain disorders are known to be associated with a group of proteins called HLAs, which form part of the body's immune system and determine a person's tissue type. HLAs are inherited, and each individual has a unique combination of them. In some people, particular HLAs increase susceptibility to certain disorders, such as ankylosing spondylitis (p.223) and systemic lupus erythematosus (p.281).

What might be done?
The underlying cause of single gene disorders cannot be treated. Gene therapy, in which a normal copy of a gene is inserted into cells, holds promise for some conditions but is technically very challenging and is still experimental. However, the symptoms of some gene disorders can be treated successfully. For example, people who have haemophilia are unable to produce a protein involved in blood clotting, and are treated with injections of the missing protein. Similarly, improved treatment for people with cystic fibrosis, has increased life expectancy. However, some single-gene disorders, such as Huntington's disease, are not easily treated and have severe consequences.

Can they be prevented?
People who have a blood relative with an inherited disorder may be able to have a genetic test to determine whether they have the altered gene, but tests are available only for certain disorders, such as cystic fibrosis and sickle-cell disease, in which the altered gene has been identified. A couple with a family history of a gene disorder may opt for genetic counselling (below) before conceiving or have antenatal genetic tests (p.509) for fetal abnormalities. Screening may be offered to whole communities in which there is a high incidence of a faulty gene. For example, Ashkenazi Jews may be screened for Tay–Sachs disease.

▶ **TEST**

Genetic counselling

Genetic counselling can help people to plan their families if there is a history of an inherited disease. Counsellors use the most up-to-date information and test results to estimate the chance that a given single gene disorder will recur in the same family. They may discuss the options available for reducing the risk of a child being born with the particular disorder.

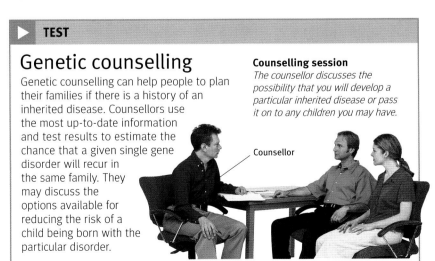

Counselling session
The counsellor discusses the possibility that you will develop a particular inherited disease or pass it on to any children you may have.

Counsellor

Cancer

Cancer is a generic term for a group of diseases that are characterized by uncontrolled growth of abnormal body cells. Of the many types of cancer, the majority form solid tumours in a specific part of the body, for example, the skin, breast, lung, bowel, or prostate gland. The disease may then spread to other parts of the body through the blood and lymphatic systems. As our understanding of cancer has advanced, changes in lifestyle, efficient screening programmes, and new types of therapy have improved prevention and treatment of the disease.

THE TERM "CANCER" comes from the Greek word for crab. The ancient Greek physician Hippocrates likened a spreading cancerous tumour to the shape of a crab's claw. Although our understanding of the disease has advanced dramatically since then, the description is still apt. An important feature of a cancerous tumour is its ability to spread within the body.

Genetic basis of cancer
The discovery in the late 1970s that damage to genetic material underlies cancer was one of the most important

breakthroughs in cancer research. Every cell contains genetic information in the form of about 20,000–25,000 genes that control the activities of cells. A cell may become cancerous when certain genes that control vital processes such as cell division become damaged. These faulty genes may be inherited or caused by carcinogens (cancer-causing agents), such as sunlight and tobacco smoke. Cells are continually exposed to carcinogens, but they rarely become cancerous for several reasons: cells can usually repair their damaged genes; more than one gene must be damaged before

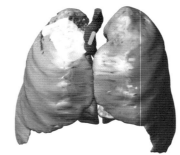

Lung cancer
The yellow and white area in this colour-enhanced CT scan of the lungs is a cancerous tumour, probably caused by smoking.

cancer develops; and the body's immune system often destroys any abnormal cells before they are able to multiply enough to form a cancerous tumour.

Aging and cancer
Cancer is most common among older people, largely because their cells have had more time to accumulate genetic damage, but also because the body's defences against cancer, particularly the cells and proteins of the immune system, gradually become less efficient with age. In addition, a cancer that began earlier in life may not be diagnosed until old age because it can take many years for some types of tumour to grow large enough to produce noticeable symptoms. Since life expectancy increased significantly in developed countries in the past few decades, cancer has become one of the leading causes of death; in the UK, it is the second most common cause (after heart and circulatory disease).

Treating cancer
For over 2,000 years, doctors have attempted to cure cancer by surgically removing visible tumours, and this is still often the first-line treatment in many cases. For some localized cancers, radiotherapy can be effective; this treatment may be combined with surgery with the aim of curing the cancer. Treatment with anticancer drugs (chemotherapy) may be used instead of or in combination with surgery and/or radiotherapy to destroy cancers that have spread around the body.

Newer treatments include biological therapies, which consist of drugs that disrupt the biological processes of cancer cells or stimulate the immune system's ability to destroy them. However, the most effective ways to lower the number of cancer deaths are prevention through a healthy lifestyle and screening to detect cancer at an early stage.

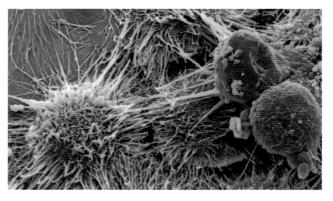

Kidney cancer cells
The pink cells in this highly magnified image are cancer cells from a kidney tumour. The threads extending from the cells are projections of the cells' cytoplasm.

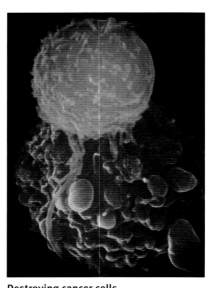

Destroying cancer cells
In this highly magnified image, a white blood cell is chemically destroying the larger cancerous cell.

➕ **DATA**

Causes of cancer

Although most cancers appear to be caused by several factors, including inherited ones, an environmental cause can sometimes be identified for a particular cancer. The most common carcinogens (cancer-causing agents), such as tobacco smoke, are avoidable. Smoking has caused a major lung cancer epidemic throughout the world.

Carcinogens in the environment
The pie chart (right) shows various environmental factors that can cause cancer, together with an estimate of the percentage of cancers for which each factor is responsible.

Occupational factors 4%
Viruses 7%
Other 10%
Sunlight 10%
Alcohol 3%
Radiation 1%
Diet 35%
Tobacco 30%

Cancerous tumours

A cancerous (malignant) tumour is a collection of many abnormal cells, most of which divide uncontrollably. Cancerous tumours infiltrate neighbouring tissues by forcing their way between normal cells and can spread to distant body parts through blood or lymph vessels. Cancerous cells are extremely irregular in shape and size and often bear little resemblance to the cells from which they arose. This characteristic irregular appearance of cancerous cells is often used to help diagnose cancer.

Migration of cancerous cells
In this magnified image, cancerous cells are migrating after separating from a tumour. Some of these cells will settle at new sites and divide to form tumours.

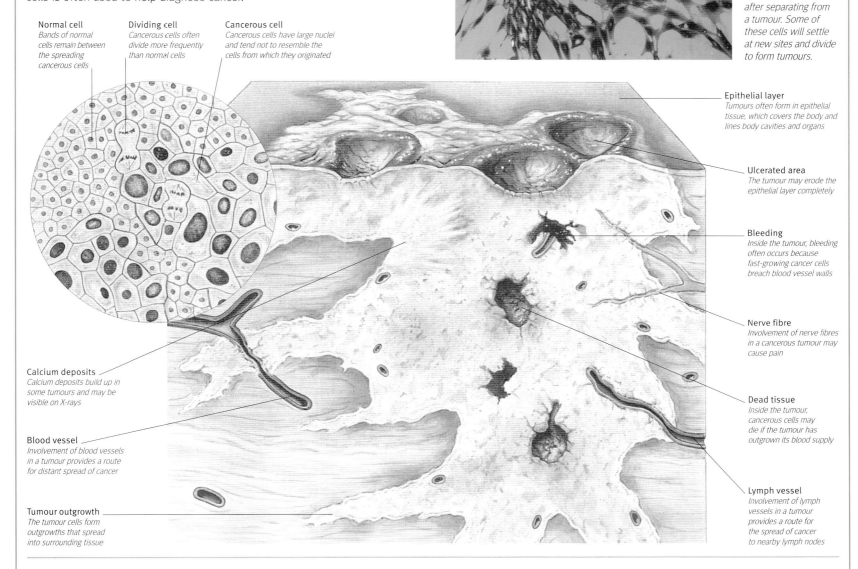

Normal cell
Bands of normal cells remain between the spreading cancerous cells

Dividing cell
Cancerous cells often divide more frequently than normal cells

Cancerous cell
Cancerous cells have large nuclei and tend not to resemble the cells from which they originated

Epithelial layer
Tumours often form in epithelial tissue, which covers the body and lines body cavities and organs

Ulcerated area
The tumour may erode the epithelial layer completely

Bleeding
Inside the tumour, bleeding often occurs because fast-growing cancer cells breach blood vessel walls

Nerve fibre
Involvement of nerve fibres in a cancerous tumour may cause pain

Dead tissue
Inside the tumour, cancerous cells may die if the tumour has outgrown its blood supply

Lymph vessel
Involvement of lymph vessels in a tumour provides a route for the spread of cancer to nearby lymph nodes

Calcium deposits
Calcium deposits build up in some tumours and may be visible on X-rays

Blood vessel
Involvement of blood vessels in a tumour provides a route for distant spread of cancer

Tumour outgrowth
The tumour cells form outgrowths that spread into surrounding tissue

Noncancerous tumours

Noncancerous (benign) tumours are common and include lipomas, which are fatty lumps beneath the skin, and many other skin lesions. These types of tumour do not invade tissue, but they may compress nearby structures as they grow. Noncancerous tumours do not spread around the body.

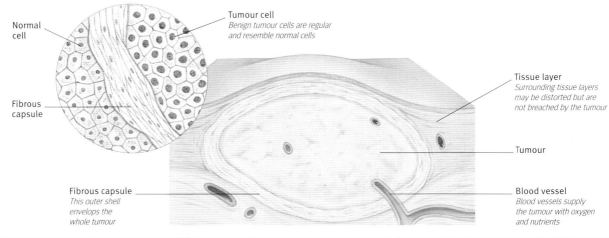

Normal cell

Tumour cell
Benign tumour cells are regular and resemble normal cells

Fibrous capsule

Tissue layer
Surrounding tissue layers may be distorted but are not breached by the tumour

Tumour

Blood vessel
Blood vessels supply the tumour with oxygen and nutrients

Fibrous capsule
This outer shell envelops the whole tumour

Structure of a noncancerous tumour
A noncancerous tumour has an outer fibrous capsule that separates it from the surrounding normal tissue.

✚ **PROCESS**

How cancer starts

Cells are continually bombarded by carcinogens (cancer-causing agents such as sunlight and certain viruses). Carcinogens damage specific genes (sections of DNA that control specific cell functions), known as oncogenes, that regulate vital processes such as cell division. Most damaged genes are repaired, but this process occasionally fails. Progressive damage to oncogenes may cause the cell to function abnormally and eventually become cancerous.

Genetic damage

Oncogenes regulate the rate at which a cell divides. They also repair damaged genes and programme faulty cells to self-destruct. In time, carcinogens may cause irreparable damage to a cell's oncogenes. As damage accumulates, the oncogenes may start to function abnormally, causing the cell to become cancerous. If a faulty oncogene is inherited, a cell may become cancerous much more quickly.

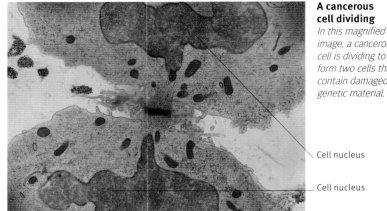

A cancerous cell dividing
In this magnified image, a cancerous cell is dividing to form two cells that contain damaged genetic material.

Cell nucleus

Cell nucleus

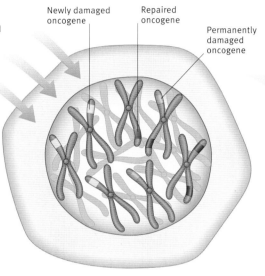

Normal oncogene

Outer cell membrane

Carcinogen

Newly damaged oncogene

Chromosome

Nucleus

1 *Carcinogens penetrate the cell and cause repeated damage to oncogenes on the chromosomes. Most newly damaged oncogenes are repaired.*

Newly damaged oncogene

Repaired oncogene

Permanently damaged oncogene

2 *The damage and repair of oncogenes continues. With time, some of the oncogenes in the cell become permanently damaged and cannot be repaired.*

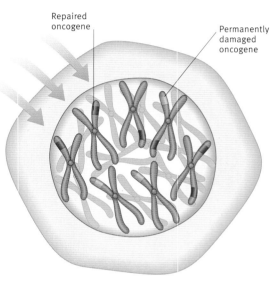

Repaired oncogene

Permanently damaged oncogene

3 *If a number of oncogenes controlling key cell functions are permanently damaged, the cell no longer functions normally and becomes cancerous.*

Formation of a tumour

A cancerous tumour begins as a single cell. If the cell is not destroyed by the body's immune system, it will multiply uncontrollably, dividing to form two cells, which in turn divide to form four, and so on. Tumour growth rates are measured by the time taken for the number of cells in a tumour to double (the "doubling time"). The doubling time of a tumour generally varies from about 1 month to 2 years.

Tumour size
A solid tumour can usually be detected after 25–30 doublings. At this stage in its growth, a tumour contains about a billion cells and has a diameter of about 13 mm (¹/₂ in).

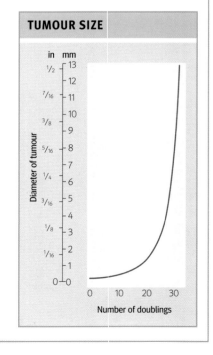

TUMOUR SIZE

in mm

Diameter of tumour

Number of doublings

Tumour doubling
After only four cell divisions, a cancerous tumour contains 16 cells. The cells double in number regularly, causing the tumour to grow larger.

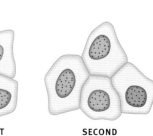

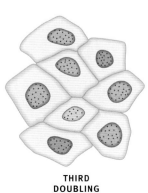

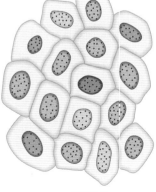

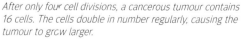

CANCEROUS CELL

FIRST DOUBLING

SECOND DOUBLING

THIRD DOUBLING

FOURTH DOUBLING

How cancer spreads

The defining feature of a cancerous tumour is its ability to spread not only locally but also to distant sites in the body by a process called metastasis. In metastasis, a cancerous cell detaches from a tumour and travels in the blood or lymph to a new location. The cell must overcome many obstacles if it is to settle in a new site and form a secondary tumour, also known as a metastasis. It must survive attacks from the immune system and stimulate the growth of blood vessels (angiogenesis) to provide oxygen and nutrients.

Spread in the lymph fluid

Cancerous cells may spread into the lymphatic system, which is a network of vessels that drains lymph fluid to nearby lymph nodes, where the fluid is filtered. A cell may become trapped in a lymph node and multiply to form a tumour. Immune cells in the lymph node attack the tumour and may halt the progression of the cancer.

1 *As a tumour grows, it invades surrounding tissues and can enter nearby lymph vessels. If some of the cancerous cells from the tumour detach themselves in the lymph vessel, they may be carried along the vessel until they reach and settle in a lymph node.*

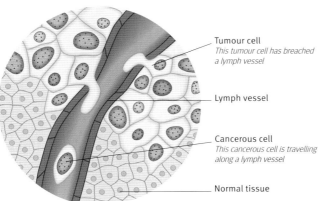

Tumour cell
This tumour cell has breached a lymph vessel

Lymph vessel

Cancerous cell
This cancerous cell is travelling along a lymph vessel

Normal tissue

2 *A cancerous cell enters a local lymph node, where it begins dividing to form a tumour. The tumour usually remains within the node, and the cells of the immune system may temporarily stop it from spreading to other parts of the body.*

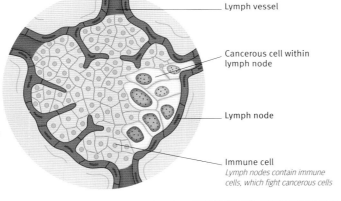

Lymph vessel

Cancerous cell within lymph node

Lymph node

Immune cell
Lymph nodes contain immune cells, which fight cancerous cells

Spread in the blood

Cancer often spreads to sites in the body that have a good blood supply, such as the liver, lungs, bone, and brain. The liver is a particularly common site since it receives blood from the heart and intestines. When cancerous cells reach very small blood vessels, they pass through the walls to invade tissues.

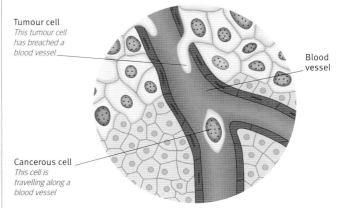

Tumour cell
This tumour cell has breached a blood vessel

Blood vessel

Cancerous cell
This cell is travelling along a blood vessel

1 *The growing tumour ruptures the walls of nearby blood vessels. Some cancerous cells detach from the tumour and pass through blood vessel walls into the blood circulation.*

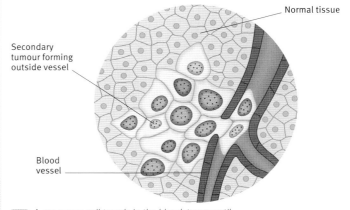

Normal tissue

Secondary tumour forming outside vessel

Blood vessel

2 *A cancerous cell travels in the bloodstream until it becomes lodged in a capillary (tiny blood vessel) at a distant site. The cell then starts dividing to form a secondary tumour.*

How tumours obtain nutrients

A cancerous cell obtains oxygen and nutrients from surrounding blood vessels by diffusion across its outer membrane, in the same way as normal cells. As the tumour enlarges, its inner cells are starved of nutrients. Enlarging tumours use two methods of acquiring nutrients – by invading existing blood vessels and by angiogenesis, the process by which a tumour stimulates new blood vessels to form. To survive and grow, a tumour must be able to stimulate angiogenesis successfully.

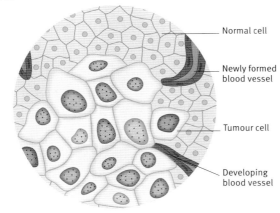

Normal cell

Newly formed blood vessel

Tumour cell

Developing blood vessel

Angiogenesis
In angiogenesis, tumour cells produce chemicals that stimulate the growth of blood vessels towards the tumour.

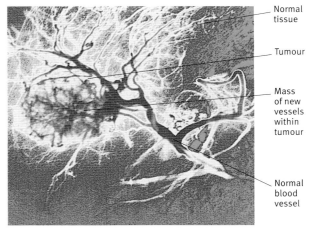

Normal tissue

Tumour

Mass of new vessels within tumour

Normal blood vessel

Angiogram of a liver tumour
This contrast X-ray of a tumour within the liver shows a large number of new blood vessels in the area of the tumour.

Living with cancer

In recent years, improved techniques in the early diagnosis and treatment of cancer have led to more cures than ever before. However, cancer is primarily a disease of old age, and, as life expectancy increases, so does the proportion of people who will eventually develop some form of cancer in later life.

Cancer is not a single disease. Tumours arising in different tissues behave in different ways and respond differently to treatment. However, all cancers have some elements in common, such as their invasive growth.

The aim of this section is to look at the general principles applied to the diagnosis, treatment, and aftercare of all cancers. Research is being carried out to produce new treatments and cures. Some modern cancer treatments are still experimental but will probably eventually increase the proportion of people who survive. Even if a cancer cannot be cured, many treatments are available to relieve symptoms and improve quality of life.

Cancers that arise in a specific part of the body are covered in the relevant body system section. For example, lung cancer (p.307) is covered in the section on lung disorders, and breast cancer (p.486) in the breast disorders section.

KEY ANATOMY

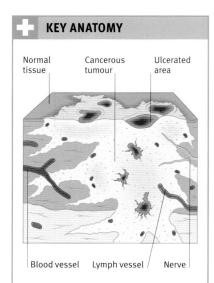

| Normal tissue | Cancerous tumour | Ulcerated area |

| Blood vessel | Lymph vessel | Nerve |

For further information about cancer, see pp.152–155.

Cancer and its management

The different causes of cancer and its management

 Age, gender, genetics, and lifestyle as risk factors depend on the type

Cancer is the second most common cause of death after heart and circulatory disease in many developed countries. In some countries, it is the leading cause of death. Although about 1 in 2 people in developed countries develops cancer at some stage in life, many people can be diagnosed early and treated successfully.

Many types of cancer produce a solid tumour that forms in an organ, such as the breast, intestine, or bladder. If not detected and treated, these cancers may spread to other body tissues. Other cancers are often widespread from early on, such as cancer of the lymph nodes (see Lymphoma, p.279) and cancer of blood-forming cells in the bone marrow (see Leukaemia, p.276).

What are the causes?
Cancer occurs when cells divide and grow in an uncontrolled manner. Cell division and cell functioning are controlled by genes, and defects in some of these genes can lead to a cell becoming cancerous. In both children and adults, these defects (mutations) in genes may be caused by environmental

factors such as chemicals (especially from smoking), viruses, ultraviolet light, or other types of radiation. In some cases, an abnormal gene is inherited from a parent. The main causes of cancer vary in different age groups.

Children and adults with reduced immunity, such as those with AIDS (see HIV infection and AIDS, p.169) or people who are taking immunosuppressants (p.585), have an increased risk of developing certain types of cancer. In such people, agents such as viruses are more likely to cause cancer.

Cancer in children Cancers in children are rare, affecting about 1 in 500 children under the age of 15 in the UK, but they are still a major cause of death in infancy. The

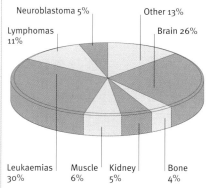

Neuroblastoma 5%		Other 13%
Lymphomas 11%		Brain 26%
Leukaemias 30%	Muscle 6%	Kidney 5%	Bone 4%

Childhood cancers
The various types of leukaemia (cancer of the bone marrow) are the most common cancers affecting children in the UK.

most common childhood cancers in the UK are leukaemia and tumours of the brain and spinal cord (see Brain and spinal cord tumours in children, p.550).

The cause of most types of cancer in children is not known. Some cancers, such as a neuroblastoma (p.550), occur primarily in children. A neuroblastoma develops in an adrenal gland or the nervous system from tissue that normally disappears during fetal development. Cancers of this type are most common during infancy. Other types of childhood cancer, such as primary bone cancer (p.220), affect older children.

Occasionally, cancer is due to an inherited abnormal gene or genes. About half of all cases of the eye cancer retinoblastoma (p.556) are mainly genetic in origin, and kidney cancer (see Wilms' tumour, p.565) sometimes runs in families. In such cases, one or more family members may have the same cancer.

The risk of cancer is increased in some genetic disorders. For example, children with Down's syndrome (p.533) are 10–20 times more likely than other children to develop leukaemia.

Some cancers in children may be caused by environmental factors. For example, certain viruses, such as the Epstein–Barr virus, are known to cause some types of cancer, including one type of childhood lymphoma.

Cancer in adults Cancer occurs much more commonly in adults than in children. In the UK, about 1 in 2 people develops cancer at some time in adult life. The most common types of cancer that occur in adults are lung cancer (p.307), skin cancer (p.199), breast cancer (p.486), colorectal cancer (p.421), and prostate cancer (p.464).

Many cancers in adults under the age of 40 have a significant inherited factor. Up to about 1 in 10 cases of cancer of the ovary (p.477), breast cancer, prostate cancer, and colorectal cancer are due in part to inheritance of abnormal genes. In older people, a combination of several factors eventually leads to cancer. The most common factors are carcinogens (cancer-causing agents), which include certain chemicals (particularly those found in tobacco smoke), dietary factors, some viruses, and specific types of radiation, including the ultraviolet light in natural sunlight.

In adults over the age of 50, the total number of newly diagnosed cancer cases roughly doubles each decade. Therefore, an 80-year-old person is eight times more likely to have cancer than a 50-year-old person. Some cancers, such as certain types of skin cancer and prostate cancer, are very common in old age, but these cancers may often be present without causing serious problems.

What are the symptoms?
Sometimes, a cancer is detected before it causes symptoms, often during a routine screening test. However, cancer is more often discovered when symptoms gradually develop and become noticeable over a period of weeks or months, prompting a person to visit a doctor. The symptoms of cancer may include:

- A lump, which may be firm and painless, in or beneath the skin or in the breast.
- Development of a new mole or changes in the appearance of an existing mole.
- Unusual breast changes.
- A nonhealing sore, ulcer, or wound.
- Blood in the urine, faeces, or sputum.
- Changes in bowel habits.
- Bleeding from the rectum.
- Unexplained vaginal bleeding.
- Persistent heartburn, indigestion, bloating, or abdominal pain.
- Unusual breathlessness.
- Persistent cough.
- Hoarseness or changes in the voice.
- Difficulty with swallowing.
- Severe, recurrent headaches.

Many cancers also produce more general symptoms, which may include:
- Weight loss.
- Unexplained tiredness.
- Loss of appetite and nausea.

If you experience one or more of these symptoms, you should consult your doctor as soon as possible. The symptoms may be caused by noncancerous conditions, but it is important to get them medically checked.

How is it diagnosed?
Routine screening (p.13) is constantly improving the early diagnosis of cancer. Screening aims to detect disease before symptoms are present. Examples are the faecal occult blood test or bowel scope screening to detect colorectal cancer (p.421). Other common screening tests include mammography (p.487) to check for breast cancer and the cervical screening test (p.480) to look for precancerous cells that may lead to cancer of the cervix (p.481).

Alternatively, cancer may be diagnosed as a result of tests to investigate symptoms. Such tests may include imaging tests, such as X-rays (p.131), ultrasound scanning (p.135), CT scanning (p.132), or MRI (p.133), or endoscopy (examination using a viewing tube). In a few cases, blood tests may be performed. For example, one test looks for proteins that indicate a particular type of tumour. To confirm a diagnosis, it is usually necessary to have a biopsy, in which a sample of abnormal tissue is removed and tested to find out if cancer is present. If cancer is present, further tests will identify the type of cell in the tissue that has become cancerous, which can give an indication of how fast the tumour is likely to grow and the best way to treat it. Once a diagnosis of cancer has been made, you will probably have tests to investigate how far the cancer has spread from its original site (see Staging cancer, opposite page).

What are the treatments?
Although cancer can develop at many different sites around the body, the general principles of treatment are the same. The chances of a cancer being curable are highest if it is detected by screening at a sufficiently early stage before it causes symptoms.

Staging cancer

If you are diagnosed with cancer, your doctor will need to know if the cancer has spread from its primary site to nearby lymph nodes or to other parts of the body. This assessment of the spread of a cancer is known as staging and may involve surgery and imaging tests. Staging allows doctors to plan the best treatment and to determine the prognosis.

Size and local spread

The first part of staging involves measuring the size of the tumour assessing the extent of its invasion into nearby tissues. A biopsy may be performed, in which a sample of tissue is taken from the tumour and examined, or the whole tumour may be removed for examination.

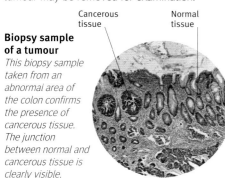

Cancerous tissue   Normal tissue

Biopsy sample of a tumour
This biopsy sample taken from an abnormal area of the colon confirms the presence of cancerous tissue. The junction between normal and cancerous tissue is clearly visible.

Lymph node involvement

If a cancer spreads, it often first affects nearby lymph nodes, causing them to enlarge. Cancer in lymph nodes can be detected by examination under a microscope after surgical removal or by imaging techniques such as CT scanning (p.132).

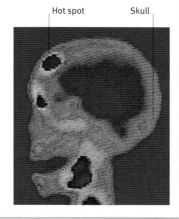

Enlarged mass of lymph nodes

Spine

Kidney

Cancer in the lymph nodes
This CT scan of the abdominal cavity shows an enlarged mass of cancerous lymph nodes. In this case, the cancer has spread from a testis.

Distant spread

If cancer cells enter the bloodstream, metastases (secondary tumours) may develop in other parts of the body. Imaging of the most common sites of metastases, such as the liver, lungs, and bones, may therefore be performed after a primary tumour is diagnosed.

Hot spot   Skull

Bone metastases
In this radionuclide scan of the skull, "hot spots" show areas of increased cell activity. Such areas indicate the presence of cancer that has spread from elsewhere in the body.

The three main techniques used to treat cancer are surgery, chemotherapy (below), and radiotherapy (p.158). Other treatments include biological and hormonal therapies.

Depending on the type and stage of cancer, treatment may be intended to cure the cancer, slow the growth of the cancer, or be palliative (in which treatment is intended to help a person live as comfortably as possible rather than to cure the cancer).

In most cases, curative treatment involves the surgical removal of a tumour. In addition to surgery, nonsurgical treatments, such as chemotherapy and radiotherapy, are often given with the aim of destroying any cancer cells that have spread beyond the obvious solid tumour. Nonsurgical treatments may also be used if a cure is not possible with the aim of slowing the growth of certain types of cancer rather than curing them.

Palliative care can control the symptoms of cancer, maximize quality of life, and provide psychological help for you and your family as you come to terms with the process of dying. Palliative care may also prolong life, although that is not its primary aim.

Treatment is tailored to the type and extent of the cancer, your age, your general health, and your wishes after discussing the outlook and options with doctors and family. For example, attempts to cure a cancer may not be appropriate in extreme old age because of the adverse effects of the treatment. Instead, treatment may be offered to relieve symptoms and to improve quality of life for the time left.

Surgery Surgical removal of a tumour is the main treatment for most common solid tumours at an early stage. During surgery, it is usual to remove some normal tissue surrounding the tumour to maximize the chances that all cancerous cells are removed from the body. Sometimes, the lymph nodes near the tumour are also removed because cancer often spreads to these nodes first. Less commonly, surgery aims to remove tumours that have spread to more distant sites in the body.

Surgery may not be appropriate if a tumour is inaccessible. For example, surgery to remove a tumour deep inside the brain may cause great damage to healthy brain tissue. Surgery may also not be the best treatment if the cancer has already spread to other parts of the

body. In such cases, other treatments, including chemotherapy or radiotherapy, may be appropriate.

Surgery may be used as a palliative treatment for certain types of cancer (*see* **Palliative surgery for cancer**, p.159). For example, surgery may be carried out to remove a tumour that is blocking the bowel or bile duct or to treat fractures of bones that have been weakened by cancer.

Treatment with anticancer drugs In chemotherapy (below), anticancer drugs (p.586) are used to kill cancerous cells. This is the principal treatment for most types of leukaemia and for other cancers that are widespread in the body. It may also be used for solid tumours that have spread to other parts of the body or to reduce the risk of further spread. Like surgery, chemotherapy may be used to cure cancer or as a palliative treatment. The side effects vary with the type of drug, but can include nausea and vomiting, temporary hair loss (*see* **Alopecia**, p.208), constipation, diarrhoea, tiredness, and rarely kidney damage or anaemia (p.271). You may be offered treatments for some of these side effects, such as antiemetic drugs (p.595) for nausea and vomiting or blood transfusions (p.272) for anaemia. The duration of treatment varies depending on the type of cancer and the aim of the treatment.

Treatment with radiation In this technique, radiation is directed at cancerous cells and tissue to destroy them or slow their growth (*see* **Radiotherapy**, p.158). It may be used curatively or palliatively. Also known as radiation therapy, radiotherapy can have serious side effects, although fewer side effects are likely to occur with modern techniques because radiation can be targeted at the cancerous area more effectively, thereby reducing the amount of radiation normal tissues receive.

Fatigue is a common general effect of radiotherapy. Other side effects that may occur vary depending on the site being treated, and any area that receives a high dose of radiation will be affected. For example, radiotherapy to the breast or head often causes redness or soreness of the skin; treatment to the scalp usually causes hair loss; and radiotherapy to the abdomen or pelvis typically causes nausea, abdominal cramps, and diarrhoea. Many side effects can be relieved with drugs and clear up after the course of radiotherapy has been completed. Radiotherapy does not make the patient radioactive.

Hormonal therapies Certain types of hormone affect the cell growth and replication of some cancers. For example, the female sex hormone oestrogen is known to stimulate the growth of many breast cancers. Hormone therapy to lower the level of oestrogen or to inhibit its effects may therefore play an important part in the management of this type of cancer (*see* **Sex hormones and related drugs**, p.602).

Biological therapies These newer types of treatment are being used increasingly to treat cancer. Unlike traditional cytotoxic drugs, which attack the cancer cells' DNA

Chemotherapy

Treatment of cancer with anticancer drugs (p.586) is known as chemotherapy. The drugs may be taken orally but are more often given directly into the bloodstream by injection into a vein. You may need to take the drugs daily, weekly, or monthly. Treatment by injection will usually be given in hospital.

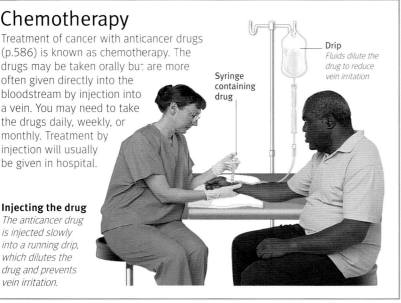

Drip
Fluids dilute the drug to reduce vein irritation

Syringe containing drug

Injecting the drug
The anticancer drug is injected slowly into a running drip, which dilutes the drug and prevents vein irritation.

or RNA (genetic material), biological therapies are drugs that disrupt specific biological processes of cancer cells or stimulate the immune system against the cancer (see **Anticancer drugs**, p.586).

Biological therapies that disrupt cancer cells' biological processes work in various ways, depending on the specific process they affect. For example, anti-angiogenesis agents (such as bevacizumab, used to treat some cases of breast cancer) inhibit the tumours' formation of new blood vessels, which are necessary to keep the tumours alive. Sunitinib, used to treat some kidney cancers, inhibits a specific enzyme (called tyrosine kinase) that is essential for tumour growth. Erlotinib, used to treat some cases of lung cancer, and cetuximab, used to treat some bowel cancers, block particular types of receptor (called epidermal growth factor receptors) and so prevent cancer cells with these receptors from growing.

Biological therapies that stimulate the immune system may involve taking drugs known as "cancer vaccines". For example, substances such as interferons, which trigger some types of white blood cell to attack abnormal cells, may be manufactured synthetically and given as interferon drugs (p.586). You may also be given synthetically created antibodies (proteins that recognize and attack foreign cells or particles in the body) that deliver a radioactive substance or anticancer drug directly to a cancer.

Although biological therapies are being used to treat an increasing range of cancers, they are not suitable in every case. Like all drug treatments, they may also cause side effects, such as fever, muscle aches, vomiting, fatigue, rash, and diarrhoea.

Supportive care A diagnosis of cancer and its treatment can be stressful and frightening. The aim of supportive care is to make life continue as normally as possible. You will be offered relief for the symptoms of cancer, such as pain (see **Pain relief for cancer**, opposite page). Side effects due to cancer treatments, such as vomiting, will also be treated. You and your family will probably be offered psychological support and advice from the medical team involved in your treatment. These specialists will help you to understand and cope with the diagnosis and treatment of the cancer. You may wish to see a counsellor to obtain advice and psychological support (see **Counselling**, p.624). Such support can boost your emotional wellbeing and self-esteem, which may be particularly affected if treatment has caused obvious physical changes, such as removal of a breast or hair loss. Research appears to show that people with a positive mental attitude survive longer than those who simply resign themselves to the disease.

Sharing problems with people who have had similar personal experiences can be reassuring, and it may be helpful to join a support group for people with cancer and their families.

What is the prognosis?

The earlier a cancer is diagnosed, the more likely it is that treatment will be successful and the cancer cured. The prognosis is usually expressed in terms of a 5-year survival rate (the percentage of people alive 5 years after the diagnosis of cancer). For many types of cancers, the outlook has improved greatly over the last few decades, especially in children. Even in cases where the cancer cannot be cured, there is still a good chance of long-term survival, often for many years after the diagnosis.

▶ **TREATMENT**

Radiotherapy

During radiotherapy, cancer cells are destroyed by using high-energy radiation. Treatment can be either external or internal depending on the site of the tumour. The dose and position of the radiation is carefully calculated so that normal cells receive as little radiation as possible, allowing them to recover with little or no long-term damage. The treatment is painless at the time, but side effects such as fatigue may develop as treatment continues. Radiotherapy may be used alone or with other cancer treatments.

External radiation

External radiation is mainly carried out using a linear accelerator, which produces X-rays or electron beams. The type of radiation used depends on the type of cancer. The skin is usually marked with ink to ensure correct positioning of the patient. Treatment may be given once, several times a week, or several times a day, depending on the cancer and type of radiation used.

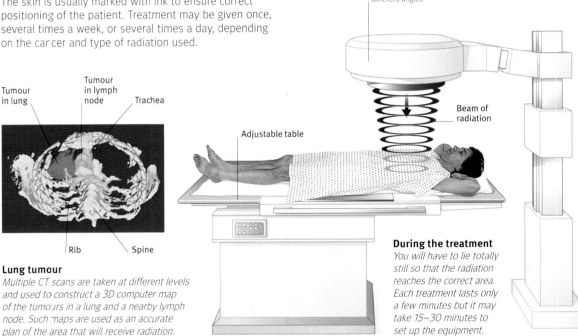

Radiation source
The machine tilts so that the cancer can be irradiated from different angles

Beam of radiation

Adjustable table

Tumour in lung · Tumour in lymph node · Trachea

Rib · Spine

Lung tumour
Multiple CT scans are taken at different levels and used to construct a 3D computer map of the tumours in a lung and a nearby lymph node. Such maps are used as an accurate plan of the area that will receive radiation.

During the treatment
You will have to lie totally still so that the radiation reaches the correct area. Each treatment lasts only a few minutes but it may take 15–30 minutes to set up the equipment.

Internal radiation

During this procedure, radioactive materials are placed directly into or around the cancer. For example, temporary radioactive implants may be placed within hollow organs, such as the uterus or vagina. Occasionally, a radioactive substance may be taken orally or injected into a body cavity. In some instances, small radioactive seeds may be placed directly into the affected organ and left in place while they gradually release radiation.

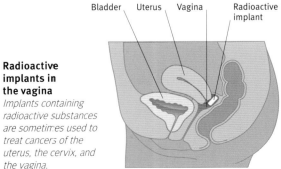

Bladder · Uterus · Vagina · Radioactive implant

Radioactive implants in the vagina
Implants containing radioactive substances are sometimes used to treat cancers of the uterus, the cervix, and the vagina.

Prostate gland · Bladder · Radioactive *seed*

Radioactive seeds in the prostate
Prostate cancer may be treated by the insertion of radioactive seeds. The seeds emit radiation for several months.

Surviving cancer

An overview of the features of life after successful treatment for cancer

 Age, gender, genetics, and lifestyle as risk factors depend on the type

Cure rates may be higher than 9 in 10 for some types of cancers and lower than 1 in 10 for others. The chances of a cure depend on various factors, including the age and general health of the affected person, the type of cancer and the stage it has reached, and the effectiveness of treatment (*see* **Cancer and its management**, p.156). Full remission occurs when all the symptoms disappear and there is no evidence of any cancerous cells in the body. If cancer does not recur for 5 years, there is a good chance that it has been cured. A relapse may be indicated by the return of symptoms or by evidence of cancer in follow-up tests.

Sometimes, treatment may damage the immune system (*see* **Acquired immunodeficiency**, p.280). Radiotherapy (opposite page) and chemotherapy (p.157) may increase the risk of a second type of cancer developing in previously normal tissue. For example, chemotherapy may increase the risk that leukaemia (p.276) or lymphoma (p.279) will develop.

Are there complications?

Cancer treatment often causes physical changes that may be psychologically difficult to deal with. For example, a breast may have been removed because of breast cancer (p.486). Mental abilities may also be affected, especially after treatment for a brain tumour (p.327).

Emotional problems after treatment may understandably include a fear that the cancer is going to recur. You may also become depressed as a reaction to the physical changes caused by the treatment (*see* **Depression**, p.343).

You may encounter discrimination at work, even though there is legislation against such discrimination. Nevertheless, some employers may be reluctant to employ or promote you if you have been treated for cancer. They may be unwilling

to invest money in you and assume that you are going to die soon or that you will claim large amounts of money from pension and health insurance plans. Employers may also have an unfounded belief that survivors of cancer are unproductive workers and may fear that you will need a long time off work. However, there are organizations that can offer emotional support and legal advice if you face discrimination.

What might the doctor do?

You will be advised to visit the doctor for follow-up evaluations once the cancer has gone into remission. Follow-up involves routine checkups at intervals after treatment. During the checkups, you may have various tests, which may include a physical examination; imaging tests, such as X-rays (p.131), MRI (p.133), CT scanning (p.132), or ultrasound scanning (p.135); endoscopy (p.138); or blood tests. However, you will probably not have all these tests at every follow-up visit. Some cancers can be successfully treated if a recurrence is detected early enough.

What can I do?

You should attend any recommended follow-up appointments and try not to feel too anxious or fearful about these checkups. They will be scheduled less frequently over time and are often required only annually after 5 years. Follow-up is carried out to maximize the chances of diagnosing and successfully treating any recurrence of cancer early.

Once your cancer has been cured, you may feel the need to improve the quality of your life by making a change in your priorities. Many cancer survivors decide to leave or change their jobs in order to fulfil lifelong ambitions or to spend more time with their families. You and your family may also wish to join a self-help organiza-

tion, usually run by cancer survivors, which can offer support and advice to other survivors and their families.

If you develop cancer before the age of about 50, it may have a genetic cause. If this genetic cause has been inherited then other family members may also be at increased risk of developing the same cancer. For example, some cases of colorectal cancer (p.421), breast cancer (p.486), cancer of the ovary (p.477), and prostate cancer (p.464) have an inherited genetic cause.

If your family has a higher than normal incidence of a particular type of cancer, it is important for relatives at risk to be regularly screened for that cancer (*see* **Screening**, p.13).

▶ TREATMENT

Palliative surgery for cancer

The aim of palliative surgery is to relieve the symptoms or to prevent complications rather than to cure the cancer. Palliative surgery may be performed to remove an unsightly growth; to relieve or remove an obstruction that is due to a tumour, particularly within the digestive or respiratory tract; to cut nerves that transmit pain signals; or to prevent fractures of bones that are weakened by cancerous deposits. Two common examples of palliative surgery for cancer are described below.

Relieving an obstruction

If narrowing of an airway or of the intestine is causing symptoms, a rigid incompressible tube, known as a stent, can help to keep the passage unblocked. Often under general anaesthesia, the stent is pushed through the obstruction to open up or widen the affected passage.

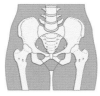

LOCATION

Tumour / **Narrowed oesophagus**

Tumour / **Stent**

BEFORE SURGERY   **AFTER SURGERY**

Oesophageal stent
The oesophagus has become narrowed by a tumour, which makes swallowing difficult. A rigid plastic tube (stent) inserted to widen the oesophagus makes swallowing easier.

Preventing fractures

If cancer spreads from elsewhere in the body to an area of the bone, the affected bone becomes weak and thin and may eventually fracture. To help to prevent fractures from occurring and allow a person to remain as active as possible, the bone may be pinned using a metal rod.

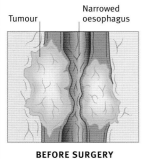

LOCATION

Femur

Tumour

BEFORE SURGERY

Metal rod

Tumour

AFTER SURGERY

Pinning the femur
Cancer has spread to the femur from elsewhere in the body. The metal rod supports the affected area of bone to prevent a fracture.

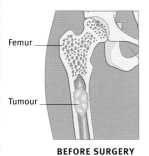 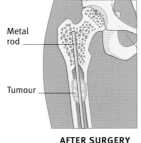

▶ TREATMENT

Pain relief for cancer

It should be possible to control pain due to cancer by using drugs. Painkillers (p.589) of increasing strength can be prescribed and most are taken orally as pills or liquids, or applied as skin patches. If pain is severe and not controlled by these types of drugs, morphine or other powerful painkillers may be injected continuously at home using a portable syringe driver, which allows a person to pursue normal activities.

Using a syringe driver
A painkiller is pumped continuously by the syringe driver through a needle inserted in the skin.

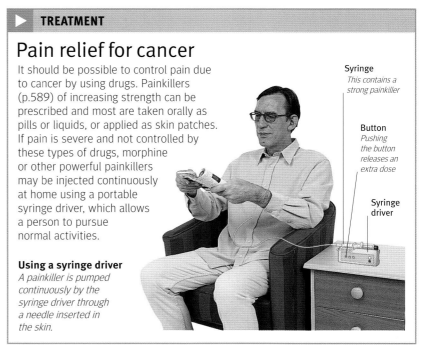

Syringe
This contains a strong painkiller

Button
Pushing the button releases an extra dose

Syringe driver

Infections and infestations

The most common cause of disease is infection by microorganisms that find their way into internal body tissues, where they multiply and disrupt normal cell function. These organisms, which are commonly known as germs, take a wide range of forms and contain the groups classified broadly as viruses, bacteria, protozoa, and fungi. Disease can also be caused by larger, more complex organisms, such as parasitic worms and their larvae, which may infest various parts of the body, especially the intestine.

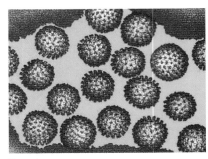

Rotaviruses
These wheel-shaped viruses are a common cause of gastrointestinal infections.

THE LIKELIHOOD OF serious illness from infectious disease is largely influenced by the environment. In the developed world, most infections can be treated effectively or prevented. However, in the developing world, where children are often malnourished, many of the common infections, such as measles, can be fatal. People living in temperate regions are rarely affected by cholera, malaria, or parasitic worms, but in the tropics such disorders are frequent causes of ill health and death.

Sometimes, an infectious disease spreads rapidly worldwide. Influenza, for example, tends to occur in annual outbreaks in all countries. Among the more recent global health threats are newer diseases, such as HIV/AIDS, as well as long-established ones, such as tuberculosis, in which organisms have become resistant to common drugs.

How infections are transmitted

The organisms that cause disease enter the body in a variety of ways. Some are breathed in or swallowed in food and water; others may gain entry through a break in the skin or be transmitted during sexual contact. An infection may spread throughout the body, affecting several organs at once. However, certain infectious organisms target and damage only one particular organ or part of the body, such as the liver, respiratory tract, or intestine.

Infections are more likely to develop if the number of infecting organisms is large or if a person's resistance to disease is reduced. Reduced resistance may be due to factors such as extremes of age, poor nutrition, or an immune system already weakened by disease.

Controlling infection

Over the last 100 years, great advances have been made in the control of infections, largely due to improvements in diet, housing, and hygiene. In addition, the increasing availability of routine immunizations and drugs such as antibiotics have made it possible to cure or even wipe out many infectious diseases. International programmes to monitor the occurrence of infections have also helped to check the spread of many often fatal diseases.

✚ **COMPARISON**

Sizes of organisms

There are vast differences in size between the various infectious organisms. However, an organism's size does not determine the severity of the disease it causes. A microscopic virus can lead to a life-threatening illness, and a tapeworm 6 m (20 ft) long may cause only mild symptoms.

Relative dimensions of organisms
Worms are the largest disease-causing organisms. In this diagram, each successive picture after worms represents a 100-fold magnification. The smallest disease-causing organisms are the viruses.

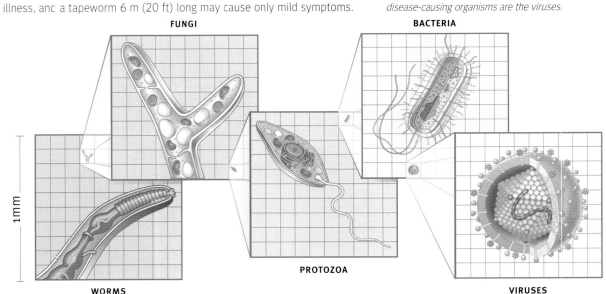

FUNGI

BACTERIA

1mm

WORMS

PROTOZOA

VIRUSES

Viruses

Viruses are the smallest infectious organisms, and they are so tiny that millions of them could fit inside a single human cell. Viruses are only capable of reproduction inside a living cell, called a host cell, that they invade. A virus consists of little more than a single or double strand of genetic material surrounded by a protein shell. However, some types of virus also have a protective outer envelope.

Capsomere
The protein shell (capsid) is made of many subunits called capsomeres

Protein shell
The shell, known as the capsid, surrounds the genetic material of the virus. Capsids have geometric shapes

⊢ 1mm ⊣
SCALE

Outer envelope
Some viruses have a protective outer layer of membrane that is acquired from the cells they have infected

Genetic material
The core of RNA or DNA contains sufficient genetic information for the virus to copy itself

Surface protein
Proteins on the surface attach to specific receptors on host cells. Viruses without envelopes also have these proteins

How viruses reproduce

To survive, viruses must reproduce inside living cells. The genetic material from an infecting virus takes over the functions of the host cell to make millions of new virus particles. The new viruses leave the host cell by bursting out of the cell or by budding out from the cell surface.

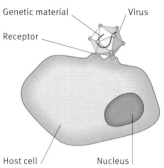

Genetic material   Virus

Receptor

Host cell   Nucleus

1 *Proteins on the virus attach to specific receptors on the surface of a host cell. The virus may enter the cell by being engulfed by the cell membrane or by fusing into the cell membrane.*

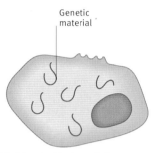

Genetic material

2 *When inside the cell, the virus sheds its protein shell. The genetic material of the virus reproduces, using substances from inside the cell.*

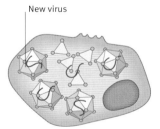

New virus

3 *Each copy of the genetic material programmes the formation of a new protein shell. Once the shells have formed, the new viruses are complete.*

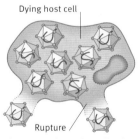

Dying host cell

Rupture

4 *The viruses leave the cell either by suddenly rupturing the cell membrane, which destroys the host cell, or by slowly budding out from the surface of the cell membrane.*

Changes in viruses

The immune system recognizes viruses by the proteins that are on their surfaces (antigens). When viruses reproduce, the antigens on the new viruses may become slightly different to prevent the immune system from recognizing the virus. This is known as antigenic drift. Much larger changes (antigenic shifts) may result in epidemics.

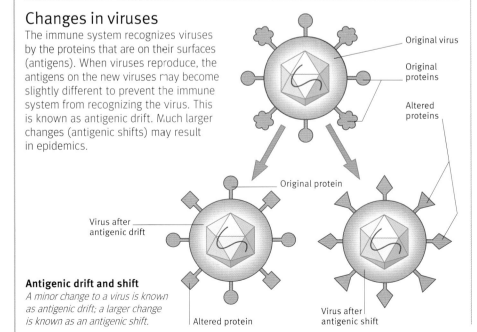

Original virus

Original proteins

Altered proteins

Original protein

Virus after antigenic drift

Virus after antigenic shift

Altered protein

Antigenic drift and shift
A minor change to a virus is known as antigenic drift; a larger change is known as an antigenic shift.

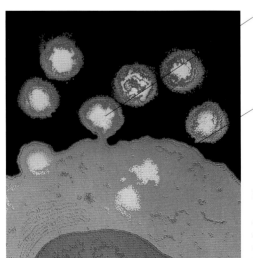

Budding virus

Host cell membrane

Budding viruses
When certain viruses bud out from their host cell, they envelop themselves in host cell surface membrane.

✚ STRUCTURE AND FUNCTION

Bacteria

Bacteria are microscopic single-celled organisms that are found in every environment. Some bacteria live in or on our bodies without causing disease. There are thousands of different types of bacterium, but relatively few of these cause disease in humans. Bacteria have a variety of shapes that are broadly classified as cocci (spheres), bacilli (rods), and spirochetes and spirilla (curved or spiral-shaped forms).

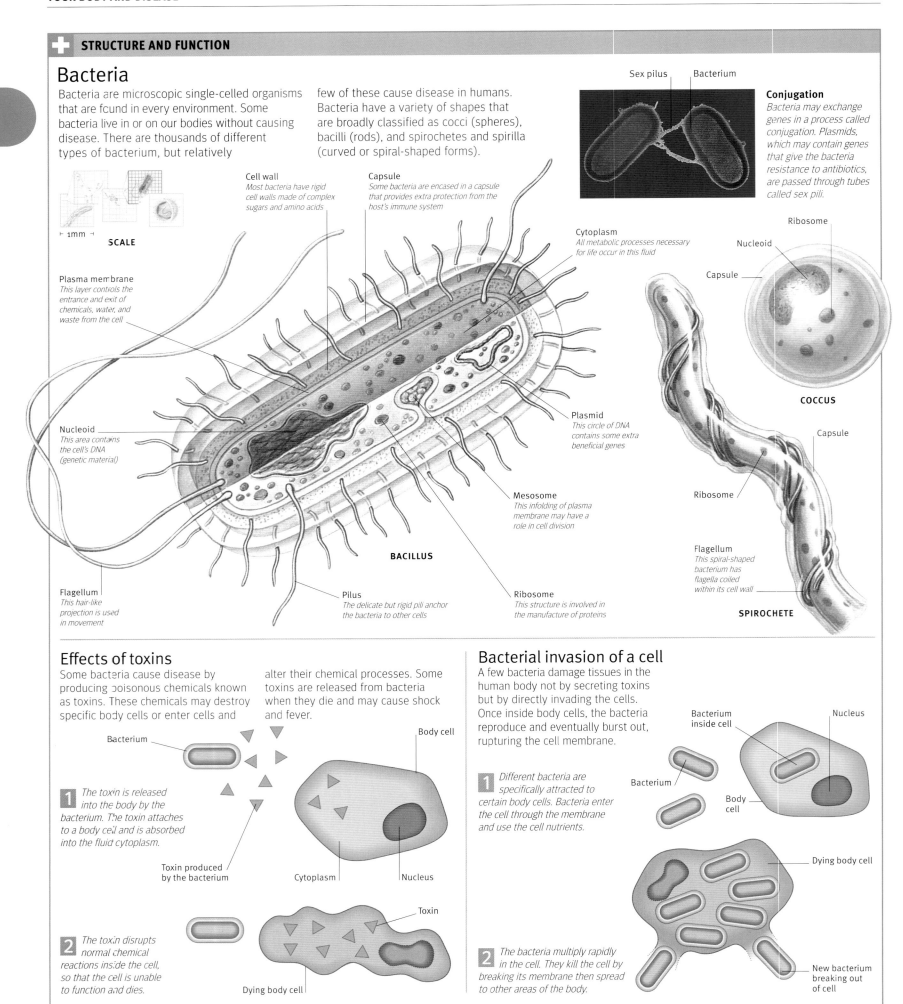

Conjugation
Bacteria may exchange genes in a process called conjugation. Plasmids, which may contain genes that give the bacteria resistance to antibiotics, are passed through tubes called sex pili.

Sex pilus
Bacterium

SCALE
⊢ 1mm ⊣

Cell wall
Most bacteria have rigid cell walls made of complex sugars and amino acids

Capsule
Some bacteria are encased in a capsule that provides extra protection from the host's immune system

Cytoplasm
All metabolic processes necessary for life occur in this fluid

Plasma membrane
This layer controls the entrance and exit of chemicals, water, and waste from the cell

Nucleoid
This area contains the cell's DNA (genetic material)

Plasmid
This circle of DNA contains some extra beneficial genes

Mesosome
This infolding of plasma membrane may have a role in cell division

BACILLUS

Flagellum
This hair-like projection is used in movement

Pilus
The delicate but rigid pili anchor the bacteria to other cells

Ribosome
This structure is involved in the manufacture of proteins

Ribosome
Nucleoid
Capsule

COCCUS

Capsule
Ribosome

Flagellum
This spiral-shaped bacterium has flagella coiled within its cell wall

SPIROCHETE

Effects of toxins

Some bacteria cause disease by producing poisonous chemicals known as toxins. These chemicals may destroy specific body cells or enter cells and alter their chemical processes. Some toxins are released from bacteria when they die and may cause shock and fever.

Bacterium
Body cell

1 *The toxin is released into the body by the bacterium. The toxin attaches to a body cell and is absorbed into the fluid cytoplasm.*

Toxin produced by the bacterium
Cytoplasm
Nucleus

2 *The toxin disrupts normal chemical reactions inside the cell, so that the cell is unable to function and dies.*

Toxin

Dying body cell

Bacterial invasion of a cell

A few bacteria damage tissues in the human body not by secreting toxins but by directly invading the cells. Once inside body cells, the bacteria reproduce and eventually burst out, rupturing the cell membrane.

Bacterium inside cell
Nucleus

1 *Different bacteria are specifically attracted to certain body cells. Bacteria enter the cell through the membrane and use the cell nutrients.*

Bacterium
Body cell

Dying body cell

2 *The bacteria multiply rapidly in the cell. They kill the cell by breaking its membrane then spread to other areas of the body.*

New bacterium breaking out of cell

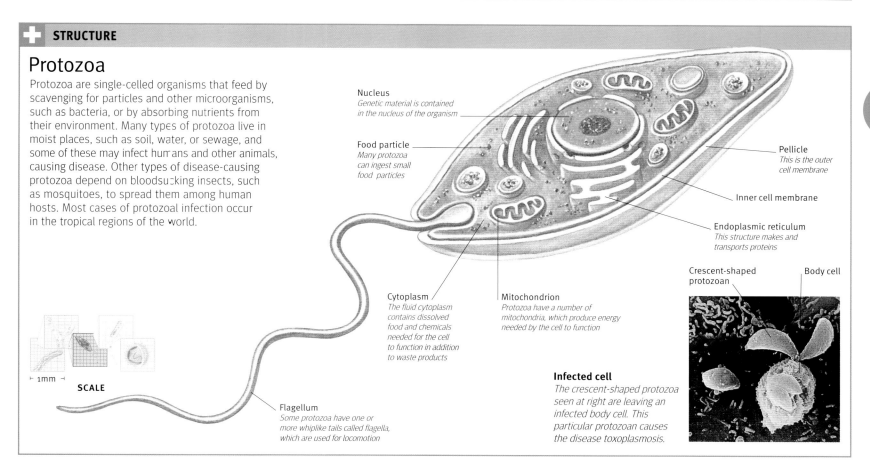

+ STRUCTURE

Protozoa

Protozoa are single-celled organisms that feed by scavenging for particles and other microorganisms, such as bacteria, or by absorbing nutrients from their environment. Many types of protozoa live in moist places, such as soil, water, or sewage, and some of these may infect humans and other animals, causing disease. Other types of disease-causing protozoa depend on bloodsucking insects, such as mosquitoes, to spread them among human hosts. Most cases of protozoal infection occur in the tropical regions of the world.

Nucleus
Genetic material is contained in the nucleus of the organism

Food particle
Many protozoa can ingest small food particles

Pellicle
This is the outer cell membrane

Inner cell membrane

Endoplasmic reticulum
This structure makes and transports proteins

Cytoplasm
The fluid cytoplasm contains dissolved food and chemicals needed for the cell to function in addition to waste products

Mitochondrion
Protozoa have a number of mitochondria, which produce energy needed by the cell to function

Crescent-shaped protozoan

Body cell

⊢ 1mm ⊣ **SCALE**

Flagellum
Some protozoa have one or more whiplike tails called flagella, which are used for locomotion

Infected cell
The crescent-shaped protozoa seen at right are leaving an infected body cell. This particular protozoan causes the disease toxoplasmosis.

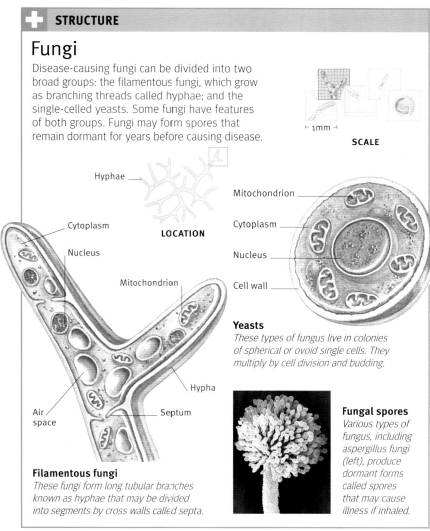

+ STRUCTURE

Fungi

Disease-causing fungi can be divided into two broad groups: the filamentous fungi, which grow as branching threads called hyphae; and the single-celled yeasts. Some fungi have features of both groups. Fungi may form spores that remain dormant for years before causing disease.

⊢ 1mm ⊣ **SCALE**

Hyphae

Cytoplasm

Nucleus

LOCATION

Mitochondrion

Mitochondrion

Cytoplasm

Nucleus

Cell wall

Hypha

Air space

Septum

Yeasts
These types of fungus live in colonies of spherical or ovoid single cells. They multiply by cell division and budding.

Filamentous fungi
These fungi form long tubular branches known as hyphae that may be divided into segments by cross walls called septa.

Fungal spores
Various types of fungus, including aspergillus fungi (left), produce dormant forms called spores that may cause illness if inhaled.

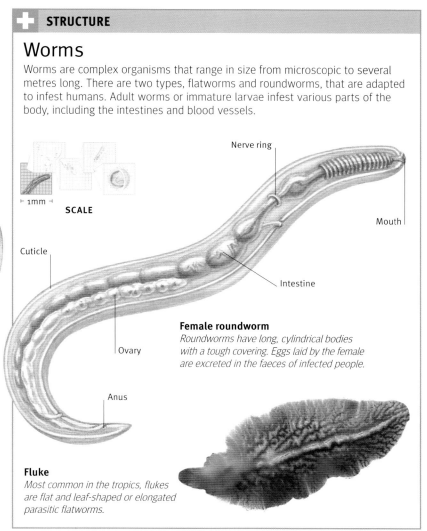

+ STRUCTURE

Worms

Worms are complex organisms that range in size from microscopic to several metres long. There are two types, flatworms and roundworms, that are adapted to infest humans. Adult worms or immature larvae infest various parts of the body, including the intestines and blood vessels.

Nerve ring

⊢ 1mm ⊣ **SCALE**

Cuticle

Mouth

Ovary

Intestine

Female roundworm
Roundworms have long, cylindrical bodies with a tough covering. Eggs laid by the female are excreted in the faeces of infected people.

Anus

Fluke
Most common in the tropics, flukes are flat and leaf-shaped or elongated parasitic flatworms.

Viral infections

Some of the most familiar minor illnesses, such as coughs, sore throats, and attacks of diarrhoea and vomiting, are often caused by viral infections. However, viruses are responsible not only for minor infections but also for potentially fatal diseases, such as rabies and some viral haemorrhagic fevers (for example, Ebola infection).

The first articles discuss frequently occurring viral infections such as the common cold and influenza, the related infections chickenpox and herpes zoster, and herpes simplex infections. The next articles describe the once-common viral infections of childhood: measles, mumps, and rubella. Until the second half of the 20th century, almost all children experienced these illnesses. Routine immunization has now made such diseases rare in developed countries. However, some of these viruses can still affect adults who have not been immunized,

producing symptoms that are often severe. Articles follow on a number of viral diseases, including yellow fever and dengue fever, that may be encountered in the developing world. The section ends with an article on HIV infection and AIDS.

Viral infections that affect only one body system are covered elsewhere in the book. For example, acute hepatitis (p.408) and chronic hepatitis (p.409) are covered in liver and gallbladder disorders, and genital herpes (p.493) and genital warts (p.493) are covered in sexually transmitted infections.

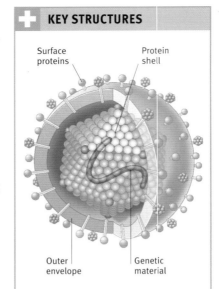

KEY STRUCTURES

Surface proteins

Protein shell

Outer envelope

Genetic material

For more information on the structure and function of viruses, *see* p.161.

Common cold

An infection of the nose and throat that can be caused by many different viruses

 More common in children

 Gender, genetics, and lifestyle are not significant factors

There are at least 200 highly contagious viruses that are known to cause the common cold, including rhinoviruses, coronaviruses, and respiratory syncytial virus (RSV). These viruses are easily transmitted in the minute airborne droplets sprayed from the coughs or sneezes of infected people. In many cases, the viruses are also spread to the nose and throat by way of hand-to-hand contact with an infected person or by way of objects that have become contaminated with the virus.

Colds can occur at any time of the year, although they are more frequent in autumn and winter. In the UK, adults typically get between two and five colds a year and children get between seven and ten. Children are more susceptible to colds than adults because they have not yet developed immunity to the most common cold viruses and also because the viruses usually spread very quickly in communities such as nurseries and schools.

What are the symptoms?
The initial symptoms of a cold usually develop between 1 and 3 days after infection. Symptoms usually intensify over 24–48 hours, unlike those of influenza (right), which usually worsen rapidly over a few hours. If you have a cold, symptoms may include:

- Frequent sneezing.
- Runny nose with a clear watery discharge that later becomes thick and green coloured.
- Mild fever and headache.
- Sore throat and, sometimes, a cough.

In some people, a common cold may be complicated by a bacterial infection such as

Airborne droplets

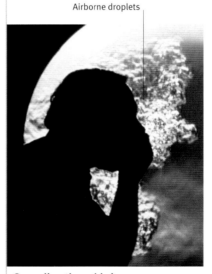

Spreading the cold virus
Cold viruses are easily spread by coughs and sneezes. This specialized photograph shows how far droplets are sprayed by a sneeze, even when a handkerchief is used.

an infection of the chest (*see* **Acute bronchitis**, p.297) or of the sinuses (*see* **Sinusitis**, p.290). Bacterial ear infections, which may cause earache, are a common complication of colds (*see* **Otitis media**, p.374, and **Acute otitis media in children**, p.557).

What can I do?
Most people recognize their symptoms as those of a common cold and do not seek medical advice.

Despite a great deal of scientific research, there is no cure for the common cold, but over-the-counter drugs (*see* **Cold and flu remedies**, p.588) can help to relieve the symptoms. These drugs include painkillers (p.589) to relieve a headache and reduce a fever, and decongestants (p.587) to help clear a stuffy nose. It is important to drink plenty of fluids, particularly if you have a fever (*see* **Bringing down a fever**, opposite page). Many people take large quantities of vitamin C to prevent infection and treat the common cold, but any benefit from this popular remedy is unproved.

If your symptoms do not improve in a week or your child is no better in 2 days, you should consult a doctor. If you have developed a bacterial infection on top of a cold, your doctor may prescribe antibiotics (p.572). (Antibiotics are ineffective against viruses so will not help the cold.)

The common cold usually clears up without treatment within 2 weeks, but a cough may last longer.

Influenza

An infection of the upper respiratory tract (airways), commonly known as flu

 Age, gender, genetics, and lifestyle are not significant factors

Influenza, also known as flu, is a contagious viral disease that tends to occur in epidemics during the winter but may occur any time of the year. The infection mainly affects the upper respiratory tract (airways).

Types of influenza
Many different viral infections can result in mild flu-like symptoms, but true influenza is caused by three types

of influenza virus: A, B, and C. These viruses can affect animals and birds as well as humans.

Type A can affect birds, pigs, and humans, and is responsible for the influenza pandemics (widespread epidemics) that occur periodically. The 1918 Spanish flu pandemic, 1957 Asian flu pandemic, 1968 Hong Kong flu pandemic, and 2009 swine flu pandemic were all caused by type A influenza.

Type B affects humans almost exclusively but can also affect seals and ferrets. It typically causes only small, localized influenza outbreaks. Type C can affect humans, dogs, and pigs but is less common than the other types and usually causes only mild disease in children.

Types A and B are constantly changing their structure (mutating) and producing new strains to which few people have immunity. That is why it is recommended that certain groups get immunized every year against the particular strain that is circulating. Swine flu and bird flu are variants of type A influenza that originated in pigs and birds, respectively, and can cause influenza in humans.

The influenza virus can be spread in several ways. Typically, it is transmitted in airborne droplets from the coughs and sneezes of infected people or by direct human-to-human contact. "Ordinary" seasonal influenza and swine flu can be spread in these ways. However, there have been very few cases of human-to-human transmission of bird flu and it seems that this type is almost always caught directly from infected birds.

What are the symptoms?
All types of influenza produce similar symptoms, which resemble those of the common cold (left) but, unlike the cold, tend to worsen rapidly over just a few hours. Symptoms of influenza may include the following:

- Fever (38°C/100.4°F or above), sweating, and shivering.
- Cough.
- Aches and pains.
- Severe exhaustion.
- Frequent sneezing, stuffy or runny nose, sore throat.
- Headache.
- Vomiting or diarrhoea.

For all types of influenza the symptoms usually last for a few days and then clear up, although tiredness and depression may be experienced after the other symptoms have disappeared.

Are there complications?
The most serious complication of influenza is infection of the lungs (*see* **Pneumonia**, p.299), which can be life-threatening to people in certain high-risk groups. These include babies and children under 5 years old; pregnant women; adults over 65; those with reduced immunity, such as people with HIV/AIDS (p.169) and those

undergoing chemotherapy or treatment with corticosteroids; people with chronic lung disease or asthma (p.295); those with heart disease, diabetes mellitus (p.437) or another metabolic disorder, chronic liver disease, cystic fibrosis (p.535), sickle-cell disease (p.272), kidney disease, or muscular dystrophy p.536); and people who have recently had a stroke (p.329) or who have a nervous system disorder such as cerebral palsy (p.548), Parkinson's disease (p.333), or multiple sclerosis (p.334).

What might be done?

The symptoms of all types of influenza can be relieved by resting in bed, drinking plenty of fluids, and following the advice for bringing down a fever (below). Paracetamol helps lower temperature and ease aches and pains; ibuprofen has the same effects but should not be taken by pregnant women. However, you should consult your doctor immediately if you are in a high-risk group or have another serious underlying illness, if you have breathing difficulty, if your condition suddenly gets worse, or if your symptoms are still worsening after 7 days (or 5 days for a child). Your doctor may prescribe the antiviral drugs oseltamivir (Tamiflu) or zanamivir (Relenza). These drugs may reduce the severity and duration of the illness. They are best taken within 48 hours of the onset of symptoms, but the earlier the better. Your doctor may also arrange for tests to check for another infection, such as pneumonia. If another infection is found, your doctor may prescribe antibiotics (p.572), and in certain cases admission to hospital may be advised.

Bringing down a fever

A fever is a body temperature that is above 38°C (100.4°F). If you or your child develops a fever, look at the symptom charts on p.45 and p.115 to check whether medical help is required. If medical help is not necessary, follow the measures described below:

- Drink plenty of fluids.
- You can take paracetamol or ibuprofen to help bring down the fever and make you feel more comfortable. For a baby or child, give paracetamol or ibuprofen at the dose recommended for his or her age.
- Make sure the room temperature is neither too hot nor too cold.
- Dress lightly. Do not "wrap up" a child who has a fever.
- Young children should be watched closely as they are susceptible to febrile convulsions if they have a high fever.
- Sponging with tepid water to bring down a fever is no longer advised.
- Do not give aspirin to anyone under 16 years old.

To reduce the spread of all types of influenza (and other infectious diseases) general hygiene measures are important: you should cover your nose and mouth with a tissue when coughing or sneezing and then dispose of the tissue promptly and carefully; wash your hands frequently with soap and water; and clean hard surfaces (such as door handles and work surfaces) frequently. You should also make sure any children in the household follow these measures. People with symptoms of influenza should stay at home until they feel better as this will also help prevent the spread of the disease.

What is the prognosis?

For normally healthy people who do not develop complications, most symptoms of influenza usually disappear after 6–7 days, although a cough may persist for over 2 weeks and tiredness may last longer. However, for a minority of people – principally those in high-risk groups – influenza may cause severe illness and serious complications, which may be fatal in some cases.

Can it be prevented?

The influenza virus mutates frequently and different strains are in circulation each year. The strains most likely to be circulating in any given year are included in the flu vaccine for that year. Immunization can therefore significantly reduce the likelihood of getting flu, although it can never guarantee complete protection because of the possibility that a new strain of influenza might arise.

Annual flu vaccination is recommended for various groups, including those over 65; pregnant women; adults with certain medical conditions or health problems; those with a weakened immune system; healthy infants and children aged 2 to 4 years old, plus those in school years 1 and 2; children with a long-term health condition; and adults at particular risk of infection, such as health care and social care workers.

Antiviral medications can reduce the severity and duration of influenza but cannot prevent it.

Chickenpox

A childhood infection that causes a fever and widespread crops of blisters

 Mainly affects unimmunized children between the ages of 2 and 10

 Gender, genetics, and lifestyle are not significant factors

Chickenpox, sometimes called varicella, is a common viral infection that mostly affects young children. The infection, with its characteristic rash of blisters, is caused by the varicella zoster virus, which also causes herpes zoster (p.166). The virus is infectious and is easily transmitted in air-

borne droplets from the coughs and sneezes of infected people or by direct contact with the blisters. You can catch chickenpox from someone who has either chickenpox or herpes zoster (shingles) if you are not immune but you cannot catch shingles from a person who has chickenpox.

The illness is usually mild in children, but symptoms are more severe in young babies, older adolescents, and adults. Chickenpox can also be more serious in people with reduced immunity, such as those with AIDS (*see* **HIV infection and AIDS**, p.169).

What are the symptoms?

The symptoms of chickenpox appear 10–21 days after infection. In children, the illness often starts with a mild fever or headache; in adults, there may be more pronounced flu-like symptoms (*see* **Influenza**, opposite page). As infection with the virus progresses, the following symptoms usually become apparent:

- Rash in the form of crops of tiny, red spots that rapidly turn into itchy, fluid-filled blisters. Within 24 hours the blisters dry out, forming scabs. Successive crops occur for 1–6 days. The rash may be widespread or consist of only a few spots, and it can occur anywhere on the head or body.
- Sometimes, discomfort during eating caused by spots in the mouth that have developed into ulcers.

A person with chickenpox is contagious from about 2 days before the rash first appears until up to 6 days after the rash has first appeared.

The most common complication of chickenpox is bacterial infection of the blisters due to scratching. Other complications include pneumonia (p.299), which is more common in adults, and, rarely, inflammation of the brain (*see* **Viral encephalitis**, p.326). Newborn babies and people with reduced immunity are at higher risk of complications. Rarely, if a

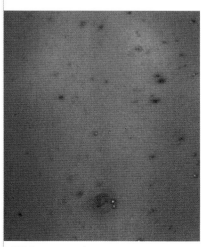

Chickenpox rash
Itchy, fluid-filled blisters are usually widespread all over the head and body in chickenpox. The blisters, seen here on the abdomen, form scabs within 24 hours.

woman develops chickenpox in early pregnancy, the infection may result in fetal abnormalities.

What might be done?

Chickenpox can usually be diagnosed from the appearance of the rash. Children with mild infections do not need to see a doctor; rest and simple measures to reduce fever (*see* **Bringing down a fever**, left) are all that are needed for a full recovery. Calamine lotion (*see* **Antipruritic drugs**, p.576) may help to relieve the itchiness of the rash. To prevent skin infections, especially in children, keep fingernails short and avoid scratching. People who are at risk of severe attacks, such as babies, older adolescents, adults, and people with reduced immunity, should be seen by their doctor immediately. An antiviral drug (p.573) may be given to limit the effects of the infection, but it must be taken in the early stages of the illness in order to be effective.

Children who are otherwise healthy usually recover within 10–14 days from the onset of the rash, but they may be left with permanent scars where the blisters have been scratched and then developed a bacterial infection. Adolescents, adults, and people who have reduced immunity take longer to recover from chickenpox.

To avoid spreading the disease, children with chickenpox should stay at home for 5–6 days. Adults should stay at home until they are no longer infectious. Infected people and those in close contact with them should avoid contact with newborn babies, pregnant women, and anybody with a weakened immune system.

Can it be prevented?

One attack of chickenpox usually gives lifelong immunity to the disease. However, the varicella zoster virus remains dormant within nerve cells and may reactivate years later, causing herpes zoster. A vaccine against chickenpox is available but is not part of the routine immunization schedule. However, it is recommended for those at high risk of severe chickenpox infection, and for those who are not immune and are at increased risk of contracting the infection (healthcare workers, for example) and passing it on to somebody at risk of developing severe infection (such as a person with reduced immunity). The vaccine should not be given to pregnant women, those with reduced immunity, or people who are seriously unwell. Women who are given the vaccine should avoid becoming pregnant within a month of vaccination.

Herpes zoster

An infection, also known as shingles, that causes a painful rash of blisters along the path of a nerve

 Most common between the ages of 50 and 70

 Gender, genetics, and lifestyle are not significant factors

Herpes zoster, often known as shingles, is characterized by a painful crop of blisters that erupts along the path of a nerve. The rash commonly occurs on only one side of the body and usually affects the skin on the chest, abdomen, or face. In older people, discomfort may continue for months after the rash has disappeared. This prolonged pain is called postherpetic neuralgia.

Herpes zoster infection is caused by the varicella zoster virus. This virus initially causes chickenpox (p.165) but then remains dormant in nerve cells. If the virus is reactivated later in life, it causes herpes zoster. The reason for reactivation is unknown, but herpes zoster often occurs at times of stress or ill health. The disorder most commonly occurs in people aged 50–70 years. People with reduced immunity, such as those with AIDS (*see* **HIV infection and AIDS**, p.169) or those undergoing chemotherapy (p.157), are more susceptible to herpes zoster. People with AIDS are particularly likely to have severe outbreaks of herpes zoster.

The varicella zoster virus is easily spread by direct contact with a blister and will cause chickenpox in a person who is not immune to the disease.

What are the symptoms?

Initially, you may experience tingling, itching, and a sharp pain in an area of skin. After a few days, the following symptoms may also develop:

- Painful rash of red spots that turn into fluid-filled blisters.
- Fever.
- Headache.
- Tiredness.

Within 3–4 days, the blisters form scabs. These scabs heal and drop off within 10 days but may leave scars in some people. If a nerve that supplies the eye is affected, it may cause a potentially serious inflammation of the cornea (*see* **Corneal ulcer**, p.356). Rarely, infection of a facial nerve causes weakness or paralysis on one side of the face (*see* **Facial palsy**, p.339).

What might be done?

Herpes zoster can be difficult to diagnose until the rash appears, and severe pain around the ribs can be mistaken for the chest pain of angina (p.244). Your doctor may prescribe antiviral drugs (p.573) to reduce the severity of the symptoms and the risk of postherpetic neuralgia. If your eyes are affected or if you have reduced immunity, you will need immediate treatment with antiviral drugs. Painkillers (p.589) may help to relieve discomfort, and amitriptyline (*see* **Antidepressant drugs**, p.592) or gabapentin (*see* **Anticonvulsant drugs**, p.590) may help to relieve the prolonged pain of postherpetic neuralgia. Most people who develop herpes zoster recover within 2–6 weeks, but up to half of all affected people over the age of 50 develop postherpetic neuralgia.

A single attack of herpes zoster does not provide immunity to the disease, and the infection may recur. A vaccine to prevent shingles is routinely offered to certain people aged 70 or over.

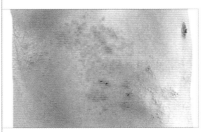

Herpes zoster rash
A rash of blisters develops along the path of a nerve in herpes zoster. The blisters often occur on the skin over the ribs on only one side of the body, as shown here.

Herpes simplex infections

Infections that can cause painful blisters on or around the lips or genitals

 Unprotected sex with multiple partners is a risk factor for genital herpes

 Age, gender, and genetics are not significant factors

The highly contagious herpes simplex viruses cause a number of different disorders characterized by small, painful blisters on the skin and mucous membranes, most commonly on or around the lips (*see* **Cold sore**, p.205) or genital area (*see* **Genital herpes**, p.493). Herpes simplex virus (HSV) infection is transmitted by contact with a blister.

Infection with HSV does not give immunity against future attacks. The viruses remain dormant in the nerves and may be reactivated by stress or illness. Outbreaks are more frequent and severe in people with reduced immunity, such as those with AIDS (*see* **HIV infection and AIDS**, p.169).

What are the types?

Several types of HSV have been identified. The two most common types are HSV1 and HSV2. HSV1 usually causes infections of the lips, mouth, and face; and HSV2 typically causes infections of the genitals. However, there is considerable overlap between the two types: conditions that are typically caused by HSV1 may sometimes be caused by HSV2 and vice versa.

Most people have been infected with HSV1 by the time they are adults. In most cases, the initial infection produces no symptoms, but some children may develop blisters on the inside of the mouth (*see* **Stomatitis**, p.401), and children with the skin disorder eczema may develop eczema herpeticum (*see* **Eczema in children**, p.538). After the initial infection, the virus becomes dormant but may reactivate periodically later in life, causing cold sores.

HSV2 is usually sexually transmitted and causes genital herpes. This condition, like cold sores, tends to recur. HSV2 can also cause a life-threatening infection in a newborn baby if the baby comes into contact with the mother's genital blisters during birth (*see* **Congenital infections**, p.530).

Both HSV1 and HSV2 can affect the eyes, causing inflammation and a discharge (*see* **Conjunctivitis**, p.355); without treatment, a corneal ulcer (p.356) may develop. In rare cases, infection with HSV results in severe inflammation of the brain (*see* **Viral encephalitis**, p.326).

What might be done?

HSV infection can be diagnosed from the appearance and site of the blisters. Mild cold sores can usually be treated with over-the-counter topical antiviral drugs (p.573). If you have genital herpes or severe or recurrent cold sores, you may be given oral antiviral drugs. The earlier these drugs are given, the more effective they are likely to be.

Infectious mononucleosis

An infection causing swollen lymph nodes and a sore throat that is common in adolescence and early adulthood

 Most common between the ages of 12 and 20

 Gender, genetics, and lifestyle are not significant factors

Infectious mononucleosis is known as the "kissing disease" of adolescence and early adulthood because it is mainly transmitted in saliva. Another name is glandular fever because the symptoms include swollen lymph nodes (glands) and a high temperature. The illness is usually characterized by tonsillitis (*see* **Pharyngitis and tonsillitis**, p.293), which may be severe.

What is the cause?

Infectious mononucleosis is usually caused by the Epstein–Barr virus (EBV), which attacks lymphocytes, the white blood cells that are responsible for fighting infection. EBV infection is very common; about 9 in 10 people have been infected by the age of 50. More than half of all infected people do not develop symptoms and, consequently, are unaware that they have been infected.

What are the symptoms?

If symptoms of infectious mononucleosis develop, they usually do so 4–8 weeks after infection and appear over several days. Symptoms may include:

- High fever and sweating.
- Extremely sore throat, causing difficulty in swallowing.
- Swollen tonsils, often covered with a thick, greyish-white coating.
- Enlarged, tender lymph nodes in the neck, armpits, and groin.
- Tender abdomen as the result of an enlarged spleen.

These symptoms are often accompanied by poor appetite, weight loss, headache, and tiredness; sometimes, there may be a rash on the trunk and face. In some people, the sore throat and fever clear up quickly, and the other symptoms last less than a month. Other people may be ill for longer and feel lethargic for months after the infection.

What might be done?

Your doctor will probably diagnose the infection from your symptoms. A blood test may be carried out to look for antibodies against EBV. A throat swab may also be taken to exclude bacterial infection, which may need treatment with antibiotics (p.572).

There is no specific treatment for infectious mononucleosis, but simple measures may help to relieve symptoms. Drinking plenty of cool fluids and taking over-the-counter painkillers (p.589), such as paracetamol, may help to control the fever and pain. Alcohol should be avoided until you have recovered fully, because the liver may be affected. Contact sports should also be avoided until at least 6–8 weeks after recovery, because the spleen may be enlarged as a result of the illness.

What is the prognosis?

Almost everyone who has infectious mononucleosis makes a full recovery eventually. However, in some people, recovery may be slow, and tiredness may last for weeks or even months after the symptoms first appear. One attack of the disease, with or without symptoms, provides lifelong protection.

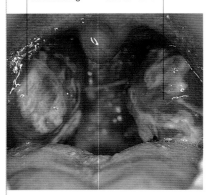

Thick coating   Swollen tonsil

Swollen tonsils
In infectious mononucleosis, the tonsils become swollen, causing a very sore throat. They may also become covered with a thick, greyish-white coating.

Cytomegalovirus infection

An infection that usually produces no symptoms but can cause fatal illness in people with reduced immunity

 Age, gender, genetics, and lifestyle are not significant factors

Infection with cytomegalovirus (CMV) is very common and affects most people at some time in their lives. However, most people do not develop symptoms and are not aware that they have been infected with the virus, although they will carry CMV for life in an inactive form. CMV is a type of herpesvirus.

People with reduced immunity, such as those who have AIDS (*see* **HIV infection and AIDS**, p.169), are at risk of serious illness from a first infection, and CMV can also be reactivated in this group. In addition, the virus can seriously affect a fetus if a woman is first infected during pregnancy (*see* **Congenital infections**, p.530).

The virus can be passed in saliva, in minute droplets from the coughs or sneezes of infected people; during sexual intercourse; through a blood transfusion; during an organ transplant; and across the placenta to a fetus if the mother becomes infected during pregnancy. In developed countries, blood that is used for transfusion to high-risk groups is screened for CMV.

What are the symptoms?

CMV infection can produce widely differing symptoms, depending on the age and general health of the person affected. Most people have no symptoms from a first infection with the virus. If symptoms are present, they are often vague and may include:

- Tiredness.
- Fever.
- Sore throat.
- Nausea, vomiting, and diarrhoea.

In teenagers and young adults, symptoms may resemble those of infectious mononucleosis (opposite page)

The symptoms of CMV infection are more severe in people with reduced immunity. In such cases, first infection or reactivation of the virus can result in a fever lasting for 2–3 weeks, a nonitchy rash, and inflammation of the liver (*see* **Acute hepatitis**, p.408), which causes yellowing of the skin and whites of the eyes (*see* **Jaundice**, p.407). In addition, the virus can cause inflammation of the brain (*see* **Viral encephalitis**, p.326) and the lungs (*see* **Pneumonia**, p.299). In people with reduced immunity, CMV can also cause retinitis (inflammation of the light-sensitive cells at the back of the eye), which may result in blindness.

If a woman is first infected with the virus during pregnancy, there is a risk that the virus will infect the fetus and the baby may

be born with jaundice, liver enlargement, and certain blood disorders. In other cases where the fetus is infected during pregnancy there are no symptoms present at birth but disorders such as hearing loss may develop later in life.

What might be done?

In a person who is otherwise healthy, CMV infection usually goes unnoticed, causes no problems, and is not treated. If your symptoms are severe and your doctor suspects CMV infection, he or she may arrange for a blood test to look for antibodies against the virus. The symptoms are often relieved by early treatment with antiviral drugs (p.573).

For people with reduced immunity, complications can be life-threatening. These people may be given antiviral drugs to protect against infection or, if a blood test shows that the virus is already present, to prevent symptoms from developing. Drugs may also be given to a pregnant woman who has the infection to help protect the fetus.

Measles

A childhood illness that causes fever and a widespread nonitchy rash

 Mainly affects unimmunized children between the ages of 1 and 5

 Gender, genetics, and lifestyle are not significant factors

Measles is a highly contagious viral illness that causes a distinctive rash and fever and mainly affects young children. Rare in the developed world because of routine immunization, the disease kills more than 100,000 unimmunized children in the developing world each year.

The measles virus is easily transmitted in minute airborne droplets from the coughs and sneezes of infected people. A child who has measles may feel very ill, and there is a small risk of complications, especially if the child has reduced immunity or is severely malnourished. Measles is contagious for 1–2 days before the rash appears and for about 5 days afterwards.

What are the symptoms?

Symptoms of measles usually develop 10 days after infection and may include:

- Fever.
- Tiny white spots with a red base, known as Koplik spots, on the insides of the cheeks.
- After 2–4 days, a red, nonitchy rash that starts on the head and spreads downwards. At first, the rash consists of separate flat spots. The spots then merge to give a blotchy appearance.
- Painful, red, watery eyes (*see* **Conjunctivitis**, p.355).
- Stuffy or runny nose.
- Hacking cough.

The most common complications of measles are bacterial infections of the middle ear (*see* **Acute otitis media in children**, p.557) and the lungs (*see* **Pneumonia**, p.299). In about 1 in 1,000 cases, the brain is affected (*see* **Viral encephalitis**, p.326), a serious complication that starts 7–10 days after the appearance of the rash.

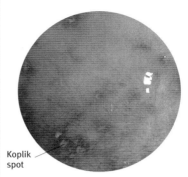

Koplik spot

Koplik spots in measles
These tiny white spots may appear on the insides of the cheeks when the symptoms of measles first develop, shortly before the onset of the rash on the head and body.

What might be done?

Your doctor will probably be able to diagnose measles from the combination of symptoms. In most children, rest and simple measures to reduce a fever (*see* **Bringing down a fever**, p.165) are all that are needed for a full recovery. If there are no complications, symptoms usually disappear in 7 days. Antibiotics (p.572) may be prescribed if a bacterial infection develops as a complication of measles, such as pneumonia.

Can it be prevented?

Babies and young children are immunized against measles with the measles, mumps, and rubella (MMR) vaccine, given at 12–13 months and again between 3 years 4 months and 5 years (*see* **Routine immunizations**, p.13). Immunization or an attack of measles usually gives lifelong immunity.

Mumps

An illness causing swelling of the salivary glands on one or both sides of the jaw

 Mainly affects unimmunized schoolchildren and young adults

 Gender, genetics, and lifestyle are not significant factors

Mumps is a mild viral infection that was common among schoolchildren until routine immunization was introduced. The mumps virus is spread in saliva and in minute airborne droplets from the coughs and sneezes of infected people. The virus causes swelling and inflammation of one or both of the parotid salivary glands, which are situated below and just in front of the ears. If both glands are affected, the child's face may have a hamster-like appearance. In adolescent boys and men, the virus may

affect the testes; rarely, this effect may result in problems with fertility (*see* **Male infertility**, p.499).

What are the symptoms?

Up to half of all people with mumps develop no symptoms, and in most other people the symptoms are mild. The main symptoms appear 2–3 weeks after infection and may include:

- Pain and swelling on one or both sides of the face, below and just in front of the ear, lasting about 3 days.
- Pain when swallowing.

A person infected with the mumps virus may also have a sore throat and fever, and the salivary glands under the chin may become painful. He or she is contagious from 2 days before the swelling first appears until 5 days after the swelling has appeared.

About 1 in 4 adolescent boys or adult men with mumps also develops painful inflammation of one or both testes (*see* **Epididymo-orchitis**, p.459). Rarely, the inflammation may result in infertility. A few people who develop mumps also develop viral meningitis (p.325), in which the membranes that surround the brain and spinal cord become inflamed. Inflammation of the pancreas (*see* **Acute pancreatitis**, p.413) is a rare complication of mumps.

What might be done?

Your doctor will probably diagnose the disorder from the distinctive swelling of the parotid glands. There is no specific treatment, but drinking plenty of cool fluids and taking over-the-counter painkillers (p.589), such as paracetamol, may relieve discomfort. Most people recover without further treatment, but adolescent boys and men who have severe inflammation of the testes may be prescribed a stronger painkiller. If complications develop, other types of treatment may be recommended.

Can it be prevented?

Babies and young children are immunized against mumps with the measles, mumps, and rubella (MMR) vaccine, given at 12–13 months and again between 3 years 4 months and 5 years (*see* **Routine immunizations**, p.13). Immunization or an attack of mumps usually gives lifelong immunity.

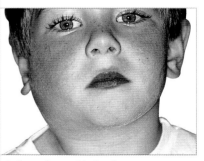

Inflamed parotid gland
The parotid glands are situated below and just in front of each ear. In the viral infection mumps, one (as shown above) or both parotid glands may become swollen.

Rubella

An illness, also known as German measles, that is usually mild but can severely damage a developing fetus

 Age, gender, genetics, and lifestyle are not significant factors

Rubella, also called German measles, usually causes little more than a mild rash. However, because it can cause serious birth defects in a fetus if the mother contracts the illness during early pregnancy, unimmunized pregnant women should avoid contact with an infected person. The disease is caused by the highly contagious rubella virus, which is transmitted through airborne droplets from the coughs and sneezes of infected people. Rubella has become less common in the developed world because of routine childhood immunization.

What are the symptoms?

The symptoms of rubella appear from 2–3 weeks after infection and may include all or some of the following:

- Swollen lymph nodes at the back of the neck and behind the ears. In some cases, lymph nodes throughout the body are swollen, including those in the armpits and groin.
- After 2–3 days, a pink, nonitchy rash, first on the face and then the body, that usually disappears within 3 days.

Children may have mild fever, but adolescents and adults can develop high fever and headache. Rarely, several joints may become inflamed for a short time (*see* **Reactive arthritis**, p.224). A person who has rubella is infectious from about 7 days before the rash appears until about 5 days after the rash has appeared.

Are there complications?

If you contract rubella in early pregnancy, there is a risk of miscarriage (p.511) or, if your baby is carried to term, he or she is at serious risk of being born with abnormalities, such as congenital deafness (p.556), congenital heart disease (p.542), clouding of the lens in the eye (*see* **Cataract**, p.357), and the nervous system disorder cerebral palsy (p.548). The greatest risk is during the first 3 months of pregnancy, and the earlier rubella is contracted, the more likely the

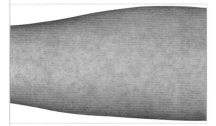

Rubella rash
The light pink rash of rubella is shown here on an arm. The rash usually first develops on the face and gradually spreads to the trunk and then to the limbs.

baby will be seriously affected. However, contracting rubella later in pregnancy also puts the baby at risk.

What might be done?

Your doctor may suspect rubella from the symptoms, but the rash is not distinctive and other viral infections can produce similar symptoms. He or she may arrange for a blood test to confirm the diagnosis. There is no specific treatment for this disease, but drinking plenty of cool fluids and taking over-the-counter painkillers (p.589), such as paracetamol, may help to reduce fever and ease discomfort. Most affected people recover in about 10 days, and one attack usually gives lifelong immunity against the virus.

If you are pregnant and have rubella or have been in contact with someone with the disease, it is important to discuss with your doctor the risk to the fetus and how best to proceed.

Can it be prevented?

Babies and young children are immunized against rubella with the measles, mumps, and rubella (MMR) vaccine, given at 12–13 months and again between 3 years 4 months and 5 years (*see* **Routine immunizations**, p.13). Immunization or an attack of rubella provides long-term immunity. Nevertheless, women who are planning a pregnancy should be tested for antibodies against rubella and should receive advice about immunization.

Fifth disease

An infection that causes a rash and inflammation of the joints

 Mainly affects children

 Gender, genetics, and lifestyle are not significant factors

Fifth disease, also known as erythema infectiosum or slapped cheek disease, is caused by a strain of parvovirus (strain B19). It mainly affects children, in whom it typically causes a mild illness, with a fever that is often unnoticed. It is rare in adults but may cause severe joint pain. Parvovirus is usually transmitted in airborne droplets from the coughs and sneezes of infected individuals but it may occasionally be transmitted through a blood transfusion or from mother to fetus. Infection causes a brief halt in red blood cell production, so can have serious effects in people with anaemia (p.271).

What are the symptoms?

Many children do not develop symptoms; in others they may appear within 7–18 days of infection:

- Bright red rash on the cheeks that may spread to the trunk and limbs.
- Mild fever.
- In rare cases, mild inflammation of the joints (*see* **Arthritis**, p.220).

Adults are likely to develop more severe symptoms that may include:

- Rash on the palms and soles.
- Severe inflammation and pain in the joints of the knees, wrists, and hands.

Some people develop a form of arthritis that can last for up to 2 years.

In people with reduced immunity, the infection may become long-term and can cause anaemia. Many pregnant women are immune to the virus. However, for women who are not immune, contracting the infection during the first 20 weeks of pregnancy increases the risk of miscarriage (p.511) and of the baby developing hydrops fetalis, a serious condition in which there is anaemia, heart failure, and tissue swelling.

What might be done?

If the parvovirus infection cannot be diagnosed from symptoms a blood test may detect antibodies against the virus. One attack of parvovirus infection provides lifelong immunity.

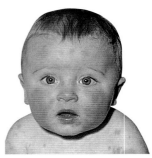

Fifth disease rash
The bright red rash on this baby's face is due to fifth disease. The condition is also known as slapped cheek disease.

Poliomyelitis

A rare infection, commonly known as polio, that can affect the nervous system

 Mainly affects unimmunized children but can affect unimmunized adults

 Travel in some parts of Asia and Africa is a risk factor

 Gender and genetics are not significant factors

Poliomyelitis is a highly infectious disease that varies in severity from a mild condition with few or no symptoms to a disease that can lead to paralysis. The polio virus is most commonly transmitted by contact with the faeces of an infected person but can also be spread through saliva and airborne droplets.

Since routine immunization began in the 1950s, polio has been virtually eliminated from developed countries. However, in some parts of Africa and Asia the disease remains a serious risk for travellers who do not have up-to-date immunization.

What are the symptoms?

For most infected people, polio produces no symptoms or results in a mild illness with a slight fever and sore throat that develops 3–21 days after infection. However, in about

1 in 75 adults and 1 in 1,000 children, the brain and spinal cord become inflamed. In a few cases, one or more limbs may be paralysed, and the muscles of the respiratory system may be affected.

What might be done?

In most cases, polio is undiagnosed and untreated. If the disease is suspected it can be confirmed by tests on the faeces. There is no specific treatment. People who have severe symptoms are admitted to hospital, and if the respiratory muscles are paralysed, mechanical ventilation may be given.

Most people make a full recovery from milder forms of the disease. Of those who become paralysed, many improve within 6 months.

Can it be prevented?

In the UK, vaccination against polio is given at ages 2, 3, and 4 months, with booster doses between the ages of 3 years 4 months and 5 years, and again at 13–18 years. The polio vaccine is combined with other vaccines and given as part of the routine childhood immunization programme (p.13). Since 2004, inactivated polio vaccine (given by injection) has been used; this is safer than the previously used live oral vaccine. Before travelling to areas where infection with polio is still a risk, adults may need a booster dose of vaccine (*see* **Travel immunizations**, p.35).

Severe acute respiratory syndrome

A potentially serious viral infection sometimes causing pneumonia

 Living in or visiting areas where the disease is known to have occurred is a risk factor

 Age, gender, and genetics are not significant factors

Severe acute respiratory syndrome (SARS) is believed to have originated in China in late 2002 from where it spread to affect areas around the world. A strain of coronavirus is the cause of the disease. It is spread by inhaling infected droplets (from a sneeze or cough, for instance), by contact with infected surfaces, or by close personal contact.

What are the symptoms?

After an incubation period of about 2–7 days, symptoms appear, including sudden onset of fever – generally over 38°C (100.4°F) – sometimes accompanied by chills, aching muscles, and headache. After a further 3–7 days, a dry (nonproductive) cough may develop. There may also be shortness of breath, which may become severe and which may indicate the development of pneumonia (p.299).

What might be done?

Various tests may be performed to confirm the diagnosis and to exclude other possible causes of pneumonia. The tests may include a blood test to check for antibodies associated with the virus, a viral culture, and a genetic test to look for viral DNA in the blood, faeces, or nasal secretions.

Treatment is mainly supportive and may include oxygen therapy, with artificial ventilation if necessary. In some cases, antibiotic and/or antiviral drugs may also be given. There is no vaccine or curative treatment at present. Control of the disease depends on physical measures, such as the use of face masks, handwashing, and isolation of infected people.

SARS is not highly infective, and most people who get the disease recover, including those who develop pneumonia. However, in some cases the illness is fatal.

Viral haemorrhagic fevers

A group of infections that cause abnormal bleeding and may be fatal

 Travel in some parts of Africa is a risk factor for some infections

 Age, gender, and genetics are not significant factors

Viral haemorrhagic fevers, which cause severe abnormal bleeding, occur predominantly in Africa. The only one with a worldwide distribution is Hantavirus infection. Marburg, Ebola, and Lassa fever occur only in localized outbreaks in Africa.

Hantavirus and Lassa fever virus are carried by rodents, and transmitted to people through contact with the animals' urine, faeces, or saliva. Marburg fever virus is carried by monkeys. The animal carrier of Ebola fever virus is probably the fruit bat. All the diseases are highly contagious and can be transmitted from person to person in body secretions.

What are the symptoms?

Symptoms typically develop slowly from a few days to about 3 weeks after infection and may include:
- Flu-like symptoms.
- Rash, which causes peeling skin in Ebola fever.
- Abnormal bleeding from the skin and mucous membranes.

Symptoms of viral haemorrhagic fevers vary from mild to severe, depending on the specific virus; Lassa fever may be symptomless. Complications of Ebola and Marburg fevers include acute kidney injury (p.450), severe breathing difficulty, and shock (p.248).

What might be done?

Viral haemorrhagic fevers are diagnosed from the symptoms and a blood test. There are no specific proven treatments for Hantavirus infection, Marburg fever, or Ebola fever. However, Lassa fever may respond to antiviral drugs (p.573) if given in the first week. The outlook depends on the type of virus and medical care available. Fatality rates vary from about 1 in 50 cases in Lassa fever up to about 9 in 10 cases in Ebola fever.

Yellow fever

An infection, mainly confined to Africa, that is transmitted by mosquitoes

 Travel to Africa and South and Central America is a risk factor

 Age, gender, and genetics are not significant factors

The tropical viral infection yellow fever was given its name because it can cause severe jaundice (p.407), in which the skin turns bright yellow. The virus is transmitted by mosquitoes from monkeys to humans and then by mosquitoes from person to person. More than 9 in 10 cases occur in Africa; the remainder occur mainly in South and Central America. The disease has become less common with routine immunization, but epidemics still occur in Africa.

The symptoms of yellow fever appear suddenly, 3–6 days after a bite from an infected mosquito. In some cases, there may be a mild flu-like illness. However, in other cases there may be abnormal bleeding, liver failure (p.411), or kidney failure (p.450). Severe bleeding may lead to shock (p.248). Rarely, the infection leads to convulsions and coma (p.323).

Diagnosis is based on the symptoms and confirmed by a blood test to look for antibodies against the virus. There is no specific treatment for yellow fever, and the disease is fatal in 2–5 out of 10 people. An attack provides lifelong immunity. Immunization gives protection for at least 10 years and is recommended for people travelling to high-risk areas (*see* Travel immunizations, p.35).

Dengue fever

An infection, also known as breakbone fever, caused by Flavivirus *and spread by mosquitoes*

 Travel to tropical and subtropical countries is a risk factor

 Age, gender, and genetics are not significant factors

Dengue fever is endemic in many tropical and subtropical areas of the world, and there are an estimated 100 million new cases every year. It can be caused by any one of four subtypes of *Flavivirus*, which are carried and transmitted by the mosquito *Aedes aegypti*. This mosquito is commonly found in pools of stagnant water and usually bites during the daytime. Since the disease causes severe pain in the muscles and joints, it is also known as "breakbone fever".

The symptoms of dengue fever appear 4–8 days after a bite from an infected mosquito. They include a high temperature, headache, severe backache, muscle pain and weakness, and joint pain. Small red spots may also develop on the skin during the first few days of the illness.

The fever often subsides for 3–4 days but then recurs before subsiding again. In severe cases, abnormal bleeding may occur from areas such as the gums and nose and from injection sites.

What might be done?

Dengue fever can usually be diagnosed from the symptoms. There is no specific treatment, but it is important to rest and drink plenty of cool fluids. Over-the-counter painkillers (p.589), such as paracetamol, may help to relieve symptoms and reduce fever. Severely affected people may need observation and treatment in hospital, but life-threatening complications are uncommon. Recovery usually takes several weeks.

An attack of dengue fever gives lifelong immunity, but only to the specific subtype of *Flavivirus* involved, and there is no vaccine against the virus. Travellers to areas where it is common should use mosquito repellents and wear clothing that completely covers the arms and legs (*see* Travel health, p.35).

Rabies

A serious infection of the nervous system, usually transmitted in saliva from a bite by an infected animal

 Travel to Africa, Asia, and South and Central America is a risk factor

 Age, gender, and genetics are not significant factors

The rabies virus mainly affects animals but can be passed to humans by an animal bite or a lick over a break in the skin. After entering the wound, the virus can travel along nerves to the brain and cause potentially fatal inflammation. Immunization against the virus and prompt medical treatment give complete protection against the disease, but, if left untreated, about half of all people bitten by a rabid animal develop rabies and almost inevitably die.

Rabies is very rare in developed countries, although only a few, including the UK, Japan, and Australia, are completely free from the disease. Africa and many parts of Asia are high-risk areas. In developed countries, most cases are due to bites from bats, and worldwide most cases result from bites by dogs that have been infected by other dogs or wild animals. Some animals infected with the rabies virus act aggressively and salivate excessively.

What are the symptoms?

An infected person may develop symptoms within 2–8 weeks of a bite, although the incubation period is very variable and the virus can lie dormant for months or longer before causing symptoms. Rabies usually starts with flu-like symptoms (*see* Influenza, p.164) that last for about 2–7 days, followed by:
- Paralysis of face and throat muscles.
- Extreme thirst.

- Painful throat spasms leading to an inability to drink and a fear of water.
- Disorientation and agitation.
- Loss of consciousness.
- Paralysis of limbs.

Once symptoms have developed, the condition is usually fatal.

What might be done?

Wash all suspect animal bites immediately with soap and water. Seek medical advice without delay because treatment must be started at once to be effective. Treatment includes injections of rabies immunoglobulin (antibodies against the virus), followed by a course of rabies vaccine to simulate production of more antibodies. If possible, the animal that inflicted the bite should be quarantined and observed.

There is no cure once symptoms have developed. Sedative drugs and painkillers may be given to help alleviate the symptoms, but the disease is almost always fatal. Diagnosis may not be obvious from the symptoms, and blood and saliva tests are usually carried out to confirm the presence of the virus.

Rabies can be prevented by a vaccine, which is recommended for people working with animals. It may also be advised for people travelling to or living in areas where rabies is endemic (*see* Travel immunizations, p.35).

HIV infection and AIDS

A long-term infection that, left untreated, results in reduced immunity to other infections

 Unprotected sex and intravenous drug use are risk factors

 Age, gender, and genetics are not significant factors

Infection with the human immunodeficiency virus (HIV), which can lead to acquired immunodeficiency syndrome (AIDS) if left untreated, has been one of the most written about and researched diseases of recent years. Despite the development of effective drugs to limit the progression of the infection, there is still no effective vaccine against the virus, and the number of people with HIV infection continues to rise, especially in developing countries, although the rate of new infections is declining in most parts of the world.

HIV is believed to have originated in Africa, where a similar virus is carried by some species of primate. The virus is thought to have spread from monkeys to humans, then around the world from person to person by sexual contact or through other exchange of body fluids. The first recognized cases of AIDS occurred in 1981, when there was an outbreak of unusual cases of pneumonia and skin cancer in young homosexual men in Los Angeles. Two years later, the causative virus was isolated and identified as HIV.

HIV infects and gradually destroys cells in the immune system, weakening the response to infections and cancers. People infected with HIV may have no symptoms for years, or may experience frequent or prolonged mild infections. When the immune system becomes severely weakened, people are susceptible to serious infections caused by organisms that are usually harmless, and also to certain types of cancer. The development of some specific diseases or cancers leads to a diagnosis of AIDS.

Who is affected?
At the end of 2013, there were an estimated 107,800 people in the UK living with HIV/AIDS, of whom about 26,100 were not aware they were infected. About 6,000 new cases of HIV infection were diagnosed in the UK in 2013. Worldwide, in 2013 there were an estimated 35 million people with HIV/AIDS, of whom about 24.7 million were living in sub-Saharan Africa; 2.1 million new cases were diagnosed in that year.

In the mid-1990s more effective antiviral drug therapy became available, as a result of which the number of deaths from HIV/AIDS in the developed world diminished significantly; in the UK, for example, deaths reduced from more than 1,700 in 1995 to 320 in 2013, and most of those who died were diagnosed in the late stage of their illness. However, antiviral therapy is complex, expensive, and requires detailed monitoring of patients, and therefore therapy was initially limited to patients in wealthier countries. More recently, access to antiviral therapy has improved in some developing countries. Nevertheless, about 1.5 million people still died from HIV/AIDS in developing countries in 2013, 1.1 million of whom lived in sub-Saharan Africa.

How is HIV transmitted?
In people infected with HIV, the virus is present in body fluids, including blood, semen, vaginal secretions, saliva, and breast milk. It is most commonly transmitted sexually, by anal, oral, or vaginal intercourse. People are at higher risk of HIV infection and more likely to transmit the virus if they have another sexually transmitted infection.

People who use intravenous drugs and share or reuse needles contaminated with the virus are at high risk of infection. Medical workers are also at risk from accidental skin punctures with contaminated needles (see **Needlestick injury**, p.207), but the risk is low.

HIV infection can be passed from an infected woman to the fetus or to the baby at birth (see **Congenital infections**, p.530) or by breast-feeding. The virus can be transmitted through organ transplants or blood transfusions, but in developed countries, routine screening of blood, organs, and tissues for HIV has made the risk of infection by these routes extremely low. HIV infection cannot be transmitted by everyday contact, such as

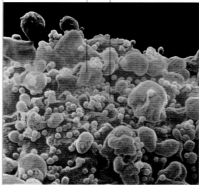
Cell surface   New HIV viruses

Human immunodeficiency virus
This highly magnified view of a white blood cell known as a CD4 lymphocyte shows tiny, newly formed HIV viruses budding out of the cell's uneven surface.

shaking hands, or by coughs or sneezes. There is no risk from working or living with an infected person.

What is the cause?
HIV enters the bloodstream and infects cells with a special structure called the CD4 receptor on their surfaces. These cells include a type of white blood cell known as a CD4 lymphocyte, which is responsible for fighting infection. The virus reproduces rapidly within the cells and destroys them in the process.

At first, the immune system is able to function normally, and symptoms may not develop for years. However, the number of CD4 lymphocytes eventually falls, causing susceptibility to other infections and some types of cancer.

What are the symptoms?
The first symptoms of HIV infection can appear within 6 weeks of the virus entering the body. Some people experience a flu-like illness that may include some or all of the following symptoms:
- Swollen lymph nodes (see **Lymphadenopathy**, p.279).
- Fever.
- Tiredness and aching muscles.
- Rash.
- Sore throat.

These symptoms usually clear up after a few weeks, and many people with HIV infection feel completely healthy. However, in some people, any of the following minor disorders may develop:
- Persistent, swollen lymph nodes.
- Mouth infections such as thrush (see **Candidiasis**, p.177).
- Furred white patches in the mouth (see **Leukoplakia**, p.402).
- Gum disease (see **Gingivitis**, p.389).
- Persistent herpes simplex infections (p.166), such as cold sores (p.205).
- Extensive genital warts (p.493).
- Itchy, flaky skin (see **Seborrhoeic dermatitis**, p.194).
- Weight loss.

The time between infection with HIV and the onset of AIDS varies and can be

between 1 and 14 years. Often, people are unaware for years that they are infected with HIV until they develop one or more serious infections or cancers known as AIDS-defining illnesses.

Are there complications?
The single complication of HIV infection is the development of AIDS. A person infected with HIV is said to have AIDS if he or she has developed a particular AIDS-defining illness. These illnesses include opportunistic infections (infections that occur only in people with reduced immunity), certain cancers, and nervous system disorders that may result in dementia (p.331), confusion, and memory loss.

Opportunistic infections These infections may be caused by protozoa, fungi, viruses, or bacteria, and can be life-threatening.

One of the most common illnesses in people with AIDS is a severe infection of the lungs by the parasite *Pneumocystis jirovecii* (see **Pneumocystis infection**, p.177). Other common diseases are the protozoal infections cryptosporidiosis (p.176), which may result in prolonged diarrhoea, and toxoplasmosis (p.176), which can affect the brain.

Candida albicans is a fungus that can cause mild superficial infections in healthy people but may produce much more serious infections in people who have developed AIDS (see **Candidiasis**, p.177). The cryptococcus fungus (see **Cryptococcosis**, p.177) may cause fever, headaches, and lung infections.

People with AIDS suffer from severe bacterial and viral infections. Bacterial infections include tuberculosis (p.300) and salmonellosis, which may lead to blood poisoning (see **Septicaemia**, opposite page). Viral infections include those caused by the herpes viruses. Herpes simplex infections can affect the brain, causing meningitis and viral encephalitis (p.326). Cytomegalovirus infection (p.167) may cause a number of severe conditions, including pneumonia, viral encephalitis, and a type of eye inflammation that can result in blindness.

Cancers The most common type of cancer that affects people with AIDS is Kaposi's sarcoma (p.201), a type of skin cancer that can also affect the inside of the mouth and internal organs, including the lungs. Other types of cancer that commonly develop in people with AIDS include lymphomas (p.279), such as non-Hodgkin's lymphoma. Cancer of the cervix (p.481) is an AIDS-defining illness in women infected with HIV.

How is it diagnosed?
If you suspect that you may have been exposed to HIV infection, you should have a blood test to check for antibodies against the virus. You may also have this blood test if you have symptoms that suggest HIV infection, and it is often offered as part of antenatal care. Consent is always obtained before the test, and counselling is given to discuss the implications of a positive result.

If your HIV test result is negative, you may be advised to have another test in a

few weeks because antibodies take time to develop. HIV infection can also be difficult to diagnose in the baby of an infected woman because the mother's antibodies may remain in the baby's blood for up to 18 months.

HIV can also be tested for by analysing a sample of saliva or a spot of blood taken by a skin prick but it may take several weeks before antibodies to the virus show up in these tests, so a negative result does not definitely mean a person is virus-free.

AIDS is diagnosed when an AIDS-defining illness, such as pneumocystis infection, develops or when a blood test shows that the CD4 lymphocyte count has dropped below a certain level.

What is the treatment?
If your HIV test result is positive, you will probably be referred to a special centre where you will receive monitoring, treatment, and advice from a team of health-care professionals.

Antiviral drug treatment (see **Drugs for HIV infection and AIDS**, p.573) may be started if there are symptoms of infection or if there are other indications that your immune system is weakened, such as a reduced CD4 lymphocyte level.

If AIDS has developed, opportunistic infections are dealt with as they occur. In some cases, there may also be long-term preventive treatment against the most common infections. Emotional support and practical advice can be obtained from the many groups and organizations that help people with HIV infection and AIDS.

What is the prognosis?
There is no cure for HIV infection, but the drug treatments available in the developed world have made it possible to regard the condition as a long-term illness rather than a rapidly fatal one. Since the introduction of antiviral drug combination therapies, deaths from AIDS in the developed world have been reduced dramatically. In the developing world, although advances have been made in delivering care, many people still have limited access to such care and HIV/AIDS remains a major cause of illness and premature death.

Can it be prevented?
HIV infection can be prevented by teaching at an early age about the risks of infection. The two main precautions that everyone can take to avoid sexual transmission are to use a condom during sexual intercourse and to avoid sex with multiple partners (see **Sex and health**, p.27). It is also recommended that both partners have an HIV test before having unprotected sex in a new relationship. Specific groups need to take special precautions. For example, people who inject drugs intravenously must use a clean needle and syringe every time.

People who are HIV positive need to take special care to prevent others from coming into contact with their blood or body fluids and should always inform dental or medical staff that they have HIV infection. Women who are HIV positive and pregnant may be given antiviral drugs to reduce the risk of transmission to the fetus, and they may also be advised to have a caesarean section (p.518) and avoid breast-feeding to reduce the risk of transmitting the virus to their babies.

Medical professionals take many steps to prevent transmission of HIV, including screening all blood products and tissues for transplant and using disposable or carefully sterilized equipment.

Extensive research is being carried out to develop a vaccine against HIV and to prevent the development of AIDS. However, although researchers are optimistic they will succeed, there will inevitably be millions more deaths worldwide before an affordable cure is found and made widely available.

Bacterial infections

A large group of diseases is caused by bacteria entering the body and multiplying too fast to be destroyed by the immune system. Some types of bacteria also release powerful poisons, known as toxins, that rapidly damage tissues. In the past, bacterial diseases were a major cause of death; today, most serious infections can be treated effectively with antibiotics.

Each of the bacterial infections covered in this section affects many areas of the body simultaneously. The most serious of these infections is septicaemia, described in the first article, which can be due to almost any bacterium. The diseases in the following articles are caused only by particular bacteria. They include both relatively recently identified infections, such as toxic shock syndrome, and those that have long been recognized, such as diphtheria and plague. The final articles describe illnesses caused by the rickettsiae bacteria, some of which may be transmitted to humans through insect bites.

Many other bacterial infections, such as pneumonia (p.299), tuberculosis (p.300), and meningitis (p.325), cause damage to certain organs, and for this reason they are covered in the sections on specific body systems.

Bacterial skin infections, such as boils, are discussed in skin infections and infestations (pp.204–207).

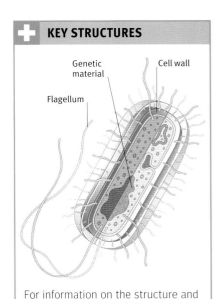

KEY STRUCTURES

Genetic material
Cell wall
Flagellum

For information on the structure and function of bacteria, *see* p.162.

What are the symptoms?

The symptoms of septicaemia and sepsis develop suddenly and include:
- High fever.
- Chills and violent shivering.

If septicaemia or sepsis are left untreated, the bacteria may produce toxins that damage blood vessels, causing a drop in blood pressure and widespread tissue damage. In this dangerous condition, called septic shock, symptoms may include:
- Faintness.
- Cold, pale hands and feet.
- Restlessness and irritability.
- Rapid, shallow breathing.
- In many cases, delirium and eventual loss of consciousness.

In some people, bacteria may lodge on the heart valves, especially if the heart has previously been damaged by disease. This serious

Bacterium   Red blood cell   White blood cell

Bacteria in blood
This magnified blood sample from a person with septicaemia shows small, rod-shaped bacteria among the blood cells.

condition is called infective endocarditis (p.256). In rare cases, septicaemia may result in a lack of the blood cells involved in blood clotting (*see* **Thrombocytopenia**, p.275), which increases the risk of excessive bleeding.

What might be done?

If your doctor suspects that you have septicaemia or sepsis, you will be admitted to hospital for immediate treatment. Intravenous antibiotics (p.572) are given first, and then blood tests are performed to identify the bacterium causing the infection. Once the bacterium has been identified, specific antibiotics are given. With prompt treatment, most people make a complete recovery.

Septicaemia

An infection, also known as blood poisoning, in which bacteria multiply in the bloodstream

 More common in children and elderly people

 Intravenous drug use is a risk factor

 Gender and genetics are not significant factors

Septicaemia, also known as blood poisoning, is a potentially fatal condition in which bacteria multiply rapidly in the bloodstream. It is common for bacteria to enter the bloodstream in small numbers through sites such as a breach in the skin or through the mouth when the teeth are brushed. The bacteria are usually destroyed by the immune system and cause no symptoms. However, if bacteria enter the bloodstream in large numbers from a major source of infection, such as a kidney infection (*see* **Pyelonephritis**, p.446), blood poisoning can result. In some cases, the bacteria in the bloodstream may trigger an exaggerated response by the immune system, causing widespread reactions (such as inflammation) throughout the body – a condition known as sepsis. Septicaemia and sepsis can develop as a complication of almost all types of serious infectious diseases.

The infection is more likely to occur in people with reduced immunity due to disorders such as diabetes mellitus (p.437) or HIV infection (*see* **HIV infection and AIDS**, p.169) or due to treatment with chemotherapy (p.157) or immunosuppressant drugs (p.585). Young children and elderly people are also more susceptible. Others at increased risk are intravenous drug users, who may introduce bacteria into their blood from contaminated needles.

Toxic shock syndrome

A rare but serious condition caused by staphylococcal or streptococcal toxins

 Most common between the ages of 15 and 20

 More common in females

 Using tampons may be a risk factor

 Genetics is not a significant factor

Toxic shock syndrome is an uncommon but potentially fatal infection caused by a toxin produced by *Staphylococcus aureus*

and some streptococcal bacteria, which enter the bloodstream from a localized site of infection.

Toxic shock syndrome mainly affects young adults, and about half of all cases occur in menstruating women. The infection may be linked to the use of tampons, which can provide a site for bacterial growth in the vagina, particularly if a tampon is left in place longer than the recommended time.

The symptoms start suddenly and may include fever, vomiting, diarrhoea, and severe muscular aches and pains. A widespread red, sunburn-like rash may appear, and confusion may occur. More serious complications can also develop, such as acute kidney injury (p.450).

Toxic shock syndrome requires immediate treatment in hospital with intravenous antibiotics (p.572). Treated promptly, 9 in 10 people recover fully.

MRSA infection

An infection with an antibiotic-resistant form of the Staphylococcus aureus *bacterium*

Hospital inpatient treatment or living in a crowded community are risk factors

Age, gender, and genetics are not significant factors

MRSA is the abbreviation for meticillin-resistant *Staphylococcus aureus*, a bacterium that is resistant to meticillin and many other common antibiotics. Because of its drug resistance, MRSA is commonly known as a "superbug". The bacterium is often found on the skin, nostrils, and throat and is usually harmless but can cause minor skin infections, such as boils. However, if it enters the body through a break in the skin such as wound, it may cause potentially life-threatening infections, such as septicaemia (left), pneumonia (p.299), or infection of the heart (*see* **Infective endocarditis**, p.256).

The bacterium is usually spread by skin-to-skin contact but can also be spread through contact with contaminated objects, such as towels, bedding, and surfaces. People staying in hospital are most of risk of infection because of their health problems, surgical wounds, or invasive devices such as catheters, and because the relatively crowded environment allows bacteria to spread more easily. The risk of infection is also greater in other close communities, such as care homes, but lower than in hospitals.

What are the symptoms?

Minor superficial infections may cause the symptoms of a boil (p.204) or abscess. If the bacteria penetrate deeper inside the body, symptoms may include:
- Fever, chills, and shivering.
- Pain and swelling in the affected area.
- Dizziness and/or confusion.

- Rapid, shallow breathing.
- Delirium and loss of consciousness.

If the infection cannot be treated successfully, it may be fatal.

What might be done?
Treatment of MRSA infection varies according to the site and severity of infection. Minor superficial infections, such as boils, may be treated simply by draining pus from the site of infection. Invasive or more serious infections are treated with antibiotics or combinations of antibiotics to which the specific strain of MRSA is sensitive.

To prevent spreading MRSA, many people are screened for the bacterium before admission to hospital and, if necessary, are treated with topical antibacterials to eliminate it. Good hygiene, including proper hand hygiene, can also significantly reduce the risk of transmitting the bacterium.

Scarlet fever

A rare streptococcal infection causing a red rash and a sore throat

 Most common between the ages of 6 and 12

 Gender, genetics, and lifestyle are not significant factors

Once a common and dangerous childhood disease, scarlet fever has become rare in developed countries since the introduction of antibiotics (p.572). This infection is caused by the bacterium *Streptococcus pyogenes*, transmitted in microscopic droplets from coughs and sneezes. A prominent feature of the condition is a widespread scarlet rash.

What are the symptoms?
About 2–5 days after infection, the following symptoms may develop:
- Sore throat and headache.
- Fever and vomiting.
- Raised, red rash, spreading rapidly on the neck, trunk, armpits, and groin.

A thick, white coating may develop on the tongue, disappearing in a few days to leave the tongue bright red with a pimpled "strawberry" appearance.

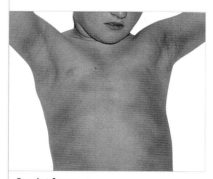

Scarlet fever
The characteristic red rash of scarlet fever begins on the trunk and is often most obvious in the armpits.

What might be done?
Scarlet fever is usually diagnosed from the symptoms. To confirm the diagnosis, a throat swab may be taken.

The infection is treated with antibiotics, and the symptoms usually begin to improve within 24–48 hours. Most people recover within a week.

Diphtheria

A rare throat infection that can cause breathing difficulties

 More common in children

 Gender, genetics, and lifestyle are not significant factors

Now rare in developed countries, diphtheria was a common cause of death in children until immunization became routine. In this disease, the bacterium *Corynebacterium diphtheriae* multiplies in the throat and may release toxins into the blood. The infection is usually transmitted through airborne droplets from coughs or sneezes of infected people.

Diphtheria bacteria may also infect the skin. This form of the disease, known as cutaneous diphtheria, is more common in tropical countries but it can affect people elsewhere. Outbreaks of diphtheria tend to occur among overcrowded communities.

What are the symptoms?
The symptoms of diphtheria may develop up to 7 days after infection and include:
- Sore throat.
- Fever.
- Swollen lymph nodes in the neck.
- In many cases, a grey membrane that grows across the throat, causing difficulty in breathing.

In the cutaneous form of the disorder, deep sores may develop. If diphtheria is not treated, bacterial toxins may spread in the blood and cause potentially fatal complications such as acute heart failure (p.247) and paralysis.

What might be done?
Diphtheria may be diagnosed from the symptoms, but a throat swab is taken for confirmation. Most people recover fully if treated immediately with antibiotics (p.572) and antitoxin injections in hospital. Routine immunization in children and young adults provides protection against diphtheria (*see* **Routine immunizations**, p.13). The diphtheria vaccine is usually combined with other vaccines and is given at 2, 3, and 4 months of age, with a booster at 3 years 4 months to 5 years and another booster at 13 to 18 years. Adults may need further booster doses for travel purposes.

Brucellosis

A rare infection, contracted from farm animals and dairy products, that may cause recurrent illness

 Working with farm animals is a risk factor

 Age, gender, and genetics are not significant factors

Brucellosis is caused by various types of brucella bacteria, which can be transmitted to humans through contact with infected farm animals and in unpasteurized milk and other dairy products. The disease rarely occurs in developed countries, where domestic animals are normally free of the infection.

The symptoms of brucellosis vary considerably from person to person. In some cases, depression and weight loss are the only signs of infection, although many people develop fever with night sweats, tiredness, headache, and pain in the joints. Left untreated, the illness can become persistent, recurring at intervals over months or sometimes years.

What might be done?
A lack of specific symptoms makes brucellosis difficult to diagnose, although the bacteria can be identified by a blood test. It is usually treated with antibiotics (p.572), which are sometimes given with corticosteroids (p.600). With treatment, most people recover within 2–3 months.

Listeriosis

An uncommon infection transmitted through contaminated food

 Eating certain foods, such as soft cheeses and meat pâté, is a risk factor

 Age, gender, and genetics are not significant factors

The bacterium that causes listeriosis, *Listeria monocytogenes*, is widespread in the soil and is present in most animal species. It can pass to humans through food products, particularly soft cheeses, milk, meat pâtés, and prepackaged salads. The risk of listeriosis is increased by incorrect storage of these foods. The bacteria multiply in the intestines and may spread in the blood (*see* **Septicaemia**, p.171) and affect other organs.

The symptoms of listeriosis vary from one person to another. The infection often goes unnoticed in healthy adults, although some people may develop flu-like symptoms such as fever, sore throat, headache, and aching muscles.

In elderly people and people with reduced immunity, such as those with HIV infection (*see* **HIV infection and AIDS**, p.169) or those taking immunosuppressant drugs (p.585), listeriosis can lead to meningitis (p.325), a potentially fatal inflammation of the membranes covering the brain. In pregnant women, infection can pass to the fetus, causing miscarriage (p.511), the birth of a baby infected with the bacteria, or stillbirth (p.520).

What might be done?
Listeriosis is usually diagnosed from a blood test. In otherwise healthy people, mild listeriosis clears up without treatment in a few days. People with serious infection, especially during pregnancy, need urgent treatment in hospital with intravenous antibiotics (p.572).

Hygienic handling and storage of food reduces the risk of listeriosis (*see* **Home safety and health**, p.33).

Typhoid and paratyphoid

Infections caused by salmonella bacteria that result in high fever, sometimes followed by a rash

 Visiting or living in areas where the disease occurs is a risk factor

 Age, gender, and genetics are not significant factors

Typhoid and paratyphoid are almost identical diseases that are caused by the bacteria *Salmonella typhi* and *S. paratyphi*, respectively. The bacteria multiply in the intestines and spread to the blood and to other organs, such as the spleen, gallbladder, and liver. The diseases are transmitted through infected faeces and most commonly occur in areas where hygiene and sanitation are poor. Infection is commonly due to food or water contaminated by unwashed hands.

What are the symptoms?
Symptoms of both diseases appear 7–14 days after infection and may include:
- Headache and high fever.
- Dry cough.
- Abdominal pain and constipation, usually followed by diarrhoea.
- Rash of rose-coloured spots appearing on the chest, abdomen, and back.

Both infections can lead to serious complications, such as intestinal bleeding and perforation of the intestines.

What might be done?
Typhoid and paratyphoid can be diagnosed by testing blood or faecal samples for the bacteria. The diseases are usually treated with antibiotics (p.572) in hospital. Symptoms normally subside 2–3 days after treatment is begun, and most people recover fully in a month.

Even with treatment, the bacteria are excreted for up to 3 months after the symptoms have disappeared. Some people who do not have treatment may become lifelong carriers of the bacteria and transmit the infection to others, although they appear to be healthy.

Scrupulous attention to personal hygiene and to food and water hygiene is the best protection against infection (*see* **Travel health**, p.35). Several vaccines (including oral vaccine) are available, and if you intend to travel to a developing country, immunization may be advisable (*see* **Travel immunizations**, p.35).

Cholera

An intestinal infection that causes profuse, watery diarrhoea

 Visiting or living in areas where the disease occurs is a risk factor

 Age, gender, and genetics are not significant factors

Cholera typically occurs in epidemics and has caused millions of deaths over the centuries. It is due to infection of the small intestine by the bacterium *Vibric cholerae*. Usually associated with areas of poor sanitation, cholera can be spread through contaminated water or food.

The illness starts suddenly, 1–5 days after infection, with vomiting and profuse, watery diarrhoea. In some cases, fatal dehydration develops.

What might be done?
Cholera is usually diagnosed from the characteristic "rice water" appearance of the diarrhoea. To confirm the diagnosis, a faecal sample may be checked for the presence of the bacteria.

Urgent hospital treatment is needed to replace lost fluids and minerals, which are given orally or intravenously. Antibiotics (p.572) may be given to reduce the risk of passing the infection to others. If treated without delay, most people make a complete recovery.

Scrupulous attention to personal hygiene and to food and water hygiene is the best protection against infection (*see* **Travel health**, p.35). An oral vaccine is available for travellers to areas where cholera is prevalent (*see* **Travel health**, p.35).

Botulism

A rare, life-threatening form of poisoning in which a bacterial toxin in food damages the nervous system, causing paralysis

 Eating home-preserved food is a risk factor

 Age, gender, and genetics are not significant factors

The toxin that causes botulism is one of the most dangerous poisons known to humanity. This toxin is produced by the

bacterium *Clostridium botulinum*, which can multiply rapidly in canned or preserved foods. If contaminated food is eaten, absorption of even minute amounts of toxin can cause severe damage to the nervous system.

Strict controls on commercial canning have made botulism caused by shop-bought products rare. The foods most commonly affected are home-preserved vegetables, fish, and fruit. Babies, who are especially susceptible to the effects of the toxin, may develop botulism after being given contaminated honey.

What are the symptoms?
The symptoms of botulism appear very suddenly, 12–36 hours after eating contaminated food. In the initial stages, the symptoms usually include:
- Nausea and constipation.
- Dry mouth.

Within 24 hours, these symptoms are followed by muscle weakness that starts in the eyes, causing blurred vision, and then progresses down the body. Without treatment, the respiratory muscles may become paralysed, causing suffocation.

What might be done?
Botulism needs immediate treatment in hospital with antitoxin drugs. For people whose breathing is affected, mechanical ventilation may be necessary. If given prompt treatment, 9 in 10 people make a full recovery.

To reduce the risk of poisoning, any bulging cans or abnormal-smelling preserved foods should be discarded, and home-preserved food should be cooked thoroughly. Babies under the age of 12 months should not be given honey.

Tetanus

A wound infection, caused by a bacterial toxin, that produces severe muscle spasms

 Age, gender, genetics, and lifestyle are not significant factors

Tetanus is caused by a toxin produced by the bacterium *Clostridium tetani*, which lives in soil and in the intestines of humans and other animals. If the bacteria enter a wound, they multiply, and an infection may develop that acts on the nerves controlling muscle activity. The condition, also called lockjaw, is rare in developed countries because most people have been immunized.

The symptoms of tetanus usually appear 3–21 days after infection. Fever, headache, and muscle stiffness in the jaw, arms, neck, and back are typical. As the condition progresses, painful muscle spasms may develop. In some people, the muscles of the throat or chest wall are affected, leading to breathing difficulties and possible suffocation.

What might be done?
Diagnosis of tetanus is based on details of the injury and on the symptoms. The disease needs immediate treatment in hospital with antitoxin injections, antibiotics (p.572), and sedatives (*see* **Antianxiety drugs**, p.591) to relieve muscle spasm. Mechanical ventilation may be needed to aid breathing. If treated promptly, most people make a complete recovery, otherwise tetanus is usually fatal.

To reduce the risk of tetanus, you should thoroughly clean wounds and treat them with antiseptic. Wounds contaminated with soil or manure and deep wounds should be seen by a doctor immediately. Anybody who has not had the full course of vaccinations should also see a doctor.

Vaccination against tetanus, usually started in early childhood (*see* **Routine immunizations**, p.13), is highly effective. The tetanus vaccine is combined with other vaccines and is given at 2, 3, and 4 months of age, with a booster at 3 years 4 months to 5 years and another booster at 13 to 18 years. A person who has had 5 injections is likely to be immune for life, but boosters may be required after a dirty wound or if travelling in an area with poor medical services.

Hansen's disease

An infection, also known as leprosy, that affects nerves and skin, causing numbness and disfigurement

 Age, gender, genetics, and lifestyle are not significant factors

Hansen's disease, commonly known as leprosy, is a long-term infection caused by the bacterium *Mycobacterium leprae*, which damages the skin and nerves. The limbs and face, in particular, may be affected. Infection is thought to be transmitted in airborne droplets produced when an infected person coughs or sneezes and through skin contact. The disease is not easily transmitted from person to person. Only people who live in prolonged, close contact with an infected person are at risk of infection. The disease is rare in developed countries and is most common in Asia, Africa, and South America. Hansen's disease develops very slowly, the first symptoms often appearing more than 5 years after infection and sometimes not for as long as 20 years. Initially, nerve damage causes numbness of the skin on the face, hands, and feet. The affected skin may also become thickened and discoloured. Lack of sensation may lead to injury or even loss of fingers and toes.

Diagnosis is based on the symptoms and examination of a sample of skin tissue to identify the bacterium. Treatment

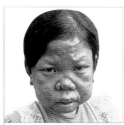

BEFORE TREATMENT

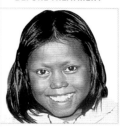

AFTER TREATMENT

Hansen's disease
At the age of 7, this girl had thickened facial skin due to Hansen's disease. After 2 years of treatment with antibiotics, her appearance had improved dramatically.

with antibiotics (p.572), for up to 2 years or longer, prevents further nerve damage and reduces areas of thickened skin. With early diagnosis and treatment, Hansen's disease is curable. However, any nerve damage that has already occurred is irreversible.

Leptospirosis

A group of infections transmitted to humans by rats and other animals

 Working on farms or with sewage is a risk factor

 Age, gender, and genetics are not significant factors

Infections caused by different types of *Leptospira* bacteria are known generally as leptospirosis. The bacteria are carried by animals such as rats or foxes and excreted in their urine. The infection is usually transmitted to humans by contact with water or soil contaminated by infected urine. In most cases the infection causes a flu-like illness. However, in its most severe form, which is known as Weil's disease, leptospirosis may be life-threatening.

Leptospirosis most commonly occurs in farmers and sewage workers, but the disease can affect anyone who comes into contact with contaminated water, such as swimmers or those taking part in watersports.

What are the symptoms?
The symptoms of leptospirosis usually appear abruptly 7–12 days after infection but can appear at any time from 2–30 days. They may include:
- Fever.
- Intense headache and muscle pain.
- Flat, red rash.
- Inflammation of the eyes and eyelids (*see* **Conjunctivitis**, p.355).

The symptoms tend to disappear after a few days but may recur if immediate treatment is not given. If the disease goes untreated, it frequently causes a potentially dangerous inflammation of the membranes covering the brain (*see* **Meningitis**, p.325).

About 1 in 10 infected people develops Weil's disease. This disorder leads to widespread internal bleeding, damage to the kidneys and liver, and jaundice (p.407), which causes the skin and the whites of the eyes to turn yellow.

What might be done?

To diagnose leptospirosis, your doctor may arrange for blood and urine tests to check for the presence of bacteria. Most cases are mild and are treated successfully with antibiotics, and painkillers to relieve symptoms. In more severe cases, hospital treatment with antibiotics and supportive measures, such as intravenous fluids, may be necessary.

As a preventive measure, workers at particular risk of infection may sometimes be given antibiotics after minor injuries such as cuts.

Lyme disease

An infection transmitted by ticks that causes a rash and flu-like symptoms

 An outdoor lifestyle during summer is a risk factor in certain regions

 Age, gender, and genetics are not significant factors

Named after Old Lyme, the North American town where the disease was first recognized, Lyme disease is caused by a bacterium called *Borrelia burgdorferi*. The infection is transmitted to humans by ticks that usually live in areas with overgrown or deep vegetation where there are animals they can feed on. If a person is bitten by an infected tick that remains attached to his or her skin, bacteria can enter the bloodstream and may then spread throughout the body. A tick may be infected with more than one type of bacterium, and as a result a single bite may cause other, similar infections at the same time.

Although Lyme disease is most widely reported in the US, the infection is also a problem in the UK, particularly in areas of woodland or parkland. People who go camping or walking in such areas during late spring or summer are most at risk of being bitten by a tick carrying Lyme disease bacteria.

What are the symptoms?

A bite from an infected tick usually produces a red lump with a scab on the skin, although some people who have been bitten may not notice this initial sign. Within 2 days to 4 weeks after the bite, the following symptoms may develop:

- Spreading circular rash at the site of the bite that may clear in the centre.
- Tiredness.
- Flu-like chills and fever.
- Headache and joint pains.

If the infection is left untreated, these symptoms may persist for several weeks. In some people who have Lyme disease,

Preventing tick bites

Ticks are tiny, spider-like parasites that are difficult to see, and their bites often go unnoticed. If you are walking or camping in tick-infested areas you should take the following precautions to minimize the risk of being bitten:

- Wear light-coloured clothes, so that ticks can be seen more easily.
- Keep your skin covered by wearing long sleeves and tucking trousers into socks.
- Use a DEET-containing insect repellent on any exposed areas of the skin and on clothing.
- Where there is vegetation, do not sit directly on the ground.
- Whenever possible, keep to well-trodden trails and pathways, and avoid walking through overgrown vegetation.
- While out walking, stop to make occasional checks for ticks, especially on children and dogs.
- Before going to bed at night, carefully examine your own and your children's skin and clothing for ticks.

dangerous complications may develop up to 2 years later that may affect the heart, nervous system, and joints.

What might be done?

Your doctor may suspect from your symptoms that you have Lyme disease and may also arrange for a blood test to confirm the diagnosis.

If they are given prompt treatment with antibiotics (p.572), most people make a complete recovery. Nonsteroidal anti-inflammatory drugs (p.578) act as painkillers and can help to relieve joint pain and discomfort. Complications of Lyme disease are extremely rare.

In regions known to be tick-infested, you should wear clothes that cover your arms and legs to reduce the risk of being bitten (*see* **Preventing tick bites**, above) and immediately remove any ticks that you find attached to your skin. Use fine-pointed tweezers or your fingernails to pull the tick out but do not apply a hot match, alcohol, or any other substance to the tick in an attempt to remove it.

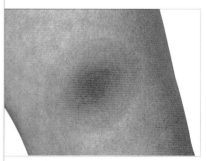

Lyme disease
A bite from a tick infected with the bacterium that causes Lyme disease typically produces an expanding circular red rash, as seen here on the thigh.

Plague

A serious infection carried by rodents and transmitted to humans by flea bites

 Age, gender, genetics, and lifestyle are not significant factors

Plague is the result of infection by the bacterium *Yersinia pestis*, which usually affects rodents but can be transmitted to humans through flea bites. During the Middle Ages, the disease caused pandemics (widespread epidemics), one of the largest of which was the so-called Black Death of the 14th century, which killed over 25 million people in Europe. Today, small outbreaks occur sporadically, mainly in Africa, South America, and Asia, but not in Europe.

The two main forms of the plague are bubonic plague, which affects the lymph nodes, and pneumonic plague, which occurs if the infection spreads to the lungs. The symptoms of both forms develop rapidly and include a high fever and chills. In bubonic plague, painful swellings known as buboes develop in the lymph nodes, usually in the groin and armpits. Pneumonic plague causes a severe cough, shortness of breath, and chest pain. Once the lungs are infected, plague can be transmitted from person to person through airborne droplets from coughs and sneezes.

Plague is diagnosed from the symptoms and by a blood test. People given immediate treatment with antibiotics (p.572) usually make a complete recovery. However, if treatment is delayed, the disease is frequently fatal.

Q fever

A bacterial infection transmitted to humans by contact with farm animals

 Working with farm animals or meat is a risk factor

 Age, gender, and genetics are not significant factors

Labelled Q for "query" before the source of the infection was identified, Q fever is caused by the rickettsia-like bacterium *Coxiella burnetii*. The bacteria are carried by livestock such as cows, sheep, and goats and can be transmitted through urine, faeces, and milk, or inhaled in dust contaminated with particles of tissue from infected animals.

Within 2–3 weeks of infection, a high fever, severe headache, muscle pain, and cough may suddenly occur. The symptoms usually disappear in 1–2 weeks, but, in some people, infection spreads and damages the heart valves (*see* **Infective endocarditis**, p.256) and the liver (*see* **Acute hepatitis**, p.408).

Q fever can be accurately diagnosed by a blood test. In mild cases, the symptoms clear up by themselves and treatment is not necessary. More severe cases may need treatment with antibiotics (p.572).

Rocky Mountain spotted fever

A rickettsial infection, transmitted to humans by animal ticks, that causes fever and a spotted rash

 An outdoor lifestyle during summer is a risk factor in certain regions

 Age, gender, and genetics are not significant factors

Despite its name, Rocky Mountain spotted fever occurs not only in the Rocky Mountain states of the US but also in eastern US states and South America. The disease is caused by the bacterium *Rickettsia rickettsii*, which is transmitted to humans through bites from infected animal ticks. Although the disease does not occur in Europe, visitors to the US who go camping or walking in woodland areas may be at risk, especially during spring and summer.

The initial symptoms appear suddenly about a week after infection and may include severe headache, muscle pains, chills, and fever. Within a few days, a rash of tiny pink spots develops, usually appearing first on the limbs and then

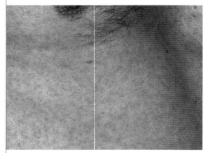

Rocky Mountain spotted fever
The rash of Rocky Mountain spotted fever often begins on the limbs and spreads over the body, as seen here on the chest.

spreading rapidly over the rest of the body. This rash gradually becomes darker. If the condition is left untreated, potentially fatal complications, such as gangrene (p.262) and kidney failure (p.450), may develop.

Rocky Mountain spotted fever is usually diagnosed from the appearance of the rash, but blood tests may be carried out. If given prompt treatment with antibiotics (p.572), most infected people make a rapid recovery.

In regions known to be infested with ticks, you should wear clothes that keep your arms and legs covered to reduce the risk of being bitten (*see* **Preventing tick bites**, left) and promptly remove any ticks that attach themselves to your skin by pulling them off with fine-pointed tweezers or your fingernails.

Typhus

A serious rickettsial infection transmitted to humans by lice, fleas, or mites

 Living in overcrowded, unhygienic conditions is a risk factor

 Age, gender, and genetics are not significant factors

There are three main forms of typhus, all of which are caused by different types of rickettsial bacteria.

Epidemic typhus is transmitted by body lice, usually in overcrowded conditions, and has resulted in hundreds of thousands of deaths in times of war or famine. Today, the disease is rare except in some areas of tropical Africa and South America. Endemic typhus, which is also known as murine typhus, is a rare disease that can be transmitted from rats to humans by fleas; a few cases occur each year in North and Central America. Scrub typhus, which is transmitted by mites, has been reported in India and Southeast Asia.

The first sign of infection with scrub typhus is a black scab over the site of the bite. In all types of typhus, flu-like symptoms may develop in 1–3 weeks of infection, followed a few days later by a widespread, blotchy pink rash. In severe cases of typhus, delirium and coma (p.323) occur. If the disease is not treated, dangerous complications such as pneumonia (p.299) or kidney failure (p.450) are also likely to develop.

What might be done?

Typhus is often diagnosed from the symptoms, but a blood test may be carried out. Treatment with antibiotics (p.572) is usually effective. Without treatment, the bacteria can lie dormant in the body for years before being reactivated and causing the disease to recur.

Protozoal and fungal infections

Protozoa and fungi are simple organisms, capable of living in many different habitats. Some protozoa and fungi are parasites of humans. They acquire all their food from our bodies and often cause disease. One protozoal infection, malaria, affects hundreds of millions of people worldwide each year and is often fatal.

Protozoal infections are discussed first, starting with malaria, the most important health hazard for visitors to the tropics. Further articles deal with other protozoal infections, including diseases that are common causes of diarrhoea, such as amoebiasis and cryptosporidiosis. The protozoal infection trichomoniasis, which is transmitted sexually, is covered with other such sexually transmitted infections (*see* **Trichomoniasis**, p.492). Fungal infections are discussed next. Like most protozoal infections, fungal infections may be serious in people with reduced immunity, such as those who have AIDS. The types of fungi described in this section can spread around the body from the initial site of infection, sometimes causing long-term illness. Common fungal infections that affect particular areas of the body, such as the skin and vagina, are covered in the sections on specific body systems.

> ### ✚ KEY STRUCTURES
>
> **FILAMENTOUS FUNGUS**
>
> **FUNGAL YEAST CELL**
>
> **PROTOZOAN**
>
> For more information on the structure of protozoa and fungi, *see* p.163.

Malaria

A parasitic infection of red blood cells spread by mosquitoes

 Visiting or living in areas where the disease occurs are risk factors

 Age, gender, and genetics are not significant factors

Malaria, a parasitic infection that leads to the destruction of red blood cells, is one of the greatest public health problems in the world. In tropical countries, where the infection is most likely to be contracted, about 200 million new cases of malaria and 600,000 deaths due to the disease occur every year. Most of those who die of malaria are children. The disease is the most serious health threat to people who visit the tropics. In the UK, there are about 1,500 cases every year, occurring in travellers returning from malaria-endemic areas.

The World Health Organization has been trying to control malaria for years but with only partial success. Malarial parasites are transmitted to humans by mosquitoes of the anopheles group, which have now become resistant to many insecticides. In many areas, the malarial parasite itself has now also become resistant to the common antimalarial drugs (p.574). Currently, no effective vaccine has been developed.

If you live in a region where malaria is common, you may have several mild episodes of infection that increase your resistance, making you less likely to develop a serious infection. However, this protection is lost within a year if you move to a malaria-free region. Therefore, if you emigrate from a malaria-affected area and later return for a holiday, you will need to take preventive measures (*see* **Preventing malaria**, right). If you become ill after a visit to the tropics, you should tell your doctor where you have been and when you went there.

Malarial parasite   Red blood cell

Infected red blood cell
The protozoa that cause malaria infect red blood cells. Attacks of the disease occur when the protozoa burst out of the cells.

What are the types?

Five species of protozoal parasites from the plasmodium group cause malaria in humans. The most dangerous type of malaria is falciparum malaria, caused by *Plasmodium falciparum*. This type of malaria results in the most deaths and is often fatal within 48 hours of the first symptoms if it is left untreated. The types of malaria caused by *Plasmodium malariae*, *Plasmodium ovale*, and *Plasmodium vivax* are less severe. The fifth type of malaria, caused by *Plasmodium knowlesi*, occurs only in Southeast Asia and is very rare.

All types of malarial parasite are transmitted to humans by a bite from an infected mosquito. Initially, the parasites multiply in the liver and are then released into the bloodstream, where they penetrate red blood cells. After 48–72 hours, depending on the species of parasite, the infected cells rupture, releasing parasites that invade other red blood cells. If a noninfected mosquito bites the infected person, the insect itself becomes infected and can then spread the disease to other people. In all types of malaria, the disease can pass from an infected pregnant woman to her fetus.

SELF-HELP

Preventing malaria

If you plan to visit an area where malaria occurs, your doctor will be able to advise you on antimalarial drugs (p.574) for that area. You may need to start taking the drugs up to 3 weeks before you leave, and continue during and for 1–4 weeks after your visit; the timings depend on the drugs taken. To protect yourself against mosquito bites:

■ Keep your body covered as much as possible.
■ Sleep under a mosquito net that is impregnated with insecticide.
■ Use insect repellent on clothes and exposed skin.

These measures against mosquito bites are especially important between dusk and dawn, when malaria-carrying mosquitoes bite.

What are the symptoms?

The symptoms of malaria usually begin between 10 days and 6 weeks after being bitten by an infected mosquito. However, in some cases, symptoms may not develop for months or years, especially if preventive drugs were being taken at the time of infection.

If not treated, malaria due to *P. vivax*, *P. ovale*, and *P. malariae* causes recurrent attacks of symptoms with each episode of red blood cell destruction by the parasites. Each attack usually lasts for 4–8 hours and may occur at intervals of 2 or 3 days, depending on the species of parasite. Symptoms of an attack include:

■ High fever.
■ Shivering and chills.
■ Heavy sweating.
■ Confusion.
■ Tiredness, headache, and muscle pain.

Between each attack, extreme tiredness may be the only symptom.

Falciparum malaria causes a continuous fever that may be mistaken for influenza (p.164). It is more severe than the other types, and attacks may lead to loss of consciousness and kidney failure (p.450) and may be fatal. *P. knowlesi* also causes severe malaria.

What might be done?

Your doctor may suspect malaria if you have an unexplained fever within a year after a trip to a malarial region. Diagnosis is confirmed by identifying the malarial parasite in a blood smear under a microscope, or by a blood test that detects malaria antigens (substances that trigger an immune response) in the blood.

If you are diagnosed with malaria, you should be given antimalarial drugs (p.574) as early as possible to avoid complications. Treatment depends on the type of malaria, how resistant the parasite is to drugs, and the severity of the symptoms. If you have falciparum malaria, you may be treated in hospital with oral or intravenous antimalarial drugs. Treatment may also involve a blood transfusion (p.272) to replace destroyed red blood cells or kidney dialysis (p.451) if kidney function is impaired. Malaria due to *P. knowlesi* is treated in the same way as falciparum malaria. Other types of malaria are usually treated on an outpatient basis with oral antimalarial drugs.

If treated early, the outlook is usually good, and most people make a full recovery. However, malaria caused by *P. vivax* and *P. ovale* may recur after treatment.

Preventive measures, including using antimalarial drugs (p.574), should be taken to reduce the risk of infection when visiting areas where malaria occurs.

Amoebiasis

An intestinal infection that causes diarrhoea and may spread to the liver

 Visiting or living in the tropics and poor personal hygiene are risk factors

 Age, gender, and genetics are not significant factors

The intestinal infection amoebiasis is caused by the protozoan parasite *Entamoeba histolytica*. Worldwide, the disease is very common, particularly in areas with poor sanitation. Usually, infection results from drinking water or eating food contaminated with the parasite, which is excreted in the faeces of infected people. In severe cases, ulcers develop in the walls of the intestine, and the condition is then known as amoebic dysentery.

What are the symptoms?
Most infected people do not develop symptoms or have only mild, intermittent symptoms, which may include:
■ Diarrhoea.
■ Mild abdominal pain.
If you develop amoebic dysentery, the symptoms usually first appear between 5 days and several weeks after the initial infection. Symptoms may include:
■ Watery, bloody diarrhoea.
■ Severe abdominal pain.
■ Fever.

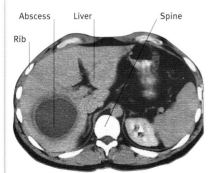

Liver abscess due to amoebiasis
In some people with amoebiasis, infection spreads to the liver and forms an abscess, as seen in the CT scan above.

In some cases, dehydration and anaemia (p.271) may develop. In addition, there is a risk of infection spreading through the bloodstream to the liver, causing high fever, painful liver abscesses, extreme tiredness, and loss of appetite.

What might be done?
Diagnosis of amoebiasis is usually made from examination of a sample of faeces under a microscope to look for the parasite. Your doctor may also arrange for you to have a blood test to look for antibodies that are produced by the body in response to the parasite. If your doctor suspects that you have liver abscesses, he or she will arrange for you to have imaging tests, such as CT scanning (p.132) or ultrasound scanning (p.135). Amoebiasis can be successfully treated with antibiotics (p.572), which usually kill the parasite within a few days. With drug treatment, most affected people make a full recovery from the infection within a few weeks.

Can it be prevented?
There are several preventive measures you can take against amoebiasis if you visit a region where the disease is common. You should drink only bottled or thoroughly boiled water to be certain that it is safe (*see* **Travel health**, p.35). You should also avoid eating raw vegetables, salads, or fruits with skins that cannot be peeled because their skins may be contaminated with the parasite.

Giardiasis

An intestinal infection with a protozoal parasite, often leading to diarrhoea

 More common in early childhood

 Poor personal hygiene is a risk factor

 Gender and genetics are not significant factors

Giardiasis is caused by a minute parasite known as *Giardia lamblia*, which infects the small intestine. Cysts (the dormant stages) of the parasite are excreted in the faeces of infected people and animals. The disease occurs mainly as a result of drinking water contaminated with cysts. The infection may also spread as a result of poor personal hygiene.

Infections are more serious in people with reduced immunity due to disorders such as HIV infection and AIDS (p.169) or treatment with immunosuppressant drugs (p.585).

Giardiasis occurs mainly in developing countries. In developed countries, the infection usually affects children, walkers who drink from contaminated streams, and people who have returned from travelling in developing countries.

What are the symptoms?
Some people may not have symptoms, but, if symptoms do develop, they usually

appear within 2 weeks of infection with the parasite and may include:
■ Diarrhoea.
■ Excessive flatulence and belching.
■ Bloating and abdominal pain.
■ Nausea.

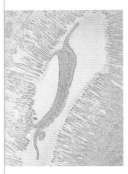

Parasite in body tissue
This highly magnified image shows the parasite Giardia lamblia *in a sample of tissue taken from the small intestine of a person with giardiasis.*

If the symptoms last longer than about a week, the infection may damage the lining of the small intestine, preventing the absorption of food and vitamins (*see* **Malabsorption**, p.415). This may result in weight loss and, in some cases, the blood disorder anaemia (p.271).

What might be done?
If your doctor suspects that you have giardiasis, you will probably be asked to provide a sample of faeces, which will be examined for the parasite cysts or tested for the presence of parasite proteins. If giardiasis is confirmed, your doctor will prescribe antibiotics (p.572), which usually kill the parasite in a few days. However, the infection may recur.

Can it be prevented?
If you are visiting a region where giardiasis occurs, you can prevent infection by boiling your drinking water for at least 5 minutes to kill the cysts. You should also follow strict standards of personal hygiene. Washing hands thoroughly after bowel movements and before preparing food should help to prevent the spread of the infection. You should avoid swimming unless you know the water is safe.

Cryptosporidiosis

An intestinal infection caused by a protozoal parasite, often leading to watery diarrhoea and fever

 More common in children

 Poor personal hygiene is a risk factor

 Gender and genetics are not significant factors

Cryptosporidiosis is caused by a protozoal parasite known as *Cryptosporidium*. It is an intestinal infection that is spread through contact with infected people or animals or by the intake of contaminated food or water. The disease occurs worldwide, but is more common

in developing countries because of poor hygiene. In developed countries, outbreaks may be due to contamination of reservoirs. Cryptosporidiosis is often severe in people who have reduced immunity, such as those with AIDS (*see* **HIV infection and AIDS**, p.169).

In some cases, there are no symptoms. In others, watery diarrhoea, abdominal pain, fever, nausea, and vomiting may develop a week after infection. The symptoms usually last 14–28 days, and most otherwise healthy people make a full recovery. However, people with reduced immunity may have persistent symptoms and develop severe malnutrition and dehydration, which can be fatal.

What might be done?
Cryptosporidiosis is usually diagnosed by examining a sample of faeces under a microscope for the parasite. There is no effective treatment to cure this infection, but, if your symptoms are severe, you may need hospital treatment with intravenous fluids and antidiarrhoeal drugs (p.597). If a local outbreak of the disease occurs, you should boil all your drinking water to kill the parasite.

Toxoplasmosis

A protozoal infection that can seriously affect fetuses and people who have reduced immunity

 Contact with cats and eating raw or undercooked meat are risk factors

 Age, gender, and genetics are not significant factors

The protozoal infection toxoplasmosis is caused by *Toxoplasma gondii*. Cysts (dormant stages) of the parasite are excreted in the faeces of infected cats and can be passed to people by direct contact with cats or by handling cat litter. Another source of infection is the raw or undercooked meat of animals that have eaten food contaminated with cysts from the faeces of infected cats. In most people, the infection does not cause symptoms because the cysts are dormant. However, people with reduced immunity, such as those with AIDS (*see* **HIV infection and AIDS**, p.169), may become seriously ill either from an initial infection or if dormant cysts are reactivated. If a woman develops toxoplasmosis while pregnant, the parasites may infect the fetus and cause abnormalities (*see* **Congenital infections**, p.530).

What are the symptoms?
Most otherwise healthy people do not develop symptoms. However, in some, mild symptoms appear 1–3 weeks after the initial infection and include:
■ Painless, enlarged lymph nodes, usually in the neck.
■ Tiredness.
■ Fever and headache.

The heart, muscles, skin, and eyes may become damaged by the infection, and, in people with reduced immunity, it may affect the brain. In such cases, the symptoms may develop suddenly or over several weeks and include:

- Fever and headache.
- Paralysis affecting a limb or one side of the body.
- Partial loss of vision.
- Confusion.
- Lethargy.

In some people with reduced immunity, toxoplasmosis causes seizures. If a fetus is infected, toxoplasmosis may damage the eyes and cause blindness.

What might be done?

Toxoplasmosis is diagnosed by microscopic examination of affected tissue, or by blood tests in those with mild symptoms. Usually, no treatment is necessary, although people with reduced immunity or those with very severe infection may be given pyrimethamine (see **Antimalarial drugs**, p.574) and antibiotics (p.572). Pregnant women may be prescribed an antibiotic alone.

Infection can be prevented by avoiding contact with cats and cat litter, and by not eating undercooked or raw meat.

Pneumocystis infection

A fungal infection that is a common cause of pneumonia in people with reduced immunity

 Age, gender, genetics, and lifestyle are not significant factors

People with reduced immunity, such as those who have AIDS (see **HIV infection and AIDS**, p.169) or those receiving chemotherapy (p.157), may develop a form of pneumonia called pneumocystis infection, caused by inhaling the *Pneumocystis jirovecii* (formerly known as *Pneumocystis carinii*) parasite. In people who have a healthy immune system, the parasite does not cause pneumonia. In developing countries, children who are malnourished often have the infection.

What are the symptoms?

The symptoms of pneumocystis infection generally develop gradually over weeks, but, in some people, they may develop quickly. Symptoms include:

- Tiredness.
- Feeling unwell.
- Fever.
- Dry cough.
- Shortness of breath on mild exertion.

As the infection progresses, shortness of breath may develop even at rest.

How is it diagnosed?

Pneumocystis infection is diagnosed by a physical examination, a chest X-ray (p.300)

or CT scan (p.132), or by examining a sample of sputum. Sometimes, the parasite is hard to isolate. In such cases, a bronchoscopy (p.308) may be performed. In this procedure, secretions from the bronchi (the main airways of the lungs) and/or a piece of lung tissue are removed and examined for evidence of pneumocystis infection.

What is the treatment?

Pneumocystis pneumonia is treated with antibiotics (p.572). Your doctor may also prescribe corticosteroids (p.600).

Once the infection has cleared up, you may need to continue taking low doses of antibiotics, depending on the cause of reduced immunity. People with AIDS require long-term antibiotics. Those receiving chemotherapy may need antibiotics until the therapy is finished.

What is the prognosis?

Fewer than 1 in 10 cases of initial pneumocystis infection are fatal. However, without treatment with preventive antibiotics, the infection may recur. In the developed world, many people with HIV infection or AIDS are now treated for pneumocystis infection before their immunity is seriously impaired.

Cryptococcosis

A rare fungal infection that most commonly affects the brain or lungs

 Age, gender, genetics, and lifestyle are not significant factors

Cryptococcosis is caused by the fungus *Cryptococcus neoformans*, which occurs in soil contaminated by bird droppings. If the fungal spores are inhaled, infection may develop in the lungs and/or the fungus may be absorbed into the blood, spreading to other parts of the body, most commonly the brain, skin, and bones.

People whose immunity is reduced, such as those who have AIDS (see **HIV infection and AIDS**, p.169) or who are undergoing chemotherapy (p.157), are most at risk from cryptococcosis. The fungus rarely causes serious illness in those individuals who are otherwise healthy.

In its most dangerous form, cryptococcosis can cause inflammation of the membranes covering the brain and spinal cord (see **Meningitis**, p.325). Symptoms may include fever, severe headache, and a stiff neck. Lung infections may result in chest pain, coughing, and shortness of breath. Infection of the skin may cause ulcers to develop. Affected bones may be painful.

What might be done?

A diagnosis of cryptococcosis is based on the presence of the fungus in blood, sputum, or body tissues. An MRI scan (p.133) may also be done to look for signs of cryptococcal infection. If meningitis is suspected,

samples of fluid from the spine will be tested (see **Lumbar puncture**, p.326). If the lungs have been affected, the levels of oxygen and other gases in the blood may be measured to assess lung function (see **Measuring blood gases**, p.306).

For severe cryptococcal infections, antifungal drugs (p.574) are given. In people with AIDS, it may be difficult to eradicate the fungus from the body, although symptoms can often be well controlled. A mild lung infection in an otherwise healthy person should clear up without treatment.

Aspergillosis

A fungal infection that can affect the lungs and spread to other organs

 Age, gender, genetics, and lifestyle are not significant factors

Aspergillosis is caused by spores of the aspergillus fungus, which occur in dust, soil, and decaying plants. The spores are harmless if a healthy person inhales them. However, the fungus can cause lung disease and other serious illnesses in people who are vulnerable to infection because of particular sensitivity, pre-existing lung damage, or reduced immune function.

What are the types?

There are several forms of aspergillosis. In some people, a sensitivity to the fungus eventually develops into a disorder known as allergic bronchopulmonary aspergillosis, the symptoms of which are similar to those of asthma (p.295).

In people who already have damaged lungs as a result of a long-term disease, such as tuberculosis (p.300) or bronchiectasis (p.303), the fungi spores may become lodged in cavities in the lung tissue caused by the disease. Eventually, the spores grow into masses known as "fungus balls". This condition usually causes a cough that may be accompanied by bloody sputum.

The fungus can also cause a serious infection of the lungs in people whose immune systems are suppressed, such as those with AIDS (see **HIV infection and AIDS**, p.169) or those receiving chemotherapy (p.157). The result of this infection is a pneumonia-like illness. In severe cases, the infection may spread to other body organs, including the heart, brain, and kidneys.

What might be done?

Aspergillosis is diagnosed by examining a sample of sputum under a microscope to look for the fungus, by a blood test for antibodies, or by a skin prick test. A chest X-ray (p.300) may also be carried out. Treatment usually involves antifungal drugs (p.574). It may be necessary to remove a fungus ball surgically. Aspergillosis is sometimes fatal in people who have impaired immunity.

Sporotrichosis

A fungal infection that usually affects only the skin but sometimes spreads to other parts of the body

 Working with plants is a risk factor

 Age, gender, and genetics are not significant factors

The fungus that causes sporotrichosis, *Sporothrix schenckii*, normally grows on plants, especially moss and tree bark. Florists and gardeners are at particular risk of infection, which usually occurs when the fungus enters the skin, for example through injury with a thorn.

If a wound has become infected with the fungus, a reddened, painless lump usually develops 1–3 months later. The infection may spread, producing small lumps beneath the skin around the wound. In people with reduced immunity, such as those with AIDS (see **HIV infection and AIDS**, p.169) or people who are taking immunosuppressant drugs (p.585), the fungus may spread to other parts of the body, including the lungs and joints.

Diagnosis is usually suspected from the appearance of lumps below the skin and can be confirmed by a skin biopsy (p.199), in which a small sample of affected skin is removed for examination. Treatment is usually treated with antifungal drugs (p.574). If the infection is widespread in people with reduced immunity, long-term drug treatment may be necessary. In such cases, the disease can be difficult to eradicate.

Candidiasis

A fungal yeast infection that usually affects only one part of the body but can be serious if it spreads around the body

 Using intravenous drugs is a risk factor

 Age and gender as risk factors depend on the type

 Genetics is rarely a significant factor

In healthy people, the yeast *Candida albicans* normally exists on the surface of certain moist areas of the body, including the mouth, throat, and vagina, and does not cause any problems. However, sometimes the fungus multiplies excessively in localized areas, causing minor forms of candidiasis such as oral thrush (p.559) and vaginal thrush (p.482). In people who have reduced immunity, such as those with AIDS (see **HIV infection and AIDS**, p.169) or diabetes mellitus (p.437), the fungus sometimes spreads into the blood and other tissues. Infection that spreads throughout the body may also occur in people who have long-term urinary catheters or intravenous catheters, or people who have had prolonged courses of antibiotics or who use intravenous drugs.

Widespread candidiasis can be diagnosed by culturing the fungus from a sample of blood or other body fluid or tissue specimens. A chest X-ray (p.300) may also be carried out to look for signs of infection in the lungs. Treatment consists of antifungal drugs (p.574), which may be given either orally or intravenously, depending on the severity of the infection. Without treatment, candidiasis can spread throughout the body and may eventually be fatal. The outlook depends on the extent of infection and on the person's general health.

Worm infestations

Most animals, including humans, can be infested with parasitic worms that derive all their nutrients from their hosts. Most of these worms live in the intestines for at least part of their life cycle. In many cases, worm infestations are long-term diseases that produce few symptoms in their early stages.

Various types of the family of worms known as roundworms can infest humans. Most affect only people in the developing world. However, some roundworms, such as threadworm, commonly affect people in developed countries. The first five articles in this section describe several types of roundworm infestation: threadworm infestation, toxocariasis, ascariasis, hookworm infestation, and tropical worm infestations, such as filariasis.

Infestations in humans that are caused by other types of worms known as flatworms, which include tapeworms and flukes, are covered in the last three articles on schistosomiasis, tapeworm infestation, and hydatid disease.

It is possible to acquire a tropical worm infestation abroad but not to experience symptoms until some months later. If you become ill after visiting the tropics, you should visit a doctor familiar with tropical diseases.

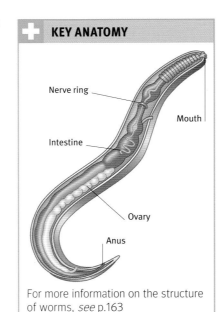

✚ KEY ANATOMY

Nerve ring

Mouth

Intestine

Ovary

Anus

For more information on the structure of worms, *see* p.163

Threadworm infestation

An infestation of thin worms that lay eggs around the anus, causing intense itching

 More common in children

 Poor sanitation and inadequate personal hygiene are risk factors

 Gender and genetics are not significant factors

Threadworm infestation is caused by the roundworm *Enterobius vermicularis* and is the most common parasitic worm infestation affecting humans in the UK. Usually, infestation occurs by ingesting worm eggs in contaminated food, on fingers, or in house dust. If they are swallowed, the eggs develop into adult threadworms in the intestine. At night, female threadworms crawl out of the anus to lay eggs around the anal region, causing intense itching. Threadworm infestation mainly affects children.

What are the symptoms?

In most cases, the symptoms of threadworm infestation include:
■ Intense itching in the anal region at night when the worms lay eggs.
■ Inflammation around the anus as a result of constant scratching.
■ In some cases, mild abdominal pain.
Sometimes, tiny, white threadworms can be seen wriggling in the faeces after a bowel movement. In rare cases, infestation causes appendicitis (p.420).

What might be done?

The diagnosis can be confirmed by identification of threadworm eggs in a swab taken from the anal region. Your doctor will probably prescribe an anthelmintic drug (p.575) to kill the worms effectively and speed recovery. Usually, the entire household is treated. Reinfection is common because the eggs can be picked up under the fingernails when scratching and accidentally swallowed. The cycle of infestation then begins again. Underwear, nightwear, and bedlinen may also be contaminated.

Threadworm infestation is usually easy to control. The risk of reinfection is reduced by scrupulous attention to personal hygiene: washing hands after going to the toilet, avoiding scratching the anal area, and washing clothes and bedlinen regularly.

Toxocariasis

The infestation of various organs with roundworm larvae, which may cause fever

 More common in children

 Owning pet dogs or cats may be a risk factor

 Gender and genetics are not significant factors

The adult forms of the roundworms *Toxocara canis* and *Toxocara cati* normally infest dogs and cats, which excrete faeces containing worm eggs. However, the larvae (immature forms) of the worms can infest humans, usually as a result of ingestion of soil contaminated with worm eggs. Children are particularly susceptible because they are more likely to play in soil and then put their fingers in their mouths.

Once the eggs have been swallowed, they hatch in the intestine into tiny larvae, which may then migrate to other parts of the body, including the lungs and liver. In rare cases, the larvae can migrate to the eyes and the brain.

What are the symptoms?

In most cases of toxocariasis, symptoms do not develop. However, in some cases, symptoms may include:
■ Mild fever.
■ Feeling unwell.
A heavy infestation of the larvae in the lungs may cause wheezing and a dry cough. If larvae reach the brain, they may cause epilepsy (p.324), and infestation of the eyes may damage the retina (the light-sensitive membrane at the back of the eye), causing blindness that is likely to be permanent.

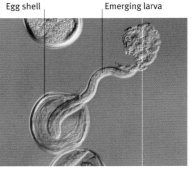

Egg shell   Emerging larva

Toxocariasis
A larva (immature form) of the worm that causes the disease toxocariasis can be seen in this highly magnified image. The larva has just hatched from the egg.

What might be done?

A diagnosis of toxocariasis can usually be made from blood tests, although a tissue biopsy (removal of a small sample of tissue for microscopic examination) may be necessary in some cases. Most people recover completely from the infestation without needing treatment. However, your doctor may prescribe an anthelmintic drug (p.575) to kill the worms. In severe cases in which the brain is affected, anticonvulsant drugs (p.590) will probably be given. Brain or eye damage due to toxocariasis is usually permanent.

It is important to deworm pets regularly to prevent toxocariasis, and dogs or cats should be prevented from defecating in places where children are likely to play, such as in a sandpit.

Ascariasis

An intestinal roundworm infestation that may cause diarrhoea and abdominal pain

 More common in children

 Poor sanitation and inadequate personal hygiene are risk factors

 Gender and genetics are not significant factors

The roundworm *Ascaris lumbricoides* is responsible for ascariasis, which is one of the most common parasitic infestations that affects humans. About 1 in 4 people in the world has ascariasis at sometime in his or her life. The disease is most common in tropical and subtropical areas, and children are affected more commonly than adults. Ascariasis is rare in developed countries such as the UK.

People usually become infested with roundworms by eating food or drinking water contaminated with the worm eggs. Poor sanitation, the use of human excrement as fertilizer and inadequate personal hygiene contribute to the spread of ascariasis among humans. Once swallowed, the worm eggs hatch into larvae in the intestine. The larvae then travel in the blood to the lungs and later return to the intestine, where they develop into adults, breed, and lay eggs.

What are the symptoms?

In most cases, ascariasis does not cause symptoms. However, in large numbers, the roundworms may cause:
■ Diarrhoea.
■ Abdominal pain.
Worm larvae in the lungs may cause wheezing and coughing. A large number of worms in the intestine may cause a blockage (*see* **Intestinal obstruction**, p.419).

What might be done?

Ascariasis is usually diagnosed by identification of the worm eggs in a sample of faeces or of the worm itself, which is pale pink and has a long cylindrical body approximately 20–30 cm (8–12 in) in length. Treatment is with anthelmintic drugs (p.575) to kill the worms. However, the infestation will recur if roundworm eggs are swallowed again after treatment.

Hookworm infestation

An infestation of small, bloodsucking roundworms that may cause abdominal pain, cough, and fever

 More common in children

 Poor sanitation and inadequate personal hygiene are risk factors

 Gender and genetics are not significant factors

The two main species of hookworms that can infest humans are *Ancylostoma duodenale* and *Necator americanus*. People are usually infested by direct contact with hookworm larvae (immature forms of the worm), which live in soil and can penetrate human skin. The larvae travel in the bloodstream to the lungs and trachea (windpipe) and then to the intestines, where they develop into adult worms that can reach up to 1 cm (½ in) in length. The adults attach themselves to the intestinal wall with hook-like teeth and feed by sucking blood from the intestinal wall. The female worms lay eggs, which pass out in the faeces of an affected person and develop into larvae in the soil.

Poor sanitation, inadequate personal hygiene, and the use of human faeces as fertilizer may increase the spread of the disorder. Hookworm is very common in tropical areas, affecting up to 1 in 2 people, especially children, at any one time. In the UK, people with hookworm have almost always acquired the infestation abroad through walking barefoot in water contaminated by sewage.

What are the symptoms?

In the early stages of hookworm infestation, the only symptom may be an itchy rash at

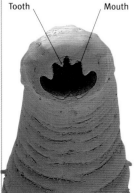

Tooth   Mouth

Hookworm
This magnified image shows the mouth of a hookworm. The "teeth" attach the worm to the wall of the intestine.

the site where the larvae have pierced the skin. As the infestation progresses, symptoms may include:

■ Dry cough and mild fever due to the presence of larvae in the lungs.

■ Abdominal pain due to the presence of worms in the intestines.

Left untreated, large numbers of worms in the intestines may cause gradual, heavy blood loss, which may lead to iron-deficiency anaemia (p.271). If the anaemia is severe, it may cause heart failure (p.247).

What might be done?

Your doctor will arrange for a sample of faeces to be examined for worm eggs if he or she suspects hookworm infestation. You will be given anthelmintic drugs (p.575) to kill the worms and, if anaemia has developed, iron supplements. Rarely, if the anaemia is severe, a blood transfusion (p.272) is necessary.

In order to prevent hookworm infestation when travelling in tropical and subtropical regions, you should wear waterproof shoes in villages and other populated areas if the ground is wet.

Tropical worm infestations

Diseases caused by parasitic roundworms that are widespread in tropical regions

 Poor sanitation and inadequate personal hygiene are risk factors

 Age as a risk factor depends on the type

 Gender and genetics are not significant factors

Parasitic worms that infest humans are most common in tropical and subtropical regions. Both poor sanitation and poor personal hygiene contribute to the spread of parasites among people, especially children. In the UK, tropical worm infestations are very rare and usually occur only in people who have visited or lived in the tropics.

What are the types?

There are four main types of roundworm infestation that normally affect only people in tropical and subtropical regions, such as Central and South America, Africa, and Southeast Asia.

Trichinosis This disease is caused by a tiny worm called *Trichinella spiralis*. People usually become infested by eating undercooked pork containing cysts (larval stages of the worm). In severe cases, symptoms may include vomiting, diarrhoea, abdominal and muscle pains, and fever. In some cases, trichinosis can cause acute heart failure (p.247) or an illness similar to meningitis (p.325).

Strongyloidiasis The minute worm *Strongyloides stercoralis* causes this condition. Infestation is usually a result of

walking barefoot on soil contaminated with larvae. If severe, infestation may result in abdominal pain and diarrhoea between periods of constipation and weight loss. Infestations may be present for years without causing symptoms, but symptoms will appear if immunity becomes reduced due to conditions such as HIV infection (*see* **HIV infection and AIDS**, p.169).

Filariasis Various types of worm or their larvae cause filariasis. The parasites are transmitted to people by certain bloodsucking insects. Different parts of the body are affected, depending on the type of worm. A severe infestation with some types may lead to a massive, painful, disfiguring swelling in the limbs or in the scrotum known as elephantiasis. Infestation with a type of worm known as *Onchocerca volvulus* sometimes results in blindness.

Trichuriasis This infestation is due to *Trichuris trichuria*, also known as whipworm, and it is most common in children. People become infested when they ingest worm eggs. Adult worms live in the intestines, and a severe case of trichuriasis may cause bloody diarrhoea, abdominal pain, and weight loss.

What might be done?

The diagnosis depends on the type of worm but is usually confirmed when eggs, larvae, or adult worms are found in a sample of faeces, blood, or tissue. Treatment also varies with the infestation, but anthelmintic drugs (p.575) are commonly prescribed. Most people make a full recovery if treated early, but reinfection is common in tropical countries. Preventive measures include not walking barefoot on soil, not eating undercooked meat or other foods that may be contaminated, and using insect repellents and mosquito nets.

Schistosomiasis

An infestation of flukes that can damage the liver and bladder

 More common in children

 Swimming in fresh water containing infested snails is a risk factor

 Gender and genetics are not significant factors

People who bathe in lakes, canals, or unchlorinated freshwater pools in the tropics are at risk of schistosomiasis, also known as bilharzia. The disease is caused by any of five species of fluke (types of flatworm) of the schistosoma group. Freshwater snails release larvae (immature forms) of the parasite, which can penetrate the skin of bathers. Once inside the body, the parasites mature into adults, and the females lay eggs, which

may cause inflammation. Schistosomiasis affects about 200 million people worldwide, mainly in developing countries. People in the UK become infested only when visiting tropical regions.

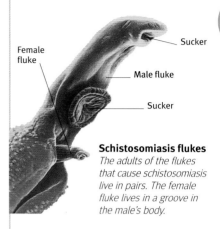

Female fluke

Sucker

Male fluke

Sucker

Schistosomiasis flukes
The adults of the flukes that cause schistosomiasis live in pairs. The female fluke lives in a groove in the male's body.

What are the symptoms?

The symptoms of schistosomiasis vary depending on the species of fluke. Most people experience itching (known as "swimmer's itch") at the site where the parasite has entered the skin. The itching usually occurs within a day of exposure to the parasite. Some people may have no further symptoms, whereas others may develop them within 4–6 weeks. Symptoms may include:

■ Fever.

■ Muscle pains.

■ Diarrhoea.

■ Coughing and vomiting.

■ Passing urine more frequently, with a burning sensation.

■ Blood in the urine, especially at the end of the stream.

Without treatment, schistosomiasis may damage the liver or the urinary system. In many cases, this damage is life-threatening. A long-standing, untreated infestation may cause enlargement of the liver and spleen, bladder tumours (p.456), and kidney failure (p.450).

What might be done?

Schistosomiasis is usually diagnosed by finding fluke eggs in a sample of either urine or faeces. Sometimes, the condition is diagnosed by a rectal biopsy, in which a sample of tissue is taken from the rectum and examined under a microscope for eggs. The biopsy is usually accompanied by a blood test to look for antibodies that the body produces against the parasite. In nearly all cases, the infestation is treated with an anthelmintic drug (p.575), which usually is effective in killing the worms. Schistosomiasis can be prevented by not swimming or wading in fresh water in the regions of the world where the infestation is known to occur.

Tapeworm infestation

*An intestinal infestation
of ribbon-shaped
parasitic flatworms that
may cause abdominal pain
and diarrhoea*

 Eating raw or undercooked meat or fish is a risk factor

 Age, gender, and genetics are not significant factors

Three types of large, adult tapeworms infest humans. These worms are the porktapeworm (*Taenia solium*), the beef tapeworm (*Taenia saginata*), and the fish tapeworm (*Diphyllobothrium latum*). Infestation usually occurs by eating raw or undercooked meat or fish that contains larvae (immature stages of the worms). Once in the intestines, the worms mature into adults, which may reach 6–9 m (20–30 ft) in length. Tapeworm eggs are passed out in the faeces and, in the case of pork tapeworm, may cause reinfection. Certain other species of tapeworm may live as slow-growing larval cysts in humans (*see* **Hydatid disease**, right).

Pork and beef tapeworm infestations occur most commonly in developing countries. Fish tapeworm infestation is most common in regions where raw fish dishes, such as sushi, are popular. These regions include Eastern Europe, Scandinavia, and Japan.

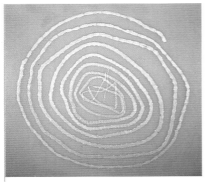

Tapeworm
*This coiled beef tapeworm was removed
from a human intestine, where it had grown
to several metres in length.*

What are the symptoms?
In many people, a tapeworm infestation does not produce any symptoms. However, you may experience:
- Mild abdominal pain.
- Diarrhoea.
- In beef and pork tapeworm infestations, an increase in appetite.

If you are infested with beef tapeworm, you may feel segments of the worm wriggling out of your anus. Rarely, fish tapeworms may cause the blood disorder megaloblastic anaemia (p.272).

A disorder called cysticercosis may develop if pork tapeworm eggs enter the stomach, either in food contaminated with eggs or if an adult worm in the intestine lays eggs that then travel to the stomach. Larvae hatch from the eggs and migrate to the intestine. They burrow through the intestinal wall and travel around the body in the blood. Epilepsy (p.324) may result if larvae reach the brain, and, if they infest the eyes, they may cause blindness (p.369).

What might be done?
A diagnosis is made if tapeworm segments or eggs are present in the faeces. To kill the worms, an anthelmintic drug (p.575) is prescribed. Tapeworm infestation can be prevented by freezing or cooking meat and fish thoroughly. To prevent reinfection and cysticercosis, wash your hands carefully after a bowel movement.

Hydatid disease

*A rare infestation of tapeworm
cysts that may affect the liver,
lungs, or other organs*

 Infestation usually occurs in children but normally becomes apparent in adults

 Owning pet dogs may be a risk factor

 Gender and genetics are not significant factors

Infestation with cysts that contain the larvae (immature stages) of the tapeworm *Echinococcus granulosus* is called hydatid disease. The cyst stage of the worm normally affects livestock such as sheep. If a dog eats raw offal containing a cyst, the larvae mature into egg-laying adults in the dog's intestines. Worm eggs pass out in the dog's faeces and can be transmitted to humans who eat food that is contaminated with eggs. The eggs hatch into larvae when they reach the human intestine. The larvae then move to the liver, lungs, bones, or other organs, where they develop into slow-growing cysts up to 20 cm (8 in) in diameter.

Hydatid disease occurs most commonly in sheep-farming regions where sheepdogs are used, such as Australia, New Zealand, and, to a lesser extent, the UK. The infestation also occurs in Middle Eastern countries.

What are the symptoms?
Infestation mainly occurs in childhood, but symptoms may not develop until adulthood because the hydatid cysts are so slow-growing. In many cases, there are no symptoms. However, a hydatid cyst in the liver may cause:
- Pain.
- Nausea.
- Yellowing of the skin and whites of the eyes (*see* Jaundice, p.407).

A cyst in the lungs may lead to chest pain and coughing, and a cyst in bone may cause pain and fractures (p.232) in the long bones of the limbs.

What might be done?
Diagnosis is made from the symptoms and by ultrasound scanning (p.135) or X-rays (p.131). The larvae can be killed by an anthelmintic drug (p.575), but cysts must be surgically removed. The spread of hydatid disease can be stopped by controlling and deworming dogs.

Serious injuries and environmental disorders

Most people know somebody who has had a potentially fatal injury, even if they have not experienced one themselves. Susceptibility to injury is linked to lifestyle, environment, and gender, with more than twice as many men as women sustaining a life-threatening injury. Age is also an important factor, and statistics show that most injuries and accidents tend to happen in adolescence and early adulthood.

IN 2014, THERE were about 19,860 deaths in England and Wales due to injury or poisoning, of which about 13,100 were accidental.

One of the most common causes of fatal serious injuries is road traffic accidents. In 2014, 1,775 people in England and Wales were killed on the roads and about 22,800 were seriously injured.

Poisoning caused about 2,800 deaths in England and Wales in 2014, and was responsible for over 171,000 hospital attendances in England alone. In adults, poisoning is most often due to a drug overdose. However, most nonfatal accidental poisonings occur in children under the age of 5

Burns, scalds, and smoke inhalation caused about 230 deaths in England and Wales in 2014 and, in England alone, resulted in more than 100,000 people needing treatment in hospital. These types of injuries occur most commonly in the very young and the elderly.

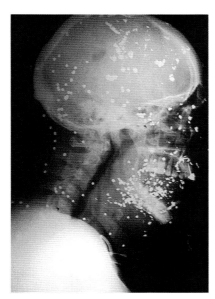

Shotgun injury
This X-ray of a skull and neck shows multiple injuries that have been caused by the pellets from a shotgun.

Environmental factors
Illness and injury that result from environmental factors, such as altitude and low temperatures, are becoming more common, particularly in young adults. Disorders such as frostbite, hypothermia, and altitude sickness can occur when young people take risks on holidays in remote areas with extreme climates. Hypothermia is a particular threat to elderly people, even at home. This is because the body's ability to regulate body temperature becomes less effective with old age. However, the most common cause of fatal injury in elderly people is a fall, which often results in one or more bone fractures. In 2014, almost 4,000 people over the age of 65 died in England and Wales as the result of falls.

Some accident statistics indicate improving trends. For example, vehicle safety features are improving survival rates for traffic accidents. The medical management of serious injuries has also improved. Paramedics and prehospital teams can now provide resuscitation at the incident scene, major trauma networks have been set up, and casualties are taken to major trauma centres where there are specialist trauma medical teams. Emergency departments are better staffed, and intensive therapy units have more effective procedures for dealing with multiple injuries and shock.

Types of injury
The nature and location of an injury determines its severity. For example, crush injuries to the torso tend to be more serious than those to the limbs because they may damage internal organs. The severity of gunshot and stab injuries depends on the location of the wounds and whether major organs or blood vessels are involved. Poisoning and drowning may affect entire systems and damage vital organs.

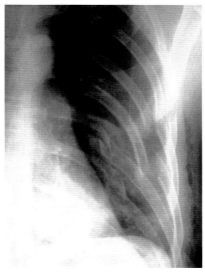

Multiple rib fractures
Crush injuries to the chest often result in multiple rib fractures, as in this X-ray. The fractured ribs may penetrate internal organs, such as the lungs.

The heart may be directly damaged by physical injuries, such as a stab wound, or its function may be impaired by toxic substances in an overdose of drugs.

When the liver is injured, a large amount of blood may be lost. Drug overdoses may also damage the liver.

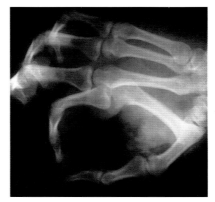

Explosives injury
In this X-ray of the right hand, the metacarpal (hand bone) of the index finger has been displaced as the result of an explosion.

The spleen may rupture following a severe blow or crush injury to the lower chest or abdomen, resulting in severe internal bleeding. A lacerated kidney may leak urine into the surrounding tissue, which causes inflammation. An injury that tears the kidney from its blood supply causes profuse bleeding. If the intestinal wall is damaged, the contents may leak into the abdomen, causing serious infection.

A lung may collapse following a penetrating wound or become inflamed by inhaled gases or smoke released in chemical incidents or fires. If the trachea (windpipe) is crushed or obstructed, asphyxia (a potentially fatal lack of oxygen) may result.

Severe burns to the skin's protective layer may cause large amounts of body fluid to be lost from the circulation, leading to potentially fatal shock.

If the spine is injured, the vertebrae may be fractured or displaced and damage the spinal cord, causing paralysis or death.

The brain may be damaged by a blow to the head, which may fracture the skull and/or cause internal bleeding or swelling of the brain. Such injuries can lead to the formation of a blood clot, which raises pressure inside the skull, causing brain tissue to become compressed and distorted.

Serious injuries

Injuries can affect any part of the body, but they are most often serious if they affect the head, chest, abdomen, or pelvis. Such injuries may be the result of an accident or a deliberate act of violence by another person. In addition to their physical impact, serious injuries may have long-term psychological effects.

The first part of this section covers serious injuries that usually have an accidental cause. Crush injuries often result from a road traffic crash. The number of deaths from traffic crashes has fallen in recent years, mainly due to safer cars and other factors such as drink–drive laws. However, every day about 5 people are killed on the roads in England and Wales. The next two articles discuss burns and electrical injuries. Burns are extremely common and may result from a wide variety of causes. Most burns are due to minor accidents and occur around the home. Severe burns often occur in industrial environments and may result in permanent scarring or even death. Electrical injuries are a specific form

of burn injury, often causing damage to internal tissues that may not be initially apparent. Such injuries may occur in the home but are more common in the electrical or construction industries. Contact with high-voltage electrical cables on railways is also an important cause of severe burns, particularly in young people. The final two articles cover injuries that are usually associated with crime: stab and gunshot injuries. These type of injuries are still relatively uncommon in the UK.

Injuries that are specific to one area of the body are covered elsewhere (see **Head injuries**, p.322, **Spinal injuries**, p.323, **Musculoskeletal injuries**, pp.231–234, and **Eye injuries**, p.363).

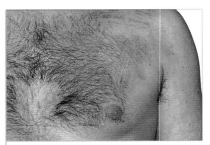

Crush injury
Skin bruising may be the only visible sign of a crush injury. This bruise is due to a seat belt pressing across the chest.

Crush injuries

Injury to any part of the body caused by compression, most frequently as a result of a road traffic accident

 More common in males

 Lifestyle as a risk factor depends on the cause

 Age and genetics are not significant factors

Crush injuries are most often caused by road traffic accidents, which accounted for 1,775 deaths in England and Wales in 2014. Accidents that occur in the construction industry and explosions can also cause crush injuries to any part of the body. This type of injury may range in severity from simple bruising to life-threatening damage to internal organs and tissues. Men are at greater risk of sustaining crush injuries because they are more likely to work in the construction industry and engage in high-risk activities.

What are the types?
Most damage caused by crushing is internal, and often the only obvious external evidence is bruising. Fractures (p.232) are common, especially to the limbs, and, if the chest is crushed, one or more ribs are likely to be broken and may puncture the lungs. Multiple rib fractures may result in a flail chest, in which breathing may become sufficiently impaired to cause respiratory failure (p.310) and shock (p.248). Crush injuries may lead to a pneumothorax (p.303) or haemothorax, in which air or blood is trapped between the two-layered membrane covering the lungs. The heart can also be damaged.

If the abdomen has been crushed, the liver, spleen, kidneys, or intestines may be damaged. If the liver or spleen is ruptured, massive internal bleeding may occur. The contents of a ruptured intestine may leak out into the abdominal cavity and cause infection (see **Peritonitis**, p.421).

In addition to specific injuries, more general complications may develop. For example, if a large proportion of the body's tissues is compressed, chemicals released from the damaged tissue may impair kidney function (see **Kidney failure**, p.450), which may be fatal. In some cases, when circulation is restored to crushed tissues after a prolonged period of entrapment, the sudden release of chemicals from the damaged tissue may lead to severe shock (p.248) and cardiac arrest (p.252).

What might be done?
Call an ambulance immediately. Anyone with a suspected crush injury should be freed as soon as possible. Find a trained first-aider to administer emergency first aid. If the person has been trapped for a prolonged period, treatment will usually be started at the scene by paramedics or other medical personnel. Once the person reaches hospital, treatment depends on the injuries sustained. General measures include emergency resuscitation and giving oxygen and intravenous fluids. Painkillers (p.589) are given as needed. If bleeding is excessive, a blood transfusion (p.272) may be necessary.

After emergency measures have been carried out, internal damage is assessed using imaging techniques, such as chest X-rays (p.300), CT scanning (p.132), and MRI (p.133). Treatment is then directed at specific injuries. For example, fractures are treated by resetting the broken bones in

their correct position and immobilizing the affected part if needed (see **Fracture treatments**, p.232). If limbs have been crushed, surgery may be done to repair blood vessels and nerves (see **Microsurgery**, p.613). Amputation may be necessary if limb damage is irreparable. A person with severe or multiple rib fractures may need mechanical ventilation to aid breathing (see **Intensive therapy unit**, p.618).

If internal bleeding into the abdominal cavity is suspected, an ultrasound scan (p.135) of the abdomen may be performed for confirmation. If the internal bleeding is life-threatening, the person may then be taken into surgery immediately so that the source of the bleeding can be located and repaired. With less serious internal bleeding, a CT scan (p.132) is usually taken to identify the specific injury and source of bleeding before surgery is carried out.

Antibiotics (p.572) are prescribed to treat peritonitis and other infections. Additional complications, such as kidney failure, are treated as they arise.

The outlook depends on the type of crush injury, the length of time that the person was crushed, and the speed with which treatment was initiated.

Burns

Areas of damage to tissue, usually skin, caused by heat, chemicals, or electricity

 More common in males

 Working with hot or caustic substances is a risk factor

 Age and genetics are not significant factors

In 2013–2014, about 109,500 people in England required hospital treatment for burns, scalds, and fire-related injuries (such as smoke inhalation), and around 230 died as a result of their injuries. Elderly people and young children are particularly vulnerable to the effects of burns.

Most burns are minor and are caused by accidents in the home, such as scalding with hot water. Although almost all minor burns heal quickly, more severe burns often require hospital treatment and can be life-threatening. The severity of a burn

depends on how deep the burn extends into tissue and the size of the area affected. Burns to sensitive areas, such as the face, hands, feet, or genitals, can be particularly serious.

Burns are usually due to heat, such as fire, hot fluids, or sunlight. However, caustic chemicals, such as certain paint strippers, and electricity (see **Electrical injuries**, opposite page) can also cause burns. These burns tend to be more common in men because they are more likely to work in chemical or electrical industries. Burns usually involve the skin, but caustic substances can produce burns in the oesophagus and stomach if they are swallowed. Hot smoke can burn the windpipe and airways.

What are the types?
The skin is made up of two layers: the surface layer, called the epidermis, and the more sensitive dermis underneath. Burns are categorized as partial thickness or full thickness, according to the depth of tissue damage. Partial-thickness burns are further divided into superficial or deep.

Superficial partial-thickness burns
These are burns that affect only the epidermis and are the least severe type of burn. The burned area may be red, slightly swollen, and sensitive to the touch, but blisters do not form. Within a few days, the skin heals and the damaged layer of skin may peel off. Sunburn (p.207) is one of the most common causes of this type of burn.

Deep partial-thickness burns These are burns that destroy the epidermis and extend down into the more sensitive dermis. They are usually very painful. The skin becomes red and covered with large blisters filled with clear fluid. After about 3 days, the pain usually decreases, and most deep partial-thickness burns should be fully healed within about 14 days.

Full-thickness burns These are the deepest and most serious type of burn. In this type, the epidermis, dermis, and the underlying fat are destroyed. Sometimes, this damage may extend into the muscle tissue.

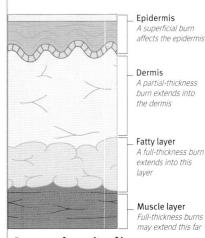

Epidermis
A superficial burn affects the epidermis

Dermis
A partial-thickness burn extends into the dermis

Fatty layer
A full-thickness burn extends into this layer

Muscle layer
Full-thickness burns may extend this far

Degrees of severity of burns
Burns are categorized depending on the extent of damage to the different layers of tissue. The more severe the burn, the more layers of tissue are affected.

The area becomes numb due to destruction of nerve endings, thickened, and discoloured. Healing is very slow since the damaged dermis cannot regenerate itself, and new skin can grow only from the edges of the damaged area.

Are there complications?
In large partial- and full-thickness burns, fluid is lost from the damaged areas, which may lead to shock (p.248) and damage to the kidneys (see **Kidney failure**, p.450). Breathing difficulties may arise if the lungs have been damaged by smoke (see **Asphyxiation**, p.188).

Burns are particularly susceptible to infection because the damaged skin can no longer act as a barrier against infection. Infection with bacteria is most common after full-thickness burns and may delay healing. If bacteria enter the bloodstream, they may multiply and cause septicaemia (p.171).

What can I do?
Seek medical assistance for all but minor burns. Large partial-thickness and all full-thickness burns require specialized hospital care, ideally in a burns unit. Seek medical advice if you have any doubt about the severity of a burn. Anyone with burns on the face or lips must be admitted to hospital immediately in case swelling of the tissues causes the airways to close up and obstructs breathing. Hospital admission is also necessary if someone has inhaled smoke.

Immediately after a minor burn or scald, cool the damaged skin by flooding it with cold water; continue flooding the burned area for at least 10 minutes or until pain is relieved. Do not apply lotions or creams because these may make the burn worse. Remove any constricting clothing, watches, or jewellery around the area then cover the burn with clingfilm. Lay the clingfilm in strips over the burned area; do not wrap it around the trunk or limbs as this may restrict breathing or circulation. Alternatively, use a sterile, non-adherent dressing and bandage it loosely in place. Check the wound daily for signs of infection, such as swelling or pus. If infection does develop, consult a doctor.

What might the doctor do?
Minor burns are cleaned and dressed. Dressings may need to be changed frequently if there is a lot of leakage from the burned area. If an infection does develop, it is usually treated with intravenous antibiotics (p.572).

If the burns are extensive, intravenous fluids, painkillers (p.589), and oxygen may be given. Mechanical ventilation (see **Intensive therapy unit**, p.618) may be needed if breathing problems develop due to smoke inhalation.

Anyone with severe burns will be monitored to make sure that his or her fluid levels are maintained and that kidney function is not affected. Skin grafting (right) will be considered to aid healing for most partial-thickness burns and for all full-thickness burns.

▶ **TREATMENT**

Skin grafting
Skin grafting involves using a section of normal skin from one part of the body (the donor site) to cover another site where the skin has been lost as a result of an injury, such as a burn, or a disorder, such as an ulcer. There are several different methods of skin grafting. The two examples shown here use small donor sites to cover large areas of missing skin.

Meshed graft
A meshed graft is used when a very large area of missing skin needs to be covered and donor sites are limited. The donor skin is removed and made into a mesh using angled cuts. The meshed graft can then be stretched to cover the large area of missing skin.

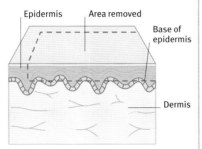
Epidermis — Area removed — Base of epidermis — Dermis

Taking the donor skin
A very thin slice of skin is shaved off the donor site. A sufficient number of cells are left at the base of the epidermis to allow the skin to regrow over the wound.

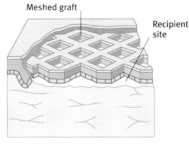
Meshed graft — Recipient site

Positioning the meshed graft
The donor skin is cut and stretched to form a mesh that fits in the larger recipient site. Once in place, new skin grows to fill the spaces around the mesh.

Pinch grafts
Pinch grafts are very small pieces of skin that are often used to help skin ulcers to heal. Multiple small grafts are pinched up and removed from the donor site. The pinch grafts are then placed over the larger area of missing skin and grow to cover the area.

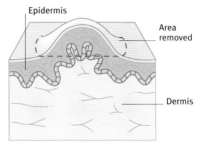
Epidermis — Area removed — Dermis

Taking the pinch grafts
Small sections of skin are pinched up at the donor site and cut using scissors or a scalpel. The donor site can heal because the removed sections are small.

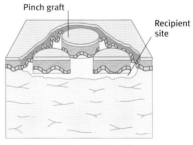
Pinch graft — Recipient site

Positioning the pinch grafts
Multiple small pinch grafts are placed on the recipient site. The grafts will gradually grow outwards to form a new sheet of healthy skin in about 10–14 days.

Scar tissue, which is fragile and sensitive, often develops following severe burns. Scarred areas should be protected from the sun with clothing or sunscreen (p.577). Scars may cause itching, which can be relieved with antipruritic drugs (p.576). Scarred areas may also become taut and inflexible, restricting movement if skin over a joint is affected, and skin grafting may be required. Physiotherapy (p.620) sometimes helps to improve movement.

What is the prognosis?
With correct treatment, minor burns usually heal within a few days; more severe burns may take several weeks. Full-thickness burns may take months to heal even if skin grafts are used, and there will be permanent scarring.

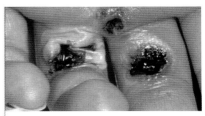

Electrical burns
These two fingers have sustained deep burns as a result of direct contact with an uninsulated electrical cable.

The current may also disrupt the normal functioning of the heart or brain and may be immediately fatal.

In 2013–2014, there were more than 9,500 attendances at hospital emergency departments in England and Wales with electricity-related injuries. Causes of electrical injuries include accidents in the home and lightning strikes. This type of injury also occurs in people who work in the electricity-generating or construction industries.

The majority of electrical injuries occur as a result of touching exposed electrical wires, faulty switches, or water that is electrified by a wire or device. The danger of receiving an electrical injury is greatly increased in the presence of water because water acts as an excellent conductor of electricity.

Men are at greater risk than women of sustaining an electrical injury because they are more likely to work in industries involving electricity.

What are the symptoms?
General symptoms that are common to many electrical injuries include:
- Loss of consciousness, which may be short-lived.
- Dazed, confused behaviour.
- Burns on the skin.
- Rapid, shallow breathing.

The severity of these symptoms depends on the voltage of the electricity and the duration of contact with the electric current. In addition, the muscles may become rigid, preventing a person from breaking contact with the electric current. Severe muscle spasms may lead to bone fractures (p.232).

Specific symptoms vary depending on the route taken by the electric current through the body. For example, if the current passes through the heart, it may disrupt the rhythm of the heartbeat (see **Arrhythmias**, p.249) and occasionally lead to cardiac arrest (p.252). If the current passes through the brainstem, which controls automatic body functions such as breathing, the shock may be fatal (see **Brain death**, p.323). If the person survives such a shock, irreversible brain damage may have occurred.

What can I do?
You should call for medical assistance for anything more than a minor electric shock. If you find someone who has had an electric shock, turn off the electricity before you attempt to touch him or her. Find a trained first-aider to carry out resuscitation and

Electrical injuries

Damage to body tissues caused by the passage of an electric current through the body

 More common in males

 Working with electricity is a risk factor

 Age and genetics are not significant factors

An electric current passing through the body can generate intense heat and burn the tissues. Although burns may occur internally, they are often most obvious on the skin (see **Burns**, opposite page).

other necessary measures; the first-aider should continue these measures until medical help arrives. You should also follow this course of action if you come across someone who has been struck by lightning.

Never attempt to rescue a person injured by high-voltage electricity (over 1,000 volts) because the electricity may jump from the victim to you. Keep at least 18 m (60 ft) from the person and call for medical assistance immediately.

What might the doctor do?
Once the person has been admitted to hospital, a full physical examination will be carried out and tissue damage will be assessed. The heartbeat may be monitored to detect an abnormal rhythm. Oxygen may be given and mechanical ventilation (*see* **Intensive therapy unit**, p.618) may be required. An irregular heart rhythm will probably be treated with an antiarrhythmic drug (p.580). Most people recover if they receive first-aid and medical treatment promptly.

Stab injuries

Penetrating injuries to any part of the body inflicted by a sharp object

 More common in young adults

 More common in males

 Living in urban areas is a risk factor

 Genetics is not a significant factor

Stab injuries resulted in about 4,500 people being admitted to hospital in England and Wales in 2011–2012; around 90 per cent of these were men, with 14 per cent being 18 or younger. Most stab wounds are inflicted by knives but other items have also been used, such as ice picks, screwdrivers, and pieces of glass. Stab wounds vary in severity, depending on the site and depth of the wound. Chest or abdominal wounds are particularly likely to cause internal bleeding, which can be life-threatening.

Medical attention is always essential after a stab injury because visible bleeding is often minor in relation to the severity of the internal injuries.

What are the types?
Shallow wounds may damage skin and muscle only. However, deeper wounds can cause significant internal bleeding, which may lead to loss of consciousness and shock (p.248).

Stab injuries may also damage specific body organs. For example, a stab wound to the chest may result in a pneumothorax (p.303), in which air enters the space between the two-layered membrane that surrounds the lungs, causing breathing difficulties. If the abdomen is wounded in a stab injury, there is a risk of the intestines

being punctured and the contents leaking into the abdominal cavity, which can result in infection (*see* **Peritonitis**, p.421).

What can I do?
Call for immediate medical assistance. Find a trained first-aider to make sure that the person is breathing and has a pulse and to try to stop any external bleeding. If the weapon is still in the body, it should be left in place until doctors can remove it safely.

What might the doctor do?
Shallow wounds may only need stitching. An injection to prevent tetanus (*see* **Vaccines and immunoglobulins**, p.571) and antibiotics (p.572) to prevent infection may be given.

Deeper stab injuries require a full assessment to check for internal damage. Emergency measures may include giving oxygen and intravenous fluids. A blood transfusion (p.272) may also be needed. An ultrasound scan (p.135) and CT scan (p.132) may be done to look for internal bleeding, and exploratory surgery may be carried out to locate and repair the site of internal bleeding. If a chest X-ray (p.300) shows a pneumothorax, a tube is inserted to allow the air to escape (*see* **Chest drain**, p.304).

The outlook depends on the type of stab injury. The victim may be offered counselling to help reduce the risk of developing post-traumatic stress disorder (p.342).

Gunshot injuries

Injuries to any part of the body inflicted by a bullet or shotgun pellets

 More common in young adults

 More common in males

 Living in urban areas is a risk factor

 Genetics is not a significant factor

The effects of a gunshot injury depend on the site of injury, the type of weapon and bullets used, and the range from which the weapon was fired. In addition to tissue damage, there is a high risk of infection. Wounds to the head or trunk are often life-threatening. In the UK, gunshot injuries are uncommon. When such injuries do occur, the victims are usually young men living in urban areas.

What are the types?
A gunshot injury to a limb may damage muscle only or cause a fracture (p.232). Such limb injuries are often not serious. However, damage to vital organs may be life-threatening. For example, a gunshot to the chest will probably cause breathing difficulties and may result in a pneumothorax (p.303), in which air enters the space between the two-layered membrane that surrounds the lungs, or a haemothorax, due

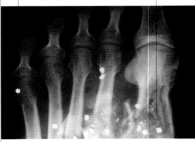
Shotgun pellet   Shattered bone

Gunshot injury
Multiple shotgun pellets can be seen in and between the bones of the toes and foot in this X-ray. The bone at the base of the big toe is also shattered.

to bleeding into that space. If the spleen or the liver is damaged, life-threatening bleeding may occur, leading to shock (p.248) and loss of consciousness. A gunshot injury to the intestines may cause their contents to leak into the abdominal cavity, which can cause infection (*see* **Peritonitis**, p.421). Gunshot injuries to the heart or the brain are often fatal.

What can I do?
If you are with someone who has been shot, call an ambulance immediately. Find a trained first-aider to check the victim's breathing and pulse, and to deal with any external bleeding or any signs of shock (such as a rapid pulse, greyish-blue lips, and sweating with cold, clammy skin). Do not leave the victim alone, except to call an ambulance.

What might the doctor do?
Anyone with a gunshot injury needs to be taken to hospital, where initial measures may include controlling blood loss and administering oxygen and intravenous fluids. If a lot of blood has been lost, a blood transfusion (p.272) may be needed. An injection to prevent tetanus (*see* **Vaccines and immunoglobulins**, p.571) and antibiotics (p.572) to prevent infection are given if necessary.

Following initial measures, the extent of internal tissue damage is investigated using imaging techniques, such as chest X-rays (p.300), CT scanning (p.132), and MRI (p.133). Almost all gunshot injuries require surgery to repair damaged organs and remove fragments of the bullet, shreds of clothing, and other debris in the wound. Once the wound has been cleaned and bleeding has been stopped, the wound is covered with sterile gauze for 4–5 days to help to prevent infection. The wound is then closed.

Certain injuries may need additional treatment. For example, if a pneumothorax develops, a chest drain (p.304) is inserted into the space between the two membranes to allow the air to escape. If breathing difficulties occur, mechanical ventilation may be necessary (*see* **Intensive therapy unit**, p.618).

With prompt treatment, many gunshot injuries do not lead to long-term physical damage. If vital internal organs are affected, the injury may be fatal.

Poisoning and environmental disorders

The natural environment can be hazardous, and, with increased travel and leisure, people today are more likely than ever to be exposed to potentially life-threatening conditions. Although the human body can adjust to some extent, it cannot cope with poisons or prolonged exposure to extremes of environment.

The first article in this section covers deliberate or accidental drug overdose and poisoning. In adults, many drug overdoses are intentional, whereas in children poisoning usually occurs as a result of the accidental ingestion of common household substances.

Disorders caused by extremes of temperature are described next. Heat exhaustion and heatstroke are almost inevitable consequences of spending too long in very high temperatures. In hypothermia, the body's temperature falls to life-threatening levels as a result of excessive cold. If the body tissues are cold enough, they may freeze. This condition is known as frostbite and is particularly likely to affect extremities that are inadequately protected.

Illness can also result from exposure to extremes of elevation, and this is described next. Altitude sickness not

only affects mountaineers but may also occur in people travelling to cities at high altitudes. Decompression sickness, more commonly known as "the bends", usually results from a rapid decrease in pressure when a person surfaces too rapidly after a deep dive underwater.

The next articles in this section deal with environmental injuries that affect oxygen supply to the brain. Drowning and near-drowning are both caused by water preventing normal breathing. The more general term of asphyxiation is used to describe oxygen deprivation that results from a wider variety of causes, such as an object in the throat or carbon monoxide poisoning.

The final articles covered here deal with poisoning from snake and spider bites and scorpion stings. Such injuries are painful but rarely serious. Most of these environmental disorders can be easily prevented by simple measures.

Drug overdose and accidental ingestion

Deliberate or unintentional consumption of potentially harmful substances

 Accidental ingestion more common in young children

 Drug overdose more common in females

 Alcohol and drug abuse are risk factors

 Genetics is not a significant factor

In England, about 171,000 people attended hospital for treatment for poisoning in 2013–2014. Most accidental poisonings occur in children under the age of 5, and many are preventable (*see* **Home safety and health**, p.33). However, poisoning in adults is commonly the result of a deliberate overdose (*see* **Attempted suicide and suicide**, p.344). Women are more likely than men to take a drug overdose.

Some substances, such as household bleach, are harmful regardless of how much is ingested. Prescribed drugs, such as sleeping drugs (p.591), usually cause harm only if the recommended dose is exceeded. Illegal substances, such as heroin, can have unpredictable effects, depending partly on the amount taken and on the person's susceptibility to the drug (*see* **Drugs and health**, p.26).

What are the symptoms?

The symptoms vary from mild to severe. They may develop immediately or over a number of days. Some common general symptoms include:

- Nausea and vomiting.
- Abdominal pain.
- Diarrhoea.
- Rapid heartbeat.
- Chest pain.
- Shortness of breath.
- Confusion.
- Seizures.
- Eventually, loss of consciousness.

There may also be local symptoms, such as burns in the mouth after swallowing caustic substances.

An overdose of certain drugs, such as tricyclic antidepressants (*see* **Anti-depressant drugs**, p.592), can disturb the action of the heart and result in an irregular heart rhythm (*see* **Arrhythmias**, p.249), faintness, and loss of consciousness. In severe cases, an arrhythmia may lead to cardiac arrest (p.252). Overdose of an opium-based drug, such as heroin, causes a reduction in breathing rate, which may be life-threatening. An overdose of some substances may also damage the liver and kidneys. For example, an overdose of paracetamol (*see* **Painkillers**, p.589) may cause liver failure (p.411).

Rarely, ingestion of certain poisons can cause a severe allergic reaction (*see* **Anaphylaxis**, p.285).

What can I do?

If the casualty is unconscious or loses consciousness, call an ambulance. Find a trained first-aider to monitor the person's breathing and pulse rate and give emergency first aid as necessary. Stay with the casualty until help arrives.

Even if there are no symptoms and the quantity of poison ingested is small, always consult your doctor or poison centre for advice. Collect as much information as possible, including bottles or containers and remains of the substance that has been taken. If vomiting has occurred, collect a sample for analysis by the doctor. If the person is unconscious or reluctant to talk, you may be needed to provide vital information. Do not give the person anything to drink or try to induce vomiting.

What might the doctor do?

The doctor needs to know what has been taken and when. He or she will examine the person and, if a drug overdose has been taken, may arrange for blood tests to measure drug levels in the circulation. Other body fluids, such as vomit, may be analysed.

In some cases, admission to an intensive therapy unit (p.618) for monitoring and treatment may be required. If tricyclic antidepressants have been taken, the heart rhythm is monitored to detect any abnormalities. After a paracetamol overdose, blood tests are carried out to look for signs of liver damage.

Various methods may be used to try to eliminate the ingested substance from the digestive tract and to prevent it from being absorbed into the circulation. Stomach washout (also called gastric lavage) is generally ineffective and potentially dangerous, so it is no longer used, except in rare instances. If the person is unconscious, a tube may be passed into the windpipe to prevent the stomach contents from entering the lungs.

If the overdose is serious, activated charcoal may be given orally, but usually only if the person receives treatment within about an hour of taking the overdose. The toxic substance binds to the charcoal in the digestive tract and is then passed out in the faeces. If very high levels of a toxic substance are present in the circulation, elimination can be increased by dialysis (p.451). Some substances can be inactivated by giving a specific antidote. For example, naloxone may be given for an opium-based overdose.

Complications are usually treated as they arise. For example, antiarrhythmic drugs (p.580) can be prescribed for an irregular heartbeat. If breathing difficulties are severe, mechanical ventilation may eventually be required.

If an overdose was taken deliberately, a psychiatric assessment will be carried out when the person is stable.

What is the prognosis?

Although poisoning may be fatal, most cases are treated successfully. However, in some cases, there may be permanent damage, such as liver damage following an overdose of paracetamol.

Heat exhaustion and heatstroke

Conditions resulting from exposure to excessive heat, in which there is loss of fluids and a rise in body temperature

 May occur at any age but most common in babies and elderly people

 Exertion in a hot environment is a risk factor

 Gender and genetics are not significant factors

In a hot environment, the body loses heat by diverting blood to the skin and by sweating. Profuse sweating may lead to an excessive loss of fluids and salts, resulting in heat exhaustion. This condition is rarely serious, but, if exposure to heat continues, heatstroke may occur as the body's normal cooling mechanisms break down and the temperature of the body rises. Heatstroke is a life-threatening medical emergency.

Heat exhaustion and heatstroke most commonly occur above 40°C (104°F). High humidity levels increase the risk of heatstroke because sweating is ineffective and heat loss is decreased.

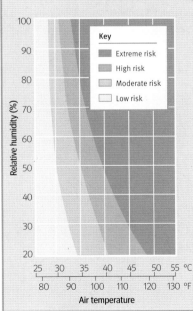

EFFECT OF HUMIDITY ON THE RISK OF HEATSTROKE

Key
- Extreme risk
- High risk
- Moderate risk
- Low risk

Relative humidity (%)

Air temperature

The risk of heatstroke
As the amount of moisture in the atmosphere (the relative humidity) increases, it becomes more and more difficult to lose heat from the body by sweating, and heatstroke may therefore occur at lower air temperatures.

Who is at risk?

Heat exhaustion and heatstroke may affect otherwise healthy people, particularly after physical exertion in a hot climate. People who come from temperate climates and travel to the tropics need time to acclimatize to the heat before they can safely exert themselves.

The body's cooling mechanisms are less efficient in infants and in elderly people, making them more susceptible to heat exhaustion and heatstroke. Diabetes mellitus (p.437), obesity (p.400), alcohol dependence (p.350), and chronic heart failure (p.247) all reduce the body's ability to lose heat. Diarrhoea (p.397) may contribute to dehydration and increase the risk of developing heat exhaustion and heatstroke.

What are the symptoms?

After prolonged exposure to hot conditions, the following symptoms of heat exhaustion may develop:

- Profuse sweating.
- Tiredness.
- Muscle cramps.
- Nausea and vomiting.
- Faintness and unsteadiness.
- Headache.

If exposure to heat continues, the body temperature rises and heatstroke may develop, causing symptoms such as:

- Fast, shallow breathing.
- Confusion and disorientation.
- Seizures.

Left untreated, heatstroke may progress to coma (p.323) in minutes. Death may be due to kidney failure (p.450), acute heart failure (p.247), or direct heat-induced damage to the brain.

What can I do?

Heat exhaustion can be treated easily. The affected person should rest in a cool place (ideally in an air-conditioned building) and drink plenty of fluids (water or a rehydration drink, such as an electrolyte sports drink) until he or she feels comfortable. Alcohol and caffeine should be avoided. If heatstroke is suspected, he or she should be admitted to hospital as soon as possible.

What might the doctor do?

Treatment for heatstroke is usually carried out in an intensive therapy unit (p.618). Body temperature is lowered by sponging the body with tepid water or loosely wrapping the person in a wet sheet and placing him or her near a fan. Intravenous fluids are given. Once the body temperature has been reduced to 38°C (100°F), these cooling procedures are stopped to prevent the development of hypothermia. Monitoring is carried out continuously to make sure that the body temperature is returning to normal levels and that vital organs are functioning normally. In some severe cases, mechanical ventilation may be required to assist breathing.

Most people with heat exhaustion recover in a few hours if they are moved to a cooler place and fluids are gradually replaced. If heatstroke is treated promptly, most people recover after a few days of bed rest, although their body temperature may fluctuate for several weeks afterwards.

Can they be prevented?
Heat-related disorders can be largely prevented by avoiding strenuous exertion in the heat of the day, spending as much time as possible in the shade, consuming large quantities of liquids, and avoiding alcoholic drinks.

Hypothermia

A fall in body temperature to a dangerously low level

 May occur at any age but most common in babies and elderly people

 Homelessness and outdoor activities in cold climates are risk factors

 Gender and genetics are not significant factors

Hypothermia is a condition that occurs when the body's temperature, normally about 37°C (98.6°F), falls below 35°C (95°F). The body normally has various warming mechanisms, including shivering, that replace lost heat. However, if the environment is too cold or if the body's warming mechanisms fail, hypothermia develops. Hypothermia may be associated with frostbite (right) and, if it is extreme, can be life-threatening.

Who is at risk?
Hypothermia is particularly common in climbers and walkers who are inadequately dressed for cold weather. People who are

EFFECT OF WIND SPEED ON THE RISK OF HYPOTHERMIA

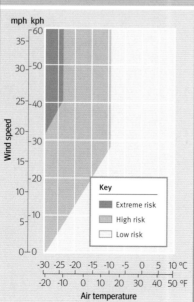

The risk of hypothermia
As the wind speed increases, heat is lost more rapidly from the body, making hypothermia more likely to occur at warmer temperatures.

homeless in cold weather are also vulnerable. In addition, people who have reduced awareness of low temperatures due to alcohol or drug abuse may not realize they need to protect themselves and may develop hypothermia.

Certain disorders increase the risk of developing hypothermia. For example, hypothyroidism (p.432) slows down the body's functions and reduces the body temperature. People whose mobility is reduced generate little body heat and are also more susceptible to hypothermia.

Elderly people are particularly at risk of developing hypothermia. As the body ages, it becomes less able to maintain its normal body temperature in cold conditions. Elderly people may also be less aware of the cold and do not always notice if their body temperature drops. In some cases, dementia (p.331) may reduce an elderly person's awareness of temperature changes.

Babies are susceptible to hypothermia because they lose heat rapidly and, like elderly people, cannot easily maintain their body temperature.

In all cases, the rate of heat loss and therefore the risk of hypothermia is increased in high winds or wet conditions, and hypothermia may develop particularly quickly when a person is immersed in cold water.

What are the symptoms?
The symptoms of hypothermia usually develop gradually over hours or days but may develop in minutes in someone immersed in cold water or exposed to high winds. The person may not feel cold. Symptoms may include:
■ Tiredness.
■ Slow, clumsy movements.
■ Confusion, impaired judgment, and slow reactions.
■ Blue, cold hands and feet.
As the body temperature drops further, these symptoms become more obvious. In addition, the lips may turn blue, delirium or loss of consciousness may develop, and the heart may develop an abnormal rhythm (*see* **Arrhythmias**, p.249) or, eventually, even stop beating (*see* **Cardiac arrest**, p.252).

What can I do?
If you are with someone who has mild hypothermia, move him or her to a warm, sheltered place. If necessary, help remove damp clothes and replace them with warm, dry clothing, including a hat. Wrap the person in a warm blanket, and, if he or she is fully conscious, give him or her a warm, nonalcoholic drink. Do not give the person alcohol because it increases heat loss from the surface of the skin and can therefore exacerbate the condition. If hypothermia is more severe, or if the person becomes unconscious, call for medical help as soon as possible.

If you are stranded in a remote place with a person with severe hypothermia, you should follow as many of the above measures as possible until help arrives. If possible, get into a survival or sleeping bag together to help warm the person up.

Avoiding hypothermia in elderly people
Elderly people are particularly susceptible to hypothermia. If you are elderly, you should take care to protect yourself against the cold. The following measures may help:
■ Keep all your windows closed in cold weather.
■ Install an easy-to-read wall thermometer. The temperature in the room where you spend most of your time should be at least 20°C (68°F).
■ Make sure that your home is warm before getting out of bed in the morning.
■ Have at least one hot meal and several hot drinks each day.
■ Try to move around at least hourly to create your own heat.
■ Wear several layers of clothing to trap warm air.
■ Wear a hat to prevent loss of body heat through the scalp.
■ If your clothes get wet, change into dry clothes as soon as possible to prevent the moisture in the clothes from conducting heat away from the body.

What might the doctor do?
The doctor will assess the degree of hypothermia using a rectal thermometer that can record low temperatures. People with severe hypothermia need rewarming in hospital, usually in an intensive therapy unit (p.618). Most people with mild to moderate hypothermia recover fully. The outlook is best for young, otherwise healthy people.

In most cases, hypothermia can be prevented by self-help measures, such as dressing warmly and keeping moving in cold weather.

Frostbite

Damage to the body tissues caused by exposure to extreme cold

 Outdoor activities in intensely cold climates are risk factors

 Age, gender, and genetics are not significant factors

Exposure to extreme cold can freeze the body tissues and damage them, a condition that is known as frostbite. If not treated, frostbite may result in tissue death and permanent damage to the affected area. Frostbite can develop at any temperature below 0°C (32°F). The lower the temperature, the more rapidly frostbite develops. The risk of frostbite is increased by windy conditions.

People who have impaired circulation, such as those with diabetic vascular disease (p.260), are at increased risk of frostbite. Certain drugs affecting circulation (*see* **Beta-blocker drugs**, p.581) may also make frostbite more likely.

The extremities are most susceptible to frostbite and are affected first. White, cold patches of skin appear, accompanied first by tingling then by numbness. When warmed, mildly affected tissues become red and swollen. If frostbite is more severe, blisters appear, and the area becomes very painful. Prolonged frostbite may lead to tissue death (*see* **Gangrene**, p.262), and the skin may appear black or dark blue. Frostbite is often associated with hypothermia (left).

What can I do?
Rapid rewarming is the single most effective treatment for frostbite. However, it should be done only if there is no possibility of refreezing. Immerse the affected part in warm water that is not too hot to touch (about 38–40°C/100.4–104°F). The water must not be allowed to get cold as this may make the frostbite worse. Do not use direct heat, such as a fire, as the skin may be burned. During the rewarming, the affected part should be actively but gently moved, if possible, but do not massage or rub it as this can cause tissue damage. Thawing usually takes about 20–40 minutes for superficial frostbite and up to 1 hour for severe frostbite. As the blood circulation returns, the affected area may become painful. Continue rewarming until the frostbitten tissue becomes flushed, soft, and can be moved easily. Remove it from the water then place gauze between the frostbitten fingers and toes, and bandage the affected areas loosely. Seek medical advice as soon as possible.

What might the doctor do?
If the affected area does not completely recover with warming, go to hospital as soon as possible. In hospital, rewarming will be completed, and sterile dressings applied to reduce the risk of infection. Physiotherapy (p.620) may also be required to promote circulation to the affected areas. In very severe cases, and after all other means have been tried, amputation of dead areas may be necessary to preserve nearby healthy tissue.

Frostbite damage usually heals within 6 months, but lasting sensitivity to the cold is common. If frostbite is severe, stiffness, pain, and numbness may persist indefinitely.

Altitude sickness

A potentially life-threatening condition experienced at high altitudes resulting from oxygen deficiency in the blood and tissues

 Rapidly ascending to high altitudes is a risk factor

 Age, gender, and genetics are not significant factors

At high altitudes, the amount of oxygen in the air is reduced. The resulting low levels of oxygen in the blood and tissues cause symptoms such as tiredness, unsteadiness, headache, and nausea. This condition is known as altitude sickness. Altitude sickness usually affects mountaineers, but people flying from sea level to a high-altitude location may experience some mild altitude sickness upon arrival. The severity of the illness depends on how high and fast a person ascends, but altitude sickness does not normally occur below about 2,400 m (8,000 ft).

What are the symptoms?
Symptoms may begin to develop about 6 hours after arriving at high altitude. Symptoms may include:
- Headache.
- Tiredness and weakness.
- Unsteadiness.
- Nausea.

These symptoms are usually mild and disappear within 1–2 days if you do not ascend further. In some people, more severe symptoms, including shortness of breath and vomiting, may develop within 36 hours. In rare cases, fluid may build up in the lungs (a condition known as high-altitude pulmonary oedema) and result in a cough with frothy sputum. Fluid may also accumulate in the brain (high-altitude cerebral oedema), causing the brain to swell, which initially results in clumsiness and difficulty in walking. If altitude sickness is left untreated, further symptoms may develop, including confusion, seizures, and coma (p.323), and the person may even die.

What can I do?
If you have mild altitude sickness, rest, painkillers (p.589), plenty of fluids, and a light diet should enable you to acclimatize to the altitude. A further ascent should not be attempted until all your symptoms have subsided.

In severe cases, a rapid descent to a lower altitude may be life-saving. Even descending only 300 m (1,000 ft) may lead to an improvement. If symptoms persist, hospital admission is necessary.

What might the doctor do?
In severe cases, immediate oxygen therapy is necessary. If the lungs and brain are affected, a delay in treatment may lead to permanent brain damage and possibly death. Bed rest will be recommended, and the drug dexamethasone (see Corticosteroids, p.600) may be given to relieve the symptoms.

Most people treated for altitude sickness recover fully within 1–3 days. Even if the lungs and brain are affected, a full recovery is likely, although in this case treatment may be needed over a longer period of several days or weeks.

Can it be prevented?
Good physical preparation and a high level of fitness are essential prerequisites for climbing at high altitudes. Ascents to high altitudes should be staged and gradual and should include intervals of a few days spent at intermediate altitudes before climbing higher.

Plenty of fluids should be taken on climbs. Occasionally, the drug acetazolamide may be prescribed beforehand to reduce susceptibility to altitude sickness.

An oxygen supply should be part of the equipment for people climbing above 3,700 m (12,000 ft) because it may be necessary for treating unforeseen cases of altitude sickness.

Decompression sickness

A condition resulting from the formation of gas bubbles in the blood and tissues following a rapid decrease in pressure

 Deep-sea diving is a risk factor

 Age, gender, and genetics are not significant factors

Decompression sickness, also known as "the bends", usually occurs when a person surfaces too quickly after a deep dive underwater. The condition may also result from working in pressurized tunnels, being exposed to sudden aircraft decompression at high altitude, or flying too soon after scuba diving.

At normal atmospheric pressure, a certain amount of gas is dissolved in the blood and other tissues. More gas accumulates in the tissues of divers due to the high-pressure gas mixture they breathe while underwater. If, during a slow ascent to the water's surface, the surrounding pressure is lowered gradually, excess gas is carried to the lungs by the blood and is exhaled. If the reduction in pressure during ascent is too rapid, gas cannot be carried away gradually and bubbles form in the blood and tissues, causing decompression sickness. Decompression sickness in people other than divers is also due to the formation of gas bubbles in blood and tissues.

What are the symptoms?
Symptoms usually occur within a few hours of the pressure being reduced but may take up to 24 hours to develop. They often include:
- Itching.
- Mottling of the skin.
- Severe pains in the larger joints, particularly the shoulders and knees.
- Headache.

Humerus   Detached bone   Shoulder
           fragment   joint

Effect of decompression sickness
A rapid reduction in atmospheric pressure may cause decompression sickness, resulting in bone damage, often near large joints.

Gas bubbles may lodge in the blood vessels that supply the heart or lungs, causing a tight pain across the chest. If bubbles lodge in the brain or spinal cord, weakness in the legs or problems with vision and balance may occur.

What might be done?
If you have symptoms of decompression sickness, you should be taken to a recompression chamber immediately. Once you are in the sealed chamber, air is pumped in to increase the pressure (recompression). The increased pressure forces the gas bubbles to redissolve into the tissues, thereby relieving the symptoms. Decompression can then be carried out slowly over several hours to prevent bubbles from forming again.

Prompt treatment usually leads to a full recovery. Serious, untreated cases may cause long-term paralysis. People who have repeated episodes of decompression sickness and recompressions may develop progressive degeneration of their bones and joints.

Drowning and near-drowning

Suffocation after submersion in water, often leading to unconsciousness and even death

 May occur at any age but most common in children and adolescents

 More common in males

 Access to unfenced water is a risk factor

Genetics is not a significant factor

In 2013, there were about 380 drowning and water-related deaths in the UK, and near-drowning is even more common. The majority of cases of drowning are the result of water activities in a strong current or after drinking alcohol. However, young children who drown often do so in swimming pools or ponds at home. The risk of drowning can be greatly reduced by taking care around water and particularly by supervising children when they are swimming or playing in water (see Safety in and around water, p.34).

When a submerged person starts to choke, the larynx (voice box) goes into spasm, preventing water from entering the lungs but blocking normal breathing. Eventually, lack of oxygen causes loss of consciousness, and the larynx usually relaxes. If the face is submerged, water may then enter the lungs. In 1 out of 10 cases, the larynx stays closed and no water enters the lungs. This condition is known as dry drowning.

People who are drowning can often be revived by first aid. However, life-threatening complications may develop, and hospital treatment is still needed even if they have apparently recovered.

Are there complications?
Lack of oxygen can lead to brain damage and death. Even if breathing is restored, water may cause inflammation of the lining of the lungs, leading to acute respiratory distress syndrome (p.309). Debris in the lungs may cause infection and lung damage, impairing the ability of the lungs to function normally.

Inhaled water may alter blood chemistry. If fresh water is inhaled, it passes from the lungs to the bloodstream and destroys the red blood cells. If salt water is inhaled, the salt causes blood to enter the tissues of the lungs.

A drowning person can survive for longer in cold water because the body's processes slow down. As a result, many people who have been resuscitated after a near-drowning experience may also have hypothermia (opposite page).

What can I do?
Call an ambulance. Shout for a trained first-aider to help you. Only attempt to rescue a drowning person if you are sure that you can do so without putting yourself at risk.

The person will need to be brought back to land before any other measures can be taken. If the person is conscious and close to you, throw him or her an object that will float, ideally with a rope attached. Alternatively, throw in one end of a stick, pole, or even an item of clothing for the person to grasp. If the person cannot reach the object, swim out only if it is safe. Otherwise, note the position of the person and call for assistance.

Once the person is on land, ask the first-aider to assess his or her condition and, if necessary, carry out emergency measures such as resuscitation.

If the person has fallen into cold water, wrap him or her in warm, dry clothing or blankets to try to reduce the risk of hypothermia. Continue resuscitating a person who is cold because nearly drowned people can survive far longer if they have hypothermia.

Even if the person seems well, medical attention should be sought to make sure that there are no complications.

What might the doctor do?
Even if the person is conscious when first seen in hospital, he or she is likely to be admitted for observation because problems can develop in the first 24–48 hours. Treatment may range from giving oxygen to monitoring and care in an intensive therapy unit (p.618). In some cases, mechanical ventilation may be needed to ease breathing difficulties. Additional treatment depends on any complications that develop. For example, corticosteroids (p.600) may be given to reduce inflammation in the lungs, and antibiotics (p.572) may be administered to counter possible lung infections.

If hypothermia has developed, the person is rewarmed slowly. Body temperature needs to be slowly returned to normal before an assessment for brain damage can be carried out.

What is the prognosis?

The outlook is improved if the water is cold, the period of submersion is short, and the person is young and otherwise healthy. About 1 in 20 people who are resuscitated later die of a complication. Those who survive may have sustained some permanent brain damage.

Asphyxiation

Failure of oxygen to reach the brain for a variety of reasons

 Age, gender, genetics, and lifestyle are not significant factors

Asphyxiation is a potentially fatal condition in which oxygen is prevented from reaching the brain. If it is not treated within a few minutes, asphyxiation leads to loss of consciousness, irreversible brain damage, and, subsequently, to death.

What are the causes?

Asphyxiation may be the result of an inability to breathe or insufficient oxygen in the inhaled air.

An inability to breathe can be due to a variety of factors. One of the most common causes is a foreign object lodged in the throat. Something held over the face may also block the airway, as may the person's tongue if he or she is unconscious. A severe head injury (p.322) or a drug overdose (p.185) may slow down breathing or even stop it completely. Severe damage to the chest wall (*see* **Crush injuries**, p.182) may prevent the lungs from inflating, particularly if one or more of the ribs has been fractured. The neck may be compressed by accidental or deliberate strangulation.

Lack of oxygen in the air can occur as a result of carbon monoxide from a car exhaust or defective gas appliance, such as a gas boiler. Even small amounts of carbon monoxide can result in severe or even fatal poisoning because it is taken up by body tissues in preference to oxygen. Smoke from a fire reduces the level of oxygen in the air, or oxygen may become depleted if a person is enclosed in an airtight space.

What are the symptoms?

Asphyxiation usually develops rapidly over a few minutes but can occur over several hours, depending on the cause. Most cases of asphyxiation lead to similar symptoms, including:

- Agitation.
- Confusion.
- Eventually, loss of consciousness.

In most cases, the skin, particularly the lips, turns blue. However, when carbon monoxide poisoning is the cause, the skin may turn a bright cherry red.

What can I do?

Call an ambulance. Only go to the aid of a person who is being asphyxiated if you are in no danger yourself. Once the person is

out of danger, ask a trained first-aider to deal with any obstruction to breathing, and, if necessary, carry out emergency resuscitation until help arrives.

What might the doctor do?

Once in hospital, medical treatment is directed at reversing the cause of the asphyxiation. For example, if the condition is due to a foreign body lodged in the throat, the object will be removed. If the object cannot be removed quickly, an incision may be made in the trachea (the windpipe) and a tube inserted to restore breathing until the airway can be cleared. Fractured ribs will be treated and painkillers (p.589) given. Drug overdoses are treated by eliminating as much of the ingested toxic substance as possible. In some severe cases in which the underlying cause of the asphyxiation cannot be treated rapidly, mechanical ventilation (*see* **Intensive therapy unit**, p.618) may be required.

The shorter the period of oxygen deprivation, the better the prognosis. Following prolonged asphyxiation, there may be permanent brain damage.

Poisonous bites and stings

Penetrating injuries from snakes, scorpions, insects, or marine life that are followed by an injection of venom

 Walking or swimming in areas where venomous biting or stinging animals live is a risk factor

 Age, gender, and genetics are not significant factors

The risk of receiving a poisonous bite or sting varies considerably in different parts of the world. The animals most commonly responsible for venomous bites and stings include snakes, spiders, scorpions, and marine animals such as jellyfish. If you are travelling abroad, it is important to seek advice about the risk of encountering venomous animals, especially if you intend to go camping, hiking, or swimming. You should also take appropriate precautions to prevent being bitten or stung (*see* **Avoiding bites and stings**, right).

What are the causes?

Worldwide, there are many species of venomous snake, but only one of these, the adder, occurs naturally in the UK. Poisonous spiders are found in parts of America and Australia. For example, black widow and brown recluse spiders occur in North America, while Australia is home to the redback and funnel web spider. Venomous scorpions are found in several parts of the world, including North Africa, South America, and India.

Poisonous marine animals, including jellyfish and sea anemones, can be found around the shores of Britain. Poisonous fish, such as stingrays and scorpion fish, are found only in tropical waters.

What are the symptoms?

If a person is bitten by a snake and there are no fang marks, no venom has been injected and there will be no symptoms. If there is venom in the wound, symptoms may appear immediately or over the next few hours. Initial symptoms occur around the bite and may include:

- Swelling and discoloration.
- Pain and a burning sensation.

Later, symptoms of widespread poisoning may begin to appear, including:

- Pale skin and sweating.
- Confusion.
- Eventual loss of consciousness.

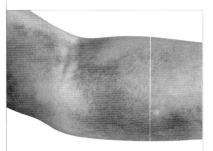

Effect of a snake bite
A bite by a poisonous snake may cause swelling and discoloration of surrounding tissues, obscuring the bite marks.

Blood pressure may fall, causing shock (p.248). Major organs may be affected, possibly resulting in respiratory failure (p.310) and acute heart failure (p.247).

Most scorpion stings are extremely painful but otherwise harmless. However, a sting from a bark scorpion, which is found in parts of America, may cause further symptoms, including sweating, restlessness, vomiting, diarrhoea, an irregular heartbeat, and muscle spasms.

The bite of a venomous spider, such as the black widow spider, usually causes generalized muscle pain, sweating, and headache and may lead to shock.

Stings by marine creatures may produce pain and swelling. Raised, red, itchy areas of skin may appear at the point of contact with a jellyfish or sea anemone. Rarely, stings from marine animals may result in symptoms such as diarrhoea, vomiting, and an irregular heartbeat.

In addition, any poisonous bite or sting may cause a life-threatening anaphylactic reaction in susceptible people (*see* **Anaphylaxis**, p.285).

What can I do?

Call an ambulance. If a person has been bitten by a snake or poisonous spider, remove any clothing or jewellery that may cause constriction if the area around the bite starts to swell. Then lay the person down with the shoulders raised. The person should not walk and should move as little as possible in order to slow down the rate at which venom is absorbed into body tissues. If he or she has been bitten on a limb, immobilize the limb. Do not interfere with the wound. Reassure the

Avoiding bites and stings

The chance of being bitten or stung when hiking can be reduced by taking the following steps:

- Apply insect repellent before setting out on a hike.
- Wear a long-sleeved shirt tucked into your waistband and long trousers tucked into socks.
- Put a rubber band where trousers and socks meet to prevent insects from getting under clothing.
- Wear strong walking boots to protect the entire foot and ankle.
- Stay in the middle of paths when you are hiking and avoid areas of dense undergrowth.
- Make noise as you walk through areas where there may be snakes.
- If you come across a snake, retrace your steps because there may be others in the vicinity.

If you are swimming, the following measures will help you to avoid being stung by a marine animal:

- Look out for signs warning of the presence of jellyfish or other hazardous marine life.
- Do not touch unfamiliar marine creatures.
- Swim near a lifeguard.

person and stay with him or her until medical help arrives. If the person has been bitten by a snake, note the time of the bite and the snake's appearance (or take a digital photograph of the snake, if possible) to help doctors identify the snake and, if necessary, give the appropriate antivenom.

Most scorpion stings need only application of a cold compress to the wound and painkillers (p.589) for pain.

If a person has been stung by a marine animal, wipe off any stingers or tentacles and wash the area with sea water before seeking medical attention.

What might the doctor do?

Hospital treatment for a snake bite may include resuscitation and intravenous fluids. Antivenom may also be given, and antianxiety drugs (p.591) may be helpful if the person is agitated. Once the person's condition has stabilized, the affected area will be elevated and immobilized until the swelling subsides.

Treatment for a spider bite, or for a sting by a scorpion or marine animal, depends on the symptoms. Oxygen may be given for breathing difficulties. If the symptoms are severe, antivenom may be given to counteract the effects of the poison. Antivenoms are available for some scorpion stings and for the more dangerous species of poisonous marine animal. Pain can be relieved by applying a local anaesthetic (p.590) to the skin.

With the appropriate treatment, most symptoms improve within a few days and there are no long-lasting effects.

Skin, hair, and nails

With an average surface area of about 2 sq. m (2½ sq. yd), the skin is one of the largest organs of the body. The skin forms a protective barrier between the harsh environment of the outside world and the body's muscles, internal organs, blood vessels, and nerves. Hair and nails grow from the skin and provide extra protection. The appearance of the skin varies widely, not only changing with factors such as increasing age but also acting as a barometer of our fluctuating emotions and general health.

THE SKIN IS a living organ. The topmost layer of the epidermis, which forms the surface of the skin, is made up of dead cells, and a person sheds about 30,000 of these cells every minute. However, live skin cells are continually produced in the lower part of the epidermis to replace them. Below the epidermis lies the dermis, which contains blood vessels, nerve endings, and glands. A layer of fat lies under the dermis and acts as an insulator, shock absorber, and energy store.

Protecting and sensing
Even though most parts of it are less than 6 mm (¼ in) thick, the skin is still a robust protective layer. The main component of its surface is a tough, fibrous protein called keratin. This substance can also be found in hair, which provides protection and warmth, and in nails, which cover the delicate

ends of the fingers and toes. The skin forms a highly effective barrier against microorganisms and harmful substances, but it is most effective when the surface remains intact. Wounds may become infected and allow bacteria, some of which live on the skin's surface, to enter the bloodstream. Sebum, an oily fluid formed in the sebaceous glands in the dermis, helps to keep the skin supple and repels water. It is because skin is waterproof that we do not soak up water like a sponge when we bathe.

Our sense of touch comes from receptors in the skin's dermis that respond to pressure, vibrations, heat, cold, and pain. Every second, billions of signals from stimuli received all over the body are sent to the brain, where they are processed to create a sensory "image" and to warn of dangers, such as a hot cooker. Some sensory areas, such as the fingertips, have a high density of receptors. The skin also plays

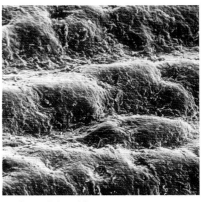

Surface of the skin
This magnified view of the hairless skin of the palm shows sweat pores arranged along ridges. The ridges help us to hold on to objects.

a major part in regulating body temperature and, when exposed to sunlight, produces vitamin D, which is essential for strong bones.

A responsive layer
Our skin responds to the life we lead. For example, the skin of a gardener's hands becomes thickened, giving extra protection. The aging process, during which the skin becomes wrinkled and less elastic, can be accelerated by smoking or excessive exposure to sun. Skin can also change colour. In direct sunlight, the epidermis and dermis produce extra melanin, a pigment that filters harmful ultraviolet rays and causes the skin to darken. People originating in areas that have strong sunlight tend to have darker skin, which does not burn as easily as lighter skin. The skin of people with fair complexions has less melanin and is more susceptible to sunburn.

STRUCTURE

Parts of a nail
Protective plates called nails cover the ends of the fingers and toes. They consist mainly of keratin, the tough protein in hair and skin. Nails grow from the matrix, which lies below a fold of skin called the cuticle, and from the lunula, the crescent-shaped area at the base of the nail.

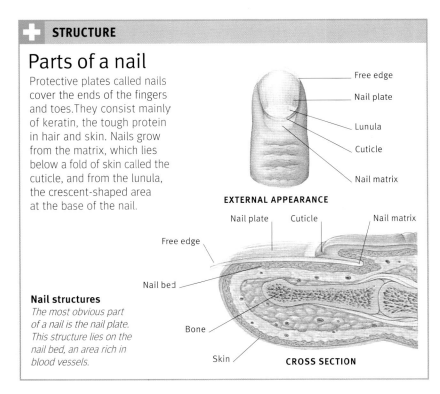

Free edge
Nail plate
Lunula
Cuticle
Nail matrix

EXTERNAL APPEARANCE

Nail plate   Cuticle   Nail matrix
Free edge
Nail bed
Bone
Skin
CROSS SECTION

Nail structures
The most obvious part of a nail is the nail plate. This structure lies on the nail bed, an area rich in blood vessels.

Skin and hair

The skin consists of two basic layers: the epidermis, which is the thin outer layer, and the dermis, which is the thick inner layer. The epidermis consists of sheets of tough, flat cells. Hair grows from hair follicles, which are modified regions of epidermis that reach into the dermis. New hair cells, made in the follicle, eventually die to form the scaly hair shaft. The dermis is made of strong, elastic tissue and contains blood vessels, glands, and nerve endings, which respond to stimuli such as heat, pressure, and pain.

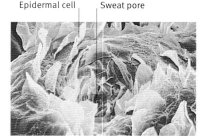

Pore surrounded by epidermal cells
Sweat from glands in the dermis reaches the skin's surface through pores such as this one. The large, upright flakes around the pore are dead epidermal cells.

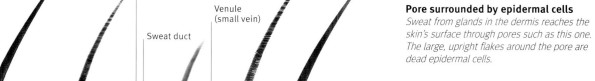

Hair shaft

Sweat pore
The pore releases sweat onto the skin surface

Venule (small vein)

Sweat duct

Meissner's ending
This nerve receptor is sensitive to vibration

Arteriole (small artery)

Scaly upper layer
The upper layer of the epidermis consists of dead, scaly cells

Epidermis

Dermis

Subcutaneous fat

Capillaries
Tiny blood vessels that supply oxygen and nutrients to tissues, while collecting waste

Basal cell layer
New skin cells are made here

Free nerve endings
Different free nerve endings respond to touch, heat, cold, and pain

Arrector pili muscle
This muscle tenses to pull the hair upright

Sebaceous gland
Waxy sebum produced by this gland moistens and waterproofs skin

Hair bulb
New hair cells are produced in the hair bulb

Hair follicle
Hairs emerge from the follicle in a continual cycle of growth, rest, and eventual loss

Eccrine sweat gland
Sweat produced by this gland is carried by the sweat duct up to the skin's surface

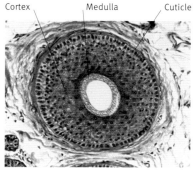

Cortex　Medulla　Cuticle

Magnified section of hair
Hair has three layers: the inner medulla (which is usually hollow), a thick pigmented cortex, and an outer cuticle.

Mucous membranes

Mucous membranes are sheets of cells that protect body areas that must not dry out. These membranes line the mouth and nose; the insides of the eyelids; and the genital, digestive, and respiratory tracts. Special cells in the membranes, called goblet cells, secrete mucus, a sticky protein that lubricates and cleans. At the opening of body cavities, mucous membranes are continuous with the skin.

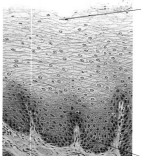

Flat surface cells

Membrane layers
The structure of mucous membranes – rapidly dividing cells in the basal layer below the layer of flat cells – is similar to that of the skin's epidermis, but lacks a thick, distinctive outer edge.

Basal cell layer

✚ **FUNCTION**

Growth and repair

The skin constantly renews itself by shedding dead cells from the surface and generating new cells below. As a result, surface cells that are lost through wear, damage, or disease are quickly replaced. New cells are made in the epidermis, the skin's upper layer, which serves as a tough, protective covering.

Skin growth

In most areas of the body, the epidermis has four layers. In the lowest, the basal layer, new cells are produced. As new cells move to the surface, they change to form intermediate layers of prickle cells and granular cells. The cells reach the surface in 1–2 months. The layer at the surface consists of dead, flat cells, which are continually shed.

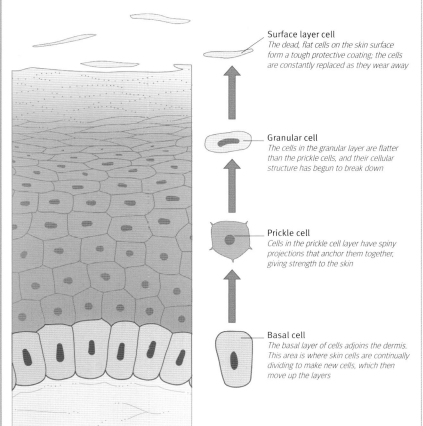

Surface layer cell
The dead, flat cells on the skin surface form a tough protective coating; the cells are constantly replaced as they wear away

Granular cell
The cells in the granular layer are flatter than the prickle cells, and their cellular structure has begun to break down

Prickle cell
Cells in the prickle cell layer have spiny projections that anchor them together, giving strength to the skin

Basal cell
The basal layer of cells adjoins the dermis. This area is where skin cells are continually dividing to make new cells, which then move up the layers

Skin repair

When the skin is injured, it responds by repairing the damaged tissue and replacing lost tissue with new cells. During the process of repair, dead or damaged tissue is initially supplanted by scar tissue and eventually by healthy new cells. In some cases, a scar remains. Skin repair takes place over a series of stages, shown below.

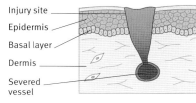

Injury site
Epidermis
Basal layer
Dermis
Severed vessel

1 *Any injury in which the skin is broken, no matter how superficial the injury, may damage the blood vessels in the dermis and cause bleeding.*

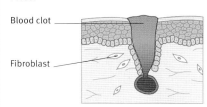

Blood clot

Fibroblast

2 *Blood seeps from the blood vessels and forms a clot. Fibroblasts and other specialized repair cells multiply and migrate to the damaged area.*

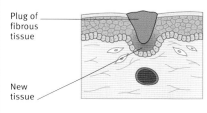

Plug of fibrous tissue

New tissue

3 *Fibroblasts produce a plug of fibrous tissue within the clot. As strands of fibrin in the plug contract, the plug shrinks. New skin tissue forms beneath.*

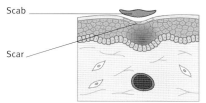

Scab

Scar

4 *The fibrous plug hardens to become a scab on the skin's surface, which falls off when new skin growth is complete. However, a scar may remain.*

Hair growth

Hair grows from a follicle, a specialized area of epidermis that grows down into the dermis. A hair is generated from rapidly dividing cells in the bulb at the base of the follicle. The papilla under the bulb contains blood vessels that carry nutrients. Each follicle has growth periods followed by rest phases. However, the phases of different follicles are not synchronized. Every day some hairs are growing while others are shed. A single hair grows between 6 mm (¼ in) and 8 mm (⅓ in) a month.

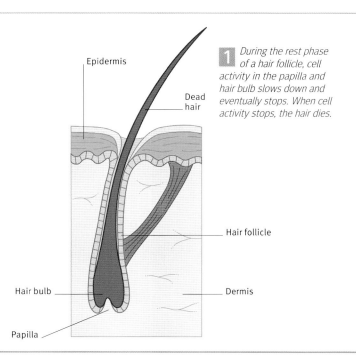

Epidermis
Dead hair
Hair follicle
Hair bulb
Dermis
Papilla

1 *During the rest phase of a hair follicle, cell activity in the papilla and hair bulb slows down and eventually stops. When cell activity stops, the hair dies.*

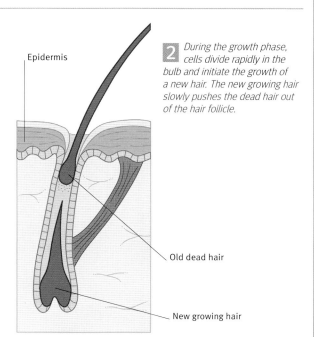

Epidermis
Old dead hair
New growing hair

2 *During the growth phase, cells divide rapidly in the bulb and initiate the growth of a new hair. The new growing hair slowly pushes the dead hair out of the hair follicle.*

Generalized skin conditions

Many skin disorders can affect several or all areas of the body surface at once. Some of these disorders have a strong inherited component, but often the cause of a particular condition is not known. Not all generalized skin problems are curable – some recur intermittently throughout life – but most can be controlled effectively with treatment and self-help measures.

Most generalized skin disorders do not pose a serious threat to health, but chronic conditions, such as psoriasis and eczema, can affect the quality of life and require long-term treatment. Other disorders cause only temporary discomfort and often clear up without treatment. Some conditions are the result of an allergy to substances such as drugs and disappear after the cause has been identified and eliminated.

The articles in this section discuss disorders that cause widespread rashes, itching, flaking, or blistering. Disorders that affect particular areas of skin are discussed elsewhere (see **Localized skin conditions**, pp.197–203, and **Skin infections and infestations**, pp.204–207). Disorders that affect the skin of children are discussed in a separate section (see **Infancy and childhood**, pp.524–529). Rashes that affect the skin as part of an infectious disease, such as rubella or measles, are also found elsewhere (see **Infections and infestations**, pp.160–163).

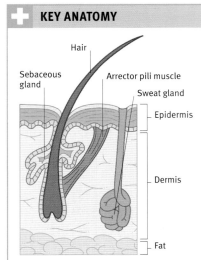

KEY ANATOMY

Hair

Sebaceous gland

Arrector pili muscle

Sweat gland

Epidermis

Dermis

Fat

For further information on the structure and function of the skin, see pp.190–191.

Psoriasis

Patches of red, thickened, scaly skin, often affecting many areas of the body

 Often runs in families

 May be aggravated by stress

 Age as a risk factor depends on the type

 Gender is not a significant factor

Psoriasis is common in Western countries, Australia and South America, and parts of Asia and Africa: it affects about 2 per cent of the UK population. There are several different types, most of which are difficult to control and flare up throughout life. Red, thickened, scaly skin occurs in all types of psoriasis. The scaly areas do not always itch, but if the condition affects many parts of the body, psoriasis may cause severe physical discomfort as well as embarrassment in public.

In areas of skin that are affected by psoriasis, new skin cells are produced at a much faster rate than dead cells are shed and the excess skin cells accumulate to form thick patches. The cause is not known, but an episode of psoriasis may be triggered or aggravated by infection, injury, or stress.

The disorder often runs in families, which suggests that a genetic factor may be involved; approximately 1 in 3 people with psoriasis has a close relative who also has the condition. The use of certain drugs, such as antidepressants (p.592), antihypertensives (p.580), beta-blockers (p.581), and antimalarial drugs (p.574), can produce psoriasis in some people.

What are the types?
There are four main types of psoriasis, each of which has a distinctive appearance. Some people may be affected by more than one type of the disorder.

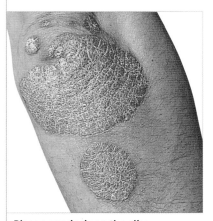

Plaque psoriasis on the elbow
The elbows are a common site for plaque psoriasis. The scaly surfaces of the patches are accumulations of dead skin cells.

Plaque psoriasis The most common form of psoriasis, plaque psoriasis is a lifelong disorder that may develop in people of any age. The condition may produce the following symptoms:
- Patches called plaques, consisting of thickened, red skin and scaly surfaces. They usually occur on the elbows, knees, lower back, and scalp; behind the ears; and at the hairline. In some cases, they develop on old scar tissue.
- Intermittent itching of affected areas.
- Discoloured nails that are covered with small pits. In severe cases, the nails lift away from the nail beds. Sometimes the nails may become thickened and the condition may be mistaken for a fungal infection.

The symptoms of plaque psoriasis tend to continue for weeks or months and may recur intermittently.

Guttate psoriasis This form most commonly affects children and adolescents and often occurs after a bacterial throat infection. Typical symptoms are:
- Numerous coin-shaped, pink patches of scaly skin, each about 1 cm ($^3/_8$ in) across, mainly on the back and chest.
- Intermittent itching of the affected areas of skin.

These symptoms usually disappear in 4–6 months and do not recur, but more than half of those affected later develop another form of psoriasis.

Pustular psoriasis This is a rare but potentially life-threatening type of psoriasis that mainly affects adults. The condition may appear abruptly, with the following symptoms:
- Small blisters filled with pus that develop on the palms of the hands and the soles of the feet.
- Widespread areas of red, inflamed, and acutely tender skin.
- Some thickening and scaling of the inflamed areas.

In severe cases, pustular psoriasis may affect the entire body and require hospital treatment.

Flexural psoriasis Elderly people are commonly affected by this type of psoriasis, in which large, moist, red areas develop in skin folds rather than over widespread body areas. The rash often affects the groin, the skin under the breasts and between the buttocks, and sometimes the armpits. Flexural psoriasis usually clears up with treatment but may recur.

Are there complications?
About 1 in 10 people with psoriasis of any type develops a form of arthritis (p.220) that usually affects the fingers or knee joints. Because of its effect on physical appearance, psoriasis may also have a psychological impact, and people with psoriasis are at increased risk of anxiety and depression. They are also at increased risk of developing heart disease, although the reason for this is not known. In pustular psoriasis, a massive loss of cells from the surface of the skin may lead to dehydration,

kidney failure (p.450), infections, and high fever. If left untreated, the condition can be life-threatening.

What might be done?
Your doctor should be able to diagnose the type of psoriasis from its appearance. If you have only mild psoriasis that does not cause problems, you may decide not to treat the skin symptoms. Otherwise, you should follow the treatment that your doctor recommends.

Topical treatments Psoriasis is commonly treated with emollients to soften the skin (see **Emollients and barrier preparations**, p.575). Other common treatments are preparations containing coal tar or a substance called dithranol, which reduce inflammation and scaling. Coal tar and dithranol are effective but coal tar smells unpleasant and both can stain clothing and bed linen. Dithranol should be applied to affected areas only because it can irritate healthy skin.

Alternatively, your doctor may prescribe a topical preparation containing either the vitamin D derivative calcipotriol (see **Vitamins**, p.598) alone or calcipotriol in combination with a topical corticosteroid (p.600). These preparations are usually applied once or twice a day, do not smell, and do not stain clothes or skin. Calcipotriol alone may take up to about 12 weeks to have maximum effect, whereas a combined calcipotriol and corticosteroid preparation often achieves faster results. However, it is important not to overuse these preparations and you should follow the advice of your doctor.

Topical corticosteroids alone may also be prescribed. However, the drugs should be used sparingly because they may cause long-term side-effects, such as thinning of the skin. If topical corticosteroids are ineffective, immunomodulator drugs called calcineurin inhibitors may be prescribed. These drugs (for example, tacrolimus and pimecrolimus) reduce the activity of the immune system and help to reduce inflammation. Applied topically, they are used primarily for psoriasis affecting sensitive areas, such as the face, scalp, and genitals.

Generalized treatments For widespread psoriasis that does not respond to topical treatments, therapeutic exposure to ultraviolet (UV) light is often effective. UV therapy is usually given without oral medications. PUVA therapy involves using UV therapy together with psoralen, an oral drug that is taken before the UV light treatment and makes the skin more sensitive to its effects. This combined treatment slightly increases the risk of skin cancer and is given only under specialist supervision.

Regular, short doses of sunlight often help to clear up psoriasis. Moderate exposure of affected areas to sunlight, if the weather is sufficiently warm, can be beneficial, but you should adopt sensible precautions to avoid sunburn (see **Safety in the sun**, p.34).

In some severe cases of psoriasis for which topical preparations or other treatments have not been effective, treatment with oral or intravenous drugs may be recommended. The drugs used for this treatment include retinoids (p.575); methotrexate (*see* **Anticancer drugs**, p.586); ciclosporin (*see* **Immunosuppressants**, p.585); and biological medications, such as etanercept, adalimumab, infliximab, or ustekinumab, which act on the immune system to reduce inflammation.

What is the prognosis?
Although there is no cure for psoriasis, treatment can relieve the symptoms and help many people with the condition to lead a normal life. If psoriasis is a long-term problem, you may find it beneficial to join a self-help group.

Eczema

Patches of red, dry, sometimes blistering, itchy skin, also known as dermatitis

 Age, gender, genetics, and lifestyle as risk factors depend on the type

The main feature of eczema is red, dry, itchy skin that may be covered with small, fluid-filled blisters. The affected skin may become thickened as a result of persistent scratching. Eczema tends to recur intermittently throughout life.

What are the types?
There are several different types of eczema. Some are triggered by particular factors, but others, such as nummular eczema, occur for no known reason.
Atopic eczema This is the most common form of eczema. It usually appears first in infancy (*see* **Eczema in children**, p.538) and may continue to flare up during adolescence and adulthood (*see* **Atopic eczema**, p.193). The cause of the condition is not known, but people who have an inherited tendency to allergies, including asthma (p.295) and hay fever (*see* **Allergic rhinitis**, p.283), are more susceptible to it.
Contact dermatitis Direct contact with an irritant substance or an allergic reaction to a substance can result in a type of eczema known as contact dermatitis (right). It can occur at any age.
Seborrhoeic dermatitis This form of eczema affects infants and adults. The precise cause of seborrhoeic dermatitis (p.194) is unknown, although the condition is often associated with a yeast-like organism on the skin.
Nummular eczema Otherwise known as discoid eczema, this form of the condition is much more common in men than in women. Itchy, coin-shaped patches develop on the arms, legs, or trunk and the affected areas of skin may ooze and become scaly or blistered. The cause is not known but may be related to atopy (allergy).
Asteatotic eczema Most common in elderly people, especially in winter, this is caused by drying of the skin that occurs with aging. The scaly rash is red and cracked.

Pompholyx eczema Also known as dyshidrotic eczema, this condition occurs where the skin is thickest, such as on the fingers, the palms, and the soles. Numerous itchy blisters develop, sometimes joining to form large, oozing areas. The cause is not known.

What is the treatment?
Try to keep your skin moist with emollients (*see* **Emollients and barrier preparations**, p.575), take short, lukewarm showers or baths, avoid using soap, and instead use moisturizer as a soap substitute. You can also use oils in the bath to help keep your skin moisturized. Topical corticosteroids (p.577) help to reduce inflammation and itching. You should avoid contact with substances that may irritate the skin. If contact dermatitis occurs, patch testing (p.194) can be carried out to identify a trigger substance. Most forms of eczema can be controlled successfully.

Atopic eczema

Itchy inflammation of the skin that appears in patches, usually in skin creases

 Usually first appears in infancy; sometimes persists into adulthood

 Often runs in families

 May be aggravated by extreme temperatures, certain foods, or stress

 Gender is not a significant factor

The intensely itchy rash that is typical of atopic eczema usually appears first in infancy and often disappears later in childhood (*see* **Eczema in children**, p.538). However, flare-ups of the rash can sometimes occur throughout adolescence and into adulthood. Atopic eczema often affects people with a family history of asthma (p.295) or other allergic disorders, such as hay fever (*see* **Allergic rhinitis**, p.283). Flare-ups in adulthood are sometimes linked to factors such as stress, temperature change, or an allergic reaction to certain foods. Often, there is no obvious trigger.

What are the symptoms?
The rash usually appears in patches, typically on the hands, as well as in skin creases in areas such as the wrists, the backs of the knees, and the insides of the elbows. The face is also often affected, especially around the eyes and behind the ears. The symptoms may include:
- Redness and swelling of the skin.
- Small, fluid-filled blisters.
- Dry, scaly, and cracked skin.
- Thickening of the skin (known as lichenification) as a result of continual scratching.
- Creases or folds below the lower eyelids (known as Morgan–Denny folds).

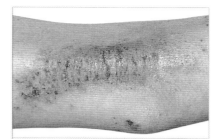

Atopic eczema
The itchy, dry, inflamed rash of atopic eczema typically develops in skin creases, such as the inside of the elbow.

Bacterial infection sometimes develops in the affected area, resulting in further swelling and discomfort.

What might be done?
Your doctor will probably be able to diagnose atopic eczema from the symptoms. He or she may suggest a topical corticosteroid (p.577) to reduce the inflammation. You should apply this sparingly and reduce the frequency of use when the rash begins to clear up. Avoid using topical corticosteroids on the face unless directed otherwise by your doctor. If topical corticosteroids cannot be used or have been used for a long period, your doctor may prescribe instead a topical preparation of a drug that modifies the functioning of the immune system (known as an immunomodulator), such as tacrolimus. Oral antihistamines may help to relieve the itching (*see* **Antipruritic drugs**, p.576). If the rash is infected, you will be prescribed oral antibiotics (p.572) or topical antibiotics (*see* **Preparations for skin infections and infestations**, p.577).

You can relieve and help prevent symptoms by using emollients (*see* **Emollients and barrier preparations**, p.575) and special

bath oil available over the counter. Self-help measures can be used between flare-ups (*see* **Managing hand eczema**, below).

What is the prognosis?
Atopic eczema can be controlled but not cured, and new patches of affected skin may appear at any time. However, the condition usually improves with age and is rare in elderly people.

Contact dermatitis

Patches of red, itchy, and flaking skin caused by irritation or allergy

 Work involving exposure to chemicals or detergents is a risk factor

 Age, gender, and genetics are not significant factors

As its name implies, contact dermatitis is inflammation of the skin caused by contact with a specific substance. There are two types: irritant contact dermatitis, which is caused by primary irritants (substances, such as bleach, that harm anyone's skin); and allergic contact dermatitis, which occurs when a person comes into contact with a particular substance to which he or she has developed a sensitivity over time.

Substances that commonly trigger irritation or allergic reactions include some cosmetics; the nickel contained in jewellery, buttons, earrings for pierced ears, watch straps, and jean studs; certain chemicals; drugs in some skin creams; and certain plants, such as ragweed and primula.

▶ **SELF-HELP**

Managing hand eczema
Eczema on the hands can be particularly persistent, painful, and unattractive. The following tips may help keep your eczema under control and reduce flare-ups:

- Avoid immersing your hands in water for long periods. If possible, wear cotton gloves inside rubber gloves for protection.
- Protect your hands with gloves or a barrier cream before cleaning, gardening, carrying out home repairs, or using irritant substances.
- Remove rings before using detergents or other irritants to prevent the chemicals becoming trapped against the skin.
- In the kitchen, avoid direct contact with foods such as onions, garlic, and citrus fruit, which contain irritant substances.
- Apply emollient creams frequently to moisturize the skin, and wash with mild soaps.

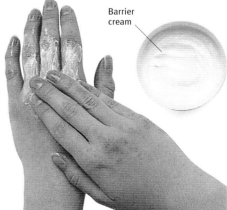

Barrier cream

Applying barrier cream
You can help prevent irritants such as detergents from coming into contact with the skin by applying a barrier cream before carrying out chores. Emollient creams, which moisturize the skin, should be used after washing.

What are the symptoms?

Contact dermatitis usually affects only the area that has been in direct contact with the substance that triggered the reaction. In irritant contact dermatitis, the skin inflammation develops soon after contact with the substance. The severity of the resulting rash depends both on the concentration of the irritant and on the duration of exposure.

Allergic contact dermatitis usually develops slowly over a period of time, and it is possible to have contact with a substance for several years without any skin inflammation occurring. However, once your skin has become sensitive to the substance, even a small amount of it or a short exposure time can trigger an allergic reaction.

In either form of contact dermatitis, the symptoms may include:
- Redness and swelling of the skin.
- Water- or pus-filled blisters that may ooze, drain, or become encrusted.
- Flaking skin, which may develop into raw patches.
- Persistent itching.

Consult your doctor if the cause of the contact dermatitis is not obvious or if the inflammation persists for a longer period of time than usual.

What might be done?

Your doctor will want to know when the skin inflammation developed and whether you have any known allergies. The site of the reaction is often a clue to its cause. For example, a patch of dermatitis on the wrist may be caused by an allergy to nickel in a watch or watch strap. People who handle chemicals at work often develop irritant or allergic contact dermatitis on their hands.

Your doctor may prescribe a topical corticosteroid (p.577) to relieve itching and inflammation. However, even with treatment, contact dermatitis may take a few weeks to clear up.

If you handle chemicals at work, it is particularly important to find the cause of your skin allergy. If the cause cannot easily be identified, you may need to have patch testing (below).

Once the trigger has been identified, try to avoid it as much as possible. If you cannot do so, you may need to cover your skin with creams (see Emollients and barrier preparations, p.575), protective clothing, or gloves before you are exposed to the trigger.

Seborrhoeic dermatitis

Patches of red, scaly, itchy skin that occur mainly on the scalp, face, and chest

 Stress can trigger an attack

Age, gender, and genetics are not significant factors

Seborrhoeic dermatitis is a rash that commonly occurs in infants and adults. In infants, either the scalp or the nappy area may be affected by the rash (see Cradle cap, p.537, and Nappy rash, p.538). In adults, the rash tends to occur on the central part of the face, the eyebrows, and the scalp, where it often leads to flaking of the skin. Seborrhoeic dermatitis can also develop in the armpits, the groin, or the middle of the chest. In men, the condition sometimes develops in the beard area.

The cause is unknown, but seborrhoeic dermatitis is sometimes linked with the overgrowth of a yeast-like substance that is present naturally on the surface of the skin. The condition can recur and flare-ups may be triggered by a period of stress or illness.

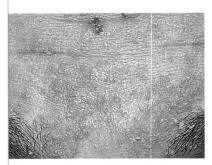

Seborrhoeic dermatitis on the forehead
The forehead and eyebrows are common sites for seborrhoeic dermatitis. Flakes of skin may become trapped in the eyebrows.

What are the symptoms?

The symptoms of seborrhoeic dermatitis may include the following:
- Scaly, red patches of inflamed skin, often with a yellow crust.
- Eyelids that are sore, red, and crusty (see Blepharitis, p.364).
- Excessive dandruff (p.208).
- Occasional itching of affected areas.

The rash may flare up intermittently over a period of months or years.

What might be done?

If a yeast overgrowth is diagnosed, your doctor may prescribe a topical corticosteroid (p.577) or an antifungal cream (p.574). If your scalp is affected, he or she may recommend an antifungal or coal tar shampoo. Both should produce a rapid improvement. However, repeat treatments may be needed if the condition recurs.

Blistering diseases

Disorders of various types that cause eruptions of blisters

Some types are due to an abnormal gene inherited from both parents

Age as a risk factor depends on the type

Gender and lifestyle are not significant factors

There are several uncommon diseases that produce eruptions of blistering on the surface of the skin. These blistering diseases may either occur in particular sites or cover widespread areas of the body. In contrast to individual blisters (p.208), which are minor skin injuries, blistering diseases can be serious. Left untreated, these diseases may eventually become life-threatening.

What are the types?

Some rare types of blistering disease are present at birth and are caused by an abnormal gene inherited from both parents in an autosomal recessive manner (see Gene disorders, p.151). These diseases cause the skin over the whole body to become very fragile and blister when rubbed. They may be fatal.

More commonly, blistering diseases are acquired in adulthood. The three main types are autoimmune disorders, in which the body produces antibodies that are damaging to the skin.

Pemphigoid The most common type of blistering disease is pemphigoid. The disorder affects people over the age of 60. It results in numerous tightly filled blisters, mainly on the legs and trunk, each measuring up to 3 cm (1¼ in) across. Initially, the blisters may itch.

Pemphigus Less common than pemphigoid, pemphigus also usually affects people over the age of 60. In this condition, blisters may appear on any part of the body but often occur around the eyes, inside the mouth, and on the scalp. The blisters are fragile and may rupture spontaneously, leaving patches of raw skin.

Dermatitis herpetiformis This disorder is associated with an allergy to gluten, the protein in wheat (see Coeliac disease, p.416). The condition results in itchy blisters, usually on the elbows, buttocks, and knees.

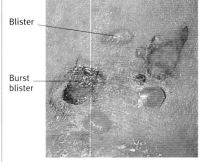

Blister

Burst blister

Blistering caused by pemphigoid
Severe blistering of the skin is the main symptom of pemphigoid, an autoimmune disorder usually affecting elderly people.

What might be done?

In all types of blistering disease, diagnosis is usually based on a skin biopsy (p.199). This procedure involves taking a sample of skin for examination.

There is no effective treatment for inherited blistering diseases. Parents of babies who have these diseases may wish to seek genetic counselling (p.151) to discuss the likelihood of further children also being affected.

If you have either pemphigoid or pemphigus, your doctor will prescribe oral corticosteroids (p.600). Some people will also need immunosuppressants (p.585) for several weeks or months. If you have severe pemphigus, you may need immediate treatment in hospital with immunosuppressants.

▶ **TEST**

Patch testing

Patch testing is carried out on people with contact dermatitis. The test is performed by a dermatologist to find out which substances provoke an allergic reaction. Possible allergens (substances that can cause an allergic reaction) are diluted and placed on small strips or discs. The test discs are then stuck to the skin using inert (nonallergenic) tape. After 48 hours, the discs are removed and the skin underneath them is examined. A red, inflamed patch indicates a positive reaction to an allergen. The tested area is examined again 2 days later to check for delayed reactions.

Inert tape   Disc of test substance

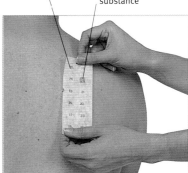

Positive reaction to patch test   Negative reaction to patch test

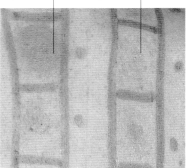

1 *Minute quantities of test substances are placed on small discs. The discs are stuck with inert tape to an inconspicuous area of the skin, usually on the back.*

2 *When the discs are removed from the skin after 48 hours, positive reactions to allergens appear as red patches. In some cases, reactions may take longer to appear.*

In most cases, dermatitis herpetiformis disappears once the affected person has adopted a gluten-free diet, but the drug dapsone may also be needed to help clear up the blisters.

What is the prognosis?
The blistering diseases that affect adults can often be controlled with treatment, but very few cases can be permanently cured. Although pemphigoid may disappear spontaneously in 2–5 years, pemphigus often needs lifelong treatment with drugs. The allergic condition dermatitis herpetiformis may recur if gluten is reintroduced into the diet.

Lichen planus

An itchy rash consisting of small, raised, flat-topped lesions that are shiny and pink or purple in colour

 More common in people over the age of 30

 Stress may increase the risk

 Gender and genetics are not significant factors

In lichen planus, small, shiny, flattened, pink or purple, itchy lesions appear in a dense cluster. Often, there is no obvious cause, but occasionally the rash may develop as a reaction to certain drugs, such as sulphonamide antibiotics (p.572) or gold-based antirheumatic drugs (p.579). Lichen planus may be associated with stress. It is more common in people over the age of 30.

What are the symptoms?
The rash can develop in patches on the lower back and on the inner surfaces of the wrists, forearms, and ankles. Lichen planus often appears suddenly and may affect more than one area, but sometimes the rash spreads gradually over a period of a few months. The symptoms of lichen planus include:
- Groups of small, shiny, pink or purple, flat-topped lesions on the skin; the surface of some may be covered by a network of fine white lines.
- Intense itching, particularly at night.

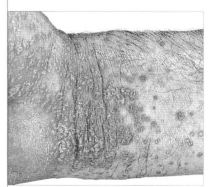

Lichen planus on the wrist
The inner surface of the wrist, shown above, is one of the areas where the itchy lesions of lichen planus may appear.

The disorder can also affect the nails and scalp. If lichen planus develops in the nails, they become ridged along their length and, in some cases, fall off (*see* **Nail abnormalities**, p.209).

If the scalp is affected, patchy hair loss with associated scarring of the scalp may occur. The lesions may also appear on the sites of skin injury such as scratches. Another form of lichen planus affects the mouth (*see* **Oral lichen planus**, p.401).

What might be done?
If the diagnosis is not obvious from the appearance of the rash, your doctor may arrange for a skin biopsy (p.199), in which a sample of skin is removed and examined under a microscope. To relieve the itching, the doctor may prescribe a strong topical corticosteroid (p.577). In addition, you can take an over-the-counter oral antihistamine (*see* **Antipruritic drugs**, p.576) for relief at night. If the rash is widespread and affects your nails or scalp, you may need oral corticosteroid drugs (p.600).

If a drug reaction is suspected, your doctor will advise you to stop taking the drug and may prescribe an alternative. Lichen planus usually persists for 12–18 months but may sometimes last for many years. It may leave patches of darkened skin where it has healed.

Erythema multiforme

A red rash usually forming concentric rings with purplish centres

 Most common in children and young adults

 More common in males

 Genetics and lifestyle are not significant factors

Erythema multiforme develops rapidly and is characterized by distinctive red spots that grow bigger over a few days. The rash is widespread, and often includes the palms of the hands and the soles of the feet. It may affect the mucous membranes, such as the lining of the mouth and nose. The rash is most common in young people and affects more males than females. The disorder is not contagious and is usually mild, although a serious form sometimes occurs.

In most cases, the cause of erythema multiforme is unknown, but the rash can be triggered by infection with a virus such as herpes simplex, the virus that produces cold sores (p.205). Other factors that can trigger the rash include taking certain drugs, such as the antigout drug allopurinol, penicillins (*see* **Antibiotic drugs**, p.572), and phenytoin (*see* **Anticonvulsant drugs**, p.590). Erythema multiforme can also be caused by cancer or by radiotherapy (p.158).

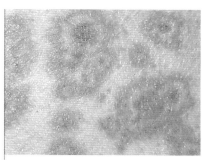

Erythema multiforme
The rash of erythema multiforme usually consists of concentric red rings, often with purplish centres (target lesions).

What are the symptoms?
The symptoms, which develop suddenly, may include:
- Many small, red spots distributed symmetrically over the body. The spots usually enlarge to form red rings with purplish centres, called target lesions. The lesions may blister in the middle.
- Itching of the affected area.
- Painful, inflamed lesions within the mouth and nose.
- Fever, headache, and sore throat.
- Occasionally, diarrhoea.

In rare instances, most of the skin and mucous membranes throughout the body become severely inflamed and ulcerated. Such cases require emergency treatment because the condition may be life-threatening if it is left untreated.

What might be done?
Your doctor will probably make a diagnosis from the appearance of the rash. If the rash appeared shortly after you started taking a prescribed drug, the doctor may prescribe an alternative treatment. If itching is a problem, he or she may suggest an oral antihistamine (*see* **Antipruritic drugs**, p.576). In the case of severe erythema multiforme, particularly if the mouth is inflamed, you may need treatment in hospital; intravenous fluids, painkillers (p.589), and corticosteroids (p.600) may be given in an intensive therapy unit.

Erythema multiforme usually disappears over a few weeks. However, there is a possibility that it may recur. If a drug is thought to be the cause, you should avoid taking it in future.

Pityriasis rosea

A rash of oval, pink, flat spots, most commonly affecting the trunk and limbs

 Mainly affects young adults

 Gender, genetics, and lifestyle are not significant factors

Pityriasis rosea produces a mild, pink rash. The condition most commonly occurs in young adults. It usually affects the trunk, arms, and upper thighs; more rarely, it

affects the feet, hands, and scalp. The condition is thought to be caused by a viral infection.

What are the symptoms?
The symptoms change over time as the condition progresses. They usually develop in the following order:
- An oval patch, 2–6 cm ($3/4$–$2^1/2$ in) in diameter, known as a herald patch, appears. This patch resembles those that occur in ringworm (p.304).
- About 3–10 days later, a number of smaller oval, pink, flat spots, 1–2 cm ($3/8$–$3/4$ in) in diameter, appears. The rash begins on the trunk, spreading across the abdomen, along the thighs and upper arms, and up towards the neck. The spots on the back usually occur in sweeping lines, resembling the shape of a Christmas tree.
- A scaly margin may appear around the edges of the patches after a week.

Itching may occur and is occasionally troublesome. Although pityriasis rosea is not serious, it is important to consult your doctor to rule out conditions such as psoriasis (p.192) and eczema (p.193).

What might be done?
The distinctive rash makes the condition easy to diagnose. It usually clears up after about 6–8 weeks without treatment and is unlikely to reappear. If itching is troublesome, your doctor may prescribe a topical corticosteroid (p.577) to relieve it.

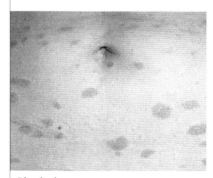

Pityriasis rosea
Oval, pink, flat spots, shown here on the abdomen, are typical of pityriasis rosea, which may affect several parts of the body.

Photosensitivity

Sensitivity of the skin to ultraviolet light, resulting in redness and discomfort

 Age, gender, genetics, and lifestyle are not significant factors

Photosensitivity is defined as an abnormal reaction of the skin to the effects of ultraviolet rays in sunlight. The condition is sometimes present at birth and sometimes develops later in life.

Various substances may cause photosensitivity, including drugs such as tetracyclines (*see* **Antibiotics**, p.572), diuretics (p.583), and, rarely, oral contraceptives. Photosensitivity may also result from the use of certain cosmetics. The condition sometimes occurs in people who have systemic lupus erythematosus (p.281), or porphyria (p.441). When there is no obvious cause, the condition is referred to as primary photosensitivity.

What are the symptoms?
The reaction occurs in areas frequently exposed to sunlight. It usually develops shortly after exposure but may be delayed for 24–48 hours. The symptoms include:
- Red, often painful rash.
- Small, itchy blisters.
- Scaly skin.

At a later stage, the nails may lift from the nail beds. Sometimes, affected people also develop generalized redness on all exposed skin. In rare cases, people with severe photosensitivity are unable to go outdoors in daylight.

What might be done?
Your doctor will probably make a diagnosis from the appearance of the rash. If the reaction is thought to be caused by a drug, the doctor may prescribe an alternative. You may also need blood and urine tests to check for underlying disorders.

To relieve the symptoms, you may need to use a topical corticosteroid (p.577) or oral antihistamine (see **Antipruritic drugs**, p.576). Severe cases are treated with controlled exposure to ultraviolet light, sometimes combined with drugs, to desensitize the skin.

You can help control the reaction by avoiding sunlight as much as possible. When outdoors, cover your skin, wear a hat, and use a high-factor sunblock.

Drug-induced rashes

Many different kinds of rash that occur in some people during or after treatment with certain drugs

 Age, gender, genetics, and lifestyle are not significant factors

Rashes are a common side-effect of drug treatment. The reaction is caused by an allergic response to the drug or to substances produced when the drug is broken down by the body.

Reactions to drugs can produce almost any type of rash, including some forms that mimic other disorders, such as lichen planus (p.195) or erythema multiforme (p.195). However, the majority of drug-induced rashes appear as raised areas of skin spread widely over the body. Drug-induced rashes may be accompanied by intense itching. Sometimes, even when a rash is mild, there may be other, more dramatic effects such as wheezing and collapse. Occasionally, people with severe reactions need hospital treatment.

The drugs that most often produce rashes are antibiotics (p.572), such as penicillin, but almost all drug treatments can cause an allergic reaction if a person becomes sensitive to them. Drug-induced rashes usually develop within the first few days of starting treatment but can also occur after a course of treatment has finished.

Sensitivity develops after at least one previous exposure to a drug. It is common for people to take a certain drug for the first time without experiencing any allergic reaction and then to develop a rash when the drug is taken in a subsequent course of treatment.

What might be done?
If you develop a rash while you are taking a drug, you should consult your doctor before the next dose is due. He or she may then stop the treatment or prescribe another drug.

If you have been taking several drugs and one of these could have caused the rash, you must tell your doctor about all the drugs you have taken recently, including over-the-counter treatments, drugs that have been prescribed in hospital, and medicines prescribed by another doctor. You should also tell the doctor about any recreational drugs or complementary remedies that you are taking.

Most drug-induced rashes disappear when the drug responsible is stopped. However, the symptoms may continue for weeks afterwards. If itching is a problem, your doctor may advise that you apply a topical corticosteroid (p.577) or take an oral antihistamine (see **Antipruritic drugs**, p.576); both types of drug are available over the counter and by prescription.

Once you know you are allergic to a drug, you should make sure you notify any doctor who treats you in future. If you have had a severe reaction to a particular drug, you should consider wearing a medical alert tag.

Itching

An irritating sensation in the skin, either localized or widespread

 Age, gender, genetics, and lifestyle as risk factors depend on the cause

Itching, also known as pruritus, is a very common symptom and is associated with many skin disorders. The irritation may be either restricted to a small area or widespread over the body. Continual scratching, which often damages the skin, aggravates the problem.

What are the causes?
Localized itching can often be the result of an insect bite. Itching may also be associated with a rash. An itchy rash is the main symptom of conditions such as urticaria (p.285), eczema (p.193), lichen planus (p.195), and parasitic skin infestations such as scabies (p.207).

Widespread itching may develop as a result of dry skin, an irritant reaction to particular bath products or detergents, or an allergic reaction to certain drugs (see **Drug allergy**, p.284). It can also occur as a symptom of a serious underlying disorder, such as liver disease or chronic kidney disease (p.451).

Persistent patches of itchy skin may develop as a result of emotional stress. The itching typically affects the limbs and neck but can also involve other areas of the body. Frequent scratching, often unconsciously, causes the skin to thicken and can increase the itching, leading to a further cycle of scratching and itching. This condition, known as lichen simplex or neurodermatitis, is more common in females.

What can I do?
There are several measures that you can take to relieve itching and stop scratching. Emollients (see **Emollients and barrier preparations**, p.575) will help to moisturize dry and itchy skin, particularly if you apply them after washing or bathing. To relieve severe itching, you may find that using over-the-counter oral antihistamines (see **Antipruritic drugs**, p.576), topical corticosteroids (p.577), or calamine is helpful.

As far as possible, you should avoid substances that are likely to irritate the skin, such as scented bath products, detergents, or woollen garments. You may benefit from wearing loose-fitting clothing made of fabric that does not irritate the skin and from keeping your fingernails cut short so that you cannot damage your skin when scratching.

You should contact your doctor if you have persistent itching for which there is no obvious cause.

Purpura

A group of disorders in which reddish-purple spots appear on the skin

 Age, gender, genetics, and lifestyle as risk factors depend on the cause

In the conditions known as purpura, reddish-purple spots or bruise-like discolorations develop on the skin. The spots or bruises, called purpuric spots, result from small areas of bleeding under the skin and may be caused by damaged blood vessels or by an abnormality in the blood. The appearance of the spots varies, and they can range from the size of a pinhead to about 2.5 cm (1 in) in diameter. Unlike many other red rashes, purpuric spots do not fade when they are pressed.

The spots themselves are harmless, but purpura is sometimes a sign of a potentially serious underlying disorder.

What are the types?
The most common type of purpura is senile purpura, which occurs mainly in elderly people. The condition gives rise to dark bruises, typically on the backs of the hands and forearms and on the thighs. Senile purpura is due to weakening of the tissues that support the blood vessels under the skin; these weakened blood vessels become susceptible to damage and bleed easily.

Very small purpuric spots, known as petechiae, often result from a reduction in the number of platelets (cells in the body that help the blood to clot). Platelet deficiency can be associated with many bone marrow disorders, such as leukaemia (p.276), or with autoimmune disorders (p.280). The condition may also occur as a side effect of treatment with some drugs, such as diuretic drugs (p.583) or antibiotics (p.572).

Purpuric spots of variable size may be a sign of a serious bacterial infection of the blood (see **Septicaemia**, p.171). In some people, the infection may be due to a type of bacterium called meningococcus, which can result in potentially life-threatening meningitis (p.325). If purpura appears in conjunction with a fever, you should seek emergency medical advice.

Henoch–Schönlein purpura (p.543) is an uncommon type of purpura occurring in childhood and caused by inflammation of small blood vessels. The spots that appear in this condition are unlike those in other forms of purpura and resemble small, raised lumps.

What might be done?
Senile purpura is usually diagnosed from the bruise-like appearance of the spots. The condition is harmless, and no treatment is needed. The spots fade gradually but are likely to recur.

Any obvious underlying disorder, such as meningitis, will be treated. If the cause of the purpura is not obvious, your doctor may arrange for blood tests to find out if the platelet levels in the blood and the ability of the blood to clot are normal.

If blood tests show an abnormality, your doctor may refer you to a specialist for further investigations. If you are found to have a very low platelet count, you may be given platelet transfusions to prevent serious internal bleeding from occurring, especially in the brain, until the underlying disorder can be diagnosed and treated. The purpura should disappear once the cause has been successfully treated. If the condition is the result of an autoimmune disorder, your doctor may prescribe corticosteroid drugs (see **Immunosuppressants**, p.585) to clear it up.

Senile purpura
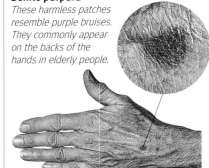
These harmless patches resemble purple bruises. They commonly appear on the backs of the hands in elderly people.

Localized skin conditions

Localized skin conditions are those that affect the skin on only one part of the body or on a small area. Many of these conditions are related to specific sites because they are associated with structures such as particular glands in the skin, or because of the localized effects of factors such as pressure or exposure to sunlight.

Acne and rosacea, two types of rash, are described first in this section. The next articles cover conditions that are associated with sweat glands or with under- or overproduction of melanin, the pigment that gives skin its colour.

Skin cancers, which are increasingly common, are given extensive coverage. It is important to be able to recognize the signs of cancerous changes in the skin, and the various types of skin cancer are described in detail to help you to identify them. Subsequent articles describe several noncancerous forms of swelling and growth. The final articles cover localized skin defects caused by factors such as friction or poor blood circulation.

Localized disorders due to infection are described in another section (*see* **Skin infections and infestations**, pp.204–207). Skin problems specific to babies are discussed elsewhere in the book (*see* **Infancy and childhood**, pp.524–529), as are minor injuries such as sunburn (*see* **Minor skin injuries**, pp.207–208).

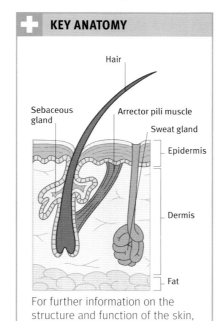

✚ KEY ANATOMY

Hair

Sebaceous gland

Arrector pili muscle

Sweat gland

Epidermis

Dermis

Fat

For further information on the structure and function of the skin, *see* pp.190–191.

Acne

A rash, usually on the face, due to blockage and inflammation of glands in the skin

- Most common in adolescents
- More common in males
- Sometimes runs in families
- Lifestyle as a risk factor depends on the type

There are various types of acne. The most common form is acne vulgaris, which is the familiar rash that affects many teenagers, although it can occur at any age. Acne vulgaris is more common and tends to be more severe in males. The condition is triggered by hormonal changes at puberty and may appear as early as the age of 10. The rash usually subsides after adolescence but may persist after the age of 30. Acne can cause great psychological distress, and teenagers may feel especially self-conscious about their appearance.

More unusual forms of acne include occupational acne, which results from exposure to certain types of industrial oil, and drug-induced acne, which is caused by some prescribed drugs, such as corticosteroids (p.600).

What are the causes?

Acne vulgaris is caused by the overproduction of sebum, an oily substance secreted by the sebaceous glands in the skin. Normally, the sebum drains into hair follicles and flows out through the follicle openings on the skin's surface, thereby keeping the skin lubricated and supple. However, when the glands produce excess sebum, the follicles become blocked. If the sebum remains clogged in the follicle openings, it hardens and becomes dark, forming plugs called blackheads. In some cases, follicles are sealed by an excess of keratin, the tough, fibrous protein produced by the skin cells. The trapped sebum then hardens into white lumps, called whiteheads, under the surface of the skin. In both types of blockage, the bacterium

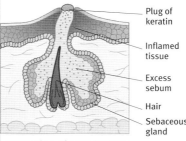

Plug of keratin

Inflamed tissue

Excess sebum

Hair

Sebaceous gland

Formation of acne lesions
Acne develops when excess sebum, and in some cases the protein keratin, blocks hair follicles. Bacteria multiply in the trapped sebum, infecting the surrounding tissues and causing various types of lesion.

Propionibacterium acnes multiplies in the sebum, causing inflammation of the surrounding tissues.

Acne starting at puberty is thought to result from increased sensitivity to androgens (male sex hormones), which are present in both boys and girls and levels of which are raised during puberty. Androgens cause the sebaceous glands to increase their output of sebum. There may be a genetic factor since acne can run in families. The use of anabolic steroids to improve performance in sports may also raise androgen levels. Other causes of acne vulgaris include hormonal disorders such as Cushing's syndrome (p.435), which is due to an excess of corticosteroid hormones.

Acne may become worse in times of stress. In girls, outbreaks may be affected by the hormonal fluctuations that occur during the menstrual cycle. The condition may also be exacerbated by the use of oil-based cosmetics.

Poor hygiene does not cause acne, but a build-up of oil and dead cells on the skin may result in blocked follicles and allow bacteria to multiply. You cannot catch acne from another person, and there is no evidence that fatty foods or sweets cause or aggravate acne.

Occupational acne is usually caused by long-term contact between the skin and oily clothes. The reasons for drug-induced acne are not known.

What are the symptoms?

Acne vulgaris occurs in areas of skin that have a high density of sebaceous glands. At puberty, the hair, face, and upper trunk normally become greasy due to increased production of sebum. However, in people with acne, oiliness is excessive. Acne tends to appear on the face, but areas such as the upper back, centre of the chest, shoulders, and neck may also be affected. The disorder is usually more severe in winter and tends to improve in summer with increased exposure to sunlight. Lesions that are caused by occupational acne may appear on parts of the body that come into close contact with oily clothes. All forms of acne may produce some or all of the following types of lesion:

- Tiny blackheads.
- Small, firm whiteheads.
- Red pimples, which often have yellow pus-filled tips.
- Painful, large, firm, red lumps.
- Tender lumps beneath the skin without obvious heads (cysts).

All these types of lesion may develop at any one time, but the severity of acne varies greatly from person to person. Deep-seated lesions may leave scars.

What is the treatment?

Self-help measures may help to clear up mild acne and prevent recurrence (*see* **Controlling acne**, right). Your doctor may also recommend a topical drug treatment, such as benzoyl peroxide or retinoid cream (*see* **Retinoid drugs**, p.575) to loosen kera-

tin that is sealing the hair follicles. The doctor may also prescribe topical antibiotics (*see* **Preparations for skin infections and infestations**, p.577). Moderate acne can often be treated successfully with a low-dose oral antibiotic (p.572), such as tetracycline or erythromycin. However, treatment often needs to be continued for 6 months or more.

If these treatments fail, you may be referred to a dermatologist. He or she may prescribe isotretinoin, an oral retinoid that acts to loosen keratin and reduce sebum secretion. However, the use of isotretinoin during pregnancy is known to result in fetal abnormalities. For this reason, sexually active women should take the drug only if they are using a reliable contraceptive. Some women may be prescribed a specific contraceptive pill containing hormones that relieve acne by counteracting the action of androgens.

There is no immediate cure for acne. However, scarring may be prevented if treatment is started at an early stage. Individual acne cysts may be treated with corticosteroid injections. If acne has already left noticeable scars, you may wish to consult a cosmetic surgeon to discuss techniques to reduce the appearance of the scars, such as laser resurfacing or dermabrasion. In these procedures, the top layer of skin is removed, leaving a more even skin surface after the skin has healed.

▶ SELF-HELP

Controlling acne

Following these simple self-help measures may help clear up acne and prevent further episodes:

- Wash your skin twice a day with warm, but not hot, water and a mild cleanser. Do not scrub your skin too vigorously.
- Do not pick at pimples because this may make the condition worse and result in scarring.
- Apply a benzoyl peroxide cream daily to the affected areas.
- If you have occupational acne, keep work clothes clean to avoid prolonged contact with oils.

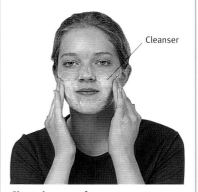

Cleanser

Cleansing your face
Wash your face with warm water and a mild cleanser. Scrubbing hard or using hot water can make the acne worse.

Rosacea

Long-term, possibly permanent, redness and pimples on the cheeks and forehead

 Most common between the ages of 30 and 55

 More common in females

 Often runs in families

 Alcohol, coffee, and spicy foods may trigger attacks

In rosacea, a rash develops on the central area of the face and often results in burning or itching. The cause of the disorder is unknown, but there may be a genetic factor because rosacea often runs in families. Women between the ages of 30 and 55 are most commonly affected. The rash may be triggered by eating a spicy meal, drinking alcohol or coffee, or entering a hot room.

What are the symptoms?
In most cases, the first symptom is red flushing, which often appears on the cheeks, nose, and forehead after exposure to one of the trigger factors. Later, a rash develops, which is intermittent at first but may become permanent. Other symptoms include:
- Red, puffy skin.
- White- or yellow-headed pimples.
- Visible tiny blood vessels.
- Stinging, burning, or itching sensation in the affected area.

If the skin of the nose is affected, it may eventually thicken, swell, and become purplish red. This condition, which is known as rhinophyma, most commonly occurs in elderly men. About 1 in 4 people who has rosacea also develops irritation of the eyes.

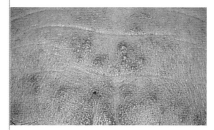

Rosacea pimples on the forehead
The white- and yellow-headed pimples resemble acne lesions and often appear on the cheeks, nose, and forehead.

What might be done?
You should avoid anything that triggers flushing, such as spicy food, alcohol, or coffee. In addition, avoid sunlight and the use of topical corticosteroids (p.577), both of which tend to aggravate rosacea.

To treat the condition, your doctor may prescribe metronidazole gel, a topical antibiotic (*see* **Preparations for skin infections and infestations**, p.577), which is usually effective. However, if the rosacea does not improve, you may be prescribed the antibiotic tetracycline (*see* **Antibiotics**,

p.572), topical azelaic acid, or an oral retinoid drug (p.575). You may need several weeks of treatment before the rash eventually clears up.

If rhinophyma develops, the area of thickened skin on the nose can be pared away under general anaesthesia. Normal skin tissue will then form to cover the treated surface of the nose.

Rosacea usually comes and goes over a period of 5–10 years before finally disappearing. Occasionally, the condition may be lifelong, especially in men.

Prickly heat

Multiple small, raised, itchy spots that appear on the skin in hot conditions

 Most common in infants and children

 Being overweight and being in a hot, humid climate are risk factors

 Gender and genetics are not significant factors

Prickly heat is an intensely itchy rash that most commonly occurs in hot weather. It develops when sweat glands are blocked by bacteria and dead skin cells. Sweat trapped in the glands then causes mild inflammation. The rash consists of tiny, red, itchy spots or blisters accompanied by a prickling or burning feeling. The most common sites are the hands, feet, armpits, and chest. Prickly heat is more likely to affect overweight people, and infants and children are more likely than adults to have the condition, in which case the rash develops in the nappy area or on the face, chest, or back.

The rash often disappears on its own in a few days. You can help this process by wearing loose clothing made from natural fibres and, in babies, by leaving nappies off as much as possible. If the rash persists, your doctor may suggest a mild topical corticosteroid (p.577), but this should not be used on the face. Consult a doctor before using a topical corticosteroid on a baby and always follow the doctor's instructions.

Hyperhidrosis

Excessive sweating in specific areas or over the whole body

 Most common between the ages of 15 and 30

 Sometimes runs in families

 Gender and lifestyle are not significant factors

Frequent and excessively heavy sweating is called hyperhidrosis. The condition usually first appears at puberty. In many cases, no cause can be found, but about half of all affected people have a family history of the condition, which suggests a

genetic factor. Hyperhidrosis can be an indication of an underlying problem, such as an overactive thyroid gland (*see* **Hyperthyroidism**, p.432) or diabetes mellitus (p.437). In some people, stress triggers sweating attacks.

Hyperhidrosis may occur in many areas of the body, particularly the feet, armpits, hands, and face. It is often accompanied by an unpleasant odour.

What might be done?
You should wash regularly, and wear loose clothing made from natural fibres that absorb sweat. Antiperspirant may help to reduce underarm sweating. If anxiety makes the problem worse, try relaxation exercises. If these methods do not help, consult your doctor.

Your doctor may prescribe a topical treatment containing aluminium chloride to reduce the activity of the sweat glands. In some cases, your doctor may suggest iontophoresis to treat hyperhidrosis of the hands and/or feet. This involves placing the affected areas in a container of water and then passing a small electric current from a special machine through the water. It may take several sessions for iontophoresis to have an effect, and then further regular sessions are needed to keep sweating under control. Iontophoresis does not work for everybody, and is not suitable if you are pregnant or have a metal implant or pacemaker. For severe hyperhidrosis, injections of botulinum toxin into the affected areas may be suggested. However, the results are not permanent and repeat treatments are usually needed.

If you have severe hyperhidrosis of the armpits or palms and other treatments have failed, your doctor may suggest endoscopic ("keyhole") surgery to cut nerves that control sweating. However, this carries the risk of potentially serious complications, is not always successful, and may result in compensatory heavy sweating in other areas.

Vitiligo

Loss of normal pigment from patches of skin, most commonly occurring on the face and hands

 More common in young adults

 Sometimes runs in families

 Gender and lifestyle are not significant factors

People who have vitiligo have irregular patches of pale skin caused by the loss of melanin, the pigment that gives the skin its colour. The disorder is more obvious in people with dark skin.

In about half of all cases, vitiligo develops before the age of 20. It does not cause physical discomfort, but some people become distressed by the discoloured appearance of their skin.

What is the cause?
It is thought that vitiligo is an autoimmune disorder in which the antibodies produced by the body react against its own tissues. In this condition, antibodies destroy the cells in the skin that produce melanin. About 1 in 3 people with vitiligo has a family history of the condition. About the same proportion also have another type of autoimmune disorder, such as pernicious anaemia (*see* **Megaloblastic anaemia**, p.272), diabetes mellitus (p.437), or autoimmune thyroiditis (p.433).

What are the symptoms?
The loss of skin colour is gradual, occurring over several months or even years. The symptoms include:
- Depigmented skin patches that may occur on any part of the body but most commonly the face and hands.
- In some cases, white hair on affected areas of skin due to loss of pigment from the hair follicles.

In most people with vitiligo, the depigmented patches of skin are distributed symmetrically over the body.

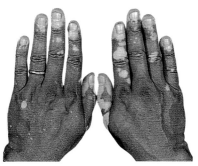

Vitiligo
The pale patches on these hands are due to vitiligo, a condition that causes a gradual loss of the skin pigment melanin.

What might be done?
The diagnosis is usually obvious, but your doctor may arrange for a skin test to exclude pityriasis versicolor (p.205), a fungal infection that may produce discoloured patches of skin. Blood tests may be done to make sure you do not have another autoimmune disorder.

In mild vitiligo, the discoloured areas can be hidden with cosmetics. No other treatment is needed. The affected areas cannot tan so you should avoid exposure to the sun and use a sunblock in direct sunlight (*see* **Safety in the sun**, p.34). Phototherapy using ultraviolet light can help but takes several months to work. Before treatment, you may be given psoralen, a drug to increase the skin's sensitivity to light. Other possible treatments include topical corticosteroids (p.577); topical immunomodulators (drugs that affect the activity of the immune system) such as tacrolimus; the vitamin D derivative calcipotriol (*see* **Vitamins**, p.598); and pseudocatalase, a substance that affects hydrogen peroxide metabolism, which is often abnormal in people with vitiligo.

Occasionally, people may lose the pigment from large areas. In these cases, the rest of the skin may be bleached so that the overall colour of the skin appears more even.

There is no cure for vitiligo. In some cases, treatment may slow down or even reverse pigmentation loss but the response to treatment varies from person to person, and the depigmented patches may continue to enlarge slowly despite treatment. However, a minority of affected people regain their natural skin colour spontaneously.

Freckles

Multiple small, brown-coloured spots on the skin that are usually harmless

 Age, gender, genetics, and lifestyle as risk factors depend on the type

Freckles result from an overproduction of melanin, the pigment that gives the skin its colour. There are two common types: children and young adults get small brown spots on areas of skin that are often exposed to the sun; and, after chronic sun exposure and/or repeated sunburn, adults and the elderly develop larger tan or brown patches on areas of skin previously exposed to the sun.

The tendency to develop freckles is usually inherited. It is more common in people with fair skin, particularly those with red hair. The patches are harmless and tend to fade during the winter, but are a sign of sensitivity to sunlight and of increased susceptibility to skin cancer (right). You should use sunscreen daily to help protect your skin.

The type of patch that develops with age is called an age spot, lentigo, or liver spot. These spots most commonly affect people over the age of 40. They can appear on covered and exposed parts of the body and do not fade in winter.

A lentigo is usually harmless, but some may eventually develop into malignant melanomas (p.201), particularly if they are on the face. A variation in colour may be a warning sign. If raised, brown lumps appear on a lentigo, consult your doctor as soon as possible so that he or she can analyse the spot and detect any cancerous changes in the cells.

Moles

Flat or raised growths on the skin that are rough or smooth and vary in colour from light to dark brown

 Increasingly common in childhood and adolescence

 Sometimes run in families

 Gender and lifestyle are not significant factors

Moles are caused by an overproduction of pigmented skin cells called melanocytes. They can form anywhere on the body,

and there are several types. Moles may appear soon after birth (*see* **Birthmarks**, p.537) or may appear during childhood and early adolescence; nearly all adults have 10–20 moles by the age of 30. Most moles are noncancerous, but in rare cases a mole may undergo changes that make it cancerous (*see* **Malignant melanoma**, p.201). Alterations in the shape, colour, or size of moles are not always a sign of cancer, and changes during puberty or pregnancy are usually normal. However, changes should always be evaluated by a doctor.

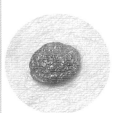

Raised mole
This noncancerous mole appears as a raised, brown spot; the area of pigmentation may extend deep into the skin.

What are the types?
Usually, moles are flat or raised growths that vary in colour from light to dark brown and measure less than 1 cm ($^3/_8$ in) in diameter. They may be rough or smooth, hairy or hairless.

One type of mole, known as a dysplastic naevus, is larger than usual and unevenly coloured. This type may appear in childhood or old age, and may develop from a smaller mole. Dysplastic naevi sometimes run in families, and are more likely to become cancerous than other moles. The risk is higher in people who have a family history of malignant melanoma or if the mole is frequently exposed to sunlight.

Blue naevi are noncancerous moles that have a bluish-black colour and occur most commonly on the face, arms, legs, and buttocks.

A halo naevus is a mole from which pigment is disappearing, leaving a ring of paler skin around a shrinking central dark spot. Eventually, the mole may disappear completely.

What might be done?
You should check your skin regularly and consult your doctor if you notice any changes that might be a cause for concern (*see* **Checking your skin**, p.200)

If your doctor suspects that a mole is cancerous, he or she may recommend that you have it removed and examined for

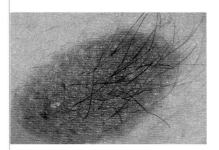

Hairy mole
Moles that are covered in hair, such as the one shown here, or moles with just a few hairs rarely become cancerous.

cancerous cells (*see* **Skin biopsy**, below). Noncancerous moles can also be removed, either for cosmetic reasons or if they are being chafed by clothing. However, removal of a mole does not always produce cosmetic improvement.

Skin cancer

Several types of cancer that originate in the skin, most of which are associated with prolonged exposure to sunlight

 Fair-skinned people are most at risk

 Exposure to the sun and the use of sunbeds are risk factors

 Age and gender as risk factors depend on the type

Skin cancer (including the non-melanoma skin cancers as well as malignant melanoma) is the most common type of cancer in the UK. In recent years, the global incidence has escalated, and the condition now affects millions of people.

The usual cause of skin cancer is prolonged exposure to the harmful ultraviolet radiation in sunlight. The risk is higher if you live or take holidays in areas with intense sun. The closer you are to the equator, the greater the risk. The recent depletion of the ozone layer is thought to play a part in increasing

the incidence of skin cancer because the ozone layer acts as a shield against harmful ultraviolet light. In addition, sunbeds, which use ultraviolet light, increase the risk of developing skin cancer.

If you work outdoors or have been sunburned (particularly in childhood), you could be vulnerable to skin cancer. People who have fair skin are especially susceptible because they have low levels of melanin, the pigment that gives the skin its colour and helps to protect it from the sun's harmful ultraviolet rays.

To reduce the risk of developing skin cancer, try to avoid exposure to the sun and protect your skin when outdoors (*see* **Safety in the sun**, p.34). Avoid the use of sunbeds altogether. You should also check your skin regularly for any unusual changes (*see* **Checking your skin**, p.200) and consult your doctor promptly if you notice any such changes

What are the types?
Skin cancer is categorized into two broad groups: malignant melanoma (p.201), and non-melanoma skin cancer (NMSC), which encompasses all the types that are not malignant melanoma, such as basal cell carcinoma (p.200), squamous cell carcinoma (p.200), and Kaposi's sarcoma (p.201).

Malignant melanoma is relatively rare in the UK, although its incidence is increasing, and about 13,300 new cases were diagnosed in 2011. It can spread rapidly to other

---

▶ **TEST**

Skin biopsy

A skin biopsy is a technique used to diagnose skin diseases, such as cancer. In this procedure, a sample of skin is removed from an anaesthetized site and sent to a laboratory to be examined under a microscope. A biopsy may be used to cut away a whole lesion from the skin, such as a mole, or to remove a small sample at the edge of a large patch of affected skin.

Abnormal area of skin   Normal skin

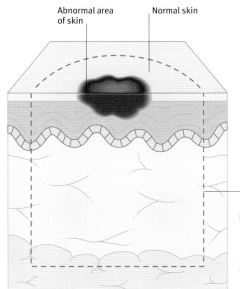

RESULTS

Pigmented cells   Surface of mole

Biopsy sample
This magnified view shows part of a removed mole. The sample confirms that the mole has no cancerous cells.

— Line of incision

Biopsy site
The biopsy site is first numbed with a local anaesthetic. A section of tissue, including skin that looks abnormal and a surrounding area of normal skin, is then removed for analysis.

parts of the body and causes more deaths than other skin cancers. NMSC is very common, with more than 100,000 new cases in the UK in 2011, although this figure is believed to be an underestimate. The most common types of NMSC are basal cell carcinoma and squamous cell carcinoma. Malignant melanoma, basal cell carcinoma, and squamous cell carcinoma are associated with overexposure to the sun and harmful ultraviolet light from sunbeds. Kaposi's sarcoma is uncommon and usually occurs only in people with AIDS (*see* **HIV infection and AIDS**, p.169).

What might be done?

Skin cancer can usually be cured if it is diagnosed early. You should consult your doctor promptly if you notice any unusual changes in your skin. You may need to have a skin biopsy (p.199). During this procedure, a small area of skin is removed and examined under a microscope for abnormal cells.

The type of skin cancer and spread of the disease determine the treatment and outlook. Sometimes, only the affected area of skin needs to be treated.

Most skin cancers can be removed surgically, but skin grafting (p.183) may be necessary if a cancer has invaded large areas of surrounding skin tissue. If the cancer spreads to other parts of the body, radiotherapy (p.158) or chemotherapy (p.157) may be needed.

Checking your skin

Most skin blemishes, such as moles, are not cancerous, but it is important to check your skin regularly so that any signs of skin cancer can be detected early and treated. You should inspect your skin about every couple of months and get to know your moles and blemishes. Ask another person to help you examine your back and scalp. You should consult your doctor promptly if you are concerned about any change to your skin or notice any of the following:

- A mole that is more than 6 mm (¼ in) in diameter and is growing rapidly.
- A mole that changes shape (no matter what size it is) or colour.
- A mole that has uneven coloration and/or a ragged edge.
- A mole that is itchy, inflamed, or crusty, or that oozes or bleeds without an obvious cause (such as having been nicked while shaving).
- A new mole that looks unusual (for example, with patchy coloration or a ragged edge).
- A blemish, lump, or sore that develops without an obvious cause (such as in insect bite) and lasts for more than a few weeks.
- Patches of skin that are itchy, flaky, tender, inflamed, ooze, or bleed without an obvious cause (such as sunburn or eczema).

Basal cell carcinoma

A skin cancer, usually affecting sun-exposed areas, that rarely spreads elsewhere in the body

 Rare in people under the age of 40; increasingly common over 40

 More common in males

 Fair-skinned people are most at risk

 Exposure to the sun and the use of sunbeds are risk factors

The most common type of skin cancer, basal cell carcinoma is also the least dangerous because it usually remains localized and rarely spreads to other parts of the body. This cancer should not be left untreated because it can destroy bone and surrounding skin.

Basal cell carcinoma is characterized by pearly lesions that can occur on any part of the body but commonly appear on the face, often at the corner of an eye, near the ear, or on the nose.

The condition is usually caused by exposure to strong sunlight, which damages cells just below the surface of the skin. Fair-skinned people over the age of 40 are most susceptible.

You can minimize your risk of developing basal cell carcinoma by avoiding prolonged exposure to sunlight, avoiding the use of sunbeds, and by protecting your skin when you are outdoors (*see* **Safety in the sun**, p.34).

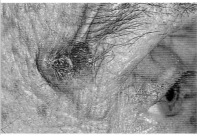

Basal cell carcinoma
This pink, shallow ulcer, with its waxy, rolled edge and central scab, is an example of an untreated basal cell carcinoma.

What are the symptoms?

Basal cell carcinoma grows slowly over months or even years. A typical lesion develops in the following way:

- A small, painless lump appears; it has a smooth surface with blood vessels, a pink to brownish-grey colour, and a waxy or pearl-like border.
- The lump gradually grows, usually spreading outwards and developing a central depression with rolled edges.

An untreated lump may form a shallow ulcer that may bleed intermittently and then form a scab but never fully heals.

You should check your skin regularly for any unusual changes (*see* **Checking your skin**, left) and consult your doctor promptly if you notice any such changes.

What might be done?

If your doctor suspects basal cell carcinoma, he or she will probably arrange for you to have a skin biopsy (p.199) to confirm the diagnosis. During this procedure, a small lesion may be scraped away or frozen off. A large lesion may need to be removed surgically. If you have several lesions or if the affected area is difficult to treat surgically (for example, if it is near the eye), you may need to have radiotherapy (p.158). If the cancer has caused damage to underlying tissue, you may need plastic surgery (p.614).

What is the prognosis?

About 9 in 10 people who develop basal cell carcinoma are successfully treated. There should be no further problems after treatment, but in a few cases the skin cancer may recur.

If you have already had an episode of basal cell carcinoma, you are more likely to develop further cancerous lesions on other parts of your body, usually within a period of 2–5 years. For this reason, you should continue to protect yourself against exposure to sunlight, avoid using sunbeds, and inspect your skin regularly. Your doctor will probably recommend that you have periodic checkups in order to detect and treat any new lesions that develop while they are still small.

Squamous cell carcinoma

A skin cancer that usually affects the face but can spread to other parts of the body

 Mainly affects people over the age of 60

 More common in males

 Fair-skinned people are most at risk

 Exposure to sun, use of sunbeds, and working with oils and tars are risk factors

Squamous cell carcinoma is a common type of skin cancer that usually affects areas that have been exposed to sunlight for prolonged periods over many years, but may also occur in other parts of the body, such as the genitals. This type of carcinoma is capable of spreading throughout the body, and for this reason early detection and treatment of the condition are essential.

What are the causes?

Squamous cell carcinoma develops on areas of skin that have been constantly exposed to sunlight over many years. Sometimes, this form of skin cancer may develop from scaly growths known as solar keratoses (opposite page). The condition is most common in fair-skinned men over the age of 60.

People who work with some industrial tars and oils are known to have a higher than normal risk of squamous cell

carcinoma, but these people are normally protected by adequate health and safety measures. The use of sunbeds also increases the risk.

Most squamous cell carcinomas can be prevented by avoiding prolonged exposure to sunlight. If this is not possible, you should take precautions to protect your skin, such as applying sunblock and wearing a hat, when you are outdoors (*see* **Safety in the sun**, p.34). You should also avoid using sunbeds.

What are the symptoms?

Squamous cell carcinoma begins as an area of thickened, scaly skin. The lesion then develops into:

- A hard, painless, gradually enlarging lump that has an irregular edge and is red to reddish brown in colour.
- Subsequently, a recurring ulcer that does not heal.

You should check your skin regularly for any unusual changes (*see* **Checking your skin**, left) and consult your doctor promptly if you notice any such changes.

What might be done?

If your doctor suspects squamous cell carcinoma, he or she may arrange for you to have a skin biopsy (p.199), in which a small piece of tissue is removed under a local anaesthetic and examined under a microscope for the presence of cancerous cells.

Squamous cell carcinoma can usually be treated surgically if the lesions are detected at an early stage. Sometimes, radiotherapy (p.158) is used as an alternative to surgery. If you have several large lesions or if the cancer has spread into underlying tissues, chemotherapy (p.157) may also be necessary.

What is the prognosis?

If the condition is detected early, about 9 in 10 people with squamous cell carcinoma are treated successfully. Lesions on the face respond particularly well to treatment. If the disease is detected late, the success of the treatment depends on how far the cancer has spread. Some lesions may recur, particularly larger ones, and your doctor will advise you to have regular checkups.

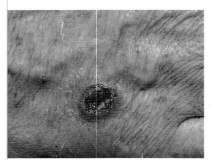

Squamous cell carcinoma
The face and hand are common sites for squamous cell carcinoma. Here, a lesion on the back of the hand has developed into an ulcer with a clearly defined edge.

Malignant melanoma

A skin cancer affecting the pigment-producing cells of the skin that can spread rapidly to other parts of the body

 Very rare in children; in adults, more common with increasing age

 More common in females

 Fair-skinned people are most at risk

 Exposure to the sun and the use of sunbeds are risk factors

Malignant melanoma is an uncommon but serious form of skin cancer. A melanoma may begin as a new growth on normal skin or may develop from an existing mole. Left untreated, the cancer can spread to other parts of the body and may be fatal. The main cause of malignant melanoma is exposure to sunlight, although use of sunbeds also increases the risk of developing the cancer.

Worldwide, the number of cases of malignant melanoma, particularly in young adults, has increased significantly over the past few years, and in 2011, about 13,000 new cases were diagnosed in the UK. The incidence of malignant melanoma increases with age, and it is more common in women, although more often fatal in men.

What is the cause?

Malignant melanoma is thought to result from damage to melanocytes (the skin cells that produce the pigment melanin) by sunlight. The cancer occurs more frequently in people with fair skin than in those with dark skin. People who are continually exposed to intense sunlight or who live in sunny climates have an increased risk of developing malignant melanoma. In particular, severe sunburn (p.207) during childhood has been shown to double the chance of developing malignant melanoma in later life. Minimizing exposure to the sun can help to decrease the risk of developing this type of cancer (*see* **Safety in the sun**, p.34), as can avoiding the use of sunbeds.

What are the symptoms?

Malignant melanomas can develop on any part of the body but appear most commonly on sun-exposed areas. Some melanomas spread across the skin in the form of an irregular, flat, pigmented patch; others appear as fast-growing dark lumps. Sometimes, a melanoma does not have any pigment (known as amelanotic melanoma). In older people, melanomas may occur on the face as freckle-like spots, known as lentigo maligna, that grow slowly over many years. If they are not removed, all of these types of melanoma will grow down into the underlying layers of the skin.

You should suspect a malignant melanoma if a quickly growing, irregular, dark-coloured spot starts to develop on your skin or if you notice any of the following changes in an existing mole:

- Increasing size.
- Irregular and asymmetrical edges.
- Itching, inflammation, or redness.
- Thickening of the surface.
- Bleeding or crusting.
- Variation in shade or colour.

You should check your skin regularly for any unusual changes (*see* **Checking your skin**, opposite page) and consult your doctor promptly if you notice any such changes.

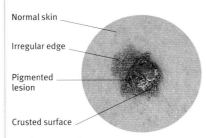

Normal skin
Irregular edge
Pigmented lesion
Crusted surface

Malignant melanoma
The uneven colour, irregularly spreading edge, and crusted surface of this raised growth are characteristic features of a malignant melanoma.

What might be done?

If your doctor suspects that you have malignant melanoma, he or she will arrange for urgent removal of the lesion (an area of surrounding skin will also be removed to decrease the risk of malignant cells remaining). The tissue will be examined under a microscope (*see* **Skin biopsy**, p.199). If the tissue is cancerous, a larger portion of skin may be removed, which may require a skin graft (p.183). Samples may also be taken from the lymph nodes near the melanoma and examined for cancerous cells, the presence of which would indicate that the cancer has spread. If it has spread, you may have chemotherapy (p.157), radiotherapy (p.158), or biological therapies (*see* **Cancer and its management**, p.156).

What is the prognosis?

Superficial melanomas that are treated early are usually cured, but melanomas are more often fatal in men, possibly because men do not always report symptoms to the doctor immediately. If melanomas are aggressive or penetrate deep into the skin, the outlook is less optimistic, and, if they spread to other areas of the body, they are often fatal.

Can it be prevented?

You can reduce the risk of developing malignant melanoma by staying out of the sun and avoiding the use of sunbeds. In particular, you should stay out of the sun between 11am and 3pm. If you have to be out in the sun, you should wear a hat with a wide brim and tightly woven clothing that at least covers your shoulders and neck (ideally, all skin should be covered). You should protect any exposed skin with a sunscreen or sunblock (p.577). Whichever you use, you should apply it liberally 15–30 minutes before you go outside and reapply it frequently.

Kaposi's sarcoma

A skin cancer, characterized by raised, pinkish-brown lesions, that is most often associated with AIDS

 More common in males

 Unprotected sex with multiple partners and intravenous drug use are risk factors in AIDS-related cases

 Age and genetics as risk factors depend on the cause

Kaposi's sarcoma used to be a very rare condition, appearing mainly in older men of Mediterranean or Jewish origin. It developed slowly and rarely spread. However, a more rapidly developing form now occurs increasingly in people with AIDS (*see* **HIV infection and AIDS**, p.169). In these cases, it is associated with infection by a herpes virus.

The lesions of Kaposi's sarcoma can occur anywhere on the skin. In AIDS-related cases, the lesions spread quickly; in severe cases, they may affect mucous membranes, especially of the palate and internal organs. Internal lesions can cause severe bleeding.

Kaposi's sarcoma can be treated effectively with radiotherapy (p.158). If the cancer is advanced, chemotherapy (p.157) may be needed. The cancer is seldom the main cause of death in people with AIDS, although it may be fatal when the internal organs are affected. Treating the underlying HIV infection is therefore also important.

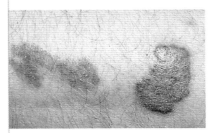

Kaposi's sarcoma
Sharply defined, pinkish-brown raised nodules and flat patches are the first signs of Kaposi's sarcoma. They may develop anywhere on the body.

Solar keratosis

A pinkish-red, scaly, rough-textured skin growth caused by prolonged exposure to sunlight; also called actinic keratosis

 More common in people over the age of 40

 More common in males

 Fair-skinned people are most at risk

 Exposure to the sun and the use of sunbeds are risk factors

Solar keratoses are small, scaly skin growths usually caused by years of exposure to sunlight. People under the age of 40 are not often affected by the condition, but the risk of solar keratoses increases after this age and is higher than normal in people (usually men) who work outdoors. The disorder is most common in fair-skinned people, who are often particularly sensitive to the sun.

The lesions are pinkish-red and have a rough texture. They most commonly appear on uncovered areas of the skin, such as the face, ears, the backs of the hands, and on bald parts of the scalp. Usually, several lesions appear at the same time. Sometimes, a solar keratosis develops into squamous cell carcinoma (opposite page), a type of skin cancer.

What might be done?

The lesions should always be removed. Various treatment options are available. Your doctor may freeze or scrape them off, or may prescribe a cream or gel to remove them. In some cases, photodynamic therapy may be suggested. This involves applying a cream that sensitizes the skin then shining a special light on to the lesions. The combination of the cream and light usually destroys the lesions. However, the lesions may recur after treatment.

To reduce the risk of developing this condition, protect your skin from exposure to the sun (*see* **Safety in the sun**, p.34) and avoid using sunbeds. People who are bald or have thin hair should wear a hat outdoors.

Discoid lupus erythematosus

A disorder in which itchy, red, scaly patches develop, usually on the face and scalp and behind the ears

 Most common between the ages of 25 and 45

 Much more common in females

 Sometimes runs in families

 Strong sunlight triggers or aggravates the condition

Discoid lupus erythematosus (DLE) is an autoimmune disorder, in which the body attacks its own tissues. It causes a red, itchy, scaly rash to appear, particularly on the face and scalp, behind the ears, and on any parts of the body that are exposed to sunlight. The disorder most commonly occurs in women between the ages of 25 and 45. The cause is unknown, but a genetic factor may be involved because DLE tends to run in families. Exposure to sunlight tends to trigger the onset of the rash or to make an existing rash worse. Over a period of several years, DLE may subside and recur repeatedly with different degrees of severity.

In some cases, the rash disappears, but it can leave behind a scarred area in which the skin is thin and discoloured.

If DLE occurs on the scalp, the damage to the skin can result in permanent loss of hair and patchy baldness of the scalp (*see* **Alopecia**, p.208).

What might the doctor do?

Your doctor will probably arrange for a small sample of skin to be removed from an affected area (*see* **Skin biopsy**, p.199) to confirm the diagnosis. If you have DLE, your doctor may prescribe a topical corticosteroid (p.577), which you apply to the affected areas of skin two or three times a day.

If the skin has not healed after the corticosteroid treatment, your doctor may prescribe a course of chloroquine, an anti-malarial drug (p.574) that often relieves the symptoms of DLE. The doctor will advise you to have regular eye examinations while you are on this drug because chloroquine may eventually cause damage to the eyes.

What can I do?

You can help control the rash by staying out of the sun or by using a sunscreen that provides full ultraviolet protection to your skin (*see* **Safety in the sun**, p.34). Concealing creams may improve the appearance of discoloured skin.

What is the prognosis?

Most cases of DLE can be successfully treated with corticosteroids, although scarring can occur. About 1 in 20 people with DLE goes on to develop a related, but frequently more serious, autoimmune disorder called systemic lupus erythematosus (p.281). This condition affects many parts of the body, including the lungs, kidneys, and joints.

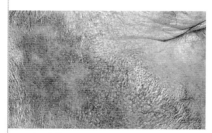

Rash of discoid lupus erythematosus
This red facial rash is characteristic of discoid lupus erythematosus. The distinct, discoloured patches are due to scarring from previous episodes of the disorder.

Erythema nodosum

Shiny, tender, red or purple swellings (nodules), usually on the shins

 Most common in young adults

 More common in females

 Genetics and lifestyle are not significant factors

Many conditions may give rise to erythema nodosum, in which tender red or purple swellings known as nodules develop, usually on the shins.

Erythema nodosum is most common in young adults, and particularly in women. It may be linked with long-standing dis-

orders such as tuberculosis (p.300) and the inflammatory disorder sarcoidosis (p.304). The condition may also be a reaction to drugs, in particular to some types of antibiotics (p.572). In children, it is often associated with a sore throat caused by a streptococcal infection. In some cases, there is no obvious cause for the condition.

What are the symptoms?

In many cases, erythema nodosum is accompanied by pains in the joints and muscles and fever. The nodules usually appear on the shins; less commonly, they develop on the forearms. They are:
■ Shiny and bright red or purple.
■ In general, between 1 cm (³/₈ in) and 15 cm (6 in) in diameter.
■ Very painful and tender.
The nodules fade over a few weeks and may begin to look like bruises.

What might be done?

A diagnosis is made from the symptoms and the appearance of the nodules. There is no specific treatment, but your doctor may advise you to rest in bed and keep your legs raised until the nodules have begun to subside. To reduce swelling, the doctor may also prescribe nonsteroidal anti-inflammatory drugs (p.578) and, occasionally, oral corticosteroids (p.600). In addition, he or she may arrange for blood tests and a chest X-ray (p.300) to be performed to check for an underlying disorder.

Most affected people recover over 4 to 8 weeks. In rare cases, the condition may be chronic or may recur.

Skin tag

A small, harmless flap of skin, usually attached by a stalk to the neck, trunk, groin, or armpit

 More common with increasing age

 Being overweight is a risk factor

 Gender and genetics are not significant factors

Tags are soft, tiny flaps of skin, sometimes darker than the surrounding area, that are attached to the body by a stalk. These skin growths usually occur spontaneously. Skin tags are found on any part of the body, typically on the neck and trunk, but they may also occur in the groin or armpit. While skin tags are harmless and usually cause no trouble, they may bleed or become sore if they are rubbed by clothing. Elderly and overweight people are especially prone to skin tags.

Consult your doctor if you are unsure whether a growth is a skin tag or if a tag is irritated by your clothes. You may have the tag removed under a local anaesthetic by burning, scraping, or snipping with surgical scissors.

Seborrhoeic keratosis

A harmless, pigmented wart-like growth that most commonly occurs on the trunk

 More common with increasing age

 Gender, genetics, and lifestyle are not significant factors

Seborrhoeic keratoses, also called seborrhoeic warts, are harmless skin growths, usually brown or black in colour. The growths occur on the trunk but may also affect the head, neck, and, less commonly, the backs of the hands and the forearms. They may appear singly or in groups. Seborrhoeic keratoses are common in elderly people.

What are the symptoms?

You may notice a seborrhoeic keratosis as a crusted patch that appears to be stuck on rather than in the skin. The growth is usually:
■ Painless but occasionally itchy. You may find that scratching the growth causes soreness.
■ Up to 2 cm (³/₄ in) in diameter.
■ Greasy and rough on the surface.
■ Brown or black in colour.
■ Either raised or flat.
In rare cases, an individual may have hundreds of seborrhoeic keratoses.

What might be done?

If you have a pigmented patch, consult your doctor to check that it is not due to a serious condition. If it is a seborrhoeic keratosis, it may be removed by scraping or cutting it off or by freezing it. The lesion is unlikely to recur, but in a person who is susceptible to seborrhoeic keratoses, new lesions may develop on other areas of the body.

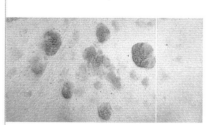

Seborrhoeic keratoses
Although they vary in colour and shape, seborrhoeic keratoses commonly take the form of rough, brown, raised patches.

Sebaceous cyst

A harmless swelling under the skin that may become infected

 More common in adults

 Gender, genetics, and lifestyle are not significant factors

A sebaceous cyst, also called an epidermoid cyst, is a smooth lump that forms under the skin due to inflammation of a hair follicle. The

sac is filled with dead skin cells and sebum, the oily secretion of the sebaceous glands. Some cysts have a dark central pore.

Sebaceous cysts commonly occur on the scalp, face, trunk, and genitals but may appear on any part of the body. Although harmless, the cysts occasionally grow large and become unsightly. A sebaceous cyst that is infected by bacteria may become inflamed and painful and eventually burst.

If a sebaceous cyst is not causing you any problems, it can safely be left untreated. However, if the cyst becomes very large or painful, it can be removed under a local anaesthetic. The cyst will usually be taken out intact because it can recur if the sac and its contents have not been completely removed. If it becomes infected, antibiotics (p.572) or incision and drainage may be required.

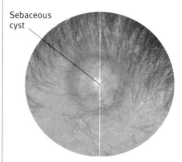

Sebaceous cyst

Sebaceous cyst on the scalp
The scalp is a typical site for a sebaceous cyst, which is a smooth, harmless lump that develops under the skin.

Calluses and corns

Areas of thickened skin on the hands or feet caused by pressure or friction

 More common in manual workers, joggers, and musicians

 Age, gender, and genetics are not significant factors

If there is prolonged pressure or friction on a small area of the hand or foot, a patch of hard, thickened skin known as a callus may develop to protect the underlying tissues. Calluses are usually painless. They commonly occur on the hands of people such as musicians due to friction. The soles of the feet may become callused by the uneven pressure of body weight during walking.

Corns are patches of thickened skin that occur on the toes. They are usually due to wearing shoes that are too tight. The patches have a hard, clear centre and can be painful and persistent.

What is the treatment?

If you have a callus, you can remove some of the hardened skin by soaking the area in warm water for 10 minutes and then rubbing the callus gently with a pumice stone. Regular application of moisturizing cream may help to keep the skin soft. If possible, keep pressure off the area to aid recovery and to prevent recurrence of the callus. It is difficult to protect calluses that have developed on the sole of the foot, but well-fitting shoes may be of some help.

To relieve pressure on corns, wear shoes that do not press on the toes, and use corn pads (small rings of sponge that are available over the counter).

Your doctor or a chiropodist may reduce the size of a thickened area by paring it down with a scalpel, usually over several sessions. Once the source of pressure has been removed, calluses and corns should not recur.

Calluses or corns may become infected and ulcerated, especially in people with diabetes mellitus (p.437). If infection or ulceration occurs, do not try to treat the lesions yourself but get advice from a doctor or chiropodist.

Keloid

A firm, raised, smooth overgrowth of scar tissue that develops after injury to the skin

 May run in families; more common in black people

 Age, gender, and lifestyle are not significant factors

A keloid is an itchy, firm, irregularly shaped overgrowth of scar tissue. Keloids are smooth and shiny, appearing pinkish red on light skin and brown on dark skin. They usually form on the surface of a wound when a defective healing process causes overproduction of the skin protein collagen. Keloids are more common in black people, and susceptibility to them may run in families. If you are prone to the growths, you may find they appear after any kind of skin damage, including cuts, burns, acne, insect bites, tattoos, piercings for jewellery, and minor surgery. Rarely, they form spontaneously with no known cause. Keloids may develop almost anywhere on the body but usually occur on the chest, shoulders, and ear lobes. The growths are harmless, although large keloids may be unsightly.

What is the treatment?
Your doctor may either inject a corticosteroid (p.600) into the scar tissue, or prescribe tape impregnated with a topical corticosteroid (p.577), which can be cut to size and placed over the keloid, causing the scar to shrink. Even with treatment, keloids often take up to a year to fade. Surgery and laser treatment are usually ineffective because the new scar tissue created forms another keloid.

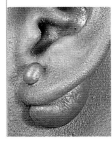

Keloid growth
An overgrowth of scar tissue called a keloid has formed on this ear lobe after ear-piercing. Susceptible people may develop keloids after even minor skin damage.

Stretch marks

Pink or purple lines on the skin, most commonly over the abdomen, buttocks, breasts, and thighs

 Sometimes occur as a result of growth spurts at puberty

 More common in females

 More common in pregnant women and overweight people

 Genetics is not a significant factor

Stretch marks, also called striae, occur when fibres of the skin protein collagen are broken due to rapid stretching of the skin or to hormonal changes that disrupt the fibres. The marks affect 3 in 5 pregnant women and are common in adolescent girls undergoing growth spurts. Overweight people may also develop them, especially if weight gain is rapid. They also occur in people with Cushing's syndrome (p.435) and in those using oral corticosteroids (p.600) or topical corticosteroids (p.577).

Stretch marks first appear as pink or purple raised lines on the abdomen, thighs, breasts, or buttocks. They vary in length and may be between 6 mm ($^1/_4$ in) and 12 mm ($^1/_2$ in) wide. Over a few months, they usually become pale and flatten, eventually becoming barely noticeable. There are no effective preventive measures or treatments.

Chilblains

Itchy, painful, reddish-purple swellings on the fingers or toes

 More common in children and elderly people

 Gender, genetics, and lifestyle are not significant factors

Chilblains result from excessive narrowing of blood vessels under the skin in cold weather. The reddish-purple swellings, which most commonly affect the fingers and toes, are painful when they are exposed to cold and are intensely itchy once the skin has become warm again.

Chilblains usually disappear without treatment but may recur. Children and elderly or inactive people in particular should wear sufficient clothing, including gloves, socks, and a hat, to keep warm and help to prevent chilblains from developing. If you are susceptible to chilblains and are exposed to cold weather, taking exercise may encourage blood flow to your hands and feet.

Leg ulcer

A persistent open sore, usually on the lower part of the leg

 More common in elderly people

 People who are of limited mobility or bedridden are at risk

 Gender and genetics are not significant factors

A leg ulcer occurs when an area of skin on the lower leg breaks down, usually as a result of poor blood circulation. An open sore may then develop, either spontaneously or following a minor injury, such as a scratch by a fingernail.

An ulcer appears as a shallow, pink area of broken skin; the surrounding skin may be swollen. Ulcers are slow to heal and often painful. They are most common in older people who have poor circulation or are not very mobile.

What are the types?
There are two main types of leg ulcer: venous ulcers and arterial ulcers. More than 9 in 10 of all leg ulcers are venous ulcers, which are caused by poor blood flow through the veins and therefore often occur in people with varicose veins (p.263). The ulcers usually form just above the ankle and may be surrounded by purplish-brown, scaly skin.

Arterial ulcers develop as a result of poor blood flow through the arteries supplying the limbs. People with diabetes mellitus (p.437) and those with sickle-cell disease (p.272) are especially susceptible to this type of ulcer. Arterial ulcers often form on the foot and are surrounded by pale, thin skin.

At the first sign of an ulcer, you should consult your doctor. Leg ulcers often become infected, and the infection may spread to the surrounding skin, causing cellulitis (p.204).

What might be done?
Your doctor may recommend Doppler ultrasound scanning (p.259) to assess blood flow in the affected leg. The ulcer should be dressed regularly and firmly bandaged to reduce swelling and improve blood circulation. Special dressings that promote healing

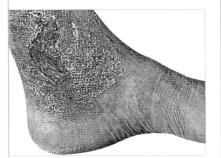

Leg ulcer on the ankle
A venous leg ulcer, such as the one shown here, consists of an open sore that is often surrounded by scaly, purplish-brown skin.

may be prescribed. Wearing support stockings, exercising regularly, and keeping the leg raised when you are resting can also help to improve the circulation of the blood. If you have an arterial ulcer, you may need surgery to improve blood flow through the arteries.

What is the prognosis?
In susceptible people, leg ulcers may take months to heal, and they often recur. Rarely, skin grafting (p.183) may be needed. You should not neglect even minor wounds. Consult your doctor at the first signs of soreness in a leg.

Pressure sores

Skin ulcers that develop in pressure spots, affecting people with limited mobility

 Most common in elderly people

 People who are of limited mobility or bedridden are at risk

 Gender and genetics are not significant factors

If people are paralysed or immobile, even for a few hours, small areas of their skin are subject to constant pressure from their own body weight. This pressure may restrict the normal supply of blood to the tissues. Sometimes, an area of tissue dies, leading to open sores, called pressure sores or bedsores. These usually affect elderly people, who are more likely to be immobile and have fragile skin. Urinary incontinence (p.454) may contribute to the development of pressure sores if it causes the skin to be continually damp.

What are the symptoms?
Common sites for pressure sores are the shoulders, hips, base of the spine, buttocks, heels, and ankles. The symptoms appear in the following stages:
- Affected areas of skin start to become red and tender.
- Painful areas become purple.
- The skin breaks down to form ulcers.
Left untreated, the sores become bigger and deeper and may become infected. Severe pressure sores may sometimes involve muscle, tendon, or bone under the damaged area of skin.

What might be done?
Bedridden people or those with limited mobility should have their skin checked regularly for signs of redness and tenderness. A bedridden person should have his or her position changed at least every 2 hours to relieve compression of the affected areas. It is important to keep the skin clean and dry. If a sore becomes infected, antibiotics (p.572) may be necessary. Usually, pressure sores gradually heal with treatment and good nutrition to improve the person's general health, but deep ulcers may take several months to clear up. If they are extensive, plastic surgery (p.614) may be necessary to promote healing.

Skin infections and infestations

The skin surface provides the body with protection from the environment and from infection, but the skin itself may become infected by bacteria, viruses, or fungi. Some of these organisms live naturally on the body and do not normally cause disease unless they breach the barrier of the skin's surface. Infestation of the skin by parasites, such as mites, may also occur.

Infectious organisms can enter the skin in various ways. Natural openings, such as a hair follicle or sweat gland, or broken skin at the site of an insect bite or a cut may provide a gateway for bacteria. Warm and moist areas, such as the skin between the toes, are more susceptible to fungal infections. Some common viral skin infections, such as warts, can be spread from one part of the body surface to another or may be passed from one person to another by direct skin contact.

In this section, bacterial skin infections are described first, followed by fungal and viral infections. The final article covers infestation by the scabies mite.

Diseases such as measles and rubella, in which a skin rash occurs due to an infection that also affects many other areas of the body, are covered elsewhere (*see* **Infections and infestations**, pp.160–163). The two common skin infestations head lice (p.539) and pubic lice (p.493) are also described in other sections of the book.

KEY ANATOMY

Hair

Sebaceous gland

Arrector pili muscle

Sweat gland

Epidermis

Dermis

Fat

For further information on the structure and function of the skin, *see* pp.190–191.

Boil

A red, painful, pus-filled swelling of the skin caused by a bacterial infection

 Age, gender, genetics, and lifestyle are not significant factors

A boil develops when a hair follicle or sebaceous gland (which secretes sebum into the hair follicle) becomes infected. The infection then spreads and pus collects in surrounding tissues. Common sites for boils are moist areas, such as the groin, or areas where friction occurs, such as under a collar. Boils are usually due to infection with the bacterium *Staphylococcus aureus*, which some people normally carry on the skin or in the nose without symptoms. A cluster of connected boils is called a carbuncle.

Boils are most common in people whose resistance to infection is lowered by a disorder such as diabetes mellitus (p.437) or AIDS (*see* **HIV infection and AIDS**, p.169), but they can occur in those without immune problems.

What are the symptoms?
The symptoms develop gradually in the following order over several days:
■ A small, red lump appears.
■ The area becomes painful and tender.

■ The lump and the tissues around it begin to swell as pus accumulates.
■ A white or yellow head of pus appears at the centre of the boil.
■ The affected area feels warm to the touch and throbs.

Boils often clear up without treatment. They may burst and release the pus or gradually subside and then disappear.

What can I do?
You can relieve pain and help the healing process by applying a cotton-wool ball or a clean cloth soaked in hot water to the area for about 30 minutes four times a day. Do not squeeze the boil because this may cause the infection to spread further. If a boil does not start to heal within a few days or it becomes large or painful, consult your doctor.

What might the doctor do?
Your doctor may drain the pus in the swelling by making a small incision in the centre of the boil with a sterile needle. You may also be prescribed oral antibiotics (p.572) to treat the cause of the infection. Large boils may need to be lanced with a surgical knife under local anaesthesia.

If you develop recurrent boils, you may have blood and urine tests to look for an underlying disorder. Your doctor may also recommend that you use antiseptic soap or cream to kill the bacteria (*see* **Preparations for skin infections and infestations**, p.577).

Impetigo

Blistering and crusting of the skin caused by a bacterial infection

 More common in children

 Gender, genetics, and lifestyle are not significant factors

The blistering skin condition impetigo is caused by bacteria entering broken skin, typically where there is a cut, an area of eczema (p.285), or a cold sore (p.306). The condition is highly contagious and is spread by physical contact. It is more common in children.

What are the symptoms?
Impetigo can appear anywhere on the body but usually occurs on the face, especially around the nose and mouth. The following symptoms usually develop over 1–2 days:
■ Initially, the skin reddens and tiny, fluid-filled blisters appear.
■ The blisters burst soon after they are formed, releasing a yellow fluid.
■ The skin underneath the burst blisters becomes red and weeping.
■ The blisters dry out to form an itchy, honey-coloured crust.
The blistered patch often spreads. Left untreated, it may become quite large.

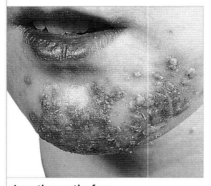

Impetigo on the face
The honey-coloured crust covering this child's chin has been formed by impetigo blisters that have burst and dried out.

What is the treatment?
Your doctor may prescribe topical antibiotics (*see* **Preparations for skin infections and infestations**, p.577) or oral antibiotics (p.572). Soaking the crusts with warm salt water helps to remove them and relieve itching. With treatment, impetigo usually clears up in a few days. To avoid spreading the condition to others, wash your hands often and do not share face flannels. Keep an affected child home from school.

Folliculitis

Inflammation of the hair follicles that produces small, yellow, pus-filled pimples

 More common in adults

 More common in males

 Shaving and hair-plucking are risk factors

 Genetics is not a significant factor

Inflammation of the hair follicles due to bacterial infection is called folliculitis. The pus-filled pimples produced by this condition may develop on any part of the body but most commonly appear on the limbs and, in men, in the beard area. Shaving, plucking, or waxing the hairs can increase the risk of inflammation. Folliculitis of the beard area is particularly common in black men, whose curly hairs often grow back into the skin and may cause an infection. The use of topical corticosteroids (p.577) may also cause folliculitis in some people.

Your doctor may prescribe topical antibiotics (*see* **Preparations for skin infections and infestations**, p.577) to treat the infection or oral antibiotics (p.572) for acute, extensive folliculitis. To avoid spreading folliculitis, wash regularly with antibacterial soap and do not share razors or towels. Men may find that growing a beard helps to prevent folliculitis from developing on the face.

Cellulitis

Bacterial infection of the skin and underlying tissues that causes redness and swelling

 More common in elderly people

 Intravenous drug use is a risk factor

 Gender and genetics are not significant factors

In cellulitis, an area of skin and the underlying tissues become infected by bacteria that enter through a small, possibly unnoticed, wound. The infection causes redness, pain, and swelling and most commonly affects the legs.

Elderly people are especially vulnerable to cellulitis because they are more likely to have poor circulation, which leads to oedema (fluid build-up in the tissues) or leg ulcers (p.203). These problems increase the risk of infection. Others who are at increased risk of cellulitis include intravenous drug users and people whose resistance to infection has been lowered by disorders such as diabetes mellitus (p.437) or AIDS (*see* **HIV infection and AIDS**, p.169).

What are the symptoms?

The symptoms appear gradually over several hours and include:

- Redness, swelling, and in some cases warmth in the affected area of skin.
- Pain and tenderness in the area.
- Occasionally, fever and chills.

If you develop these symptoms, consult your doctor without delay. Left untreated, cellulitis may cause septicaemia (p.171), a serious blood infection.

What might be done?

If you have an obvious wound, your doctor may take a swab from the area to identify the bacterium that is causing the infection. The doctor will probably prescribe oral antibiotics (p.572), which should take effect within 48 hours. In severe cases, you may need hospital treatment with intravenous antibiotics. If your leg is affected, you should keep it elevated to help to reduce the swelling. Cellulitis may recur if you have a persistent immune or circulatory problem, and long-term antibiotics may be needed in such cases.

Ringworm

A fungal infection that produces itchy, red, circular patches on the scalp, groin, or elsewhere on the skin

 Age, gender, and lifestyle as risk factors depend on the type

 Genetics is not a significant factor

Despite the name, ringworm is caused not by worms but by fungi that infect the skin and cause itchy, red, ring-shaped patches. There are a number of common forms of the disorder, including scalp ringworm (tinea capitis), body ringworm (tinea corporis), and ringworm of the groin (tinea cruris).

Scalp ringworm, which is more common in children, can spread from one person to another or be acquired from cats and dogs. Ringworm of the groin mainly affects men, particularly those who have other fungal infections, such as athlete's foot (right). All forms of ringworm are especially common in people with reduced immunity to infection due to disorders such as diabetes mellitus (p.437) or AIDS (*see* **HIV infection and AIDS**, p.169).

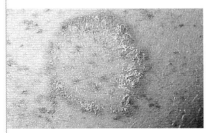

Ringworm on the body
The patch of ringworm shown here has already begun to spread, leaving a scaly, itchy, red ring surrounding normal skin.

What are the symptoms?

In all forms of ringworm, the following symptoms develop gradually over days or sometimes weeks:

- Initially, a small, round, scaly, itchy, red patch appears.
- After 1–2 weeks, more patches appear.
- Each patch grows larger and forms a scaly, red ring around a central area of normal skin.

In scalp ringworm, hairs may break off just above the surface of the skin, leading to irregular patches of stubble (*see* **Alopecia**, p.208). In ringworm of the groin, the rash occasionally spreads further to affect the skin on the inside of the thighs and the buttocks.

What might be done?

Your doctor will probably recognize ringworm from its appearance and may confirm the diagnosis by taking a skin scraping. The removed skin is examined under a microscope to confirm the presence of fungal infection.

Topical antifungal drugs may be obtained by prescription from your doctor or over the counter (*see* **Preparations for skin infections and infestations**, p.577). If the ringworm affects your scalp or is widespread, you may be prescribed oral antifungal drugs (p.574), which you will need to take for several weeks to clear up the infection completely. If you have ringworm of the groin, you can help to prevent a recurrence by keeping the area clean and dry.

Athlete's foot

A fungal infection of the foot that produces cracked, sore, itchy skin between the toes

 Most common in teenagers and young adults; rare in children

 Wearing enclosed footwear for long periods is a risk factor

 Gender and genetics are not significant factors

Athlete's foot, also called tinea pedis, is a common fungal infection of the feet that particularly affects the skin between the toes. The condition can be caused by several types of fungi that thrive in warm, humid conditions.

Athlete's foot often affects teenagers and young adults, who tend to sweat more and wear enclosed footwear, such as trainers, for long periods. It is rare in children. Athlete's foot can be picked up by walking barefoot in communal areas that are warm and humid, such as changing rooms and poolsides.

What are the symptoms?

Athlete's foot most commonly occurs between the fourth and fifth toes and produces the following symptoms:

- Cracked, sore, and itchy areas of skin.
- Flaking, white, soggy skin.

Sometimes, the infection spreads on to the sole or the sides of the foot or affects the toenails, which then become yellowish, thickened, and brittle. People who have athlete's foot are more susceptible to ringworm (left) of the groin, another fungal infection.

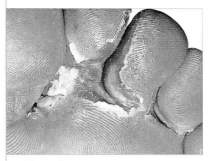

Athlete's foot
Toes affected by the fungal skin infection athlete's foot may become white and soggy, and the skin between and under them may peel away to leave painful raw areas.

What is the treatment?

The affected area can be treated using an over-the-counter antifungal preparation, which should be applied at least twice a day (*see* **Preparations for skin infections and infestations**, p.577). It is important that you continue to apply the preparation to affected areas for a few days after the symptoms have cleared up to make sure that the infection is eradicated. If over-the-counter preparations do not help or you are unsure of the diagnosis, consult your doctor, who can give you further advice about treatment or prescribe a stronger antifungal drug (p.574).

To prevent the infection from recurring, you should wash your feet at least once a day, more frequently if they become sweaty, and dry them thoroughly between the toes. At home, it may help to wear open-toed shoes or go barefoot.

Pityriasis versicolor

A fungal infection that produces patches of discoloured skin on the trunk

 More common under the age of 50

 More common in males

 Hot and humid conditions are a risk factor

 Genetics is not a significant factor

Pityriasis versicolor, also called tinea versicolor, is a patchy skin condition caused by a fungus living in the hair follicles of the body. The fungus does not normally produce symptoms, but in hot and humid conditions, when the skin becomes moist, it grows and colonizes the outer layer of skin. If the skin is oily, the fungus is more likely to spread to the surface of the skin. The infection is more common in men, particularly those under the age of 50.

What are the symptoms?

The only symptom is the appearance of painless, discoloured patches on the skin. The upper trunk area, including the neck, chest, shoulders, and back, is usually affected. The patches are:

- Of variable size, round, and flat with clearly defined edges.
- Pinkish-brown in colour on pale skin, becoming more noticeable if the surrounding skin tans. On dark skin, the patches are pale. In some people, affected areas are darkly pigmented.

Left untreated, the patches may become widespread and persist indefinitely.

What might be done?

Your doctor will probably be able to diagnose pityriasis versicolor from the appearance of the patches. To confirm the presence of the fungus, he or she may shine an ultraviolet light onto the patches, which will fluoresce yellow-green if the fungus is present, and may also take skin scrapings for laboratory analysis.

Treatment usually consists of washing the affected area regularly with an over-the-counter shampoo containing selenium sulphide, an antifungal drug (p.574). With thorough treatment, the infection usually clears up in 2–3 weeks, but it may take several more weeks for your skin to return to its normal colour. If you miss a patch of affected skin when applying the shampoo, the infection will recur. In persistent cases, your doctor may prescribe oral antifungal drugs.

Cold sore

A painful cluster of tiny blisters, usually near the lips, caused by a viral infection

 Cold wind, sunburn, and stress are risk factors

 Age, gender, and genetics are not significant factors

Cold sores are painful clusters of blisters usually caused by herpes simplex virus type 1 (HSV-1). Most people have been infected with HSV-1 at least once by the time they reach adulthood. The initial infection often goes unnoticed but may cause blisters in the mouth. The virus then remains dormant in the nerve cells, but in some people it is reactivated and produces cold sores. Trigger factors include cold wind, sunburn, tiredness, stress, the common cold, menstruation, and fever. Some people have recurrent cold sores.

What are the symptoms?

Cold sores often develop on the skin around the lips. The symptoms usually appear in the following order:

- The affected site begins to tingle.
- One or more clusters of tiny, painful blisters develop, and the surrounding skin becomes inflamed.
- The blisters burst and become crusty.

■ Usually, the blisters subside within 10–14 days.

If cold sores recur, the blisters usually reappear in the same areas on the face.

What might be done?

You may be able to prevent individual outbreaks by using an over-the-counter antiviral cream such as aciclovir (*see* **Preparations for infections and infestations**, p.577), but you must apply the cream as soon as the first symptoms develop. In some cases, oral antiviral drugs (p.573) may be prescribed. Although prompt treatment can prevent individual outbreaks, the virus remains in the system and symptoms may recur. If you have recurrent cold sores, try to protect your skin from trigger factors such as sunburn or cold wind. To minimize the risk of spreading the virus, do not touch the blisters and avoid kissing. Sometimes, oral sex can transmit the virus from the mouth to the genitals (*see* **Genital herpes**, p.493).

Warts

Firm, skin-coloured or darker growths on the skin caused by a viral infection

 Most common in children and young adults

 Warm, moist conditions are a risk factor

 Gender and genetics are not significant factors

Warts, also called verrucas, are small growths caused by human papillomaviruses. The viruses invade skin cells and encourage them to multiply, thus creating thickened areas of skin. Warts usually occur on the hands or feet and are generally harmless. However, some types affect the genitals and are more serious (*see* **Genital warts**, p.493).

Warts are transferred by direct contact with an infected person or from virus particles on recently shed flakes of skin. The infection is commonly spread in warm, moist conditions.

Most people have at least one wart by the age of 20, but in some people warts recur. People with reduced immunity due to a disease such as AIDS (*see* **HIV infection and AIDS**, p.169) may develop large numbers of warts.

What are the types?

There are three main types of wart. These types are classified according to their appearance and the different sites on the body on which they occur.

Common warts These warts most frequently occur on the hands. They are:
■ Firm with a rough, raised surface.
■ Usually round.
■ Dotted with tiny black spots.
The black spots are small blood vessels. Common warts often grow in groups, which are known as crops.

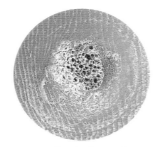

Appearance of a plantar wart
This wart on the sole of the foot has been flattened by the body's weight and has developed a thickened surface.

Plantar warts These warts occur on the soles of the feet. Although plantar warts are the same as common warts, they grow into the skin because they are continually under pressure from the weight of the body. A group of plantar warts that have joined together is called a mosaic wart. Plantar warts are:
■ Flattened into the sole of the foot.
■ Firm, with a thickened surface.
■ Usually painful to walk on.
■ Dotted with tiny black spots.
The virus that causes plantar warts is usually picked up from walking barefoot in communal areas, such as changing rooms and swimming pools.

Flat warts Verruca plana, also known as flat warts, commonly occur on the wrists, backs of the hands, and face. Flat warts vary in size and are:
■ Skin-coloured.

SELF-HELP

Treating a wart

You can treat common and plantar warts by using over-the-counter gels or lotions containing salicylic acid, which dissolves the thickened layer of skin. Apply the treatment daily for several weeks until the warts have disappeared (see below). Alternatively, you can try over-the-counter wart freezing treatments, which usually make the warts fall off in 10–14 days. However, these treatments are not suitable in all cases and you should consult your pharmacist before using them. You should keep all equipment for treating warts away from other bath items to avoid spreading the virus, and you should not share bath items.

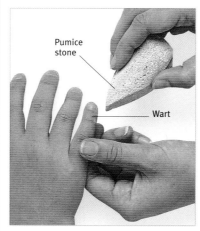

1 Soak the wart in water to soften it. Then gently rub it with a pumice stone or an emery board to remove as much of the thickened skin as possible.

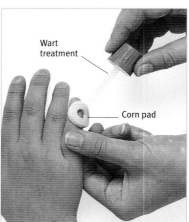

2 Shield the surrounding skin with a corn pad or petroleum jelly. Carefully apply the wart treatment to the wart and cover the area with an adhesive bandage.

■ Flat-topped and very slightly raised.
■ Often itchy.
These warts often occur in lines where the virus has spread along a scratch.

What might be done?

Most warts disappear without treatment, but this can take months or years. Many over-the-counter wart treatments are available (*see* **Treating a wart**, below). If a wart persists despite self-help measures or if you are unsure whether a lesion is a wart, consult your doctor. You should tell your doctor if a wart is painful, is on the face or genitals, or affects a child under the age of 5. The doctor may remove a wart by freezing, scraping, or burning it off. Sometimes, warts may recur.

Molluscum contagiosum

A viral infection producing multiple shiny, pearly-white pimples

 More common in children

 Close skin contact and, in some cases, sexual contact with an infected person are risk factors

 Gender and genetics are not significant factors

Molluscum contagiosum is a viral skin infection in which pimples appear in clusters on the trunk and at the tops of the arms and legs. The condition is harmless but contagious and is spread by close skin contact. It is common in children, especially in those with atopic eczema, probably because they scratch their skin, and this allows the virus to enter (*see* **Eczema in children**, p.538). In adults, molluscum contagiosum is usually spread through sexual contact. In such cases, the pimples tend to occur on the lower abdomen, genitals, and thighs. The condition is more common and often more severe in people whose immune systems are weakened by disorders such as AIDS (*see* **HIV infection and AIDS**, p.169) or by treatment with immunosuppressants (p.585).

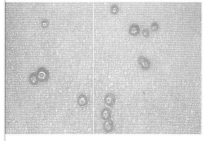

Molluscum contagiosum
These clusters of tiny, itchy, dome-shaped pimples are produced by the viral skin infection molluscum contagiosum.

What are the symptoms?

The symptoms of molluscum contagiosum begin 2–8 weeks after infection. A single, itchy pimple appears, and the infection then spreads to form a cluster of pimples. The pimples are:
■ Approximately 3–6 mm ($\frac{1}{8}$–$\frac{1}{4}$ in) in diameter.
■ Smooth and pearly-white or pink.
■ Dome-shaped with a tiny depression in the centre.
Molluscum contagiosum is not painful, but large pimples may bleed if they become caught on clothing.

What might be done?

Children with molluscum contagiosum are usually not treated because treatment may leave small scars and can be painful. The condition usually clears up by itself within 12 months. In adults, the pimples may be removed for cosmetic reasons. Your doctor may pierce them with a small probe, squeeze them with a pair of forceps, or scrape away a thin layer of skin under the pimples.

To prevent spread across the body, do not scratch the pimples. Avoid close physical contact and do not share towels or face flannels so that others are not infected. The condition can recur if you are re-exposed to infection or if your immune system becomes weakened.

Scabies

A mite infestation of the skin causing distinctive brown lines and an itchy rash

 Most common in children and young adults

 Living in overcrowded conditions is a risk factor

 Gender and genetics are not significant factors

The skin infestation scabies is caused by a mite that burrows into the outer layer of skin to lay its eggs. For several weeks there are no symptoms, but as the larvae hatch and grow into mites the skin becomes sensitive to the faeces of the mites and intense itching develops.

Scabies can affect people of any age but is most common in children and young adults. It is highly contagious and is spread by close physical contact, especially in overcrowded living conditions. It can be passed on by sexual contact or by prolonged hand-holding.

What are the symptoms?
The symptoms of scabies appear within 4–6 weeks of infestation and include:
- A rash of raised, pinkish-red spots up to 1 cm (³/₈ in) in diameter.
- Widespread itching, which is particularly severe at night.
- Light brown lines (burrows), which most often occur between the fingers and toes. In babies, they sometimes appear on the palms and soles.

The itching may occur before the rash appears, and it may persist for up to 3 weeks after the rash has disappeared.

What might be done?
Your doctor will probably be able to make a diagnosis from the appearance of the rash. To confirm the diagnosis, he or she may take a skin scraping for microscopic examination. Scabies is usually treated with an antiparasitic lotion that is applied to the entire body (including the scalp, face, and neck) and washed off after a set period (*see* **Preparations for infections and infestations**, p.577). A topical corticosteroid (p.577) may be prescribed to relieve itching. To prevent reinfection, people in close contact with you should be treated too. Clothing and bedding should be washed thoroughly at 50°C (120°F) or above or dry-cleaned. Items that cannot be washed or dry cleaned should be put in a sealed plastic bag for at least 72 hours to contain the mites until they die.

Minor skin injuries

The skin is remarkably resistant to the wear and tear of everyday life, but from time to time it may be affected by minor injury. Hands and feet are especially vulnerable to cuts, scrapes, and blisters. In a healthy person, superficial skin injuries normally heal rapidly, and most do not need attention from a doctor.

The most common types of skin injury are minor cuts and scrapes, in which the outer layer of the skin is broken. These types of wound are usually trivial, although they may be painful and there is a risk of infection entering the damaged site.

Sunburn is another common minor skin injury but one that is usually avoidable. Damage to the skin caused by overexposure to sunlight may not always appear serious, but, in the long term, sunburn increases the risk of potentially dangerous skin cancers. Friction and burns can cause damage to tissues beneath the surface of the skin, which often remains unbroken. Leaking blood and other fluids from this damage are trapped under the skin and appear as bruises or blisters. Although minor burns and scalds can be painful, most heal well within a few days if treated promptly.

Simple self-help measures are often the only treatment needed for minor skin injuries. Burns (p.182), which can be serious, are discussed elsewhere in the book.

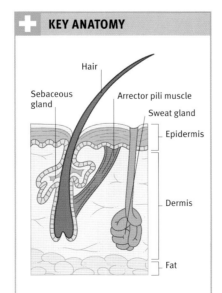

+ KEY ANATOMY

Hair

Sebaceous gland

Arrector pili muscle

Sweat gland

Epidermis

Dermis

Fat

For further information on the structure and function of the skin, *see* pp.190–191.

Cuts and scrapes

Broken areas on the surface of the skin caused by minor injuries

 Age, gender, genetics, and lifestyle are not significant factors

From time to time, the surface of the skin may be broken by small cuts and scrapes. Most of these minor injuries bleed to some extent, particularly those that are on the scalp or the palm of the hand.

A cut in the skin may be irregular or, if it results from injury caused by a sharp-edged implement such as a knife, clearly demarcated. Scrapes occur when the top layer of the skin rubs against a rough surface and is damaged. These superficial abrasions do not necessarily bleed but may ooze clear fluid.

What can I do?
Clean a cut or scrape as soon as you possibly can with soap and water and make sure that no dirt or foreign bodies are embedded in the wound. To control bleeding, press a clean gauze pad firmly over the area. Small injuries may heal more quickly if left uncovered, but, if dirt is likely to enter the wound, you should protect the area with an antiseptic cream and a sterile dressing.

What might the doctor do?
Minor injuries usually do not need medical attention. However, if a wound is slow to heal, becomes more swollen, red, and painful, or contains pus, it may be infected. You may need oral antibiotics (p.572) or topical antibiotics (*see* **Preparations for skin infections and infestations**, p.577) from your doctor.

If a wound is deep or dirty, you may need an antitetanus injection. Severe wounds may need stitches.

Needlestick injury

Accidental puncture of the skin by a used hypodermic needle

 Working in health centres and visiting public leisure areas are risk factors

 Age, gender, and genetics are not significant factors

Although a minor skin puncture with a used hypodermic needle may cause little pain or bleeding, a needlestick injury may have particularly serious implications for your health. Any needlestick injury needs to be investigated because of the risk that the needle carries organisms such as HIV, the virus that causes AIDS (*see* **HIV infection and AIDS**, p.169), or the hepatitis B or hepatitis C viruses (*see* **Acute hepatitis**, p.408).

Needlestick injuries may occasionally occur among hospital staff. People who visit public areas, such as parks or beaches, may be at risk from needles discarded by intravenous drug abusers.

If you have a needlestick injury, you should wash the wound using soap and water and consult a doctor as soon as you can. If possible, take the needle with you because your doctor may be able to check for the presence of viruses in the blood remaining in the needle.

You may need to have blood tests to find out if you have had previous exposure to hepatitis B or C; if you are already immune to hepatitis B; or if you are HIV-positive. If a course of immunization is started immediately, hepatitis B can usually be prevented. Your doctor may also suggest treatment with antiviral drugs to reduce the chance of HIV infection (*see* **Drugs for HIV infection and AIDS**, p.573). Blood tests for hepatitis B and C and HIV are usually done again after 3 months, and may be repeated at 3-month intervals for up to 12 months. The tests will determine whether you are clear of infection.

Sunburn

Inflammation of the skin caused by overexposure to the sun

 More common in fair-skinned people

Outdoor activities are risk factors

Age and gender are not significant factors

Sunburn occurs when the ultraviolet rays in sunlight damage cells in the outer layer of the skin, causing soreness, redness, and blistering. Damage is most likely to occur in the middle of the day when the sun is at its highest, but sunlight at any time of day can be harmful. It is possible for sunburn to occur even when the sky is overcast because ultraviolet rays can penetrate the cloud cover. Sunlight reflected off water or snow is especially damaging because its effects are intensified.

Fair-skinned people are more susceptible to sunburn because their skin produces only a small amount of the protective pigment melanin.

Sunburn or long-term exposure to the sun can cause the skin to age prematurely and increase the risk of developing skin

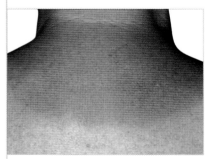

Sunburn
Even a short period of exposure to the sun can damage the surface of the skin, resulting in reddening and soreness.

cancer (p.199). To prevent sunburn and to protect the skin from the damaging effects of ultraviolet (UV) radiation, use sunscreens regularly (see **Sunscreens and sunblocks,** p.577). You should also avoid excessive exposure to the sun (see **Safety in the sun,** p.34).

What are the symptoms?

Sunburn can occur after just 30 minutes of exposing the skin to the sun. The symptoms may take a few hours to develop and include:

- Sore, red, hot skin.
- Swelling of the affected area.
- In severe cases, blistering.

A few days after the initial sunburn, the skin may become dry and start to peel. Severe sunburn may be associated with heatstroke, which is a potentially fatal condition (see **Heat exhaustion and heatstroke,** p.185).

What is the treatment?

If you develop sunburn, stay in the shade and drink plenty of fluids. You may be able to relieve symptoms by applying aloe-based gels or calamine lotion. Cool baths and compresses may also help. Severe sunburn needs immediate medical attention, and you should consult your doctor

as soon as possible. If you are severely burned and you also have heatstroke, you will need urgent treatment in hospital.

Blister

A collection of fluid beneath the surface of the skin

 Age, gender, genetics, and lifestyle are not significant factors

A blister forms when fluid leaks from blood vessels in the skin, usually after minor injury, and collects to form a small, raised area just beneath the outer layer of skin. The most common causes of single blisters are friction, such as that caused by a badly fitting shoe, and burns, including sunburn (p.207). Widespread blistering may be caused by eczema (p.193), or it may occur in some viral infections, such as chickenpox (p.165) and shingles (see **Herpes zoster,** p.166). The bacterial skin infection impetigo (p.204) may cause pus-filled blisters. There are also a number of much less common but potentially life-threatening conditions that result in blistering either on specific areas of skin or over the whole of the body (see **Blistering diseases,** p.194).

Blistering caused by minor damage usually heals rapidly without treatment. New skin develops beneath the blister, the fluid is gradually absorbed, and the top layer of skin dries and peels away. If the skin is broken, or if the blistered site is likely to be damaged further, you should protect the area with a dry, sterile dressing. Blistering due to disease or infection may need drug treatment.

You should not prick a blister to release the fluid because the skin acts as a barrier against infection. If the blisters are filled with pus or you notice spreading redness in the surrounding skin, consult your doctor.

Bruise

A discoloured area of skin caused by bleeding in underlying tissues

 Most common in children and elderly people

 Gender, genetics, and lifestyle are not significant factors

If the blood vessels beneath the skin are damaged by a blow or a fall, blood may leak into the surrounding tissues. This internal bleeding, even if it occurs deep in a muscle,

will eventually show through the surface of the skin as black or blue patches called bruises. Over a period of a few days after the injury, the red cells in the leaked blood break down and the bruises gradually change colour, fading to green, light brown, or yellow. The discoloration normally disappears completely within a week.

After receiving an injury, you can reduce blood loss beneath the skin by applying firm pressure to the area with an ice pack. You should maintain the pressure for at least 5 minutes.

Children and elderly people bruise more easily than young and middle-aged adults. If severe bruising appears for no obvious reason at any age, you should consult your doctor because it may be a sign of a bleeding disorder such as Von Willebrand's disease (p.275).

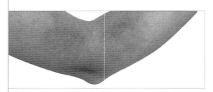

Bruising around the elbow
Prominent areas of the body, such as the elbow and knee, are vulnerable to injury and are common sites for bruises.

Hair and nail disorders

Hair and nails, like the outer layers of skin, are made of dead cells that grow from a living base. The dead parts that show above the skin's surface can be cut or damaged without causing pain, but damage to the living roots is painful. The condition of the hair and nails often reflects general health. Changes in the nails, in particular, may indicate an underlying disease.

Most hair and nail disorders are not a health threat but may be unsightly and cause embarrassment. However, some are caused by serious health problems. For example, excessive growth of body hair may be due to a hormonal imbalance, and spoon-shaped nails suggest iron deficiency. In these cases, treating the underlying disorder often improves the condition. Hair disorders may be due to factors such as drug treatments and localized skin diseases. Many nail abnormalities are usually due to minor injury or infection but they can be difficult to treat because topical preparations do not penetrate the nail. A damaged nail will not appear normal until it grows out, so the condition of the nails is sometimes an indication of past rather than present health.

This section begins by describing several disorders that affect scalp or body hair. The remaining articles describe abnormalities of the nails and the skin that surrounds them. Some common scalp problems are discussed elsewhere, including head lice (p.539) and seborrhoeic dermatitis (p.194).

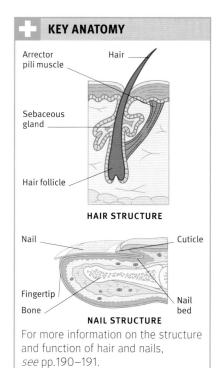

✚ **KEY ANATOMY**

Arrector pili muscle
Hair
Sebaceous gland
Hair follicle

HAIR STRUCTURE

Nail
Cuticle
Fingertip
Nail bed
Bone

NAIL STRUCTURE

For more information on the structure and function of hair and nails, see pp.190–191.

Dandruff

Excessive shedding of flakes of skin from the scalp

 More common in young adults

 Gender, genetics, and lifestyle are not significant factors

Dandruff is a harmless condition that involves an acceleration in the normal shedding of dead skin cells from the scalp. This dead skin accumulates as white flakes in the hair and sometimes causes itching. The condition is most common in young adults and may be a source of embarrassment.

Dandruff is most often caused by a yeast organism that grows in the scalp. Extensive dandruff is known as seborrhoeic dermatitis (p.194), a disorder that causes inflammation and scaling of the skin in other areas of the body, such as the face, chest, and back. Dandruff may be associated with inflammation of the eyelids (see **Blepharitis,** p.364). You can treat dandruff by washing your hair three to four times a week with a tar-based shampoo or a shampoo that contains an antiyeast agent, such as selenium sulphide or ketoconazole (see **Antifungal drugs,** p.574).

If the dandruff persists despite treatment, you should consult your doctor because you may have developed a skin condition, such as eczema (p.193) or psoriasis (p.192), that also affects the scalp. These disorders may require specific treatment with prescription drugs.

Alopecia

Loss of part or all of the hair, most commonly the hair on the scalp

 Age, gender, genetics, and lifestyle as risk factors depend on the type

Alopecia, or hair loss, can occur in any body area but is particularly noticeable when it affects the scalp. The condition may be localized, in which hair is lost in patches, or generalized, in which there is thinning or total hair loss over the whole scalp. Hair loss can be temporary or permanent. Alopecia is not always associated with ill health, but it may cause embarrassment.

What are the causes?

The most common cause of alopecia in men is oversensitivity to the hormone testosterone, producing a characteristic pattern of hair loss (see **Male-pattern baldness,** opposite page).

Patchy hair loss is usually due to alopecia areata, an autoimmune disorder that causes bald patches to appear on the scalp. These bald areas are surrounded by short, broken hairs. The hair usually regrows within 6 months, but in rare cases alopecia areata can cause permanent loss of all body hair.

Hairstyles that pull on the scalp are a common cause of patchy hair loss; if the pulling is continuous, hair loss may be permanent. Patchy hair loss may be the result of a rare psychological disorder in which

▶ **TREATMENT**

Hair transplant

Baldness can be treated surgically by several different methods of hair transplantation. In the method shown here, a strip of skin and hair is taken from a donor site, usually at the back of your scalp or behind your ears. The removed hairs and their attached follicles are then inserted into the bald area on the scalp, which is called the recipient site. You will usually be given a mild sedative, and both the donor and recipient sites on the scalp are anaesthetized before the procedure is carried out.

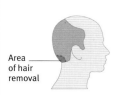

Area of hair removal

DONOR SITE

During the procedure
A strip of skin containing hairs with attached follicles is taken from the donor site, usually at the back of the scalp. The surgeon then makes numerous tiny incisions in the area that is to receive transplanted hair.

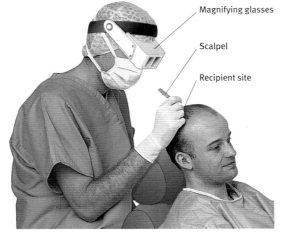

Magnifying glasses

Scalpel

Recipient site

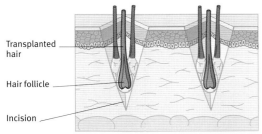

Transplanted hair

Hair follicle

Incision

Transplanted hairs
The hairs from the donor site are inserted into the incisions using tweezers. The hairs themselves fall out shortly afterwards, but new hair starts to grow from the follicles 3 weeks to 3 months later. The donor site heals in about 5 days.

the hair is compulsively pulled. Burns or skin disorders, such as ringworm (p.304), which scar the scalp may cause patchy hair loss.

Generalized hair loss is normal in elderly people. It may also occur temporarily after pregnancy and is a common side effect of chemotherapy (p.157). Other causes of thinning hair include acute illness, stress, and malnutrition.

What is the treatment?
Your doctor will probably be able to diagnose alopecia areata by the appearance of your scalp. This condition does not usually require treatment, but corticosteroids injected into the hairless patches may be effective in promoting regrowth. In most other cases of hair loss, the hair usually regrows once the underlying cause has been treated. Hair lost during pregnancy usually regrows about 3 months after childbirth.

If your scalp has patchy scarring, you may need a skin biopsy (p.199) to diagnose the underlying cause. Scarred areas may be treated with topical corticosteroids (p.577) or antifungal drugs (p.574), but if the damage is severe and has affected the hair follicles it is unlikely that new hair will grow.

Male-pattern baldness

Progressive loss of hair from the scalp, often in a characteristic pattern

 More common over the age of 30

 Much more common in males

 Often runs in families

 Lifestyle is not a significant factor

In male-pattern baldness, also called androgenic alopecia, hair is lost over several years, first from the temples and then from the crown, leaving a rim of hair around the scalp. The condition is very common in men over the age of 30 but may develop much earlier. In rare cases, it begins during puberty. This type of male-pattern baldness is often progressive and is thought to be caused by hypersensitivity of the follicles to the male sex hormone testosterone. There may be a family history of baldness in the male relatives on the mother's side.

Male-pattern baldness also occurs in women but is less common. Hair loss in women is usually due to hormonal disturbances, in particular those that take place after the menopause. In these cases, thinning is more generalized.

Your doctor may arrange for you to have tests to look for an underlying health problem (*see* **Alopecia,** opposite page). Over-the-counter solutions containing the substance minoxidil may stimulate regrowth temporarily, but new hair disappears when treatment is stopped. A more permanent way to replace hair in male-pattern baldness is by having a hair transplant (left).

Excessive hair

Excessive growth of hair or hair growth in areas that would not normally have hair

 Occurs only after puberty; more common with increasing age

 More common in females

 Sometimes runs in families

 Lifestyle is not a significant factor

There are two types of excessive hair growth: hirsutism and hypertrichosis. Hirsutism affects women only. In this condition, excessive hair develops particularly on the face, trunk, and limbs. This type of excessive growth is more common in women over the age of 60, especially in those of Mediterranean, Asian, Hispanic, or Arab descent.

The second type of excessive hair growth, hypertrichosis, can affect both males and females. In this condition, hair grows all over the body, even in areas that do not normally have hair.

What are the causes?
Mild hirsutism in women is often considered normal, especially following the menopause. In some cases, it may be a result of an increase in normally occurring male hormones in the female body (*see* **Virilization,** p.474), which may be caused by disorders such as polycystic ovary syndrome (p.477).

Hypertrichosis can occur with anorexia nervosa (p.348) or as a side effect of immunosuppressants (p.585) or antihypertensive drugs (p.580).

What might be done?
If you are a young woman with hirsutism, your doctor may arrange for a blood test to measure your male hormone levels. If these are high, you may be given a drug to block the hormones' effects and be treated for the underlying disorder. For example, polycystic ovary syndrome may be treated with hormones or surgery. If hypertrichosis is a side effect of a drug, stopping the treatment often reverses the condition.

You can deal with hirsutism yourself by bleaching, shaving, plucking, waxing, or using depilatory creams. The only way to remove hair permanently is by electrolysis, but it is a slow process. Laser treatment may also be helpful.

Pilonidal sinus

A pit, often containing hairs, at the top of the cleft between the buttocks

 Most common in young adults

 More common in males

 Genetics and lifestyle are not significant factors

A pilonidal sinus is a small, enclosed pit beneath the skin at the top of the cleft between the buttocks. The condition occurs most commonly in men with a lot of body hair. The exact cause is unknown but may be a defect in the development of that area. Hair growth at the site tends to be directed inwards, which may cause infection in the sinus and result in a painful abscess.

Prompt action at the first signs of infection may prevent an abscess from forming. You should soak the area in warm water to relieve discomfort and consult your doctor as soon as possible. You may be prescribed oral antibiotics (p.572) to treat the infection. If pus has built up, the abscess will need to be drained under general anaesthesia and left open to heal. In most cases, the infection is unlikely to recur.

Nail abnormalities

Changes in the shape, colour, or texture of the nails, often due to injury, infection, or underlying disease

 Age, gender, genetics, and lifestyle as risk factors depend on the type

The nails are particularly susceptible to damage. Injury is the most common cause of abnormalities in the shape, colour, or texture of the nails. Changes in general health and in the health of the skin at the nail bed may also lead to abnormalities. In addition, infection of the nail itself may alter its appearance.

What are the types?
Some forms of nail abnormality need treatment only if they are unsightly or painful; others may be signs of underlying health problems that may require medical investigation.

White spots Small white marks that appear on one or more nails occur naturally and are due to minor damage, such as from a knock or blow.

Thickening Thickening of the nails, a condition known as onychogryphosis, may be due to neglect or a fungal infection or occur for no apparent reason. Distortion of the nail may result. The toenails are most likely to be affected.

Ridges The occurrence of ridged lines running from the base of the nail to the tip is normal in people who are elderly. In younger people, these ridges may be a sign of rheumatoid arthritis (p.222) or of the skin conditions lichen planus (p.195) and eczema (p.193).

Pitting Multiple pits the size of a pinhead on the nail surface often indicate a general skin disorder, such as psoriasis or eczema (p.193). Pitting may also be associated with the hair disorder alopecia areata (*see* Alopecia, p.208).

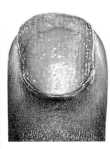

Pitted fingernail
Many small pits can be seen all over the surface of the fingernail. In this case, the pitting is caused by the skin disorder psoriasis.

Nail separation If a nail is damaged as a result of injury, it can lift away from the nail bed (a condition called onycholysis) and eventually fall off. Separation of the nail from the nail bed may also occur in some people who have psoriasis or lichen planus or in those with certain types of thyroid problem. Nail separation makes the nail bed susceptible to infection, which causes the lifted nail to appear green.

Yellowing Yellow, crumbly nails may be due to a fungal infection (onychomycosis). Sometimes, heavy smoking causes discoloration of the nails.

Clubbing Increased curvature of the nails and broadening of the fingertips is called clubbing. This condition often indicates a serious underlying disorder of the lungs, particularly cystic fibrosis (p.535), bronchiectasis (p.303), or lung cancer (p.307). Alternatively, clubbing of the nails may be a sign of liver disease, congenital heart disease (p.542), thyroid disease, or certain bowel disorders, such as Crohn's disease (p.417).

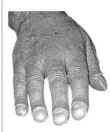

Clubbing of the fingernails
Increased curvature of the nails, known as clubbing, may result in loss of the normal indentation at the nail bed.

Spoon-shaped nails In this form of abnormality, known as koilonychia, the nails have a concave and spoon-shaped appearance. This condition is usually caused by a severe iron deficiency.

What might be done?
Minor nail abnormalities that are not associated with underlying disorders, such as white spots caused by minor injury, are unlikely to need treatment. However, if the colour, shape, or general condition of your nails changes when no obvious damage has occurred, you should consult your doctor to find out if the problem is caused by a disease. Clubbing that has existed from childhood is probably due to a hereditary defect. This form of clubbing is irreversible and need not be investigated. However, you should consult a doctor if you develop clubbing as an adult. Once the cause of an underlying disorder has been treated, the nails should begin growing normally again, and healthy nail will gradually replace the abnormal tissue. The process is slow; abnormal fingernails may take between 6 and 9 months to grow out, and toenails take even longer. In the meantime, the appearance of the damaged fingernails may be improved by having regular manicures, and a chiropodist may be able to treat distorted toenails.

Paronychia

Infection of the skin fold around a nail, causing a painful swelling

 Repeated immersion of the hands in water is a risk factor

 Age, gender, and genetics are not significant factors

Infection of the fold of skin surrounding a fingernail or toenail (nail fold) is called paronychia. The infection causes pain and swelling, which may develop either suddenly (acute paronychia) or gradually over several months (chronic paronychia), depending on the underlying cause. One or more nails may be affected by the condition.

What are the causes?
Acute paronychia is usually the result of a bacterial infection entering the nail fold through a cut or break in the skin. Chronic paronychia is common among people such as cooks who repeatedly immerse their hands in water. The skin around the nail separates from the nail, softens, and becomes infected, usually by a yeast organism. A secondary bacterial infection may then occur, resulting in acute paronychia. Some people with decreased resistance to infection, such as those with diabetes mellitus (p.437), are at increased risk of paronychia.

What are the symptoms?
Usually, the symptoms of acute paronychia become apparent about 24 hours after infection and include:
- Pain and swelling on one side of the nail fold.
- Build-up of pus around the nail.

If acute paronychia is left untreated, the nail may separate from the nail bed and eventually fall away. The symptoms of chronic paronychia develop over several months.

The condition may cause some discomfort and swelling but does not usually produce a build-up of pus. Eventually, the affected nail thickens slightly and develops horizontal ridges and brownish discoloration.

What is the treatment?
Your doctor may prescribe oral antibiotics (p.572) for acute paronychia. In severe cases, pus may be drained under local anaesthesia. Chronic paronychia may be treated with an over-the-counter cream containing an antifungal drug (p.574), but if there is a secondary infection your doctor may prescribe stronger antifungals and oral antibiotics. Acute paronychia often clears up in a few days with treatment. Chronic paronychia may take several weeks.

To prevent chronic paronychia, you should dry your hands thoroughly after washing and wear cotton-lined rubber gloves when your hands are in water.

Ingrown toenail

Painful inward growth of the edges of a toenail into the surrounding skin

 Most common in teenagers and young adults

 More common in males

 Tight or badly fitting shoes increase the risk

 Genetics is not a significant factor

An ingrown toenail curves under on one or both sides and cuts into the surrounding skin, causing inflammation and sometimes infection. The condition, which most commonly affects the big toe, is often due to ill-fitting shoes pressing on an incorrectly cut nail. In some cases, injury can cause the skin around the nail to overgrow and engulf part of the nail. Poor foot hygiene can also increase the risk of infection, leading to inflammation.

What are the symptoms?
The symptoms of an ingrown toenail may include the following:
- Pain, redness, and swelling around the toenail.
- Broken skin at the nail edge, which oozes clear fluid, pus, or blood.

You should consult your doctor as soon as you notice a toenail that has become ingrown because it is possible that your toe may be infected.

What is the treatment?
You can relieve the pain of an ingrown toenail by bathing your foot in warm salt water daily and taking painkillers (p.589). You should protect the affected toe by keeping it covered with a clean, dry gauze. If there is no improvement within a few days, you should consult your doctor. If your toenail is infected, he or she may pre-

scribe oral antibiotics (p.572) or topical antibiotics (*see* **Preparations for skin infections and infestations**, p.577).

To help to prevent an ingrown toenail from recurring, keep your feet clean and wear correctly fitting shoes. Your toenails should be cut straight across, rather than along a curve, to prevent them from growing into the skin. If the problem recurs, your doctor may suggest that you have part or all of the toenail removed to stop it growing into the toe (*see* **Removal of an ingrown toenail**, below).

▶ TREATMENT

Removal of an ingrown toenail

Minor surgery may be needed for an ingrown toenail. Your toe will be anaesthetized and cleaned with antiseptic, and a tourniquet will be applied to its base. The nail, or part of it, will be removed, and phenol will be applied to the exposed nail bed to kill it and prevent regrowth. You should be comfortable enough to walk within 24 hours of surgery, and the wound should heal within a week.

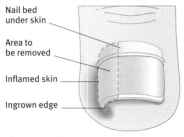

Nail bed under skin

Area to be removed

Inflamed skin

Ingrown edge

The operation
A vertical cut is made along the toenail. The ingrown part is removed and the nail bed treated to prevent regrowth.

Musculoskeletal system

Every day we use our muscles and joints to carry out voluntary movements. Many of these actions, such as walking, demand very little concentration, but complex tasks, such as playing the piano, require more conscious effort, supported by a subconscious system of coordination learned when the skill was first mastered. All movements are based on mechanical changes in the muscles, which contract or relax, making specific bones pivot, hinge, rotate, or glide at the joints.

SKELETAL MUSCLES MOVE the body at its joints by contracting. In addition, they maintain a steady tension, or tone, that gives the body the support it needs to maintain its posture, such as keeping the head upright on the neck. This postural tone is automatic but does require alertness. Unlike horses, people cannot sleep standing up.

There are two other types of muscle in the body: cardiac muscle, found only in the heart; and smooth muscle, occurring in hollow organs such as the intestines. Most muscle of these types is not under conscious control.

Types of bone
Bones come in many shapes and sizes, ranging from the flat bones found in the skull to the long bones of the limbs. The outer layer of each bone is made of dense, heavy, compact bone. The inner layer consists of spongy bone that is made up of numerous trabeculae (struts) arranged in such a way that they provide maximum support without excessive weight.

Bone gives the body shape and supports the body's structure. It is a living tissue, which is constantly being renewed. Bone also serves as a reservoir for various minerals, such as calcium and phosphorus. Bone marrow, the soft, fatty substance that fills the cavities in bones, produces most of the body's blood cells (see **Formation of blood cells**, p.265).

Movement
Joints, which are formed where bones meet, are covered with lubricated cartilage that allows smooth

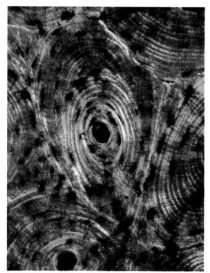

Structure of compact bone
The structural units of compact bone are called osteons (shown here in cross section). Osteons consist of rings of collagen (protein) around central canals.

➕ FUNCTION

How the body moves
Movement of the body depends on the interaction of muscles, bones, and joints in response to signals from the brain and nerves. A muscle typically connects two bones and crosses the joint between them. When a muscle contracts, it pulls on the bones to which it is attached and produces movement. Muscles can only pull, not push. Therefore, many muscles are arranged in pairs, one on each side of a joint, so that they produce opposing movements. An example is the pairing of the triceps and biceps muscles in the upper arm.

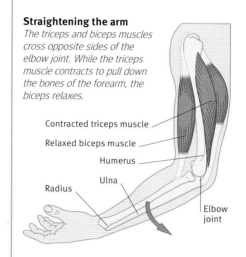
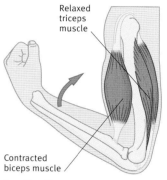

Straightening the arm
The triceps and biceps muscles cross opposite sides of the elbow joint. While the triceps muscle contracts to pull down the bones of the forearm, the biceps relaxes.

Contracted triceps muscle
Relaxed biceps muscle
Humerus
Ulna
Radius
Elbow joint

Relaxed triceps muscle
Contracted biceps muscle

Bending the arm
To bend the arm, the biceps muscle contracts to pull up the bones of the forearm, while the triceps relaxes.

movement. The range of movement of the joints is determined both by their structure and by the ligaments that stabilize and support them; the hip joint, for example, moves less freely than the shoulder. In contrast, the joints in the wrist, foot, and spine sacrifice mobility for stability; their bones are joined by strong, inflexible ligaments that allow little movement. Most of the skull bones fuse together and become immobile once growth has ceased.

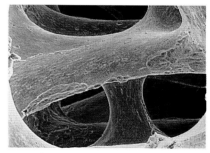

Struts in spongy bone
The trabeculae (struts) that form spongy bone make it light but strong.

IN THIS SECTION

The body's skeleton

The adult human skeleton is a bony framework that supports the body and gives it shape. It also protects the internal organs and anchors the body's muscles. The skeleton is composed of 206 bones and is divided into two parts. The axial skeleton – the skull, spine, and rib cage – consists of 80 bones and protects the brain, spinal cord, heart, and lungs. The appendicular skeleton has 126 bones and consists of the bones of the limbs, the collarbones, the shoulder blades, and the bones of the pelvis.

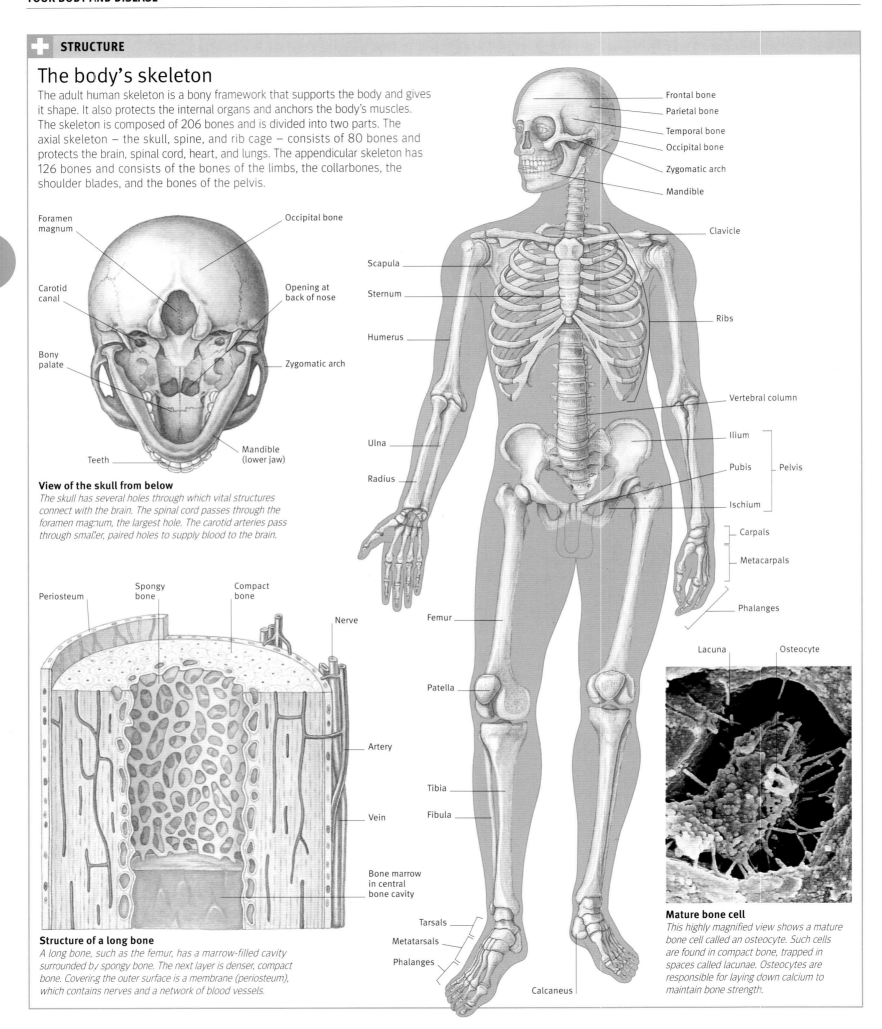

View of the skull from below

The skull has several holes through which vital structures connect with the brain. The spinal cord passes through the foramen magnum, the largest hole. The carotid arteries pass through smaller, paired holes to supply blood to the brain.

Structure of a long bone

A long bone, such as the femur, has a marrow-filled cavity surrounded by spongy bone. The next layer is denser, compact bone. Covering the outer surface is a membrane (periosteum), which contains nerves and a network of blood vessels.

Mature bone cell

This highly magnified view shows a mature bone cell called an osteocyte. Such cells are found in compact bone, trapped in spaces called lacunae. Osteocytes are responsible for laying down calcium to maintain bone strength.

STRUCTURE

The backbone

The spine, also known as the vertebral column, holds the body upright, supports the head, and encircles the spinal cord. It consists of 33 bones called vertebrae. Joints and discs of fibrous tissue between most of the vertebrae make the spine flexible, while ligaments and muscles stabilize it and control movement.

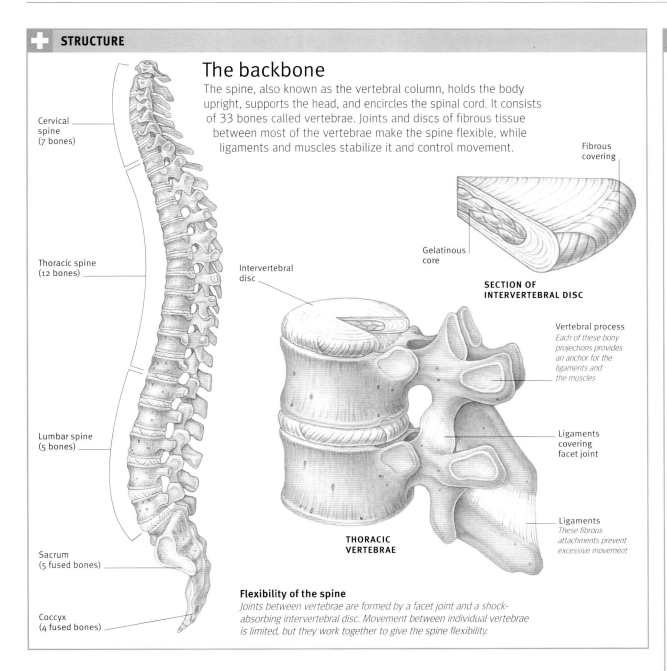

Cervical spine (7 bones)

Thoracic spine (12 bones)

Lumbar spine (5 bones)

Sacrum (5 fused bones)

Coccyx (4 fused bones)

Intervertebral disc

Fibrous covering

Gelatinous core

SECTION OF INTERVERTEBRAL DISC

Vertebral process
Each of these bony projections provides an anchor for the ligaments and the muscles

Ligaments covering facet joint

Ligaments
These fibrous attachments prevent excessive movement

THORACIC VERTEBRAE

Flexibility of the spine
Joints between vertebrae are formed by a facet joint and a shock-absorbing intervertebral disc. Movement between individual vertebrae is limited, but they work together to give the spine flexibility.

STRUCTURE AND FUNCTION

The joints

Joints are formed where two or more bones meet. Most joints, including those of the limbs, move freely and are known as synovial joints. They are lubricated by synovial fluid secreted by the joint lining. In contrast, semi-movable joints, such as those in the pelvis and spine, are less flexible but give greater stability. A few joints, such as those of the skull, are fixed and allow no movement.

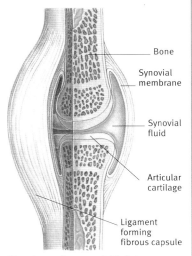

Bone

Synovial membrane

Synovial fluid

Articular cartilage

Ligament forming fibrous capsule

Structure of a synovial joint
The bones of synovial joints are held together by ligaments that form a fibrous capsule. The synovial membrane lining the capsule secretes a lubricating fluid, and articular cartilage on the bone ends provides a smooth surface for movement.

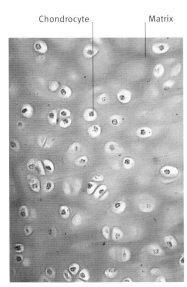

Chondrocyte

Matrix

Composition of articular cartilage
Articular cartilage is composed of cells (chondrocytes) located in cavities in a tough matrix of collagen, forming a smooth, flexible surface.

FUNCTION

How bone repairs itself

A broken bone and any damaged blood vessels start to repair and heal themselves immediately. A fracture in a long bone, such as the collarbone, normally takes about 6 weeks to heal in an adult. However, some injured bones may not regain their full strength for several months, and healing may need to be aided by a plaster or resin cast or by mechanical fixation. In children, fractured bones usually heal more quickly.

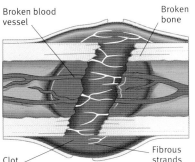

Broken blood vessel

Broken bone

Clot

Fibrous strands

1 *A clot forms to seal broken blood vessels. Gradually, a mesh of fibrous tissue forms and starts to replace the clot.*

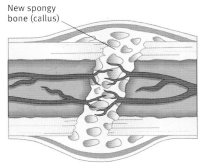

New spongy bone (callus)

2 *New, soft, spongy bone called callus develops on the framework provided by the fibrous tissue, joining the broken ends.*

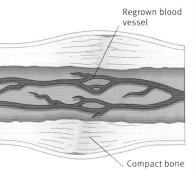

Regrown blood vessel

Compact bone

3 *Dense, compact bone gradually replaces the callus, and blood vessels regrow. Eventually, the bone regains its shape.*

The joints (continued)
Types of joint

Illustrated here are six examples of synovial joints, each of a different type, and one fixed and one semi-movable joint. Synovial joints are classified according to how their articular surfaces (where bones meet) fit together and the movements each permits. The diagram accompanying each synovial joint illustrates its range of movement.

Joint between uppermost bones of neck

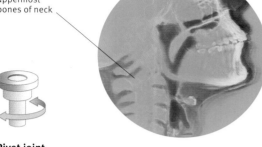

Pivot joint
In a pivot joint, one bone rotates within a collar formed by another. The pivot joint between the atlas and the axis, the uppermost bones of the neck, allows the head to turn to either side.

Joint at base of thumb

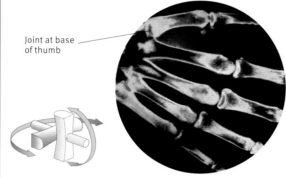

Saddle joint
Saddle-shaped bone ends that meet at right angles form a saddle joint. The bones can rotate a little and move sideways and back and forth. The body's only saddle joint is at the base of the thumb.

Foot joint

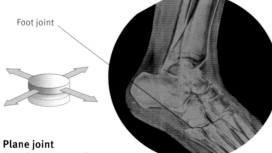
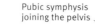

Plane joint
In a plane joint, surfaces that are almost flat slide over each other, back and forth and sideways. Some joints in the foot and wrist are plane joints.

Pubic symphysis joining the pelvis

Semi-movable joint
In a semi-movable joint, the articular surfaces are fused to a tough pad of cartilage that allows only a little movement. Examples are the pubic symphysis, which joins the front halves of the pelvis, and the joints of the spine.

Joint of skull (suture)

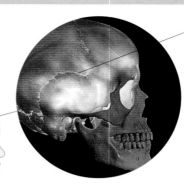

Fixed joint
In a fixed joint, the bones are bound together by fibrous tissue, allowing little or no movement. The fixed joints between the bones of the skull are called sutures.

Shoulder joint

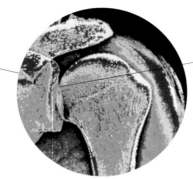

Ball-and-socket joint
In a ball-and-socket joint, the ball-shaped end of one bone fits into a cup-shaped cavity in another, allowing movement in all directions. The shoulder and hip are ball-and-socket joints.

joint between the scaphoid and radius bones

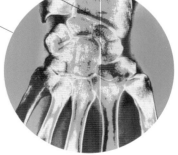

Ellipsoidal joint
The oval end of one bone fits into the oval cup of another in an ellipsoidal joint, allowing movement in most directions and limited rotation. The wrist is an ellipsoidal joint.

Knee joint

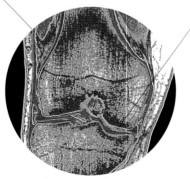

Hinge joint
The cylindrical surface of one bone fits into the groove of another to form a hinge joint. This type of joint either bends or straightens a limb. The knee, elbow, and finger joints are all examples of hinge joints.

+ STRUCTURE

The body's muscles

Muscles consist of tissue that can contract powerfully to move the body, maintain its posture, and work the various internal organs, including the heart and blood vessels. These functions are performed by three different types of muscle (p.216), of which skeletal muscle makes up the greatest bulk. (Many of the body's skeletal muscles are identified, right.) Usually each end of a skeletal muscle is attached to a bone by a tendon, a flexible cord of fibrous tissue. The skeletal muscles may be controlled consciously to produce movement.

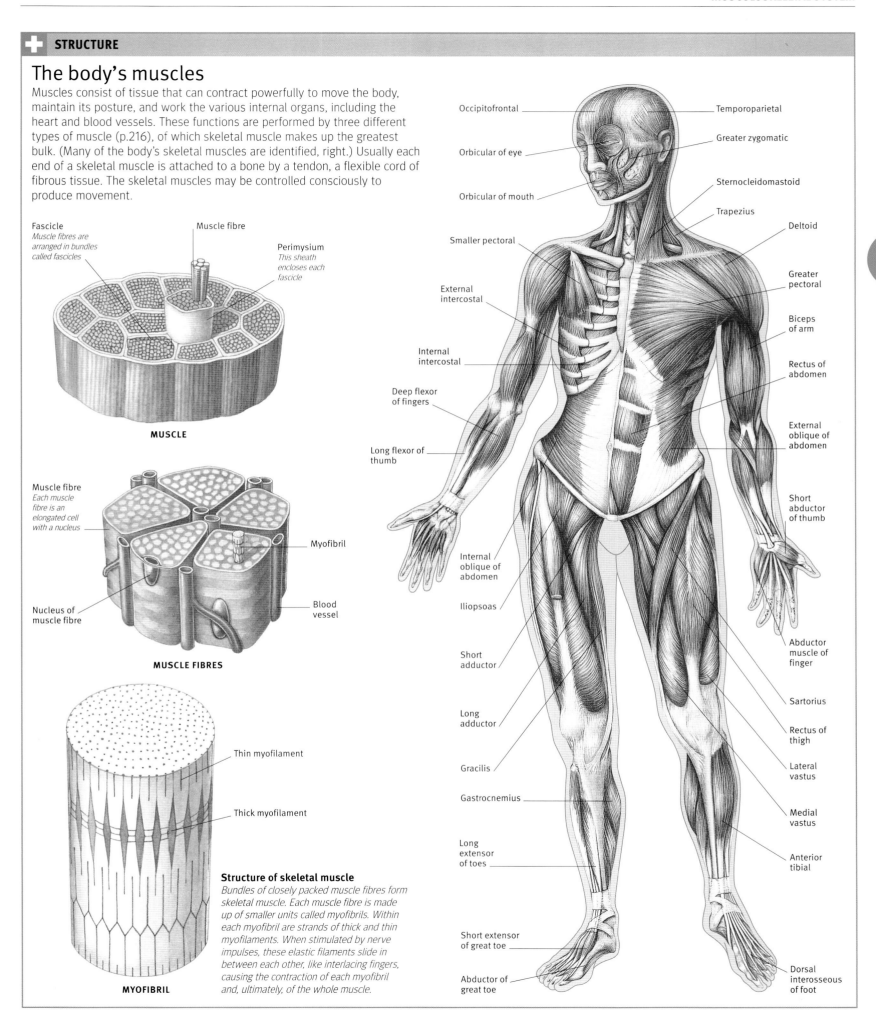

Fascicle
Muscle fibres are arranged in bundles called fascicles

Muscle fibre

Perimysium
This sheath encloses each fascicle

MUSCLE

Muscle fibre
Each muscle fibre is an elongated cell with a nucleus

Myofibril

Nucleus of muscle fibre

Blood vessel

MUSCLE FIBRES

Thin myofilament

Thick myofilament

Structure of skeletal muscle
Bundles of closely packed muscle fibres form skeletal muscle. Each muscle fibre is made up of smaller units called myofibrils. Within each myofibril are strands of thick and thin myofilaments. When stimulated by nerve impulses, these elastic filaments slide in between each other, like interlacing fingers, causing the contraction of each myofibril and, ultimately, of the whole muscle.

MYOFIBRIL

Occipitofrontal

Orbicular of eye

Orbicular of mouth

Smaller pectoral

External intercostal

Internal intercostal

Deep flexor of fingers

Long flexor of thumb

Internal oblique of abdomen

Iliopsoas

Short adductor

Long adductor

Gracilis

Gastrocnemius

Long extensor of toes

Short extensor of great toe

Abductor of great toe

Temporoparietal

Greater zygomatic

Sternocleidomastoid

Trapezius

Deltoid

Greater pectoral

Biceps of arm

Rectus of abdomen

External oblique of abdomen

Short abductor of thumb

Abductor muscle of finger

Sartorius

Rectus of thigh

Lateral vastus

Medial vastus

Anterior tibial

Dorsal interosseous of foot

✚ **STRUCTURE**

The body's muscles (continued)

Occipitofrontal

Orbicular of eye

Brachioradial

Platysma

Temporoparietal

Semispinalis of head

Splenius of head

Trapezius

Deltoid

Greater rhomboid

Latissimus dorsi

Triceps of arm

Extensor of fingers

Ulnar extensor of wrist

Infraspinous

Erector of spine

Gluteus minimus

Quadrate of thigh

Great adductor

Semimembranous

Popliteal

Long peroneal

Posterior tibial

Short peroneal

Long flexor of great toe

Plantar interosseous of hand

Gluteus maximus

Biceps of thigh

Gastrocnemius

Soleus

Long extensor of toes

Achilles tendon

Short extensor of toes

Types of muscle

The three types of muscle are skeletal muscle, which covers and moves the skeleton; cardiac (heart) muscle, which pumps blood around the body; and smooth muscle, which is found in the walls of the digestive tract, blood vessels, and the genital and urinary tracts. Smooth muscle performs the unconscious actions of the body, such as propelling food along the digestive tract.

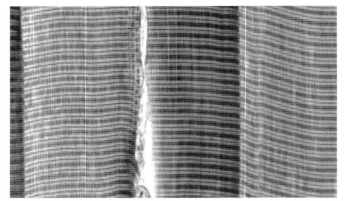

Skeletal muscle
This type of muscle is formed of long, strong, parallel fibres, which are able to contract quickly and powerfully, but can do so only for short periods of time.

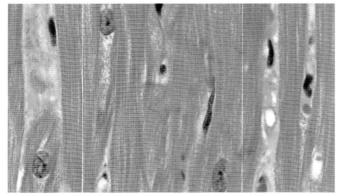

Cardiac muscle
Short, branching, interlinked fibres form a network within the wall of the heart. Cardiac muscle contracts rhythmically and continually without tiring.

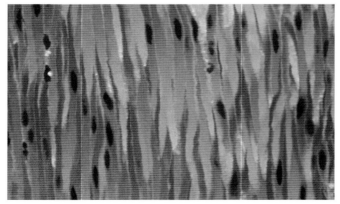

Smooth muscle
These fibres are short, spindle-shaped, and thinner than skeletal muscle fibres. Smooth muscle cells form sheets of muscle that can contract for prolonged periods.

Bone disorders

Bone consists of a resilient protein framework strengthened by calcium and phosphate deposits. While people often think of bone as lifeless and unchanging, it is actually a living tissue, supplied with nerves and blood vessels, that is continually being broken down and rebuilt. Bone can be weakened by nutritional and hormonal factors and by certain long-term disorders.

This section starts by discussing the bone disorder osteoporosis, which is common in elderly people. This disorder affects the natural processes of bone breakdown and replacement, causing bones to become brittle and fracture more easily. The section also covers the other main disorders that affect bone formation, including osteomalacia and rickets, both of which are due to lack of vitamin D, and Paget's disease of the bone, the cause of which has yet to be established. Kyphosis, lordosis, and scoliosis, bone disorders that affect the curvature of the spine, are described next. Further articles discuss the bone infection osteomyelitis and noncancerous and cancerous tumours of the bones. Defects in the bone marrow are covered elsewhere in the book (*see* **Blood disorders**, pp.271–278).

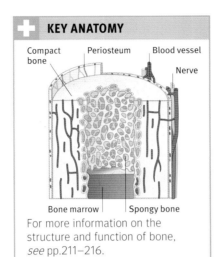

KEY ANATOMY

Compact bone · Periosteum · Blood vessel · Nerve · Bone marrow · Spongy bone

For more information on the structure and function of bone, *see* pp.211–216.

Osteoporosis

Loss of bone tissue, resulting in bones that are brittle and susceptible to fracture

 Common over the age of 50

 More common in females

 Sometimes runs in families; more common in white and Asian people

 Poor diet, lack of exercise, smoking, and alcohol are risk factors

As people get older, their bones become thinner and lighter. By the age of 70, most people's skeletons are about a third lighter than they were at the age of 40. This loss of bone density, known as osteoporosis, is the result of an imbalance between the natural breakdown and replacement of bone. Eventually, all elderly people are affected by osteoporosis, but the severity of the condition varies from person to person. People who are thin, who do little exercise, and whose relatives have osteoporosis are likely to develop the condition to a greater degree than others.

Many people do not realize that they have osteoporosis until they fracture a wrist or hip as a result of a minor fall. In the UK, thousands of fractures occur each year in people aged 65 or over. Osteoporosis is a major cause of these fractures, the hip being the most common site. In elderly people, hip fractures are often life-threatening or result in immobility.

What are the causes?

Sex hormones are necessary for bone replacement. In both men and women, osteoporosis begins to develop as sex hormone production declines with age. Any condition that causes this decline to accelerate can increase the severity of age-related osteoporosis. In women, production of the sex hormone oestrogen declines rapidly at the menopause. Early menopause increases the risk of osteoporosis. In men, untreated hypogonadism (p.466) results in low levels of the sex hormone testosterone early in life and a low bone density.

Osteoporosis may occur as a result of long-term treatment with oral corticosteroids (p.600). People with rheumatoid arthritis (p.222), an overactive thyroid gland (*see* **Hyperthyroidism**, p.432), or chronic kidney disease (p.451) are also at increased risk of osteoporosis.

Exercise is essential to maintain bone health. The density of bones declines rapidly in people who are confined to bed and in those whose daily activity is reduced, for example, by disorders such as arthritis (p.220) or multiple sclerosis (p.334).

Osteoporosis sometimes runs in families. Women who have a close relative with osteoporosis are more likely to develop the disorder themselves. White and Asian women, especially those who have a slight build, are at increased risk of developing the condition.

Can it be prevented?

Measures to prevent osteoporosis are most effective if they are started early in life. Teenagers and young adults should eat a balanced diet rich in calcium and vitamin D (*see* **A healthy diet**, p.16) and maintain it throughout life. Calcium is essential for bone strength, and vitamin D aids calcium absorption in the body. Extra calcium is needed during pregnancy, while breast-feeding, and during and after the menopause; it may be advisable to take a supplement at such times (*see* **Vitamin and mineral supplements**, p.598). Vitamin D is mainly produced in the skin in response to sunlight. People who are exposed to little sunlight may need to take vitamin D supplements.

Walking and other weight-bearing exercise help to increase bone density. Not smoking and limiting the intake of alcohol also reduce the risk of developing osteoporosis.

Anyone thought to be at increased risk of osteoporosis, such as having a family history of the disorder, can have his or her bone density measured (*see* **Bone densitometry**, p.218). Bone density testing is often used to assess a person's likelihood of having bone loss and also to monitor people who are taking preventive treatment.

What are the symptoms?

Some physical changes associated with aging are, in fact, often due to osteoporosis. These include:

■ Gradual loss of height.
■ Rounding of the back.

For many people, the first evidence of osteoporosis is a painful fracture (p.232) of a bone after minor stress or injury. An example is sudden, severe back pain due to a compression fracture of the body of a vertebra (bone of the spine). In severe osteoporosis, a fracture may occur spontaneously.

What might be done?

The diagnosis of osteoporosis is made from your medical history, a physical examination, and bone densitometry. Blood tests are also commonly carried out to look for conditions that can cause osteoporosis, such as hyperthyroidism.

If you have back pain due to a fracture, your doctor may recommend that you take painkillers (p.589) or use a heat pad on the affected area. Underlying disorders will be treated if possible. For example, you may

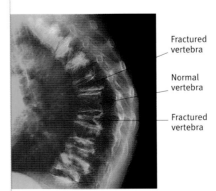

Fractured vertebra

Normal vertebra

Fractured vertebra

Spine affected by osteoporosis
This colour-enhanced X-ray shows severe curvature of the upper spine due to compression fractures of vertebrae that have been weakened by osteoporosis.

be prescribed drugs to treat an overactive thyroid gland (*see* **Drugs for hyperthyroidism**, p.602).

To slow the progression of osteoporosis it is important to follow the advice given above for taking preventive measures. In addition, your doctor may prescribe calcium and vitamin D supplements, and bisphosphonate drugs (*see* **Drugs for bone disorders**, p.579) to help prevent bone loss and reduce the risk of fractures. If bisphosphonates are not suitable, your doctor may prescribe alternative medications, such as strontium ranelate or raloxifene. In certain severe cases, parathyroid hormone or a drug called teriparatide may be prescribed. Hormone replacement therapy (HRT) is not generally recommended as a first-line treatment for osteoporosis but it may be considered for postmenopausal women when other treatments have been ineffective or are unsuitable. Women who have gone through a premature menopause (before 45 years of age) may be advised to have HRT to protect against their higher risk of osteoporosis. In men with osteoporosis due to low levels of male sex hormones, testosterone may be prescribed. However, even if these measures are taken, some bone loss is inevitable in later life.

Osteomalacia and rickets

Disorders due to lack of vitamin D, resulting in weak, soft bones that become distorted or fracture easily

 Osteomalacia develops in adults; rickets develops in children

 In some cases, the cause is inherited

 Minimal exposure to sunlight and vegan or fat-free diets are risk factors

 Gender is not a significant factor

The minerals calcium and phosphate give bone its strength and density. A deficiency of vitamin D results in poor absorption of calcium from the diet, leading to weak and soft bones that are easily deformed or fractured. In adults, the condition is called osteomalacia; in children, it is known as rickets.

What are the causes?

Healthy people obtain the vitamin D they need partly from their diet (from eggs, fish, fortified fat spreads, milk, and some cereals) and partly from vitamin D production in the skin on exposure to sunlight. A deficiency of vitamin D, therefore, is most common in people who eat a restricted diet and receive little direct sunlight. In tropical countries, vitamin D deficiency is almost unknown, except in women who are required to cover their entire bodies. At higher latitudes, deficiency may occur in elderly, housebound people.

▶ **TEST**

Bone densitometry

Also known as a DEXA scan, this procedure uses low-dose X-rays to measure the density of bone. The test is carried out to screen for and diagnose osteoporosis. The varying absorption of X-rays as they pass through the body is interpreted by a computer and displayed as an image. The computer calculates the average density of the bone and compares it with the normal range for the person's age and sex. The procedure typically takes about 10–20 minutes and is painless.

Bone densitometry of the spine
You will be asked to lie still with your legs raised and your back flat. The X-ray generator and detector move along the length of your spine and transmit information to a computer.

Foam cube
This is used to raise the legs and keep the spine flat

X-ray generator
A beam of low-dose X-ray radiation is emitted here and passes through the body

X-ray detector
The X-rays that have not been absorbed by the body are detected here

Monitor
The scan appears on the screen

RESULTS

Low-density bone

Medium-density bone

High-density bone

Spinal bone density scan
This is a colour-coded, computerized representation of the relative densities of bone in different areas of the spine.

Some people cannot absorb vitamin D from food due to intestinal surgery or coeliac disease (p.416). Less commonly, osteomalacia and rickets may be caused by inherited disorders of vitamin D metabolism or chronic kidney disease (p.451). In rare cases, drugs used to treat epilepsy (*see* **Anticonvulsant drugs**, p.590) interfere with vitamin D metabolism and cause osteomalacia or rickets.

What are the symptoms?
The symptoms of osteomalacia develop over months or years and may include:
■ Painful, tender bones, most often the ribs, hips, and bones of the legs.
■ Difficulty in climbing stairs or in getting up from a squatting position.
■ Bone fractures after a minor injury.
A child with rickets may experience similar symptoms, and may also have:
■ Retarded growth.
■ Swelling and tenderness at the growing ends of the bones.
■ Prominence of the ribs where they join the breastbone.
Left untreated, bow legs or knock-knees may develop in affected children.

What might be done?
Your doctor may suspect osteomalacia or rickets from your symptoms and a physical examination. He or she may arrange for blood tests to check for low levels of calcium, phosphate, and vitamin D. A bone biopsy, in which a bone sample is taken for analysis, or X-rays (p.131) can confirm the diagnosis.

If you have a vitamin D deficiency, you should eat foods rich in vitamin D (*see* **A healthy diet**, p.16) and increase your exposure to sunlight. If you have a disorder that prevents absorption of the vitamin from food, you may need to have vitamin D injections (*see* **Vitamins**, p.598). Calcium supplements (*see* **Minerals**, p.599) may also be required.

After treatment, most people make a full recovery, although deformities that occur in childhood may be permanent.

Paget's disease of the bone

A disorder of bone maintenance and repair, leading to weakened, distorted, and occasionally painful bones

 Rare under the age of 40; increasingly common over the age of 50

 More common in males

 Sometimes runs in families; rare in people of Asian or African origin

 Lifestyle is not a significant factor

In a healthy person, bone is continually being broken down and replaced by new bone to maintain the normal bone structure. However, in Paget's disease of the bone (also known as osteitis deformans), the processes involved in the normal breakdown and replacement of bone tissue become disrupted in some parts of the skeleton. The condition may affect any bone in the body, but the pelvis, collarbone, vertebrae (bones of the spine), skull, and leg bones are those most commonly involved. The affected bones become larger and structurally abnormal, which progressively weakens them and makes them more liable to fracture.

Paget's disease usually develops after the age of 50 and affects 1 in 10 people over the age of 80. The disorder tends to run in families and affects more men than women. Paget's disease is most common in Europe, North America, and Australia. It is rare in people of Asian or African origin.

What are the symptoms?
Frequently, Paget's disease produces no symptoms and may be diagnosed only by chance when an X-ray has been taken for some other reason. If symptoms are present, they may include:
■ Bone pain that is worse at night.
■ Joint pain, especially in those joints near affected bones.
■ Bone deformities, such as bow legs or enlargement of the skull.
■ Fractures (p.232) that occur after a minor injury.
Long-standing Paget's disease may also lead to the following complications:
■ Numbness, tingling, or weakness in the affected area if the bone presses on adjacent nerves.
■ Hearing loss.

In rare cases, a further complication of Paget's disease is the development of a type of bone cancer (*see* **Primary bone cancer**, p.220).

What might be done?
If your doctor suspects you have Paget's disease, he or she may arrange for you to have X-rays (p.131) to confirm the diagnosis. You may also have blood and urine tests to check for abnormal levels of substances involved in the formation and breakdown of bone. If your hearing is affected, you will probably have hearing tests (p.377).

Treatment is not necessary if you have no pain or other symptoms and are unlikely to be at risk of fractures. If you are in discomfort, your doctor will prescribe painkillers (p.589) or a nonsteroidal anti-inflammatory drug (p.578). If these drugs are inadequate then specific treatment may be needed. The most common treatment is with bisphosphonates, such as zoledronic acid; less commonly, the hormone calcitonin may be prescribed (*see* **Drugs for bone disorders**, p.579). Your response to these drugs may be monitored by blood tests.

Although drug treatment will not reverse any bone deformity that may have already developed, it will slow the progress of the disease.

Kyphosis and lordosis

Excessive outward curvature at the top of the spine (kyphosis) or inward curvature in the lower back (lordosis)

 Being overweight is a risk factor

 Age, gender, and genetics as risk factors depend on the cause

Viewed from the side, a normal spine has two main curves along its length. If you have kyphosis or lordosis, these natural curves may become exaggerated. In kyphosis, there is an excessive outward curve at the top of the back, which results in a rounded back, or "hunchback". Lordosis affects the spine in the lower back, leading to an exaggerated "hollow back". Kyphosis and lordosis often occur together, resulting in excessive curvature both at the top and in the small of the back.

If kyphosis occurs in childhood, the cause is often not known. In adults, disorders that limit mobility, such as osteoarthritis (p.221), or that weaken the vertebrae (bones of the spine), such as osteoporosis (p.217), are the most common causes of kyphosis. Poor posture may also lead to kyphosis.

Kyphosis often leads to lordosis because the lower spine compensates for the imbalance of the curve at the top of the spine. Lordosis may also develop in people with weak abdominal muscles and poor posture. People who are very

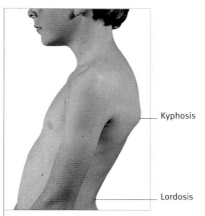

Kyphosis and lordosis
The child in this photograph has kyphosis, in which the back below the neck is curved out and rounded, and lordosis, in which the lower back is excessively hollow.

overweight are more likely to develop lordosis since they tend to lean backwards to improve their balance. Your doctor may advise you on ways to improve your posture. He or she will probably recommend that you avoid strenuous activity and lose any excess weight. Posture can be improved by physiotherapy (p.620), which strengthens the muscles supporting the spine.

People with abnormal curvature of the spine have a predisposition to other spinal problems in later life, such as a prolapsed or herniated disc (p.227).

Scoliosis

Abnormal curvature of the spine to the left or right

 More common in females

 Sometimes runs in families

 Age and lifestyle are not significant factors

The spine normally forms a straight, vertical line when viewed from the back. Scoliosis is an abnormal sideways curvature of the spine, most commonly affecting the spine in the chest area and the lower back region. Scoliosis is more common in females. Early diagnosis is important because, if left untreated, the deformity can become worse.

What are the causes?
In most cases, the cause of scoliosis is unknown. Genetic factors may be involved since the condition tends to run in families. In some cases, scoliosis is congenital (present from birth). Rarely, the curvature is the result of muscle weakness around the spine or due to a neuromuscular disease such as cerebral palsy (p.548) or poliomyelitis (p.168). Scoliosis may also be due to skeletal defects, such as unequal leg length. In rare cases, temporary scoliosis occurs as a result of muscle spasm following a spinal injury (p.323).

What are the symptoms?
Unless the condition is congenital or the result of a spinal injury, the symptoms develop gradually, usually during childhood or adolescence. The symptoms may include:
■ Visible curving of the spine to one side, which is more obvious when bending forwards.
■ Back pain.
■ Abnormal gait.
If scoliosis is severe, the ribcage may become deformed, sometimes leading to heart and lung problems.

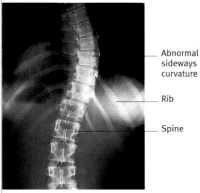

Scoliosis
In this X-ray, the upper spine curves to one side, a condition known as scoliosis. Left untreated, the curvature may increase.

What might be done?
The doctor will probably diagnose scoliosis from a physical examination and X-rays (p.131). If possible, treatment is aimed at the underlying condition. For example, if your legs are of unequal length, your doctor may recommend wearing corrective shoes.

If there is no underlying cause and the spinal curvature is slight, you will probably only need regular checkups to monitor your condition. If scoliosis is severe or is progressing rapidly, it may be necessary for you to wear a spinal brace to limit further curvature. Surgery may be necessary to fuse the affected vertebrae or to straighten the spine with metal rods and wires.

Coccydynia

Severe, sharp pain in the coccyx, the small triangular bone at the base of the spine

 Poor posture when sitting is a risk factor

 Age, gender, and genetics are not significant factors

Pain in the coccyx, or coccydynia, may be due to injury, a baby pushing against the mother's coccyx during birth, or prolonged pressure due to poor posture while sitting. Often, no cause is found.

Before making a diagnosis, your doctor may carry out a rectal examination to rule out a tumour in the rectum. Women may also have a vaginal examination to look for a tumour in the uterus. Your doctor

may also arrange for you to have an MRI scan (p.134) of the lower spine to look for signs of injury.

Coccydynia may be relieved with a painkiller (p.589) or a nonsteroidal anti-inflammatory drug (p.578). You may also be able to ease the pain by applying heat to the area with a heat pad or cold with an ice pack. A local injection with a corticosteroid drug (*see* **Locally acting corticosteroids**, p.578), often in combination with an anaesthetic, can sometimes provide relief. Usually no further treatment is necessary.

Osteomyelitis

Infection of bone, causing pain and damage to surrounding tissue

 Most common in young children and elderly people but can occur at any age

 Use of intravenous drugs is a risk factor

 Gender and genetics are not significant factors

Osteomyelitis is infection of bone, usually due to bacteria. The condition is most common in young children, but elderly people are also at risk. In other age groups, the condition is most common in people with reduced immunity, such as those with sickle-cell disease (p.272) or diabetes mellitus (p.437). In young children, the vertebrae (spinal bones) or one of the long bones of the limbs are usually affected. In adults, osteomyelitis most commonly affects the vertebrae or the pelvis.

What are the causes?
There are two forms of osteomyelitis: one that comes on suddenly (acute), and the other that develops more gradually and is long-term (chronic).

The acute form of osteomyelitis is usually a consequence of infection with *Staphylococcus aureus* bacteria. These bacteria normally live harmlessly on the skin but they can enter the bloodstream and result in osteomyelitis if they infect the bone tissue as a result of a wound, fracture (p.232), joint replacement (p.223), or intravenous injection with a contaminated needle.

The chronic form of osteomyelitis may be caused by tuberculosis (p.300) or, in rare cases, by a fungal infection. In some cases, acute osteomyelitis may develop into the chronic form.

What are the symptoms?
The symptoms of acute osteomyelitis develop suddenly and may include:
■ Swelling of the skin and severe pain in the affected area.
■ Fever.
■ In young children, not wanting to move an affected arm or leg.
Chronic osteomyelitis develops more slowly. Its symptoms include:
■ Weight loss.

■ Mild fever.
■ Persistent pain in the affected bone.
Pus may form in the bone and can make its way to the skin's surface, causing a discharging opening (a sinus).

How is it diagnosed?
If your doctor suspects that you have osteomyelitis, he or she may arrange for X-rays (p.131), radionuclide scanning (p.135), or MRI (p.133) to locate the infected area of bone. If pus is present, a sample may be aspirated (removed from the bone through a fine needle) for examination to identify the organism that is causing the disease.

What is the treatment?
Treatment with intravenous antibiotics (p.572) is usually begun in hospital and may continue after you return home. You may then need to continue taking antibiotics orally for a period of several months. When osteomyelitis is caused by tuberculosis, antituberculous drugs (p.573) may be prescribed for a period of 12–18 months.

In some cases, surgery may be necessary to remove infected bone. If a large area of bone is removed, you may need a bone graft, in which the infected bone is replaced by new bone taken from elsewhere in the body or from a donor. If the infection is associated with a joint replacement, the artificial joint will be removed, the infection treated, and a new joint put in its place.

The acute form of osteomyelitis is usually treated successfully, but the chronic form may take several months or years to clear up. In some cases, it may be necessary to take antibiotics indefinitely to suppress the infection.

Noncancerous bone tumours

Noncancerous growths that may cause pain and deformity in a bone

 Most common in childhood or adolescence; rare over the age of 40

 Gender, genetics, and lifestyle are not significant factors

Noncancerous bone tumours may occur in any part of a bone. These tumours develop most commonly in the long bones of the limbs, such as the femur (thighbone). The bones of the hands are another common site. Noncancerous bone tumours most often develop during childhood or adolescence. They are rare in people over the age of 40.

Although the presence of a tumour normally causes no symptoms, sometimes there may be pain in the affected area, or the bone may become enlarged and deformed. Affected bone is more likely to fracture from even a minor injury. Occasionally, a tumour may press on nerves, causing a tingling sensation or numbness. In some cases, movement may be restricted,

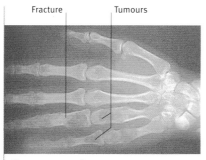

Fracture   Tumours

Noncancerous bone tumours
This X-ray shows several noncancerous tumours in the bones of the fingers. Some bones have become enlarged as a result of the tumours, and one has a fracture.

or pain may be felt on movement if the tumour presses on nearby tendons (fibrous bands that connect muscles to bones).

A bone tumour is usually diagnosed from X-rays (p.131), MRI (p.133), or radionuclide scanning (p.135). To confirm that the tumour is noncancerous, your doctor may arrange for a biopsy of the bone, in which a small piece of the affected bone is removed for analysis.

A tumour may be removed surgically if it is painful, causes deformity of the bone, or grows rapidly. You may subsequently need a bone graft, in which artificial bone or bone taken from elsewhere in your body or from a donor is used. Generally, surgery is successful in removing noncancerous tumours, although occasionally these recur and may require further surgery.

Primary bone cancer

Cancerous tumours that originate within the bone tissue

 Most common in childhood and adolescence

 Sometimes runs in families

 Gender and lifestyle are not significant factors

Cancers originating in bone, known as primary bone cancers, are rare. They usually develop in children and teenagers. The causes are unknown, but some cases are associated with genetic factors. The most common site of primary bone cancer is the leg, either just above or just below the knee.

The first symptom is often painful, tender swelling of the affected area. If the cancer affects a bone in the leg, you may experience pain on standing or while you are at rest, and the pain may become worse at night. The diseased bone may fracture easily.

What might be done?
To confirm the diagnosis, your doctor will probably arrange for you to have X-rays (p.131) and possibly CT scanning (p.132) or MRI (p.133). He or she may also arrange for you to have chest X-rays (p.300) and radionuclide scanning (p.135) to check if the cancer has spread to other parts of the body.

Radiotherapy (p.158) may reduce the size of the tumour. However, in most cases the tumour is removed surgically. Removed bone is replaced by artificial bone or by bone taken from elsewhere in the body or from a donor.

Following surgery, radiotherapy or chemotherapy (p.157) may be given to destroy any remaining cancerous cells. Amputation of a limb is rarely necessary. Most people treated for primary bone cancer have only a small chance of recurrence in the first 5 years. After this period, recurrence is unlikely.

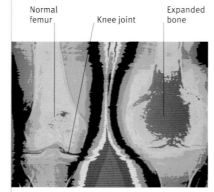

Normal femur   Knee joint   Expanded bone

Primary bone cancer in the leg
This colour-enhanced CT scan of both legs reveals a primary bone cancer of one femur (thighbone) and associated swelling.

Bone metastases

Cancerous tumours in bone that have spread from a cancer elsewhere in the body

 More common in elderly people

 Risk factors depend on the type

 Gender and lifestyle are not significant factors

Bone metastases, also known as secondary bone cancer, are tumours that have spread from another part of the body. Metastases most often develop in the ribs, pelvis, skull, or spine. The condition occurs much more commonly than primary bone cancer, especially in older people, who are more likely to have cancer elsewhere in their body. The cancers that most often spread to bone are those originating in the breast, the lung, the thyroid gland, the kidney, and the prostate gland.

What are the symptoms?
Bone metastases may cause the following symptoms in addition to those of the main cancer:
- Gnawing bone pain that may become worse at night.
- Swelling of the affected area.
- Tenderness over the affected area.

The affected bones fracture easily, often after minor injury.

What might be done?
If you already have a cancer somewhere else in your body, you may have X-rays (p.131) or radionuclide scanning (p.135)

to check whether the cancer has spread to the bones. If the site of the primary cancer is unknown, you may need further tests to find out where the metastasis came from. For example, women may have a breast X-ray (*see* **Mammography**, p.487) to look for evidence of breast cancer.

Your doctor will probably direct treatment at your original cancer. He or she may also make arrangements for

you to have a course of chemotherapy (p.157), radiotherapy (p.158), or hormonal therapy to relieve bone pain.

The outlook for people with bone metastases usually depends on the site of the original cancer and how successfully it can be treated. However, the best that can usually be achieved after bone metastases is a period of remission.

Joint and ligament disorders

Joints occur where bones meet, and they allow our bodies to be flexible. Lubricated tissue called cartilage lines the ends of bones and prevents friction during movement, and fibrous ligaments surrounding the joint give strength and support. Joints may be damaged by arthritis, injury, infection, or degeneration of bone, cartilage, and ligaments caused by aging or disease.

Joint disorders are a significant cause of disability and immobility, but the treatment of long-term joint disorders has greatly improved in recent years, due partly to the availability of safe, reliable artificial joints and partly to new medications for some forms of arthritis.

The first article describes the many types of arthritis, a general term for disease of one or more joints. This is followed by separate articles on the most common types, including osteoarthritis, rheumatoid arthritis, gout, and reactive arthritis. Septic arthritis, which in the past was a major cause of crippling joint disease, is now usually curable with antibiotics. Next in this section is a detailed look at lower back pain, together with self-help measures to help prevent it. The section ends with articles on nonarthritic conditions such as bursitis, in which the fluid-filled cushions around the joints become swollen and inflamed.

There is a similar but distinct form of rheumatoid arthritis that can develop in children (*see* **Juvenile chronic arthritis**, p.541).

KEY ANATOMY

Ligament   Bone

Synovial membrane

Articular cartilage   Synovial fluid

For more information on the structure and function of joints and ligaments, *see* pp.213–214.

Arthritis

Pain, inflammation, and stiffness in one or more joints

 Age, gender, genetics, and lifestyle as risk factors depend on the type

The term arthritis covers a group of inflammatory and degenerative conditions that cause stiffness, swelling, and pain in the joints. Arthritis may also be linked with disorders such as psoriasis (p.192) and Crohn's disease (p.417).

What are the types?
There are several different types of arthritis, each having different characteristics. The most common form is

osteoarthritis (opposite page), which most often involves the knees, hips, and hands and usually affects middle-aged and older people. Cervical spondylosis (p.222) is a form of osteoarthritis that affects the joints in the neck.

Rheumatoid arthritis (p.222) is a damaging condition that causes inflammation in the joints and in other body tissues, such as the membranous heart covering, lungs, and eyes. The disorder has different effects in children (*see* **Juvenile chronic arthritis**, p.541). Ankylosing spondylitis (p.223) is a chronic form of arthritis that initially affects the spine and the joints between the base of the spine and the pelvis. Other tissues, such as the eyes, may also be affected. The disorder may eventually cause the vertebrae to fuse.

Reactive arthritis (p.224) typically develops in susceptible people after they have had an infection, most commonly of the genital tract or intestines. Reactive arthritis most often causes inflammation in an ankle or a knee.

Both gout (p.224) and pseudogout (p.225) are types of arthritis in which crystals are deposited in a joint, resulting in swelling and pain.

Septic arthritis (p.225) is a relatively rare condition that can develop when infection enters a joint either through a wound or from the bloodstream.

Treatment depends on the type of arthritis. Painkillers (p.589), such as paracetamol, and nonsteroidal anti-inflammatory drugs (p.578) may relieve symptoms. Physiotherapy (p.620) may keep joints mobile and strengthen surrounding muscles. Severely damaged joints may be replaced surgically (see Joint replacement, p.223).

Osteoarthritis

Gradual degeneration of the cartilage covering the bone ends within joints

 Rare under the age of 45; increasingly common over the age of 60

 Twice as common in females

 Sometimes runs in families

 Past injuries and being overweight are risk factors

In a joint affected by osteoarthritis, the protective cartilage found at the ends of bones is worn away. As the condition develops, the bone around the affected joint thickens, and bony growths called osteophytes form. If the synovial tissue that lines the joint capsule becomes inflamed, fluid may accumulate within the joint. These changes cause pain, swelling, and stiffness of the joints, reducing their mobility.

Osteoarthritis is most common in weight-bearing joints, such as the knees and hips. However, the hands, feet, and shoulders may also be affected, as may the bones of the neck (see Cervical spondylosis, p.222). Nearly everyone has developed a degree of osteoarthritis by the age of 70, but only some people have symptoms. Women are more commonly affected by osteoarthritis than men, and their symptoms are more severe. This form of arthritis sometimes develops in younger people, particularly in those who have had joint injuries.

What are the causes?

There is often no obvious cause for the onset of osteoarthritis, but there are known factors that may increase the risk of developing the disorder. Wear occurs most often in joints that have been damaged by repeated strenuous activity or by repeated minor injuries. For example, the pressure that ballet dancers exert on their feet makes them susceptible to developing osteoarthritis of the ankle. Osteoarthritis is also common in former athletes.

Damage to a joint early in life may lead to osteoarthritis later on. Excessive weight can also increase a person's risk of developing the condition because of the extra stress it places on the joints. Another risk factor is damage to cartilage caused by another joint disorder, such as septic arthritis (p.225). Finally, if a close member of your family has osteoarthritis, you are more likely to develop the condition yourself.

What are the symptoms?

Initially, the symptoms are mild, but they may slowly get worse. Often only one or

---

▶ SELF-HELP

Living with arthritis

If you have long-term arthritis, you may be able to manage your symptoms so that you can maintain an active lifestyle. Consult your doctor about pain relief and keeping joints mobile. Organizations concerned with arthritis can also provide you with valuable information and support.

Mobility

Gentle, regular exercise helps to relieve stiffness and improve mobility. Physical activity also helps to strengthen the muscles that support joints. However, if exercise causes swelling or pain, stop the activity and consult your doctor.

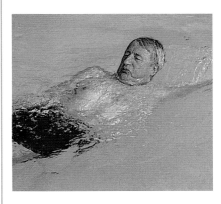

Exercising
Regular swimming is an ideal sport for maintaining your joint flexibility and stamina. Since the water supports your body, muscles can be exercised without straining your joints.

Pain relief

To relieve severe joint pain, apply heat or cold to the affected area. Heat increases blood flow, and cold helps to reduce swelling. Both decrease sensitivity to pain.

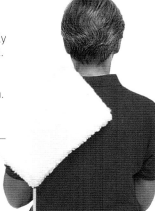

Electric heat pad

Using a heat pad
You can use a heat pad to provide a steady supply of heat to an aching joint.

Specialized equipment

Your doctor or a physiotherapist may be able to suggest specially adapted pieces of equipment to help you with household tasks. The equipment may have particular features, such as handles that are easy to grip or extending arms to help you reach objects without bending down.

Eating and drinking
If arthritis restricts the movement in your hands, use cutlery with thick handles and glasses with wide stems that will be easier to grip. A plate with a rim may keep food from spilling, and a nonslip mat will help to hold your plate still during a meal.

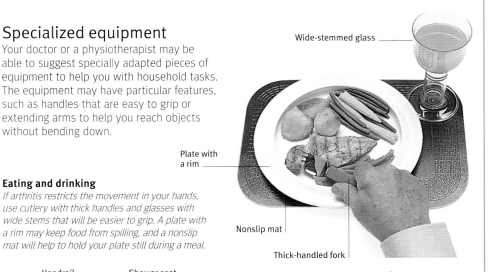

Wide-stemmed glass

Plate with a rim

Nonslip mat

Thick-handled fork

Handrail   Shower seat

Taking a shower
A fixed seat in the shower cubicle allows you to sit down while you wash. Handrails and a nonslip floor surface reduce the risk of falls.

Picking up objects
Tongs enable you to pick up objects that are out of your reach without bending or stretching. Some types of tongs have a trigger mechanism that operates pincers at the end of the arm.

Trigger mechanism

Arm

Pincers

two joints are badly affected, but sometimes osteoarthritis is more widespread. The symptoms may include:
- Pain and tenderness that worsen with activity and are relieved by rest.
- Swelling around the joint.
- Stiffness lasting a short time after a period of inactivity.
- Restricted joint movement.
- Enlarged, distorted finger joints if the hands are affected.
- Crackling noise (called crepitus) on moving the affected joint.

Referred pain, which is felt in areas remote from the site of damage but on the same nerve pathway as the affected joint, may develop. For example, an arthritic hip may cause referred pain in the knee. The pain may become worse towards the end of the day.

If movement is severely restricted, an affected person may be confined to the home. Lack of mobility may lead to weakness and wasting of muscles and sometimes to weight gain.

What might the doctor do?
Your doctor may suspect that you have osteoarthritis from your symptoms, a history of joint problems, and a physical examination. It is often possible to confirm a diagnosis of osteoarthritis, while at the same time ruling out other types of arthritis, by means of blood tests and X-rays (p.131).

Osteoarthritis cannot be cured, but with treatment most symptoms can be relieved. Your doctor may recommend that you take painkillers (p.589), such as paracetamol, or a nonsteroidal anti-inflammatory drug (p.578). If you experience a severe flare-up of pain and inflammation in a single joint, your doctor may inject a corticosteroid drug directly into the affected joint in order to reduce the swelling and relieve pain (see **Locally acting corticosteroids**, p.578).

To improve muscle function around joints affected by osteoarthritis, your doctor may refer you for physiotherapy (p.620). If osteoarthritis is very severe, surgery may be necessary to repair or replace an affected joint (see **Joint replacement**, opposite page).

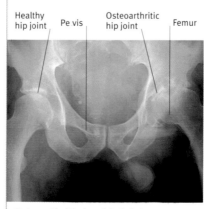

Osteoarthritis in a hip joint
In the hip joint seen on the right of this X-ray, the head of the femur (thighbone) has become worn where it fits into the pelvis, causing pain and stiffness.

What can I do?
If you have mild osteoarthritis, you may be able to participate in most everyday activities by adapting your lifestyle (see **Living with arthritis**, p.221). If you are overweight, ask your doctor for dietary advice to enable you to lose weight and reduce further wear on your joints. If possible, take gentle exercise to help to lose weight, maintain muscle tone, and delay the progression of the disease. Supportive shoes with rubber soles will absorb shock and reduce further wear. If you have a painful hip or knee, use a walking stick for support. Massage, warm baths, or a heat pad may ease joint pain and increase mobility.

Cervical spondylosis

A disease of bones and cartilage in the neck, which may lead to pain and stiffness

 Increasingly common over the age of 45

 More common in males

 Genetics and lifestyle are not significant factors

Cervical spondylosis is osteoarthritis (p.221) affecting the upper spine. In this disorder, the vertebrae (bones of the spine) and the discs of cartilage between them begin to show signs of disease. The bones thicken, and bony outgrowths called osteophytes develop on the vertebrae. Inflamed joints and osteophytes may press on spinal nerves or compress blood vessels in the neck.

The condition is increasingly common over the age of 45 and affects more men than women. Rarely, it is triggered by injury and affects younger people.

What are the symptoms?
Many people do not have symptoms or may develop only very mild symptoms. When symptoms do become apparent, they may include:
- Restricted neck movement that may be painful.
- Pain at the back of the head.
- Aching or shooting pain that travels from the shoulders to the hands.
- Numbness, tingling, and muscle weakness in the hands and arms.

Sometimes, if the head is moved too quickly, the deformities in the upper spine may suddenly compress blood vessels that carry blood to the brain, resulting in dizziness, unsteadiness, or double vision (see **Vertigo**, p.379).

In rare cases, joints that have severely degenerated may put prolonged pressure on the spinal cord, causing tingling and muscle weakness or paralysis in the legs or, sometimes, difficulty controlling bladder or bowel function. Such cases require emergency medical treatment.

How is it diagnosed?
Some people may not have symptoms and cervical spondylosis may be recognized only when an X-ray (p.131) is taken for another reason. However, if you experience neck pain or dizziness, consult your doctor, who may arrange for X-rays to look for signs of cervical spondylosis. If your doctor thinks that your symptoms may not be due solely to cervical spondylosis, he or she may arrange further tests to look for other causes, such as a prolapsed or herniated disc (p.227). You may also undergo nerve conduction studies and EMG (see **Nerve and muscle electrical tests**, p.337) to assess nerve activity in your arms and hands. CT scanning (p.132) or MRI (p.133) may also be carried out to see if there have been any changes affecting the bones, discs of cartilage, or tissues of the spine.

What is the treatment?
Changes in the spine are not inevitably progressive. There may be little deterioration for many years, and sometimes symptoms improve. To relieve symptoms in mild cases, your doctor may recommend painkillers (p.589) or prescribe nonsteroidal anti-inflammatory drugs (p.578). Once the initial pain has been relieved, the doctor may also suggest some simple exercises to maintain mobility and increase the strength of muscles in your neck.

If cervical spondylosis has damaged a nerve, surgery may be recommended to prevent the symptoms from getting worse. In this operation, the surgeon widens the natural opening between the vertebrae through which the nerve passes when it branches off the spinal cord. In a few rare cases, surgery may also be carried out to stabilize the spine by fusing together affected vertebrae.

Rheumatoid arthritis

A chronic disorder that can cause the joints to become painful, swollen, stiff, and deformed

 Most common over the age of 40

 Three times more common in females

 May run in some families

 Lifestyle is not a significant factor

In rheumatoid arthritis, the affected joints become stiff and swollen as a result of inflammation of the synovial membrane, which encloses each joint. If the inflammation persists, it may damage both the ends of the bones and the cartilage that covers them. Tendons and ligaments, which support the joints, may also become worn and slack, and deformity of the joints occurs.

In most cases, rheumatoid arthritis affects several joints. The disorder usually appears first in the small joints of the hands and feet but may develop in any joint. It usually tends to appear in similar areas on both sides of the body. Tissues in other parts of the body, such as the eyes, the lungs, the membranous sac around the heart, and blood vessels, may also be affected by the inflammation.

Rheumatoid arthritis is a chronic disease and usually recurs in episodes lasting for several weeks or months with relatively symptom-free periods in between. The disorder affects about 1 in 100 people and is three times more common in women than in men. A similar but distinct arthritic disorder can develop in children (see **Juvenile chronic arthritis**, p.541).

Rheumatoid arthritis is an autoimmune disorder (p.280) in which the body produces antibodies that attack the synovial membrane and, in some cases, other body tissues. Genetic factors may be involved since the condition is common in some families.

What are the symptoms?
Rheumatoid arthritis usually develops slowly, although sometimes the onset of the inflammation can be abrupt. General symptoms associated with the condition may include tiredness, poor appetite, and loss of weight. Specific symptoms may include:
- Painful, swollen joints that are stiff on waking in the morning.
- Painless, small bumps (nodules) on areas of pressure, such as the elbows.

Since the condition can be both painful and debilitating, depression (p.343) is common in people with rheumatoid arthritis. In women, the symptoms of rheumatoid arthritis may improve during pregnancy but may then flare up again after the baby is born.

Are there complications?
Over time, thinning of the bones (see **Osteoporosis**, p.217) and a greater susceptibility to fractures may develop in people with rheumatoid arthritis. This results partly from the disease itself and partly from reduced mobility.

The general symptoms of rheumatoid arthritis are partly due to anaemia (p.271), caused by a failure of the bone marrow to manufacture enough new red blood cells. Bursitis (p.229) may develop, in which one or more of the fluid-filled sacs around a joint become inflamed. Swelling that compresses the median nerve in the wrist may lead to a tingling feeling and pain in the fingers (see **Carpal tunnel syndrome**, p.338). Spasm or narrowing of the walls of the arteries that supply the fingers and toes results in Raynaud's phenomenon (p.262), in which the digits become pale and painful on exposure to cold.

A less common complication is when the spleen and the lymph nodes enlarge (see **Lymphadenopathy**, p.279). Inflammation may affect the membranous sac that surrounds the heart (see **Pericarditis**, p.258) and also the lungs (see **Pulmonary fibrosis**, p.304). In some cases, there may

▶ **TREATMENT**

Joint replacement

Joints that have been severely damaged by a disorder such as arthritis or by an injury may be surgically replaced with artificial joints made of metal, ceramic, or plastic. The joints that are most commonly replaced are the hips, knees, and shoulders; ankle, elbow, and wrist joints, and small joints in the hands and feet, are also routinely replaced. During the operation, the ends of damaged bones are removed and the artificial components are fixed in place. The operation usually relieves pain and increases the range of movement in the affected joint, and is often associated with significant improvement in the quality of life.

Hip replacement

The most commonly replaced joint in the body is the hip. During the operation, both the pelvic socket and the head of the femur (thighbone), which fits into the socket, are replaced. The operation is carried out under general anaesthesia and involves a short stay in hospital.

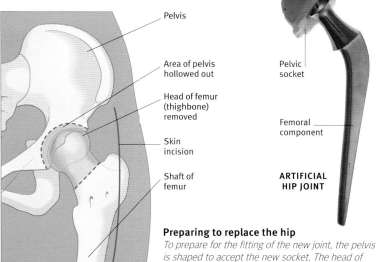

Pelvis

Area of pelvis hollowed out

Head of femur (thighbone) removed

Skin incision

Shaft of femur

Pelvic socket

Femoral component

ARTIFICIAL HIP JOINT

Preparing to replace the hip
To prepare for the fitting of the new joint, the pelvis is shaped to accept the new socket. The head of the femur is removed, and the centre of the bone shaped to fit the femoral component.

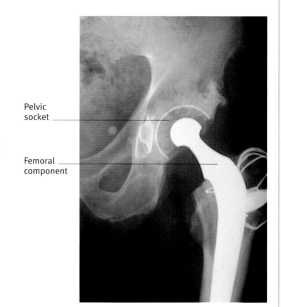

Pelvic socket

Femoral component

Artificial hip in position
This X-ray shows an artificial hip joint in place, with the femoral component fitted into the femur (thighbone) and the socket fitted into the pelvis.

Other joints

Many different types of joint in the body can be replaced, from tiny finger joints to large joints such as the knees.

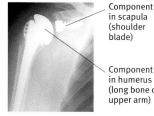

Component in scapula (shoulder blade)

Component in humerus (long bone of upper arm)

Artificial shoulder joint
This replacement shoulder joint has components fitted in the humerus and the scapula.

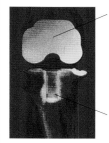

Component in femur (thighbone)

Component in tibia (shinbone)

Artificial knee joint
This replacement knee joint has artificial components fitted both in the femur (thighbone) and in the tibia (shinbone).

---

be inflammation of the white of the eye (*see* Scleritis, p.357), or the eyes may become very dry (*see* Sjögren's syndrome, p.281).

How is it diagnosed?
The diagnosis is usually based on your medical history and a physical examination. Your doctor may arrange for blood tests to check for the presence of antibodies known as rheumatoid factors or anti-CCP, which are usually associated with rheumatoid arthritis. You may also have blood tests to measure the severity of the inflammation. X-rays (p.131) of the affected joints may be taken to assess the degree of damage.

What is the treatment?
There is no cure for rheumatoid arthritis. The aim of treatment is to control symptoms and limit further joint damage by slowing the progression of the disease.

In most cases, rheumatoid arthritis is treated with disease-modifying antirheumatic drugs (DMARDs), which are started as soon as possible after diagnosis (*see* Antirheumatic drugs, p.579). These drugs modify the disease process of rheumatoid arthritis, which leads to a reduction in symptoms and can also limit further joint damage. Treatment with DMARDs is started under specialist supervision, and before you are prescribed the drugs you may have tests to

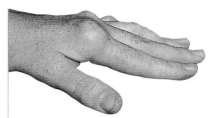

Swelling in rheumatoid arthritis
The swollen knuckles of this hand are caused by rheumatoid arthritis, a condition in which the joints become inflamed and may be damaged.

check whether any specific drug is unsuitable for you. DMARDs may have to be taken for several months before the full benefits are felt and therefore you may be prescribed painkillers (p.589), nonsteroidal anti-inflammatory drugs (p.578) and/or corticosteroids (p.600) to relieve symptoms in the interim, and also to control any later flare-ups of symptoms. DMARDs can sometimes cause serious side effects, such as kidney, liver, blood, or eye problems, so the doctor will closely monitor your condition. If DMARDs alone are ineffective, you may also be prescribed biological therapy with drugs such as etanercept, infliximab, or adalimumab. These medications are usually prescribed in addition to DMARDs and, like DMARDs, modify the disease process to reduce symptoms.

In addition to medication, your doctor may also advise you to use a splint or brace to support a particularly painful joint and to slow down the development of deformities. Gentle, regular exercise may help to keep your joints flexible and prevent supporting muscles from weakening. Physiotherapy (p.620) may be given to improve joint mobility and help increase muscle strength. Hydrotherapy and heat or ice treatments may provide pain relief.

An intensely painful joint may be eased if your doctor injects it with a corticosteroid drug (*see* Locally acting corticosteroids, p.578). If a joint is severely damaged, surgery to replace the damaged joint with an artificial one (*see* Joint replacement, above) or to fuse the joint may be suggested.

What is the prognosis?
Many people with rheumatoid arthritis are able to lead a near-normal life (*see* Living with arthritis, p.221), but lifelong drug treatment may be needed to control the symptoms. About 1 in 10 people becomes severely disabled as repeated attacks destroy the joints. To monitor progression of the disease and your response to treatment, regular blood tests will be needed. Sometimes, the attacks gradually cease, and the disease is said to have burned itself out, but some disability may remain.

Ankylosing spondylitis

Persistent inflammation and stiffening of the joints, usually affecting the spine and pelvis

 Usually begins in late adolescence or early adulthood; onset rare over the age of 45

 About three times more common in males

 Sometimes runs in families

 Lifestyle is not a significant factor

In ankylosing spondylitis, persistent joint inflammation affects the sacroiliac joints (the joints between the spine and back of the pelvis) and the vertebrae (bones of the spine) in particular. If the spine is severely diseased, new bone grows between the vertebrae, which eventually fuse together. In some cases, ankylosing spondylitis may also affect other joints, such as the hips.

This form of arthritis is about three times more common in men than in women. A variant of ankylosing spondylitis is associated, in some cases, with the persistent skin disorder psoriasis (p.192) or with inflammatory bowel disease, such as Crohn's disease (p.417).

What are the causes?

The cause of ankylosing spondylitis is unknown, but about 9 in 10 affected people have a particular antigen (a substance capable of stimulating an immune response) called HLA-B27 on the surface of most cells. This antigen is inherited, which helps to explain why ankylosing spondylitis runs in some families. Most people with HLA-B27 do not develop the condition, and a bacterial infection is thought to trigger ankylosing spondylitis in those who are predisposed.

What are the symptoms?

Symptoms usually appear in late adolescence or early adulthood and develop gradually over a period of months or even years. Men are usually more severely affected. The main symptoms include:

■ Lower back pain, which may spread down into the buttocks and thighs.
■ Lower back stiffness that may be worse in the morning and improves with exercise.
■ Pain in other joints, such as the hips, knees, and shoulders.
■ Pain and tenderness in the heels.
■ Tiredness, weight loss, and mild fever.

If left untreated, ankylosing spondylitis can distort the spine (see **Kyphosis and lordosis**, p.218), resulting in a stooped posture. If the joints between the spine and the ribs are affected, expansion of the chest becomes restricted. In some people, ankylosing spondylitis causes inflammation or damage to tissues in areas other than the joints, such as the eyes (see **Uveitis**, p.357).

How is it diagnosed?

Your doctor may suspect that you have ankylosing spondylitis from the pattern of your symptoms. He or she will perform a physical examination and may arrange for an X-ray (p.131) to look for evidence of fusion in the joints of the pelvis and the spine. Your doctor may also arrange for you to have blood tests to measure the level of inflammation and look for the HLA-B27 antigen.

What is the treatment?

Treatment of ankylosing spondylitis is aimed at relieving symptoms and preventing the development of spinal deformity. Your doctor may prescribe a painkiller (p.589), such as a nonsteroidal anti-inflammatory drug (p.578), to control pain and inflammation. Occasionally, a short course of oral corticosteroids (p.600) may be prescribed for short-term relief of symptoms, and injection of a corticosteroid into a severely affected joint may sometimes be given to ease pain in the joint. In severe cases, drugs such as infliximab or adalimumab may be given. These work by inhibiting a natural chemical called tumour necrosis factor-alpha that promotes inflammation. If joints other than those in the spine are affected, disease-modifying antirheumatic drugs (DMARDS, see **Antirheumatic drugs**, p.579) may be prescribed to relieve pain and inflammation.

In addition to medication, your doctor may refer you for physiotherapy (p.620), which may include breathing exercises and exercises to help improve your posture, strengthen the back muscles, and prevent deformities of the spine (see **Preventing back pain**, p.226). You may also benefit from regular physical activity, such as swimming, which may help to relieve pain and stiffness. If a joint such as a hip is affected, you may eventually need to have it replaced surgically (see **Joint replacement**, p.223). If your mobility is severely reduced, you may need occupational therapy (p.621). The therapist may suggest using specially designed equipment and furniture to make your life easier.

What is the prognosis?

Ankylosing spondylitis is not curable, but most people with the condition are only mildly affected. In many cases, early treatment and regular exercise help to relieve pain and stiffness of the back and prevent deformity of the spine. However, about 1 in 20 people with ankylosing spondylitis may eventually become disabled and have difficulty in carrying out many routine activities.

Reactive arthritis

Inflammation of joints as a result of an abnormal immune response to a recent infection elsewhere in the body

 Most common between the ages of 20 and 40

 More common in males

 Sometimes runs in families

 Lifestyle as a risk factor depends on the cause

Reactive arthritis is usually a short-term disorder that develops after a bacterial infection of the genital tract, such as chlamydial infection (p.492) or nongonococcal urethritis (p.491), or the intestinal tract (see **Gastroenteritis**, p.398). Any of these infections may stimulate an abnormal immune response that causes tissues in the joints, usually the knee or ankle, to become inflamed.

About 8 in 10 people who develop reactive arthritis have a particular antigen (a substance capable of stimulating an immune response in the body) known as HLA-B27. Although reactive arthritis is induced by infection, it usually develops in people who have a genetic predisposition to the condition. The disorder may therefore run in families.

What are the symptoms?

Depending on the infection that has triggered reactive arthritis, you may experience symptoms of a genital infection, such as pain on passing urine, or symptoms of gastroenteritis, such as diarrhoea. However, some people have no initial symptoms.

Reactive arthritis typically develops 3–30 days after the initial infection. The symptoms may include:

■ Painful, red, tender joints.
■ Swelling around the joints.

Although the knees or ankles are most commonly affected, other joints may also be involved. In addition to symptoms affecting the joints, you may also develop:

■ Sore, red eyes (see **Conjunctivitis**, p.355, and **Uveitis**, p.357).
■ Pain on passing urine and a discharge from the penis or vagina.

Less commonly, complications such as mouth ulcers (p.401), inflammation of the penis (see **Balanitis**, p.461), lower back pain (opposite page), and skin lesions on the hands and feet may develop.

What might be done?

Your doctor may diagnose reactive arthritis from your medical history and symptoms. He or she will probably take swabs from your urethra or cervix or collect a stool sample to try to establish the source of infection. Further tests may include a blood test to detect signs of inflammation and an X-ray (p.131) to look for joint damage.

If you are still affected by a genital or intestinal infection, your doctor may prescribe oral antibiotics (p.572). To relieve pain in your joints, he or she may recommend a nonsteroidal anti-inflammatory drug (p.578). If the pain is very severe and there is no infection present in the joint itself, you may be given a corticosteroid drug, injected directly into the joint (see **Locally acting corticosteroids**, p.578). If symptoms persist despite these treatments, you may be prescribed a disease-modifying antirheumatic drug (see **Antirheumatic drugs**, p.579).

What is the prognosis?

The symptoms of reactive arthritis usually last for less than 6 months, and most people make a full recovery. However, some people continue to have symptoms for a year or longer, and a few have long-term joint problems. The condition may also recur after another infection.

Gout

A type of arthritis in which crystalline deposits of uric acid form within joints, particularly at the base of the big toe

 Most common between the ages of 30 and 60

 Twenty times more common in males

 Often runs in families

 Being overweight and excessive intake of alcohol are risk factors

Gout causes sudden pain and inflammation, usually in a single joint. The base of the big toe is the most common site, but any joint may be affected. The disorder affects many more men than women. In women, gout rarely appears before the menopause.

What are the causes?

An attack of gout is usually caused by raised blood levels of uric acid (a waste product of the breakdown of cells and proteins). An excess of uric acid may be caused by the overproduction and/or decreased excretion of uric acid and may lead to uric acid crystals being deposited in a joint. The underlying cause of gout is unknown, but the condition is often inherited. A few people with gout also develop kidney stones (p.447) formed from excess uric acid.

Gout may occur spontaneously or be triggered by surgery, being overweight, drinking alcohol, treatment with diuretics (p.583), or excess cell destruction associated with chemotherapy (p.157).

What are the symptoms?

The symptoms of gout usually flare up suddenly. They may include:

■ Redness, tenderness, swelling, and warmth around the affected area.
■ Pain, which may be severe, in the affected joint or joints.
■ Mild fever.

In long-standing gout, deposits of uric acid crystals may collect in the earlobes and the soft tissues of the hands or feet, forming small lumps called tophi.

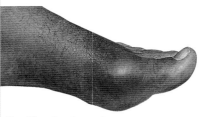

Swelling due to gout
As a result of an attack of gout, in which uric acid crystals form in a joint, the joint at the base of this big toe has become painful and swollen.

What might be done?

Your doctor may suspect that you have gout from your symptoms and arrange for blood tests to measure your uric acid levels. To confirm the diagnosis, he or she may arrange for you to have a joint aspiration (opposite page), in which fluid is withdrawn from the affected joint and examined for uric acid crystals.

Gout may subside by itself after a few days. To reduce severe pain and inflammation, you may be treated with a nonsteroidal anti-inflammatory drug (p.578), with colchicine, or with oral corticosteroids (p.600). If gout persists, your doctor may give you a corticosteroid injection directly into the affected joint (see **Locally acting corticosteroids**, p.578).

If you have recurring gout, you may need lifelong treatment with drugs to reduce the production of uric acid (such as allopurinol), or to increase the excretion of uric acid (such as benzbromarone).

To reduce the likelihood of attacks, your doctor may recommend lifestyle changes, such as reducing alcohol consumption and avoiding foods that can trigger attacks, such as offal, yeast extracts, and meat extracts. You may be able to reduce the frequency and severity of attacks by losing excess weight (see **Controlling your weight**, p.19).

Gout is painful and can disrupt normal activities, but attacks can usually be controlled with drugs and changes in lifestyle. Repeated attacks may damage the joint.

Pseudogout

A type of arthritis in which crystals of calcium pyrophosphate or other chemicals are deposited in joints

 Usually develops after the age of 60; more common with increasing age

 More common in females

 Sometimes runs in families

 Lifestyle is not a significant factor

In pseudogout, crystals of calcium pyrophosphate or similar chemicals are deposited in joints, causing attacks of pain and stiffness. Usually, a single joint is affected. The most common sites are the knee and wrist, but crystals may be deposited in any joint. Although the process of formation and deposition of the crystals may start earlier, symptoms are less common before the age of 60.

In most people, the cause of pseudogout is unknown, although attacks may be triggered by surgery, infection, or injury. Pseudogout is often associated with other joint disorders, particularly osteoarthritis (p.221). Pseudogout may also be linked to hyperparathyroidism (p.434), a hormonal condition that leads to high blood levels of calcium, or haemochromatosis (p.441), a disorder in which the body is overloaded with iron. Pseudogout is more common in women and may run in families.

What are the symptoms?

Symptoms are similar to those of gout (opposite page). Attacks may cause:
■ Severe pain, stiffness, swelling, and redness of the affected joint.
■ Mild fever.
Some people have no pain between attacks, while others experience persistent pain and stiffness.

What might be done?

If your doctor suspects pseudogout, he or she may arrange for X-rays (p.131) of the affected joint. You may also need joint aspiration (right), in which fluid is removed from a joint for analysis and to relieve swelling.

The symptoms of pseudogout may be relieved by simply removing fluid from the affected joint. In severe cases, a corticosteroid drug may be injected directly into the joint during the same procedure (*see* **Locally acting corticosteroids**, p.578). You may also need nonsteroidal anti-inflammatory drugs (p.578). Once treatment starts, symptoms usually clear up within 48 hours.

There is no cure for pseudogout, but if the underlying cause is treated many people can lead normal lives. Physiotherapy (p.620) can help to increase joint mobility and muscle strength.

Septic arthritis

A type of arthritis resulting from infection of a joint

 Most common in children and elderly people

 Intravenous drug use is a risk factor

 Gender and genetics are not significant factors

Septic arthritis is an infection in the synovial fluid or tissues of a joint, such as a hip or a knee. The condition is usually caused by bacteria that have entered the joint through a nearby open wound or have travelled through the bloodstream from an infection elsewhere in the body. For example, the bacteria that cause gonorrhoea (p.491) may spread from the genital tract through the bloodstream. The risk of developing septic arthritis is increased in people who have rheumatoid arthritis (p.222), who have been fitted with an artificial joint, or who use intravenous recreational drugs.

What are the symptoms?

The symptoms of septic arthritis usually appear suddenly and may include:
■ Fever.
■ Swelling, tenderness, redness, and warmth around the affected joint.
■ Severe pain and restricted movement of the affected joint.
If pus builds up in an infected area, the joint may be damaged permanently. If you develop the above symptoms, consult your doctor immediately.

What might be done?

Your doctor may arrange for you to have a sample of fluid taken from the affected joint (*see* **Joint aspiration**, below). The fluid is analysed to look for evidence of infection and to try to establish its cause.

Septic arthritis caused by bacteria is initially treated with intravenous antibiotics (p.572) for at least 4 weeks. Your doctor may then prescribe oral antibiotics for several weeks or months.

To help to relieve pain and inflammation, pus may be drained from the infected joint several times. Your doctor may also prescribe a nonsteroidal anti-inflammatory drug (p.578). You should rest the joint until the inflammation has completely subsided. Gentle movement is allowed and is important later on to prevent the joint becoming stiffened by shrinkage of the surrounding tissues. If the infected joint is an artificial joint, it may need to be replaced with a new one.

What is the prognosis?

If treatment is started early, the symptoms of septic arthritis should begin to subside within a few days, and eventually the inflammation may disappear completely. However, left untreated, the infection may be life-threatening and lead to irreversible joint damage.

Lower back pain

Pain in the back, below the waist, that may be sudden and sharp or persistent and dull

 Age, gender, genetics, and lifestyle as risk factors depend on the cause

Lower back pain affects about 6 in 10 adults during the course of a year. More working days are lost due to back pain than to any other medical condition. In most cases, the pain lasts for only a week or so, but many people find that their problem recurs. In a minority of people, persistent lower back pain causes long-term disability.

Lower back pain is usually caused by minor damage to the ligaments and muscles in the back. The lower back is vulnerable to these problems because it supports most of the body's weight and is under continual stress from movements such as bending and twisting. Less commonly, lower back pain may be a result of an underlying disorder such as a prolapsed or herniated disc (p.227) in the spine.

What are the causes?

Lower back pain may come on suddenly (acute) or develop gradually over a period of weeks (chronic).

Acute back pain is often caused by a physical injury due to lifting heavy objects or to activities such as digging in the garden. The pain is commonly caused by a strained muscle or ligament. The injury may be aggravated by subsequent activity. In most cases, symptoms subside within 2–14 days.

Back pain that is more persistent may be a result of poor posture, for example, while sitting at a desk or driving a car.

▶ **TEST AND TREATMENT**

Joint aspiration

During joint aspiration, fluid is withdrawn from a swollen joint with a needle and syringe, possibly under local anaesthesia. The fluid is then examined to find the cause of the swelling. Joint aspiration may also be carried out to relieve swelling due to excess fluid and to diagnose or treat disorders such as gout, pseudogout, and rheumatoid arthritis.

Tibia   Patella   Needle

Fluid   Femur

INSIDE THE JOINT

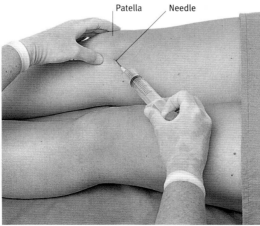

Patella   Needle

Knee joint aspiration
You will be asked to keep your knee relaxed so that the needle can be inserted easily. The patella is held still while the needle is passed into the space under the patella and fluid is withdrawn.

RESULTS

Fluid sample
A fluid sample withdrawn from a swollen joint is examined under a microscope to look for any visible abnormalities. This magnified view of the fluid reveals the presence of uric acid crystals, which are indicative of gout.

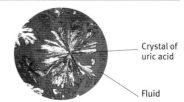

Crystal of uric acid

Fluid

Preventing back pain

Back pain is often due to poor posture, weak abdominal or back muscles, or sudden muscle strain. You can improve your posture by wearing comfortable shoes, sitting and standing properly, and choosing an appropriate mattress for your bed. Regular exercises strengthen abdominal and back muscles; losing weight will relieve stress on the back; and lifting objects safely can help to prevent back strain. Ask your doctor or physiotherapist for advice on posture, exercises, and diet.

Correct body posture

To break bad postural habits, you should be constantly aware of the way in which you stand, sit, move, and even sleep. The pictures on this page show how to carry out everyday activities comfortably, with minimal strain on your spine and back muscles.

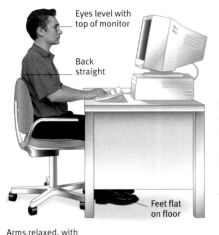

Eyes level with top of monitor

Back straight

Feet flat on floor

Sitting position
Sit with your back straight and both feet flat on the floor. Use a chair that supports the small of your back. When using a computer, position the monitor so that your eyes are level with the top of it.

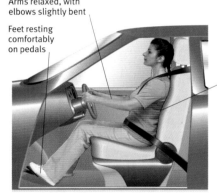

Arms relaxed, with elbows slightly bent

Feet resting comfortably on pedals

Spine supported by seat

Driving position
Angle your seat backwards a little to support your spine, and position the seat so that you can reach the hand and foot controls easily.

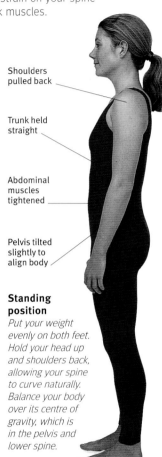

Shoulders pulled back

Trunk held straight

Abdominal muscles tightened

Pelvis tilted slightly to align body

Standing position
Put your weight evenly on both feet. Hold your head up and shoulders back, allowing your spine to curve naturally. Balance your body over its centre of gravity, which is in the pelvis and lower spine.

Lifting a heavy object

When lifting, pushing, or pulling a heavy object, keep the object close to you so that you can use your full strength to move it. To lift an object, hold the bottom edge so that you support the full weight of the object and keep your body balanced as you lift to avoid straining your spine.

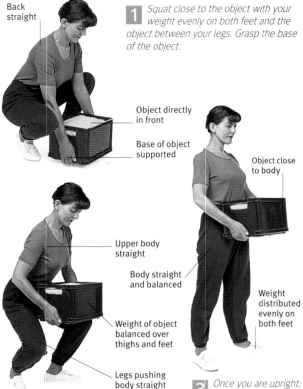

Back straight

1 *Squat close to the object with your weight evenly on both feet and the object between your legs. Grasp the base of the object.*

Object directly in front

Base of object supported

Object close to body

Upper body straight

Body straight and balanced

Weight distributed evenly on both feet

Weight of object balanced over thighs and feet

Legs pushing body straight upwards

2 *Keep your back straight and lean forwards slightly. Stand up in a single, smooth movement, pushing yourself up with your leg muscles and keeping the object close to you.*

3 *Once you are upright, keep the weight close to your body. Keep your back straight and head up, so that your body is balanced over its centre of gravity.*

Back-strengthening exercises

You can help to prevent back pain by gently exercising the muscles in your back and abdomen. See a doctor or ask for a referral to a physiotherapist before starting a programme of exercise. You should not continue to do any exercise that causes you pain. The movements shown below should make your back muscles stronger and your spine more flexible. Repeat each one 10 times if you can, and try to exercise daily. Do the exercises on a comfortable but firm, flat surface, such as a mat laid on the floor.

Hump and sag
The movements in this exercise should increase suppleness in the joints and muscles of the back. Support yourself on your hands and knees with your knees slightly apart. Tuck your chin into your chest, then gently arch your back. Hold for about 5 seconds. Look up, allowing your back to sag, and hold again for about another 5 seconds.

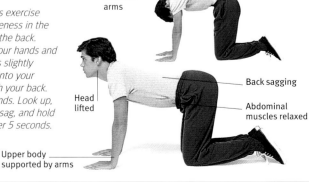

Head tucked between arms

Back arched

Head lifted

Back sagging

Abdominal muscles relaxed

Upper body supported by arms

Lower back stretch
This stretch may relieve aching joints and muscles in the lower back. Lie on your back with your feet flat on the floor and with your knees bent. Lift your knees towards your body. With your hands, pull your knees into your chest. Hold for 7 seconds and breathe deeply. Keeping your knees bent, lower your feet to the floor one at a time.

Pelvic tilt
This movement helps to stretch the muscles and ligaments of the lower back. Lie on your back with your knees bent and your feet flat on the floor. Press the small of your back into the floor. Tighten your abdominal and buttock muscles so that your pelvis tilts upwards and your buttocks rise slightly off the floor. Hold for 6 seconds and then relax.

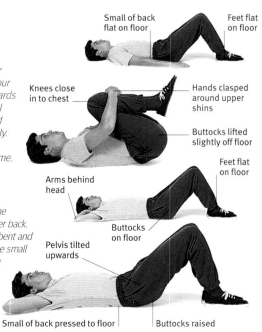

Small of back flat on floor

Feet flat on floor

Knees close in to chest

Hands clasped around upper shins

Buttocks lifted slightly off floor

Arms behind head

Feet flat on floor

Pelvis tilted upwards

Buttocks on floor

Small of back pressed to floor

Buttocks raised

Being overweight can also be a causative factor, because of the heavier load on the back. Pain may be aggravated by emotional stress and excessive muscle tension. Lower back pain may also occur during pregnancy, due both to changes in posture because of the extra weight of the baby and to softening of ligaments supporting the spine caused by hormonal changes.

Another cause of lower back pain is a prolapsed or herniated disc exerting pressure on a spinal nerve or the spinal cord. Back pain of this type may have a gradual or sudden onset and is accompanied by sciatica (p.338), in which severe shooting pain extends down the back of one or both legs.

Persistent lower back pain may be caused by joint disorders. In people over the age of 45, the most common joint problem is osteoarthritis (p.221), while in younger people the problem may be ankylosing spondylitis (p.223), which affects the joints of the spine. Less often, back pain results from bone disorders, such as Paget's disease of the bone (p.218), or cancer that has spread to bone from a tumour elsewhere in the body (see **Bone metastases**, p.220).

In some cases, disorders affecting internal organs can lead to pain in the lower back. Examples include certain disorders of the female reproductive system, such as pelvic inflammatory disease (p.475), and of the urinary system, such as prostatitis (p.463).

What are the symptoms?
Pain in the lower back can take various forms. You may experience:
- Sharp pain localized to a small area of the back.
- More general, aching pain in the back and buttocks, which is made worse by sitting and relieved by standing.
- Back stiffness and pain on bending.
- Pain in the back that radiates to the buttock and leg, sometimes accompanied by numbness or tingling.

Back pain that is associated with weight loss or difficulty in controlling your bowel or bladder may be due to a serious underlying disorder. You should consult your doctor immediately if you develop any of these symptoms.

What can I do?
In most cases, you should be able to treat lower back pain yourself by taking an over-the-counter painkiller (p.589), such as paracetamol. If the pain persists, additional relief may be provided by a heat pad or wrapped hot-water bottle and sometimes by an ice pack placed against your back. Some people find that changing their sleeping position can help to reduce the pain. You should try to continue your normal activities as much as possible, even if this initially causes some discomfort. However, you should stop any activity that makes the pain worse. Resting in

bed used to be recommended for back pain but it has been found that remaining active is likely to lead to a faster recovery. If the pain does not improve within a few days, worsens, or is so severe that you cannot move, you should consult your doctor.

Once the pain has subsided, you can help to prevent recurrence if you pay attention to your posture, lose any excess weight, learn to lift correctly, and do regular exercises to strengthen the muscles of your back and make your spine more flexible (see **Preventing back pain**, opposite page).

What might the doctor do?
Your doctor will probably carry out a physical examination to assess your posture, the range of movement in your spine, and any areas of local tenderness. Your reflexes, the strength of different leg muscles, and the sensation in your legs may also be tested to look for evidence of pressure on spinal nerves or the spinal cord. A pelvic or rectal examination may be necessary if you have symptoms that are associated with the female reproductive organs or with the bowels.

You may have various blood tests and X-rays (p.131) to look for underlying causes of the pain, such as joint inflammation or bone cancer. If there is evidence of pressure on the spinal cord or spinal nerves, MRI (p.133) or CT scanning (p.132) may be carried out to detect abnormalities that require additional treatment, such as a prolapsed or herniated disc.

Unless there is a serious underlying cause for your back pain, your doctor will probably advise you to continue taking a painkilling drug. In some cases, he or she may prescribe a stronger painkiller or, if you are experiencing muscle spasms in your back, a muscle relaxant drug (p.579). If you have had back pain for several weeks, your doctor may also advise special exercise classes; manual therapy, such as physiotherapy (p.620) or osteopathy to mobilize stiff and painful joints between the vertebrae; or you may be referred to a specialist pain clinic. Spinal surgery is not usually recommended unless all other treatments have failed and the pain is so severe that it interferes with normal daily activities.

What is the prognosis?
Most episodes of lower back pain clear up without treatment, but the problem may recur. Improving posture and lifting techniques reduces the risk.

In a few cases, lower back pain may be a long-standing condition, severely disrupting work and social life and sometimes leading to depression (p.343). Effective pain control is essential, and maintaining physical activity, despite some pain, reduces disability. People who become depressed because of their condition may benefit from treatment with antidepressant drugs (p.592).

▶ TREATMENT

Microdiscectomy
Microdiscectomy is a surgical procedure used to treat a prolapsed or herniated disc pressing on a spinal nerve or the spinal cord. The protruding part of the disc is removed through an incision in the fibrous outer coat of the disc. The operation is performed under general anaesthesia and requires a brief stay in hospital.

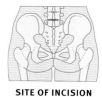

SITE OF INCISION

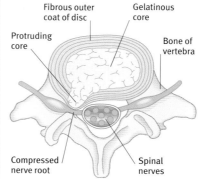

Before the operation
The soft core of the disc is pushed outwards, distorting (and sometimes rupturing) the outer coat. The protruding tissue presses on the spinal cord.

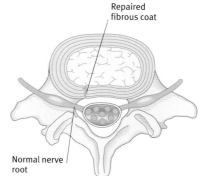

After the operation
The protruding tissue has been removed, and the incision in the outer coat of the disc has been closed up. The spinal cord is no longer compressed.

Prolapsed or herniated disc

Protrusion of one of the shock-absorbing pads that lie between the vertebrae of the spine, also known as a "slipped disc"

 Most common between the ages of 25 and 45

 Slightly more common in males

 Being overweight and lifting objects incorrectly are risk factors

 Genetics is not a significant factor

The shock-absorbing discs between the vertebrae (bones of the spine) consist of a strong, fibrous outer coat and a soft, gelatinous core. A prolapsed disc occurs when the core pushes outwards, distorting the shape of the disc. If the outer coat of the disc ruptures, the condition is termed a herniated disc. When a disc prolapses or herniates, the surrounding tissues become inflamed and swollen. Then, together with the protruding part of the disc, the tissues may press on a spinal nerve or the spinal cord, causing symptoms such as pain, tingling, numbness, or weakness in a limb. The discs in the lower back are most commonly affected but prolapse or herniation can affect any of the vertebrae, including those in the neck or, rarely, the upper back.

People between the ages of 25 and 45 are most vulnerable to disc prolapse or herniation. The disorder is slightly more common in men.

What are the causes?
With age, the discs begin to dry out. They also become more vulnerable to prolapse or herniation as a result of the normal stresses of daily life and minor injuries. Sometimes, a disc is damaged by bending forwards or a sharp twisting movement, or by lifting a heavy object incorrectly.

What are the symptoms?
Symptoms of a prolapsed or herniated disc may develop gradually over a period of weeks or may appear suddenly. They may include:
- Dull pain in the affected area.
- Muscle spasm and stiffness around the affected area that makes movement difficult.

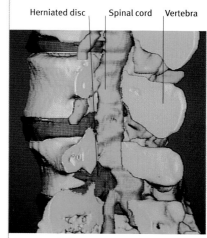

Herniated disc
This 3D CT scan shows a herniated disc in the spine. The soft core of the disc is protruding through the fibrous outer coat and pressing against the spinal cord.

If the disc presses on a spinal nerve, you may also have the following symptoms:
- Severe pain, tingling, or numbness in a leg (*see* Sciatica, p.338) or, if the neck is affected, in an arm.
- Weakness or restricted movement in the leg or arm.

The pain is frequently relieved by rest but may be made worse by sitting, coughing, sneezing, bending, or bowel movements. Impaired bladder or bowel function may indicate pressure on the spinal cord, and you should consult a doctor urgently in such cases.

What might be done?

Diagnosis is usually made from your symptoms and a physical examination. Your doctor may also arrange for you to have an X-ray (p.131), to rule out other causes of back pain, and MRI (p.133) or CT scanning (p.132), which can locate the position of the prolapsed or herniated disc accurately.

Although the disc is permanently damaged, the pain usually improves over 6–8 weeks as the swelling subsides. You should try to keep active, even though movement may initially be difficult, but you should avoid activities and exercises that put too much strain on your back. Your doctor will probably suggest ways in which you can modify physical activities to avoid further stress on your back. He or she may also recommend painkillers (p.589) and refer you for physiotherapy (p.620), which can help to reduce muscle spasms and speed recovery. In some cases, your doctor may also prescribe a muscle relaxant drug to relieve muscle spasms. Injection of a corticosteroid drug (*see* **Locally acting corticosteroids**, p.578) around the compressed nerve may sometimes be carried out to decrease swelling.

In a few cases, surgery may be recommended but usually only if other treatments have been ineffective, if bladder or bowel function is impaired due to pressure on a nerve or the spinal cord, or if there is severe pain or muscle weakness. The surgery involves removing the protruding material and repairing the disc (*see* **Microdiscectomy**, p.227).

Spondylolisthesis

A disorder in which a vertebra (bone of the spine) slips forwards over one beneath it

 Age, gender, genetics, and lifestyle as risk factors depend on the cause

In spondylolisthesis, a vertebra (bone of the spine) slides forwards to project over the vertebra below, distorting the spinal canal. Spondylolisthesis usually affects the vertebrae in the lower part of the back. The disorder may be caused by a deformity of the spine present from birth or a stress fracture due to excessive load on the bone, especially in people who take part in sports, such as cricketers and rowers. In elderly people, particularly women, spondylolisthesis may be the result of a joint disorder such as osteoarthritis (p.221). In rare cases, the condition is caused by a severe injury.

Many people with spondylolisthesis have no symptoms. However, sometimes pain and stiffness may be felt in the affected area of the spine. Pressure on the spinal roots of the sciatic nerve may lead to sciatica (p.338), a condition in which pain is felt in the lower back and travels down the leg.

A diagnosis of spondylolisthesis will need to be confirmed by X-rays (p.131). Procedures such as MRI (p.133) or CT scanning (p.132) may also be needed to exclude other possible causes of back pain such as a prolapsed or herniated disc (opposite page). Treatment may include painkillers (p.589), exercises or physiotherapy (p.620) to strengthen the muscles supporting the affected vertebrae, and sometimes injection of a corticosteroid drug (p.578) and local anaesthetic (p.590). Rarely, surgery may be needed to fuse the affected vertebrae together. Normal activity can often be resumed about 6 months after treatment.

Frozen shoulder

Pain and restriction of movement in the shoulder joint

 More common over the age of 40

 More common in females

 Genetics and lifestyle are not significant factors

Pain and stiffness in a shoulder joint, severely restricting its movement, is known as frozen shoulder. The condition may be due to inflammation resulting from an injury to the shoulder region. Frozen shoulder can also sometimes occur if the shoulder is kept immobilized for a long period of time, such as following a stroke (p.329). However, in many cases, frozen shoulder develops for no apparent reason. The condition occurs most frequently in people over the age of 40 and is more common in women. People who have diabetes mellitus (p.437) are more susceptible to the condition.

What are the symptoms?

The symptoms of frozen shoulder often begin gradually over a period of weeks or months. They may include:
- Pain in the shoulder, which is severe in the early stages of the condition and is often worse at night.
- With time, gradually decreasing pain but increasing stiffness and restricted joint movement.
- In severe cases, pain travelling down the arm to the elbow.

If you have pain in the shoulder that lasts for more than a few days, you should consult your doctor.

What might be done?

Your doctor will probably diagnose frozen shoulder from the symptoms and an examination of your shoulder. A painkiller (p.589) or a nonsteroidal anti-inflammatory drug (p.578) may be prescribed to relieve the discomfort and reduce inflammation.

If the pain persists or is severe, you may be given a corticosteroid drug by means of a direct injection into the shoulder joint (*see* **Locally acting corticosteroids**, p.578). You may also be referred for physiotherapy (p.620). Despite these measures, your shoulder may remain stiff for up to about a year.

Even when the stiffness has disappeared, recovery is usually slow and may take up to a further 6 months.

Chondromalacia

Pain in the front of the knee due to an abnormality of the cartilage at the back of the kneecap

 Most common in teenagers and young adults

 Sometimes runs in families

 Strenuous exercise can trigger symptoms

 Gender is not a significant factor

Chondromalacia, also referred to as patellofemoral pain syndrome, occurs when the cartilage surface of the back of the patella (kneecap) is damaged. The underlying cause of the condition is not known, but it can be triggered by strenuous exercise or repeated knee injuries. In teenagers, chondromalacia may be caused by increased weightbearing on the knee joint during a growth spurt. The condition may also be associated with a misaligned or a recurrently dislocated patella or with muscle weakness in the upper leg.

What are the symptoms?

Symptoms vary in severity from person to person but may include:
- Pain in the knee when the leg is bent and straightened (such as when going up or down stairs).
- Stiffness after prolonged sitting.
- Crepitus (a crackling noise) during knee movement.

Chondromalacia usually occurs in only one knee, although the condition does sometimes develop in both knees.

What might be done?

Your doctor will examine your knee and press down on the patella to see if your symptoms worsen. He or she may arrange

---

▶ **TEST AND TREATMENT**

Arthroscopy

In arthroscopy, the inside of a joint is inspected with a viewing instrument called an arthroscope. The procedure is most commonly used to inspect the inside of the knee joint and to treat disorders such as a damaged cartilage. It is usually performed under general anaesthesia. The arthroscope is inserted into the joint through a small incision in the skin. Surgical instruments can then be passed down through the arthroscope or through the incisions. During the examination, the surgeon can remove or repair tissue, such as damaged cartilage, or shave the surface of the patella (kneecap).

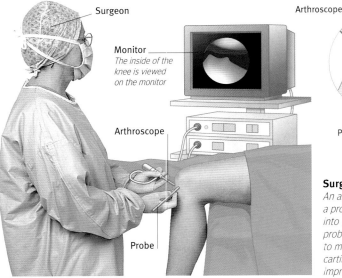

Surgeon

Monitor
The inside of the knee is viewed on the monitor

Arthroscope

Probe

Arthroscope

Probe / Cartilage
INSIDE THE KNEE

Surgical procedure
An arthroscope and a probe are inserted into the joint. The probe can be used to manipulate the cartilage and improve the view.

for X-rays (p.131) of the knee and back of the patella. In severe cases, arthroscopy (opposite page) may be performed to examine the interior of the knee joint and remove damaged cartilage.

Your doctor may advise you to take a painkiller (p.589) or a nonsteroidal anti-inflammatory drug (p.578) and to apply ice packs for pain relief. He or she may also advise exercise to strengthen thigh and knee muscles and reduce stress on the knee joint. You may be advised to wear a knee support as a temporary measure. In rare cases, surgery is necessary to realign the patella.

What is the prognosis?

Chondromalacia often improves over time and most people are not disabled, although they may have mild recurrences of pain in the knee. Regular exercise to strengthen the muscles of the thigh and the ligaments around the knee will reduce the risk of developing osteoarthritis (p.221) in later life.

Bursitis

Inflammation of a bursa, one of the fluid-filled sacs located around joints

 More common in adults

 Occupations involving repeated stress on a joint are risk factors

 Gender and genetics are not significant factors

Bursae act as friction-reducing cushions around joints. Inflammation of a bursa, called bursitis, may occur if it s put under prolonged or repeated stress. The bursa becomes tender and swollen, and movement of the joint is restricted.

The knee is most commonly affected, especially as a result of frequent kneeling, but the elbow or other joints may also be affected. Bursitis may also follow injury or unaccustomed exercise. Certain joint diseases, such as rheumatoid arthritis (p.222) and gout (p.224), increase the risk of bursitis. Rarely, the condition is due to a bacterial infection.

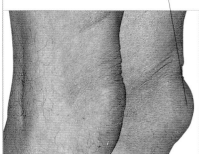
Swollen knee

Bursitis in the knee
The knee seen on the right is swollen due to a fluid-filled, inflamed bursa, which can be caused by prolonged kneeling.

Your doctor will probably diagnose bursitis from a physical examination. Treatment includes resting the affected joint. Your doctor may also recommend a nonsteroidal anti-inflammatory drug (p.578) and application of ice packs. However, if symptoms persist, he or she may drain the bursa and inject it with a corticosteroid drug (*see* **Locally acting corticosteroids**, p.578) to reduce inflammation. If a bacterial infection is present, antibiotics (p.572) will be prescribed, in which case the symptoms usually subside within a few days. If bursitis is persistent or recurrent, surgical removal of the bursa may be necessary.

Bunion

Inflamed, thickened soft tissue and bony overgrowth at the base of the big toe

 Most common in young adults and older people

 More common in females

 Sometimes runs in families

 Wearing tight, pointed shoes, especially with high heels, is a risk factor

A bunion is a thickened lump at the base of the big toe. It often becomes inflamed and painful, making walking difficult. The underlying cause is usually a minor bone deformity, called hallux valgus, in which the joint at the base of the big toe develops an abnormal projection, which forces the tip of the toe to turn towards the other toes. The cause of hallux valgus itself is not known, but the condition runs in some families. As a result of pressure on the deformity, the surrounding tissues thicken. The term bunion refers to the thickened lump that is due to the combination of the bony deformity and thickening of the soft tissue around it. The condition is particularly common in young women who wear tight, pointed shoes with high heels.

In rare cases, the constant rubbing of tight shoes on the skin over a bunion may cause an abrasion, which then leads to a bacterial infection. People with diabetes mellitus (p.437) are particularly susceptible to infected bunions because the sensation in their feet may be reduced (*see* **Diabetic neuropathy**, p.336). In such people, damage to the skin tends to heal more slowly.

Without attention, a bunion may gradually worsen. Pain may be alleviated by wearing comfortable shoes or using a bunion pad or a special bunion splint that straightens the big toe. However, if a bunion causes severe discomfort, your doctor may suggest that you have surgery to correct the underlying deformity by realigning the bone (*see* **Bunion surgery**, above). If the bunion becomes infected, your doctor will prescribe antibiotics (p.572). A bunion increases the chance of developing osteoarthritis (p.221) of the toe joint in later life.

▶ TREATMENT

Bunion surgery

Surgery to treat a bunion is aimed at correcting the underlying bone deformity, known as hallux valgus. One common type of surgical procedure used to treat a bunion involves reshaping and realigning the deformed bone at the base of the big toe. The operation is performed under general anaesthesia and may require a brief stay in hospital. After surgery, your foot may be swollen for several months and you may not be able to wear normal shoes for about 6 months.

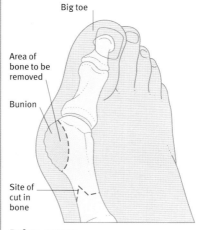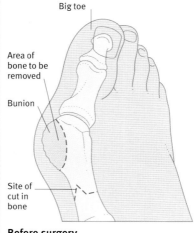

Before surgery
The big toe is turned towards the other toes. The bone has become obviously deformed, and the soft tissue around it has thickened, forming a painful bunion.

After surgery
The protruding part of the bone has been removed and a V-shaped cut made in the lower part of the bone. The big toe is straight due to realignment of the bone.

Muscle and tendon disorders

Skeletal muscles contract and relax to move the body and are connected to bones by fibrous tissue known as tendons. Both muscles and tendons can be temporarily or permanently damaged by injury, overexertion, infection, or other disorders, causing pain, weakness, restricted movement, and tiredness.

Skeletal muscles account for half the weight of the body but are only rarely affected by disease. Injury to a muscle or tendon, either through strenuous exercise or as a result of a repetitive physical activity, is the cause of some of the disorders described in this section, including muscle cramps, torticollis, repetitive strain injury, and tennis and golfer's elbow. The next articles discuss inflammation of a tendon (tendinitis) or tendon sheath (tenosynovitis) and ganglia, which are fluid-filled cysts that commonly arise on the wrist or the back of the hand.

Some disorders that affect the skeletal muscles are covered in other parts of the book. These conditions include the immune system disorders polymyalgia rheumatica (p.282) and polymyositis (p.282) and the inherited disease muscular dystrophy (p.536). Musculoskeletal injuries (pp.231–234) are also covered elsewhere.

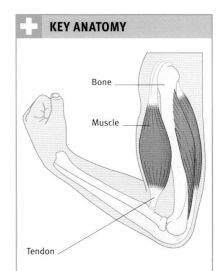

✚ KEY ANATOMY

Bone

Muscle

Tendon

For more information on the structure and function of muscles and tendons, *see* pp.215–216.

Muscle cramps

Sudden painful spasms in a muscle or group of muscles

 Age, gender, genetics, and lifestyle are not significant factors

Muscle cramps affect almost everyone from time to time. Painful spasms, often lasting only a few minutes, make the affected muscle become hard and tender. Muscle cramps may occur in any muscle in the body but they are most common in leg muscles. When abdominal muscles are affected, the condition is also known as a "stitch".

Muscle cramps often develop during physical exercise, possibly as a result of reduction in the oxygen supply to the muscles or a build-up of chemical waste produced by muscles during exercise. Another possible cause is the loss of salt and water that occurs due to heavy sweating during hot weather or strenuous exercise. Muscle cramps may also develop if you have been sitting or lying in an awkward position for a long time. Sometimes, there is no obvious cause.

Cramps are not the only cause of attacks of muscle pain. If you develop recurrent muscle pain in your calves when walking, you should consult your doctor; the cause may be lower limb ischaemia (p.261), a disorder in which the arteries that supply blood to the leg muscles become narrowed.

The immediate self-help treatment for muscle cramps is to stretch and rub the affected area and to apply a heat pad. You should drink plenty of fluids and eat something salty. If you regularly have cramps at night, your doctor may prescribe a low dose of quinine, an antimalarial drug (p.574) that effectively relieves the symptoms.

Torticollis

Muscle spasm in the neck causing twisting of the head; also known as wry neck

 Age, gender, genetics, and lifestyle are not significant factors

In torticollis, the muscles on one side of the neck contract and cause the head to be pulled over to one side. The condition is typically accompanied by pain and stiffness in the neck.

Torticollis may develop in babies after a difficult birth involving neck muscle damage. In children, the disorder may be a result of swollen glands in the neck caused by an infection. Torticollis in adults is often caused by physical injury to muscles or by sleeping in an awkward position. The disorder can also be a side effect of certain drugs, such as some antipsychotic drugs (p.592). Rarely, it results from torsion dystonia, a neurological disorder that causes involuntary muscle contractions, or cervical spondylosis (p.222).

Your doctor may make the diagnosis from a physical examination. Torticollis in babies will gradually get better with physiotherapy (p.620). In adults and older children, painkillers (p.589), local heat, and massage may help to relieve the muscle spasm. Recovery usually takes only a few days but if torticollis persists, a local injection of botulinum toxin (*see* **Muscle relaxants**, p.579) may be given. If the disorder is caused by a particular drug, it will improve once the drug is stopped.

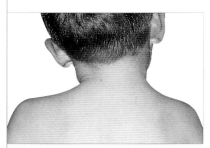

Torticollis
Muscle contraction on one side of the neck has caused this child's head to tip to the side. This condition is called torticollis.

Fibromyalgia

Pain, stiffness, and tiredness associated with muscle tenderness

 Occurs mainly in adults

 More common in females

 Stress may be a risk factor

 Genetics is not a significant factor

Fibromyalgia is a disorder that causes widespread muscle pain and tenderness. The condition has no particular cause, and no visible abnormality has ever been identified in the muscle tissue. However, fibromyalgia commonly develops during periods of stress.

What are the symptoms?
The symptoms of fibromyalgia develop slowly over weeks and occur in a distinct pattern around the body. They may include the following:
- Muscle pain in the upper back, head, thighs, abdomen, and hips.
- Particularly tender areas of muscle, typically at the base of the skull and near the shoulder blades and back.

Fibromyalgia is commonly associated with headaches, tiredness, depression (p.343), anxiety disorders (p.341), and disturbed sleep patterns. Some people have irregular bowel movements (*see* **Irritable bowel syndrome**, p.415). All of these symptoms usually become worse with increased stress.

What might be done?
The diagnosis of fibromyalgia is often based on the symptoms and a physical examination, but your doctor may arrange for blood

tests to rule out other disorders, such as rheumatoid arthritis (p.222). Treatment is aimed at relieving symptoms. However, no one treatment is effective for everybody so you may have to try several to find the best for you. Treatment options include medication, such as painkillers (p.589), antidepressants (p.592), and muscle relaxants (p.579); psychological therapies, such as cognitive–behavioural therapy (p.623); relaxation techniques (p.32); and individually tailored exercises. Fibromyalgia is often long-standing, but many people learn to manage their symptoms effectively.

Repetitive strain injury

Symptoms associated with repetitive physical activity

 Activities that involve repeated movements are risk factors

 Age, gender, and genetics are not significant factors

Prolonged, repeated movements of one part of the body, particularly if the movements are rapid and forceful, can cause symptoms described as repetitive strain injury (RSI). Overuse injury and cumulative trauma disorder are other names for the same condition. RSI most commonly affects the muscles and tendons in the arms. The condition may be associated with stress in the workplace or the home.

People who often carry out repeated movements as part of their everyday work, such as those using a keyboard, are particularly at risk of RSI. Musicians and athletes are also susceptible. Other disorders that cause pain in the muscles and tendons, such as tendinitis and tenosynovitis (opposite page) or carpal tunnel syndrome (p.338), can cause symptoms similar to those of RSI.

What are the symptoms?
The symptoms of RSI develop gradually and at first may occur only while performing the repetitive activity. The symptoms may include:
- Pain, aching, and tingling.
- Restricted movement in the affected part of the body.

In the early stages of RSI, the symptoms may disappear when the affected area is rested. Later, you may have symptoms at rest. If you develop RSI, you should consult your doctor without delay since the condition is more difficult to treat once it has become long-standing.

What might the doctor do?
Your doctor will ask about your lifestyle and any repetitive physical activities. Diagnosis is usually made after a physical examination. However, you may also have X-rays (p.131) and blood tests to rule out disorders such as rheumatoid arthritis (p.222). Your doctor may also recommend a painkiller (p.589) or nonsteroidal anti-inflammatory drug (p.578) to relieve discomfort.

What can I do?
If you believe the symptoms are related to your occupation, you should inform your employer and seek advice from an occupational doctor or nurse. He or she can give you advice about posture changes and special equipment, such as adjustable seating, that may help you to avoid unnecessary strain. You should also make sure you take regular breaks from repetitive tasks. Rarely, a change in work or leisure activities may be advisable.

What is the prognosis?
If RSI is recognized at an early stage and steps are taken to reduce stress at work, you should make a complete recovery. A physiotherapist will probably be able to give you advice on how to use your muscles and build up their strength (*see* **Physiotherapy**, p.620).

Tennis elbow and golfer's elbow

Inflammation of a tendon at its attachment to the bone at the elbow

 More common over the age of 30

 Common among recreational tennis players and golfers and among people carrying out repetitive activities

 Gender and genetics are not significant factors

Tennis elbow and golfer's elbow both occur when the tendon attachment of the muscle to the bone at the elbow becomes damaged. In tennis elbow, the tendon on the outer side of the elbow is injured; in golfer's elbow, the tendon on the inner side of the elbow is affected.

Both conditions are caused by vigorous and repeated use of the forearm against resistance, which can occur when playing certain sports, such as tennis, or using a screwdriver. The tendon is repeatedly pulled at the point at which it is attached to the bone, which may cause small tears to develop. The resulting damage leads to tenderness and pain in the affected arm.

You should rest the affected painful arm as much as possible. Physiotherapy (p.620), ice packs, simple exercises to stretch and strengthen the muscles, and ultrasound treatment may help to relieve symptoms. You may also find that a nonsteroidal anti-inflammatory drug (p.578) helps. If the condition does not improve within 2–6 weeks, your doctor may inject a corticosteroid drug into the affected area (*see* **Locally acting corticosteroids**, p.578), although such treatment is often not effective in the long term. Once the symptoms have subsided, you should seek advice on ways to change your technique before resuming the sport or activity that gave rise to the condition.

Tendinitis and tenosynovitis

Painful inflammation of a tendon (tendinitis) or of a tendon sheath (tenosynovitis)

 More common in adults

 More common in athletes

 Gender and genetics are not significant factors

Tendinitis is inflammation of a tendon, the fibrous cord that attaches a muscle to a bone. Tenosynovitis is inflammation of the sheath of tissues that surrounds a tendon. These two conditions usually occur together. Tendons around the shoulder, elbow, wrist, fingers, thigh, knee, or back of the heel are most commonly affected.

Both conditions may be caused by injury of a particular tendon or, rarely, by an infection. Inflammation of the Achilles tendon between the heel and the calf may be the result of a sports injury (below) or of wearing ill-fitting shoes. Tenosynovitis may be associated with rheumatoid arthritis (p.222). In some cases, the cause is unknown.

What are the symptoms?
You may notice the following symptoms in the affected area, particularly during movement:
- Pain and/or mild swelling.
- Stiffness and restricted movement in the affected area.
- Warm, red skin over the tendon.
- A tender lump over the tendon.

Occasionally, you may feel a crackling sensation (known as crepitus) when the affected tendon moves.

What might be done?
Diagnosis is based on the symptoms and a physical examination. Your doctor will treat any underlying disorder. To reduce the pain and inflammation, he or she may recommend nonsteroidal anti-inflammatory drugs (p.578). You may also require an injection of a corticosteroid drug (*see* **Locally acting corticosteroids**, p.578) into the tendon sheath. If the condition is due to an infection, a course of antibiotics (p.572) will be prescribed. In some cases, a tendon will heal more quickly if it is splinted. Tendinitis and tenosynovitis improve with treatment.

Dupuytren's contracture

Thickening and shortening of tissues in the palm of the hand, resulting in deformity of the fingers

 More common over the age of 50

 Much more common in males

 Sometimes runs in families

 Alcohol abuse is a risk factor

In Dupuytren's contracture, the fibrous tissue in the palm of the hand becomes thickened and shortened. As a result, one or more fingers, often the fourth and fifth fingers, are pulled towards the palm into a bent position. Sometimes, painful lumps develop on the palm, and the overlying skin becomes puckered. In about half of all cases, both hands are involved. Rarely, the disorder affects the soles of the feet and the toes. The tissue changes in Dupuytren's contracture develop slowly over several months or years. The cause is unknown, but the condition occurs more commonly in men over the age of 50, in people with diabetes mellitus (p.437) or epilepsy (p.324), and in people who abuse alcohol. About 1 in 10 people with Dupuytren's contracture has a relative with the disorder.

What might be done?
In mild cases of Dupuytren's contracture, no treatment may be needed. If your fingers are slightly bent, you may benefit from stretching exercises or short-term splinting. If you have painful lumps in your palm, a corticosteroid may be injected into the area (*see* **Locally acting corticosteroids**, p.578). In severe cases, it may be necessary to surgically remove the thickened tissue in the palm in order to allow the fingers to straighten. Further treatment may be needed if the disorder recurs.

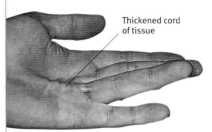
Thickened cord of tissue

Dupuytren's contracture
The fourth finger of this hand is pulled towards the palm by fibrous tissue that has thickened and shortened. This is known as Dupuytren's contracture.

Ganglion

A fluid-filled cyst that most commonly develops on the wrist or back of the hand and sometimes the foot

 Age, gender, genetics, and lifestyle are not significant factors

A ganglion is a cyst that develops under the skin near a joint and is filled with a jelly-like fluid. The ganglion is usually an outgrowth from the capsule surrounding a joint or from the sheath of a tendon, the fibrous cord that attaches muscle to bone. The fluid inside the ganglion is derived from the synovial fluid that lubricates tendons and joints.

Ganglia are extremely common and are usually painless. They most commonly occur on the wrist or the back of the hand but occasionally they develop on the foot. They vary in size from that of a small pea to that of a plum.

A ganglion may be felt as a lump under the skin and may be present for several years without causing a problem. However, some ganglia become very uncomfortable or even painful. A ganglion may disappear spontaneously, or it can be removed surgically under local anaesthesia. Ganglia sometimes recur.

Musculoskeletal injuries

The bones, joints, muscles, and connective tissues of the body's musculoskeletal system are susceptible to injury from the stresses and strains placed on them during routine and leisure activities. The healing of minor injuries is usually rapid and complete, but major ones require expert treatment to avoid permanent damage.

Today, many people are aware of the health benefits of exercise and use part of their leisure time to pursue athletic activities. However, such pursuits may lead to musculoskeletal injuries if care is not taken. The first article in this section gives an overview of the main types of sports injury, the treatment of which has now become a specialized branch of medicine.

Injury may result in bone fractures of various types and these are covered next. The treatment of fractures has changed a great deal in the past 25 years as a result of various technical innovations,

particularly for more complicated fractures in which the damaged bone is fragmented.

Injuries occurring in other parts of the musculoskeletal system, including joints, ligaments, muscles, and tendons, are also discussed. As with fractures, these injuries may cause long-term disability if not treated properly.

Damage to the musculoskeletal system may also occur as part of more widespread damage to the body following serious trauma, such as a motor vehicle accident (*see* **Serious injuries**, pp.182–184).

KEY ANATOMY

- Bone
- Muscle
- Synovial membrane
- Synovial fluid
- Cartilage
- Ligament
- Tendon

For more information on the structure of the musculoskeletal system, *see* pp.212–216.

Sports injuries

Damage to any part of the body as a result of athletic activity

 Older participants may be more likely to be injured and injuries heal more slowly

 More common in males

 Playing sports, especially contact sports, is a risk factor

 Genetics is not a significant factor

Sports injuries often occur in people who are new to a sport, begin to exercise after prolonged inactivity, or do not warm up properly before exercise. Men are at greater risk because they play more contact sports.

What are the types?
Any part of the musculoskeletal system may be injured while playing sports. In some sports, there is an increased risk of injury to a specific part of the body.

Bone injuries Many sports activities can cause damage to the bones, either through repetitive actions or as a result of an impact with another person, the ground, or equipment, such as a bat or a ball. Bones may be broken or cracked (*see* **Fractures**, right) during contact sports such as rugby. The repetitive jarring of bones of the lower limbs of runners may cause stress fractures.

Joint injuries The bones that form a joint may partially or completely pull apart (*see* **Dislocated joint**, opposite page) during sports that put them under great strain, such as javelin throwing. Dislocation is also a risk in all contact sports. A common injury among football players is damage to the cartilage pads in the knee joint (*see* **Torn knee cartilage**, p.234).

Ligament and tendon injuries The fibrous bands of tissue that hold the structures of the musculoskeletal system together are often injured during sports activities. Ligaments, which hold the bones together, may become damaged by a sudden twisting movement or during a fall (*see* **Ligament injuries**, opposite page). Tendons, which attach muscle to bone, may become torn during athletic activities, such as jumping, that involve a sudden muscle contraction (*see* **Ruptured tendon**, p.234).

Muscle injuries Most sports rely on strength and suppleness of the muscles, and damage to muscles is common in athletes (*see* **Muscle strains and tears**, p.234). For example, calf strain, overstretching of the muscles in the calf region, is a common injury in basketball players. Muscle injury is frequently caused by sudden, strenuous movements and lifting heavy objects.

Can they be prevented?

Many sports injuries could be prevented by warming up correctly before starting exercise (*see* **Warming up and cooling down in your exercise routine**, p.22). Adequate preparation can increase flexibility and reduce stiffness in the muscles and joints. In sports such as running, you should start gently, gradually increasing your pace to prevent placing too much strain on your body. Wear clothes and footwear designed for your type of sport and use recommended safety equipment.

What might be done?

Many minor injuries to ligaments, tendons, and muscles can be treated using basic techniques, such as applying a cold compress or an ice pack to the affected areas, and nonsteroidal anti-inflammatory drugs (p.578). If a sports injury is causing intense or persistent pain, you should consult a doctor. He or she will examine you and may arrange for you to have an X-ray (p.131) to check whether you have sustained a fracture.

If you have a fracture, it may be necessary to immobilize the injured area by using a cast (*see* **Fracture treatments**, right). Surgery may be required for some injuries, such as a ruptured tendon. You may also need physiotherapy (p.620). You should not participate in any sports until you are free of pain.

Fractures

Breaks or cracks in bones anywhere in the body from a variety of causes

 Age, gender, genetics, and lifestyle as risk factors depend on the cause

Any bone in the body can be fractured. Most fractures are caused by an injury such as a direct impact or a twisting movement, which may occur during an athletic activity or a fall.

Susceptibility to fractures increases with the bone disorder osteoporosis (p.217), which mainly affects women after the menopause and results in brittle bones. Fractures that occur in bones affected by tumours are called pathological fractures and may occur after minor injury or even spontaneously.

The most common sites of fracture in elderly people are the neck of the femur (thighbone) and the lower end of the radius bone of the forearm near the wrist. A fracture at the end of the radius, known as a Colles' fracture, may occur if a person trips and breaks his or her fall with an outstretched arm.

What are the types?

There are two main types of fracture: closed (simple), in which the broken bone does not break through the overlying skin; and open (compound), in which the bone pierces the skin and is exposed. Open fractures are more serious because of the risk of infection and an increased risk of damage to nerves

---

▶ **TREATMENT**

Fracture treatments

Although some broken bones do not need immobilization, most have to be returned to their correct position (reduction) and held in place so that the fractured ends are able to heal and join together properly. The method of immobilization chosen for a particular fracture depends on the type, location, and severity of the fracture.

Immobilization in a cast

The simplest form of immobilization is a cast, a rigid casing that is applied to a limb and left in position for several weeks to hold the fractured bone ends together and prevent movement. Casts are usually made from plaster, plastic, or resin. They are removed using an electric saw, which cuts through the cast.

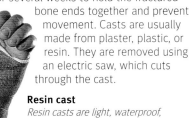

Resin cast
Resin casts are light, waterproof, and durable. The cast is applied as a bandage to fit the affected limb. It then sets and provides support without restricting the blood supply.

Internal fixation

Bones that are severely fractured may need metal plates, screws, nails, wires, or rods to be inserted surgically to hold the broken bone ends together. A cast may not be required. Internal fixation is often used for fractures at the ends of bones.

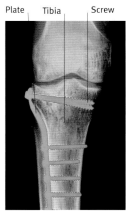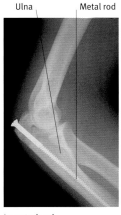

Plate   Tibia   Screw   Ulna   Metal rod

Plate and screws
A fracture in the tibia (shinbone) may be immobilized by a metal plate secured by screws.

Inserted rod
A fractured ulna (lower arm bone) may be held together by a metal rod inserted into the bone.

External fixation

A specialized technique known as external fixation is often required to repair bones that are fractured in several places. In this technique, pins are inserted through the skin into the bone fragments. The pins are held in place by an external metal frame, which allows the affected limb to be used normally within a few days. The frame and pins are removed when the bone has healed.

Repairing a broken tibia
This photograph shows a fractured tibia (shinbone) immobilized by external fixation. The diagram below shows the positions of the metal pins in the bone. They have been inserted through the skin and are attached to two external metal rods. The pins are inserted and removed under a general anaesthetic and are painless when in place.

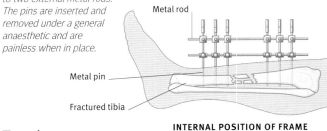

Metal pin   Metal rod

EXTERNAL POSITION OF FRAME

Metal rod

Metal pin

Fractured tibia

INTERNAL POSITION OF FRAME

Traction

Traction is used for the temporary immobilization of a fracture until further treatment of the injury can be carried out. The technique is often used for fractures in the shaft of the femur (thighbone). Weights are used to maintain alignment because the powerful muscles in the thigh would normally pull on the ends of the broken bone, forcing them out of alignment.

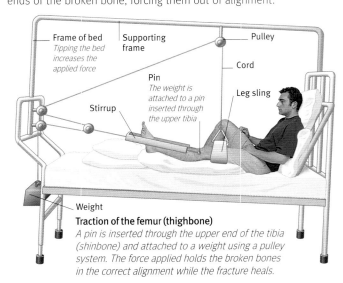

Frame of bed
Tipping the bed increases the applied force

Supporting frame

Pulley

Cord

Pin
The weight is attached to a pin inserted through the upper tibia

Leg sling

Stirrup

Weight

Traction of the femur (thighbone)
A pin is inserted through the upper end of the tibia (shinbone) and attached to a weight using a pulley system. The force applied holds the broken bones in the correct alignment while the fracture heals.

and blood vessels. Open and closed fractures may be further subdivided according to their shape and pattern.

Transverse fracture In a transverse fracture, there is a straight break across a bone. Transverse fractures, often in a long bone in the arm or leg, are usually due to a powerful blow, such as that sustained in a collision during a traffic accident.

Spiral fracture This type of fracture is also known as an oblique fracture. Spiral fractures are usually caused by sudden, violent, rotating movements, such as twisting the leg during a fall. Spiral fractures usually occur in arm and leg bones.

Greenstick fracture If a long bone in the arm or leg bends, it may crack on one side only, producing a break called a "greenstick" fracture. This type of fracture occurs only in children, whose bones are still growing and flexible.

Comminuted fracture In a comminuted fracture, the bone is broken into small fragments, which increases the likelihood of damage to soft tissues surrounding the broken bone. These fractures are usually caused by severe, direct forces.

Torn-off bone

Tendon

Avulsion fracture In this type of fracture, a piece of bone is pulled away from the main bone by a tendon, a fibrous band that attaches muscle to a bone. It usually results from a sudden violent twisting injury.

Compression fracture

Compression fracture A compression fracture occurs if spongy bone, like that in the vertebrae of the spine, is crushed. This type of fracture is often due to osteoporosis.

Fractures caused by repeated jarring of a bone are called stress fractures. They may occur in the feet or shinbones of long-distance runners. In the elderly, fractures may result from minor stress such as a cough, which can break a rib.

What are the symptoms?
The symptoms of a fracture depend on its type and may include:
- Pain and tenderness, which may limit movement of the affected area.
- Swelling and bruising.
- Deformity in the affected area.
- Crackling noise (crepitus) caused by grating of the ends of the bones on movement or pressure.
- In an open fracture, damage to skin, bleeding, and visible bone.

All fractures cause a certain amount of internal bleeding because of damage to blood vessels in the bone. The broken bone ends may cause further bleeding by damaging tissues and blood vessels in the injured area. In some fractures, blood loss may be severe and can occasionally lead to shock (p.248).

Various complications may be associated with a fracture. For example, if you fracture a rib, there is a risk that the broken rib may puncture a lung (*see* Pneumothorax, p.303). An open fracture may become infected.

Delay in treating a fracture properly may result in failure of the bone to heal and permanent deformity or disability. Consult a doctor immediately if you think that you have a fracture.

How is it diagnosed?
Your doctor will arrange for you to have X-rays (p.131) of the affected area to reveal the type and extent of the fracture. CT scanning (p.132) or MRI (p.133) may be needed to investigate complex fractures. If a fracture was not due to injury, your doctor may check for a possible underlying disorder that may have weakened your bones.

What is the treatment?
If the broken ends of the bone have been displaced, they will need to be returned to their original position to restore normal shape. This process is known as reduction. Depending on the location and severity of the fracture, a broken bone may be manipulated back into its correct position under a local or general anaesthetic, either without an incision (closed reduction) or through an incision in the skin (open reduction). The fractured bone may be held in place until it has healed fully by using one of several methods (*see* Fracture treatments, opposite page).

In some cases, it may not be appropriate to immobilize a broken bone. For example, a broken rib is generally not immobilized because the chest needs to expand normally during breathing. This is important to reduce the risk of pneumonia (p.299), which can develop as a result of shallow breathing and an impaired ability to cough. As a preventive measure, you may be asked to take deep breaths regularly.

Occasionally, healing is slowed down because not enough blood can reach the fracture site or because the broken bone has not been immobilized effectively. In such cases, surgery may be needed; the splintered bone is removed and bone taken from a different part of the body is grafted in its place. A broken bone, such as a fracture in the femur close to the hip joint, may be replaced with an artificial substitute, in this case comprising either part of the femur or the entire hip joint (*see* Joint replacement, p.223).

You may need to have physiotherapy (p.620) after the fracture has healed to restore mobility to a nearby joint and strengthen the surrounding muscles.

What is the prognosis?
In adults, most fractures take 6–8 weeks to heal. Fractures in children generally heal much more quickly. Fractures in babies may heal in a couple of weeks.

Dislocated joint

Displacement of the bones in joints, usually as a result of injury

 More common in males

 Sometimes runs in families

 Playing contact sports, such as rugby, is a risk factor

 Age is not a significant factor

A dislocated joint occurs when a bone has been displaced from its normal position. As a result of pain and the dislocation itself, movement of the joint is severely restricted. The ligaments that hold the bones in place are often torn during the process of dislocation (*see* Ligament injuries, right), and the capsule that surrounds the joint may be damaged. Sometimes the bones within the joint also fracture (opposite page). Shoulder and finger joints are particularly susceptible to dislocation.

What are the causes?
Any powerful force acting against a joint may cause a dislocation. Contact sports, such as rugby, and heavy falls are common causes in men. Abnormally loose joints that are susceptible to dislocation may be an inherited condition. Dislocation may also be associated with a joint disorder, such as rheumatoid arthritis (p.222). Dislocation of the hip may be present from birth (*see* Developmental dysplasia of the hip, p.540).

What are the symptoms?
If you dislocate a joint, the symptoms will appear suddenly and may include:
- Severe pain in the affected area.
- Deformity of the joint.
- Swelling around the joint.
- Bruising of the skin around the joint.

Displaced bones may cause damage to nearby nerves, tendons, and blood vessels, resulting in reduced circulation in tissues beyond the affected area.

If you think that you may have dislocated a joint, you should consult a doctor promptly. If a back injury causes dislocation of the vertebrae (bones of the spine), there may be damage to the spinal cord and consequent paralysis.

What might be done?
Diagnosis of a dislocated joint is usually obvious from the symptoms and a physical examination. However, you may have an X-ray (p.131) to confirm the dislocation and to check for a fracture. Dislocated joints can usually be manipulated back into position by a doctor. You may be given a painkiller (p.589) to relieve discomfort or, in some cases, a sedative to relieve muscle spasm while the joint is being manipulated. If manipulation is unsuccessful, you may need surgery to reposition the joint.

After treatment, the affected joint may be immobilized for 3–6 weeks and you may need physiotherapy (p.620) to help you start to use the joint again. There may be an increased risk that the joint will dislocate again. Joints that dislocate repeatedly may require surgical treatment to stabilize them.

Ligament injuries

Damage to ligaments, the fibrous bands of tissue that hold bones together at a joint

 More common in males

 Playing sports is a risk factor

 Age and genetics are not significant factors

Ligaments attach bones to each other within joints and help to keep joints stable. Ligaments are only slightly elastic and are easily damaged if they are overstretched. Possible injuries range from minor tears, also called sprains, to complete rupture. The most common cause of a ligament injury is a sudden twisting or wrenching movement due to a fall, playing sports, or exercising excessively. Such injuries occur more commonly in men because they exercise more vigorously. Failure to warm up properly before starting exercise is another cause of ligament injury. The ankle and knee are injured most often.

What are the symptoms?
Symptoms usually develop suddenly in the affected joint and may include:
- Pain, particularly on movement.
- Swelling and bruising.
- An abnormal range of movement at the joint.

If you are unable to use a joint after injuring it, you should consult your doctor promptly because tearing a ligament may lead to a dislocation of the bones within the affected joint (*see* Dislocated joint, left).

What might be done?
Most ligament injuries heal well within 8 weeks without treatment, but you can help speed up recovery of a mild sprain using measures such as applying a cold compress to the affected area. To relieve pain, you may be given nonsteroidal anti-inflammatory drugs (p.578). If the pain is severe, you may have an X-ray (p.131) to rule out a fracture (opposite page). Physiotherapy (p.620) is often needed after severe injuries, and surgery may also be necessary. Sometimes, the ruptured ligament is beyond repair. In such cases, the ligament may be replaced with a nearby tendon or a donor graft.

Torn knee cartilage

Damage to the cartilage pads (menisci) in the knee joints

 More common in males

 Playing contact sports, such as football, is a risk factor

 Age and genetics are not significant factors

Damage to cartilage commonly occurs in the knee joint, where two cartilage discs, known as menisci, act as shock absorbers between the femur (thighbone) and tibia (shinbone). These discs help to distribute body weight in the joint. A torn cartilage often occurs in football players and is therefore more common in men. The injury is usually caused by a sudden twisting of the leg, often with the knee bent and the foot on the ground. A cartilage can tear without sudden injury, and people whose occupation involves squatting down and placing strain on the knees are at risk.

If you do tear a cartilage abruptly, you will feel a sharp pain and may hear a noise at the time of the injury. Pain usually becomes worse on moving the joint, and swelling may develop immediately or several hours later. You will probably be unable to straighten the joint. A torn cartilage may prevent the leg from supporting your body weight.

What might be done?

Your doctor will examine your knee and probably arrange for an X-ray (p.131) to check for bone damage. The diagnosis may be confirmed by examining the knee using MRI (p.133) or arthroscopy (p.228). Sometimes, damaged knee cartilage is repaired surgically under a general anaesthetic, and most people are able to use the injured joint 2–3 weeks afterwards. Physiotherapy (p.620) may be needed to help to mobilize the affected joint. There is a risk that torn knee cartilage may lead to early development of osteoarthritis (p.221), a degenerative disorder of the joints.

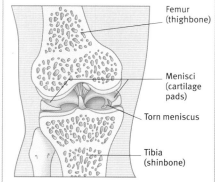

Cartilage in the knee
In the knee joint, two menisci (cartilage pads) act as cushions between the femur and tibia. The menisci are vulnerable to tearing, often as a result of acute injury.

Muscle strains and tears

Injuries of varying severity resulting from the overstretching of a muscle

 More common with increasing age

 Intensive athletic training and lifting heavy weights are risk factors

 Gender and genetics are not significant factors

Muscle strain occurs when a muscle is overstretched, damaging some of its fibres. A tear occurs when the damage is severe and affects many muscle fibres. Both conditions are usually caused by sudden, strenuous movements and occur most often in people who play sports. Abdominal and back muscles may be injured by lifting heavy objects. Athletes are particularly susceptible to these injuries. Symptoms may include pain, swelling, and bruising.

Muscle strains and tears may be prevented by preparing adequately before sports activities (*see* **Warming up and cooling down in your exercise routine**, p.22). If you do strain or tear a muscle, consult your doctor. To speed recovery, apply a cold compress or ice pack. When the pain and swelling subside, usually within 2 days, you can exercise the muscle gently. However, if pain remains, consult your doctor.

Your doctor may suggest that you take a nonsteroidal anti-inflammatory drug (p.578). He or she may also advise you to rest the affected muscle and receive physiotherapy (p.620). If the injury is severe, you may have an X-ray (p.131) to rule out a fracture (p.232). Rarely, surgery may be needed to repair a muscle that has been badly torn.

Ruptured tendon

A complete tear in one of the tough, fibrous bands that attach muscle to bone

 Intensive sports training and lifting heavy weights are risk factors

 Age, gender, and genetics are not significant factors

A tendon may rupture when the muscle to which it is attached contracts suddenly and powerfully, usually during vigorous physical activity such as playing sports or lifting a heavy object. Athletes tend to carry out these activities more often and are therefore more likely to sustain injury. A ruptured tendon may also result from a severe blow, deep cut, or fracture (p.232). In some cases, a ruptured tendon can occur spontaneously as a complication of long-term joint disease such as rheumatoid arthritis (p.222). The tendons in the limbs, particularly the Achilles tendon (which runs from the calf muscle to the heel bone) and those in the hands, are most susceptible to rupture.

You may feel a snapping sensation in the injured area at the time that the tendon ruptures. Other symptoms include pain, impaired movement, and swelling of the affected area.

What might be done?

Diagnosis is usually obvious from the symptoms and physical examination of the affected area. Your doctor may prescribe nonsteroidal anti-inflammatory drugs (p.578). In some cases of Achilles tendon rupture, surgery will be needed to join the torn ends of the tendon. Whether or not you have surgery for an Achilles tendon injury, the injured area will be immobilized by the successive application of different casts. The first cast holds the heel up and the toes down, to avoid stretching the tendon. Subsequent casts are used to flatten the foot gradually and return it to its normal position. You may also be advised to have physiotherapy (p.620) to help to strengthen the muscles in the injured area around the tendon.

The time taken for recovery varies, but motion is usually fully restored in 4–12 months. If an Achilles tendon was involved, you may be vulnerable to further injury on the opposite side.

Cardiovascular system

The cardiovascular system and the blood contained in its vessels are the body's transport system. The heart pumps blood around two circuits of blood vessels. The main (systemic) circuit carries blood that contains oxygen, vital nutrients, and hormones to every cell. The second (pulmonary) circuit takes blood to the lungs, where oxygen is absorbed and the waste product carbon dioxide is eliminated. Other waste products are taken to the liver for processing and finally eliminated by the kidneys.

THE HEART PUMPS the body's total volume of blood (about 5 litres or 9 pints) around the entire body about once a minute. In the systemic circulation, blood containing oxygen and vital nutrients is pumped to tissues and organs through blood vessels called arteries. Body cells absorb the oxygen and nutrients, while the blood absorbs waste products from the cells before returning to the heart through blood vessels called veins. The deoxygenated blood is then pumped to the lungs in the pulmonary circulation. After oxygen has been absorbed and carbon dioxide eliminated, the blood returns to the heart. During exercise, the rate of circulation may increase several times to meet the body's demand for oxygen. The blood supply to some muscles may increase twelvefold while that to the digestive system falls by a third.

The heart and its chambers
About the size of a clenched fist, the heart is a muscular organ that lies in the centre of the chest, slightly to the left. It is divided into two halves, each of which contains an upper chamber (the atrium) and a lower chamber (the ventricle). The atria collect blood from various parts of the body, while the ventricles pump blood out of the heart. Each of the four chambers is joined to one or more blood vessels. The largest of these vessels, the aorta, is about the diameter of a garden hose. Forceful contractions of the ventricles pump blood out of the heart about 70 times per minute at rest.

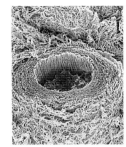

A small artery
The multi-layered wall of the artery seen in this highly magnified image contains muscle and elastic fibres. Individual red blood cells inside the artery are also visible.

This pumping rate is called the heart rate and is measured in beats per minute. With each beat, a pressure wave travels along the arteries, causing their walls to expand. This wave, or pulse, can be felt where the arteries are close to the skin's surface.

Heart muscle (myocardium) must work continuously for 24 hours a day without rest. Therefore, myocardial cells contain more and larger energy-producing units (mitochondria) than other types of body cell.

Heart rate and blood pressure
Heart rate is regulated by electrical impulses from the heart's pacemaker, the sinoatrial node, which is a small area of nervous tissue in the wall of

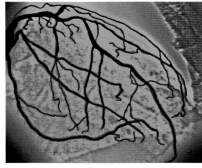

Blood supply to the heart
The extensive network of arteries that surround the heart and supply oxygenated blood to its muscle can be seen in this contrast X-ray.

the right atrium. Each impulse causes a rapid sequence of contractions, first in the atria and then in the ventricles, that corresponds to one heartbeat.

Blood pressure depends on the rate and force of the heart's contractions, the volume of blood pumped out, and the resistance to blood flow in the blood vessels, which varies with their size. Heart rate and blood pressure are controlled by the nervous system in the short term and by hormones, which act over a longer period.

✚ FUNCTION

Blood flow through the heart
Blood flows through veins into the heart's upper chambers (atria) and is pumped into the arteries by the lower chambers (ventricles). Deoxygenated blood collects in the right atrium and flows into the right ventricle, which pumps it to the lungs. Oxygenated blood returns from the lungs to the left atrium. The left ventricle then pumps this blood around the body.

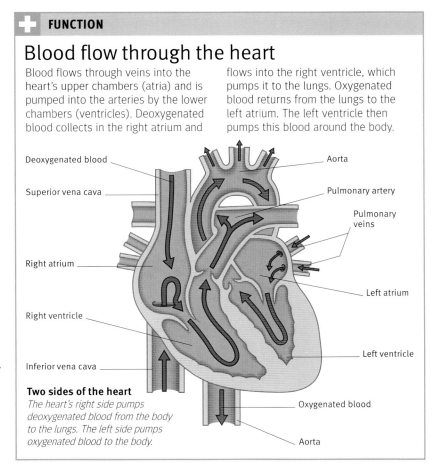

Deoxygenated blood
Superior vena cava
Right atrium
Right ventricle
Inferior vena cava
Aorta
Pulmonary artery
Pulmonary veins
Left atrium
Left ventricle
Oxygenated blood
Aorta

Two sides of the heart
The heart's right side pumps deoxygenated blood from the body to the lungs. The left side pumps oxygenated blood to the body.

+ STRUCTURE AND FUNCTION

The blood vessels

The cardiovascular system includes three types of blood vessel: arteries, veins, and capillaries. Placed end to end, they would circle the Earth nearly four times. The smallest vessels, the capillaries, make up 98 per cent of this length. The largest artery, the aorta, emerges from the heart and branches into a network of progressively smaller arteries that carry blood to every part of the body. The smallest arteries join capillaries, which in turn join a network of tiny veins that merge into larger veins as they return blood to the heart.

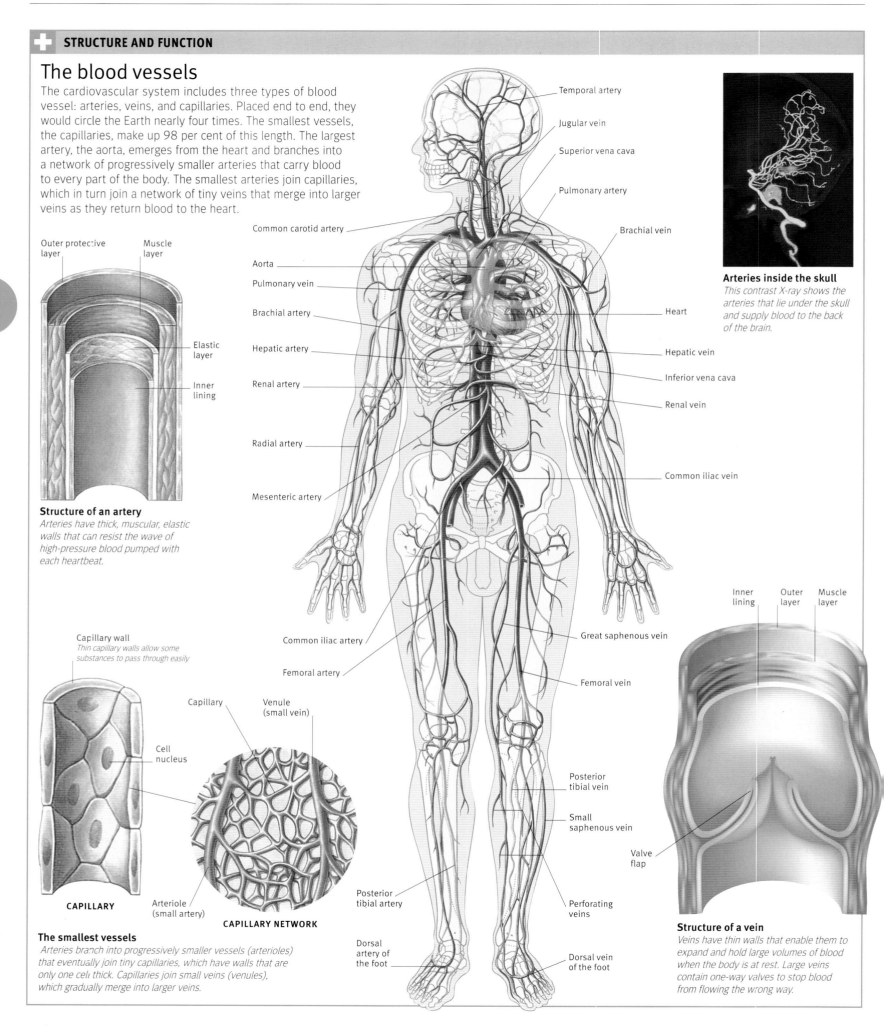

Arteries inside the skull
This contrast X-ray shows the arteries that lie under the skull and supply blood to the back of the brain.

Structure of an artery
Arteries have thick, muscular, elastic walls that can resist the wave of high-pressure blood pumped with each heartbeat.

Outer protective layer
Muscle layer
Elastic layer
Inner lining

Common carotid artery
Aorta
Pulmonary vein
Brachial artery
Hepatic artery
Renal artery
Radial artery
Mesenteric artery
Common iliac artery
Femoral artery

Temporal artery
Jugular vein
Superior vena cava
Pulmonary artery
Brachial vein
Heart
Hepatic vein
Inferior vena cava
Renal vein
Common iliac vein

Great saphenous vein
Femoral vein
Posterior tibial vein
Small saphenous vein
Perforating veins
Dorsal vein of the foot

Posterior tibial artery
Dorsal artery of the foot

The smallest vessels
Arteries branch into progressively smaller vessels (arterioles) that eventually join tiny capillaries, which have walls that are only one cell thick. Capillaries join small veins (venules), which gradually merge into larger veins.

Capillary wall
Thin capillary walls allow some substances to pass through easily

Cell nucleus

CAPILLARY

Capillary
Venule (small vein)
Arteriole (small artery)

CAPILLARY NETWORK

Structure of a vein
Veins have thin walls that enable them to expand and hold large volumes of blood when the body is at rest. Large veins contain one-way valves to stop blood from flowing the wrong way.

Inner lining
Outer layer
Muscle layer
Valve flap

STRUCTURE

Structure of the heart

The heart is a hollow muscular pump consisting mainly of myocardium, a type of muscle that can work without resting. The interior of the heart is divided into two halves, each of which consists of an upper chamber and a lower chamber (the atrium and the ventricle). Each chamber connects to one or more blood vessels. Blood flow through these chambers is controlled by one-way valves.

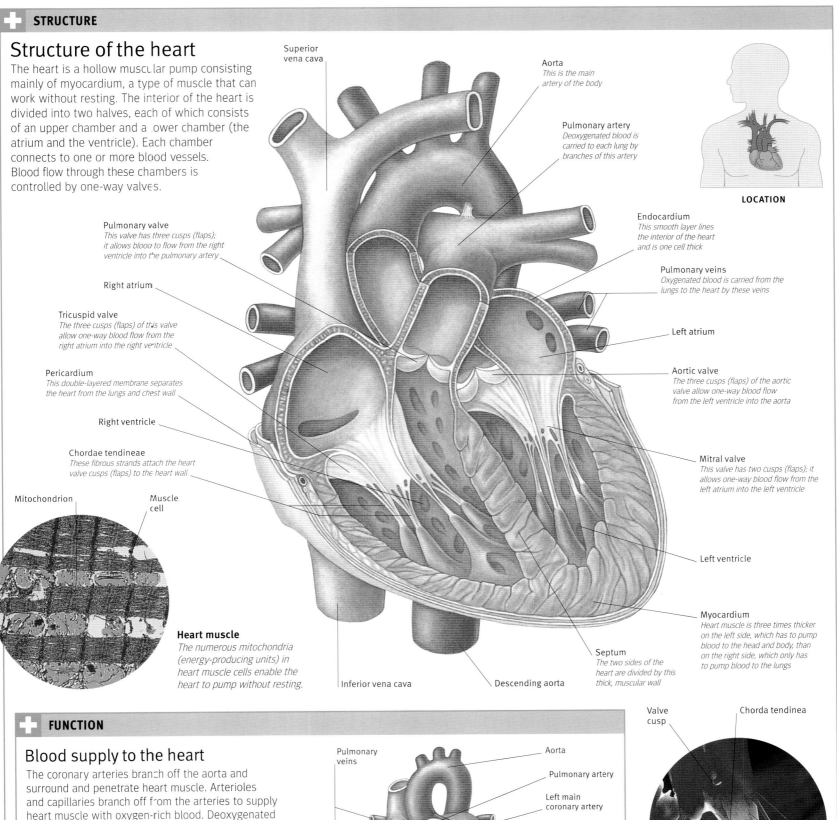

LOCATION

Superior vena cava

Aorta
This is the main artery of the body

Pulmonary artery
Deoxygenated blood is carried to each lung by branches of this artery

Endocardium
This smooth layer lines the interior of the heart and is one cell thick

Pulmonary valve
This valve has three cusps (flaps); it allows blood to flow from the right ventricle into the pulmonary artery

Pulmonary veins
Oxygenated blood is carried from the lungs to the heart by these veins

Right atrium

Left atrium

Tricuspid valve
The three cusps (flaps) of this valve allow one-way blood flow from the right atrium into the right ventricle

Aortic valve
The three cusps (flaps) of the aortic valve allow one-way blood flow from the left ventricle into the aorta

Pericardium
This double-layered membrane separates the heart from the lungs and chest wall

Right ventricle

Mitral valve
This valve has two cusps (flaps); it allows one-way blood flow from the left atrium into the left ventricle

Chordae tendineae
These fibrous strands attach the heart valve cusps (flaps) to the heart wall

Mitochondrion

Muscle cell

Left ventricle

Heart muscle
The numerous mitochondria (energy-producing units) in heart muscle cells enable the heart to pump without resting.

Septum
The two sides of the heart are divided by this thick, muscular wall

Myocardium
Heart muscle is three times thicker on the left side, which has to pump blood to the head and body, than on the right side, which only has to pump blood to the lungs

Inferior vena cava

Descending aorta

FUNCTION

Blood supply to the heart

The coronary arteries branch off the aorta and surround and penetrate heart muscle. Arterioles and capillaries branch off from the arteries to supply heart muscle with oxygen-rich blood. Deoxygenated blood drains into the coronary veins, which carry it back into the heart's right atrium.

The coronary arteries
There are two main coronary arteries, the left and the right. The left one branches to form the left circumflex artery and the left anterior descending artery.

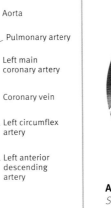

Pulmonary veins

Aorta

Pulmonary artery

Left main coronary artery

Coronary vein

Right main coronary artery

Left circumflex artery

Left anterior descending artery

Vena cava

Valve cusp

Chorda tendinea

Anchoring the valves
String-like chordae tendineae anchor each valve cusp (flap) to the heart wall to prevent it from being turned inside out.

How the heart beats

A single pumping action of the heart is called a heartbeat. A healthy adult heart beats at a rate of 60–80 beats per minute at rest and at up to 200 beats per minute during strenuous exercise. One-way valves inside the heart prevent blood from being pumped in the wrong direction. The rhythmic "lub-dub" sound of the heart is due to the heart valves shutting tightly.

The heart cycle

A heartbeat has three phases. In diastole, the heart relaxes. During atrial systole, the atria contract, and in ventricular systole, the ventricles contract. The sinoatrial node (the heart's pacemaker) regulates the timing of the phases by sending electrical impulses to the atria, from where they pass to the ventricles.

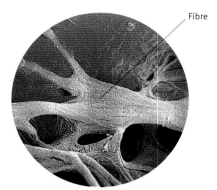

Fibre

Conducting fibres
Specialized muscle fibres in the walls of the heart conduct electrical impulses that regulate the heartbeat.

Heart valves

Heart valves consist of two or three cup-shaped cusps (flaps). The cusps consist mainly of collagen, a tough protein, and are covered in endocardium, a thin layer of tissue that lines the inside of the heart and joins the lining of the blood vessels.

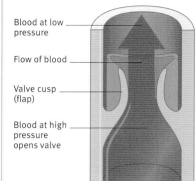

Blood at low pressure

Flow of blood

Valve cusp (flap)

Blood at high pressure opens valve

Open heart valve
When a heart chamber contracts, the high pressure of the blood inside it pushes open the valve cusps, and blood flows through to the other side of the valve.

Diastole

The heart muscle relaxes, and blood flows into the atria and ventricles from the pulmonary veins and venae cavae. Near the end of this phase, the sinoatrial node emits an electrical impulse.

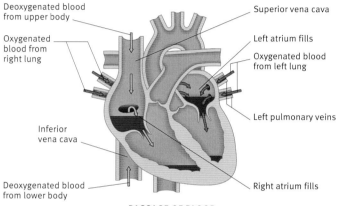

Deoxygenated blood from upper body

Oxygenated blood from right lung

Inferior vena cava

Deoxygenated blood from lower body

Superior vena cava

Left atrium fills

Oxygenated blood from left lung

Left pulmonary veins

Right atrium fills

PASSAGE OF BLOOD

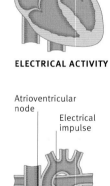

Sinoatrial node

Electrical impulse

ELECTRICAL ACTIVITY

Atrial systole

The electrical impulse spreads through both atria. The impulse causes their muscular walls to contract and push blood into the ventricles. By the end of atrial systole, the impulse reaches the atrioventricular node, which is in the right atrium.

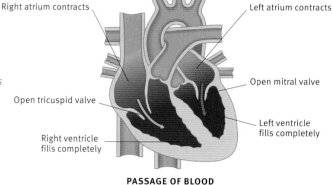

Right atrium contracts

Open tricuspid valve

Right ventricle fills completely

Left atrium contracts

Open mitral valve

Left ventricle fills completely

PASSAGE OF BLOOD

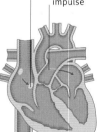

Atrioventricular node

Electrical impulse

ELECTRICAL ACTIVITY

High-pressure blood closes valve

Valve cusp

Low-pressure blood

Closed heart valve
The pressure of blood on the other side of the valve rises and snaps shut the valve cusps. The closed valve prevents backflow.

Ventricular systole

The impulse reaches the atrioventricular node, where it is momentarily delayed before it spreads throughout the walls of the ventricles. The impulse causes the ventricles to contract, pushing blood out into the aorta and the pulmonary arteries.

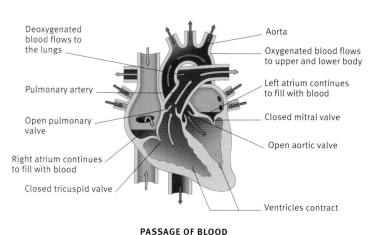

Deoxygenated blood flows to the lungs

Pulmonary artery

Open pulmonary valve

Right atrium continues to fill with blood

Closed tricuspid valve

Aorta

Oxygenated blood flows to upper and lower body

Left atrium continues to fill with blood

Closed mitral valve

Open aortic valve

Ventricles contract

PASSAGE OF BLOOD

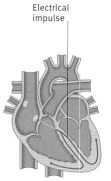

Electrical impulse

ELECTRICAL ACTIVITY

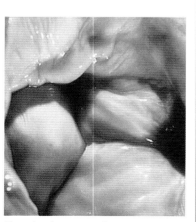

Closed pulmonary valve
The pulmonary valve has three cusps with rounded undersides that are attached to the inner wall of the pulmonary artery.

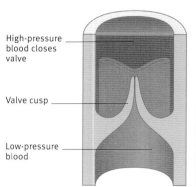

✚ **FUNCTION**

The blood circulation

Blood circulates in two linked circuits: the pulmonary, which carries blood to the lungs to be oxygenated, and the systemic, which supplies oxygenated blood to the body. Arteries carrying blood from the heart divide into smaller vessels called arterioles and then into capillaries, where gas, nutrient, and waste exchange occurs. Capillaries join up to form venules, which in turn join to form veins that carry blood back to the heart. The portal vein does not return blood to the heart but carries it to the liver.

A double circuit

The heart powers the pulmonary and the systemic circulations. In the pulmonary circulation, deoxygenated blood (blue) travels to the lungs, where it absorbs oxygen before returning to the heart. This oxygenated blood (red) is pumped around the body in the systemic circulation. Body tissues absorb oxygen, and deoxygenated blood returns to the heart to be pumped to the lungs again.

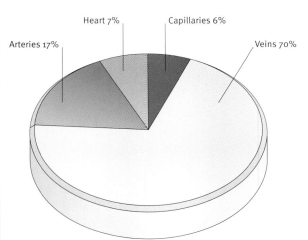

Distribution of blood in the circulation
At rest, the veins act as a reservoir for blood, holding most of the body's blood volume. If an increase in blood supply is needed, the veins constrict and return more blood to the heart.

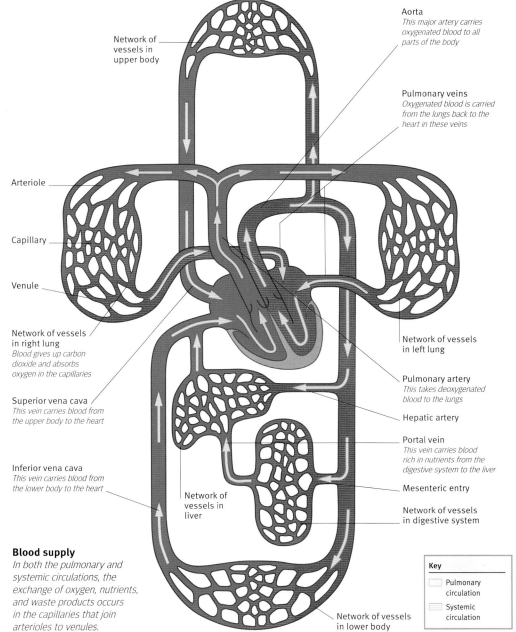

Network of vessels in upper body

Aorta
This major artery carries oxygenated blood to all parts of the body

Pulmonary veins
Oxygenated blood is carried from the lungs back to the heart in these veins

Arteriole

Capillary

Venule

Network of vessels in right lung
Blood gives up carbon dioxide and absorbs oxygen in the capillaries

Superior vena cava
This vein carries blood from the upper body to the heart

Inferior vena cava
This vein carries blood from the lower body to the heart

Network of vessels in liver

Blood supply
In both the pulmonary and systemic circulations, the exchange of oxygen, nutrients, and waste products occurs in the capillaries that join arterioles to venules.

Network of vessels in left lung

Pulmonary artery
This takes deoxygenated blood to the lungs

Hepatic artery

Portal vein
This vein carries blood rich in nutrients from the digestive system to the liver

Mesenteric entry

Network of vessels in digestive system

Network of vessels in lower body

Key	
☐	Pulmonary circulation
☐	Systemic circulation

Venous return

The blood pressure in the veins is about a tenth of that in the arteries. Various physical mechanisms ensure that there is adequate venous return (blood flow back to the heart). Many deep veins lie within muscles. When the muscles contract, they squeeze the veins and force blood back to the heart. The action of inhalation during breathing also draws blood to the heart. In addition, venous return from the upper body is assisted by gravity.

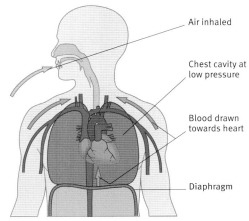

Air inhaled

Chest cavity at low pressure

Blood drawn towards heart

Diaphragm

Respiratory pump during inhalation
While inhaling, the chest cavity expands, lowering the pressure in the chest. Higher pressure in the rest of the body pushes blood in the veins towards the heart.

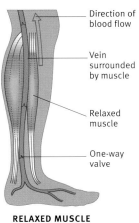

Direction of blood flow

Vein surrounded by muscle

Relaxed muscle

One-way valve

Direction of increased blood flow

Squeezed vein

Contracted muscle

RELAXED MUSCLE   **CONTRACTED MUSCLE**

Muscular pump
Muscles contract and relax as we move, squeezing the veins that pass through them and pushing blood back to the heart. One-way valves prevent backflow.

✚ **FUNCTION**

Control of blood pressure

Blood pressure in the arteries must be regulated to ensure an adequate supply of blood, and hence oxygen, to the organs. If arterial blood pressure is too low, not enough blood reaches body tissues. If it is too high, it may damage blood vessels and organs. Rapid changes in blood pressure trigger compensatory responses from the nervous system within seconds. These autonomic nervous responses do not involve the conscious parts of the brain. Longer-term changes are largely regulated by hormones that affect the volume of fluid excreted by the kidneys. Hormonal responses work over several hours.

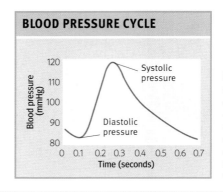

BLOOD PRESSURE CYCLE

Systolic and diastolic pressure
Arterial pressure is low while the heart fills with blood (diastolic pressure) but rises as the heart pumps blood out (systolic pressure). The units of pressure are millimetres of mercury (mmHg).

Short-term control of blood pressure

Heavy bleeding or a sudden change in posture may cause a rapid change in blood pressure, to which the nervous system immediately responds. Baroreceptors (stretch receptors in the walls of the major arteries) detect pressure changes and send signals along sensory nerves to the brain. A reflex autonomic response adjusts the heart rate, volume of blood pumped, and arterial diameter to restore normal pressure.

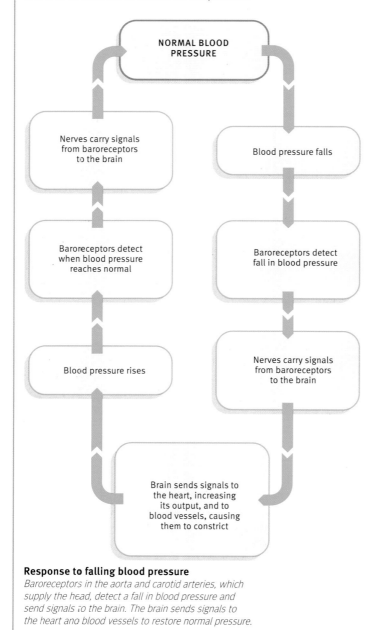

Response to falling blood pressure
Baroreceptors in the aorta and carotid arteries, which supply the head, detect a fall in blood pressure and send signals to the brain. The brain sends signals to the heart and blood vessels to restore normal pressure.

Long-term control of blood pressure

Blood pressure is controlled in the long term by the action of hormones. The kidneys respond to low blood pressure by secreting renin. This hormone promotes the generation of angiotensin, which constricts arteries and raises blood pressure. The adrenal glands, hypothalamus, and heart also respond to high or low pressure by secreting aldosterone, vasopressin, and natriuretic hormone, respectively. These hormones alter the amount of fluid excreted by the kidneys, which affects the volume of blood in the body and hence the blood pressure.

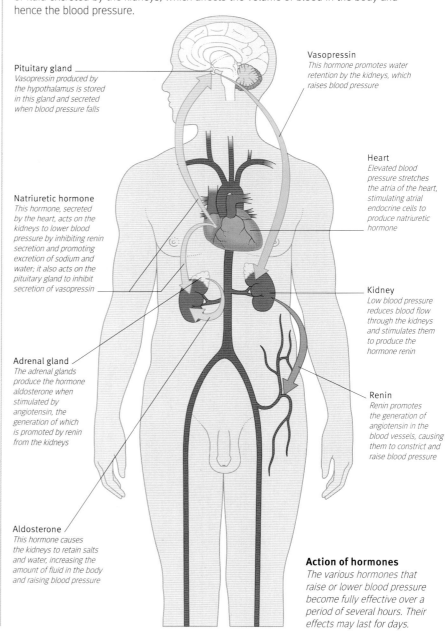

Pituitary gland
Vasopressin produced by the hypothalamus is stored in this gland and secreted when blood pressure falls

Natriuretic hormone
This hormone, secreted by the heart, acts on the kidneys to lower blood pressure by inhibiting renin secretion and promoting excretion of sodium and water; it also acts on the pituitary gland to inhibit secretion of vasopressin

Adrenal gland
The adrenal glands produce the hormone aldosterone when stimulated by angiotensin, the generation of which is promoted by renin from the kidneys

Aldosterone
This hormone causes the kidneys to retain salts and water, increasing the amount of fluid in the body and raising blood pressure

Vasopressin
This hormone promotes water retention by the kidneys, which raises blood pressure

Heart
Elevated blood pressure stretches the atria of the heart, stimulating atrial endocrine cells to produce natriuretic hormone

Kidney
Low blood pressure reduces blood flow through the kidneys and stimulates them to produce the hormone renin

Renin
Renin promotes the generation of angiotensin in the blood vessels, causing them to constrict and raise blood pressure

Action of hormones
The various hormones that raise or lower blood pressure become fully effective over a period of several hours. Their effects may last for days.

Major cardiovascular disorders

By the middle of the 20th century, cardiovascular disease was the leading cause of death in northern Europe. Coronary artery disease was the most common cause, although rheumatic fever and high blood pressure also claimed lives. The number of deaths caused by cardiovascular disease peaked by the early 1980s, and over the last 25–35 years preventive treatments have brought about a steady decline in cardiovascular disease deaths in many developed countries.

This section covers the major disorders affecting the heart and the circulation. The first articles overlap to a certain extent because some cardiovascular disorders can lead to the development of others. Smoking, an unhealthy diet, being overweight, and lack of exercise are risk factors for the development of hypertension (high blood pressure) and atherosclerosis, in which the arteries are narrowed. Narrowing of the coronary arteries that supply the heart muscle can cause coronary artery disease, which itself is the major cause of angina and heart attacks. If the heart is damaged by coronary artery disease or a heart attack, it may be too weak to pump blood efficiently around the rest of the body, resulting in heart failure. Heart failure can develop suddenly, or it may be a chronic disorder that develops over several years.

The last articles in the section cover hypotension, the medical term for low blood pressure, and shock. Shock is a medical emergency that requires immediate treatment in hospital.

KEY ANATOMY

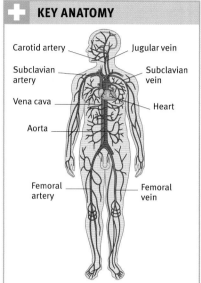

Carotid artery
Jugular vein
Subclavian artery
Subclavian vein
Vena cava
Heart
Aorta
Femoral artery
Femoral vein

For further information on the structure of the cardiovascular system, *see* pp.235–240.

Atherosclerosis

Accumulation of cholesterol and other fatty substances in the walls of arteries, causing them to narrow

 More common with increasing age

 More common in males until the age of 60, then equal incidence

 Sometimes runs in families

 Smoking, an unhealthy diet, lack of exercise, and excess weight are risk factors

Atherosclerosis is a disease that results in the arteries becoming narrowed. The condition can affect arteries in any area of the body and is a major cause of stroke (p.329), heart attack (*see* **Myocardial infarction**, p.245), and poor circulation in the legs (*see* **Lower limb ischaemia**, p.261). The arteries become narrowed when fatty substances, such as cholesterol, that are carried in the blood accumulate on the inside lining of the arteries and form yellow deposits called atheroma. These deposits restrict the blood flow through the arteries. In addition, the muscle layer of the artery wall becomes thickened, narrowing the artery even more.

Platelets (tiny blood cells responsible for clotting) may collect in clumps on the surface of the deposits and initiate the formation of blood clots. A large clot may completely block the artery, resulting in the organ it supplies being deprived of oxygen.

Atherosclerosis is much more common in northern Europe than in developing countries in Africa and Asia. The condition becomes more common with increasing age and tends to run in families. Autopsies on young men who have died in accidents reveal that many have already developed some atheroma in their large arteries, and most people who die in middle age are found to have a degree of atherosclerosis. However, the condition rarely causes symptoms before the age of 45–50, and many people are unaware that they have it until they have a heart attack or a stroke.

The incidence of atherosclerosis is much lower in women before the menopause than in men. However, by the age of 60 a woman's risk of developing atherosclerosis is the same as a man's. Although it is likely that the female sex hormone oestrogen contributes to the lower risk in premenopausal women, hormone replacement therapy in postmenopausal women does not reduce the risk of heart disease and may increase the risk of certain cancers.

What are the causes?

The risk of developing atherosclerosis is determined largely by the level of cholesterol in the bloodstream, which depends on dietary and genetic factors. Since cholesterol levels are closely linked with diet, atherosclerosis is most common in Western countries where many people eat a diet high in refined and processed foods and unhealthy fats. Some disorders, such as diabetes mellitus (p.437), can be associated with a high cholesterol level regardless of diet. Certain inherited lipid disorders also result in a high level of fats in the blood (*see* **Inherited hyperlipidaemias**, p.440).

In addition to high blood cholesterol, factors that make atherosclerosis more likely are smoking, lack of regular exercise, high blood pressure (*see* **Hypertension**, p.242), and being overweight, especially if there is a concentration of fat around the waist.

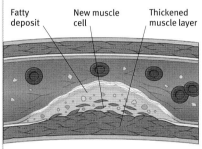

Fatty deposit
New muscle cell
Thickened muscle layer

How atherosclerosis develops
Fatty substances gradually accumulate in the lining of the artery wall, and the muscle layer thickens as new muscle cells form in the fatty deposit. As a result, the artery becomes progressively narrowed and blood flow is restricted.

What are the symptoms?

There are usually no symptoms in the early stages of atherosclerosis. Later, symptoms are caused by the reduced or total absence of a blood supply to the organs supplied by the affected arteries. If the coronary arteries, which supply the heart muscle, are partially blocked, symptoms may include the chest pain of angina (p.244). If there is a complete blockage in a coronary artery, there may be a sudden, often fatal, heart attack. Many strokes are a result of atherosclerosis in the arteries that supply blood to the brain. If atherosclerosis affects the arteries in the legs, the first symptom may be cramping pain when walking caused by poor blood flow to the leg muscles. If atherosclerosis is associated with an inherited lipid disorder, fatty deposits may develop on tendons or under the skin in visible lumps.

How is it diagnosed?

Since atherosclerosis has no symptoms until blood flow has been restricted, it is important to screen for the disorder before it becomes advanced and damages organs. Routine medical checkups include screening for the major risk factors of atherosclerosis, particularly raised blood cholesterol levels, high blood pressure, and diabetes mellitus. It is recommended that adults who have

cardiovascular disease or are at high risk of developing it, or who have a family history of high blood cholesterol, should have their cholesterol levels checked regularly.

If you develop symptoms of atherosclerosis, your doctor may arrange tests to assess the damage both to the arteries and to the organs they supply. Blood flow in affected blood vessels can be imaged by Doppler ultrasound scanning (p.259) or coronary angiography (p.245). If your doctor thinks that the coronary arteries are affected, an ECG (p.243) may be carried out to monitor the electrical activity of the heart and imaging techniques, such as angiography and radionuclide scanning (p.135), may be used to look at the blood supply to the heart. To check how the heart functions when it is put under stress, some of these tests may be done as you exercise (*see* **Exercise testing**, p.244) or after you have been given a drug to stress the heart.

What is the treatment?

The best treatment is to prevent atherosclerosis from progressing. Preventive measures include following a healthy lifestyle by eating a good-quality diet, not smoking, exercising regularly, and maintaining the recommended weight for your height. These measures lead to a lower than average risk of developing significant atherosclerosis.

If you have been found to have a high blood cholesterol level but are otherwise in good state of health, you will be advised to adopt a diet that is low in unhealthy fats and to avoid refined and processed foods. You may also be given drugs that decrease your blood cholesterol level (*see* **Lipid-lowering drugs**, p.603). For people who have had a heart attack or are at high risk of having one, research has shown that there may be a benefit in lowering blood cholesterol, even if the person's cholesterol level is within the average range for healthy people.

If you have atherosclerosis and are experiencing symptoms of the condition, your doctor may prescribe a drug such as aspirin to reduce the risk of blood clots forming on the artery lining (*see* **Drugs that prevent blood clotting**, p.584). Your doctor may also prescribe drugs to relieve the symptoms, such as drugs for angina (p.244).

If you are thought to be at high risk of severe complications, your doctor may recommend that you undergo an invasive treatment, such as coronary angioplasty and stenting (p.246), in which a balloon is inflated inside the artery to widen it and improve blood flow. In most cases, a stent (a tubular scaffold device) will be inserted in the artery to help keep it open. If blood flow to the heart is severely obstructed (*see* **Coronary artery disease**, p.243), you may be advised to have a bypass operation (*see* **Coronary artery bypass graft**, p.247) to restore blood flow.

What is the prognosis?

A healthy diet and lifestyle can slow the progress of atherosclerosis in most people. If you do have a myocardial infarction or a stroke, you can reduce the risk of developing further complications by taking preventive measures (*see* **Life after a heart attack**, p.246).

Hypertension

Persistent high blood pressure that may damage the arteries and the heart

 More common with increasing age

 Slightly more common in males

 Often runs in families; more common in people of African or Caribbean origin

 Stress, alcohol abuse, a high-salt diet, and excess weight are risk factors

In the UK, an estimated 30–40 per cent of adults have high blood pressure, also known as hypertension. The condition puts strain on the heart and arteries, resulting in damage to delicate tissues. If it is left untreated, hypertension may eventually affect the eyes, brain, and kidneys. The higher the blood pressure, the greater the risk that complications such as heart attacks (*see* **Myocardial infarction**, p.245), coronary artery disease (opposite page), and stroke (p.329) will develop.

Blood pressure varies naturally with activity, rising during exercise or stress and falling during rest. It also varies among individuals, gradually increasing with age and weight. Blood pressure is expressed as two values given in units of millimetres of mercury (mmHg). The blood pressure of a resting, healthy young adult should not be more than 120/80 mmHg. In general, a person is considered to have hypertension when his or her blood pressure is persistently higher than 140/90 mmHg, even at rest.

Hypertension does not usually cause symptoms, but, if your blood pressure is very high, you may have headaches, dizziness, or blurred vision. However, usually the only symptoms that develop are those due to the damage caused by hypertension. By the time these arise and hypertension becomes evident, irreversible damage to arteries and organs has usually occurred. Hypertension is sometimes called the "silent killer" because individuals may have a fatal stroke or heart attack without warning.

In recent years, health education and screening programmes have led to many more people being diagnosed with hypertension at an early stage before symptoms occur. Early diagnosis and improved treatments have substantially reduced the incidence of heart attacks and strokes caused by hypertension.

What are the causes?

In about 9 in 10 people with hypertension, there is no obvious cause for the condition. However, both lifestyle and genetic factors

▶ TEST

Blood pressure measurement

Blood pressure measurement is a routine part of having a physical examination. A measuring device called a sphygmomanometer gives a blood pressure reading as systolic pressure (the higher figure) when the heart contracts and diastolic pressure when the heart relaxes. A healthy young adult has a blood pressure of about 120/80 mmHg. Your blood pressure may be taken when you are sitting, standing, or lying down.

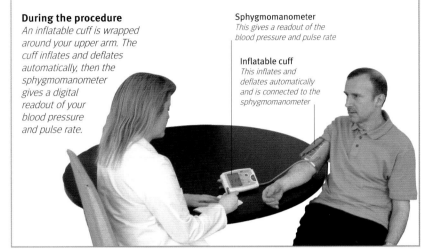

During the procedure
An inflatable cuff is wrapped around your upper arm. The cuff inflates and deflates automatically, then the sphygmomanometer gives a digital readout of your blood pressure and pulse rate.

Sphygmomanometer
This gives a readout of the blood pressure and pulse rate

Inflatable cuff
This inflates and deflates automatically and is connected to the sphygmomanometer

may contribute. The condition is most common in middle-aged and elderly people because the arteries become more rigid with age. It is also marginally more common in men. People who are overweight or who drink excessive amounts of alcohol are more likely to develop hypertension, and a stressful lifestyle may aggravate the condition. Although hypertension occurs most often in developed countries, it is now a significant problem in the developing world too. The tendency to develop hypertension is thought to be inherited, and people of African or Caribbean origin are more susceptible to the condition. Hypertension is rare in countries where people are typically not overweight, physically active, and have a low-salt diet, this last factor suggesting that salt may be a contributing factor.

In a minority of cases, an underlying cause is found, such as kidney disease or the hormonal disorders hyperaldosteronism, (p.436), Cushing's syndrome (p.435), or phaeochromocytoma (p.436). Some drugs, such as combined oral contraceptives and corticosteroids (p.600), can cause hypertension.

When hypertension develops during pregnancy, it can be associated with the development of the potentially life-threatening conditions pre-eclampsia and eclampsia (p.513). Although the elevated blood pressure usually returns to normal after the birth, women who have hypertension in pregnancy are at a slightly increased risk of developing it later in life.

Are there complications?

The risk of damage to the arteries, heart, and kidneys rises with the severity of hypertension and the length of time for which it is present. Arteries that have been damaged are at greater risk of becoming narrowed by atherosclerosis (p.241), in which fatty deposits build up in vessel walls, causing them to narrow and restricting blood flow.

Atherosclerosis is more likely in people with high blood pressure who also smoke or who have high blood cholesterol levels. Atherosclerosis of the coronary arteries may lead eventually to chest pain (*see* **Angina**, p.244) or to a heart attack. In other arteries in the body, atherosclerosis may result in disorders such as aortic aneurysm (p.259) or stroke. Hypertension puts strain on the heart that may eventually lead to chronic heart failure (p.247). Damage to the arteries in the kidneys may result in chronic kidney disease (p.451). Hypertension may also damage arteries supplying the retina in the eye (*see* **Retinopathy,** p.360) and reduce blood flow to the brain, which may lead to dementia (p.331).

How is it diagnosed?

Healthy adults should have their blood pressure checked every 3–5 years from about the age of 40 (*see* **Blood pressure measurement**, above). In the UK, all adults aged 40–74 are offered blood pressure measurement as part of a routine health check. If you already have high blood pressure or a condition such as diabetes mellitus, you should have more frequent checks. If your blood pressure is more than 140/90 mmHg, your doctor may ask you to return in a few weeks so that he or she can check it again. Some people become anxious when visiting their doctor, which may cause a temporary rise in blood pressure; this phenomenon is known as "white coat hypertension".

Consequently, a diagnosis of hypertension is usually not made unless you have elevated blood pressure on three separate occasions. If your readings are variable, you may be offered a portable device to measure your blood pressure at home.

If you have hypertension, your doctor may arrange for tests that check for organ damage. Tests for heart damage include echocardiography (p.255) or electrocardiography (*see* **ECG**, opposite page). Your eyes may be examined to look for damaged blood vessels, and your urine may be tested to check for kidney damage. You may also have tests to look for other factors, such as a high blood cholesterol level, that may increase your risk of a heart attack.

If you are young or have severe hypertension, you may have tests to find the underlying cause. For example, you may have urine and blood tests and ultrasound scanning (p.135) to look for kidney disease or a hormonal disorder.

What is the treatment?

Hypertension cannot usually be cured but can be controlled with treatment. If you have mild hypertension, changing your lifestyle is often the most effective way of lowering your blood pressure. You should reduce your salt and alcohol consumption and try to keep your weight within the ideal range (*see* **Are you a healthy weight?**, p.19). If you smoke, you should give up.

If self-help measures are not effective in reducing your blood pressure, your doctor may prescribe antihypertensive drugs (p.580). These drugs work in different ways, and you may be prescribed one type of drug or a combination of several. The type of drug and the dosage are tailored to the individual, and it may take some time to find the right combination and dosage. If you develop side effects, consult your doctor so that your medication can be adjusted. He or she may recommend that you measure your blood pressure regularly yourself to help evaluate your treatment. You can now buy small electronic blood pressure machines for use at home, but seek advice from your doctor first.

If your hypertension has an obvious underlying medical cause, such as a hormonal disorder, treatment of this disorder may result in your blood pressure returning to a normal level.

What is the prognosis?

The outlook depends on how high your blood pressure is and how long it has been high. For most people, lifestyle changes and drug treatment can control blood pressure and reduce the risk of complications from hypertension. These measures usually need to be maintained for life. Long-standing, severe hypertension carries the greatest risk of complications.

Coronary artery disease

Narrowing of the coronary arteries that supply the heart muscle with blood, leading to heart damage

 More common with increasing age

 More common in males until the age of 60, then equal incidence

 Sometimes runs in families

 Smoking, an unhealthy diet, lack of exercise, and excess weight are risk factors

The coronary arteries, which branch from the main artery in the body, the aorta, supply the heart muscle with oxygen-rich blood. In coronary artery disease (CAD), also known as coronary heart disease, one or more of the coronary arteries is narrowed. Blood flow through the arteries is restricted, which can lead to heart muscle damage. Heart disorders, including heart attacks (*see* **Myocardial infarction**, p.245) and the chest pain of angina (p.244), are usually caused by CAD. This condition is therefore a leading cause of death in many developed countries. The number of deaths from CAD reached its peak in the UK in the late 1970s, with about 85 people per 100,000 dying each year. The death rate from CAD has since fallen by more than half as a result of health education about smoking and diet and the introduction of more effective treatments. However, in many parts of the world, including some developing countries, mortality from CAD is rising as a result of changing lifestyle factors.

What are the causes?
Coronary artery disease is usually due to atherosclerosis (p.241), in which fatty deposits accumulate on the inside of arteries. These deposits narrow the arteries and restrict blood flow. If a blood clot forms or lodges in the narrowed area of an artery, the vessel can become completely blocked. CAD caused by atherosclerosis is more likely if your blood cholesterol level is high and you eat a poor-quality diet high in refined and processed foods and unhealthy fats. CAD is also linked to smoking, obesity, lack of exercise, diabetes mellitus (p.437), and high blood pressure (*see* **Hypertension**, opposite page).

In premenopausal women, the risk of CAD is lower, possibly because of the effects of the female hormone oestrogen. After the menopause, oestrogen levels fall, and by the age of 60 women have the same risk of developing CAD as men, although their mortality remains lower. Hormone replacement therapy (HRT) does not reduce mortality from CAD in postmenopausal women and is likely to increase the risk of certain cancers.

Rarely, the coronary arteries are damaged by inflammation, which may be due to the autoimmune disorder polyarteritis nodosa (p.283). Temporary narrowing of the coronary arteries can be caused by spasm in the artery wall, which, in rare cases, may cause a heart attack.

What are the symptoms?
In the early stages of CAD, there are often no symptoms. In the later stages of CAD, the first symptom is usually either pain in the chest on exertion, a condition known as angina, or a heart attack. Some people with CAD develop an abnormality of the heart rhythm (*see* **Arrhythmias**, p.249), which may cause palpitations (awareness of heartbeats), light-headedness, and, sometimes, loss of consciousness. Some severe forms of arrhythmia can cause the heart to stop pumping completely (*see* **Cardiac arrest**, p.252), which accounts for most of the sudden deaths from CAD.

Coronary artery disease may lead to a condition called chronic heart failure (p.247), in which the heart gradually becomes too weak to provide adequate circulation of blood around the body. This is more common in elderly people. Chronic heart failure may then lead to the accumulation of excess fluid in the lungs and tissues, causing additional symptoms such as shortness of breath and swollen ankles.

How is it diagnosed?
CAD is usually diagnosed only when a person develops symptoms of the disease. Sometimes, a heart attack is the first sign. If you have symptoms such as chest pain, your doctor may arrange a series of tests to detect and establish the severity of the problem. These tests include an ECG (right) to monitor the heart's electrical activity and radionuclide scanning (p.135) to show whether the blood supply to the heart muscle is adequate. You may have exercise testing (p.244) to see how the heart performs under stress, and echocardiography (p.255), an ultrasound technique that images the heart muscle and valves. The imaging techniques of high-resolution CT scanning (p.132) and MRI (p.133) are increasingly used to detect heart and coronary artery abnormalities.

If these tests suggest that the blood supply to your heart is inadequate, you may be referred for coronary angiography (p.245), in which a dye is injected into the bloodstream to enable arteries to be seen on an X-ray. Angiography detects blocked or seriously narrowed sections of an artery and provides your doctor with the information needed to decide whether surgical treatment is required.

What is the treatment?
Treatment for CAD falls into three categories: lifestyle changes and protective drug treatment – for example, with lipid-lowering drugs (p.603) – to reduce the risk of CAD becoming worse; drug treatments to improve the function of the heart and help to relieve symptoms; and surgical procedures, such as coronary angioplasty (p.246), that improve the blood supply to the heart muscle.

▶ **TEST**

ECG

ECG (electrocardiography) is used to record the electrical activity of the heart. The procedure is frequently used to diagnose abnormal heart rhythms and to investigate the cause of chest pain. Several electrodes are attached to the skin to transmit the electrical activity of the heart to an ECG machine. Several traces are produced at the same time. Each trace shows electrical activity in different areas of the heart. The test usually takes several minutes to complete and is safe and painless.

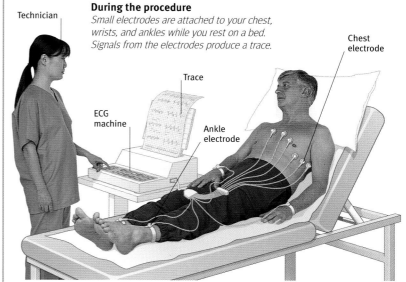

During the procedure
Small electrodes are attached to your chest, wrists, and ankles while you rest on a bed. Signals from the electrodes produce a trace.

Technician · ECG machine · Trace · Chest electrode · Ankle electrode

RESULTS

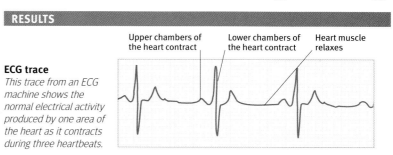

Upper chambers of the heart contract · Lower chambers of the heart contract · Heart muscle relaxes

ECG trace
This trace from an ECG machine shows the normal electrical activity produced by one area of the heart as it contracts during three heartbeats.

If you are diagnosed with CAD, you should adopt a healthier lifestyle, with regular exercise and a good-quality diet that is low in refined and processed foods and unhealthy fats. If you smoke, you should stop.

The drugs used to treat CAD depend on your symptoms and their severity and on the cause of the disorder. If tests show that you have a high blood cholesterol level, you will be treated with lipid-lowering drugs (p.603). These drugs are usually prescribed even if you eat a healthy diet and your cholesterol levels are within the acceptable range. This is because treatment with lipid-lowering drugs slows the progression of CAD and, as a consequence, reduces the risk of a heart attack.

Angina may be treated with drugs, such as nitrate drugs (p.581) and beta-blocker drugs (p.581), that improve the blood flow through the arteries and help the heart to pump effectively. Other drugs that may be used to treat angina include calcium channel blockers (p.582), which relax the arteries and thereby improve blood flow, and ivabradine, which slows the heart rate and so reduces the heart's oxygen and energy requirements. An abnormal heart rhythm is often treated using antiarrhythmic drugs (p.580).

If treatment fails to relieve the symptoms or if there is extensive narrowing of the arteries, your doctor will discuss other treatment options with you. If only small segments of the artery are affected, you may be offered coronary angioplasty and stenting (p.246), in which a balloon is inflated in the narrowed area of the affected blood vessel to widen it. During the procedure, a stent (a tubular scaffold device) will usually be inserted into the affected artery to keep it open. Alternatively, your doctor may suggest a coronary artery bypass graft (p.247). In this procedure, blockages in one or more coronary arteries are bypassed using an artery on the inside of the chest wall or veins taken from a leg.

What is the prognosis?
Coronary artery disease affects people in middle to old age and is more easily prevented than treated. The chance of

▶ **TEST**

Exercise testing

Exercise testing may be done when coronary artery disease is suspected. It is used to assess the function of the heart when it is put under stress. The test typically involves raising your heart rate by exercising, often using an adjustable treadmill or exercise bicycle, and monitoring the heart's activity with an ECG. Instead of exercise, medication may sometimes be used to raise the heart rate. During stress testing, the heart may also be imaged by radionuclide scanning (p.135) or echocardiography (p.255). The ECG and imaging results from stress testing are compared with those at rest to assess heart function.

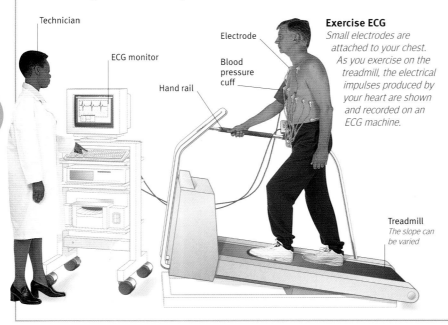

Technician

ECG monitor

Hand rail

Electrode

Blood pressure cuff

Exercise ECG
Small electrodes are attached to your chest. As you exercise on the treadmill, the electrical impulses produced by your heart are shown and recorded on an ECG machine.

Treadmill
The slope can be varied

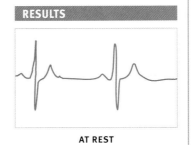

RESULTS

AT REST

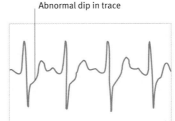

Abnormal dip in trace

DURING EXERCISE

ECG tracing
These traces are from a person with coronary artery disease. At rest, the ECG trace is normal (top). During exercise, when the heart beats faster and requires more oxygen, the trace becomes abnormal (bottom), showing an exaggerated downward dip.

developing the disease can be reduced by following a healthy lifestyle. More efficient methods of diagnosing CAD and screening for risk factors also make it possible to begin treatment early in the course of the disease. Effective drugs to prevent the progression of CAD and the success of both coronary angioplasty and bypass grafting have greatly improved the prognosis for CAD.

For an individual with CAD, the outlook depends on the number of blood vessels involved and how extensively the heart muscle is damaged.

Angina

Pain in the chest, usually brought on by exertion and relieved by rest

 More common with increasing age

 More common in males until the age of 60, then equal incidence

 Sometimes runs in families

 Smoking, an unhealthy diet, lack of exercise, and excess weight are risk factors

Angina is chest pain that originates in the heart muscle during physical activity and is quickly relieved by rest. The pain is due to an inadequate supply of blood to the heart muscle. Angina affects both sexes but is less common in women under 60 because the hormone oestrogen protects against it. This protection gradually disappears when levels of oestrogen drop after the menopause.

Over the last 40 years, angina has become progressively less common in western Europe, mainly due to more healthy lifestyles. At the same time, treatment with drugs and surgery has also improved the outlook for people who have the condition.

What are the causes?

The most common cause of angina is coronary artery disease (p.243), a narrowing of the arteries that supply the heart muscle. This narrowing is usually the result of fatty deposits building up on the inside of the artery walls (*see* **Atherosclerosis**, p.241). The blood flow through the arteries may be sufficient for the heart while it is at rest but becomes inadequate during exertion. If the supply of oxygen-rich blood is insufficient, the heart muscle is starved of oxygen and toxic substances build up in the heart muscle, causing a constrictive, cramp-like pain. People who have a high blood cholesterol level (*see* **Hypercholesterolaemia**, p.440), persistently high blood pressure (*see* **Hypertension**, p.242), or diabetes mellitus (p.437) have an increased risk of developing atherosclerosis and angina.

Having a close relative with the disorder also increases the risk of angina, as does smoking.

Angina can also be caused by temporary spasm of the coronary arteries, in which the arteries narrow for a short time, or by a damaged heart valve that causes a reduction in the blood flow to the heart muscle (*see* **Aortic stenosis**, p.254). Occasionally, angina is caused or made worse by anaemia, in which the ability of the red blood cells to carry oxygen is impaired, thus reducing the supply of oxygen to the heart.

What are the symptoms?

The chest pain of angina varies from mild to severe. It usually starts during exertion and is relieved after a short rest. The features of angina are:

■ A dull, heavy, constricting sensation in the centre of the chest.

■ A discomfort that spreads into the throat and down one or both arms, more often the left arm.

Angina usually occurs predictably at a particular level of exertion. For example, if you regularly walk uphill or climb stairs, it will develop at about the same stage of the activity each time. Angina caused by outdoor exertion often occurs more rapidly in cold or windy weather.

If you experience this type of chest pain for the first time or if your angina becomes more frequent, more severe, or develops at rest, you should contact your doctor immediately. Worsening angina can be a warning that a blood clot has formed in the coronary artery, which may completely block it and cause a heart attack (*see* **Myocardial infarction**, opposite page). A prolonged and very severe attack of angina may be due to a heart attack.

How is it diagnosed?

Your doctor will usually make a diagnosis of angina from your symptoms. However, in some circumstances it may be difficult for your doctor to be certain that the pain is actually angina and is not caused by another problem such as gastro-oesophageal reflux disease (p.403) or pain from the chest wall.

Your doctor will measure your blood pressure to see if you have hypertension (p.242). He or she may also arrange for you to have blood tests to check for anaemia or raised cholesterol levels. You will probably have an ECG (p.243) to monitor the electrical activity of the heart. You may also have various other tests. These may include a myocardial perfusion scan, a type of radionuclide scan (p.135) that shows how well blood is reaching your heart; stress echocardiography (p.255), in which an ultrasound scan of the heart is taken after you have been given a drug to increase the heart rate; and a coronary CT scan (p.132) to image the coronary arteries. If the tests confirm that there is a significant problem with blood flow to the heart, you may need coronary angiography (opposite page), in which dye is injected into the coronary arteries so that narrowed areas can be detected on an X-ray.

What is the treatment?

The treatment of angina depends on its severity. Drugs are used to relieve acute episodes of pain and also to reduce the number and severity of attacks. Drug treatment of an acute attack usually includes nitrate drugs (p.581) to widen coronary arteries. Fast-acting nitrates can be administered in the form of a spray or soluble under-tongue tablets. Longer-acting nitrates can be taken on a regular basis to prevent attacks. Other drugs that may be used to widen the coronary arteries and improve blood flow to the heart include calcium channel blockers (p.582). In addition, drugs may be used to reduce the heart's need for oxygen, such as beta blockers (p.581) or ivabradine. Doctors also advise a daily low dose of aspirin (*see* **Drugs that prevent blood clotting**, p.584) because this reduces the risk of clots forming in an artery. If there is an underlying disorder contributing to angina, such as aortic stenosis, hypertension, or diabetes mellitus, it will be treated.

Lifestyle changes can prevent worsening of angina and increase the level of exercise that you can achieve without experiencing pain. It is imperative that you stop smoking; cutting down is not sufficient. A diet

▶ **TEST**

Coronary angiography

Coronary angiography is used to image the arteries that supply the heart muscle with blood. Angiography can image narrowed or blocked coronary arteries, which are not visible on a normal X-ray. A local anaesthetic is injected, and a fine, flexible catheter is passed into the femoral artery, through the aorta, and into a coronary artery. Contrast dye is injected through the catheter, and a series of X-rays is taken. The procedure is painless, but you may feel a flushing sensation as the dye is injected.

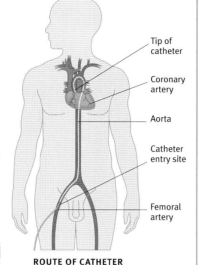

- Tip of catheter
- Coronary artery
- Aorta
- Catheter entry site
- Femoral artery

ROUTE OF CATHETER

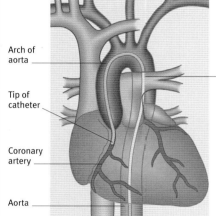

- Arch of aorta
- Catheter
- Tip of catheter
- Coronary artery
- Aorta

During the procedure
The catheter is positioned in the heart so that its tip rests in a coronary artery, and contrast dye is then injected. The artery and the small vessels leading from it are visualized by a series of X-rays. The catheter may be repositioned and the procedure repeated to check all the coronary arteries.

RESULTS

Coronary artery disease
This angiogram of the heart shows a section of coronary artery that has become narrowed by coronary artery disease, restricting blood flow.

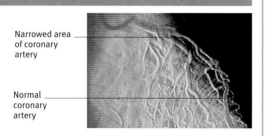

- Narrowed area of coronary artery
- Normal coronary artery

that is low refined and processed foods and unhealthy fats is important, and, if necessary, you should try to lose weight (*see* **Controlling your weight**, p.19). You may also be prescribed drugs to lower your blood cholesterol level (*see* **Lipid-lowering drugs**, p.603), even if it is within the normal range, because these drugs slow down the progress of coronary artery disease. You should take as much regular exercise as you can within the limits prescribed by your doctor. Walking as little as 1.5–3 km (1–2 miles) every day can be enough to reduce the risk of a fatal heart attack.

If angina becomes more severe in spite of drug treatment, your doctor may advise an invasive procedure to improve blood flow to the heart, such as coronary angioplasty (p.246). Usually a stent (a tubular scaffold device) is inserted to help keep the artery open, although this

may not be possible if the artery is very narrow or convoluted. In about 5 per cent of people who have coronary angioplasty and stenting, the artery narrows again within about 6 months. However, new stents have been developed that are coated with slow-release drugs that reduce the risk of arterial renarrowing (called drug-eluting stents). If you have had a conventional stent inserted, you may be prescribed clopidogrel, an antiplatelet drug (p.584) that reduces the chance of a clot forming at the site of the stent. If you have had a drug-eluting stent inserted, you may be prescribed both clopidogrel (or an alternative, such as prasugrel) and aspirin.

Angioplasty and stenting is rarely suitable if several coronary arteries are narrowed, in which case you will probably be advised to have a coronary artery

bypass graft (p.247), in which an artery inside the chest wall or a vein taken from a leg is used to bypass the diseased areas in the arteries. Coronary artery bypass grafting is a major surgical procedure that requires a brief stay in an intensive therapy unit (p.618) because it carries a small risk of complications. You will need 2–3 months of convalescence.

What is the prognosis?
The outlook depends on the extent of coronary artery disease. If you have mild angina, the outlook is good provided that you make sensible lifestyle changes and follow treatment advice. People often experience no further symptoms once treatment has started, and many are able to live a normal life apart from some restrictions on exercise. If you are otherwise in good health, you have a 1 in 2 chance of surviving for at least 10–12 years.

Myocardial infarction

Loss of blood supply to part of the heart muscle due to a blockage in a coronary artery, commonly known as heart attack

 More common with increasing age

 More common in males until the age of 60, then equal incidence

 Sometimes runs in families

 Smoking, an unhealthy diet, lack of exercise, and excess weight are risk factors

Heart attack or "coronary" are common terms for the disorder myocardial infarction. The term means death of part of the heart muscle following a blockage in its blood supply. Myocardial infarction is one of the major causes of death in developed countries such as the UK. However, the mortality rates have fallen significantly since the early 1980s due to recent improvements in treatment and an increasing awareness that following a healthier lifestyle helps to prevent heart attacks.

What are the causes?
Myocardial infarction is usually a result of coronary artery disease (p.243). In this condition, the coronary arteries, which supply the heart muscle with fresh oxygenated blood, become narrowed. This narrowing is usually due to atherosclerosis (p.241), in which droplets of fatty substances, such as cholesterol, build up on the inside of the artery wall. These substances form deposits called atheroma, which then become covered with a fibrous layer that may rupture or become roughened. Blood cells called platelets can stick to the rough or damaged area and trigger the formation of a blood clot. Once formed, the clot may completely block blood flow through the artery, leading to a heart attack.

If you have a family history of coronary artery disease (CAD), you are at increased risk of having a heart attack, especially if one or more members of your family developed CAD or had a heart attack under the age of 60. The risk of having a heart attack is also increased if you have raised blood pressure (*see* **Hypertension**, p.242) or diabetes mellitus (p.437).

What are the symptoms?
The symptoms of a heart attack usually develop suddenly and may include:
- Severe, heavy, crushing pain in the centre of the chest that may spread up to the neck and into the arms, especially the left arm.
- Pallor and sweating.
- Shortness of breath.
- Nausea and, sometimes, vomiting.
- Anxiety, sometimes accompanied by a fear of dying.
- Restlessness.

If you develop these symptoms, you should assume that you are having a heart attack and require urgent medical attention. Do not delay calling an ambulance to "see how things go" because this delay may be fatal. A well-equipped emergency ambulance is the most appropriate means of transportation to hospital because life-saving treatment may be required on the journey. While waiting for the ambulance, you should chew an aspirin tablet (300 mg) if possible. Aspirin reduces the stickiness of the blood to prevent further clotting.

Sometimes, a myocardial infarction may cause a different pattern of symptoms. If you have been suffering from the chest pain of angina (opposite page), your pain may have been getting steadily worse and may have been occurring at rest as well as on exertion. An episode of angina that does not respond to your usual treatment or one that lasts longer than 10–15 minutes may be a myocardial infarction and needs immediate emergency hospital treatment.

About 1 in 5 people does not have chest pain in a heart attack. However, there may be other symptoms, such as breathlessness, faintness, sweating, and pale skin. This pattern of symptoms is known as a "silent infarction". This type of heart attack is more common in elderly people and those with diabetes.

Are there complications?
In the first few hours and days after a heart attack, the main risks are the development of heart rhythm problems, which may be life-threatening and lead to cardiac arrest (p.252). Although the risk of cardiac arrest is greatest close to the time of a heart attack, there is an increased long-term risk of heart rhythm problems, particularly if the heart attack causes a large amount of damage to the heart muscle. Depending on the extent and site of the damaged muscle, other problems may develop. For example, in the weeks or months after the attack, the pumping action of the heart muscle may be too weak, leading to a condition called heart

▶ **TREATMENT**

Coronary angioplasty and stenting

Coronary angioplasty is used to widen coronary arteries that are narrowed or blocked by fatty deposits. A special catheter is passed through the femoral artery in the groin, or through an artery in the arm, and into the coronary artery. A guidewire is passed through this catheter and across the narrowed segment of artery. A balloon catheter is threaded over the wire and the balloon is inflated in the narrowed segment of artery to widen it. In most cases a stent (a tubular scaffold device) is inserted afterwards to keep the artery open.

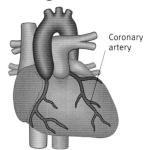

Coronary artery

LOCATION

Catheter
Deflated balloon
Narrowed area
Fatty deposit

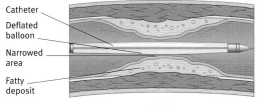

1 *A catheter with a deflated balloon attached to its tip is threaded into the artery. The catheter is placed precisely so that the balloon is inside the narrowed area of the coronary artery.*

Inflated balloon
Compressed fatty deposit

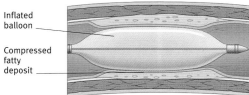

2 *The balloon is inflated and deflated in order to compress the fatty deposits and widen the narrowed segment of artery. The balloon is then withdrawn.*

Partly inflated balloon
Partly expanded stent

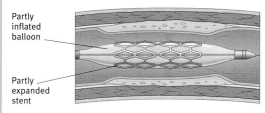

3 *A stent, mounted on a balloon, is threaded into the artery, and positioned at the site of narrowing. The balloon is inflated, expanding the stent so that it presses against the artery wall.*

Fully expanded stent in position
Compressed fatty deposit

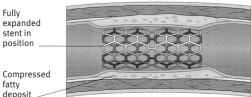

4 *The balloon is then deflated and removed from the artery. The stent remains expanded in position and holds the artery open.*

RESULTS

Blocked artery

Widened artery

Effect of treatment
X-rays using contrast dye are taken before and after coronary angioplasty. These images show that the blocked artery has been widened successfully and blood flow improved.

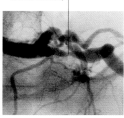

BEFORE TREATMENT

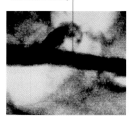

AFTER TREATMENT

failure (*see* **Acute heart failure**, and **Chronic heart failure**, opposite page). Less common complications include damage to one of the heart valves (*see* **Mitral incompetence**, p.254); development of a ventriculoseptal defect (a hole in the septum between the heart's two lower chambers); or inflammation of the membrane covering the heart's

surface (*see* **Pericarditis**, p.258). These conditions may also lead to the development of heart failure.

How is it diagnosed?

In many cases, the diagnosis is obvious. An ECG (p.243), which is a tracing of the electrical activity of the heart, often shows changes

that confirm myocardial infarction. The ECG can be valuable in assessing which part and how much of the heart muscle has been damaged and will establish whether the heart rhythm is still normal. To confirm the diagnosis, blood samples may be taken to measure the levels of particular chemicals that leak into the blood from damaged heart muscle.

What is the treatment?

The immediate aims of treatment are to relieve pain and restore the blood supply to the heart muscle to minimize the amount of damage and prevent further complications. These aims are best achieved by immediate admission to an intensive therapy unit (p.618), where you can be monitored continuously. If you have severe chest pain, you will probably be given a powerful painkilling drug (p.589), such as morphine.

Within the first 6 hours of the attack, you may also be given a "clot-busting" thrombolytic drug (p.584) to dissolve the blood clot blocking the coronary artery. Alternatively, you may have immediate coronary angioplasty (left), usually with the insertion of a stent (a tubular scaffold device) to reopen and widen the blocked artery. The sooner blood flow to the heart can be restored, the greater the chance of a full recovery.

While you are in the coronary care unit, your heartbeat is monitored, and treatment is given if arrhythmias or symptoms of heart failure develop. If your progress is satisfactory, you will be allowed out of bed briefly after 24–48 hours. Soon afterwards, you should begin a rehabilitation programme, during which you are encouraged to spend gradually longer periods out of bed.

Once you have recovered, the condition of your coronary arteries and heart muscle is assessed. Tests such as echocardiography (p.255) and exercise electrocardiography (*see* **Exercise testing**, p.244) are often used to help to decide on further treatment. For example, if the heart's pumping action is impaired, you may be prescribed an ACE inhibitor (p.582) and/or a diuretic drug (p.583). If a coronary artery is narrowed or blocked, you may need angioplasty and stenting (left) or bypass surgery at a later stage (*see* **Coronary artery bypass graft**, opposite page). If tests reveal a persistent slow or abnormal heart rhythm, you may need to have a pacemaker fitted (*see* **Cardiac pacemaker and ICD**, p.251).

Certain drugs taken long-term can reduce the risk of another heart attack. You may be prescribed a beta-blocker drug (p.581), an ACE inhibitor (p.582), and aspirin plus another antiplatelet drug (p.584), such as clopidogrel, to reduce the risk of blood clots. You will also be advised to adopt a diet low in refined and processed foods and unhealthy fats, and, in most cases, to take a statin (*see* **Lipid-lowering drugs**, p.603) to lower your blood cholesterol level. Statins reduce the risk of another heart attack even if your cholesterol level is not elevated. You will also be advised to eat oily fish 2–4 times a week and may be prescribed a purified omega-3 supplement.

What can I do?

It is important to follow your doctor's advice about how soon to return to normal activities and to continue to take your prescribed medication. It is natural to feel worried about your health, and many people feel mild depression (p.343). It is important to avoid becoming disabled by the fear of having another heart attack. After a heart attack, you are likely to be invited to attend a cardiac rehabilitation course. This is a structure programme, led by a multidisciplinary team of healthcare professionals, that provides education, a graded exercise regimen, and psychological and social support. Such a programme can help you to return to as normal a life as possible and to maintain a healthy level of physical activity and lifestyle changes that will help reduce your long-term risk of further heart problems.

What is the prognosis?

If you have not had a previous myocardial infarction, you are treated quickly, and there are no complications, the outlook is good. After 2 weeks, the risk of another heart attack is considerably reduced, and you have a good chance of living for another 10 years at least. The outlook is better if you stop smoking, reduce alcohol intake, exercise regularly, and follow a healthy diet.

If you have had a previous heart attack or suffered a significant amount of heart damage, the outlook depends on the amount of heart muscle that was damaged and whether you have additional complications. However, many people who have surgery or angioplasty live for 10 years or more.

SELF-HELP

Life after a heart attack

Making changes in your lifestyle after a heart attack can help to speed your recovery and to reduce the risk of another attack:

■ Stop smoking. This is the single most important factor in preventing a further attack.

■ Eat a healthy diet and try to keep your weight within the ideal range for your height and build (*see* **Diet and health**, p.16).

■ If you drink alcohol, take only moderate amounts. You should have no more than 1–2 small glasses of wine or beer a day.

■ Together with your doctor, agree on a programme of increasing exercise until you are able to engage in moderate exercise, such as swimming regularly, for 30 minutes or more at a time.

After a period of recovery, you can make a gradual return to your normal daily routine:

■ You will probably be able to return to work within 8–12 weeks, or sooner if you have a desk job. You might consider working part-time at first.

■ Try to avoid stressful situations.

■ You should be able to drive a car within 4 weeks.

■ You can resume having sexual intercourse about 4 weeks after a heart attack.

Coronary artery bypass graft

During this procedure, one or more narrowed coronary arteries are bypassed using blood vessels from the chest or, sometimes, from the legs. The operation takes about 2 hours. In most cases, the heart is stopped and a heart–lung machine is used to take over the function of the heart during surgery (*see* **Surgery using a heart–lung machine**, p.615). However, an increasing number of operations are performed without stopping the heart (sometimes known as "off-pump" coronary artery bypass grafting), and less invasive techniques using endoscopic surgery are also being used more commonly. After surgery, you will be monitored in an intensive therapy unit for several days.

Mammary artery bypass graft

One of the internal mammary arteries within the chest, usually the left artery, is used to create the coronary artery bypass. Artery grafts are preferable to vein grafts because they are better able to take the pressure of the blood that normally flows through the coronary arteries and are less likely to become blocked over time.

SITE OF INCISION

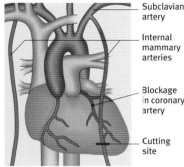

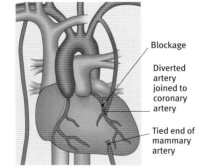

Subclavian artery
Internal mammary arteries
Blockage in coronary artery
Cutting site

Blockage
Diverted artery joined to coronary artery
Tied end of mammary artery

1 *The left internal mammary artery is cut where shown above. The upper end is left attached to the subclavian artery and the lower end is tied off.*

2 *The free end of the mammary artery is connected to the coronary artery at a point beyond the blockage to supply blood to the heart muscle there.*

Saphenous vein bypass graft

If more than one blockage in a coronary artery needs to be bypassed or if the internal mammary artery is not suitable, sections of the saphenous vein may be used. Often, the vein is used in addition to the mammary artery. Because veins tend to become obstructed more quickly than arterial grafts, sometimes the radial artery from the forearm is used to create the bypass graft.

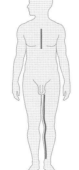

SITES OF INCISION

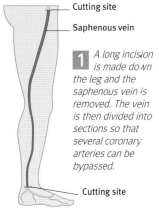

Cutting site
Saphenous vein

1 *A long incision is made down the leg and the saphenous vein is removed. The vein is then divided into sections so that several coronary arteries can be bypassed.*

Cutting site

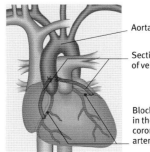

Aorta
Sections of vein
Blockages in the coronary arteries

2 *Sections of the saphenous vein are used to bypass the blockages. One end of each section is attached to the aorta, and the other is attached to the coronary artery beyond a blockage.*

Acute heart failure

Sudden deterioration in the pumping action of the heart, usually leading to accumulation of fluid in the lungs

 More common over the age of 65

 Slightly more common in males

 Genetics and lifestyle as risk factors depend on the cause

Heart failure is the term used when the heart's ability to pump efficiently is reduced. In acute heart failure, the condition develops suddenly, often due to a severe heart attack. In most cases, only the left side of the heart is affected. This side receives oxygen-rich blood directly from the lungs and pumps it to the rest of the body. If acute heart failure develops, a back-up of blood occurs in the blood vessels leading from the lungs to the heart. Back pressure then causes a build-up of fluid in the lungs, known as pulmonary oedema. If it is not treated immediately, it may be life-threatening.

What are the causes?

Acute heart failure often develops in people with chronic heart failure (right) if the weakened heart is put under strain. For example, a severe infection, such as pneumonia (p.299), may increase the workload on the heart and lead to acute heart failure. Other common causes of acute heart failure are severe myocardial infarction (p.245); valve problems, including infective endocarditis (p.256); and rhythm problems, such as complete heart block (p.251) or tachycardia (p.250).

Right-sided acute heart failure is rare. It is usually due to a blood clot blocking the pulmonary artery, which leads from the lungs to the right side of the heart (*see* **Pulmonary embolism**, p.302).

What are the symptoms?

The symptoms of acute heart failure usually develop rapidly and include:

■ Severe shortness of breath.
■ Wheezing.
■ Cough with pink, frothy sputum.
■ Pale skin and sweating.

If acute heart failure is caused by a heart attack, you may have additional symptoms such as intense, prolonged chest pain and feelings of anxiety. If heart failure is caused by a pulmonary embolism, you may cough up blood and have sharp chest pain that is worse when inhaling. If acute heart failure is not treated, it can cause dangerously low blood pressure (*see* **Shock**, p.248), and the condition may then be fatal.

What might be done?

Acute heart failure is an emergency and needs immediate hospital treatment. You will be treated sitting up and may be given oxygen through a face mask. You may also

---

be given several drugs intravenously, including diuretics (p.583), morphine (*see* **Painkillers**, p.589), and nitrates (p.581) to make you more comfortable and to help remove fluid from the lungs. You are likely to have electrocardiography (*see* **ECG**, p.243) and echocardiography (p.255) to help determine the cause of heart failure. A chest X-ray (p.300) is usually done to assess the size and shape of your heart and confirm the presence of fluid in the lungs. You may also have coronary angiography (p.245) to look for narrowing or blockages in the coronary arteries.

Longer-term treatments will focus on the underlying cause. For example, blockage of the coronary arteries may be treated with coronary angioplasty and stenting (opposite page). If the cause cannot be fully treated and chronic heart failure develops, drugs such as ACE inhibitors (p.582) and digitalis drugs (p.582) may be given to help reduce recurrences of acute heart failure and slow deterioration in heart function. However, in spite of these treatments, the condition may be progressive and ultimately fatal.

Chronic heart failure

Long-standing inefficient pumping action of the heart, leading to poor circulation of blood and accumulation of fluid in tissues

 More common over the age of 65

 Slightly more common in males

 Genetics and lifestyle as risk factors depend on the cause

In chronic heart failure, the heart is unable to pump blood around the body effectively. This problem leads to a gradual build-up of fluid in the lungs and body tissues. Chronic heart failure is a common progressive condition that may be so mild at first that symptoms go unnoticed. It mostly affects people over 65.

Although the term "chronic heart failure" may appear to imply a life-threatening disorder, it can often be treated, and people who have mild chronic heart failure can live for many years. However, the condition may limit physical activity.

At first, one side of the heart may be predominantly affected, and, in these circumstances, the condition is termed right- or left-sided heart failure. Right-sided heart failure leads to ankle swelling and accumulation of fluid throughout the body. Left-sided heart failure causes fluid to accumulate in the lungs. Fluid in the lungs due to left-sided failure usually rapidly leads to right-sided failure, and the combination of the two, known as congestive heart failure, is the most common form of chronic heart failure.

What are the causes?

Any condition that causes damage to the heart can lead to chronic heart failure. Whether the right or left side of the heart is first affected depends on the cause. In 8 out of 10 cases, chronic heart failure is caused by coronary artery disease (p.243), in which the blood supply to the heart muscle is reduced. Persistent high blood pressure (*see* **Hypertension**, p.242) can lead to chronic heart failure because the heart works harder to pump blood through vessels in which pressure is abnormally high. These disorders initially produce left-sided heart failure.

Failure of the right side of the heart is a common complication of chronic lung disease, particularly chronic obstructive pulmonary disease (p.297).

Other possible causes of chronic heart failure are heart valve disorders (p.253) and dilated cardiomyopathy (p.257). In rare cases, chronic heart failure may be due to anaemia (p.271), the hormone disorder hyperthyroidism (p.432), or extreme obesity (p.400). People who have diabetes mellitus (p.437) are also at risk of developing the condition.

What are the symptoms?
The symptoms develop gradually, are often vague, and may include:
- Tiredness.
- Palpitations (awareness of an abnormal heartbeat).
- Shortness of breath that is worse during exertion or when lying flat.
- Loss of appetite.
- Nausea.
- Swelling of the feet and ankles.
- In some cases, confusion.

People with chronic heart failure may also have sudden attacks of acute heart failure (p.247), with symptoms of severe shortness of breath, wheezing, and sweating. These attacks usually occur during the night. Occasionally, acute heart failure develops if the heart is put under additional strain due to a heart attack or an infection. Acute heart failure needs immediate hospital treatment.

How is it diagnosed?
If chronic heart failure is suspected, you may have electrocardiography (*see* **ECG**, p.243) to assess the electrical activity of your heart. You may also have a blood test for a substance called brain natriuretic peptide (BNP), levels of which are raised in heart failure, and echocardiography (p.255) to image the heart and check its function. A chest X-ray (p.300) may show signs of heart failure, such as an abnormally large heart or excess fluid in the lung tissue.

Your doctor may arrange for further tests to investigate the underlying cause of heart failure. For example, you may have coronary angiography (p.245) to diagnose narrowing of the coronary arteries or blood tests to check for anaemia or an overactive thyroid gland.

What can I do?
If you have chronic heart failure, you should avoid strenuous exercise and stress. Regular gentle exercise, such as walking, should help if you have mild or moderate chronic heart failure. If you smoke, stop immediately. If necessary, try to lose excess weight to avoid putting unnecessary strain on your heart (*see* **Are you a healthy weight?**, p.19). You should also avoid salty foods, which can encourage fluid retention.

How might the doctor treat it?
Your doctor will probably prescribe diuretics (p.583), which help to remove excess fluid and salt from your body by stimulating the kidneys to increase urine production. He or she will probably also prescribe ACE inhibitor drugs (p.582) or angiotensin II blockers (p.582), which cause blood vessels to widen and reduce the workload on the heart, as well as reducing salt and water retention; and a beta-blocker (p.581) to improve the efficiency of your heart muscle in the longer term (although you may not be prescribed a beta-blocker if you have asthma or arterial disease in your legs). You may also be prescribed an aldosterone blocker drug, such as spironolactone or eplerenone; these drugs work in a similar way to diuretics but can prevent excessive loss of potassium due to diuretics and may help reduce heart damage. In addition, you may be treated with digoxin (*see* **Digitalis drugs**, p.582) or other drugs, which also increase the efficiency of the heart. If diagnostic tests show narrowing of the coronary arteries, your doctor may advise coronary angioplasty and stenting (p.246).

You may also be treated to help prevent progression of any underlying disorder. For example, if you have coronary artery disease, you may be advised to take a daily dose of aspirin (*see* **Drugs that prevent blood clotting**, p.584), which reduces the risk of a heart attack. If you have an irregular heart rhythm or if your heart is severely enlarged, you may be treated with warfarin or another anticoagulant drug to reduce the risk of blood clots forming in the heart. If an ECG shows the electrical activity of your heart's conducting system is very slow, your doctor may recommend that you have a special type of pacemaker called a biventricular pacemaker (*see* **Cardiac pacemaker and ICD**, p.251) fitted. This type of pacemaker increases the efficiency of the heart by improving the synchronization of contractions of the heart chambers. Whatever the details of your treatment, your doctor will monitor your heart condition and adjust your medication as needed.

In some cases, drug treatment may not be effective, and a heart transplant (p.257) may be considered if a person is otherwise in good health.

What is the prognosis?
Treatment is usually initially successful in relieving symptoms and improving quality of life. However, in most cases, the underlying cause cannot be treated effectively. As a result, heart failure becomes increasingly severe, and symptoms are then difficult to control with drugs. In about half of these cases, the condition is fatal within 2 years.

Hypotension

Lower than normal blood pressure due to a variety of causes

 Age, gender, genetics, and lifestyle as risk factors depend on the cause

Hypotension is the medical term for low blood pressure. The pressure with which the blood is pumped around the circulation varies between individuals and throughout the day. The normal range is that which is adequate to supply all of the organs and body tissues with blood. Blood pressure at the lower end of the normal range is not likely to produce symptoms. However, if the pressure in the circulation falls below the level needed to provide the brain with enough blood, light-headedness or fainting may occur.

A common type of hypotension is postural hypotension, in which suddenly standing or sitting up leads to light-headedness and fainting.

What are the causes?
In many people, low blood pressure occurs as a result of dehydration following loss of large amounts of fluid or salts from the body. For example, heavy sweating, loss of blood, or profuse diarrhoea or vomiting may all cause hypotension.

Disorders that reduce the efficiency of the heart's pumping action are common causes of low blood pressure. These disorders include heart failure (*see* **Acute heart failure**, p.247, and **Chronic heart failure**, p.247), heart attack (*see* **Myocardial infarction**, p.245), and an irregular heartbeat (*see* **Arrhythmias**, opposite page).

Hypotension may also be caused by an abnormal widening of the blood vessels, which may occur as a result of an infection in the bloodstream (*see* **Septicaemia**, p.171) or a severe allergic reaction (*see* **Anaphylaxis**, p.285).

Postural hypotension may be caused by disorders in which the nerve supply to the blood vessels is damaged, such as diabetic neuropathy (p.336) or peripheral neuropathies (p.336). Hypotension may also sometimes be the result of an adverse effect of certain drugs, particularly those used in the treatment of high blood pressure (*see* **Antihypertensive drugs**, p.580) and certain types of antidepressant drugs (p.592).

What are the symptoms?
You may not have symptoms of hypotension unless your blood pressure is very low. Symptoms may include:
- Tiredness.
- General weakness.
- Light-headedness and fainting.
- Blurred vision.
- Nausea.

These symptoms are usually temporary, and blood pressure rises when the cause is treated. However, if blood pressure is too low to provide an adequate blood supply to vital organs, it can be fatal (*see* **Shock**, below).

What might be done?
Your blood pressure will be measured while you are lying down and then standing (*see* **Blood pressure measurement**, p.242). There may be an obvious reason for your low blood pressure. For example, you may be dehydrated and need treatment with intravenous fluids. If your doctor suspects an underlying disorder, such as a heart condition, you may be admitted to hospital for tests and treatment. If your medication is causing hypotension, your doctor will probably advise a change of drug or dosage.

Shock

A severe reduction in blood pressure causing poor blood supply to major organs

 Age as a risk factor depends on the cause

 Gender, genetics, and lifestyle are not significant factors

Shock is a potentially life-threatening condition that necessitates immediate medical attention. The medical term shock describes the cold, pale, collapsed state that results from low blood pressure due to serious injury or illness. Left untreated, the reduced blood supply deprives the vital organs and body tissues of oxygen and is eventually fatal.

The condition is unrelated to the psychological and emotional distress that may follow a traumatic experience.

What are the causes?
Shock may develop as a result of any situation in which the heart is unable to pump blood effectively or in which there is too little blood for the heart to pump. The heart is unable to function normally if it is damaged following a heart attack (*see* **Myocardial infarction**, p.245) or if the heart rhythm is abnormal (*see* **Arrhythmias**, opposite page).

Shock due to insufficient blood circulating around the body may be the result of major blood loss, such as bleeding from the digestive tract (p.399) or from a serious injury. The volume of blood circulating in the body may also be reduced by fluid loss due to severe burns or profuse diarrhoea.

Some conditions, such as severe allergic reactions (*see* **Anaphylaxis**, p.285) or a blood infection (*see* **Septicaemia**, p.171), may cause the blood vessels in the body to widen, resulting in a significant drop in blood pressure and shock.

What are the symptoms?
Shock may not develop until hours after the injury or illness, but as soon as blood pressure falls, the symptoms develop suddenly. Symptoms may include:
- Confusion or agitation.
- Cold, clammy skin and sweating.

- Rapid, shallow breathing.
- Fast heartbeat.
- Loss of consciousness.

Symptoms of the underlying cause may also be present, such as prolonged chest pain due to a heart attack.

If shock is not treated immediately, the internal organs may be damaged, leading to various disorders including kidney failure (p.450) and acute respiratory distress syndrome (p.168).

What might be done?
A person in shock requires emergency admission to an intensive therapy unit (p.618) for treatment and careful monitoring.

The priority is to restore the blood and oxygen supply to the body's major organs regardless of the initial cause of shock. Immediate treatment usually includes oxygen therapy and intravenous fluids, blood or blood products, and drugs to increase blood pressure.

Once the cause of shock has been established, specific treatment can be given. For example, antibiotics (p.572) may be prescribed to treat septicaemia. Surgery may be needed to stop severe bleeding. However, for treatment to be successful, the blood supply to the internal organs must be restored before permanent damage occurs.

Heart rate and rhythm disorders

Disorders of heart rate and rhythm are caused by disturbances in the heart's electrical system and are very common, particularly in elderly people. These disorders do not always cause symptoms and are sometimes detected only during routine health checkups. Treatment usually consists of drugs, although therapeutic techniques that use controlled electric currents are also used.

A healthy adult has a resting heart rate of 60–80 beats per minute, although this rate rises during exercise. Children have a higher resting heart rate, while that of very fit adults and the elderly may be as low as 50 beats per minute. Disorders that affect the pumping action of the heart may increase or decrease the heart rate, alter its rhythm, or, in cardiac arrest, stop the heart pumping altogether. Many of these disorders have coronary artery disease (p.243) or heart failure (p.247) as an underlying cause. The first article in this section describes ectopic beats, which are extra, isolated heartbeats. This article is followed by an overview of arrhythmias, which are abnormal heart rates and rhythms, and a discussion of individual types of arrhythmias. The final article discusses cardiac arrest, which is the sudden and complete failure of the heart to pump blood caused by a disturbance in its electrical system. Cardiac arrest is a potentially fatal condition and requires emergency medical treatment.

KEY ANATOMY

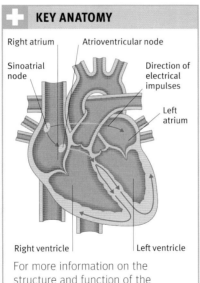
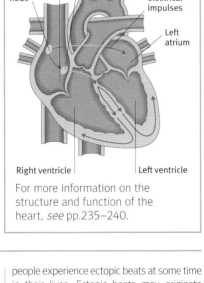

Right atrium — Atrioventricular node
Sinoatrial node — Direction of electrical impulses
— Left atrium
Right ventricle — Left ventricle

For more information on the structure and function of the heart, *see* pp.235–240.

Ectopic beats

Contractions of the heart that are out of the normal rhythmic pattern

 More common in young people and elderly people

 Smoking and consumption of alcohol and caffeine are risk factors

 Gender and genetics are not significant factors

An ectopic beat is an isolated, extra heartbeat that rapidly follows a normal one. The interval between an ectopic beat and the next normal beat may be longer than usual, producing a transient irregularity of the heart rhythm. Most

people experience ectopic beats at some time in their lives. Ectopic beats may originate either in the atria (the upper chambers of the heart) or in the ventricles (the lower chambers of the heart). Atrial ectopic beats are usually harmless. They typically occur in young people and are often associated with the use of nicotine and the consumption of caffeine and alcohol. Ventricular ectopic beats occur less frequently, usually in elderly people, and may indicate the presence of a more serious underlying disorder, such as coronary artery disease (p.243). They may also occur after a heart attack (*see* **Myocardial infarction**, p.245). Ectopic beats may be symptomless or may cause a thumping sensation in the chest as the heart briefly beats more strongly than usual.

What might be done?
Ectopic beats in young people are likely to be atrial and harmless. They may disappear if you stop smoking and reduce your intake of coffee and alcohol. If they persist, visit your doctor. Ectopic beats that are frequent or accompanied by light-headedness, shortness of breath, or chest pain, or that occur at an older age, are likely to be ventricular. They may have a serious underlying cause, requiring urgent medical attention.

Since ectopic beats are intermittent, your doctor may arrange for your heart to be monitored continuously over 24 hours or more (*see* **Ambulatory ECG**, below). Tests may be carried out to look for an underlying cause.

The treatment of ventricular ectopic beats depends on the underlying cause. Antiarrhythmic drugs (p.580) may occasionally be prescribed. If the ectopic beats follow a heart attack, beta-blocker drugs (p.581) lower the risk of cardiac arrest (p.252).

Arrhythmias

Abnormal rates and/or rhythms of the heartbeat

 More common in elderly people

 Genetics and lifestyle as risk factors depend on the type

 Gender is not a significant factor

The normal resting adult heart rate is 60–80 beats per minute. Both heart rate and rhythm may be affected in arrhythmias, which may involve both the atria (upper

heart chambers) and the ventricles (lower heart chambers). There are two types of arrhythmias: tachycardias, in which the heart rate is too high, and bradycardias, in which the rate is too low. Tachycardias may arise in the atria or ventricles and can be regular or irregular. When tachycardias occur in the ventricles, they can deteriorate into ventricular fibrillation, a serious arrhythmia that can lead to cardiac arrest (p.252). Bradycardias include sick sinus syndrome (p.251) and complete heart block (p.251). Most arrhythmias are caused by disorders of the heart and its blood vessels. A heart rate outside the usual range is not always a cause for concern. An elevated rate is normal during exercise and pregnancy, and exceptionally fit people have a resting heart rate that is lower than normal.

Arrhythmias may reduce the pumping efficiency of the heart, causing too little blood to reach the brain. Although arrhythmias may cause alarming symptoms, such as a thumping heartbeat, the different types vary in seriousness.

What are the causes?
Most arrhythmias are caused by heart disease. The most common underlying cause is coronary artery disease (p.243). Other common causes include heart failure and disorders of the electrical system that controls heart rate. Less common causes include various heart valve disorders (pp.253–258) and inflammation of the heart muscle (*see* **Myocarditis**, p.256). Some types of arrhythmia present from birth are due to a defect of the heart, such as an abnormal electrical pathway between the atria and the ventricles. However, these arrhythmias typically cause symptoms later in life.

▶ TEST

Ambulatory ECG

Ambulatory electrocardiography (ECG) is carried out using a wearable device called a Holter monitor that records the electrical activity of the heart using a number of electrodes attached to the chest. The device is usually worn for 24 hours and detects intermittent arrhythmias (abnormal heart rates and rhythms). An event monitor is a similar device that can be worn for longer periods but records only when it is activated by the user.

Using a Holter monitor
You press a button on the device to mark times when symptoms occur. A doctor can check if these markings coincide with periods of arrhythmia.

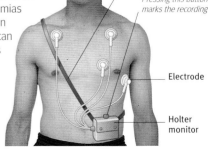

Shoulder strap
Marker button
Pressing this button marks the recording
Electrode
Holter monitor

RESULTS

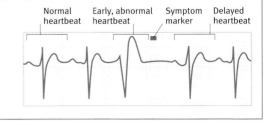

Normal heartbeat | Early, abnormal heartbeat | Symptom marker | Delayed heartbeat

ECG trace
This trace shows normal heartbeats interrupted by an isolated abnormal beat, which coincides with a symptom marker.

Some arrhythmias occur in people with otherwise healthy hearts. Causes include an imbalance of thyroid hormones (*see* Hyperthyroidism, p.432), or of blood chemistry, such as an excess of potassium. Some drugs, such as bronchodilators (p.588) and digitalis drugs (p.582) may cause arrhythmias, as may caffeine and tobacco, but sometimes their cause is unknown.

What are the symptoms?
Symptoms do not always develop, but, if they do, their onset is usually sudden. The symptoms may include:
- Palpitations (awareness of an irregular, abnormally rapid, or heavy heartbeat).
- Light-headedness, sometimes leading to loss of consciousness.
- Shortness of breath.
- Pain in the chest or neck.

Complications include stroke (p.329), acute heart failure (p.247), and chronic heart failure (p.247).

What might be done?
Your doctor may suspect an arrhythmia from your symptoms and by checking your pulse. He or she may arrange for you to have electrocardiography (*see* ECG, p.243) to monitor electrical activity in the heart. Since some arrhythmias occur only intermittently, you may need to have a continuous ECG over 24 hours or be fitted with an event monitor (*see* Ambulatory ECG, p.249). You may also have tests to detect abnormalities that affect electrical pathways of the heart (*see* Cardiac electrophysiological studies, right).

In some cases, antiarrhythmic drugs (p.580) can be used to treat arrhythmias. In other cases, electric shock treatment may be given to restore a normal heartbeat (*see* Cardioversion, p.252). Abnormal electrical pathways in the heart can be destroyed using a technique called radiofrequency ablation (also known as catheter ablation), which is carried out at the same time as electrophysiological studies. If the heart rate is too low, a cardiac pacemaker (opposite page) may be fitted to stimulate an increase in the heart rate. For some arrhythmias, a device called an implantable cardioverter defibrillator (ICD) may be fitted (*see* opposite page). This is similar to a pacemaker but sends a larger electric shock to the heart to restore normal rhythm when the heart beats at a dangerously abnormal rate. In some cases, a device containing both a pacemaker and an ICD may be fitted.

The outlook for an arrhythmia depends on the type. Supraventricular tachycardia usually is not serious and does not affect life expectancy, whereas ventricular arrhythmias are potentially fatal and need emergency medical treatment.

Supraventricular tachycardia

Recurrent episodes of rapid heart rate arising in the upper chambers of the heart

 Most common in children and young adults

 Sometimes runs in families

 Exertion and consumption of alcohol and caffeine may trigger attacks

 Gender is not a significant factor

Supraventricular tachycardia (SVT) is a type of arrhythmia caused by a fault in the electrical pathway that regulates the heart rate. During an episode of SVT, which may last up to several hours, the heartbeat is rapid but regular. The heart rate rises to 140–180 beats per minute and sometimes climbs even higher. In a heart that is working normally, each heartbeat is triggered by an electrical impulse from the sinoatrial node (the heart's pacemaker), located in the right atrium (one of the heart's upper chambers). The impulse passes to a second node, the atrioventricular node, which relays it to the ventricles. In SVT, the heartbeat is not controlled by the sinoatrial node. This problem may occur either because an abnormal pathway develops, causing an impulse to circulate continuously between the atrioventricular node and the ventricles, or because an extra area of cells develops and sends out pacemaking impulses.

SVT may first appear in childhood or adolescence, although it can occur at any age. In some cases, SVT is caused by an inherited abnormality in the heart's electrical pathways. Episodes generally occur for no apparent reason, but they may be triggered by exertion and by caffeine and alcohol.

What are the symptoms?
The symptoms of SVT usually develop suddenly. They last from a few seconds to several hours and include:

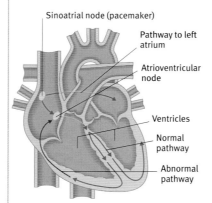

Supraventricular tachycardia (SVT)
Impulses from the sinoatrial node normally control heart rate. One cause of SVT is an abnormal electrical pathway, which allows an impulse to circulate continuously in the heart, taking over from the sinoatrial node.

Labels: Sinoatrial node (pacemaker); Pathway to left atrium; Atrioventricular node; Ventricles; Normal pathway; Abnormal pathway

- Palpitations (awareness of an irregular, abnormally rapid, or heavy heartbeat).
- Light-headedness.
- Pain in the chest or neck.

In rare cases, a prolonged episode of SVT may reduce blood pressure to a life-threatening level.

What might be done?
If your doctor suspects that you have SVT, you will probably have electrocardiography (*see* ECG, p.243) to record the electrical activity of your heart. This investigation may last 24 hours or more (*see* Ambulatory ECG, p.249) because SVT occurs only intermittently. You may have further tests to look for abnormalities in the heart's electrical pathways (*see* Cardiac electrophysiological studies, above).

A prolonged and severe episode of SVT requires emergency hospital treatment. In hospital, you may be given oxygen and an intravenous injection of an antiarrhythmic drug (p.580). In some cases, an electric shock may be given to restore the heart to its normal rate and rhythm (*see* Cardioversion, p.252).

People who have occasional, brief episodes of SVT can control the symptoms by stimulating the vagus nerve, to slow the heart rate. One way to stimulate the nerve is to rub the area over the carotid artery in the neck, although this is not recommended in adults over the age of 50 because it may precipitate a stroke. Other techniques include plunging your face into ice-cold water or straining as if moving one's bowels. Your doctor can teach you these techniques.

▶ TEST AND TREATMENT

Cardiac electrophysiological studies

Cardiac electrophysiological studies (EPS) are used to pinpoint abnormal pathways in the heart's electrical conducting system. A catheter that has electrodes at its tip is introduced into the heart and manipulated to record the electrical activity at different sites. Once an abnormal pathway is located, it can be destroyed by sending a current through the electrodes in a procedure known as radiofrequency ablation or catheter ablation. This procedure can provide a permanent cure for some disorders and has a high success rate.

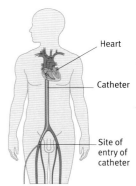

Labels: Heart; Catheter; Site of entry of catheter

ROUTE OF CATHETER

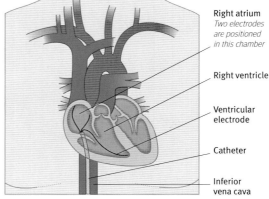

Labels: Right atrium — *Two electrodes are positioned in this chamber*; Right ventricle; Ventricular electrode; Catheter; Inferior vena cava

During EPS
A catheter is inserted into a vein in the groin under local anaesthesia and threaded into the heart. Electrodes at the tip of the catheter detect electrical activity and can be used to deliver a current to destroy abnormal pathways.

Troublesome episodes of SVT may be treated with long-term antiarrhythmic drugs. SVT may be cured by radiofrequency ablation, a treatment carried out during cardiac electrophysiological studies. This treatment destroys abnormal electrical pathways but carries a very small risk of causing complete heart block (opposite page), in which the heart's electrical system fails. In most cases, SVT does not affect life expectancy.

Atrial fibrillation

Rapid, uncoordinated contractions of the atria, the upper chambers of the heart

 Most common in people over the age of 60

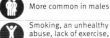 More common in males

 Smoking, an unhealthy diet, alcohol abuse, lack of exercise, and excess weight are risk factors

Genetics is not a significant factor

Atrial fibrillation is the most common type of rapid, irregular heart rate. It most often occurs in people over 60, and up to 1 in 20 very elderly people in the UK may be affected. In atrial fibrillation, the atria contract weakly and in an uncoordinated way at 300–500 beats per minute. Some of the electrical impulses that cause this rapid beating are conducted through the heart to the ventricles (the lower chambers), which also beat more rapidly than normal, at up to 160 beats per minute. Since the atria and ventricles are not beating in rhythm, the strength and timing of the heartbeat become irregular and less blood is pumped.

The most dangerous complication of atrial fibrillation is stroke (p.329), the risk of which increases with age. Since the atria do not empty properly during contractions, blood stagnates in them and may form a clot. If a part of the clot breaks off and enters the bloodstream, it may block an artery anywhere in the body (see **Thrombosis and embolism**, p.259). A stroke occurs when part of a clot blocks an artery supplying the brain.

What are the causes?
Atrial fibrillation may occur for no apparent reason, especially in the elderly, but it is usually due to an underlying disorder that causes the atria to enlarge. Such disorders include heart valve disorders (p.253), coronary artery disease (p.243), and high blood pressure (see **Hypertension**, p.242). Smoking, lack of exercise, an unhealthy diet, and being overweight are risk factors for many of these disorders. Atrial fibrillation is also common in people with an overactive thyroid gland (see **Hyperthyroidism**, p.432) or low potassium levels in the blood. It may occur in people who drink excessive amounts of alcohol.

What are the symptoms?
Symptoms do not always develop, but, if they do, their onset is usually sudden. The symptoms may be intermittent or persistent and typically include:
- Palpitations (awareness of an irregular or abnormally rapid heartbeat).
- Light-headedness.
- Shortness of breath.
- Chest pain.
Stroke and acute or chronic heart failure (pp.247–248) may be complications.

What might be done?
Your doctor may suspect atrial fibrillation if you have a fast, irregular pulse. To confirm the diagnosis, you will have electrocardiography (see **ECG**, p.243). You may have blood tests to look for an underlying cause such as hyperthyroidism. If a cause is found, treating it often cures the arrhythmia. If atrial fibrillation is diagnosed early, it may be treated successfully using cardioversion (p.252) in which a brief electric shock is applied to the heart.

Atrial fibrillation is usually treated with antiarrhythmic drugs (p.580) such as beta-blockers (p.581), diltiazem (see **Calcium channel blocker drugs**, p.582), or digitalis drugs (p.582). These slow the conduction of electrical impulses from the atria to the ventricles, giving the ventricles time to fill with blood between heartbeats. Other antiarrhythmics may then be used to treat the irregular rhythm. You may also be prescribed warfarin, which reduces the risk of clots (see **Drugs that prevent blood clotting**, p.584) and thus lowers the risk of a stroke. If drug treatment is ineffective, your doctor may suggest a cardiac electrophysiological study (opposite page) with radiofrequency ablation, which can permanently cure certain cases of atrial fibrillation.

Complete heart block

Failure of the system that conducts electrical impulses from the atria to the ventricles

 More common in elderly people

 Smoking, an unhealthy diet, lack of exercise, and excess weight are risk factors

 Gender and genetics are not significant factors

In complete heart block, damage to the heart's conductive tissue prevents electrical impulses from the atria (upper chambers) from reaching the ventricles (lower chambers), so that the ventricles cannot contract normally. Heart muscle contracts automatically in the absence of a regulating signal. In complete heart block, the ventricles contract at about 40 beats per minute or less instead of the usual rate of 60–80 beats per minute, which greatly reduces the heart's efficiency. In some cases, the heart may stop beating altogether for up to 20 seconds.

The tissue damage that causes complete heart block is more common in elderly people and is linked with coronary artery disease (p.243), for which lifestyle factors such as smoking increase the risk. Sudden complete heart block, which may be either temporary or permanent, may follow a heart attack (see **Myocardial infarction**, p.245).

What are the symptoms?
The symptoms may come on gradually or suddenly and typically include:
- Palpitations (awareness of an irregular abnormal or heavy heartbeat).
- Light-headedness, and loss of consciousness if the heart stops beating.
- Shortness of breath.
- Chest pain.
If it is left untreated, complete heart block may lead to acute heart failure (p.247), chronic heart failure (p.247), stroke (p.329), shock (p.248), and even death.

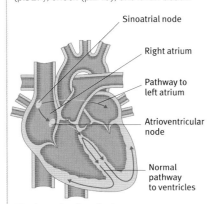

The heart's electrical system
Normally, electrical impulses pass from the sinoatrial node to the atrioventricular node and then to the ventricles. In complete heart block, the pathways to the ventricles are blocked and impulses cannot reach them.

Sinoatrial node
Right atrium
Pathway to left atrium
Atrioventricular node
Normal pathway to ventricles

What might be done?
Complete heart block is usually suspected if you have a very slow heartbeat and is confirmed by electrocardiography (see **ECG**, p.243).

The initial treatment of complete heart block may involve temporary insertion of a pacing wire into the heart; the wire transmits electrical impulses that restore a normal heartbeat until a permanent cardiac pacemaker and ICD (below) can be fitted. The general outlook depends on whether there is an underlying disorder, such as coronary artery disease.

Sick sinus syndrome

Abnormal function of the sinoatrial node, the heart's natural pacemaker

 Most common in elderly people

 Smoking, an unhealthy diet, lack of exercise, and excess weight are risk factors

 Gender and genetics are not significant factors

In sick sinus syndrome, the sinoatrial node, the heart's natural pacemaker, becomes faulty, causing the heart to beat too slowly or miss a few beats. Often, the heart rate

---

▶ **TREATMENT**

Cardiac pacemaker and ICD

Cardiac pacemakers stimulate the heart with electrical impulses to maintain a regular heartbeat. They are used to treat disorders in which the heart's electrical conducting system is faulty, such as complete heart block. Most pacemakers sense the heart rate and send an impulse when it falls too low. An ICD (implantable cardioverter defibrillator) is similar to a pacemaker but delivers an electric shock to the heart to restore normal rhythm only when the rhythm becomes dangerously abnormal. Some implanted devices contain both a pacemaker and an ICD.

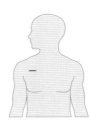
SITE OF INCISION

Insertion of a pacemaker
A pacemaker is inserted just under the skin and stitched into position in the chest wall, usually under local anaesthesia. Two wires from the pacemaker are passed into the large vein above the heart (superior vena cava). One wire is guided into the right atrium and the other into the right ventricle.

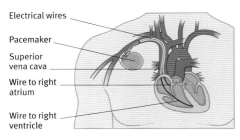

Electrical wires
Pacemaker
Superior vena cava
Wire to right atrium
Wire to right ventricle

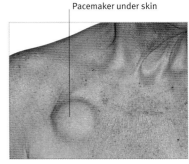
Pacemaker under skin
EXTERNAL VIEW

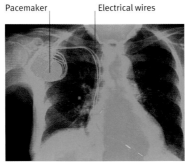
Pacemaker | Electrical wires
X-RAY IMAGE

Pacemaker in place
The pacemaker is implanted into the chest and appears as a small bulge under the skin. An X-ray image reveals the wires that lead from the pacemaker to the right atrium and ventricle of the heart.

Biventricular pacemaker

People who have heart failure and whose ECG shows that electrical activity of the heart's electrical conducting system is very slow may be treated by implantation of a special type of pacemaker called a biventricular pacemaker. This device is inserted and positioned in the same way as a standard pacemaker (above) and similarly has one wire running to the right atrium and another wire running to the right ventricle. A biventricular pacemaker also has a third wire, which runs to the outside surface of the left ventricle. This type of pacemaker delivers an impulse simultaneously to the left and right ventricles, which improves the efficiency of the heart by causing the heart chambers to contract in a more coordinated way (known as resynchronization).

alternates between runs of slow and fast beats. Sick sinus syndrome is caused by the degeneration of cells in the sinoatrial node and is most common in elderly people. Often, the underlying cause is coronary artery disease (p.243). Sick sinus syndrome may also be due to heart muscle disease (*see* **Dilated cardiomyopathy**, p.257). Typically, it is a progressive condition with episodes becoming more frequent and prolonged over time.

What are the symptoms?

Symptoms have a sudden onset and are intermittent. They may include:
- Palpitations (awareness of an irregular, abnormally rapid, or heavy heartbeat).
- Brief attacks of light-headedness.
- Loss of consciousness.
- Shortness of breath.

Many of the symptoms are caused by decreased oxygen levels to the brain due to the reduced efficiency of the heart.

What might be done?

If your doctor suspects you have sick sinus syndrome, he or she will probably arrange for you to have electrocardiography (*see* **ECG**, p.243). Because the symptoms are intermittent, you may need to have your heartbeat monitored for 24 hours or more while you carry out your everyday activities (*see* **Ambulatory ECG**, p.249). Your doctor may also recommend that you have further tests, such as echocardiography (p.255), to look for signs of underlying heart disease.

Treatment of sick sinus syndrome usually involves inserting a pacemaker to stimulate the heart when it is beating too slowly (*see* **Cardiac pacemaker and ICD**, p.251). If the heart is alternating between fast and slow rates, antiarrhythmic drugs (p.580) may also be given in order to slow down the fast heart rate and stabilize the rhythm. If a pacemaker has been fitted, you will need regular checkups with a doctor or pacemaker technician, who will check the battery life and make any necessary adjustments to the pacemaker. These checks and adjustments are done from outside the body and so are not invasive or painful.

Sick sinus syndrome can usually be treated successfully with a cardiac pacemaker and/or drugs. However, the general outlook depends on the underlying cause of the condition.

▶ **TREATMENT**

Cardioversion

In cardioversion, sometimes known as defibrillation, a brief electric shock is given to the heart using a device called a defibrillator. The shock can return the heartbeat to its normal rhythm. The defibrillator produces an electric current that passes between two metal plates, or paddles, which are placed on the patient's chest. Cardioversion is performed under general anaesthesia to treat some arrhythmias (abnormal heart rates and rhythms). It is also often performed as an emergency treatment for cardiac arrest. An automatic defibrillator has been developed that can diagnose heart rhythm problems and deliver the correct therapy, without the need for a medically trained operator.

Emergency cardioversion
Emergency treatment of cardiac arrest involves giving one or more electric shocks to the heart through the chest wall. Breathing is maintained by inflating the lungs using a breathing bag. The person using the bag temporarily stops and lets go each time a shock is delivered.

Paddle
An electric current passes through the chest between the paddles

Jelly pad
These pads prevent the skin from being burned

Blood-pressure cuff

Defibrillator
This device delivers the electric shock that is applied to the heart

Trace

Breathing bag
Squeezing the bag inflates the lungs with oxygen

Drip

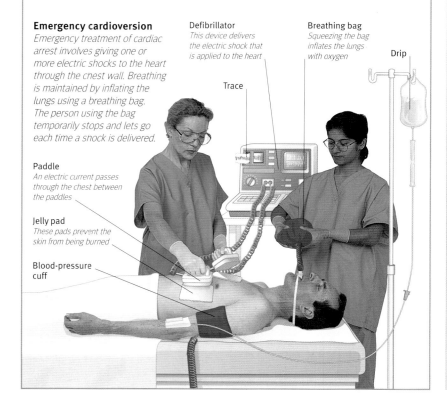

Cardiac arrest

Sudden failure of the heart to pump blood, which is often fatal

 More common with increasing age

 More common in males

Smoking, an unhealthy diet, lack of exercise, and excess weight are risk factors

 Genetics is not a significant factor

During cardiac arrest, the heart stops pumping. As a result, the brain and other organs no longer receive oxygenated blood, without which they cannot function. Within about 3 minutes of cardiac arrest, the brain will have sustained some damage. Death is likely to occur within about 5 minutes if the pumping action of the heart is not restored by emergency treatment or if circulation is not maintained by external cardiac massage.

What are the causes?

Cardiac arrest is commonly caused by one of two types of electrical problem in the heart: ventricular fibrillation, the more common type, and asystole. During ventricular fibrillation, the ventricles (lower chambers of the heart) rapidly contract in an uncoordinated manner, preventing the heart from pumping out blood. Ventricular fibrillation may occur suddenly in people with coronary artery disease (p.243), for which lifestyle factors such as smoking and an unhealthy diet increase the risk. It is also a frequent complication of a heart attack (*see* **Myocardial infarction**, p.245), usually occurring shortly after the attack. Ventricular fibrillation may also be caused by electrical injuries (p.183), drowning (p.187), and dilated cardiomyopathy (p.257), in which a disease of the heart muscle reduces its pumping efficiency.

Asystole is an electrical problem of the heart in which there is a total failure of the heart muscle to contract, leading to cardiac arrest. Asystole may be due to suffocation or to disorders or injuries that cause massive bleeding.

What are the symptoms?

Within seconds of a cardiac arrest, these symptoms usually occur:
- Collapse.
- Loss of consciousness.
- Blue lips, fingers, and toes.

An affected person has no pulse and has stopped breathing.

What might be done?

If you are with a person who has had a cardiac arrest, send for medical help immediately. If you are alone with the affected person, shout for help. At the same time, you should begin resuscitation to maintain blood flow to the brain.

While continuing cardiopulmonary resuscitation, the paramedic team may conduct electrocardiography (*see* **ECG**, p.243) to establish whether the cause of cardiac arrest is asystole or ventricular fibrillation. They will then administer the appropriate treatment. Ventricular fibrillation can be treated effectively with a device called an electric defibrillator (*see* **Cardioversion**, below, left), which delivers electric shocks to the heart to restore its normal rhythm and rate. Asystole may sometimes be treated successfully by an injection of epinephrine (adrenaline) into a large vein or directly into the heart to start it pumping again.

After resuscitation, monitoring in an intensive therapy unit will determine if a heart attack has occurred and, if so, whether it was the cause of the cardiac arrest. Monitoring will also detect a recurrence of cardiac arrest. A person with ventricular fibrillation may be prescribed antiarrhythmic drugs (p.580) on a long-term basis or have an implantable cardioverter defibrillator (ICD) fitted (*see* **Cardiac pacemaker and ICD**, p.251).

What is the prognosis?

If resuscitation has been performed without delay, the chances of survival depend on the underlying cause. In a person who has ventricular fibrillation as a complication of a heart attack, a complete recovery may be possible if the normal heartbeat is restored by prompt cardioversion, particularly if the heart attack has not resulted in major damage to the heart muscle. Afterwards, the person will be carefully assessed and may have an ICD implanted to prevent further episodes of ventricular fibrillation. The outlook for cardiac arrest caused by asystole depends on whether rapid, effective treatment can be given for the underlying cause and whether the normal heartbeat can be re-established. People are more likely to survive a cardiac arrest that occurs in hospital than one that takes place elsewhere because recognition of the condition and access to emergency treatment is more rapid.

Heart valve and muscle disorders

Healthy heart valves and muscle are essential for the heart to pump blood efficiently. Heart valve disorders are less common today in the UK than in the past because a major cause, rheumatic fever, is now rare. Heart muscle disorders often used to be fatal but have a better outlook now because of improved treatments.

The first articles in this section cover heart valve disorders. Blood is pumped around the body at very high pressure by the left side of the heart. The valves on this side, called the aortic and mitral valves, are therefore the ones most often affected by disorders. If a heart valve does not work properly, blood cannot circulate efficiently, and the heart has to pump harder or faster in order to compensate. The next articles discuss disorders of the heart muscle and the lining of the heart (the endocardium). Any disorder that affects the heart muscle reduces the heart's efficiency and may eventually be fatal. The last article discusses rheumatic fever, a disorder that may damage the heart valves after many years.

Other disorders of the heart muscle, such as heart attack and heart failure, are discussed elsewhere in the book (see **Major cardiovascular disorders**, pp.241–249). Congenital heart disease (p.542) is covered in the section on infancy and childhood.

✚ KEY ANATOMY

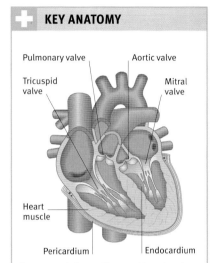

For more information on the structure and function of the heart valves and muscle, see pp.235–240.

Heart valve disorders

Abnormalities of the heart valves, which may impair blood flow through the heart

👤 Age, gender, genetics, and lifestyle as risk factors depend on the cause

There are four valves in the heart that ensure that blood flows in one direction by opening to let blood through and then closing tightly when the heart muscle contracts. If a heart valve is damaged, blood flow through it may be restricted or blood may leak backwards because a valve fails to close completely. As a result, the heart then

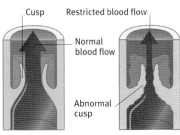

NORMAL   **STENOSED**

Valve stenosis
If a heart valve is healthy, blood flows through easily when the valve is open. In stenosis, the valve cusps (flaps) do not open fully and blood flow is restricted.

has to work harder in order to pump blood around the body. Disorders of the heart valves often do not cause symptoms, but sometimes they result in tiredness and shortness of breath on exertion. Since the efficiency of the heart is impaired, a severe heart valve disorder may result in chronic heart failure (p.247) or an arrhythmia (p.249), in which the heart beats abnormally. Damaged valves are also more susceptible to infection (see **Infective endocarditis**, p.256).

Some heart valve disorders are present at birth. Heart valves may also be damaged later in life by changes due to aging, infection of the heart lining, or a heart attack (see **Myocardial infarction**, p.245). Rheumatic fever (p.258) was once a major cause of heart valve damage but is now rare in developed countries such as the UK.

What are the types?
The cusps (flaps) inside a heart valve may not open fully, making the opening of the valve too narrow (see **Mitral stenosis**, p.255, and **Aortic stenosis**, p.254). Alternatively, a valve may not form a tight seal when closed, allowing blood to leak back through it (see **Mitral incompetence**, p.254, and **Aortic incompetence**, p.254). In some cases, both stenosis and incompetence occur in the same valve. Mitral valve prolapse (p.256) is a common, but usually harmless, cause of incompetence;

in this condition, the mitral valve bulges backwards when it is closed and allows slight leakage of blood.

What might be done?
Valve disorders may be diagnosed in a routine examination or after symptoms have developed. Your doctor listens for sounds, called heart murmurs, that are made by turbulent blood flow through abnormal valves. You may have an ECG (p.243) to check the electrical activity of the heart. Chest X-rays (p.300) may also be taken, and the imaging technique echocardiography (p.255) may be used to view the interior of the heart and its blood flow.

If treatment is needed, you may be given drugs to control the heartbeat or relieve the symptoms. In severe valve disorders, surgery may be needed to repair or replace the

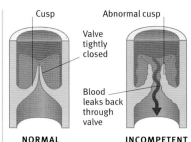

NORMAL   **INCOMPETENT**

Valve incompetence
Normally, the valve cusps (flaps) meet to stop blood from flowing backwards. An incompetent valve does not close completely and blood leaks backwards.

valve (see **Heart valve replacement**, below). An abnormal or replacement heart valve is more susceptible to infection (see **Infective endocarditis**, p.256) than a normal valve.

▶ TREATMENT

Heart valve replacement

Heart valves may need to be replaced if it is not possible to repair them. Replacement valves made of tissue may come from a human donor or from a pig. Valves may also be mechanical. Replacing heart valves usually involves open heart surgery. During the operation, the heart is stopped, and its function is taken over by a heart–lung machine (p.615). You may need to stay in hospital for 7–14 days after surgery. If a mechanical valve is used, drugs that prevent blood clotting (p.584) are taken for life to reduce the risk of clots forming on the valve. If you need aortic valve replacement and are too ill for open heart surgery, the valve may be replaced using a minimally invasive procedure called transcatheter aortic valve implantation (TAVI).

LOCATION OF VALVES

Aortic valve replacement
Replacing the aortic valve by conventional surgery involves opening the chest and making an incision in the aorta to gain access to the valve. The diseased valve is cut out, and the replacement aortic valve is then stitched in place. Alternatively, a TAVI procedure may be used. This involves using a catheter (thin tube), threaded through blood vessels, to insert a replacement valve in the heart.

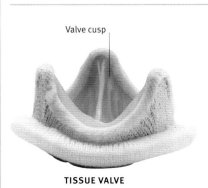

TISSUE VALVE

MECHANICAL AORTIC VALVE

Replacement valves
Tissue valves have three cusps that open and close to control blood flow. In one type of mechanical valve, blood flow pushes a ball into a cage to allow blood through the valve.

Your doctor will advise you to maintain good oral hygiene to reduce the risk of infection. You will also be told how to recognize symptoms of infective endocarditis so that treatment can be given promptly if it does develop.

Aortic incompetence

Leakage of blood back through the aortic valve of the heart

 More common in males

 In some cases, the condition is inherited

 Age and lifestyle are not significant factors

The aortic valve separates the left lower chamber of the heart (the left ventricle) from the aorta, which is the main artery leading from the heart. This valve normally stops blood from flowing back into the heart from the aorta. In aortic incompetence, the valve cusps (flaps) do not close tightly, letting blood leak back from the aorta. As a result, the heart has to pump harder and faster to circulate blood around the body, and this may eventually lead to the development of chronic heart failure (p.247).

What are the causes?
About 1 in 50 boys and 1 in 100 girls are born with an aortic valve with two cusps instead of the normal three. Another cause of aortic incompetence is the rare genetic disorder Marfan's syndrome (p.534). A possible cause of valve damage later in life is infection (*see* **Infective endocarditis**, p.256). Sometimes, long-standing high blood pressure (*see* **Hypertension**, p.242) can cause the root of the aorta to stretch so that the cusps of the aortic valve do not close tightly and the valve leaks. The aortic valve flaps may also become leaky as a result of the rare inflammatory joint disorder ankylosing spondylitis (p.223). Other causes of aortic incompetence include rheumatic fever (p.258) and syphilis, but these diseases are now rare in developed countries due to the widespread use of effective antibiotics.

What are the symptoms?
If aortic incompetence is mild, it may not cause symptoms for years. If symptoms do develop, they may include:
■ Tiredness.
■ Shortness of breath during exertion.
■ Awareness of the heart beating strongly.
In severe aortic incompetence, heart failure may eventually develop, leading to symptoms such as constant shortness of breath and swollen ankles.

What might be done?
If there are no symptoms, aortic incompetence is usually discovered during a routine examination. Your doctor may then arrange for electrocardiography (*see* **ECG**, p.243) to

evaluate the electrical activity of the heart. In addition, the heart may be imaged by echocardiography (opposite page), which looks at the interior of the heart and can evaluate the movement of the valves. A chest X-ray (p.300) may also be taken to see if the heart has enlarged.

If the aortic incompetence is mild, often no treatment is needed. However, if you have symptoms or if chronic heart failure develops, you may need treatment with drugs such as ACE inhibitors (p.582), which reduce the work that the heart has to do.

You may also be evaluated to see whether surgery to repair or replace the defective valve will help (*see* **Heart valve replacement**, p.253). In some cases, valve replacement surgery may be recommended if tests show that the valve is leaking severely and the heart has started to enlarge, even though there may be no external symptoms or signs of heart failure. In all cases where surgery is performed, it is likely to be more successful if it is done before heart failure becomes advanced.

An abnormal or replacement aortic valve is more susceptible to infection (*see* **Infective endocarditis**, p.256) than a normal valve. Your doctor will advise you to maintain good oral hygiene to reduce the risk of infection. You will also be told how to recognize symptoms of infective endocarditis so that treatment can be given promptly if it does develop.

Once the damaged aortic valve has been repaired or replaced, the outlook for the affected person is good and life expectancy should be normal.

Aortic stenosis

Narrowing of the aortic valve, reducing the flow of blood into the circulation

 May be present at birth but most common in people over the age of 70

 More common in males

 Genetics and lifestyle are not significant factors

The aortic valve separates the left lower chamber (left ventricle) of the heart and the main artery of the body, the aorta. The valve opens to allow blood to flow out of the heart. In aortic stenosis, the opening of the valve is narrowed, reducing the flow of blood through it. The heart then has to pump harder to compensate. Aortic stenosis is the most common valve disorder requiring valve replacement in the UK.

What are the causes?
In young people living in developed countries, aortic stenosis is usually the result of a heart abnormality that is present at birth (*see* **Congenital heart disease**, p.542). In elderly people, aortic stenosis is often caused by calcium deposits on the aortic

valve, which naturally build up over time. Rheumatic fever (p.258) was once a common cause of aortic stenosis. However, rheumatic fever is now rare in developed countries, mainly due to the use of effective antibiotics.

What are the symptoms?
In mild cases of aortic stenosis, there are often no symptoms. In some cases of mild stenosis, tiredness may be the only symptom. Other symptoms may develop in more severe cases, such as:
■ Dizziness and fainting.
■ Chest pain during exertion.
If the opening through the aortic valve is very narrow, the flow of blood to the coronary arteries that supply blood to the heart muscle is reduced, and the heart also has to work harder to pump blood around the body. This will eventually lead to breathlessness due to chronic heart failure (p.247). Abnormal heart rhythms may also develop (*see* **Arrhythmias**, p.249), and infection of the valves is more likely.

How is it diagnosed?
Often, mild aortic stenosis is detected during a routine examination. If your doctor suspects that you have aortic stenosis, he or she may arrange for echocardiography (opposite page) to image the interior of the heart, including the aortic valve. You may also have a chest X-ray (p.300) because, if there is stenosis, calcium deposits on the valve may be visible on the X-ray. If these investigations are not conclusive, a procedure called cardiac catheterization may be performed. In this procedure, a flexible catheter is inserted into an artery in the arm or groin and passed into the heart. A small device on the catheter then measures the pressures on either side of the valve.

What is the treatment?
Mild stenosis is often treated with drugs such as diuretics (p.583), which relieve breathlessness by removing excess fluid from the lungs. However, a heart valve replacement (p.253) is often needed eventually. If you have a certain type of congenital aortic stenosis, you may be advised to have a balloon valvuloplasty, in which a balloon is inflated in the valve to widen it. The outlook is good if you are

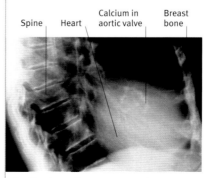

Spine   Heart   Calcium in aortic valve   Breast bone

Aortic stenosis
This chest X-ray, taken from the side, shows calcium deposits that have formed in a narrowed aortic valve. The deposits make the valve visible on the X-ray.

given treatment before the heart muscle becomes badly damaged. A stenotic or replacement valve is more susceptible to infection (*see* **Infective endocarditis**, p.256). Your doctor will advise you to maintain good oral hygiene to reduce this risk and will also tell you how to recognize symptoms of infective endocarditis so that it can be treated promptly if it does develop.

Mitral incompetence

Leakage of blood back through the mitral valve of the heart

 In some cases, the condition is inherited

 Age, gender, and lifestyle as risk factors depend on the cause

The mitral valve sits between the upper chamber (atrium) and the lower chamber (ventricle) on the left side of the heart. In mitral incompetence, the valve fails to close properly and allows blood to leak back into the atrium. This increases the pressure in the blood vessels leading to that chamber. The left side of the heart has to work harder to pump blood around the body, and eventually chronic heart failure (p.247) develops. Mitral incompetence can occur in conjunction with mitral stenosis (opposite page).

What are the causes?
In rare cases, mitral incompetence is present at birth, sometimes as a result of the rare genetic disorder Marfan's syndrome (p.534). Any condition that damages the mitral valve can lead to mitral incompetence. Rheumatic fever (p.258) was once a major cause of the disorder but is now rarely seen in developed countries, mainly because of the widespread use of antibiotics. A more common cause is an infection of the valve (*see* **Infective endocarditis**, p.256). Hypertrophic cardiomyopathy (p.257), in which the wall of the left ventricle is thickened, may distort the valve, causing incompetence. The condition can also be a consequence of a heart attack if the heart muscle attached to the valve is affected (*see* **Myocardial infarction**, p.245). In some cases, mitral incompetence occurs in conjunction with mitral valve prolapse (p.256).

What are the symptoms?
Symptoms of mitral incompetence usually develop gradually over months or years but may appear suddenly if the cause is a heart attack or valve infection. The symptoms include:
■ Unexplained tiredness.
■ Shortness of breath during exertion.
■ Palpitations (awareness of an irregular or abnormally rapid heartbeat).
Eventually, symptoms of chronic heart failure may occur, such as shortness of breath at rest as well as during exertion, due to fluid in the lungs. The build-up of fluid in the body tissues also causes swelling of the ankles.

Are there complications?

The backward blood flow into the left atrium may enlarge it, leading to an irregular heartbeat (*see* **Atrial fibrillation**, p.250). If the atrium is so large that it cannot empty fully with each heartbeat, a blood clot may form. If a clot passes into an artery supplying the brain and blocks it, the result may be a stroke (p.329). Another potential complication is infection of the leaky mitral valve after dental treatment or surgery on the digestive or urinary tracts.

What might be done?

Your doctor may suspect mitral incompetence if he or she hears characteristic sounds known as heart murmurs. Tests to assess the function of the heart and lungs may be carried out, including an ECG (p.243) to monitor the electrical activity of the heart and a chest X-ray (p.300). The interior of the heart may be imaged by echocardiography (below right) to confirm the diagnosis. This procedure can show the movements of the mitral valve.

If heart failure develops, drugs such as diuretics (p.583) may be prescribed to relieve the symptoms. If the left atrium becomes enlarged, you may also be given drugs that prevent blood clotting (p.584) to lessen the risk of clots in the atrium. Severe mitral incompetence may need to be treated surgically to repair the valve or implant a heart valve replacement (p.253). An abnormal or replacement mitral valve is more susceptible to infection (*see* **Infective endocarditis**, p.256) than a normal valve. Your doctor will advise you to maintain good oral hygiene to reduce the risk of infection. You will also be told how to recognize symptoms of infective endocarditis so that treatment can be given promptly if it does develop.

The outlook for people with mitral incompetence is good if treatment is given before the heart has become badly damaged.

Mitral stenosis

Narrowing of the mitral valve, resulting in a decrease in blood flow within the heart

 More common after the age of 40

 More common in females

 Genetics and lifestyle are not significant factors

The mitral valve sits between the upper chamber (atrium) and lower chamber (ventricle) on the left side of the heart. In mitral stenosis, the opening of this valve is narrowed, restricting the blood flow through the atrium. The heart works harder to pump blood through the narrow valve, and chronic heart failure (p.247) may eventually develop. Mitral stenosis is more common in females and sometimes occurs with mitral incompetence (opposite page).

What are the causes?

Mitral stenosis is almost always due to damage to the valve caused by an earlier attack of rheumatic fever (p.258). This condition is now rare in developed countries, and, in the UK, mitral stenosis is most often found in middle-aged or elderly people who had rheumatic fever during their childhood. In rare cases, mitral stenosis is present at birth.

What are the symptoms?

Symptoms usually develop gradually in adulthood and may include:
- Unexplained tiredness.
- Shortness of breath, occurring during exertion at first but later also at rest.
- Palpitations (awareness of an irregular or abnormally rapid heartbeat).

As the stenosis becomes worse, the symptoms of heart failure may develop, including swelling of the tissues due to a buildup of fluid, which is most noticeable in the ankles and feet.

Are there complications?

Sometimes, the atria beat irregularly and rapidly (*see* **Atrial fibrillation**, p.250). Blood clots may also form on the wall of the left atrium because it does not empty fully. If fragments of clots break off, they may block a blood vessel elsewhere in the body. If a blood clot blocks an artery supplying the brain, the result may be a stroke (p.329).

How is it diagnosed?

Your doctor will examine you and will probably arrange for an ECG (p.243) to assess the electrical activity of the heart. The inside of the heart may be imaged by echocardiography (below). Special types of echocardiography, such as transoesophageal and Doppler echocardiography, may also be carried out to check the functioning of the heart and heart valves and to assess blood flow through the heart. You may also have a chest X-ray (p.300). The severity of the mitral stenosis can be estimated by echocardiography but occasionally it may need to be more accurately assessed by a procedure in which a thin tube called a cardiac catheter is inserted through blood vessels into the heart. The catheter is attached to a device that measures the pressure on either side of the mitral valve.

What is the treatment?

In most cases of mitral stenosis, drug treatments are used to help to relieve the symptoms. For example, diuretics (p.583) may be prescribed to remove excess fluid from the body and to relieve shortness of breath. Antiarrhythmic drugs (p.580) may be given to help correct an abnormal heart rhythm. If the abnormal rhythm is atrial fibrillation, drugs that prevent blood clotting (p.584) are often prescribed to reduce the risk of blood clots forming in the heart.

If drug treatment is ineffective, a balloon valvuloplasty may be performed. In this procedure, a balloon-tipped catheter is passed into the heart, the balloon is inflated and deflated several times inside the stenosed valve to widen it, and then the catheter is removed. Alternatively, the valve may be repaired or replaced by surgery (*see* **Heart valve replacement**, p.253).

A stenotic or replacement mitral valve is more susceptible to infection (*see* **Infective endocarditis**, p.256) than a normal valve. Your doctor will advise you to maintain good oral hygiene to reduce the risk of infection. You will also be told how to recognize symptoms of infective endocarditis so that treatment can be given promptly if it does develop.

Mitral stenosis may recur after a balloon valvuloplasty, often within about a year. However, a heart valve replacement is often effective for 10 years or more.

▶ **TEST**

Echocardiography

Echocardiography uses ultrasound waves to image the interior of the heart. The test looks at the size and function of the heart and is used to diagnose disorders of the heart and the heart valves. The test is usually performed using an ultrasound transducer (probe) placed on the skin of the chest directly over the heart. In some cases, a small probe is passed down the oesophagus instead so that it is close to the back of the heart; this procedure is known as transoesophageal echocardiography. It produces a moving image of the beating heart with its valves and chambers. Another variation of this test (called Doppler echocardiography) may sometimes be carried out to assess blood flow in different parts of the heart.

During the procedure
A gel is placed on the skin of the chest, and an ultrasound probe is moved over the area. An image of the moving heart is displayed on a monitor screen and is also recorded.

Doctor

Monitor

Ultrasound transducer

RESULTS

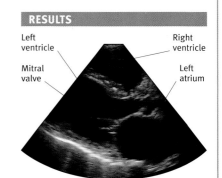

Left ventricle

Right ventricle

Mitral valve

Left atrium

Echocardiography of the heart
This image shows structures inside the heart. The chambers and valves seen here are normal.

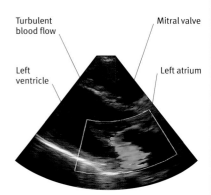

Turbulent blood flow

Mitral valve

Left ventricle

Left atrium

Doppler echocardiography
Different colours show variations in blood flow. Here, turbulent flow back into the left atrium indicates a mitral valve leak.

Mitral valve prolapse

An abnormality of the mitral valve, also known as floppy mitral valve

 Most common between the ages of 20 and 40

 More common in females

 In some cases, the condition is inherited

 Lifestyle is not a significant factor

The mitral valve sits between the upper chamber (atrium) and the lower chamber (ventricle) on the left side of the heart. This valve normally closes tightly when the heart contracts to pump blood out into the circulation. In the disorder called mitral valve prolapse, the valve is slightly deformed and bulges back into the left atrium. This prolapse may allow a small amount of blood to leak back into the atrium (see **Mitral incompetence**, p.254). Mitral valve prolapse is common, occurring in up to 1 in 20 people. This condition occurs most commonly in young or middle-aged women, but often the cause is not known. In some cases, mitral valve prolapse is associated with the rare genetic disorder Marfan's syndrome (p.534).

What are the symptoms?
Mitral valve prolapse usually causes no symptoms, and most people are unaware that they have the condition. If symptoms do occur, they are usually intermittent and may include:
■ Light-headedness.
■ Fainting.
■ Sharp, left-sided chest pains.
■ Palpitations (awareness of an irregular or abnormally rapid heartbeat).
There is also an increased chance that a floppy valve may become further damaged by an infection (see **Infective endocarditis**, right), particularly following dental procedures or surgery on the digestive or urinary tracts.

How is it diagnosed?
Your doctor may suspect mitral valve prolapse if he or she hears a characteristic clicking sound when listening to your heart with a stethoscope. He or she may arrange for you to have tests, including an ECG (p.243), which monitors the electrical activity of the heart. A diagnosis of mitral valve prolapse is usually confirmed by echocardiography (p.255), which examines the movements of the valves. If you have palpitations, your heart rhythm may also be monitored over a period of 24 hours while you perform your normal activities (see **Ambulatory ECG**, p.249).

What is the treatment?
Most people with mitral valve prolapse do not need treatment, although regular monitoring with echocardiography (p.255) may be needed to check there has been no worsen-

ing of the condition. If symptoms such as an irregular heartbeat cause problems, an anti-arrhythmic drug (p.580) may be prescribed.

The disorder usually has no effect on life expectancy, but occasionally mitral incompetence develops, leading to chronic heart failure (p.247). Heart valve repair or replacement (p.253) may then be needed, but the outlook is still good. An abnormal or replacement mitral valve is more susceptible to infection (see **Infective endocarditis**, below) than a normal valve. Your doctor will advise you to maintain good oral hygiene to reduce the risk of infection. You will also be told how to recognize symptoms of infective endocarditis so that treatment can be given promptly if it does develop.

Infective endocarditis

Inflammation of the lining of the heart, particularly affecting the heart valves, caused by an infection

 Intravenous drug abuse increases the risk

 Age, gender, and genetics are not significant factors

The internal lining of the heart, the endocardium, may become infected if microorganisms enter the bloodstream and reach the heart. Infection causes the lining, especially over the heart valves, to become inflamed, and bacteria and blood clots can collect over the inflamed areas. The valves are particularly prone to infection if they are already damaged or if they are replacement valves (see **Heart valve replacement**, p.253).

In most cases, infective endocarditis is a chronic (long-term) disorder that develops over weeks or months and causes only vague symptoms, such as a fever and aching joints. Rarely, endocarditis is an acute disorder that may rapidly damage one or more of the heart valves. Within days acute endocarditis may cause acute heart failure (p.247), which may be life-threatening.

What are the causes?
The most common causes of infective endocarditis are bacteria and, less often, fungi. Normally harmless microorganisms may enter the blood during dental procedures, especially tooth extraction, and operations on the digestive or urinary tracts. The condition can also occur after a medical procedure, such as the insertion of a catheter into the bladder or from long-term treatment using an indwelling intravenous catheter, such as a skin-tunnelled catheter (p.277). Rarely, infective endocarditis develops after cardiac surgery, especially if artificial materials, such as replacement heart valves, are inserted into the heart. A person with a suppressed immune system is particularly susceptible to infective endocarditis because his or her body is less able to fight the infection. For example, anyone with HIV infection or AIDS (p.169) or who is

undergoing treatment with anticancer drugs (p.586) is at increased risk of developing the disorder. People who abuse intravenous drugs are also susceptible because microorganisms can be injected into the bloodstream and travel to the heart. There is an even greater risk of infection if needles are shared. Body piercing and tattooing also carry an increased risk of infection.

What are the symptoms?
The symptoms of chronic endocarditis are often generalized and unrelated to heart damage. They may include:
■ Abnormal tiredness.
■ Fever and night sweats.
■ Aching joints.
■ Weight loss.
Infected material from the valve may break off and block a vessel elsewhere in the body. For example, small clots may lodge in veins under the fingernails or skin, causing tiny splinter-like haemorrhages. If a clot blocks an artery that supplies blood to the brain, it may result in a stroke (p.329).

The symptoms of acute endocarditis develop suddenly and may include:
■ High fever.
■ Palpitations (awareness of an irregular or abnormally rapid heartbeat).
These symptoms can rapidly worsen. If acute heart failure develops, there may be other symptoms, such as severe shortness of breath and wheezing.

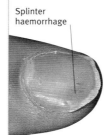

Splinter haemorrhage

Effect of infective endocarditis
Bleeding under the fingernail, resulting in so-called splinter haemorrhages, can occur in association with the heart disorder infective endocarditis.

How is it diagnosed?
Chronic infective endocarditis is difficult to diagnose because the symptoms are often unrelated to heart damage. Your doctor may suspect the disorder if he or she hears a new heart murmur or a change in an existing heart murmur. The diagnosis may be confirmed by echocardiography (p.255) to image the interior of the heart and detect infected material on the surface of the valves. Blood tests may be done to identify the organism responsible for the infection.

What is the treatment?
If you have infective endocarditis, you will usually need treatment with intravenous antibiotics (p.572) for about 6 weeks. You will have regular blood tests to confirm that the infection is clearing up. This treatment is successful in up to 4 in 5 cases. If a valve is badly damaged or if the infection cannot be controlled with drugs, heart valve replacement (p.253) may be necessary.

If you have a valve disorder or already have a replacement valve, you are at increased risk of developing endocarditis and

should be aware of the symptoms. Contact your doctor immediately if any become apparent. Once you have had one episode of the disorder, you have an increased risk of developing it again. For this reason, you may be advised to take a single dose of an antibiotic (p.572) before operations on the digestive or urinary tracts.

Myocarditis

Inflammation of the muscle tissue of the heart, usually due to an infection

 Age, gender, genetics, and lifestyle are not significant factors

Myocarditis is inflammation of the heart muscle, usually due to an infection Frequently, the condition goes unrecognized because there are no obvious symptoms. However, severe inflammation of the heart muscle may develop, causing chest pain and leading eventually to heart enlargement and chronic heart failure (p.247).

The most common cause of the disorder is a viral infection, usually with the coxsackie virus. Myocarditis may also be due to rheumatic fever (p.258), although this is now rare in developed countries, mainly due to the widespread use of antibiotics (p.572). Some autoimmune disorders, such as systemic lupus erythematosus (p.281), in which the body attacks its own tissues, may also cause myocarditis.

What are the symptoms?
Myocarditis often causes no symptoms. However, if symptoms do occur, they usually develop over a number of hours or days and may include:
■ Fever.
■ Tiredness.
■ Aching in the chest.
■ Palpitations (awareness of an irregular or abnormally rapid heartbeat).
Eventually, breathlessness and swelling of the ankles may develop due to heart failure. Rarely, myocarditis causes sudden death during vigorous exertion.

What might be done?
If your doctor suspects that you have myocarditis, he or she will probably arrange for an ECG (p.243) to monitor the electrical activity of the heart and a chest X-ray (p.300) to see if the heart is enlarged. You may have echocardiography (p.255) to image the interior of the heart. Blood tests may be carried out to check for infection and for the presence of enzymes that can indicate whether or not the heart muscle is damaged.

Myocarditis is usually mild, and the heart should recover within 2 weeks. If severe heart failure does develop, a heart transplant (opposite page) may give the best chance of a return to normal health.

Dilated cardiomyopathy

Damaged heart muscle, leading to enlargement of the heart

 More common over the age of 45

 More common in males

 Alcohol abuse increases the risk

 Genetics is not a significant factor

Healthy heart muscle is vital for the heart to pump blood effectively. In dilated cardiomyopathy, the muscular walls of the heart become damaged. The weakened muscle then stretches, making the heart larger. This weakening and the enlargement of the heart muscle reduces the heart's pumping action, leading to chronic heart failure (p.247). In some cases, dilated cardiomyopathy is caused by alcohol abuse. It may also be due to an autoimmune disorder, in which the body attacks its own tissues, or it may occur after a viral illness or after treatment with some anticancer drugs. Often, the underlying cause is not found.

The symptoms of dilated cardiomyopathy are similar to those of chronic heart failure. Therefore, before making a diagnosis, your doctor may carry out tests that exclude other disorders that cause heart failure, such as coronary artery disease (p.243) and heart valve disorders. Dilated cardiomyopathy is more common over the age of 45 and in men.

What are the symptoms?

In many mild cases, there are no symptoms. If symptoms do occur, they usually develop gradually over a number of years and may include:

- Tiredness.
- Shortness of breath during exertion.
- Palpitations (awareness of an irregular or abnormally rapid heartbeat).
- Swelling of the ankles.

As the disorder progresses the heart's pumping efficiency decreases and symptoms, such as shortness of breath, worsen. The heart enlargement may stretch the valves, causing them to become leaky, and may eventually lead to the development of chronic heart failure or an abnormal heart rhythm (*see* **Arrhythmias**, p.249). If the chambers in the heart cannot empty fully because they are too large, a blood clot can form, which may break off and block a vessel elsewhere in the body.

How is it diagnosed?

Diagnosis involves a number of tests, many of which are used to exclude other possible causes of your symptoms, such as coronary artery disease. You may have an ECG (p.243) to monitor the heart's electrical activity and echocardiography (p.255) to image the interior of the heart. You may also have a chest X-ray (p.300) or MRI scan (p.133) to detect enlargement of the heart. Coronary angiography (p.245) is used to exclude coronary artery disease. To evaluate valve function, a cardiac catheter may be passed from an artery into the heart to measure blood pressure inside it. If you have palpi-tations, an ECG may be carried out over a 24-hour period to monitor your heartbeat while you carry out your normal daily activities (*see* **Ambulatory ECG**, p.249).

What is the treatment?

If the cause of dilated cardiomyopathy is unknown, no specific treatment can be given. If alcohol abuse is the cause, you must stop drinking. Symptoms of heart failure may be relieved by drugs such as digoxin (*see* **Digitalis drugs**, p.582) to improve heart function, diuretic drugs (p.583) to remove excess fluid, and beta-blockers (p.581) and ACE inhibitors (p.582), which may help to prevent deterioration. You may also have drugs that prevent blood clotting (p.584). However, if heart failure worsens in spite of drug treatment, a heart transplant (below left) may be considered. Without a transplant, only about 3 in 10 people survive for more than 5 years.

Hypertrophic cardiomyopathy

Abnormal thickening of the muscular walls of the heart, which reduces its pumping efficiency

 Usually develops in adolescence but may be delayed until middle age

 In most cases, the condition is inherited

 Gender and lifestyle are not significant factors

In hypertrophic cardiomyopathy, the walls of the heart are excessively thick. This thickening prevents the heart from filling properly and may partially block the passage of blood from the heart, both of which reduce the pumping efficiency of the heart. The condition is usually inherited and is caused by a faulty gene involved in the formation of heart muscle. The disorder may cause sudden death in apparently healthy young people, but sometimes symptoms do not develop until middle age.

What are the symptoms?

Symptoms of the disorder usually develop in adolescence. They first occur during exertion and may include:

- Fainting.
- Shortness of breath.
- Chest pain.
- Palpitations (awareness of an irregular or abnormally rapid heartbeat).

As the disorder progresses, shortness of breath may be present at rest. In some cases, a life-threatening abnormal heart rhythm develops (*see* **Arrhythmias**, p.249). Hypertrophic cardiomyopathy may also distort the valve that sits between the left upper and lower chambers of the heart, causing it to leak (*see* **Mitral incompetence**, p.254). In severe cases, the thickened heart walls may obstruct blood flow out of the heart, causing an inadequate blood supply to the rest of the body that may be fatal.

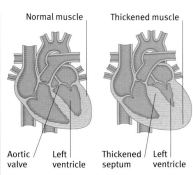

Normal muscle | Thickened muscle

Aortic valve / Left ventricle | Thickened septum / Left ventricle

NORMAL | **ABNORMAL**

Hypertrophic cardiomyopathy
In this condition, the septum and the muscular wall of the left ventricle become abnormally thick. This thickening prevents the left ventricle from filling properly and obstructs the outflow to the aortic valve.

How is it diagnosed?

If your doctor suspects that you may have hypertrophic cardiomyopathy, he or she may arrange for an ECG (p.243) to measure the heart's electrical activity. You may also have echocardiography (p.255) to image the heart. This shows the size of the heart and the thickness of the walls and is used to assess the degree to which output of blood from the heart is restricted. You may also have an exercise ECG (*see* **Exercise testing**, p.244) and monitoring of your heart rhythm for 24 hours while you carry out your normal activities (*see* **Ambulatory ECG**, p.249).

What is the treatment?

Treatment of hypertrophic cardiomyopathy is aimed at improving the filling capacity of the heart using drugs such as beta-blockers (p.581) and calcium channel blockers (p.582). If you have an abnormal heart rhythm, it may be treated with anti-arrhythmic drugs (p.580). Some of the thickened muscle may be removed surgically. Alternatively, septal ablation may be recommended. In this procedure, a small amount of alcohol is injected into one of the arteries supplying blood to the thickened heart muscle. The alcohol causes part of the thickened muscle to die and shrink to a more normal size, reducing the amount of obstruction to blood flow out of the heart. In rare cases, a heart transplant (left) may be considered.

Hypertrophic cardiomyopathy increases your risk of developing infection of the lining of the heart or heart valves (*see* **Infective endocarditis**, opposite page). Your doctor will advise you to maintain good oral hygiene to reduce the risk of infection. You will also be told how to recognize symptoms of infective endocarditis so that treatment can be given promptly if it does develop.

The disorder is usually inherited. For this reason, relatives of anyone with hypertrophic cardiomyopathy should be screened to see if they have the condition.

About 1 in 25 affected people die each year. The outlook is better if the symptoms are diagnosed and treated early.

▶ **TREATMENT**

Heart transplant

A heart transplant is sometimes the best treatment option if the heart is severely damaged and can no longer pump blood effectively. During the operation, the heart's normal function is taken over by a heart–lung machine (*see* **Surgery using a heart–lung machine**, p.615). Afterwards, you will need lifelong drug treatment to prevent the body from rejecting the donor heart. Because of the shortage of donor hearts, there may be a long wait before a suitable one is available. As an interim measure, a device called a left ventricular assist device (LVAD) may be implanted. This is a type of artificial heart pump that supports the heart until a transplant is possible.

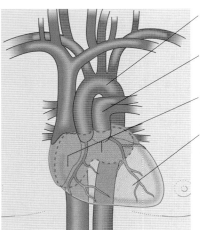

Aorta

Pulmonary artery

Remaining back walls of atria

Area to be replaced

SITE OF INCISION

The procedure
Most of the diseased heart is removed, but the back walls of the upper chambers (atria) are left in place. The lower chambers (ventricles) of the donor heart are then attached to the remaining areas of the recipient's heart.

Pericarditis

Inflammation of the pericardium, the double-layered membrane around the heart

 Age as a risk factor depends on the cause

 Gender, genetics, and lifestyle are not significant factors

The pericardium is a two-layered membrane that surrounds the heart. In pericarditis, this membrane becomes inflamed, usually due to infection. The inflammation is usually acute with symptoms that are often mistaken for a heart attack (*see* **Myocardial infarction**, p.245). The inflammation usually subsides after about a week. However, rarely, the inflammation persists and causes the pericardium to become scarred and thickened and to contract around the heart. As a result, the constricted heart is unable to fill and pump normally. This serious long-term condition is called constrictive pericarditis. In both acute and long-term disorders, fluid may accumulate between the two layers of the pericardium and stop the heart from pumping effectively. This is called a pericardial effusion and may lead to acute heart failure (p.247) or chronic heart failure (p.247).

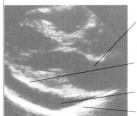

Ventricle of heart

Inner layer of pericardium

Fluid

Outer layer of pericardium

Pericardial effusion
This echocardiogram shows fluid between the two layers of the pericardium, the membrane that surrounds the heart.

What are the causes?

In young adults, pericarditis is usually due to a viral infection, although pericarditis may develop as a complication of bacterial pneumonia (p.299). Tuberculosis (p.300) is an important cause of pericarditis in some countries. A heart attack can cause pericarditis if the muscle on the surface of the heart is affected. Pericarditis may also develop when a cancerous tumour elsewhere in the body spreads to the pericardium.

Inflammation of the pericardium is also associated with autoimmune disorders, in which the body attacks its own tissues. For example, the conditions rheumatoid arthritis (p.222) and systemic lupus erythematosus (p.281) may sometimes cause pericarditis.

What are the symptoms?

The symptoms of acute pericarditis develop over a few hours and last for about 7 days. They include:
■ Pain in the centre of the chest, which worsens when taking a deep breath and is relieved by sitting forwards.

■ Pain in the neck and shoulders.
■ Fever.

In chronic constrictive pericarditis or when excess fluid builds up in the pericardium, the heart may be unable to fill with blood and pump it around the body effectively. Poor circulation may then lead to further symptoms that develop over a few months, such as breathlessness and swelling of the ankles and abdomen. An irregular heartbeat may also develop (*see* **Atrial fibrillation**, p.250).

What might be done?

Pericarditis requires assessment and treatment in hospital. The doctor will probably arrange for you to have a chest X-ray (p.300) and an ECG (p.243) to monitor the heart's electrical activity. Echocardiography (p.255) may be carried out to image the interior of the heart. This technique allows the thickness of the pericardium to be measured and can detect fluid around the heart. Blood tests can check for infection or autoimmune disease. You will probably be given nonsteroidal anti-inflammatory drugs (p.578) to relieve chest pain and to help reduce the inflammation.

When pericarditis is caused by a viral infection, the infection should clear up within a week without further treatment. In other cases, the treatment is directed at the underlying cause. For example, antibiotics (p.572) may be prescribed for bacterial infections, corticosteroids (p.600) for autoimmune disorders, and antituberculous drugs (p.573) to treat tuberculosis infection.

Fluid in a pericardial effusion may be withdrawn through a needle passed through the chest wall. If the effusion recurs, a piece of pericardium may be removed surgically, allowing the fluid to drain continuously. In chronic constrictive pericarditis, surgery may be needed to remove most of the pericardium and allow the heart to fill and pump freely.

What is the prognosis?

Most people who have viral pericarditis recover within a week, but about 1 in 10 has a recurrence in the first few months afterwards. Pericarditis may recur if it is due to an autoimmune disorder. Surgery for chronic constrictive pericarditis is successful in only a minority of cases.

Rheumatic fever

Inflammation of the heart, joints, and skin following bacterial infection

 Most common in people aged 5–15, but effects often not seen until adulthood

 Overcrowded living conditions and inadequate nutrition are risk factors

 Gender and genetics are not significant factors

Fifty years ago, rheumatic fever was a major childhood illness in Europe and North America that left thousands of people with damaged heart valves. The effects of the damage are now being seen in elderly people as heart valve disorders, most commonly as mitral stenosis (p.255). Rheumatic fever is now rare in developed countries, mainly due to the use of antibiotics (p.572) and to improved standards of living. In the UK, it is estimated that the incidence of rheumatic fever is less than 1 case per 100,000 people per year. However, the disease still affects many people in developing countries.

Rheumatic fever develops after an infection, usually of the throat, caused by streptococcal bacteria. The condition is caused by the immune system attacking the body's tissues in response to the infection.

What are the symptoms?

Rheumatic fever develops 1–4 weeks after the sore throat has cleared up. Symptoms may include:
■ High fever.
■ Aching and swelling of larger joints, such as the knees, elbows, and ankles.
■ Characteristic blotchy pink rash on the trunk and limbs.

If the heart muscle is affected, there may be shortness of breath and chest pain for a few weeks until the inflammation settles. Inflammation of a heart valve causes permanent damage that may lead to thickening and scarring of the valve years later. Valve damage causes symptoms such as excessive tiredness.

What might be done?

If rheumatic fever is suspected, a swab is taken from the throat and a blood test carried out to look for streptococcal infection. A chest X-ray (p.300) may be taken to look at the size of the heart to see if it is inflamed. An ECG (p.243) may be performed to monitor electrical activity in the heart and echocardiography (p.255) to image the interior of the heart and the valves.

Rheumatic fever is treated with antibiotics to clear up the infection and complete bed rest for about 2 weeks. Nonsteroidal anti-inflammatory drugs (p.578) may be used to reduce fever and joint inflammation, and corticosteroids (p.600) may be prescribed to reduce inflammation of the heart. Low-dose antibiotics often need to be taken for up to 5 years to avoid recurrence.

About 1 in 100 people dies during an initial attack of rheumatic fever. The risk of a recurrence is highest in the first 3 years after the initial infection in young adults and people with damaged heart valves. After 10 years, 2 in 3 people have a detectable heart valve disorder.

Peripheral vascular disorders

The peripheral blood vessels carry blood from the heart to the rest of the body and back to the heart, providing oxygen and nutrients to all parts of the body. If the blood vessels are diseased, oxygen supply to the tissues is reduced, leading to possible tissue damage and even tissue death. Many peripheral vascular disorders are more common in people who smoke and have an unhealthy diet.

All of the blood vessels that carry blood around the body, apart from those in the heart and the brain, are known collectively as the peripheral vascular system. The peripheral vascular system consists of arteries, which carry blood away from the heart, and veins, which carry blood towards the heart.

This section begins by discussing aortic aneurysm, which is a potentially life-threatening disorder of the largest artery in the body. The second article examines thrombosis and embolism, in which a peripheral artery or vein becomes blocked. The most common cause of these disorders is a build-up of fatty deposits on the artery walls, which is a factor that also contributes to the development of diabetic vascular disease. All of these disorders reduce blood supply to the tissues, leading to conditions such as lower limb ischaemia and gangrene. Disorders that affect the small blood vessels in the hands and feet are then considered.

The section ends with a discussion of disorders of the peripheral veins. The veins may be blocked by a blood clot, as occurs in deep vein thrombosis and superficial thrombophlebitis, or may develop structural abnormalities, as occurs in varicose veins.

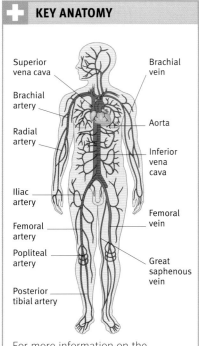

KEY ANATOMY

Superior vena cava

Brachial vein

Brachial artery

Radial artery

Aorta

Inferior vena cava

Iliac artery

Femoral vein

Femoral artery

Popliteal artery

Great saphenous vein

Posterior tibial artery

For more information on the structure and function of arteries and veins, *see* pp.235–236.

Aortic aneurysm

Enlargement of a section of the aorta due to weakness in the artery wall

 More common over the age of 65

 More common in males

 Sometimes runs in families

 Smoking, an unhealthy diet, lack of exercise, and excess weight are risk factors

If a section of an artery wall becomes weakened, the pressure of blood in the artery may cause it to bulge out. The bulging section of the artery is called an aneurysm. An aneurysm may occur in any artery in the body, but the aorta, the major artery that transports blood away from the heart, is most commonly involved. Three-quarters of all aortic aneurysms occur in the abdominal section of the aorta below the kidneys, and this type of aneurysm tends to run in families. Aortic aneurysms may also develop in the chest. The risk of having an aneurysm increases with age, and the condition most commonly occurs in men over the age of 65.

Small aortic aneurysms do not usually produce symptoms, although large ones may cause localized pain. In some enlarged aneurysms, known as dissecting aneurysms, the inner layer of the arterial wall tears and peels away from the outer layer, allowing blood to collect in the space between the two. The larger an aneurysm is, the more likely it is to rupture, causing internal bleeding that can rapidly prove fatal.

What are the causes?

The cause of most aneurysms is uncertain, but they are often associated with atherosclerosis (p.241), in which fatty deposits build up in the artery walls. The risk of developing atherosclerosis is increased by some lifestyle factors, such as smoking, eating a diet high in refined and processed foods and unhealthy fats, excess weight, and taking little exercise. Aneurysms are also more common in males and people with high blood pressure (*see* **Hypertension**, p.242).

In rare cases, an injury or an inherited weakness in the artery wall leads to the development of an aneurysm. For example, the genetic disorder Marfan's syndrome (p.534) may lead to the formation of multiple aneurysms.

What are the symptoms?

Symptoms vary according to the site and usually develop when an aneurysm enlarges. The symptoms of an abdominal aneurysm may include:
- Pain in the abdomen that may spread to the back and can be relieved temporarily by leaning forwards.
- Pulsating sensation in the abdomen.

An aneurysm in the chest may produce symptoms such as:
- Pain in the chest or in the upper back between the shoulder blades.
- Severe cough and wheezing.
- Difficulty swallowing and hoarseness.

If you have symptoms of this kind, you should seek emergency medical help.

Are there complications?

Sometimes, a blood clot forms at the site of the aneurysm and may obstruct the passage of blood through the aorta. In the case of a dissecting aneurysm, the torn part of the artery wall may block arteries that branch from the aorta close to the aneurysm. In the abdomen, such blockages may result in a reduced blood supply to the intestines or kidneys. If the obstruction occurs in the chest, branches of the aorta leading to the neck or the arms may be affected.

Pressure in the aorta may eventually cause an aneurysm to rupture, allowing blood to leak from the vessel and causing worsening pain. If rupture occurs suddenly, you may have severe pain accompanied by loss of consciousness, a fast pulse, and shock (p.248). Without immediate medical treatment, a ruptured aneurysm is likely to be fatal.

How is it diagnosed?

If there are no symptoms, an aneurysm may be detected during a routine physical examination. An abdominal aortic aneurysm may also be detected during routine screening for the condition, which is offered to all men in their 65th year. Sometimes, an aneurysm is seen on an X-ray of the chest or abdomen carried out to check for another disorder. Ultrasound scanning (p.135) may be carried out at intervals to measure the diameter of the aorta and see if the aneurysm is enlarging. CT scanning (p.132), MRI (p.133), or, rarely, angiography (*see* **Contrast X-rays**, p.132), may also be performed to image the aorta.

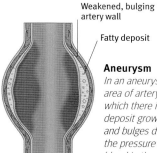

Weakened, bulging artery wall

Fatty deposit

Aneurysm
In an aneurysm, an area of artery wall in which there is a fatty deposit grows weak and bulges due to the pressure of blood in the vessel.

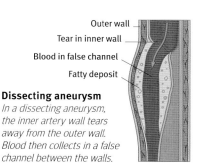

Outer wall

Tear in inner wall

Blood in false channel

Fatty deposit

Dissecting aneurysm
In a dissecting aneurysm, the inner artery wall tears away from the outer wall. Blood then collects in a false channel between the walls.

What is the treatment?

An aneurysm may be treated by surgery, the aim of which is to repair the artery before the aneurysm dissects or ruptures. Your doctor will consider your age and general state of health, as well as the size and site of the aneurysm, when deciding whether surgery is necessary. Surgery for larger aneurysms involves removing the weakened area of arterial wall and replacing it with a graft of synthetic material. To prevent complications from developing while you are waiting for surgery, you may be given beta-blockers (p.581) or other antihypertensive drugs (p.580) to lower blood pressure in the artery. For a dissecting or ruptured aneurysm, you may need to have emergency surgery.

In some cases, an aneurysm may be treated by implanting a large stent (tube) covered with an impermeable lining across the aneurysm, a procedure called an EVAR (endovascular aortic repair). The stent is inserted via a small incision in the femoral artery (the main artery in the leg) and passed up inside the artery to the area of the aneurysm, where it is fixed in place.

If you are a smoker, you should give up immediately and completely. For anyone who has already had an aneurysm, a healthy diet (p.16) and regular exercise will help to slow the progress of atherosclerosis and thus reduce the risk of further aneurysms.

What is the prognosis?

Surgery or EVAR offers a good chance of recovery provided the aneurysm has not yet dissected or ruptured. If the aneurysm has dissected or ruptured, between 15 and 50 per cent of people survive, depending on the location of the aneurysm.

Thrombosis and embolism

Obstruction of blood flow in a vessel by a blockage that has formed in that vessel or has travelled from elsewhere in the body

 Rarely, runs in families

 Smoking, an unhealthy diet, lack of exercise, and excess weight are risk factors

 Age and gender as risk factors depend on the cause

Both thrombosis and embolism can be serious and potentially fatal conditions. In thrombosis, a blood clot, known as a

---

▶ **TEST**

Doppler ultrasound scanning

Doppler ultrasound scanning is an imaging technique commonly used to measure the blood flow through a blood vessel in circulatory disorders such as thrombosis and embolism (above). It may also be used to measure blood pressure in the limbs.

The technique produces an image of the blood flow through the vessel so that narrowing and blockages of the vessel can be detected. A routine Doppler ultrasound scan can take up to 20 minutes to perform and is completely painless and safe.

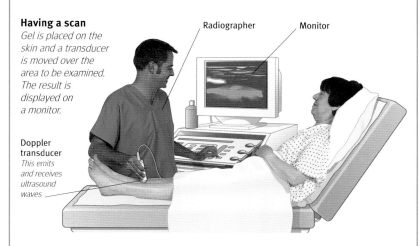

Having a scan
Gel is placed on the skin and a transducer is moved over the area to be examined. The result is displayed on a monitor.

Radiographer

Monitor

Doppler transducer
This emits and receives ultrasound waves

RESULTS

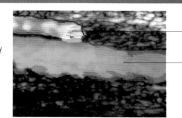

Doppler scan
This ultrasound image shows blood flow through vessels in the leg and confirms a blockage in the artery. Doppler ultrasound scans allow the precise position and severity of a blockage to be determined.

Blocked artery

Healthy vein

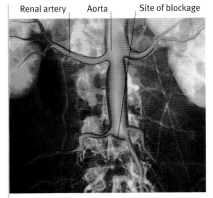

Renal artery Aorta Site of blockage

Arterial thrombosis
This contrast X-ray shows blood flow in the aorta and adjacent arteries. A blood clot in the aorta is blocking the flow of blood below the site of the obstruction.

thrombus, forms in a blood vessel and obstructs the flow of blood. Any blood vessel in the body may become blocked by a thrombus, but thrombosis is more serious in arteries and in deep veins in the legs (*see* **Deep vein thrombosis**, p.263). In embolism, a plug of material called an embolus travels through the bloodstream until it becomes lodged in an artery. Although some emboli consist of substances such as tissue or fat, most are pieces of blood clot that have become detached from a larger clot elsewhere in the body.

If an artery is blocked by either a thrombus or an embolus, and blood cannot reach the tissues beyond the blockage by an alternative route, those tissues are deprived of oxygen. Unlike thrombosis, which often develops gradually, the effects of embolism usually develop immediately and may be severe if the blood vessel becomes completely obstructed. Blockage of the arteries that supply the brain (*see* **Stroke**, p.329), the lungs (*see* **Pulmonary embolism**, p.302), or the heart (*see* **Myocardial infarction**, p.245) often proves fatal.

What are the causes?
Blood flowing through an artery is normally under pressure so that clots are unlikely to form. If the flow of blood slows down, a clot is more likely to develop. Decreased blood flow through an artery may be caused by narrowing of the vessel due to a gradual build-up of fatty deposits in its walls, known as atherosclerosis (p.241). The long-term risk of developing atherosclerosis, and therefore thrombosis, is increased by factors such as smoking and an unhealthy diet.

Thrombosis is more likely to develop if there is an increase in the natural tendency of the blood to clot, a condition known as hypercoagulability (p.275). In rare cases, the condition is inherited. Hypercoagulability may also occur as a result of taking a combined oral contraceptive (*see* **Contraception**, p.28) or hormone replacement therapy (p.605), being pregnant, or having surgery.

Blood clots sometimes form in the heart when the heartbeat is weak and irregular because the upper chambers (atria) are not totally emptied of blood at each beat (*see* **Atrial fibrillation**, p.250). These blood clots may then be released from the atria into the arteries supplying the brain, body, or limbs.

What are the symptoms?
The symptoms caused by thrombosis or embolism vary depending on which blood vessel is blocked. If the blockage affects blood supply to the legs, symptoms may develop within a few hours, and they may be more severe if there is already a reduction in blood supply to this region (*see* **Lower limb ischaemia**, opposite page). Symptoms include:
- Pain in the legs, even at rest.
- Pale, cold feet.

If the arteries supplying the intestines are affected, symptoms may include:
- Severe abdominal pain.
- Vomiting.
- Fever.

Left untreated, the reduction in blood supply may eventually result in tissue death, which may be life-threatening. The affected tissues will change colour over several days, eventually becoming black (*see* **Gangrene**, p.262). If you develop these symptoms, you should seek emergency medical attention.

What might be done?
If your doctor suspects that you have thrombosis or embolism, he or she will have you admitted to hospital immediately. The blood flow through your blood vessels may be measured using pulse volume recording and imaging, such as Doppler ultrasound scanning (p.259). Angiography (*see* **Contrast X-rays**, p.132), sometimes combined with MRI (p.133), may be used to obtain detailed images of the blood vessels and look for obstruction.

Depending on the site and size of the clot, you may be given drugs to dissolve it and prevent further clots from forming (*see* **Drugs that prevent blood clotting**, p.584). Emergency surgery may be necessary to remove the clot or to bypass it using a graft made from synthetic material. Alternatively, the affected artery may be widened by angioplasty, a procedure in which a balloon mounted on the tip of a catheter is passed into the artery and then inflated to widen the obstructed area.

After the thrombosis or embolism has been treated, you may need to continue medication for several months to prevent further blood clots from forming. For example, you may be advised to take a low dose of aspirin daily, and possibly also an antiplatelet drug such as clopidogrel; in some cases, an anticoagulant such as warfarin may be prescribed. If you smoke, you should stop immediately. You should also try to eat a healthy diet (p.16) and exercise regularly. If you are taking a combined oral contraceptive or hormone replacement therapy, you may be advised to stop.

Diabetic vascular disease

Damage to large and small blood vessels throughout the body that can occur in people who have diabetes mellitus

 The underlying condition sometimes runs in families

 Smoking, an unhealthy diet, lack of exercise, and excess weight are risk factors

 Age and gender are not significant factors

Vascular disease is a common long-term complication of diabetes mellitus (p.437), a condition that tends to run in families. There are two types of vascular disease that are more likely to affect people who have diabetes: atherosclerosis (p.241) and small vessel disease.

In atherosclerosis, fatty deposits gradually build up in the walls of larger blood vessels, making these vessels narrower. This condition, which develops to some degree in most people as they become older, is likely to occur earlier and more extensively in people with diabetes.

Diabetic small vessel disease is not fully understood, but it is thought to involve thickening of the walls of the smaller blood vessels as a result of certain chemical changes. This thickening reduces the amount of oxygen passing from blood in the vessels into the surrounding body tissues.

These vascular conditions frequently occur together and each of them may lead to serious complications. The risk of developing either type of diabetic vascular disease is higher the longer a person has had diabetes mellitus. Lifestyle factors such as smoking and an unhealthy diet increase the risk of developing diabetic vascular disease, as does poor control of blood sugar

---

▶ **TEST**

Femoral angiography

Femoral angiography is a contrast X-ray technique, sometimes combined with MRI (p.133), that is used to diagnose narrowing or blockage of arteries in the legs. During the procedure, which is carried out under local anaesthesia, a contrast medium is injected into the femoral artery. The medium spreads in the circulation to other vessels in the leg. X-rays are then taken of one or more sites. The procedure takes about 30 minutes, and you should be able to return home within 6 hours.

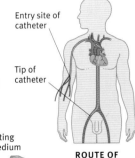

Entry site of catheter

Tip of catheter

ROUTE OF CATHETER

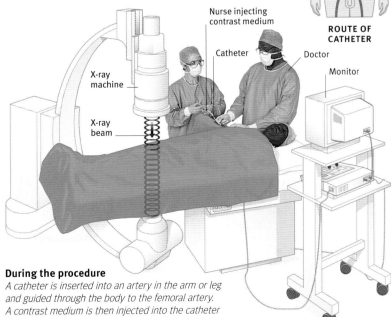

Nurse injecting contrast medium

Catheter

Doctor

Monitor

X-ray machine

X-ray beam

During the procedure
A catheter is inserted into an artery in the arm or leg and guided through the body to the femoral artery. A contrast medium is then injected into the catheter so that the artery can be seen on an X-ray.

RESULTS

Angiogram of the leg
This contrast X-ray shows a blockage in the main artery in the leg, restricting blood flow to the tissues of the lower leg. If this blockage is not treated, the tissues will be permanently damaged.

Blockage in artery   Bone

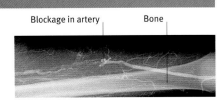

levels, and it is therefore important that your diabetes is managed effectively (*see* **Living with diabetes**, p.438).

Are there complications?

Atherosclerosis may eventually lead to blockage of the arteries, causing potentially life-threatening complications, in particular stroke (p.329), heart attack (*see* **Myocardial infarction**, p.245), and lower limb ischaemia (right).

Damage to small blood vessels may occur in many parts of the body. Small blood vessels in the eyes are commonly damaged (*see* **Diabetic retinopathy**, p.361), leading to blurred vision and sometimes even blindness. If the small vessels in the eyes are damaged, similar changes will have occurred in vessels throughout the body. If the blood vessels in the kidneys are affected, kidney function will be impaired (*see* **Diabetic kidney disease**, p.450). Kidney damage often leads to high blood pressure (*see* **Hypertension**, p.242).

Small vessel disease may also lead to nerve damage, most commonly in the feet (*see* **Diabetic neuropathy**, p.336). Such damage can reduce sensation in the affected area so that an injury goes unnoticed at first. In addition, the reduced supply of blood slows healing, and persistent skin ulcers (*see* **Leg ulcers**, p.203) and even gangrene (p.262) may develop. Some people already have these complications when they are first diagnosed as having diabetes mellitus. In other cases, complications may not develop for many years after diagnosis.

What might be done?

It is essential that diabetes mellitus is diagnosed promptly and managed well. In order to prevent or reduce the effects of diabetic vascular disease on blood vessels, you should try to maintain effective control of your blood sugar levels (*see* **Monitoring your blood glucose**, p.439), follow a healthy diet (p.16), and avoid smoking. If you have diabetes, your doctor will regularly measure your blood pressure (*see* **Blood pressure measurement**, p.242) and the level of cholesterol in your blood to assess your susceptibility to atherosclerosis. Samples of your urine may be tested for protein, the presence of which may be the first sign of kidney disease, and blood tests may be performed to find out if your kidneys are functioning normally. In addition, regular eye checks, using ophthalmoscopy (p.360) and sometimes retinal photography, are carried out to ensure that retinal

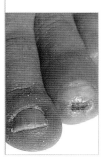

Ulcerated toe
If diabetic vascular disease affects the arteries in the leg, the tissues of the feet may become deprived of oxygen, eventually leading to the formation of a skin ulcer.

damage is detected as early as possible since early detection increases the chances of successful treatment.

If you have a high blood cholesterol level, your doctor may prescribe drugs to prevent atherosclerosis from worsening (*see* **Lipid-lowering drugs**, p.603). If protein is found in your urine, you may be prescribed ACE inhibitor drugs (p.582), which help to counteract the progression of small vessel damage in the kidneys. Treatment for high blood pressure will be given if necessary (*see* **Antihypertensive drugs**, p.580).

What is the prognosis?

Diabetic vascular disease is the most common cause of death in people who have diabetes mellitus, and the risk of developing it increases with time.

A person with diabetes is about 10 times more likely to develop lower limb ischaemia than someone without diabetes, four times more likely to have a heart attack, and twice as likely to have a stroke. Damage to small blood vessels in the eyes occurs in about 8 in 10 people with long-term diabetes. However, eye damage is often reversible if it is treated in the early stages. Kidney damage occurs in about 4 in 10 people who have had diabetes mellitus for longer than 15 years. About 3 in 10 people with diabetes develop nerve damage, but only 1 in 10 has severe symptoms.

If your diabetes mellitus is carefully managed and your blood pressure, cholesterol, and blood sugar levels are well controlled, the progress of diabetic vascular disease will be slowed and the risk of complications will be reduced.

▶ **TREATMENT**

Femoral artery bypass graft

This procedure is used to treat blocked or narrowed arteries in the leg, which can cause lower limb ischaemia (below). During the operation, the blocked artery is bypassed using a section of vein from the same leg or, less commonly, an artificial graft. The blocked artery is left in place, but, because blood can flow freely through the bypass, the blood supply to the limb is restored. The cut ends of the vein used for the graft are tied and remain in place, and blood is diverted up other veins in the leg. The operation is performed in hospital under general anaesthesia.

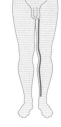

SITE OF INCISION

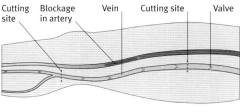

Cutting site | Blockage in artery | Vein | Cutting site | Valve

Before surgery
An obstruction in an artery in the leg prevents blood from reaching the lower leg. A small section of a vein from the same leg can be used to create a bypass around this blockage.

Tied vein | Vein bypass | Blockage | Reversed valve

After surgery
A length of vein has been removed and attached above and below the blockage, forming a bypass channel. The vein is reversed so that its valves allow arterial blood flow.

Lower limb ischaemia

A reduced oxygen supply to the tissues of the legs as a result of a poor blood supply

 More common over the age of 40

 More common in males

 Sometimes runs in families

 Smoking, an unhealthy diet, lack of exercise, and excess weight are risk factors

If blood flow to the legs is reduced, the leg tissues may become deprived of oxygen, which may led to a cramp-like pain on exertion (called claudication). Reduced blood flow is usually due to atherosclerosis (p.241), a build-up of fatty deposits in artery walls, whose effects are often most noticeable on the lower limbs. People who have an inherited tendency towards high cholesterol levels (*see* Inherited hyperlipidaemias, p.440) are more likely to develop atherosclerosis, as are those who have had diabetes mellitus (p.437) for a long time. An unhealthy diet and smoking also increase the risk. About 9 in 10 people with lower limb ischaemia smoke.

What are the symptoms?

The symptoms of lower limb ischaemia usually develop gradually over months or years. Symptoms may affect one leg more than the other. In the initial stages of the condition, blood flow to the legs may be adequate to supply the tissues when at rest but not on

exertion. The main symptom is a cramp-like pain in the legs (known as claudication) with the following features:

- Affects one or both calves when walking and may be severe.
- Consistently appears after walking a particular distance.
- Comes on sooner when walking uphill or in cold temperatures.
- Is relieved by rest and usually disappears after several minutes.

As the disease progresses, the distance a person is able to walk before experiencing pain gradually decreases, so that eventually pain may be present at rest. Additional symptoms of lower limb ischaemia may then include:

- Pale, cold feet.
- Persistent leg or foot ulcers.

If a blockage occurs in blood vessels in the pelvic region, blood flow is reduced to the whole of the lower body, and as a result there may be pain in the buttocks and, in men, erectile dysfunction. If the blood vessel suddenly becomes completely blocked by a clot (*see* **Thrombosis and embolism**, p.259), the symptoms may worsen rapidly. Without immediate treatment, death of tissues in the feet and legs may occur (*see* **Gangrene**, p.262).

What might be done?

Your doctor may suspect that you have lower limb ischaemia from your symptoms and by examining the strength of the pulses in your legs. He or she may arrange for tests such as pulse volume recording and Doppler ultrasound scanning (p.259) to measure the blood flow in your legs and angiography (*see* **Femoral angiography**, opposite page), which produces detailed images of the vessels, to look for atherosclerosis.

Treatment is aimed at increasing the blood flow to the tissues in the legs. Affected arteries may be widened using a technique known as angioplasty, in which a balloon on the tip of a catheter is passed into the artery and inflated. Sometimes, a stent (rigid tube) may then be inserted into the artery to help keep it open. In some cases, surgery is carried out to bypass affected arteries (*see* **Femoral artery bypass graft**, above).

Taking a low dose of aspirin daily may help to prevent blood clots from developing. If a clot has formed, you may be given drugs to dissolve it and to prevent more clots from forming (*see* **Drugs that prevent blood clotting**, p.584). In some cases, the clot needs to be removed surgically or by using a special catheter. If gangrene has developed, amputation of part or all of the affected limb may be necessary.

If you smoke, it is vital that you stop immediately. The nicotine in cigarettes causes blood vessels to constrict, further reducing blood supply to the legs. Even one cigarette can produce a constricting effect that lasts for several hours, and you need to give up smoking completely to improve the outlook once lower limb ischaemia is diagnosed. If you continue to smoke, the disease is likely to progress, and surgery may be required.

In addition, you should follow a healthy diet (p.16) and try to walk for longer periods each day to build up the amount of exercise you can do without feeling pain (*see* **Taking regular exercise**, p.21). Adopting these measures may enable you to prevent the condition from worsening.

Gangrene

Tissue death as a result of an inadequate blood supply or infection of a wound

 Smoking, an unhealthy diet, lack of exercise, and excess weight are risk factors

 Age, gender, and genetics as risk factors depend on the cause

Gangrene involves death of the tissues in a particular area of the body, most commonly the legs and feet, and is a potentially life-threatening condition.

There are two types of gangrene: dry and wet. Dry gangrene occurs when the tissues become deprived of oxygen as a result of a reduced blood supply. Tissue death is localized and does not spread from the affected site. Wet gangrene is less common and occurs when tissue that has been damaged by a wound or by dry gangrene becomes infected with bacteria. Infection is often due to clostridia, which are bacteria that thrive in dead tissues where there is no oxygen and produce a foul-smelling gas. The infection may spread to surrounding healthy tissues and can be fatal.

The reduction in blood supply that leads to gangrene is most often due to a blood clot forming in an artery (*see* **Thrombosis and embolism**, p.259), which may already be narrowed by the accumulation of fatty deposits on vessel walls, known as atherosclerosis (p.241). The tissues in the legs and feet are most commonly affected by these underlying conditions (*see* **Lower limb ischaemia**, p.261). The risk of an artery becoming blocked is increased by certain lifestyle factors, such as smoking and an unhealthy diet. People with diabetes mellitus (p.437) are more likely to develop gangrene as a result of progressive damage to the small blood vessels (*see* **Diabetic vascular disease**, p.260). Frostbite (p.186) may also lead to the development of gangrene.

What are the symptoms?
The symptoms of dry gangrene may develop gradually or may appear over a few hours, depending on how quickly the blood supply is reduced. If the legs are affected, symptoms include:
■ Pain in the leg and foot.
■ Pale, cold skin, which becomes red and hot before turning purple and eventually black over several days.
If the gangrene is due to an infection, additional symptoms may be present, including pus around the affected area and fever. Infection may spread to the bloodstream (*see* **Septicaemia**, p.171).

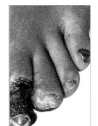

Gangrene
An inadequate supply of blood to the feet may lead to tissue death, also known as gangrene, which causes the toes to turn black. Left untreated, the dead tissue may become infected.

What might be done?
Your doctor will probably be able to diagnose gangrene from its appearance. He or she may arrange for you to have pulse volume recording or Doppler ultrasound scanning (p.259) to measure blood flow in the limb. You may require contrast X-rays (p.132), sometimes combined with MRI (p.133) or CT scanning (p.132), to look for a blocked artery.

If you have gangrene, you will be admitted to hospital without delay. Intravenous antibiotics (p.572) will be given to prevent or treat infection and, if possible, the blood supply to the gangrenous tissue will be restored. If an artery is obstructed, the vessel may be widened using angioplasty, in which a balloon on the tip of a catheter is passed into the narrowed area and then inflated. Alternatively, surgery may be carried out to remove or bypass the blockage (*see* **Femoral artery bypass graft**, p.261). The gangrenous tissue will be removed, and, if it has become infected, some of the living tissue around the gangrenous area will also be removed to prevent the infection from spreading. In some cases, amputation of a limb is necessary. If you develop wet gangrene, you may be placed in a chamber containing high-pressure oxygen to help destroy the bacteria.

The earlier gangrene is diagnosed, the better the outlook, because blood supply to the affected tissues is more likely to be restored. A good blood supply promotes tissue healing after surgery. Gangrene is fatal in about 1 in 5 people, usually because of infection in the bloodstream.

Buerger's disease

Severe inflammation of the small arteries that is triggered by smoking

 Most common between the ages of 20 and 40

 Three times more common in males

 Sometimes runs in families; more common in Asians and Eastern Europeans

 Smoking is a risk factor; exposure to cold aggravates symptoms

Buerger's disease is a rare condition that most frequently affects men who smoke. The condition tends to run in families and is more common in people of Asian or Eastern European descent. The cause is not fully understood, but it is thought that, in people genetically susceptible to the disease, smoking triggers an autoimmune response,

in which the immune system produces antibodies that attack the body's own tissues. The arteries in the legs and sometimes those in the arms become inflamed, reducing blood supply to the tissues.

What are the symptoms?
The initial symptoms of Buerger's disease are often intermittent and include:
■ Pale hands or feet, particularly after exposure to the cold.
■ Pain in the hands or feet, which may be severe at night and after exercise.
■ Numbness, tingling, or a sensation of burning in the fingers or toes.
With time, these symptoms usually become more severe and skin ulcers or gangrene (left) may develop on the tips of the toes or fingers.

What might be done?
If you have the symptoms listed above, your doctor will take your pulse to check if it is weak or absent. If this is so, he or she may suspect Buerger's disease and arrange for Doppler ultrasound scanning (p.259) and angiography (*see* **Contrast X-rays**, p.132) to assess blood flow in the small arteries in the hands or feet.

There is no cure for Buerger's disease, and the aim of treatment is to prevent progression of the condition and control any symptoms. If you are diagnosed with Buerger's disease, the single most important action you can take to improve the outlook is to stop smoking. In people who continue to smoke, the disease is likely to progress so that amputation of the affected limb may eventually become necessary. If you get any infection of the skin of your hands, it should be treated promptly. Your doctor may also recommend painkillers to control pain in the hands or feet.

Raynaud's phenomenon and Raynaud's disease

Sudden, intermittent narrowing of the arteries in the hands or, rarely, the feet

 More common in females

 Sometimes runs in families

 Smoking and exposure to cold trigger attacks

 Age as a risk factor depends on the cause

During an attack of Raynaud's phenomenon, the arteries in the hands or feet become narrowed as a result of muscle spasm in the artery walls. This narrowing restricts blood supply to the fingers or toes, causing them to become pale. Numbness or tingling may also develop in the affected fingers or toes.

In about half of all people with Raynaud's phenomenon, the condition is the result of an underlying disorder, particularly the autoimmune disorders scleroderma (p.281),

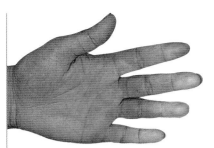

Raynaud's phenomenon
An attack of Raynaud's phenomenon in the hand restricts the blood supply to the tips of the fingers, turning them white.

rheumatoid arthritis (p.222), or Buerger's disease (left), all of which can run in families. In some people with Raynaud's phenomenon, the condition is linked with hand–arm vibration syndrome (opposite page). Certain drugs, such as beta-blockers (p.581), are known to produce the symptoms of Raynaud's phenomenon as a side effect.

If there is no apparent cause for the condition, it is known as Raynaud's disease. This disorder is most common in women aged between 15 and 45 and is usually mild. Episodes are triggered by smoking because the nicotine in cigarettes constricts the arteries. Exposure to cold and handling frozen items can also trigger an attack.

What are the symptoms?
The symptoms of Raynaud's phenomenon and Raynaud's disease affect the hands or feet, last from a few minutes to a few hours, and include:
■ Numbness and tingling in the fingers or toes that may worsen and progress to a painful burning sensation.
■ Progressive change of colour in the fingers or toes, which initially turn pale, then blue, and later red again as blood returns to the tissues.
There may be a marked colour difference between the affected area and the surrounding tissues. In severe cases, skin ulcers or gangrene (left) may form on the tips of the fingers or toes.

What might be done?
Your doctor will carry out tests to look for an underlying cause of your symptoms. For example, blood tests may be performed to look for evidence of an autoimmune disorder.

Immunosuppressant drugs (p.585) may be prescribed to treat an autoimmune disorder. Your doctor may also recommend that you take drugs that dilate the blood vessels during an attack (*see* **Calcium channel blocker drugs**, p.582). If you smoke, you should stop immediately. Wearing thermal gloves and socks in cold weather helps to avoid the onset of symptoms. If symptoms are severe, surgery may be needed to cut the nerves that control arterial constriction.

Hand–arm vibration syndrome

Painful, pale fingers associated with the use of vibrating tools

 More common in males

 Affects people who use vibrating machinery; smoking and exposure to cold aggravate symptoms

 Age and genetics are not significant factors

Hand–arm vibration syndrome, formerly known as vibration white finger, causes pain and numbness in parts of the body that are repeatedly exposed to intense vibration from machinery. As the name of the condition implies, the hands, arms, and in particular the fingers are most commonly affected. Prolonged exposure to vibration from the use of mechanical tools causes localized constriction of the small blood vessels and nerve damage. Smoking and exposure to cold, which also constrict the small blood vessels, may trigger or aggravate the symptoms of hand–arm vibration syndrome.

About 3 in 100 people in employment, most of them men, are exposed to machine vibration that may lead to hand–arm vibration syndrome. In the past, the mining and engineering industries were responsible for the majority of cases. The use of chainsaws in the forestry industry s another common cause.

What are the symptoms?

The symptoms of hand–arm vibration syndrome do not appear immediately after exposure to vibration but tend to develop slowly over several years of exposure. Symptoms are often more severe in one hand than the other and may include:
■ Pain, numbness, and tingling in the fingers, hands, or arms.
■ Pale or blue fingers.
■ Difficulty manipulating small objects, such as picking up coins, buttoning clothes, or tying shoelaces.
At first, the symptoms of the syndrome tend to occur intermittently, but they become more frequent and persistent as the condition progresses.

What might be done?

If you have the symptoms described above and you have been working with vibrating machinery, your doctor may suspect hand–arm vibration syndrome. Once the disorder has been diagnosed, you should avoid exposure to vibration. Your doctor may advise you to change jobs. You should also avoid anything that makes the symptoms worse, such as smoking and exposure to cold. There is no specific treatment, but, if you have severe symptoms, your doctor may prescribe calcium channel blocker drugs (p.582), which dilate the blood vessels.

If you use vibrating machinery, make sure that it is in good working order and that you know how to operate it correctly and safely.

In addition, you should always wear approved protective gloves. If you manage to avoid further exposure to vibrating machinery, the symptoms of hand–arm vibration syndrome may improve. However, once persistent numbness has developed, the condition is usually irreversible.

Deep vein thrombosis

Formation of a blood clot within a deep-lying vein

 More common over the age of 40

 Slightly more common in females

 Sometimes runs in families

 Prolonged immobility and excess weight are risk factors

Deep vein thrombosis is a condition in which a blood clot forms in a large vein in a muscle, usually in the leg or pelvic region. It affects an estimated 1 in 1,000 people in the UK each year, many of them over 40.

The formation of a clot in a deep vein is usually not dangerous in itself. However, there is a risk that a fragment of the clot may break off and travel through the heart in the circulation. If the fragment lodges in a vessel supplying the lungs, a potentially fatal blockage called a pulmonary embolism (p.302) occurs.

What are the causes?

Deep vein thrombosis is usually caused by a combination of slow blood flow through a vein, an increase in the natural tendency of the blood to clot, and damage to the wall of the vein.

Several factors may slow blood flow and thus increase the risk of deep vein thrombosis. Long periods of immobility, such as those experienced during long flights or car journeys or while bedridden, especially during an illness or after surgery, are a common cause of slow blood flow. Other causes include compression of a vein by the fetus during pregnancy or by a tumour. Leg injury may also slow blood flow and cause a clot to form in the deep veins of the leg.

The blood may clot more easily as a result of an injury, surgery, pregnancy, or taking a combined oral contraceptive (*see* **Contraception**, p.28) or hormone replacement therapy (p.605). Some people have an inherited tendency for the blood to clot too readily (*see* **Hypercoagulability**, p.275).

What are the symptoms?

If a blood clot has formed in a deep-lying vein, it may produce symptoms that include the following:
■ Pain or tenderness in the leg.
■ Swelling of the lower leg or thigh.
■ Enlarged veins beneath the skin.
Pulmonary embolism occurs in a small proportion of cases of deep vein thrombosis. The symptoms that occur with pulmonary

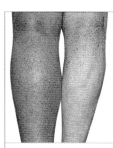

Deep vein thrombosis
The leg on the left is visibly swollen and red compared to the leg on the right, indicating that a blood clot has formed in a deep vein within the leg muscle.

embolism usually include shortness of breath and chest pain that is made worse with breathing. If a large proportion of the blood supply to the lungs is blocked, the condition is potentially life-threatening.

In some cases, thrombosis causes permanent damage to the vein and varicose veins (right) may appear later.

What might be done?

Your doctor may need to carry out various tests urgently to confirm the diagnosis of deep vein thrombosis because the symptoms are often similar to those of other conditions, such as cellulitis (p.204). You may have Doppler ultrasound scanning (p.259) to measure blood flow through the veins and sometimes a venogram, in which dye is injected into a vein and then X-rays are taken to reveal blood clots (*see* **Contrast X-rays**, p.132). MRI (p.133) may also be used. A sample of your blood may be taken and analysed to assess how easily it clots.

Thrombolytic drugs (p.584) may be prescribed to dissolve the blood clot in the vein and reduce the risk of a pulmonary embolism. You may also be given injections of anticoagulants to prevent further clots. Although treatment can take place in hospital, you may be able to administer anticoagulant drugs yourself at home. Rarely, surgery is required to remove the clot.

After you have had the initial treatment, your doctor will prescribe drugs to reduce the risk that the condition will recur (*see* **Drugs that prevent blood clotting**, p.584).

Can it be prevented?

Certain surgical procedures carry a risk of deep vein thrombosis, and your susceptibility to developing the condition will be assessed beforehand. If there is a high risk, low doses of short-acting anticoagulant drugs will probably be given before and after surgery to prevent the blood from clotting. Your doctor may also advise you to wear special elastic stockings for a few days after the operation to help maintain blood flow in the veins of the leg. Women who use a combined oral contraceptive or hormone replacement therapy may be advised to stop for a period of around 4 weeks before surgery.

The risk of deep vein thrombosis can be reduced by avoiding long periods of inactivity. If you are confined to bed, you should regularly stretch your legs and flex your ankles. Your doctor may also recommend that you wear compression stockings. During a flight, walk around at least once an

hour, and, during a long drive, stop regularly to stretch your legs. It is also important to keep well hydrated.

What is the prognosis?

Usually, if deep vein thrombosis is diagnosed in its early stages, treatment with thrombolytic drugs and anticoagulants is successful. However, if the affected vein is permanently damaged, persistent swelling of the leg or varicose veins may develop and there is a risk that deep vein thrombosis may recur.

Varicose veins

Visibly swollen and distorted veins that lie just beneath the skin, mainly in the legs

 Rare before the age of 20; more common in elderly people

 More common in females

 Often runs in families

 Pregnancy, excess weight, and prolonged standing are risk factors

Varicose veins affect about 3 in 10 adults and are more common with increasing age. Although the condition may cause discomfort and appear unsightly, it is not usually harmful to health.

Varicose veins mainly affect the legs. Normally, blood in the legs collects in the superficial veins just below the skin. These veins empty the blood into deep-lying veins through small perforating veins. The deep-lying veins carry blood back towards the heart. Contraction of the leg muscles helps to pump the blood in the veins upwards to the heart, even when you are standing, and the veins have one-way valves to stop blood from flowing backwards into the legs. If the valves in the perforating vein do not close adequately, the blood flows back into the superficial veins. The pressure of returning blood eventually causes these veins to become swollen and distorted, and they are then known as varicose veins. If left untreated, the condition often worsens.

Varicose veins can develop in other parts of the body as a complication of chronic liver disease, which raises blood pressure in the portal veins in the abdomen (*see* **Portal hypertension and varices**, p.410). The rise in blood pressure may cause veins to become swollen at the lower end of the oesophagus, and, in some cases, around the rectum (*see* **Haemorrhoids**, p.422).

What are the causes?

Varicose veins may be associated with an inherited weakness of the valves in the veins. The female hormone progesterone, which causes the veins to dilate, may encourage the formation of varicose veins, and the condition is therefore more common in women, especially during pregnancy (see **Common complaints of normal pregnancy**, p.506). In addition, increased pressure is placed on the veins in the pelvic region during pregnancy as the uterus gradually grows larger. Other factors that increase the risk of developing varicose veins include being overweight and having an occupation that involves standing for long periods with little walking.

Sometimes, varicose veins are caused by a blood clot blocking a deep vein (see **Deep vein thrombosis**, p.263).

What are the symptoms?

If you develop varicose veins in the legs, you may have the following symptoms:

- Easily visible, blue, swollen, distorted veins that bulge beneath the skin and are more prominent when standing.
- Aching or pain in the affected leg, especially after prolonged standing.

In severe cases, the skin over a varicose vein, usually in the ankle area, becomes thin, dry, and itchy. Eventually, ulceration may occur (see **Leg ulcer**, p.203).

How are they diagnosed?

Your doctor will examine the affected area while you are standing, when the veins are usually more prominent and easily

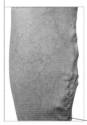

Varicose veins
Abnormal backflow of blood into the superficial veins that lie just beneath the surface of the skin has caused these veins to become swollen and distorted.

Varicose vein

Coping with varicose veins

If you have troublesome symptoms caused by varicose veins, the following measures may help:

- Avoid prolonged standing.
- Take regular walks to exercise the leg muscles and keep blood flowing in the legs.
- Keep your legs elevated when sitting, if possible.
- If your doctor has recommended that you wear compression stockings, put them on before you get out of bed in the morning while your legs are still elevated.
- Avoid wearing any clothing that may restrict the flow of blood at the top of the legs.
- If you are overweight, you should try to lose weight.

visible. You may have Doppler ultrasound scanning (p.259) to assess the direction of blood flow in the veins of the leg. If the veins are varicose, the blood will appear to flow backwards.

What is the treatment?

In the majority of cases, varicose veins do not require medical treatment, and you may be able to relieve discomfort using self-help measures (see **Coping with varicose veins**, above).

Treatment is usually carried out only if the veins become painful or especially unsightly or if the skin over an affected vein becomes ulcerated. There are several different ways of treating varicose veins, including dividing the perforating veins that connect superficial veins to deep

ones; removing the varicose veins entirely; or sealing off the varicose veins. (see **Treating varicose veins**, below). Some techniques may be more suitable than others in your particular case, so it is advisable to discuss the options with your doctor. However, even after treatment, varicose veins may recur and treatment may need to be repeated.

Superficial thrombophlebitis

Inflammation of a superficial vein (a vein just beneath the surface of the skin) that may cause a blood clot to form

	More common over the age of 20
	More common in females
	Sometimes runs in families
	Intravenous drug abuse is a risk factor

In superficial thrombophlebitis, a blood clot develops in an inflamed superficial vein. The condition is rarely serious, but it may be painful. Thrombophlebitis can affect any superficial vein but usually occurs in varicose veins (p.263) in the leg. Superficial thrombophlebitis tends to run in families and is more common in adult women.

Inflammation leading to clot formation may result from damage to a vein, which may be sustained during intravenous drug injection or surgery. The develop-

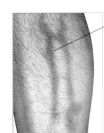

Inflamed vein

Superficial thrombophlebitis
The skin overlying the affected vein is red and inflamed. The outline of the swollen vein can be seen beneath the surface of the skin.

ment of blood clots in superficial veins is more common in people who have cancer. In some cases, superficial thrombophlebitis is associated with an increase in the tendency of blood to clot (see **Hypercoagulability**, p.275). For example, blood may clot more easily in women who are pregnant or who take a combined oral contraceptive (see **Contraception**, p.28). or hormone replacement therapy (p.605). In most cases, however, the cause is unclear.

What are the symptoms?

The symptoms associated with superficial thrombophlebitis usually develop over 24–48 hours and include:

- Redness of the skin overlying a vein.
- A painful, tender, swollen vein that may feel hard like a cord.
- Mild fever.

Inflammation is usually localized in the area of the blood clot and may spread to the overlying skin. However, in rare cases, thrombophlebitis extends into a deep-lying vein, usually in the leg, leading to deep vein thrombosis (p.263).

What might be done?

Your doctor will probably be able to diagnose superficial thrombophlebitis from your symptoms and the appearance of the vein and the overlying skin.

Most cases improve in a few days without treatment. You may be able to relieve pain by taking a painkiller, such as ibuprofen (see **Nonsteroidal anti-inflammatory drugs**, p.578), and by keeping the area rested and raised. Warm, moist compresses can also ease discomfort. If the condition is due to hypercoagulability or has resulted in a deep vein thrombosis, your doctor may recommend that you take drugs that prevent blood clotting (p.584). Superficial thrombophlebitis is likely to recur in susceptible people.

▶ **TREATMENT**

Treating varicose veins

There are various methods of treating varicose veins, including injection therapy, conventional surgery, laser therapy (using a laser to seal off the varicose veins), and radiofrequency ablation (sealing the varicose veins using radiofrequency alternating electric current). Injection therapy is mainly used to treat small varicose veins below the knee, and surgery is performed to treat larger veins. Surgery may be used to divide faulty perforating veins responsible for the formation of the varicose veins or to remove an entire varicose vein.

Division of perforating veins

Blood normally flows from the superficial veins into the deep veins along perforating veins. If the valves in the perforating veins are not working properly, there is a backflow of blood into the superficial veins, which leads to the formation of varicose veins. During the surgical division of faulty perforating veins, these veins are tied off and cut. Surgery is usually performed in hospital under general anaesthesia.

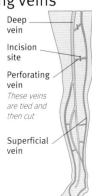

Deep vein

Incision site

Perforating vein
These veins are tied and then cut

Superficial vein

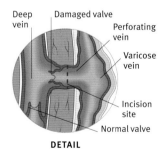

Deep vein

Damaged valve

Perforating vein

Varicose vein

Incision site

Normal valve

DETAIL

During the procedure
Small incisions are made in the leg, usually in the groin, behind the knee, and sometimes also in the lower leg. The perforating veins are then tied and cut.

Injection therapy

Injection therapy may be used to treat small varicose veins below the knee. The procedure uses a mild irritant to make the walls of the varicose veins stick together and stop blood from entering them. For a week after the procedure, an elastic bandage is worn around the leg in order to compress the veins and help the vessel walls to stick together.

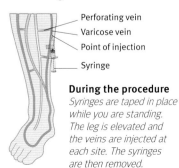

Perforating vein

Varicose vein

Point of injection

Syringe

During the procedure
Syringes are taped in place while you are standing. The leg is elevated and the veins are injected at each site. The syringes are then removed.

Blood and the lymphatic and immune systems

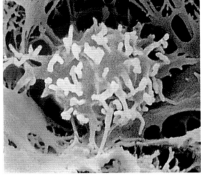

White blood cell
Some white blood cells, such as the one shown, play a particularly important part in the body's defences.

Blood is the body's internal transport system, constantly flowing around the body delivering oxygen, nutrients, and other substances to the tissues and removing waste products from them. Running almost parallel with the blood's circulation is the lymphatic system, which collects excess fluid from the tissues and returns it to the blood. Both the blood and the lymphatic system form part of the body's immune system.

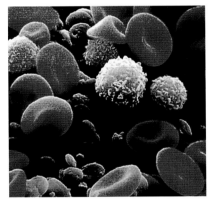

The cells in blood
A magnified view of a drop of blood reveals the various blood cells present: different types of white blood cell, together with red blood cells and platelets.

BODY TISSUES, such as muscle, brain, heart, and other internal organs, need to have a constant supply of energy to function. The energy is obtained from glucose and oxygen, which are carried to body tissues by the blood in the circulation. Blood circulates around the body in about 1 minute at rest and 20 seconds during vigorous exercise.

Circulatory transport
Glucose, a simple sugar that is derived from the breakdown of many foods, is dissolved in the blood and carried in the circulation to every cell within the body. To release its energy, glucose must be "burned" inside the cells, which requires oxygen (a process known as oxidation). The oxygen is transported by red blood cells from the lungs to the body cells, where it is released.

In addition to glucose, the body cells require proteins, fats, vitamins and minerals, and lipids such as cholesterol. These substances are carried in the watery plasma to every cell in the body.

As body cells carry out their various functions, grow, reproduce, and repair damage, they release waste products into the bloodstream. These waste products include carbon dioxide produced from the oxidation of glucose, protein wastes such as urea, and bilirubin from the breakdown of the pigment haemoglobin. The carbon dioxide is eliminated from the blood in the lungs, while the other waste products are mostly processed in the liver before being excreted in the faeces or transported to the kidneys for excretion in the urine.

The body's defences
Blood contains colourless cells known as white cells. These are the main components of the immune system, which protects the body against infection, against toxins produced by bacteria, and against some cancers.

Other essential components of the immune system transported in the blood are proteins called antibodies, which help to destroy microorganisms. Blood also contains billions of small cells called platelets, which, together with substances called clotting factors, seal injured blood vessels through blood clotting.

The lymphatic system also forms part of the immune system and helps to protect the body by filtering out and destroying "foreign" particles, such as infectious organisms and cancer cells.

➕ **FUNCTION**

Formation of blood cells

Bone marrow, the soft fatty tissue inside bone cavities, is the source of all the red blood cells and platelets and most of the white blood cells. In adults, blood cells are formed mainly in the bone marrow of flat bones, such as the shoulder blades, ribs, breastbone, and pelvis. All the blood cells are derived from a single type of cell called a stem cell. Production of mature blood cells from stem cells is controlled by hormones, including erythropoietin, which is produced by the kidneys; thyroid hormones; corticosteroids secreted by the adrenal glands; and growth hormones from the pituitary gland.

Red blood cell   Fat cell   Sinusoid   White blood cell

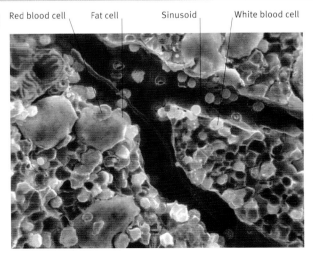

Cells in bone marrow
Blood cells, such as red and white cells, and fat cells are found in bone marrow. Tiny blood vessels called sinusoids supply nourishment and carry away wastes.

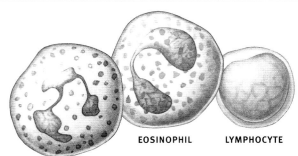

NEUTROPHIL   EOSINOPHIL   LYMPHOCYTE

➕ **STRUCTURE**

Components of blood

The average person has about 5 litres (9 pints) of blood, which consists of cells and fluid (plasma). Red blood cells, the most numerous blood cells, transport oxygen in the body. White blood cells destroy bacterial organisms, cells infected by viruses, and cancer cells. Platelets are the smallest blood cells; after an injury to a blood vessel, they rapidly clump together to seal the damaged lining. Plasma is mostly water but contains other important substances.

Dissolved substances (10% of plasma)

Water (90% of plasma)

Plasma (55% of blood volume)

White blood cells and platelets (4% of blood volume)

Plasma
Plasma consists of water, nutrients, salts, hormones, and proteins, including the dissolved protein fibrinogen, which has a key role in blood clotting.

Red blood cells (41% of blood volume)

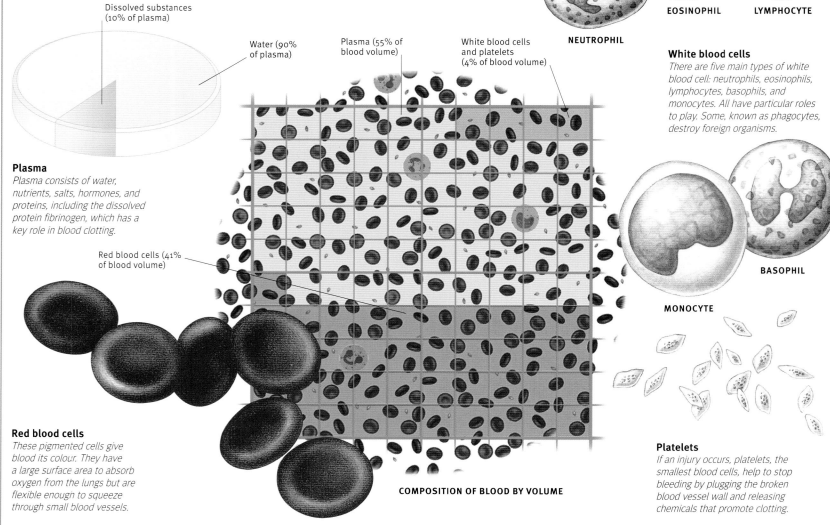

COMPOSITION OF BLOOD BY VOLUME

White blood cells
There are five main types of white blood cell: neutrophils, eosinophils, lymphocytes, basophils, and monocytes. All have particular roles to play. Some, known as phagocytes, destroy foreign organisms.

BASOPHIL

MONOCYTE

Red blood cells
These pigmented cells give blood its colour. They have a large surface area to absorb oxygen from the lungs but are flexible enough to squeeze through small blood vessels.

Platelets
If an injury occurs, platelets, the smallest blood cells, help to stop bleeding by plugging the broken blood vessel wall and releasing chemicals that promote clotting.

➕ **STRUCTURE**

Blood groups

Each person's red blood cells have proteins called antigens on their surface, which categorize the blood into various groups. Antibodies in the blood are produced against any antigens foreign to the red cells. The ABO system of blood grouping is important when assessing the compatibility of blood to be used in transfusions; if a recipient's blood contains antibodies to antigens in the donor blood, a reaction occurs. The Rhesus (Rh) system is another important method of typing blood.

Blood group A
This group has A antigens on the surface of the red blood cells and anti-B antibodies in the blood.

A antigen

Anti-B antibody

A antigen

B antigen

Blood group AB
The rarest blood group, AB, has both antigens on the red cells and neither antibody in the blood.

Blood group B
People in this group have red blood cells with B antigens, and anti-A antibodies in their blood.

B antigen

Anti-A antibody

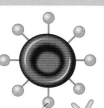

Anti-A antibody

Blood group O
The most common group, O, has no red cell antigens, and anti-A and anti-B antibodies in the blood.

Anti-B antibody

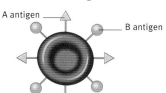

✚ **FUNCTION**

The roles of blood

One of the main functions of blood is to transport oxygen, cells, proteins, hormones, and other substances around the body to the organs and tissues. Oxygen is carried from the lungs to the body cells, and the waste product carbon dioxide is transported from the cells to the lungs. Blood also has a clotting mechanism that acts to seal damaged blood vessels and prevents internal and external blood loss.

Transporting oxygen

Each red blood cell contains millions of molecules of haemoglobin, each made up of four protein chains (two alpha- and two beta-globin) and four haeme, an iron-bearing red pigment. Haemoglobin combines with oxygen from the lungs to give arterial blood its bright red colour. Once oxygen is released in the tissues, the blood becomes darker, a distinctive feature of venous blood.

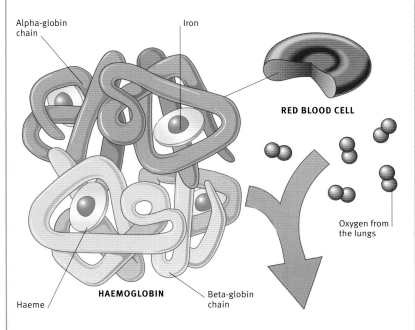

Alpha-globin chain

Iron

RED BLOOD CELL

Oxygen from the lungs

Haeme

HAEMOGLOBIN

Beta-globin chain

Alpha-globin chain

Released oxygen
Oxygen is released into cells in all the tissues of the body

Oxygen bound to iron in haeme

OXYHAEMOGLOBIN

Beta-globin chain

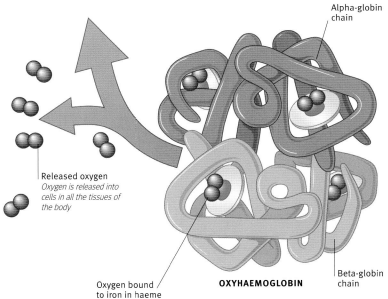

How haemoglobin carries oxygen
The oxygen from the lungs enters the red blood cells in the bloodstream. The oxygen then combines chemically with the haeme within the haemoglobin to form oxyhaemoglobin, which is carried around the body. In areas that need oxygen, the oxyhaemoglobin releases its oxygen and reverts to haemoglobin.

Blood clotting

When a blood vessel is cut or torn, the damage triggers a series of chemical reactions that lead to the formation of a blood clot to seal the injury. Clot formation depends on blood cells called platelets, which adhere at the site of injury. The platelets then clump together and release chemicals that activate proteins, called clotting factors.

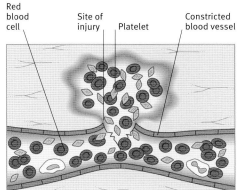

Red blood cell

Site of injury

Platelet

Constricted blood vessel

1 *When a blood vessel is damaged, it constricts at once. Platelets that come into contact with the damaged blood vessel walls are activated. They become sticky and start to adhere to the blood vessel walls near the site of the injury.*

Platelets clumped together

Released chemicals

2 *The platelets clump together. Damaged tissue and activated platelets release chemicals that start a "coagulation cascade", a complex series of reactions involving clotting factors. At each stage, more clotting factors are activated.*

Trapped red blood cell

Fibrin strand

Trapped platelet

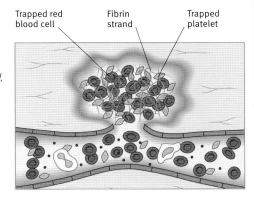

3 *The final stage is conversion of the protein fibrinogen, which is dissolved in the fluid part of the blood, to insoluble fibrin strands. The sticky fibrin threads form a tangled mesh that traps red cells and other blood cells, forming a clot.*

Fibrin strand

Red blood cell

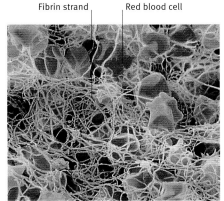

Blood clot
This magnified view shows red blood cells trapped in a mesh of sticky fibrin strands, forming a blood clot. An injured blood vessel is plugged by the clot, which becomes denser as more fibrin strands form. Eventually, the clot will solidify. When the blood vessel has healed, the clot will dissolve naturally.

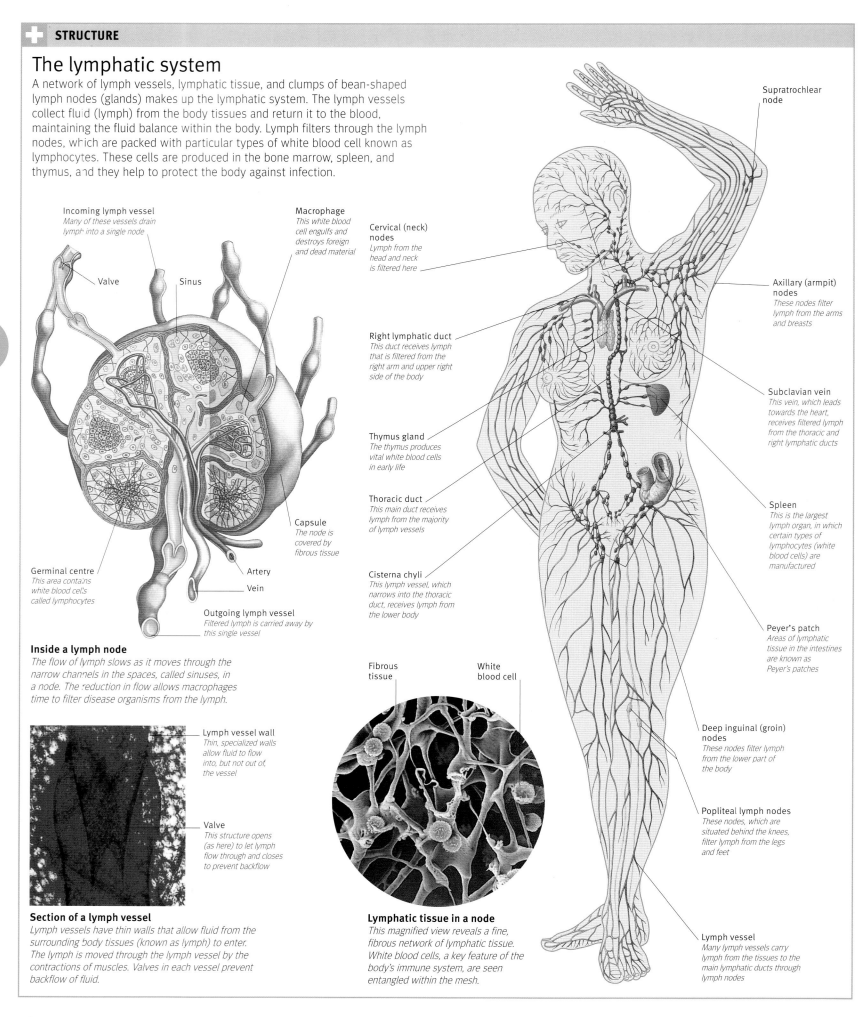

STRUCTURE

The lymphatic system

A network of lymph vessels, lymphatic tissue, and clumps of bean-shaped lymph nodes (glands) makes up the lymphatic system. The lymph vessels collect fluid (lymph) from the body tissues and return it to the blood, maintaining the fluid balance within the body. Lymph filters through the lymph nodes, which are packed with particular types of white blood cell known as lymphocytes. These cells are produced in the bone marrow, spleen, and thymus, and they help to protect the body against infection.

Incoming lymph vessel
Many of these vessels drain lymph into a single node

Valve

Sinus

Macrophage
This white blood cell engulfs and destroys foreign and dead material

Capsule
The node is covered by fibrous tissue

Germinal centre
This area contains white blood cells called lymphocytes

Artery

Vein

Outgoing lymph vessel
Filtered lymph is carried away by this single vessel

Inside a lymph node
The flow of lymph slows as it moves through the narrow channels in the spaces, called sinuses, in a node. The reduction in flow allows macrophages time to filter disease organisms from the lymph.

Lymph vessel wall
Thin, specialized walls allow fluid to flow into, but not out of, the vessel

Valve
This structure opens (as here) to let lymph flow through and closes to prevent backflow

Section of a lymph vessel
Lymph vessels have thin walls that allow fluid from the surrounding body tissues (known as lymph) to enter. The lymph is moved through the lymph vessel by the contractions of muscles. Valves in each vessel prevent backflow of fluid.

Fibrous tissue

White blood cell

Lymphatic tissue in a node
This magnified view reveals a fine, fibrous network of lymphatic tissue. White blood cells, a key feature of the body's immune system, are seen entangled within the mesh.

Cervical (neck) nodes
Lymph from the head and neck is filtered here

Right lymphatic duct
This duct receives lymph that is filtered from the right arm and upper right side of the body

Thymus gland
The thymus produces vital white blood cells in early life

Thoracic duct
This main duct receives lymph from the majority of lymph vessels

Cisterna chyli
This lymph vessel, which narrows into the thoracic duct, receives lymph from the lower body

Supratrochlear node

Axillary (armpit) nodes
These nodes filter lymph from the arms and breasts

Subclavian vein
This vein, which leads towards the heart, receives filtered lymph from the thoracic and right lymphatic ducts

Spleen
This is the largest lymph organ, in which certain types of lymphocytes (white blood cells) are manufactured

Peyer's patch
Areas of lymphatic tissue in the intestines are known as Peyer's patches

Deep inguinal (groin) nodes
These nodes filter lymph from the lower part of the body

Popliteal lymph nodes
These nodes, which are situated behind the knees, filter lymph from the legs and feet

Lymph vessel
Many lymph vessels carry lymph from the tissues to the main lymphatic ducts through lymph nodes

✚ **FUNCTION**

The body's defences

Several barriers and responses work together to protect the body against infection and the development of cancer. Physical and chemical barriers and the inflammatory response form the first two lines of defence. If invading organisms break through these general lines of defence, the body's immune system fights back with two extremely effective immune responses that are specific to different invaders.

Physical and chemical barriers

The skin and the mucous membranes, which line the body openings and the internal passages, are effective barriers against invading organisms. Saliva, tears, mucus, sebum, sweat, and acid aid these barriers in protecting the different parts of the body.

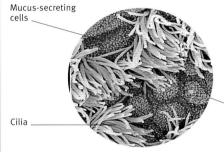

Mucus-secreting cells

Cilia

Respiratory tract
The lining of the respiratory tract produces mucus, which traps organisms. Tiny hairs (cilia) move mucus to the throat.

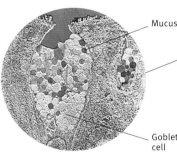

Mucus

Goblet cell

Intestines
Goblet cells in the lining of the intestines produce mucus, which protects the lining from digestive chemicals and harmful organisms.

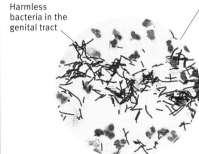

Harmless bacteria in the genital tract

Genital and urinary tracts
Harmless bacteria within the genital tract and the flushing action of urine in the urinary tract both help to prevent the growth of harmful organisms.

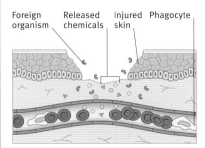

Tear-collecting duct

Glandular tissue

Eyes
Tears from glands in the eyelids wash away dirt and contain an antiseptic substance.

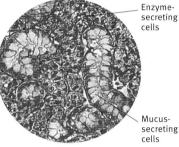

Enzyme-secreting cells

Mucus-secreting cells

Mouth
Glands in the mouth produce saliva, a mixture of mucus and enzymes that cleans the mouth.

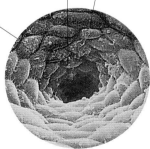

Opening of gastric gland

Stomach lining

Stomach
Glands in the stomach lining produce hydrochloric acid, a powerful agent that kills most invading organisms.

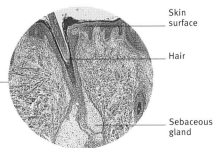

Skin surface

Hair

Sebaceous gland

Skin
The skin is protected by an oily substance, sebum, produced by sebaceous glands and by sweat. Both of these are mildly antiseptic.

The inflammatory response

If foreign organisms such as bacteria overcome the body's physical and chemical barriers, the next line of defence is the inflammatory response, characterized by redness, pain, heat, and swelling at the damaged site.

Foreign organism   Released chemicals   Injured skin   Phagocyte

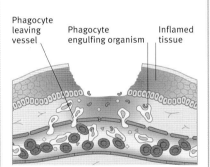

1 *Foreign organisms invade the body through skin that has been broken due to injury. Instantly, the damaged tissue releases specific chemicals that attract specialized white blood cells called phagocytes.*

Phagocyte leaving vessel   Phagocyte engulfing organism   Inflamed tissue

2 *The chemicals cause the underlying blood vessel to widen and the flow of blood to increase, leading to symptoms of inflammation. The vessel walls become slightly porous, allowing phagocytes to reach, engulf, and destroy the foreign organisms.*

Phagocyte   Foreign organism

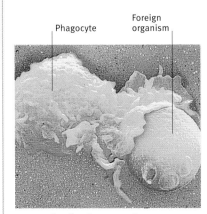

Destroying foreign organisms
Here, a white blood cell called a phagocyte has started to engulf a foreign organism. To destroy the organism, the phagocyte releases enzymes that help to break it down.

The body's defences (continued)

The antibody immune response

This specific immune response targets invading bacteria and relies on white blood cells called B-lymphocytes or B-cells. These cells recognize proteins (antigens) of invading bacteria and multiply to produce antibodies. The antibodies seek out the bacteria and lock on to them, causing their destruction.

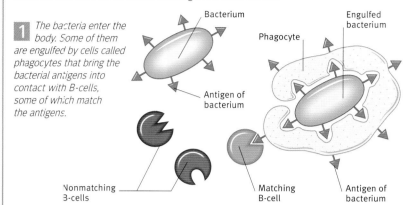

Bacterium

Engulfed bacterium

Phagocyte

Antigen of bacterium

1 *The bacteria enter the body. Some of them are engulfed by cells called phagocytes that bring the bacterial antigens into contact with B-cells, some of which match the antigens.*

Nonmatching B-cells

Matching B-cell

Antigen of bacterium

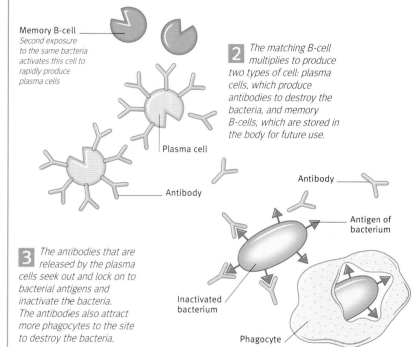

Memory B-cell
Second exposure to the same bacteria activates this cell to rapidly produce plasma cells

2 *The matching B-cell multiplies to produce two types of cell: plasma cells, which produce antibodies to destroy the bacteria, and memory B-cells, which are stored in the body for future use.*

Plasma cell

Antibody

Antibody

Antigen of bacterium

3 *The antibodies that are released by the plasma cells seek out and lock on to bacterial antigens and inactivate the bacteria. The antibodies also attract more phagocytes to the site to destroy the bacteria.*

Inactivated bacterium

Phagocyte

The cellular immune response

This type of specific immune response targets viruses, parasites, and cancer cells. It depends on white blood cells called T-lymphocytes or T-cells. After recognizing a foreign protein (antigen), T-cells multiply and engage in a direct battle against infected cells or cancer cells.

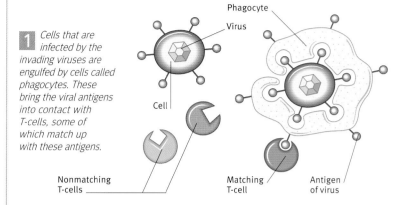

Phagocyte

Virus

Cell

1 *Cells that are infected by the invading viruses are engulfed by cells called phagocytes. These bring the viral antigens into contact with T-cells, some of which match up with these antigens.*

Nonmatching T-cells

Matching T-cell

Antigen of virus

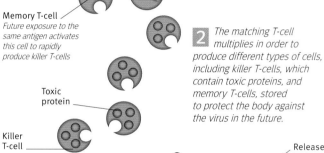

Memory T-cell
Future exposure to the same antigen activates this cell to rapidly produce killer T-cells

2 *The matching T-cell multiplies in order to produce different types of cells, including killer T-cells, which contain toxic proteins, and memory T-cells, stored to protect the body against the virus in the future.*

Toxic protein

Killer T-cell

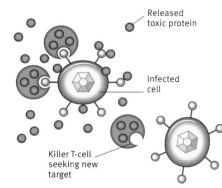

Released toxic protein

Infected cell

3 *Killer T-cells lock on to the infected cell bearing the recognized antigen and release their toxic proteins. These proteins then destroy the infected cell. Killer T-cells may then go on to seek out other infected cells.*

Killer T-cell seeking new target

Allergic reactions

An allergy is an inappropriate immune response to a normally harmless substance, called an allergen. On initial exposure to the allergen, the immune system becomes sensitized to it. During subsequent exposures, an allergic reaction occurs. Mast cells, located in the skin, nasal lining, and other tissues, are destroyed, releasing a substance called histamine that causes an inflammatory response, irritating body tissues and producing allergy symptoms. Allergic reactions tend to get worse with repeated exposure to the allergen.

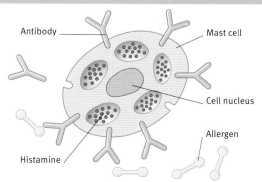

Antibody

Mast cell

Cell nucleus

Allergen

Histamine

1 *On repeat exposure to an allergen, antibodies previously produced in response to it bind to the surface of mast cells, which contain histamine.*

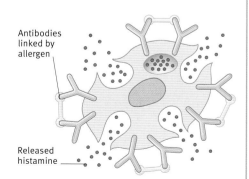

Antibodies linked by allergen

Released histamine

2 *The allergens bind to and link two or more antibodies, causing the cell to burst and release the histamine within. Histamine causes the symptoms of allergy.*

Blood disorders

Blood transports oxygen and nutrients to all parts of the body and carries away carbon dioxide and other waste materials. Oxygen is carried inside red blood cells, which make up almost half the volume of blood. Other components of blood include white blood cells, which combat infections, and platelets, tiny cells that help to form blood clots to seal damaged blood vessels.

Disorders of the blood may be caused by an abnormality in the number, content, or form of one or more of the different types of blood cell. The first articles in this section deal with the different types of anaemia and with sickle-cell disease. In these disorders, haemoglobin, the oxygen-carrying pigment in red blood cells, is deficient or abnormal, or red cells are destroyed at an accelerated rate. Disorders in which the blood either fails to clot or clots too readily are then discussed. Some of these disorders are inherited, such as the bleeding disorders haemophilia and von Willebrand's disease. In these disorders, the genes that are responsible for producing specific clotting factors are either absent or abnormal. Various cancers of the blood, called leukaemias, are also discussed. These disorders result from an overproduction of white blood cells, which suppresses the production of the normal blood cells in the body. The final article in this section deals with polycythaemia, a condition in which too many red blood cells are produced.

✚ KEY ELEMENTS

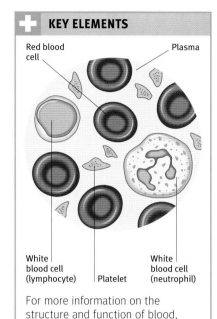

Red blood cell

Plasma

White blood cell (lymphocyte)

Platelet

White blood cell (neutrophil)

For more information on the structure and function of blood, *see* pp.265–270.

Anaemia

Disorders in which haemoglobin (the oxygen-carrying pigment in red blood cells) is deficient or abnormal

 Age, gender, genetics, and lifestyle as risk factors depend on the type

Anaemia is a deficiency or an abnormality of haemoglobin, the component of red blood cells that binds with oxygen from the lungs and carries it through the circulation to the body tissues. The oxygen-carrying capacity of the blood is thus reduced, and the tissues of the body may not receive sufficient oxygen.

Red blood cells are manufactured in the bone marrow (at the rate of more than a million every second) and circulate in the bloodstream for about 120 days before they are broken down in the spleen. In a healthy person, the production and destruction of red blood cells are balanced. Anaemia occurs if this balance is upset, reducing the number of healthy cells or if the haemoglobin is abnormal.

What are the types?

There are four main types of anaemia. The first type is due to a deficiency of one or more of the substances that are essential for the formation of healthy red blood cells. By far the most common form of this type of anaemia is iron-deficiency anaemia (right), which results from low levels of iron in the body. A much rarer form is megaloblastic anaemia (p.272), which is usually the result of low levels of either vitamin B_{12} or another vitamin, folic acid, in the body.

The second type of anaemia results from inherited abnormalities of haemoglobin production. Examples of this type include sickle-cell disease (p.272) and thalassaemia (p.273). The haemoglobin is abnormal from shortly after birth, but symptoms of anaemia may not develop until later in childhood.

The third type of anaemia is caused by excessively rapid destruction of red blood cells (haemolysis) and is called haemolytic anaemia (p.273).

The fourth type of anaemia, called aplastic anaemia (p.273), is caused by failure of the bone marrow to produce sufficient numbers of red blood cells and often of other types of blood cell as well.

Anaemia may be due to a combination of different causes, and sometimes the exact cause of the condition is not known. In some cases, anaemia develops during a long-term illness, such as cancer or rheumatoid arthritis (p.222).

What are the symptoms?

If your anaemia is mild, your body may be able to make up for a slight reduction in the oxygen-carrying capacity of blood by increasing the blood supply to the tissues. In this case, there may not be any symptoms. Symptoms of more severe anaemia may include:

■ Tiredness and a feeling of faintness.
■ Pale skin.
■ Shortness of breath on mild exertion.

You may also have a rapid heart rate because the heart has to work harder to increase blood supply to the rest of the body. Stress on the heart may result in chronic heart failure (p.247), common symptoms of which are swollen ankles and increasing shortness of breath.

What might be done?

Anaemia is usually confirmed by blood tests to measure the level of haemoglobin and to establish the type and cause of the anaemia. A bone marrow aspiration and biopsy (p.274) may be carried out to obtain tissue samples for examination under a microscope.

Most anaemias respond well to treatment. Severe cases may require blood transfusion (p.272).

Iron-deficiency anaemia

A type of anaemia caused by inadequate levels of iron in the body

 More common in females

 A vegan diet is a risk factor

 Age and genetics are not significant factors

Iron-deficiency anaemia is the most common form of anaemia (a deficiency of the oxygen-carrying pigment haemoglobin in red blood cells). Iron is an essential component of haemoglobin in the production of blood. If insufficient iron is available, the production of haemoglobin and its incorporation into red blood cells in the bone marrow are reduced. As a result, there is less haemoglobin to bind with oxygen in the lungs and to carry the oxygen to the tissues of the body. Consequently, the tissues may receive insufficient oxygen.

What are the causes?

Iron-deficiency anaemia is most commonly caused by the loss of significant quantities of iron through persistent bleeding. This type of anaemia mainly affects women who experience regular blood loss over a period of time from heavy menstrual bleeding (*see* **Menorrhagia**, p.471). Persistent loss of blood may also be due to stomach ulcers (*see* **Peptic ulcer**, p.406). Prolonged use of aspirin or long-term use of nonsteroidal anti-inflammatory drugs (p.578) is a possible cause of bleeding from the lining of the stomach. In people over the age of 60, a common cause of blood loss is a bowel disorder, such as infection, inflammation, or cancer of the bowel (*see* **Colorectal cancer**, p.421). Bleeding in the stomach or upper intestine may go unnoticed, while blood lost from the lower part of the intestine or rectum may be visible in the faeces.

The second cause of iron-deficiency anaemia is insufficient iron in the diet. People whose diet contains little or no iron, such as vegans, may be at particular risk of developing the condition.

Iron-deficiency anaemia is also more likely to develop when the body needs higher levels of iron than normal and these extra demands are not met by the existing diet. For example, children who are growing rapidly, especially adolescents, and women who are pregnant have an increased risk of developing iron-deficiency anaemia if their diet does not contain plenty of iron.

Some other causes of iron-deficiency anaemia include disorders that prevent absorption of iron from the diet. In the body, iron is absorbed from food as it passes through the small intestine; conditions that cause damage to the small intestine, such as coeliac disease (p.416) or surgery on the small intestine, sometimes result in iron deficiency.

What are the symptoms?

In addition to any specific symptoms associated with an underlying disorder, you may experience the general symptoms of anaemia, which include:

■ Tiredness and a feeling of faintness.
■ Pale skin.
■ Shortness of breath on mild exertion.

You may also have symptoms that are due to a marked deficiency of iron:

■ Brittle, concave-shaped nails.
■ Painful cracks in the skin at the sides of the mouth.
■ A smooth, reddened tongue.

If your anaemia is severe, you may be at risk of chronic heart failure (p.247) because your heart has to work harder to supply blood to the rest of the body.

What might be done?

Your doctor will arrange for blood tests to measure the levels of haemoglobin and iron in your blood. If the cause of the iron deficiency is not obvious, other tests may be arranged to look for evidence of internal bleeding. These tests may include upper digestive tract endoscopy (p.407) and colonoscopy (p.418).

If there is an underlying disorder, this will be treated. Your doctor may prescribe iron tablets (syrup for children) or, less commonly, iron injections to replace iron stores (*see* **Minerals**, p.599). Your doctor may also recommend vitamin C (abundant in citrus fruits and citrus fruit juices) with meals because this vitamin aids absorption of iron. Severe anaemia may require blood transfusion (p.272).

▶ **TREATMENT**

Blood transfusion

A blood transfusion is carried out to treat severe anaemia, to replace blood lost by bleeding, or to treat certain blood disorders, such as thalassaemia. It is performed in hospital, sometimes on a day-patient basis. The amount of blood required depends on the severity of the condition. Sometimes only a particular component of blood is transfused, such as red blood cells or platelets. Before a transfusion is given, a sample of your blood is taken to check that it is compatible with the donor blood (a process called cross matching). Matched donor blood is then transfused into a vein (usually in your arm) through a plastic cannula (a tube with a smooth tip). Typically, a unit of blood (about 500 ml/1 pint) is given over a period of 30 minutes to 4 hours, although in an emergency a unit may be given within a few minutes. During the procedure, your blood pressure, pulse, and body temperature are monitored. To minimize the risk of transmitting a potentially serious infection, all donor blood is screened for infectious organisms such as HIV and hepatitis viruses.

Megaloblastic anaemia

A type of anaemia caused by a lack of vitamin B₁₂ or folic acid

 More common over the age of 40

 Gender, genetics, and lifestyle as risk factors depend on the cause

Two major vitamins, B_{12} and folic acid, play an essential role in the production of healthy red blood cells. Deficiency of either vitamin may lead to megaloblastic anaemia, in which large, abnormal red blood cells (megaloblasts) are produced by the bone marrow, and the production of normal red blood cells is reduced. The blood may thus be unable to carry sufficient oxygen to the tissues.

What are the causes?

Lack of vitamin B_{12} is often due to an autoimmune disorder in which antibodies are produced that damage the stomach lining and prevent it from forming intrinsic factor, which is essential for the absorption of vitamin B_{12} from food in the intestines. This type of megaloblastic anaemia, called pernicious anaemia, tends to run in families and is more common in women and in people with other autoimmune disorders, such as Hashimoto's thyroiditis (*see* **Thyroiditis**, p.433). Intestinal disorders, such as coeliac disease (p.416), or abdominal surgery can also interfere with vitamin B_{12} absorption. Because vitamin B_{12} occurs naturally only in foods of animal origin, vegans are at risk of deficiency and, therefore, of developing megaloblastic anaemia unless they take supplementary vitamin B_{12}.

Folic acid deficiency is often due to a poor diet. People who abuse alcohol are at particular risk because alcohol interferes with the absorption of folic acid in the intestines. Pregnant women may also be at risk of deficiency because folic acid requirements are higher in pregnancy.

Disorders causing a rapid turnover of cells, including severe psoriasis (p.192), may also cause folic acid deficiency. In rare cases, the deficiency is a side effect of certain drugs, such as anticonvulsants (p.590) and anticancer drugs (p.586).

What are the symptoms?

The initial symptoms of megaloblastic anaemia, which are common to all anaemias, develop slowly and may include:
- Tiredness and a feeling of faintness.
- Pale skin.
- Shortness of breath on mild exertion.
These symptoms of megaloblastic anaemia may worsen over time. Although lack of folic acid does not produce additional symptoms, lack of vitamin B_{12} may eventually damage the nervous system, possibly leading to:
- Tingling in the hands and feet.
- Weakness and loss of balance.
- Loss of memory and confusion.
People who have pernicious anaemia may also notice a yellow tinge to their skin due to jaundice (p.407).

What might be done?

The diagnosis of megaloblastic anaemia requires blood tests to look for megaloblasts and also to measure the levels of vitamin B_{12}, folic acid, and iron. You may also have a bone marrow aspiration and biopsy (p.274) to obtain tissue samples for further examination.

Megaloblastic anaemia caused by an inability to absorb vitamin B_{12} may be improved by treating the underlying disorder, but some people, such as those who have pernicious anaemia and malabsorption caused by surgery, require lifelong regular injections of vitamin B_{12} (*see* **Vitamins**, p.598). Symptoms should subside within days, but existing damage to the nervous system may be irreversible.

If megaloblastic anaemia is caused by dietary deficiency, the condition usually disappears with an improved diet. Vegans may need to take vitamin B_{12} supplements.

Sickle-cell disease

An inherited blood disorder in which red blood cells become sickle-shaped

 Present from birth; first symptoms appear after about 6 months

 Due to an abnormal gene inherited from both parents; most commonly occurs in people of African or Caribbean descent

 Strenuous exercise and high altitudes may trigger symptoms

 Gender is not a significant factor

Sickle-cell disease is the result of an abnormality of haemoglobin, the pigment within red blood cells that binds to oxygen in the lungs and carries it to body tissues. When the amount of oxygen that is bound to the abnormal haemoglobin is reduced, the red blood cells become distorted into an elongated sickle shape. Because these sickle-shaped cells are rigid, they can become lodged in small blood vessels and obstruct the flow of blood, depriving the tissues of oxygen. Sickle-shaped red cells are fragile and may be destroyed prematurely, which can lead to anaemia (p.271).

In the UK, most cases of sickle-cell disease occur in people of African or Caribbean descent.

What are the causes?

Sickle-cell disease is a genetic disorder in which an abnormal gene is inherited from both parents in an autosomal recessive manner (*see* **Gene disorders**, p.151). If an abnormal gene is inherited from only one parent, a condition called sickle-cell trait results. Sickle-cell trait does not usually produce symptoms or require treatment. Having one abnormal gene (sickle cell trait) confers a small degree of protection against malaria (p.175) but having two abnormal genes (sickle-cell disease) does not.

Can it be prevented?

In communities in which sickle-cell disease is particularly common, genetic testing may be recommended for couples planning to have children. If both partners are found to carry the sickle-cell gene, genetic counselling (p.151) will be offered. Pregnant women may be offered a blood test in early pregnancy to screen for sickle-cell disease in their unborn baby. If the test is positive, counselling will be offered. Shortly after birth, all newborn babies are routinely screened for sickle-cell disease as part of the blood spot screening tests (p.561).

What are the symptoms?

The symptoms of sickle-cell disease are highly variable, even among affected individuals in the same family. In children, the symptoms first appear from about 6 months of age and may include intermittent painful swelling of the fingers and toes and delayed growth.

Distinct episodes of illness, known as sickle-cell crises, occur intermittently throughout childhood and into adult life. These crises may be precipitated by infections, but they can also occur after strenuous exercise, on exposure to cold, or at high altitude. Sickle-cell crises can produce different groups of symptoms, which may include:
- Pallor, tiredness, and faintness due to severe anaemia.
- Severe pain and swelling around a bone or joint.
- Breathlessness and chest pain.
- Abdominal pain.
- Blood in the urine.
Sickle-cell crises usually require urgent admission to hospital for treatment, and they can be life-threatening.

Are there complications?

People who have sickle-cell disease are more susceptible to serious infections, such as pneumococcal infection (*see* **Pneumonia**, p.299), and any infection can trigger a sickle-cell crisis. Gallstones (p.412) may develop. The abnormal cells can cause problems by blocking and damaging small blood vessels throughout the body, which may lead to kidney damage (*see* **Chronic kidney disease**, p.451). The risk of transient ischaemic attacks (p.328) and stroke (p.329) is also increased. Women with sickle-cell disease may have decreased fertility, and those who become pregnant face an increased risk of miscarriage (p.511).

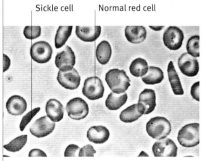

Sickle cell   Normal red cell

Sickle-shaped red blood cells
In sickle-cell disease, some of the red blood cells become distorted into a distinctive and fragile sickle shape.

What might be done?

To confirm the diagnosis, your doctor may take a sample of blood to look for sickle-shaped cells under a microscope and to test for defective haemoglobin.

If sickle-cell disease is mild, folic acid (*see* **Vitamins**, p.598), which is necessary for the production of red blood cells, may be prescribed. If the disease is more severe, you may require long-term drug treatment with hydroxyurea, which reduces the proportion of abnormal red cells in the blood. You may also need to take a preventive antibiotic (p.572) continually and to be vaccinated against pneumococcal infection.

Immediate hospital admission is usually necessary for sickle-cell crises. You may be given intravenous fluids to treat dehydration, antibiotics for underlying infections, and painkillers (p.589). People who have recurrent sickle-cell crises may be given exchange transfusions, in which some of their blood is replaced with blood from a healthy donor. In some cases, a stem cell transplant (p.276) may be considered.

Thalassaemia

An inherited type of anaemia affecting production of haemoglobin, the oxygen-carrying pigment in red blood cells

 Present from birth; age at first appearance of symptoms depends on type

 Due to one or more abnormal genes inherited from one or both parents

 Gender and lifestyle are not significant factors

In thalassaemia, an inherited genetic defect prevents the normal formation of haemoglobin, the oxygen-carrying pigment inside red blood cells. Red cells containing the defective haemoglobin carry less oxygen than normal and are destroyed prematurely, reducing oxygen transport to the body tissues.

The body tries to compensate by producing additional red blood cells throughout the bone marrow and in the liver and spleen, where red blood cells are not normally formed. The marrow expands due to overactivity, which may lead to thickening of the bones of the skull and face. The liver and spleen may become enlarged as they produce and, in the case of the spleen, destroy large numbers of the abnormal red blood cells. Thalassaemia mainly affects people from Mediterranean countries, the Middle East, Southeast Asia, and Africa.

What are the causes?
A normal haemoglobin molecule contains four protein (globin) chains: two alpha and two beta chains. Different genes are responsible for the production of each type of chain. Thalassaemia is caused by one or more genetic defects and results in a failure to produce sufficient quantities of either the alpha or the beta globin chains.

Beta-thalassaemia, due to abnormal beta chains, is more common in the UK. A person inherits two copies of the gene for haemoglobin beta chains, one copy from each parent. If one of those genes is defective, the individual will typically have no symptoms and is termed a carrier. If both genes are defective, the individual will have symptoms of thalassaemia.

Alpha-thalassaemia, due to abnormal alpha chains, is comparatively rare in the UK. A person inherits four copies of the genes for haemoglobin alpha chains, two from each parent. If one or two of those genes are defective, the individual will typically be a carrier with no symptoms, although occasionally there may be mild anaemia. If three genes are defective, the individual will usually have symptoms, such as anaemia. If all four genes are

defective, the fetus will die before birth unless blood transfusions are given while the fetus is still in the uterus and continued after birth. However, such treatment is not always successful.

Can it be prevented?
Genetic testing is available for women or couples planning to have children and, if a defective gene is identified, they may want to consider genetic counselling (p.151). In addition, pregnant women may be offered a blood test in early pregnancy to screen for thalassaemia. If testing indicates that the fetus has thalassaemia, counselling will be offered.

What are the symptoms?
Carriers of beta-thalassaemia do not usually have symptoms. However, if an individual inherits two defective genes for beta-thalassaemia, symptoms of severe anaemia usually appear between 4 and 6 months of age. These symptoms may include:
■ Pale skin
■ Shortness of breath on mild exertion.
■ Swelling of the abdomen due to an enlarged liver and spleen.
Affected children have slow growth, and sexual development is delayed. The bones of the skull and face may thicken as the bone marrow expands.

Carriers of alpha-thalassaemia (with one or two defective genes) often have no symptoms, although some individuals with two defective genes may have mild anaemia. For those with three defective genes, the symptoms are similar to those of beta-thalassaemia, although they may not appear until later in childhood or early adulthood.

Prominent forehead   Thickened skull

Enlarged skull bones in thalassaemia
In severe thalassaemia, increased bone marrow activity causes the bones of the skull to expand and become thickened, altering the appearance of the face.

What might be done?
If the thalassaemia is mild, treatment may not be needed, although folic acid supplements (*see* **Vitamins**, p.598) may be recommended to help stimulate the production of red blood cells. If the condition is severe, regular blood transfusions (opposite page) may be needed for life. However, frequent blood transfusions can lead to a build-up of iron in the heart, liver, and pancreas, causing progressive damage to these

organs. To counteract this build-up, treatment with desferrioxamine, desferasirox, or deferiprone (drugs that allow the kidneys to excrete more iron than usual) may be needed. If the spleen is enlarged, it may need to be removed. In severe cases, a stem cell transplant (p.276) may be considered.

What is the prognosis?
People with mild thalassaemia have a normal life span. Some people who have severe thalassaemia die early in childhood, but life expectancy can be greatly improved with regular transfusions.

Haemolytic anaemia

A type of anaemia caused by excessive destruction of red blood cells

 Genetics as a risk factor depends on the cause

 Age, gender, and lifestyle are not significant factors

Haemolytic anaemia occurs when the red cells in the blood are broken down more rapidly than they can be replaced. Red blood cells usually have a lifespan of about 120 days before they are destroyed in the spleen, a process known as haemolysis. The premature destruction of red blood cells may be caused by abnormal immune reactions, inherited disorders, or infections. If the bone marrow cannot replace the red blood cells rapidly, haemolytic anaemia results.

What are the causes?
Haemolytic anaemia is commonly due to an abnormal immune reaction in which the body produces antibodies that attack red blood cells and encourage their destruction in the spleen. This reaction is often triggered by drugs, including penicillin (*see* **Antibiotics**, p.572), methyldopa (*see* **Antihypertensive drugs**, p.580), or quinine (*see* **Antimalarial drugs**, p.574). Antibodies that attack red blood cells may also occur in people who have chronic lymphocytic leukaemia (p.277) or an autoimmune disorder such as systemic lupus erythematosus (p.281).

Inherited disorders that affect the red blood cells' biochemical make-up or shape may also promote haemolysis. One such biochemical abnormality, affecting more than 100 million people worldwide, is lack of G6PD (glucose-6-phosphate dehydrogenase), an enzyme in red blood cells that helps to protect them against chemical damage. People with the disorder are usually well but infection and certain drugs can trigger haemolysis. In one form of G6PD deficiency, which mostly affects people of Mediterranean origin, severe haemolysis is triggered by a chemical found in broad beans (favism).

Other inherited disorders that can lead to haemolytic anaemia include thalassaemia (left), sickle-cell disease (opposite page),

and hereditary spherocytosis. In thalassaemia, large numbers of abnormal red blood cells are destroyed by the spleen. In sickle-cell disease, the sickle-shaped red blood cells are abnormally fragile and may be destroyed prematurely. In spherocytosis, the red blood cells change to a spherical shape and are destroyed prematurely in the spleen. All of these disorders may lead to continuous haemolysis from childhood.

Red blood cells may also be destroyed as a result of infections such as malaria (p.175) in which the infective organism multiplies within the red blood cells. Rarely, haemolytic anaemia is due to damage to the red blood cells caused by an artificial heart valve.

What are the symptoms?
If you have haemolytic anaemia, you may notice the following symptoms, which are common to all anaemias:
■ Tiredness and a feeling of faintness.
■ Pale skin.
■ Shortness of breath on mild exertion.
You may also have symptoms that occur as a result of haemolysis, including:
■ Yellowing of the skin and whites of the eyes (*see* **Jaundice**, p.407).
■ Swelling of the abdomen caused by enlargement of the spleen as it filters out many damaged red blood cells.
Over a period of several years, you may develop gallstones (p.412), which form from bilirubin, a product of the breakdown of red blood cells.

What might be done?
Haemolytic anaemia can be diagnosed from blood tests that reveal numerous immature red blood cells and, in some cases, fragmented, abnormally shaped red blood cells. Your doctor may also measure your blood levels of bilirubin, and he or she may arrange for blood tests to look for antibodies to red cells to identify the cause of the anaemia.

Underlying disorders, such as an infection or autoimmune disease, will be treated and any drugs that are causing haemolysis will be stopped. Corticosteroids (p.600) may be given for haemolytic anaemia due to an immune reaction. In some cases of haemolytic anaemia, surgical removal of the spleen is necessary.

Aplastic anaemia

A type of anaemia caused by failure of the bone marrow to generate new blood cells of all types

 Rarely due to an abnormal gene

 Exposure to chemicals such as benzene is a risk factor

 Age and gender are not significant factors

The blood normally contains red blood cells, white blood cells, and platelets. These components are produced either entirely or mostly in the bone marrow. However, in aplastic anaemia, the bone marrow does not produce stem cells, the initial form of these components, resulting in abnormally low numbers of all these blood cells.

What are the causes?

In many cases of aplastic anaemia, the cause is unknown. However, the condition may result from an autoimmune disorder (p.280) in which antibodies are produced by the immune system that act against and destroy the body's own stem cells. In rare cases, aplastic anaemia is due to an inherited abnormal gene. When the cause of the condition has been established, the term secondary aplastic anaemia is used.

Secondary aplastic anaemia sometimes occurs following a severe viral infection, such as a hepatitis virus infection (see **Acute hepatitis**, p.408). The disorder may also develop after chemotherapy (p.157) or radiotherapy (p.158), as both treatments may reduce the production of blood cells by the bone marrow. Exposure to certain chemicals, such as benzene, and to some antibiotics (p.572), such as sulphonamides, may also trigger secondary aplastic anaemia.

What are the symptoms?

Aplastic anaemia may lead to the following symptoms, common to all anaemias and due to the lack of red blood cells:

■ Tiredness and a feeling of faintness.
■ Pale skin.
■ Shortness of breath on mild exertion.

Lack of platelets, the tiny cells involved in blood clotting, may cause symptoms such as easy bruising and excessive bleeding, often from the gums or nose. A deficiency of white blood cells, which form an important part of the immune system, may increase susceptibility to bacterial and fungal infections, which may become life-threatening due to the inadequate immune response.

What might be done?

To confirm the diagnosis, your doctor may arrange for blood tests to measure blood cell levels and a bone marrow aspiration and biopsy (right) to obtain cell samples for examination.

Treatment of the underlying cause may allow the bone marrow to recover. Immunosuppressant drugs (p.585) or corticosteroids (p.600) may be used to treat autoimmune disorders. During recovery, blood transfusions (p.272) and antibiotics (p.572) may be needed to prevent or treat infection. If these treatments are ineffective, you may be offered a stem cell transplant (p.276).

What is the prognosis?

If treated early, a person with aplastic anaemia may make a complete recovery. However, in some cases the condition may be fatal. A successful stem cell transplant can be life-saving.

▶ **TEST**

Bone marrow aspiration and biopsy

Bone marrow aspiration and biopsy is used to diagnose various disorders of the blood, such as leukaemia and severe anaemias. In this procedure, two types of tissue sample are taken for examination: in a bone marrow aspiration, cells are withdrawn with a fine needle and syringe; in a bone marrow biopsy, a core of bone with marrow inside is taken with a large needle. The site may be tender for a few days afterwards. This procedure is usually carried out in hospital, often on an outpatient basis.

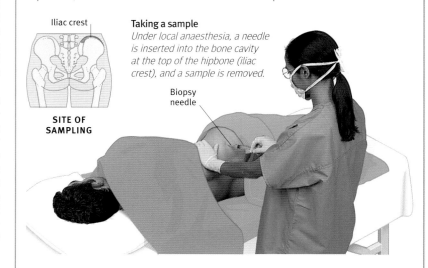

Iliac crest

SITE OF SAMPLING

Taking a sample
Under local anaesthesia, a needle is inserted into the bone cavity at the top of the hipbone (iliac crest), and a sample is removed.

Biopsy needle

RESULTS

Bone marrow biopsy sample
This magnified image of a bone marrow sample reveals large numbers of abnormal white blood cells. Chronic myeloid leukaemia is a possible cause of this type of blood cell abnormality.

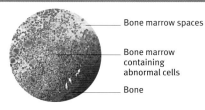

Bone marrow spaces

Bone marrow containing abnormal cells

Bone

Bleeding disorders

A group of disorders that result in excessive or prolonged bleeding

 Age, gender, genetics, and lifestyle as risk factors depend on the cause

Normally, when there is bleeding a blood clot forms to seal the damaged vessel and prevent further blood loss. The clotting process relies on an interaction between blood cells called platelets, circulating proteins in the blood known as clotting factors, and the vessel wall. A lack of clotting factors or platelets will disrupt the clotting process, which may lead to easy bruising, prolonged or severe bleeding after even minor injury, or internal bleeding into muscles, organs, and joints.

Many disorders that cause excessive bleeding are inherited, the most important being haemophilia (right) and the related disorder von Willebrand's disease (opposite page). These conditions occur when the gene that is responsible for a particular clotting factor is abnormal, resulting in either low levels or a complete absence of the clotting factor in the blood.

In thrombocytopenia (opposite page), there are too few platelets in the blood. This condition can occur as a complication of bone marrow disorders, such as leukaemia (p.276) and aplastic anaemia (p.273), or as a side effect of certain drugs, such as the anticancer drugs used in chemotherapy (p.157). Low platelet levels may result from infections, such as HIV infection (see **HIV infection and AIDS**, p.169) or sepsis (see **Septicaemia**, p.171). Occasionally, there are normal numbers of platelets but they function abnormally, causing excessive bleeding and other symptoms associated with low platelet levels. In some cases, abnormally functioning platelets may be present at birth. They may also develop as a result of certain medications (such as aspirin) or natural remedies (garlic and fish oils, for example).

Disorders of the liver, where clotting factors are produced, or the intestines, where vitamin K (an essential component of clotting factors) is absorbed, may also result in abnormal bleeding.

What might be done?

Bleeding disorders due to an absence of one or more clotting factors may be treated by regular injections of the missing factors.

If the bleeding disorder is due to a drug, the use of that drug may be stopped. In other cases, treatment is aimed at the underlying disorder.

Haemophilia

Inherited deficiency of blood clotting factors, causing excessive bleeding

 Affects males almost exclusively

 Due to abnormal genes, which in some cases are inherited

 Age and lifestyle are not significant factors

Normally, a cut or internal injury stops bleeding within a few minutes, unless it is very serious. In haemophilia, even a small cut may bleed for hours or days, and there are sometimes episodes of spontaneous bleeding. Haemophilia occurs almost exclusively in males. In rare cases, some females may be affected, although they usually have only mild symptoms.

What are the causes?

Haemophilia is due to deficiency of a protein involved in blood clotting. There are two main types of haemophilia: haemophilia A, in which there is a deficiency of the blood protein Factor VIII, and haemophilia B (previously known as Christmas disease), in which there is a deficiency of Factor IX. Haemophilia A is more common than haemophilia B, but the symptoms are very similar. In both types of haemophilia, the deficiency is the result of a faulty gene. The particular gene involved is different in the two disorders.

In both types of haemophilia, the abnormal gene is inherited in a recessive manner and is located on the X chromosome – known as X-linked recessive inheritance (see **Gene disorders**, p.151). The disorders usually affect males only because they have only one X chromosome. Females who carry the abnormal gene on one of their two X chromosomes are usually unaffected, although a few may have mild symptoms, such as heavy periods. Women carriers of a faulty gene may pass on the gene to their children. Each son of a woman who carries the abnormal gene has a 1 in 2 chance of being affected.

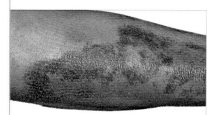

Bruising in haemophilia
In people with haemophilia, severe bruising, as seen on the arm above, can develop after even minor injury because the blood does not clot normally.

In about a third of all cases of haemophilia A and B, the cause is a spontaneous gene abnormality and there is no family history of the disorders.

What are the symptoms?

The symptoms are highly variable, and their severity depends on how much Factor VIII or IX is produced. People who produce very little or no Factor VIII or IX usually develop symptoms in infancy. Those with only moderately reduced levels may not develop symptoms until later in life. The symptoms may include:

- Easy bruising even after minor injury.
- Sudden, painful swelling of muscles and joints due to internal bleeding.
- Prolonged bleeding after an injury or a minor surgical operation.
- Blood in the urine.

Without treatment, prolonged episodes of bleeding into the joints may result in long-term damage and, eventually, may lead to deformity of the joints.

What might be done?

Your doctor will arrange for tests to see how long your blood takes to clot and to measure the level of Factor VIII or IX.

The aim of treatment is to maintain the clotting factors at a high enough level to prevent bleeding. If you have a severe form of either condition, you will probably need regular intravenous injections of Factor VIII or IX to boost the levels of these factors in the blood. If you have a mild form of either condition, you may need injections only after an injury or before surgery. You may also be prescribed desmopressin, which contains a pituitary hormone, to boost the level of Factor VIII in your blood (*see* **Pituitary drugs**, p.603).

Some people develop antibodies (known as inhibitors) to Factor VIII supplements, which makes treatment difficult. These people may need to take an immunosuppressant drug (p.585) to destroy the inhibitors.

What is the prognosis?

If you have haemophilia A or B, you can lead an active life but need to avoid sustaining any injuries. Activities such as swimming, running, and walking are beneficial, but contact sports, such as wrestling and football, should be avoided. Regular dental care is necessary to avoid the risk of bleeding from inflamed gums.

If you have a family history of either disorder, you should obtain medical advice when planning a pregnancy (*see* **Genetic counselling**, p.151). In the past, some people with haemophilia contracted acute or chronic hepatitis (p.409) or HIV (*see* **HIV infection and AIDS**, p.169) after receiving clotting factors contaminated with hepatitis B or C viruses or HIV. Synthetic Factor VIII and Factor IX clotting factors are now available and these eliminate the risk of infection with these viruses.

Von Willebrand's disease

An inherited lifelong bleeding disorder similar to haemophilia

 Due to an abnormal gene, usually inherited from one parent

 Age, gender, and lifestyle are not significant factors

In von Willebrand's disease, a substance called von Willebrand factor is either entirely absent from the blood or is present in only low levels. Von Willebrand factor binds to a protein in the blood called Factor VIII, which is needed for blood clotting. A deficiency of von Willebrand factor may therefore lead to excessive or prolonged bleeding.

Von Willebrand's disease is usually caused by a faulty gene that is inherited in an autosomal dominant manner (*see* **Gene disorders**, p.151): a person needs to inherit the gene from only one parent to develop the condition. However, in some cases, the faulty gene is inherited in an autosomal recessive manner: a person needs to inherit the gene from both parents to develop the condition.

The symptoms of the condition vary according to the level of von Willebrand factor present in the blood. They include easy bruising, frequent nosebleeds, bleeding gums, heavy menstrual periods in women, and prolonged bleeding from even minor cuts.

What might be done?

A diagnosis is usually made by determining how long your blood takes to clot and measuring the levels of clotting factors in your blood.

In mild cases, treatment is not usually necessary. If you bleed often or are due to have major surgery, you may be prescribed the drug desmopressin (*see* **Pituitary drugs**, p.603), which raises the levels of von Willebrand factor and Factor VIII in your blood. Women may be advised to take an oral contraceptive to prevent heavy menstrual periods. If bleeding is severe, a blood extract rich in clotting factors may be given intravenously.

Thrombocytopenia

Reduced levels of blood cells called platelets, causing bleeding into the skin and internal organs

 Age, gender, genetics, and lifestyle are not significant factors

Thrombocytopenia is the medical term for a reduction in the number of platelets in the blood circulation. Platelets are small blood cells, made in the bone marrow, that play a vital part in blood clotting, and a reduction in their numbers leads to a tendency to excessive bleeding.

Thrombocytopenia may be caused either by a failure of the bone marrow to produce platelets or by excessive destruction of platelets in the spleen. Platelet production in the bone marrow may be reduced by disorders such as leukaemia (p.276) or aplastic anaemia (p.273) or by chemotherapy (p.157). An excessive destruction of platelets is usually due to an abnormal immune reaction in which the body produces antibodies that attack platelets (immune thrombocytopenia). The cause is often unknown, but it may be triggered by blood transfusions (p.272) or by drugs such as quinine (*see* **Antimalarial drugs**, p.574) and rifampicin (*see* **Antituberculous drugs**, p.573). In children, the condition is often triggered by a viral infection.

Thrombocytopenia may occur as a result of infection, such as HIV (*see* **HIV infection and AIDS**, p.169), or an autoimmune disorder such as systemic lupus erythematosus (p.281). In some cases, it is associated with cancer.

What are the symptoms?

The symptoms of thrombocytopenia are often mild and may include:

- Easy bruising.
- A rash of many tiny red dots or large purple patches, neither of which fade when pressed (*see* **Purpura**, p.196).
- Bleeding gums and heavy nosebleeds.
- In women, heavy menstrual bleeding.

If you have very low levels of platelets, you may be at increased risk of stroke (p.329) due to bleeding in the brain.

What might be done?

If your doctor suspects from your symptoms that you have thrombocytopenia, he or she may arrange for you to have a blood test to measure your platelet levels. Your doctor may also arrange for you to have a bone marrow aspiration and biopsy (opposite page) in order to obtain tissue samples for examination under the microscope.

Mild thrombocytopenia triggered by a viral infection often clears up without treatment. Bleeding due to extremely low platelet levels may be treated with intravenous platelet infusions while the cause is investigated. If you have drug-induced thrombocytopenia, you will be prescribed an alternative drug that does not affect platelets; the level of platelets in the blood should promptly return to normal. When the condition is due to an immune disorder (immune thrombocytopenia), an oral corticosteroid (p.600) may be prescribed. In severe or recurrent cases due to increased destruction of platelets, removal of the spleen may be necessary for a lasting cure.

Hypercoagulability

An abnormal tendency for blood to clot inside blood vessels

 Gender, genetics, and lifestyle as risk factors depend on the cause

 Age is not a significant factor

Blood clotting normally occurs only when a blood vessel is damaged. The clotting process relies on blood cells called platelets and on proteins in the blood known as clotting factors. Other substances in the blood prevent spontaneous blood clotting or help to dissolve clots. Excessive clotting (hypercoagulability) may result if the balance of clotting and anticlotting mechanisms is upset or if blood flow is slowed down.

Increased blood clotting may be life-threatening. A clot that forms in a vein (*see* **Deep vein thrombosis**, p.263) may travel to the lungs and block an artery (*see* **Pulmonary embolism**, p.302). Clots may also block an artery in the heart, causing a heart attack (*see* **Myocardial infarction**, p.245), or in the brain, causing a stroke (p.329).

What are the causes?

Hypercoagulability may be caused by inherited conditions in which a particular anticlotting substance (proteins C or S, or antithrombin) is deficient, or an abnormal form of a blood clotting factor is produced (as occurs with the inherited gene mutations known as Factor V Leiden and prothrombin ZOZIO).

Another cause of hypercoagulability is increased "stickiness" of platelets due to abnormal platelets being produced by the bone marrow. In women, the disorder may also be a result of changes in the levels of female sex hormones, as may occur in pregnancy, while taking the combined contraceptive pill, and with hormone replacement therapy (HRT).

Raised levels of red blood cells (*see* **Polycythaemia**, p.278) can increase the thickness of the blood, leading to hypercoagulability. Immobility, such as may occur during a long flight or when confined to bed, can also increase the likelihood of hypercoagulability.

What might be done?

If you have a family history of hypercoagulability or develop a blood clot, your doctor may arrange for you to have blood clotting tests. Many people have minor variations from normal in their test results and these do not usually need treatment. Some people have more significant variations from normal, in which case their doctor may prescribe drugs that prevent blood clotting (p.584) and may also advise genetic counselling. Whatever the cause, you should avoid smoking or taking drugs that contain oestrogen, such as combined oral contraceptives and HRT.

Leukaemia

A group of bone marrow cancers in which abnormal white blood cells multiply uncontrollably

 Age, gender, genetics, and lifestyle as risk factors depend on the type

In leukaemia, cancerous white blood cells multiply rapidly and accumulate within the bone marrow, where all types of blood cell are normally produced. This reduces the production of normal white blood cells, red blood cells, and platelets within the bone marrow.

A reduction in the number of red blood cells reduces the oxygen-carrying capacity of blood (*see* **Anaemia**, p.271). If levels of normal white blood cells are reduced, infection becomes a risk, while reduced levels of platelets (which play a vital role in blood clotting) may result in abnormal bleeding (*see* **Thrombocytopenia**, p.275). In most leukaemias, the cancerous white blood cells spread via the blood, causing the lymph nodes, liver, and spleen to become enlarged.

What are the types?
The two main types of leukaemia are acute leukaemia, in which the symptoms develop rapidly, and chronic leukaemia, in which the symptoms can take years to develop. Adults may develop either type of leukaemia, but children usually have the acute form. Acute leukaemia (right) can be divided into acute lymphoblastic and acute myeloid leukaemia, depending on the type of white blood cell involved. Chronic leukaemia also takes two forms: chronic lymphocytic leukaemia (opposite page) and chronic myeloid leukaemia (opposite page).

All leukaemias produce the usual symptoms of anaemia: tiredness, pale skin, and shortness of breath on mild exertion. Other symptoms may include weight loss, fever, night sweats, excessive bleeding, and recurrent infections.

Leukaemia may be diagnosed from a blood test and a bone marrow aspiration and biopsy (p.274). Treatment usually involves chemotherapy (p.157) and, in some cases, radiotherapy (p.158). Blood transfusions (p.272) may also sometimes be necessary. The outlook varies depending on the type of leukaemia and its severity.

Acute leukaemia

A cancer in which large numbers of immature, or abnormal, white blood cells are produced by the bone marrow

 Previous exposure to radiation or toxic chemicals is a risk factor

 Age and gender as risk factors depend on the type

 Genetics is not a significant factor

Acute leukaemia is the most common childhood cancer. Until the 1960s, it was almost always fatal, but now most children survive because of better treatment.

In acute leukaemia, cancerous immature white blood cells multiply rapidly and accumulate in the bone marrow, disrupting the production of normal white blood cells, red blood cells, and platelets. A decrease in the number of normal white blood cells makes the body susceptible to infection. A deficiency of red blood cells leads to a reduction in the oxygen-carrying capacity of the blood (*see* **Anaemia**, p.271). A reduced number of platelets, which help to seal damaged blood vessels, may result in abnormal bleeding (*see* **Thrombocytopenia**, p.275).

There are two main types of acute leukaemia. In acute lymphoblastic leukaemia (ALL), the abnormal type of white blood cell involved is an immature lymphocyte (lymphoblast). In acute myeloid leukaemia (AML), the type of white blood cell that is abnormal is an immature myeloid cell (myeloblast).

ALL is the most common cancer in children; it occurs more often in boys. AML is more common in people over the age of 60, affecting men and women equally. Left untreated, acute leukaemia can be fatal within a few weeks.

What are the causes?
In most cases of acute leukaemia, no cause can be identified. However, there are some factors that have been found to increase the risk of developing the disorder. For example, previous exposure to high levels of radiation, such as from radiotherapy (p.158), or exposure to some anticancer drugs (*see* **Chemotherapy**, p.157) may increase the future risk of acute leukaemia. Exposure to certain toxic chemicals, such as benzene in petrol, may also be a risk factor.

▶ **TREATMENT**

Stem cell transplant

In a stem cell transplant, cancerous or abnormal blood-producing cells (haemopoietic stem cells) are replaced with healthy ones. Before a stem cell transplant, the recipient is given chemotherapy and radiotherapy to eliminate his or her own, abnormal, stem cells; immunosuppressant drugs may also be given to prevent rejection of the donated stem cells. The healthy stem cells may have been supplied by a donor or by the patient when the underlying disease was inactive. The healthy stem cells are usually obtained directly from the blood using a procedure similar to that of a normal blood donation. Healthy stem cells may also sometimes be obtained from the bone marrow, in which case the transplant procedure is usually known as a bone marrow transplant.

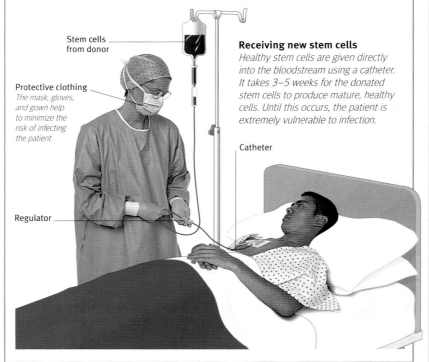

Stem cells from donor

Protective clothing
The mask, gloves, and gown help to minimize the risk of infecting the patient

Regulator

Catheter

Receiving new stem cells
Healthy stem cells are given directly into the bloodstream using a catheter. It takes 3–5 weeks for the donated stem cells to produce mature, healthy cells. Until this occurs, the patient is extremely vulnerable to infection.

People who have myelodysplasia, which is a precancerous abnormality of the bone marrow, or those who have certain chromosomal abnormalities, such as Down's syndrome (p.533), also have an increased risk of developing acute leukaemia.

What are the symptoms?
The symptoms of acute leukaemia are caused by abnormal white blood cells overcrowding the bone marrow, which reduces the numbers of normal blood cells of all types. Symptoms are also caused by the invasion of abnormal blood cells into the bloodstream, where they multiply and spread easily to other organs and tissues in the body. The symptoms of acute leukaemia may develop rapidly and include:
- Tiredness, pale skin, and shortness of breath on exertion due to anaemia.
- Easy bruising and excessive bleeding, often from the gums.
- Bone pain.
- Swelling in the neck, armpits, and groin due to enlarged lymph nodes.
- Swelling of the abdomen due to an enlarged liver and spleen.

Since only immature, nonfunctioning white blood cells are produced, and the cancerous cells are abnormal, susceptibility to infections is increased.

How is it diagnosed?
Your doctor may arrange blood tests to look for abnormal white blood cells, low platelet levels, and reduced numbers of red blood cells. The diagnosis is confirmed by a bone marrow aspiration and biopsy (p.274), a procedure in which tissue samples are obtained for examination under a microscope. You may also need a lumbar puncture (p.326), in which a fluid sample is taken from around the spinal cord, to find out if the disease has spread to the nervous system.

What is the treatment?
If you have acute leukaemia, you will be admitted to hospital, where repeated courses of chemotherapy will be given to kill the abnormal cells in the bone marrow. The aim of this treatment is to induce a remission, a period of time during which the leukaemia is inactive.

You may be given blood transfusions (p.272) to boost the numbers of normal blood cells and antibiotics (p.572) to prevent infection. Some people may need to have radiotherapy to destroy leukaemic cells in the brain.

A stem cell transplant (left) may be offered if a suitable stem cell donor can be found. Before the procedure, you will be given chemotherapy and radiotherapy.

What is the prognosis?
Acute leukaemia is curable, and the outlook for children is better than for adults. Most children treated for acute leukaemia make a full recovery. However, in adults, only about 1 in 3 under the age of 50 who is treated survives for longer than 5 years.

Chronic lymphocytic leukaemia

A bone marrow cancer in which there is uncontrolled production of mature white blood cells called lymphocytes

 Rare under the age of 50; most common between the ages of 60 and 80

 More common in males

 Genetics and lifestyle are not significant factors

Chronic lymphocytic leukaemia (CLL) is the most common type of leukaemia in the UK. It mainly affects people over the age of 50 and is more common in men. The cause is unknown.

In CLL, white blood cells called lymphocytes become cancerous as they mature and multiply uncontrollably in the bone marrow, disrupting the production of normal blood cells. Reduced levels of normal white blood cells leads to increased susceptibility to infection. Although cancerous white blood cells are present in increased numbers, they do not function normally. In addition, fewer red blood cells reduces the oxygen-carrying capacity of blood (*see* **Anaemia**, p.271) and reduced levels of platelets may cause prolonged bleeding (*see* **Thrombocytopenia**, p.275). The abnormal cells may spread to other tissues in the body, such as the lymph nodes, liver, and spleen.

What are the symptoms?
The severity of the disease depends on the white blood cell level and the degree of enlargement of the liver and spleen. Initially, there are often no symptoms, and a diagnosis of CLL is often made from a blood test carried out for some other reason. When symptoms do occur, they usually develop gradually and may include:
- Painless swellings in the armpits, neck, and groin as a result of enlargement of the lymph nodes.
- Swelling of the abdomen due to an enlarged liver and spleen.
- Fever and night sweats.
- Tiredness, pale skin, and shortness of breath on exertion due to anaemia.

As the disease progresses, easy bruising and prolonged episodes of bleeding may occur. If you have CLL, you may be prone to recurrent infections such as shingles (*see* **Herpes zoster**, p.166).

What might be done?
Following an examination, your doctor may arrange for blood tests to measure your levels of red cells and normal and abnormal white cells. He or she may also arrange for a bone marrow aspiration and biopsy (p.274) to obtain tissue samples for microscopic examination.

Treatment of CLL is often not necessary in the early stages. Some people live for many years without developing symptoms or needing specific treatment for CLL, although any infections that develop should be treated promptly. If the disease is advanced, you may need chemotherapy (p.157). You may also be treated with monoclonal antibodies (synthetic antibodies designed to attach to leukaemia cells and help destroy them) or drugs called protein kinase inhibitors, which block the production of leukaemia cells.

Most people with mild CLL survive for more than 10 years after diagnosis. People who are severely affected by this form of leukaemia typically survive for about 1–3 years after diagnosis.

Chronic myeloid leukaemia

A bone marrow cancer in which there is uncontrolled production of mature white blood cells called granulocytes

 More common over the age of 60

 Slightly more common in males

 Almost all cases are linked to an abnormal chromosome

 Previous exposure to radiation is a risk factor

Chronic myeloid leukaemia (CML) develops when the precursors of white blood cells known as granulocytes become cancerous and multiply. The cancerous cells are produced mostly in the bone marrow, but also in the liver and the spleen. All of the granulocytes produced function almost normally in fighting infection.

Chronic myeloid leukaemia is more common in people over the age of 60 and is slightly more common in men.

What are the causes?
The underlying cause of CML is not known, but in almost all cases the cancerous cells contain an abnormal chromosome (known as the Philadelphia chromosome) in which part of one chromosome becomes attached to another. This, in turn, causes two genes (the BCR and ABL genes) to be brought together to form a "fusion" BCR-ABL gene, which is responsible for the formation of abnormal proteins that cause the symptoms of the disease. Rarely, CML is linked with past exposure to radiation, such as that used in radiotherapy (p.158).

What are the symptoms?
There are two phases of CML: a chronic phase and an acute phase. In the chronic phase, you may experience:
- Tiredness, pale skin, and shortness of breath due to anaemia (p.271).
- Swelling of the abdomen due to an enlarged liver and spleen.
- Joint pains due to gout (p.224), which results from the breakdown of excessive numbers of white blood cells.

In the acute phase, CML suddenly transforms into a condition similar to acute leukaemia (opposite page).

What might be done?
CML is usually diagnosed during the chronic phase, often by chance when a blood test is carried out for another reason. If you have CML, the test will show abnormally high levels of granulocytes and their precursors. To confirm the diagnosis, you will have a blood test to look for the BCR-ABL fusion gene. You may also have a bone marrow aspiration and biopsy (p.274) to obtain tissue samples for examination.

Treatment for CML usually involves drugs called protein kinase inhibitors, which stop the BCR-ABL fusion gene from producing abnormal proteins. Most people who receive this treatment during the chronic phase revert to making normal blood cells (which lack the Philadelphia chromosome) and have an excellent chance of long-term survival. If treatment with protein kinase inhibitors is not effective, a stem cell transplant (opposite page) usually produces a cure.

If CML develops into the acute phase, you may be admitted to hospital to have intravenous chemotherapy treatment. Anticancer drugs may be injected directly into the bloodstream through a skin-tunnelled catheter (below). However, treatment rarely succeeds and the condition is usually fatal within a year.

Multiple myeloma

A bone marrow cancer in which abnormal antibody-producing white blood cells multiply in an uncontrolled manner

 Increasingly common over the age of 40; most common around the age of 70

 Gender, genetics, and lifestyle are not significant factors

Multiple myeloma is one of the commonest cancers of the bone marrow and affects plasma cells, the white blood cells that produce antibodies against infection. A plasma cell undergoes a cancerous change, multiplies excessively, and disrupts the production of normal red and white blood cells and platelets. These abnormal, cancerous plasma cells are known as myeloma cells.

The myeloma cells produce abnormal antibodies, and fewer normal antibodies are produced, thereby increasing the risk of infection. The myeloma cells also destroy bone tissue, leading to bone pain, fractures, and release of excess calcium into the bloodstream.

Low numbers of red blood cells may reduce the oxygen-carrying capacity of the

---

▶ **TREATMENT**

Skin-tunnelled catheter

A skin-tunnelled catheter is a flexible plastic tube passed through the skin of the chest or upper arm and inserted into the subclavian vein, which leads to the heart. It is often used in people who have leukaemia or other cancers and need regular chemotherapy (p.157) and blood tests. Using the catheter, drugs can be injected directly into the bloodstream and blood samples can be obtained easily.

The catheter is inserted under local anaesthesia and can remain in position for months. The external end is plugged when not in use. Because the catheter is inserted through the skin some distance away from the site of entry into the vein, the risk of infection is reduced.

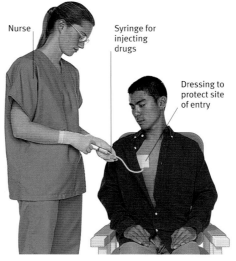

Nurse / Syringe for injecting drugs / Dressing to protect site of entry

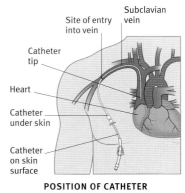

Site of entry into vein / Subclavian vein / Catheter tip / Heart / Catheter under skin / Catheter on skin surface

POSITION OF CATHETER

Using the catheter
The catheter is tunnelled under the skin and enters the subclavian vein to lie with its tip in the heart. A syringe can be attached to inject drugs.

blood (see **Anaemia**, p.271) and reduced numbers of platelets may lead to abnormal bleeding (see **Thrombocytopenia**, p.275).

What are the symptoms?

The symptoms of myeloma include:

- Tiredness, pale skin, and shortness of breath on exertion due to anaemia.
- Bone pain, most often in the spine, as myeloma cells multiply in the bone marrow and spread within the skeleton.
- Repeated infections.
- Easy bruising without injury.
- Thirst, frequent need to pass urine, and constipation due to high calcium levels in the blood.

The loss of calcium from bone tissue may lead to brittle bones that fracture easily. Increased levels of calcium and abnormal antibodies in the blood may lead to kidney failure (p.450).

What might be done?

You may have blood tests to measure levels of blood cells and look for abnormal antibodies. Your urine may also be tested for abnormal antibodies and you may have a bone marrow aspiration and biopsy (p.274). You may have X-rays (p.131) or an MRI scan (p.133) to look for skeletal damage.

There is no cure for multiple myeloma. The aim of treatment is to control the disease so that it goes into remission; that is, so that there are no signs of active disease in your body. There are various treatment options for multiple myeloma and the treatment that will be recommended for you will depend on factors such as your age, general health, symptoms, and how far the disease has progressed. If you have no symptoms, your doctor may suggest simply close monitoring. For people who do have symptoms, the initial treatment is usually with a combination of chemotherapy (p.157) and corticosteroid drugs (p.600). Other treatment options include new drugs for multiple myeloma, such as thalidomide and bortezomib. For people who are fit enough, further intensive treatment with high-dose chemotherapy and a stem cell transplant (p.276) may be suggested.

Radiotherapy (p.158) may be given for severe bone pain. You may need blood transfusions (p.272) for severe anaemia, although the anaemia may be improved and the need for transfusions reduced by injections of erythropoietin (a hormone that stimulates red blood cell production). Infections may be treated with antibiotics (p.572). You may be given bisphosphonates (see **Drugs for bone disorders**, p.579) to treat high calcium levels; these drugs also slow the progress of skeletal damage. Drinking plenty of fluids will also help to lower calcium levels and reduce the risk of kidney damage.

The outlook varies according to the age of the person affected and the severity of the disorder. Survival has improved in recent years and most people live for up to 5 years after diagnosis, while some have survived for more than 10 years.

Polycythaemia

A blood disorder in which there is an increased concentration of red blood cells

 Sometimes due to an abnormal gene

 Age and lifestyle as risk factors depend on the type

 Gender is not a significant factor

In polycythaemia (also known as erythrocytosis), the concentration of red blood cells is increased. The condition may be due to increased red blood cell production or decreased volume of the fluid part of blood (plasma), leading to a high concentration of red cells.

What are the types?

There are four types of polycythaemia: primary, secondary, stress, and idiopathic erythrocytosis.

In primary polycythaemia, which is also known as true polycythaemia or polycythaemia vera, the production of red blood cells in the bone marrow is increased as a result of a mutation (change) in a gene called the JAK2 gene, which is involved in the regulation of red blood cell production. This type of polycythaemia is rare and usually only affects people over the age of 60.

In secondary polycythaemia, there is also increased production of red cells by the bone marrow. In this case, the cause is a low oxygen level in the blood, which can occur for several reasons. For example, it can develop in people living at high altitudes, where oxygen levels are naturally low. It may also occur if the uptake of oxygen by the blood is impaired due to heavy smoking or lung disorders such as chronic obstructive pulmonary disease (p.297).

In stress polycythaemia, production of red cells is normal but the volume of blood plasma is decreased. This change in the composition of blood may result from

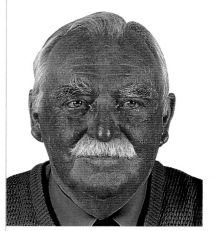

Effect of polycythaemia
This man's ruddy complexion is due to polycythaemia, an abnormally high concentration of red cells in the blood.

dehydration. It may also occur in people who are obese or abuse alcohol.

In idiopathic erythrocytosis, the cause of the increased concentration of red blood cells is unknown.

What are the symptoms?

All types of polycythaemia cause similar symptoms. They may include:

- A ruddy complexion, together with bloodshot eyes.
- Headache and ringing in the ears (see **Tinnitus**, p.378).
- Blurred vision and dizziness.

Primary polycythaemia may also produce itching, especially after a hot bath. The spleen may enlarge, causing abdominal discomfort and there may also be prolonged bleeding or increased blood clotting.

What might be done?

Your doctor may arrange for a blood test to measure the concentration of red cells in the blood and to check for the presence of a mutated JAK2 gene. You may also have tests to look for lung disease, such as a chest X-ray (p.300), and an ultrasound scan (p.135) of your abdomen to look for enlargement of the spleen.

If you have secondary or stress polycythaemia, the treatment is directed at the underlying cause, although venesection (removal of blood from a vein) may sometimes be used.

Venesection may also be used to treat primary polycythaemia or idiopathic erythrocytosis. At least 300 ml (10 fl oz) of blood are removed from the circulation at each treatment session to control the number of red blood cells. People with primary polycythaemia are likely to need more venesection and initially may have weekly sessions. Those with primary polycythaemia may also be treated with low-dose aspirin. In some cases, low-intensity chemotherapy (p.157) may also be used to reduce the production of red blood cells.

With treatment, most people live for 10–15 years after diagnosis. Rarely, primary polycythaemia may develop into another bone marrow disorder, such as acute leukaemia (p.276).

Disorders of the lymphatic system

The lymphatic system consists of lymph nodes, or glands, connected by a network of lymphatic vessels that extends to all parts of the body. The system drains a fluid called lymph from the body's tissues back into the bloodstream. It also protects the body against infection and the development of cancer by filtering out infectious organisms and cancerous cells from the lymph.

Lymph, a fluid that contains white blood cells called lymphocytes, fats, and protein, flows along the network of lymphatic vessels and ultimately re-enters the bloodstream from which it originally came. Along the way, lymph is filtered through the lymph nodes, which are located in clusters close to the skin's surface in the neck, armpits, and groin. Nodes are also found deep within the abdomen and chest. The lymph nodes contain large numbers of lymphocytes, white blood cells that can destroy infectious organisms or cancer cells. Lymphocytes can also develop into cells that produce antibodies, which help other white blood cells trap and destroy infectious organisms and cancer cells throughout the body.

The first article in this section covers lymphadenopathy, in which the lymph nodes become enlarged. A painful swelling of the lymph nodes is not often a cause for concern, but painless swelling may be a sign of a serious underlying disorder, such as cancer. The next articles cover lymphangitis, in which lymphatic vessels are inflamed, and lymphoedema, in which lymph cannot drain from a limb, causing the limb to swell. In developed countries, a common cause of lymphoedema is surgery or radiotherapy for cancer. The final article discusses lymphomas, a group of cancers that may develop in one or more lymph nodes.

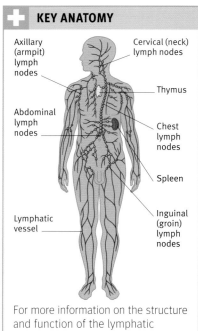

KEY ANATOMY

Axillary (armpit) lymph nodes

Cervical (neck) lymph nodes

Thymus

Abdominal lymph nodes

Chest lymph nodes

Spleen

Lymphatic vessel

Inguinal (groin) lymph nodes

For more information on the structure and function of the lymphatic system, see pp.265–270.

Lymphadenopathy

Enlarged lymph nodes, also known as swollen glands, which usually develop as a response to infection

 Age, gender, genetics, and lifestyle as risk factors depend on the cause

Swelling of the lymph nodes is a common symptom of many conditions. A single node, a group of nodes, or all the lymph nodes may be affected. Lymph nodes most commonly become swollen in response to a bacterial or viral infection. You are more likely to notice a swollen lymph node in the neck, groin, or armpit, because the nodes in these areas lie closest to the skin.

Swelling of a single node or group of lymph nodes is often due to a localized bacterial infection. For example, swollen lymph nodes in the neck are commonly caused by throat infections. In most cases of lymphadenopathy due to an infection, the swelling usually subsides when the infection clears up. Swollen lymph nodes that are the result of an infection are often painful.

Persistent swelling of many, or all, of the lymph nodes may be a result of some types of cancer, such as breast cancer (p.486), lymphoma (right), or leukaemia (p.276). Swollen lymph nodes due to cancer are not normally painful.

In the UK, long-term infections, such as tuberculosis (p.300) and HIV infection (*see* **HIV infection and AIDS**, p.169), are an uncommon cause of persistent lymphadenopathy.

You should consult your doctor if a swelling is persistent or if you are worried about accompanying symptoms.

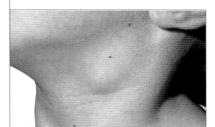

Lymphadenopathy in the neck
A throat infection may cause swelling of the lymph nodes. Here, a swollen lymph node is visible on the side of the neck.

Lymphangitis

Inflammation of the lymphatic vessels as a result of a bacterial infection

 Age, gender, genetics, and lifestyle are not significant factors

Lymphangitis develops when bacteria spread into lymphatic vessels close to the site of an infection, possibly as a result of

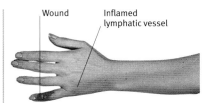

Wound   Inflamed lymphatic vessel

Lymphangitis of the arm
Inflamed lymphatic vessels (lymphangitis) have produced a red streak on the skin. The inflammation is due to bacteria that have spread from a wound on the finger.

an injury. The condition usually affects lymphatic vessels in an arm or a leg and may be accompanied by fever, headache, and a general sense of feeling unwell. The infected lymphatic vessels become inflamed and tender, and hot, red streaks may appear on the skin over the inflamed vessels. Lymph nodes near to the affected area sometimes become swollen (*see* **Lymphadenopathy**, left). If you develop any of these symptoms following an injury, you should consult your doctor immediately.

In some cases, ulcers form in the skin over an infected lymph vessel. Without treatment, the infection may spread into the blood (*see* **Septicaemia**, p.171), which can be life-threatening.

If your doctor suspects that you have lymphangitis from your symptoms and after a physical examination, he or she may take a sample of your blood, which will be tested in a laboratory to check whether the infection has spread into the blood. Antibiotics (p.572) will be prescribed to treat the lymphangitis. The symptoms of the condition usually begin to clear up within about 24 hours of starting antibiotic treatment.

Lymphoedema

A localized accumulation of fluid in the lymphatic vessels, causing painless swelling of a limb

 More common in females

 Sometimes runs in families

 Age and lifestyle are not significant factors

Lymphoedema occurs when a defect in the lymphatic vessels prevents drainage of lymph from a limb. Most commonly, lymphoedema is caused by damage to the lymphatic vessels following surgery or radiotherapy (p.158), for example in the treatment of breast cancer (p.486). Rarely, the condition may be due to the blockage of a lymphatic vessel by a cancerous growth in a lymph node.

Lymphoedema can be inherited, in which case it results from incomplete development of the lymphatic vessels. This type is more common in women.

Although the symptoms of lymphoedema may be present from birth, they usually first occur at puberty. The main

symptom is painless swelling of a limb. The skin over the affected limb often becomes rough and thickened. Injury to a limb affected by lymphoedema may result in a rapid spread of infection through the tissues. You should contact your doctor immediately if you injure a limb affected by lymphoedema.

In most cases, lymphoedema is a lifelong disorder and treatment is aimed at relieving the symptoms. You can reduce swelling by keeping the affected limb elevated; wearing an elastic stocking or sleeve helps to prevent further swelling.

Lymphoma

Any of several types of cancer arising in the lymphatic system

 Sometimes runs in families

 Age as a risk factor depends on the type

 Gender and lifestyle are not significant factors

The lymphomas are a group of diseases in which immune cells become cancerous and multiply uncontrollably in a lymph node. Initially, a single node may be affected, but the cancer may spread to other nodes and to other tissues, such as the bone marrow.

Lymphomas can be divided into two main categories: Hodgkin's and non-Hodgkin's lymphomas. In Hodgkin's lymphoma, a particular type of cancer cell is present. All the other types of lymphoma are classified as non-Hodgkin's lymphoma. Non-Hodgkin's lymphoma is about three times more common than Hodgkin's lymphoma, and it usually develops in people over the age of 50. Hodgkin's lymphoma most commonly occurs in people who are between the ages of 15 and 30 and the ages of 55 and 70. Different types of lymphoma grow and spread at different rates.

What are the causes?

The cause of lymphoma is not known but the condition sometimes runs in families, suggesting that a genetic factor is involved. Lymphomas are more common if immunity is reduced, such as in people with AIDS (*see* **HIV infection and AIDS**, p.169) or those who are taking immunosuppressant drugs (p.585). Some lymphomas may be triggered by a viral or bacterial infection. For example, Burkitt's lymphoma, which is common in children in equatorial Africa, is associated with the Epstein–Barr virus, and lymphomas of the stomach are associated with infection with the *Helicobacter pylori* bacterium (p.405).

What are the symptoms?

The symptoms of lymphoma, common to all types, may include:

■ One or more persistent and painless swellings in the neck, armpits, or groin caused by enlarged lymph nodes.

■ Fever and sweating at night.
■ Weight loss.
■ Abdominal swelling and discomfort due to enlarged lymph nodes or an enlarged spleen.

Some people with lymphoma develop anaemia (p.271), which causes symptoms such as tiredness, pale skin, and shortness of breath on mild exertion.

What might be done?

Your doctor may suspect lymphoma from your symptoms and following a physical examination. He or she may arrange for a blood test to check for anaemia. A tissue sample may also be taken from a swollen node to find out whether cancerous cells are present.

If lymphoma is diagnosed, further tests may be needed to find out how far the disease has progressed. These may include imaging techniques, such as CT scanning (p.132), to assess the size of lymph nodes in the chest and abdomen. You may also have bone marrow aspiration and biopsy (p.274) to determine whether your bone marrow is affected.

Treatment depends on the type of lymphoma and how far it has spread. However, in general, if only one node or one group of nodes is affected, the lymphoma may be treated with local radiotherapy (p.158) alone. When more than one group of lymph nodes is affected, the usual treatment is chemotherapy (p.157), which may be combined with corticosteroid drugs (p.600) or radiotherapy. In many cases, biological therapy is also used. This involves treatment with monoclonal antibodies (synthetic antibodies designed to attach to lymphoma cells and help destroy them) or with protein kinase inhibitors (drugs that block the production of lymphoma cells). In some cases, a stem cell transplant (p.276) may be recommended.

What is the prognosis?

The prognosis depends on the type of lymphoma and how far it has spread. If the cancer is not detectable following treatment, the disease is said to have gone into remission. However, lymphomas sometimes recur, and further courses of treatment may be necessary. If remission continues for 5 years or more, the risk of recurrence is small.

After treatment for Hodgkin's lymphoma, at least 8 in 10 people enter a long-term period of remission and can be assumed to be cured. About half of all people treated for non-Hodgkin's lymphoma enter long-term remission and are considered to be cured.

Immune disorders

Our immune systems protect us from the threat of infection by microorganisms, such as bacteria and viruses, and parasites, such as worms. The immune system also protects us from certain cancers and helps to repair damaged tissues. We are born with certain built-in defence mechanisms, but much of our immunity is acquired as we are exposed to the organisms that cause disease.

This section begins with an overview of acquired immunodeficiency, one of the major disorders of the immune system. Acquired immunodeficiency is a condition, developing after birth, in which the immune system fails to function properly and is unable to combat microorganisms that invade the body. Such immunodeficiency develops for a variety of reasons. The most widely publicized form of acquired immunodeficiency is AIDS, which develops after infection with the human immunodeficiency virus (see **HIV infection and AIDS**, p.169).

A temporary, mild form of acquired immunodeficiency may appear after infection with other viruses, such as measles (p.167), and may also develop following certain drug treatments.

The second overview article covers autoimmune disorders, which occur when a person's immune system functions abnormally and starts to attack the body's own tissues, causing certain organs to become inflamed and damaged. Individual autoimmune disorders that affect more than one organ are covered next. Such disorders can occur at any age and can lead to persistent poor health. Their causes are not fully understood, although a combination of genetic and environmental factors seem to be involved. Overall, women are affected much more commonly and severely by autoimmune disorders.

Autoimmune disorders that affect specific organs or sites in the body are considered in the relevant sections of this book. For example, rheumatoid arthritis (p.222), which primarily affects the joints, is dealt with in the musculoskeletal disorders section and Hashimoto's thyroiditis (see **Thyroiditis**, p.433), which causes the underproduction of hormones from the thyroid gland, is covered in the section dealing with metabolic disorders. Immunodeficiency that is present from birth is covered in the section of the book dealing with children's disorders (see **Congenital immunodeficiency**, p.536).

Acquired immunodeficiency

Complete or partial failure of the immune system, developing after birth

 Age, gender, genetics, and lifestyle as risk factors depend on the cause

Immunodeficiency is the term used for failure of the immune system to combat infections effectively. As a result of immunodeficiency, infections develop more frequently than normal and are a greater threat to health. Infections that would not normally seriously affect a healthy person may be life-threatening in someone who has immunodeficiency. They include viral infections, such as shingles and chickenpox (p.165), both of which are caused by herpes zoster (p.166) and cause only mild illnesses if the immune system is normal.

Immunodeficiency may be present from birth, in which case it is often inherited (see **Congenital immunodeficiency**, p.536). More commonly, the deficiency in a person's immune system develops later in life, and in such cases the condition is given the name acquired immunodeficiency.

Worldwide, acquired immunodeficiency is most often associated with malnutrition or with infection with the human immunodeficiency virus (see **HIV infection and AIDS**, p.169).

What are the causes?

In AIDS, the human immunodeficiency virus (HIV) destroys a particular type of white blood cell, and this causes progressive immunodeficiency.

Infections such as influenza (p.164) or measles (p.167) damage the body's ability to fight infection. They do this partly by reducing the number of white blood cells involved in fighting the infection. Usually, this type of immunodeficiency is mild, and the immune system returns to normal once the person has recovered from the infection.

A mild form of immunodeficiency may occur in some long-term disorders, including diabetes mellitus (p.437) and rheumatoid arthritis (p.222). This may occur partly because these diseases put stress on the immune system, reducing its ability to resist other diseases.

Certain types of cancer, particularly tumours of the lymphatic system (see **Lymphoma**, p.279), may cause a more severe form of immunodeficiency by damaging the cells of the immune system and by reducing the production of normal white blood cells.

The long-term use of corticosteroids (p.600) suppresses the immune system and has the inevitable effect of causing immunodeficiency. Immunosuppressant drugs (p.585), which may be given to prevent the rejection of an organ following transplant surgery (p.614), also produce immunodeficiency and affect the body's ability to fight infections. Chemotherapy (p.157) can damage the bone marrow, where the majority of blood cells are made, and may also lead to acquired immunodeficiency.

Immunodeficiency may also develop after surgical removal of the spleen, an organ in which some of the white blood cells are produced. Splenectomy may be performed if the spleen has been damaged by an injury, or it may be carried out to treat various disorders including hereditary spherocytosis, which is a type of haemolytic anaemia (p.273).

There are many other types of acquired immunodeficiency, the causes of which are not clear. One type is immunoglobulin A (IgA) deficiency, in which levels of immunoglobulin A antibodies are lower than normal.

What might be done?

Your doctor may suspect immunodeficiency if you have recurrent infections. To confirm the diagnosis of acquired immunodeficiency, you may need to have blood tests that measure the levels of white blood cells and antibodies.

If immunodeficiency is due to drug treatment, it may be possible to reduce the dose or stop taking the drug. If the underlying cause cannot be cured or reversed, treatment is aimed at reducing the risk of infection and combating infections as they occur. Your doctor may suggest regular intravenous infusions of immunoglobulin; continual low doses of antibiotics (p.572), antiviral drugs (p.573), and/or antifungal drugs (p.574); and various immunizations, such as the pneumococcus vaccine (see **Vaccines and immunoglobulins**, p.571) to protect against pneumococcal pneumonia.

The effects of immunodeficiency can usually be controlled by treatment, although immunodeficiency due to HIV infection may worsen over time.

Autoimmune disorders

Disorders in which the immune system malfunctions and reacts against the body's own tissues

 More common in adults. Less common in childhood and in old age

 More common in females

 Sometimes run in families

 Lifestyle is not a significant factor for most disorders

If a person is healthy, the cells of the immune system are able to distinguish between the body tissues and foreign organisms such as bacteria and viruses. If someone has an autoimmune disorder, the immune system mistakenly interprets the body's own tissues as foreign. As a result, antibodies or white blood cells are formed that attack the body tissues and try to destroy them.

The underlying cause of this abnormal immune reaction is unclear, but it can run in families. Certain factors, such as some viral infections and reactions to particular drugs, may trigger an autoimmune reaction in susceptible people. Hormonal factors may also play a part, since these disorders occur more often in women than in men.

What are the types?

In some autoimmune disorders, the tissues of a single organ are damaged, preventing normal function. Examples of organs that may be affected by these disorders include the thyroid gland in Hashimoto's thyroiditis (see **Thyroiditis**, p.433), the pancreas in diabetes mellitus (p.437), the adrenal glands in Addison's disease (p.436), and various joints in rheumatoid arthritis (p.222).

A second group of autoimmune disorders affects connective tissue (the material that holds together the structures of the body) and the blood vessels that supply this tissue (see **Scleroderma**, opposite page, and **Systemic lupus erythematosus**, opposite page). In these disorders, the immune system may react against connective tissue anywhere in the body.

What might be done?

If your doctor suspects an autoimmune disorder, he or she may arrange for blood tests to assess immune function and look for evidence of inflammation. The treatment of autoimmune disorders depends on which organs are affected. In Hashimoto's thyroiditis or Addison's disease, damage to the affected organs leads to a deficiency in the hormones they normally produce. Replacement of deficient hormones often restores health. In other cases, the aim of treatment is to block the abnormal immune reactions with drugs such as immunosuppressants (p.585) or corticosteroids (p.600) or reduce symptoms with nonsteroidal anti-inflammatory drugs (p.578).

The outlook for people who have autoimmune disorders depends on the amount of damage to the body's tissues and organs. Autoimmune disorders are usually lifelong, but the symptoms can often be controlled with drugs. In some cases, serious complications such as kidney failure (p.450) may develop.

Systemic lupus erythematosus

Inflammation of the body's connective tissues and the blood vessels that supply them, causing damage to the skin, joints, and internal organs

 Most common between the ages of 16 and 55

 Much more common in females

 Sometimes runs in families; more common in some ethnic groups

 Stress and sunlight may be risk factors

In systemic lupus erythematosus (SLE), the body produces antibodies that react against its own connective tissues. These tissues, which surround body structures and hold them together, become inflamed and swollen. SLE may affect only a few parts of the body or many, and symptoms may range from mild to severe.

The cause of the abnormal immune reaction that occurs in SLE is not known, but it may be triggered by factors such as a viral infection, stress, or sunlight. Hormonal factors may also be involved because many more women than men are affected. SLE sometimes runs in families and appears to be more common in black and Asian women, which suggests that a genetic factor is involved. Symptoms similar to those of SLE may be caused by certain drugs, such as hydralazine (*see* **Antihypertensive drugs**, p.580) and chlorpromazine (*see* **Antipsychotic drugs**, p.592).

What are the symptoms?

In typical cases of SLE, the symptoms flare up intermittently for periods of weeks and then become less severe, sometimes for months or even years, but they rarely disappear completely.

People who have SLE may have widely varying symptoms. Some people suffer from mild symptoms that appear gradually, whereas others report a wide range of more severe symptoms that develop rapidly. The most common symptoms are:

- Aching, swollen joints, which may become increasingly painful.
- Skin rashes – characteristically a raised, red, butterfly-shaped rash on the nose and cheeks.
- Increased sensitivity to sunlight.
- Tiredness and fever.
- Mild depression.

Additionally, there may be less common symptoms of SLE, which include:

- Shortness of breath and chest pain if the membrane covering the lungs is inflamed (*see* **Pleurisy**, p.301).
- Headaches, seizures, or strokes due to involvement of the nervous system.
- Constant chest pain if the membrane that covers the heart is inflamed (*see* **Pericarditis**, p.258).

- Hair loss.
- Pale skin.
- Painless mouth ulcers.

Women who have SLE may find that their symptoms become worse while they are taking oral contraceptive pills or during pregnancy, as a result of hormonal changes.

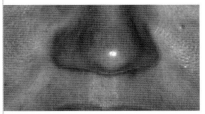

Butterfly-shaped rash in SLE
A common symptom of systemic lupus erythematosus is a red, raised rash that spreads across the nose and the cheeks in a shape that resembles a butterfly.

Are there complications?

SLE may cause damage to the kidneys, which can lead to high blood pressure (*see* **Hypertension**, p.242) and eventually kidney failure (p.450). SLE also increases the risk of cardiovascular disease. In severe cases, problems with painful, swollen joints may cause deformity. SLE may occur in association with Sjögren's syndrome (right) and rheumatoid arthritis (p.222).

Although many women with SLE have successful pregnancies, the risk of having an early miscarriage (p.511) is increased. If you have SLE and are planning a pregnancy, you ask your doctor for advice.

What might be done?

Since the symptoms of SLE are so varied, they often mimic those of other disorders. However, if your doctor suspects that you may have SLE, he or she may arrange for blood tests to look for antibodies associated with the condition. You may also need to have specific tests to determine whether particular organs have been affected.

There is no cure for SLE; treatment is aimed at relieving the symptoms and slowing the progression of the condition. However, if you have SLE-like symptoms that are triggered by a particular drug, your doctor will prescribe an alternative treatment if possible, and your symptoms should gradually disappear within a few weeks or months.

If your joints are painful, your doctor may recommend a nonsteroidal anti-inflammatory drug (p.578). You may also be given the drug hydroxychloroquine (*see* **Antimalarial drugs**, p.574), which is often used to control the symptoms of SLE. A corticosteroid (p.600) may be given to suppress severe inflammation. If corticosteroids are ineffective, an immunosuppressant drug (p.585) may be prescribed. Physiotherapy (p.620) may be suggested for joint problems. Your doctor may also advise you to avoid direct exposure to the sun and to ensure that infections are treated promptly.

Most people with SLE can lead an active life. However, in more severe cases, life expectancy may be shortened.

Scleroderma

Thickening and hardening of the connective tissues in the skin, joints, and internal organs

 Most common between the ages of 30 and 50

 More common in females

 Sometimes runs in families

 Lifestyle is not a significant factor

Scleroderma, also known as systemic sclerosis, is a rare disorder in which the connective tissues that hold together the structures of the body become inflamed, damaged, and thickened. The tissues, particularly those in the skin, then contract and harden.

This condition is an autoimmune disorder in which the body produces antibodies that attack and damage its own connective tissues. The reason for this reaction is unknown, but genetic factors may play a part since the condition may sometimes run in families. Scleroderma is approximately four times more common in women than it is in men and occurs most commonly in adults under the age of 50.

What are the symptoms?

Scleroderma commonly affects the skin and the joints, but other organs may be involved. Symptoms vary from mild to severe and may include:

- Fingers or toes that are sensitive to the cold, becoming white and painful (*see* **Raynaud's phenomenon and Raynaud's disease**, p.262).
- Ulcers and small, hardened areas that appear on the fingers.
- Swollen fingers or hands.
- Pain in the joints, especially the joints in the hands.
- Thickening and tightening of the skin, which is most severe on the limbs but may affect the trunk and face.
- Muscle weakness.
- Difficulty swallowing due to stiffening of the tissues of the oesophagus.

If the lungs are affected, shortness of breath may develop. In some people, scleroderma causes high blood pressure (*see* **Hypertension**, p.242) and eventually kidney failure (p.450).

What might be done?

Your doctor may be able to make a diagnosis from your symptoms and from a physical examination. He or she may also arrange for blood tests to look for certain antibodies. A small skin sample may also be taken for examination.

There is no cure for scleroderma, but treatment can slow progression of the condition, reduce the damage to body organs, and relieve symptoms. If the lungs are affected, an immunosuppressant drug

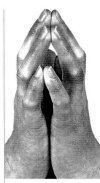

Effects of scleroderma
In a person with scleroderma, the skin on the fingers and hands may become thickened and swollen, making it difficult to straighten the fingers.

(p.585) may be prescribed. Calcium channel blockers (p.582) may be prescribed to treat Raynaud's phenomenon, and your doctor may also advise you to keep your fingers and toes warm. If your muscles or joints are affected, a corticosteroid (p.600) may be prescribed. ACE inhibitors (p.582) may also be prescribed to protect your kidneys.

The course of scleroderma is variable. Scleroderma that mainly affects the skin tends to be milder, with the internal organs being less severely affected. However, when several organs are affected, the condition tends to be more severe and can be life-threatening.

Sjögren's syndrome

Damage to glands, including the tear and salivary glands, causing dryness of the eyes and mouth

 Most common between the ages of 40 and 60

 More common in females

 Sometimes runs in families

 Lifestyle is not a significant factor

Sjögren's syndrome is a lifelong disorder in which damage to the tear and salivary glands causes the eyes and mouth to become very dry. Glands that lubricate the skin, nasal cavity, throat, and vagina may also be affected.

The syndrome is an autoimmune disorder in which gland tissues are attacked by the body's own antibodies and become inflamed and damaged. The cause is not known, but genetic factors may play a role. The condition is nine times more common in women and usually occurs between the ages of 40 and 60.

The main symptoms usually develop over several years and include gritty, red, dry eyes and dry mouth. Lack of saliva often leads to difficulty swallowing dry foods and to dental problems (*see* **Dental caries**, p.384). Some people develop joint problems similar to rheumatoid arthritis (p.222).

What might be done?

Your doctor may be able to make a diagnosis from your symptoms and an examination. He or she may arrange for blood tests to

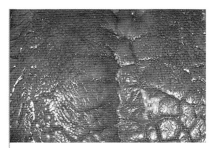

Dry tongue in Sjögren's syndrome
The salivary glands become inflamed in Sjögren's syndrome, preventing normal saliva production. As a result, the mouth and the tongue become very dry.

look for antibodies. You may also need to have tests to measure the quantity of tears your eyes produce, and a small sample of tissue may be removed from your salivary glands to look for damaged cells.

There is no cure for this disorder, but symptoms can be controlled, usually with lifelong treatment. Artificial tears may be prescribed or, occasionally, tear ducts will be plugged by an ophthalmologist to decrease tear drainage. You will be advised to drink plenty of liquids and to visit your dentist regularly. If symptoms are severe, a corticosteroid (p.600), an immunosuppressant (p.585), or the drug hydroxychloroquine (*see* **Antimalarial drugs**, p.574) may be given to reduce the inflammation.

Polymyositis and dermatomyositis

Muscle inflammation (polymyositis), sometimes with a rash (dermatomyositis)

 Most common in children aged 5–15 and adults aged 40–60

 More common in females

 Sometimes runs in families

 Lifestyle is not a significant factor

In polymyositis, inflammation of the muscles causes muscle weakness and wasting, particularly around the shoulders and pelvis. If a rash also occurs, the disorder is known as dermatomyositis. Both conditions are rare autoimmune disorders in which tissues are attacked by the body's own antibodies. The cause of this abnormal immune reaction is not known, although its onset may be triggered by a viral infection. These diseases can occur in association with other autoimmune disorders, such as rheumatoid arthritis (p.222). In adults, dermatomyositis may be associated with cancer. Polymyositis and dermatomyositis sometimes run in families, which suggests that genetic factors may be involved. Both disorders are more common in females and tend to occur in childhood and middle age.

What are the symptoms?
The symptoms of polymyositis and dermatomyositis may develop rapidly, particularly in children; in adults, the symptoms usually develop over several weeks. Symptoms may include:
- Weakness of affected muscles, leading, for example, to difficulty raising the arms or getting up from a sitting or squatting position.
- Painful, swollen joints.
- Tiredness.
- Difficulty swallowing if the muscles of the throat are affected.
- Shortness of breath if the heart or chest muscles are involved.

In dermatomyositis, the above symptoms may be preceded, accompanied, or followed by:
- A red rash, often on the face, chest, or backs of the hands over the knuckles.
- Swollen, reddish-purple eyelids.

About half of all children who have dermatomyositis develop skin ulcers.

What might be done?
If polymyositis or dermatomyositis is suspected, your doctor may arrange for blood tests to investigate inflammation and to look for antibodies that are specific to these conditions. You may also have electromyography (*see* **Nerve and muscle electrical tests**, p.337) to measure electrical activity in the muscle, and a muscle biopsy, in which a sample of muscle tissue is removed for examination. An ECG (p.243) may be carried out to check for involvement of the heart muscle. You may also have a chest X-ray (p.300) and other tests to exclude the possibility of an underlying cancer.

There is no cure for polymyositis or dermatomyositis. However, the symptoms can usually be controlled. You will probably be prescribed high doses of corticosteroids (p.600) to help to reduce the inflammation. If there is no marked improvement, an immunosuppressant drug (p.585) or a drug that is normally used to treat cancer (*see* **Anticancer drugs**, p.586), may be given to slow the progression of the disorder. If dermatomyositis does not respond to these drugs, injections of immunoglobulins (antibodies) may be given. Physiotherapy (p.620) may help to prevent muscle stiffness and restore strength.

What is the prognosis?
The outlook for both polymyositis and dermatomyositis is better in children than in adults. About 7 in 10 affected children recover completely in 2 years. Adults with polymyositis or dermatomyositis may need corticosteroid drugs for several years. In people who have cancer, the autoimmune disorder may improve if the cancer can be treated.

Polymyalgia rheumatica

Pain and stiffness in the muscles around the shoulders and hips

 Rare under the age of 60

 Twice as common in females

 Sometimes runs in families

 Lifestyle is not a significant factor

In polymyalgia rheumatica, inflammation of tissues causes pain and stiffness in the neck, shoulders, hips, and lower back as well as a general sense of feeling unwell and loss of energy.

Polymyalgia rheumatica is an autoimmune disorder in which the immune system attacks the body's own tissues. The condition is relatively common in those over 60, affects more women than men, and can run in families. It may occur in association with the disorder giant cell arteritis (right).

What are the symptoms?
The symptoms usually appear over a few weeks but sometimes develop suddenly. They may include:
- Painful, stiff muscles, especially first thing in the morning.
- Tiredness.
- Fever and night sweats.
- Weight loss.
- Depression (p.343).

The symptoms may be accompanied by those of giant cell arteritis, such as severe headaches on one or both sides of the head and tenderness of the scalp.

What might be done?
Your doctor will probably be able to make a diagnosis based on your symptoms, a physical examination, and the results of blood tests to look for inflammation. In some cases, additional blood tests may be performed to exclude other disorders, such as rheumatoid arthritis (p.222).

Your doctor will probably prescribe an oral corticosteroid (p.600) to reduce the inflammation. If you also have giant cell arteritis, the initial doses of this drug may be higher. In either case, the dose will be reduced to a maintenance level once the symptoms subside.

Symptoms are usually relieved soon after starting corticosteroid treatment. However, polymyalgia rheumatica may persist for years, in which case you need to continue taking low doses of a corticosteroid to control symptoms.

Giant cell (temporal) arteritis

Inflammation of the blood vessels around the head and scalp

 Rare under the age of 55; increasingly common with age

 More common in females

 Sometimes runs in families; more common in white people

 Lifestyle is not a significant factor

In giant cell arteritis, also called temporal arteritis, particular arteries become inflamed and narrowed, reducing the blood flow through them. The disorder mainly affects blood vessels in the head and scalp, such as the temporal arteries (the arteries on the sides of the forehead). In some cases, the arteries that supply blood to the eyes are affected.

The cause of giant cell arteritis is not known, but it may be due to an autoimmune reaction in which the immune system attacks the arteries. Giant cell arteritis may occur with polymyalgia rheumatica (left), may sometimes run in families (suggesting that genetic factors may be involved), and is more common in women and older people.

What are the symptoms?
If you have giant cell arteritis, you may notice the following symptoms:
- Severe headaches affecting either one or both sides of the head.
- Tenderness of the scalp.
- Pain in the sides of the face, which becomes worse on chewing.
- Prominent, tender temporal arteries.
- Tiredness.
- Loss of appetite and weight loss.

These symptoms may be accompanied by those of polymyalgia rheumatica, such as pain and stiffness in the muscles of the shoulders and hips. In rare cases, a stroke (p.329) may occur. If you also develop visual disturbances, you should consult your doctor at once because untreated giant cell arteritis can lead to loss of an area of vision or even blindness.

What might be done?
Your doctor may be able to diagnose giant cell arteritis from your description of the headache and by a physical examination. He or she may arrange for an urgent blood test to look for inflammation. You may also have a biopsy of the temporal artery, in which a tissue sample is taken for examination.

To reduce inflammation, a high dose of an oral corticosteroid (p.600) will be prescribed immediately. The symptoms of giant cell arteritis usually improve within 24 hours of starting treatment. Once the condition improves, the initial high dose of corticosteroid will be reduced, but you may need to continue taking smaller doses for 2–3 years.

Your doctor will probably recommend that you have regular blood tests to monitor the course of the disorder. He or she may prescribe an immunosuppressant (p.585) as an alternative drug if there is little or no improvement in your condition or if you develop side effects with the corticosteroid.

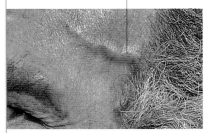
Temporal artery

Giant cell arteritis
The temporal artery shown above is prominent and inflamed due to giant cell arteritis. Headaches and tenderness of the scalp are common with this disorder.

What is the prognosis?
In some cases, giant cell arteritis may clear up completely with treatment, but in other cases the symptoms may recur. If you already have vision impairment due to giant cell arteritis, your sight may not improve with treatment. However, it may be possible to prevent further deterioration of your vision.

Polyarteritis nodosa

Widespread tissue damage as a result of patchy inflammation of the arteries

 Can occur at any age, but most common between the ages of 40 and 60

 Twice as common in males

 Genetics and lifestyle are not significant factors

In polyarteritis nodosa, segments of small- to medium-sized arteries are inflamed, reducing the blood supply to skin, muscles, joints, and many of the internal organs. If the arteries that supply the heart or kidneys are affected, the condition may be life-threatening.

Polyarteritis nodosa is an autoimmune disorder in which the immune system attacks the body's own arteries. The cause of the abnormal immune reaction is not known, but the hepatitis B and C viruses (*see* **Acute hepatitis**, p.408) have been found in some people who have polyarteritis nodosa, suggesting that these viruses may trigger the disorder. Polyarteritis nodosa is more common in middle-aged men.

What are the symptoms?
The number and severity of symptoms vary. They may include:
- Tiredness.
- Weight loss.
- Fever.
- Abdominal pain or discomfort.
- Joint pain and muscle weakness.

- Tingling and numbness in the fingers and toes.
- A red-purple patchy rash on the skin that does not fade with pressure.
- Skin ulcers.

Polyarteritis nodosa commonly leads to an increase in blood pressure (*see* **Hypertension**, p.242) caused by kidney damage. In some people, the damage to the kidneys is severe and leads to kidney failure (p.450). Less commonly, polyarteritis may cause lung damage or a heart attack (*see* **Myocardial infarction**, p.245).

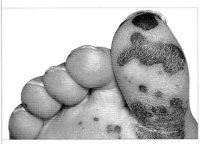

Lesions of polyarteritis nodosa
These lesions are due to polyarteritis nodosa, in which the blood vessels are inflamed and blood flow to the tissues is restricted.

How is it diagnosed?
Your doctor may arrange for you to have blood tests to check for inflammation and to look for the hepatitis B or C viruses. To confirm the diagnosis, you may have a biopsy, in which a sample of an affected artery or organ is removed and examined under a microscope. You may also have angiography, in which an X-ray of the arteries is taken to look for abnormal areas in the blood vessels (*see* **Femoral angiography**, p.260).

What is the treatment?
Polyarteritis nodosa can be effectively treated to relieve symptoms and prevent tissue damage. Your doctor may initially prescribe a high dose of a corticosteroid (p.600), which will be reduced once the symptoms subside. If there is no improvement, an immunosuppressant drug (p.585) may be prescribed. Without treatment, the condition may be life-threatening; with treatment, life expectancy is normal in about half of all cases.

Behçet's syndrome

An inflammatory disorder producing recurrent mouth and genital ulcers

 Most common between the ages of 20 and 40

 More common in males

 Sometimes runs in families; more common in some ethnic groups

 Lifestyle is not a significant factor

Behçet's syndrome is a rare disorder that varies in severity. The effects range from difficulty in eating to significant disability.

Painful ulcers usually recur in the mouth and on the genitals. Other symptoms include eye inflammation (*see* **Uveitis**, p.357), an acne-like rash, and small, tender lumps on the shins. The brain, spinal cord, and joints (*see* **Arthritis**, p.220) may be affected, and the blood has an increased tendency to clot.

Behçet's syndrome is an autoimmune disorder in which the body produces antibodies that attack its own tissues. The cause of this abnormal immune reaction is unknown, but it may be triggered by viral infection. The syndrome sometimes runs in families and occurs more often in people of Mediterranean or Japanese origin, which suggests that genetic factors may be involved. Behçet's syndrome is twice as common in men as in women and most often occurs in people under the age of 40.

What might be done?
Your doctor may suspect Behçet's syndrome from your symptoms and a physical examination. It may take some time to confirm the diagnosis because there are no specific tests for the condition and many other disorders with similar symptoms need to be excluded. Some of the symptoms may disappear without treatment, but your doctor may prescribe a topical corticosteroid (p.577) or colchicine for the ulcers and eyedrops for eye inflammation (*see* **Drugs acting on the eye**, p.594). In severe cases, oral corticosteroids (p.600) and/or immunosuppressants (p.585) may be needed.

Behçet's syndrome is a lifelong condition with symptom-free periods that may last weeks, months, or even years. It rarely affects life expectancy.

Allergies

An allergy is an abnormal reaction of the body's immune system to a foreign substance. In most people, the substance produces no symptoms, but in a susceptible person it triggers an allergic reaction. Most allergies are mild and merely unpleasant, and they are easily treated with drugs and self-help remedies. However, sometimes allergies can be life-threatening.

In this section, allergic reactions due to foreign substances such as pollen, food, and certain drugs are discussed first. The trigger substance (allergen) causes no symptoms on initial contact. However, the immune system begins to form antibodies against the allergen, and certain types of white blood cells become sensitive to it. Later contact with the allergen may stimulate specialized cells called mast cells to release histamine, the chemical that triggers the allergic response. Allergic reactions may lead to urticaria or angioedema, which are dealt with next. The last article covers anaphylaxis, a potentially life-threatening reaction to an allergen. Allergies often develop in childhood and may either persist or disappear in adulthood. Conditions such as asthma (p.295) and eczema (p.193), which may have an allergic basis, are dealt with in the sections that cover the relevant body systems.

KEY ANATOMY

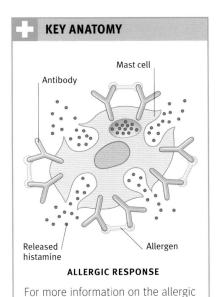
Mast cell
Antibody
Released histamine
Allergen

ALLERGIC RESPONSE

For more information on the allergic response, *see* p.397.

Allergic rhinitis

Inflammation of the membrane lining the nose due to an allergic reaction

 Sometimes runs in families

 Age, gender, and lifestyle are not significant factors

Allergic rhinitis is a condition in which the membrane lining the nose becomes inflamed. It affects people who experience an allergic reaction after they inhale specific airborne substances (allergens). Allergic rhinitis may occur only in the spring and summer, in which case it is known as seasonal allergic rhinitis or hay fever, or it may be perennial and occur all year round. Allergic rhinitis is more common in people who also have other allergic disorders, such as asthma (p.295).

What are the causes?
Seasonal allergic rhinitis is usually due to grass, tree, flower, or weed pollens, as well as mould spores. It occurs mostly during the spring and summer when pollen counts are high. The

common allergens that provoke perennial allergic rhinitis are house dust mites, animal fur and dander, and feathers.

What are the symptoms?
The symptoms of both forms of allergic rhinitis usually appear soon after contact with the allergen. They include:
- Itchy sensation in the nose.
- Frequent sneezing.
- Blocked, runny nose.
- Itchy, red, watery eyes.
- Itchy throat.

Some people may develop a headache. If the lining of the nose is severely inflamed, nosebleeds may occur.

What might be done?
Your doctor will probably recognize allergic rhinitis from your symptoms, particularly if you are able to identify the substance that triggers a reaction. A skin prick test (below right) may be carried out to identify the allergen that causes the allergic rhinitis. In some cases, the allergen cannot be found.

If you are able to avoid the allergens that affect you, your symptoms will probably subside (see **Preventing allergic rhinitis**, below). Many antiallergy drugs (p.585) are available over the counter or on prescription. For example, allergies can be blocked by nasal sprays that contain corticosteroid drugs (see **Corticosteroids for respiratory disease**, p.588) but may take a few days to work. Nasal sprays containing sodium cromoglicate are an alternative. Nasal sprays containing decongestants (p.587) can relieve the symptoms

Preventing allergic rhinitis
The following measures are all aimed at maintaining an allergen-free environment in your home. Tips on preventing perennial allergic rhinitis include:
- Avoid keeping furry animals as pets if you are allergic to them.
- Replace pillows and quilts containing animal materials such as duck feathers with those containing synthetic stuffing.
- Cover mattresses with plastic.
- Remove dust-collecting items such as upholstered furniture and curtains if possible.

To help prevent the symptoms of seasonal allergic rhinitis, also known as hay fever, the following measures may be effective:
- Avoid areas with long grass or where grass is being cut.
- In summer, keep doors and windows closed and spend as much time as possible in air-conditioned buildings.
- Try to stay inside during late morning and early evening when the pollen count is highest.
- Make sure your car is fitted with an effective pollen filter.
- When outside, wear sunglasses to help to prevent eye irritation.

but should not be used regularly. Oral antihistamines (p.585) or an antihistamine nasal spray may relieve inflammation and itching. Eyedrops may help to relieve eye symptoms. Rarely, if symptoms are severe, your doctor may prescribe an oral corticosteroid (p.600).

The most specific treatment for allergic rhinitis is immunotherapy, in which you are given gradually increasing doses of allergen with the aim of desensitizing the immune system. This treatment, which typically takes as long as 3–4 years, may be effective for people who are severely affected.

Food allergy

An abnormal reaction of the immune system to certain foods

 Affects all ages, but most common in infants and children

 Sometimes runs in families

 Gender and lifestyle are not significant factors

Food allergy is a condition in which the immune system reacts in an inappropriate or exaggerated way to a specific food or foods, causing various symptoms such as an itchy, red rash and swelling of the lips, mouth, and throat. This condition should not be confused with food intolerance (p.416), which often causes abdominal discomfort and indigestion but does not involve the immune system.

What are the causes?
Although allergic reactions can occur in response to any food, nuts (especially peanuts) are probably the most common cause. Other relatively common causes of food allergy include seafood, strawberries, and eggs. Food colourings and preservatives rarely cause reactions, but intolerance to the food additive monosodium glutamate (MSG) is common.

Wheat may cause a condition known as coeliac disease (p.416) and an allergic reaction to the protein in cows' milk is especially common in infants and young children (see **Cows' milk protein allergy**, p.560). These conditions differ from immediate sensitivity to nuts or other foods in that they produce less severe but more persistent symptoms.

Food allergy is more common in people with other allergy-related conditions such as asthma (p.295), eczema (p.193), or allergic rhinitis (p.283). The tendency to develop a food allergy may sometimes run in families.

What are the symptoms?
Symptoms may appear almost immediately after eating the food or develop over a few hours. They may include:
- Itching and swelling affecting the lips, mouth, and throat.
- An itchy, red rash anywhere on the body (see **Urticaria**, opposite page).
- Nausea, vomiting, and diarrhoea.

If you have a severe reaction, the following symptoms may also be present:
- Nonitchy swelling anywhere on the body, especially the face, mouth, and throat (see **Angioedema**, opposite page).
- Shortness of breath or wheezing.

Sometimes, food allergy may lead to anaphylaxis (opposite page), a life-threatening allergic response that causes sudden difficulty in breathing and collapse. If you develop the symptoms of a severe reaction, seek immediate medical help. If you develop anaphylaxis and have a syringe of injectable epinephrine (adrenaline), inject immediately, then call an ambulance.

What might be done?
You may be able to diagnose food allergy yourself if symptoms occur soon after eating a particular food, but you should consult your doctor, who may arrange for a blood test and skin prick test (below) to find the cause. Your doctor may advise you to follow an exclusion diet, often for 1 or 2 weeks If your symptoms improve substantially while you are on the diet, this may indicate that you have one or more allergies to the excluded foods. You can then gradually add foods to the exclusion diet, but if symptoms recur when a particular food is introduced, you should avoid it. You should not embark on an exclusion diet without first consulting your doctor and you should not follow a restricted diet for more than 2 weeks.

Avoiding the problem food is the only effective treatment. Always ask about ingredients when eating out, and check labels. Consult a diet or nutrition counsellor if you need to exclude a food that is a major part of a normal diet. If a major permanent dietary change is needed, be sure to maintain a balanced diet.

What is the prognosis?
Many food allergies in adults, particularly nut allergies, tend to be permanent, and people with such allergies must therefore avoid the relevant foods throughout their lives. However, in some cases, a food allergy may disappear spontaneously. Children under the age of 4 who avoid problem foods, such as wheat, for 2 years have an excellent chance of outgrowing their allergy.

Drug allergy

An abnormal reaction to a drug, most commonly an antibiotic

 Age, gender, genetics, and lifestyle are not significant factors

Both over-the-counter and prescription drugs can cause various problems. Most symptoms, such as nausea or diarrhoea, are not allergies but side effects that can affect anyone taking the drug. A drug allergy occurs when the immune system produces an abnormal reaction to a specific drug. Often, the reactions are mild, but some can be life-threatening.

What are the causes?
A drug may provoke an allergic reaction the first time you use it. It is also possible to develop an allergic reaction to a drug that you have been taking for some time. In the latter case, your body will gradually become more and more sensitive to the drug. Allergic reactions may occur with any drug but are most common with antibiotics (p.572). Your doctor will ask you about any known allergies before prescribing drugs.

Skin prick test

A skin prick test is a simple and painless procedure undertaken to find out which substances (allergens) cause allergic reactions in an affected person. Dilute solutions are made from extracts of allergens, such as pollen, dust, dander, and food, that commonly cause allergic reactions.

A drop of each solution is placed on the skin, which is then pricked with a needle. The skin is observed for a reaction, which usually occurs within 30 minutes of applying the solution. Antihistamines should not be taken on the day of the test because they may prevent any reaction.

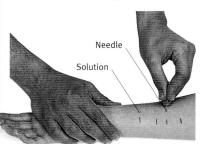

Needle

Solution

1 *Drops from 8–10 solutions containing different allergens are placed on the skin. The skin underneath is then pricked with a needle and observed for a reaction.*

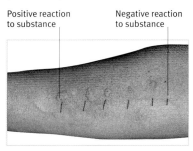

Positive reaction to substance   Negative reaction to substance

2 *If a person is allergic to one of the substances applied to the skin, a red lump, indicating a positive reaction, appears at the site of the needle prick.*

What are the symptoms?

An allergic reaction to a drug may give rise to the following symptoms:

■ Wheezing.

■ Swelling anywhere on the body, but typically affecting the face and throat (see Angioedema, right).

■ Nausea and diarrhoea.

■ An itchy rash consisting of red, raised areas and, occasionally, white lumps (see Urticaria, below).

If you develop these symptoms and suspect that they are due to a prescription or over-the-counter drug, contact your doctor at once before taking the next dose. Rarely, a drug allergy may lead to a severe and potentially fatal reaction called anaphylaxis (right).

What might be done?

If your doctor suspects that you are allergic to a particular drug, he or she will advise you to stop taking it and may prescribe an alternative. Usually, mild symptoms disappear without treatment within a few days of stopping the drug. Itchy rashes can be treated with over-the-counter products such as calamine lotion or oral antihistamines (p.585). A drug allergy is usually lifelong. It is therefore important to inform any doctor who treats you that you have an allergy to a certain drug. If the reaction was severe, you will be advised to carry a card or bracelet with you at all times to alert other people to your drug allergy in case you need emergency treatment.

Urticaria

Areas of swelling on the skin, often known as hives, that occur as the result of an allergic reaction

 Sometimes runs in families

 Age, gender, and lifestyle are not significant factors

Urticaria, also known as hives, is an intensely itchy rash that may affect the whole body or just a small area of skin. The rash consists of raised, red areas and, sometimes, white lumps. The inflamed areas usually vary in size and may merge to involve very large areas of skin. Urticaria typically lasts for only a few hours (acute urticaria), but in some cases it may persist for up to several months (chronic urticaria). Both the acute and chronic forms of urticaria may recur. Sometimes,

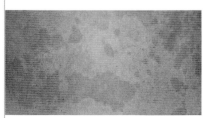

Urticaria

This rash, known as urticaria, consists of white lumps and red, inflamed areas. It is usually caused by an allergic reaction.

urticaria occurs at the same time as the more serious condition called angioedema (below) or is sometimes an early symptom of anaphylaxis (right).

What are the causes?

Urticaria can occur as a result of an allergic reaction to a particular food (see Food allergy, opposite page). It may also be due to a drug allergy (opposite page) or an allergy to plants, or it may develop after an insect bite or sting. Urticaria may sometimes be associated with a viral infection or other disorder or a physical stimulus, such as pressure or a change in temperature. However, when it occurs for the first time, it is often difficult to identify the cause. The tendency to develop urticaria may sometimes run in families.

What might be done?

Acute urticaria usually disappears without any treatment within a few hours. The chronic form of the condition may take several weeks or months to clear up. Over-the-counter products such as calamine lotion and oral antihistamines (p.585) may help to relieve itching.

If your symptoms persist or recur and the cause of the problem is not obvious, you should consult your doctor. He or she may arrange for a skin prick test (opposite page) to try to identify the substances to which you are allergic (allergens). When the substance causing your urticaria has been identified, you should avoid that substance in future.

Angioedema

Swelling of body tissues, particularly around the face, usually due to an allergic reaction

 Sometimes runs in families

 In some cases, stress is a trigger factor

 Age and gender are not significant factors

Angioedema is a condition in which the mucous membranes and tissues under the skin suddenly become swollen. The face and neck are usually affected.

The most common cause of angioedema is an allergic reaction to a type of food, such as seafood, nuts, or strawberries (see Food allergy, opposite page). Less commonly, the condition may result from an allergic reaction to a drug (see Drug allergy, opposite page), most often to an antibiotic (p.572). Angioedema may also develop after an insect bite.

Rarely, a person may inherit a tendency to develop angioedema that is unrelated to an allergy. In such cases, episodes of unexplained angioedema may begin in childhood and may be triggered by stressful events, such as an injury or a dental extraction.

It is not unusual for people to have only a single episode of angioedema, for which no cause can be determined.

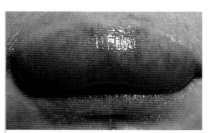

Angioedema of the upper lip

Sudden, severe swelling of the face, lips, or neck is known as angioedema, which is usually caused by an allergic reaction.

What are the symptoms?

Swelling usually develops within a few minutes and is often asymmetrical; for example, only one side of a lip may be affected. The main symptoms are:

■ Swelling of any part of the body, most commonly the face and lips.

■ Sudden difficulty in breathing, speaking, or swallowing due to swelling of the tongue, mouth, and airways.

■ In about half of all cases, an itchy rash affecting areas that are not swollen (see Urticaria, left).

The swelling may affect the larynx (voice box) and can be life-threatening if the airway becomes blocked. Angioedema may occur at the same time as anaphylaxis (below), a potentially fatal allergic reaction that requires urgent medical attention. If you develop the symptoms of angioedema above or you experience difficulty in breathing, you should seek medical help immediately.

What might be done?

Severe angioedema requires an urgent injection with the drug epinephrine (adrenaline), followed by observation in hospital. In milder cases, a corticosteroid (p.600) or an antihistamine (p.585) may be given to reduce the swelling; this may take hours or days to subside.

Your doctor may carry out tests to determine the cause of the angioedema. If a food allergy is suspected, a skin prick test (opposite page) or blood test, and/or an exclusion diet may be used to identify the substances to which you are allergic. If you suffer from severe angioedema, your doctor may teach you how to self-inject epinephrine (see Emergency aid for anaphylaxis, right).

Anaphylaxis

A severe, potentially fatal allergic reaction to certain substances

 Sometimes runs in families

 Age, gender, and lifestyle are not significant factors

Anaphylaxis, also known as anaphylactic shock, is a rare and severe type of allergic reaction that occurs in people who have developed an extreme sensitivity to a specific substance (allergen). The reaction occurs throughout the body, causing a

sudden drop in blood pressure and narrowing of the airways, and it can be fatal unless immediate treatment is available. Anaphylaxis is often triggered by insect stings or by certain drugs such as the antibiotic penicillin (see Drug allergy, opposite page). Foods such as nuts or strawberries may also trigger this serious form of allergic reaction (see Food allergy, opposite page).

What are the symptoms?

If you have an extreme sensitivity to a substance, you may experience some or all of the following symptoms as soon as you are exposed to it:

■ Sudden feeling of extreme anxiety.

■ Swollen face, lips, and tongue.

■ Wheezing and difficulty breathing.

■ In some cases, an itchy, red rash (see Urticaria, left) and flushing of the skin.

■ Light-headedness or, in some cases, loss of consciousness.

If either you or anyone you are with develops these symptoms, you should call an ambulance immediately.

What is the treatment?

Emergency treatment for anaphylaxis is an immediate injection of epinephrine (adrenaline). Antihistamines (p.585) or corticosteroids (p.600), together with fluids, may also be given intravenously.

You should avoid any substance to which you are sensitive, especially if you have had a previous anaphylactic reaction. You may be given epinephrine to self-inject (see Emergency aid for anaphylaxis, below). You will also be advised to carry an emergency card or bracelet to alert others to your allergy.

▶ TREATMENT

Emergency aid for anaphylaxis

If you have previously experienced anaphylaxis or severe angioedema, your doctor may provide you with syringes of injectable epinephrine (adrenaline). Keep one at home and one at work, and carry one with you at all times. In the event of anaphylaxis, inject epinephrine immediately, then call for an ambulance.

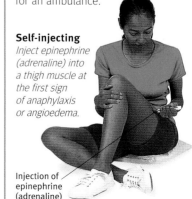

Self-injecting

Inject epinephrine (adrenaline) into a thigh muscle at the first sign of anaphylaxis or angioedema.

Injection of epinephrine (adrenaline)

Respiratory system

Every living cell in the body needs a constant supply of oxygen to survive. Cells must also dispose of their primary waste product, carbon dioxide. The role of the respiratory system, together with the circulatory system, is to deliver oxygen from the lungs to the cells and to remove carbon dioxide and return it to the lungs to be exhaled. This exchange of oxygen and carbon dioxide is very effective because of the combination of the vast surface area of the lungs, which is about 40 times greater than that of the body, and the fact that all of the blood passes through the lungs every minute.

THE EXCHANGE OF oxygen and carbon dioxide between the air, blood, and body tissues is known as respiration. Air enters and leaves the body by the respiratory system, which is made up of the mouth, nose, throat, branching airways, and lungs. The circulatory system, which consists of the heart and blood vessels, ensures that oxygen is delivered to the cells and carbon dioxide is carried away.

Respiratory processes

Healthy lungs take in about 500 ml (1 pint) of air 12–15 times each minute. Breathing is an automatic process that is controlled by the respiratory centre in the brain; we only become aware of breathing when it is difficult, such as during exercise. When we inhale, air enters the body through the mouth or nose and is warmed and moistened.

Air passes down the pharynx (throat) and larynx (voice box) and into the trachea (windpipe). A small flap of cartilage called the epiglottis covers the trachea during swallowing to prevent food from entering the airways.

In the lungs, oxygen from the air passes into the surrounding blood vessels. There, it binds to the molecule haemoglobin in the red blood cells. The oxygen-rich blood then travels from the lungs to the heart and the body tissues, where oxygen is released. At the same time, carbon dioxide waste from the tissues passes into the blood and dissolves in the plasma, the fluid part of blood. This carbon dioxide is returned to the lungs and exhaled.

Sometimes, infectious organisms or foreign particles enter the body when we inhale. The respiratory system has several ways of protecting the lungs from damage. Situated in the walls of the pharynx are the tonsils and adenoids.

In young children, these help to destroy some infectious organisms as they travel towards the lungs. Airborne particles may also be trapped by mucus in the airways and then directed away from the lungs by tiny hairs called cilia. Finally, foreign particles or excess mucus that irritate the airways or lungs can be expelled by a sneeze or a cough.

Speech production

The respiratory system also contains the vocal cords, the organs that are responsible for speech production. Sounds are formed when the vocal cords are partially closed and air from the lungs causes them to vibrate. Using these vibrations, we can produce a remarkable range of sounds.

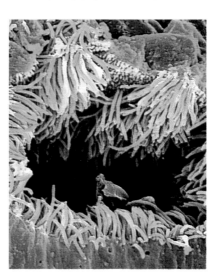

A filtering system
Fine hair-like strands, known as cilia, line the airways and trap foreign particles as the air passes through

---

✚ STRUCTURE

Sinuses

Several air-filled cavities, known as sinuses, are situated in the skull bones around the nose and the eyes. The size and shape of these sinuses vary between individuals. Sinuses are not present at birth but gradually develop throughout childhood. They help to lighten the skull bones and give the voice resonance. Within the lining of the sinuses are many mucus-secreting glands. Mucus passes continuously through narrow channels that lead from the sinuses to the back of the nose. The mucus traps small airborne particles and moistens inhaled air as it passes though the airways.

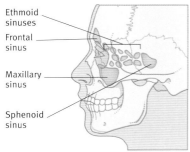

Frontal sinus
Ethmoid sinuses
Maxillary sinus
Sphenoid sinus

Front view of the sinuses
Sinuses are named after the bones in which they are found. The sinuses in the front of the skull are the frontal and maxillary sinuses.

Ethmoid sinuses
Frontal sinus
Maxillary sinus
Sphenoid sinus

Side view of the sinuses
The two sphenoid sinuses are situated deep in the skull. In front of them lie the numerous ethmoid sinuses.

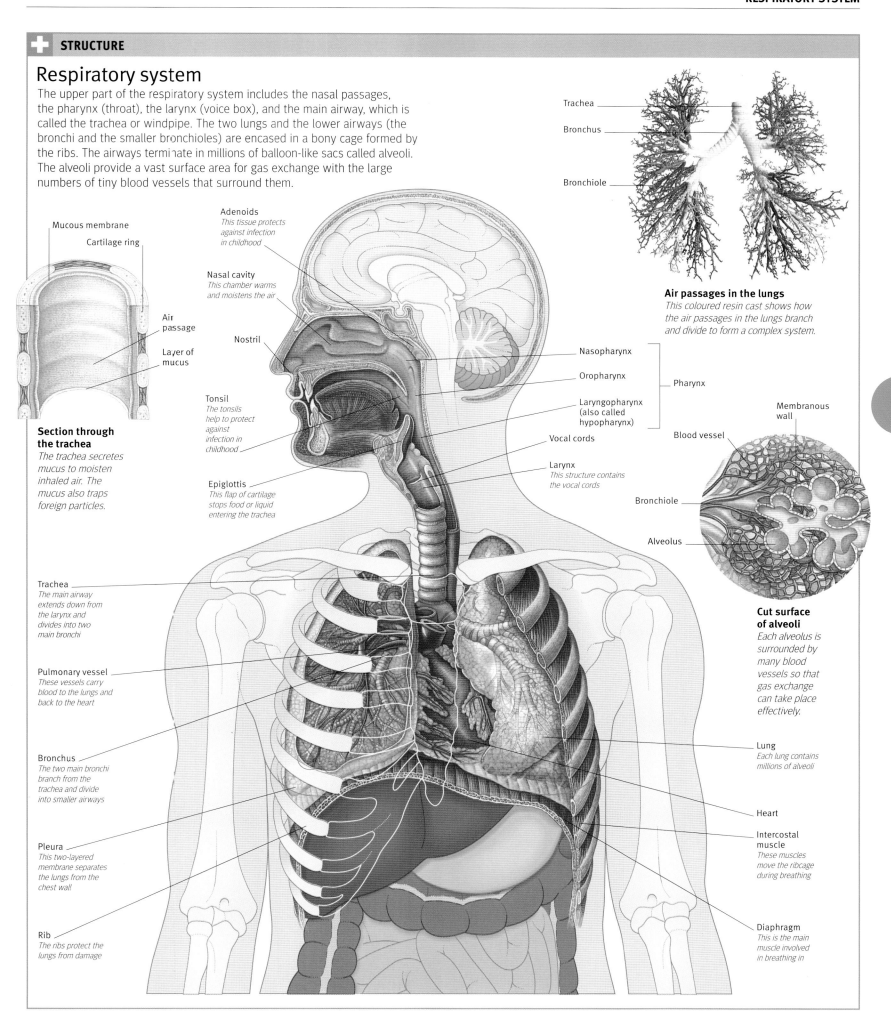

✚ STRUCTURE

Respiratory system

The upper part of the respiratory system includes the nasal passages, the pharynx (throat), the larynx (voice box), and the main airway, which is called the trachea or windpipe. The two lungs and the lower airways (the bronchi and the smaller bronchioles) are encased in a bony cage formed by the ribs. The airways terminate in millions of balloon-like sacs called alveoli. The alveoli provide a vast surface area for gas exchange with the large numbers of tiny blood vessels that surround them.

Trachea

Bronchus

Bronchiole

Air passages in the lungs
This coloured resin cast shows how the air passages in the lungs branch and divide to form a complex system.

Mucous membrane

Cartilage ring

Air passage

Layer of mucus

Section through the trachea
The trachea secretes mucus to moisten inhaled air. The mucus also traps foreign particles.

Adenoids
This tissue protects against infection in childhood

Nasal cavity
This chamber warms and moistens the air

Nostril

Tonsil
The tonsils help to protect against infection in childhood

Epiglottis
This flap of cartilage stops food or liquid entering the trachea

Nasopharynx

Oropharynx

Laryngopharynx (also called hypopharynx)

Pharynx

Vocal cords

Larynx
This structure contains the vocal cords

Blood vessel

Bronchiole

Alveolus

Membranous wall

Cut surface of alveoli
Each alveolus is surrounded by many blood vessels so that gas exchange can take place effectively.

Trachea
The main airway extends down from the larynx and divides into two main bronchi

Pulmonary vessel
These vessels carry blood to the lungs and back to the heart

Bronchus
The two main bronchi branch from the trachea and divide into smaller airways

Pleura
This two-layered membrane separates the lungs from the chest wall

Rib
The ribs protect the lungs from damage

Lung
Each lung contains millions of alveoli

Heart

Intercostal muscle
These muscles move the ribcage during breathing

Diaphragm
This is the main muscle involved in breathing in

✚ FUNCTION

Breathing and respiration

Air constantly enters and leaves the lungs, enabling the tissues of the body to receive an adequate supply of oxygen and to dispose of their waste product, carbon dioxide. Breathing is controlled by the respiratory centre in a part of the brain known as the medulla. The respiratory centre stimulates the intercostal muscles around the chest cavity to contract and relax so that we breathe in and out.

How breathing works

During breathing, air moves from areas of high pressure to areas of low pressure. When the pressure in the lungs is lower than the pressure in the atmosphere, air enters the airways. If the pressure in the lungs increases, air moves out of the lungs and is then exhaled.

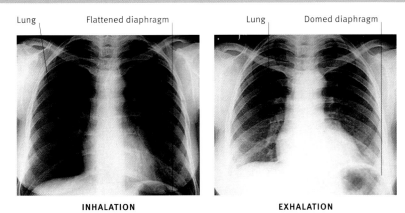

INHALATION · EXHALATION

Chest X-rays
These normal chest X-rays show the volume of air in the lungs during inhalation and exhalation, which is achieved by changes in the position of the ribs and diaphragm.

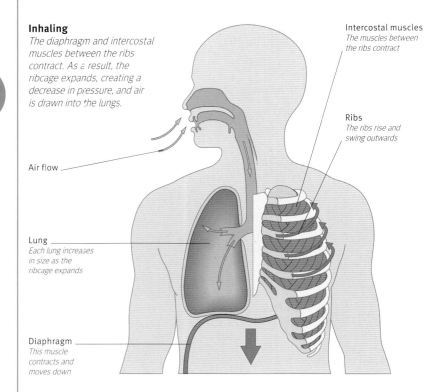

Inhaling
The diaphragm and intercostal muscles between the ribs contract. As a result, the ribcage expands, creating a decrease in pressure, and air is drawn into the lungs.

Air flow

Lung
Each lung increases in size as the ribcage expands

Diaphragm
This muscle contracts and moves down

Intercostal muscles
The muscles between the ribs contract

Ribs
The ribs rise and swing outwards

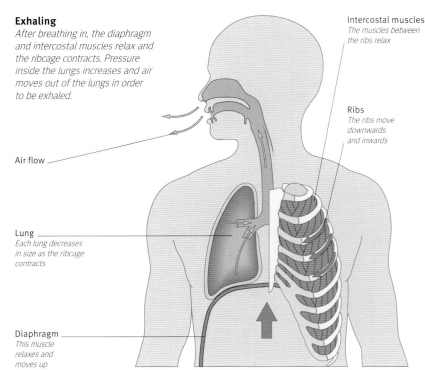

Exhaling
After breathing in, the diaphragm and intercostal muscles relax and the ribcage contracts. Pressure inside the lungs increases and air moves out of the lungs in order to be exhaled.

Air flow

Lung
Each lung decreases in size as the ribcage contracts

Diaphragm
This muscle relaxes and moves up

Intercostal muscles
The muscles between the ribs relax

Ribs
The ribs move downwards and inwards

✚ FUNCTION

How breathing is regulated

Even while we sleep, our basic breathing rhythm is controlled by a collection of nerve cells in the brain called the respiratory centre. From there, messages travel down nerves to the diaphragm and rib muscles and stimulate them so that we continue breathing. As activity changes, so does the amount of carbon dioxide in the blood. Receptors in some of the large arteries detect the changes and send instructions to the brain.

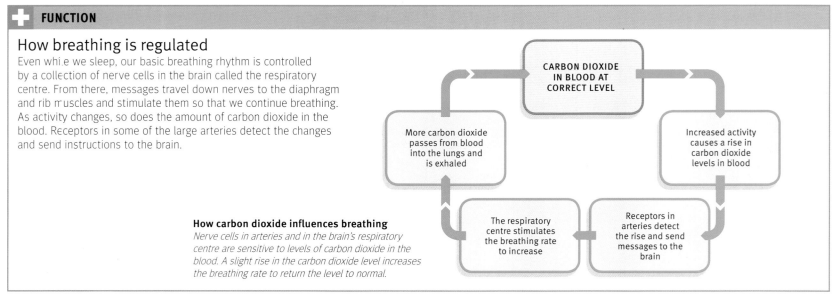

How carbon dioxide influences breathing
Nerve cells in arteries and in the brain's respiratory centre are sensitive to levels of carbon dioxide in the blood. A slight rise in the carbon dioxide level increases the breathing rate to return the level to normal.

CARBON DIOXIDE IN BLOOD AT CORRECT LEVEL

More carbon dioxide passes from blood into the lungs and is exhaled

Increased activity causes a rise in carbon dioxide levels in blood

The respiratory centre stimulates the breathing rate to increase

Receptors in arteries detect the rise and send messages to the brain

Gas exchange in the body

The exchange of oxygen and carbon dioxide gases occurs constantly throughout the body. In the lungs, oxygen crosses the delicate walls of the alveoli (air sacs) and enters tiny blood vessels (capillaries), where it binds to the molecule haemoglobin in the red blood cells. At the same time, carbon dioxide is released from the blood into the alveoli and exhaled through the mouth or nose. In tissue cells, blood from the lungs exchanges its supply of oxygen for carbon dioxide.

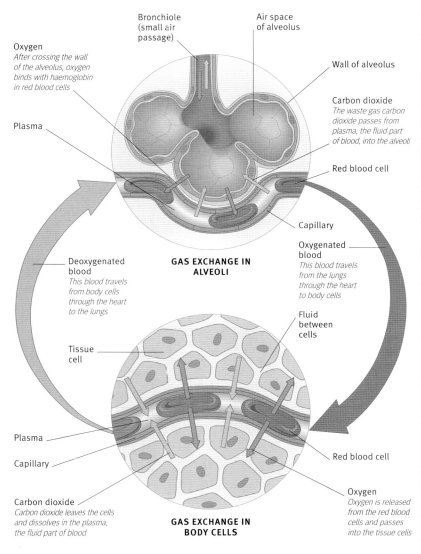

Oxygen
After crossing the wall of the alveolus, oxygen binds with haemoglobin in red blood cells

Plasma

Bronchiole (small air passage)

Air space of alveolus

Wall of alveolus

Carbon dioxide
The waste gas carbon dioxide passes from plasma, the fluid part of blood, into the alveoli

Red blood cell

GAS EXCHANGE IN ALVEOLI

Deoxygenated blood
This blood travels from body cells through the heart to the lungs

Oxygenated blood
This blood travels from the lungs through the heart to body cells

Capillary

Fluid between cells

Tissue cell

Plasma

Capillary

Carbon dioxide
Carbon dioxide leaves the cells and dissolves in the plasma, the fluid part of blood

GAS EXCHANGE IN BODY CELLS

Red blood cell

Oxygen
Oxygen is released from the red blood cells and passes into the tissue cells

Exchange of gases
Body cells require a constant supply of oxygen in order to obtain energy to survive. In addition, waste products from the body cells, mainly carbon dioxide, must be transported away from the cells.

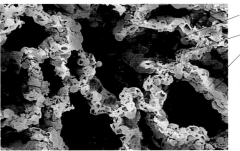

Air space

Blood vessel

Membranous wall

Cross section of alveoli
This magnified view of lung tissue shows the alveolar air spaces and their thin walls. The tiny holes seen in the walls are blood vessels.

FUNCTION

Speech
The larynx (voice box) is responsible for voice production. Sounds are made when air from the lungs passes across two fibrous bands within the larynx, known as vocal cords. The sounds produced by the vibrating cords are formed into speech by the mouth and tongue.

LOCATION

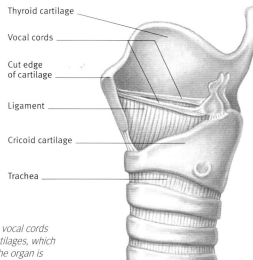

Thyroid cartilage

Vocal cords

Cut edge of cartilage

Ligament

Cricoid cartilage

Trachea

Side view of the larynx
The larynx is composed of the vocal cords and the thyroid and cricoid cartilages, which are connected by ligaments. The organ is located in the neck, above the trachea.

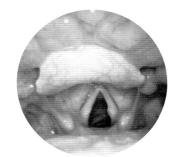

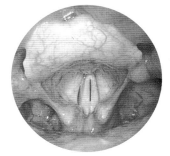

OPEN VOCAL CORDS

CLOSED VOCAL CORDS

Movements of the vocal cords
The vocal cords are held open during breathing, but during speech they pull together and vibrate as air from the lungs passes between them. Sounds vary according to the exact position of the cords.

FUNCTION

The cough reflex
If substances such as dust or excess mucus irritate the lungs or airways, they may be removed by the familiar reaction known as a cough. The irritation stimulates nerve cell receptors in the airways, sending signals to the brain, which then triggers the cough reflex.

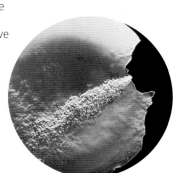

The cough
During a cough, air, moisture, and foreign particles are noisily and forcefully expelled. This reflex action helps to clear irritant material from the airways, preventing it from causing damage.

Nose and throat disorders

The upper part of the respiratory system is made up of the nose and throat and structures associated with them. These include the sinuses (the air-filled cavities in the front of the skull) and the larynx, also known as the voice box. The upper respiratory system can be affected by a variety of disorders ranging from common complaints, such as nosebleeds, snoring, and laryngitis, to rare conditions such as cancers of the throat and larynx.

Disorders that affect the nose and the sinuses are covered first in this section. These conditions include nosebleeds, which are often a symptom of a minor injury but are sometimes due to a serious underlying disorder, and sinusitis, inflammation of the sinuses, which is usually caused by a viral infection such as the common cold.

Obstruction in the nasal passages may cause problems with sleep, and two such disorders, snoring and sleep apnoea, are covered here. Articles follow on common conditions that involve inflammation of the throat or larynx, such as pharyngitis, tonsillitis, and laryngitis. Finally, noncancerous growths in the larynx, known as vocal cord nodules, and cancers of the throat and larynx are discussed.

Infections that affect the nose and the throat are described elsewhere (*see* **Infections and infestations**, pp.160–180), as is allergic rhinitis (p.283), a common disorder of the nose. Disorders of the nose and throat that are common in children, such as enlarged adenoids, are covered in another section (*see* **Infancy and childhood**, pp.524–565).

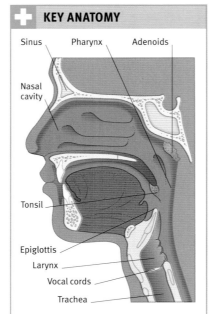

✚ KEY ANATOMY

For further information on the structure and function of the nose and throat, see pp.290–294.

Nosebleed

Bleeding from the nose, usually from one nostril only

 Most common in children and in adults over the age of 50

 Gender, genetics, and lifestyle are not significant factors

Nosebleeds are common in children, but the bleeding usually stops by itself and is minor. Nosebleeds are also common, but sometimes serious, in people over the age of 50. In this age group, bleeding may come from the back of the nose and be hard to stop. If the blood is swallowed, bleeding may not be seen.

What are the causes?
Nosebleeds commonly occur spontaneously. In dry environments or during winter months, the membranes lining the nose may become dry and cracked, causing bleeding to occur. Nosebleeds may also occur if the lining of the nose is injured by a blow to the nose or by nose-picking or forceful nose-blowing. In children, nosebleeds often occur as a result of rough play. A foreign body in the nose or

an infection in the upper respiratory tract may also result in a nosebleed. In people over the age of 50, the small blood vessels in the nose may be more fragile and therefore more likely to rupture and cause bleeding.

In rare cases, nosebleeds may be associated with cancer in the passage connecting the nose to the throat (*see* **Cancer of the nasopharynx**, p.293) or may indicate another underlying disease, such as the bleeding disorder thrombocytopenia (p.275) or a liver disease that affects blood clotting. Nosebleeds may also be caused by drugs that prevent blood clotting (p.584). A nosebleed is more likely to be prolonged if you have high blood pressure (*see* **Hypertension**, p.242).

What can I do?
If you have a nosebleed, you should put direct pressure on the soft part of your nose by pressing both sides together for at least 10–15 minutes while breathing through your mouth. You should try to avoid sniffing and/or blowing your nose afterwards because you may dislodge the blood clot that has formed and cause another nosebleed. Self-help measures are usually successful in stopping a nosebleed. If bleeding persists for half an hour or more, you should seek medical attention. If membranes in the nose

are dry and cracked, rubbing water-based ointment in your nose a few times a day or using a saline spray may help to prevent recurrent nosebleeds.

What might the doctor do?
A persistent nosebleed will probably require hospital treatment. The doctor may pack your nose with nasal sponges, which are left in place for about a day. Alternatively, a flexible tube with a small balloon at the tip may be inserted into the back of your nose and inflated to stop the bleeding by applying pressure to leaking vessels. Bleeding vessels may also be cauterized (sealed using heat or a chemical) under local anaesthesia.

If the cause is not obvious, your doctor may arrange for you to have endoscopy of the nose (*see* **Endoscopy of the nose and throat**, opposite page), in which an optical instrument is passed into each nostril in turn to look for ruptured vessels or a tumour. Rarely, CT scanning (p.132) or MRI (p.133) may be carried out to rule out a tumour. Blood tests may also be arranged to check how efficiently the blood clots.

Recurrent bleeding that is not caused by a tumour may be investigated by taking contrast X-rays (p.132) of the blood vessels in the nose. A special substance is then injected into the leaking blood vessel to block it and prevent further blood loss. In other cases, endoscopic surgery may be required to place a clip on a bleeding vessel.

Sinusitis

Inflammation of any of the sinuses (the air-filled cavities in the bones around the nose)

 More common in adults

 Genetics as a risk factor depends on the cause

 Gender and lifestyle are not significant factors

The sinuses are air-filled cavities in the skull situated behind the nose and eyes and in the cheeks and forehead. They are lined with a mucus-secreting membrane and are connected to the nasal cavity by a number of narrow channels. Inflammation of the sinuses, known as sinusitis, may be acute (developing and clearing up rapidly) or chronic (long-term). Sinusitis rarely occurs in children under the age of 5, partly because their sinuses are not fully developed.

What are the causes?
The most common cause of sinusitis is a viral infection, such as the common cold (p.164). If the channels connecting the nose to the sinuses become blocked due to the viral infection, mucus collects in the sinuses. In some cases, the mucus becomes infected with bacteria.

Blockage of the channels is more likely in people with an abnormality in the nose, such as a deviated nasal septum (p.291) or nasal

polyps (p.291). In addition, people with allergic rhinitis (p.283) or a disorder such as the inherited condition cystic fibrosis (p.535) are more likely to develop sinusitis. Rarely, the channels are blocked by a tumour (*see* **Cancer of the nasopharynx**, p.293). People with reduced immunity and those taking immunosuppressant drugs, are more susceptible to infections that lead to sinusitis.

What are the symptoms?
Symptoms depend on which sinuses are affected and may include:
■ Headache.
■ Pain and tenderness in the face that tends to worsen when bending down.
■ Toothache, if the sinuses behind the cheeks are affected.
■ Discoloured nasal discharge.
■ Nasal congestion or obstruction.
In a few cases, the infection spreads and may cause redness and swelling of the tissue around an eye.

What can I do?
In many cases, sinusitis clears up without treatment. Painkillers (p.589) and decongestants (p.587), both available over the counter, may alleviate symptoms. Steam inhalation (opposite page), which usually helps to clear the nose, may also relieve symptoms. If symptoms become worse or do not improve within 3 days, you should consult a doctor.

What might the doctor do?
Your doctor may prescribe antibiotics (p.572) to clear up secondary bacterial infection. If sinusitis recurs or does not clear up completely, you may have X-rays (p.131) to look for thickening of the lining of the sinuses and excess mucus. Your doctor may also perform endoscopy of the nose (*see* **Endoscopy of the nose and throat**, opposite page) and arrange for CT scanning (p.132) to look for a specific cause, such as nasal polyps or a tumour. Surgery may be necessary to enlarge drainage channels from the sinuses to the nose or create new ones. Acute sinusitis usually clears up in a few days, but the symptoms of chronic sinusitis may last for a couple of months.

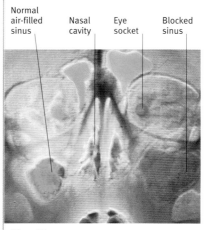

Normal air-filled sinus   Nasal cavity   Eye socket   Blocked sinus

Sinusitis
This colour-enhanced facial X-ray shows a normal air-filled sinus and a sinus filled with mucus, indicating sinusitis.

► SELF-HELP

Steam inhalation

Inhaling steam from a bowl of hot water can be used to relieve some of the symptoms of colds, sore throats, sinusitis, and laryngitis. The moisture in the steam helps to loosen secretions in congested lungs and in the nose and throat, making them easier to clear. Alternatively, you can run hot water while you are in the bathroom and inhale the steam. Children should not carry out steam inhalation unless they are supervised by an adult.

Towel
Pull the towel completely over your head to keep vapour in

Hot water

Inhaling steam
Fill a bowl one-third full with hot water. Lean forwards, pull a towel completely over your head and the bowl, and inhale steam for several minutes.

Deviated nasal septum

An abnormality of the partition that separates the nostrils

 Often present at birth

 More common in males

 Playing contact sports, such as football, is a risk factor

 Genetics is not a significant factor

Sometimes, the wall of cartilage and bone that divides the nostrils, called the nasal septum, is slightly misshapen or deviated but causes no problems. However, in some people, the nasal septum is very misshapen and blocks one side of the nose, impairing breathing. The defect is sometimes associated with snoring (right).

A mildly deviated nasal septum is often present from birth. In other cases, the condition results from a blow to the nose, usually due to a fall or a sports injury. A deviated septum occurs more commonly in men because men are more likely to participate in contact sports that may lead to this type of injury. A severely deviated nasal septum may increase the risk of infections in the sinuses (*see* **Sinusitis**, opposite page).

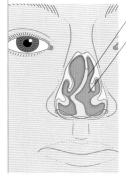

Misshapen septum

Nasal cavity

Deviated nasal septum
A misshapen nasal septum is not usually a problem, but a severe deviation may obstruct breathing.

If you have a deviated septum that causes recurrent sinusitis or breathing difficulties, your doctor may recommend surgery. Carried out under general anaesthesia, the operation involves straightening the septum by realigning or removing the deviated area of cartilage and bone.

Nasal polyps

Fleshy growths of the mucus-secreting lining of the nose

 More common in adults

 Genetics as a risk factor depends on the cause

 Gender and lifestyle are not significant factors

Growths that develop in the mucus-secreting lining of the nose are known as nasal polyps. The exact cause of nasal polyps is not known. However, they are more common in people who have asthma (p.295) or rhinitis, a condition in which the membrane that lines the nose and throat becomes inflamed. Although polyps rarely occur in children, they do sometimes develop in children who have the inherited condition cystic fibrosis (p.535).

What are the symptoms?
The symptoms of nasal polyps often develop gradually over months. The severity of the symptoms depends on the number and the size of the polyps. Symptoms may include:
- Blocked nose due to obstruction by the polyps.
- Decreased sense of smell.
- In some cases, a runny nose due to excess secretion of mucus.

Nasal polyps may lead to recurrent sinusitis (opposite page) if the narrow channels that drain mucus from the sinuses become blocked by the polyps and the sinuses become inflamed.

What might be done?
If your doctor suspects that you have nasal polyps but cannot see them easily, he or she may arrange for you to have endoscopy of the nose (*see* **Endoscopy of the nose and throat**, below). You may also have CT scanning (p.132) if the number and size of the polyps cannot be assessed with an endoscope. If there is a single polyp, a small sample of the polyp may be removed and examined under a microscope to exclude cancer.

Small nasal polyps may be treated by using a corticosteroid nasal spray or drops, which shrink the polyps over a few weeks. Larger polyps may be removed during an endoscopic procedure. A corticosteroid spray may also be necessary for several months after surgery to help prevent the polyps from recurring. In more severe cases, a course of oral corticosteroids (p.600) may also be prescribed.

Snoring

Noisy breathing during sleep, which may be a symptom of the more serious disorder sleep apnoea

 Most common in children and in adults between the ages of 40 and 60

 More common in males

 Being overweight, drinking alcohol, and smoking are risk factors

 Genetics is not a significant factor

Snoring is the sound made by the vibration of the soft tissues at the back of the mouth. Although it is often considered to be an insignificant problem, snoring can be distressing both to the people who are affected and their partners. Loud snoring may also be an early symptom of sleep apnoea (p.292). The condition is most common in children and adults between the ages of 40 and 60, and particularly affects men.

What are the causes?
Vibration of the soft palate may be caused by an obstruction or narrowing of the nasopharynx (the passage leading from the back of the nasal cavity to the throat). The nasopharynx may become obstructed if you are overweight. Sleeping on your back can make snoring worse because the nasopharynx is more likely to become partly blocked if you lie in this position.

Other causes of snoring include narrowing of the nasopharynx caused by relaxation or swelling of the tissues of the soft palate. Relaxation may be the result of drinking alcohol or taking sedatives. Swelling may be caused by a throat infection or irritation of the soft palate by tobacco smoke.

Snoring also occurs because of congestion due to a common cold (p.164). In some cases, an anatomical abnormality such as a deviated nasal septum (left) may be associated with snoring. In children, the condition usually occurs as a result of enlarged tonsils and adenoids (p.546).

► TEST

Endoscopy of the nose and throat

Endoscopy can be used to look at the internal structures of the nose and throat as well as to diagnose disorders such as nasal polyps or cancer of the larynx. During the procedure, an endoscope is inserted up each nostril in turn and into the nasal cavity. The instrument may be flexible or rigid; flexible endoscopy is mainly used to examine the back of the throat and the larynx. Endoscopy is carried out under local anaesthesia. The procedure can be repeated easily to monitor the progress of a disorder or treatment.

During the procedure
The endoscope is used to examine the nasal cavity and sometimes also the larynx. Instruments inserted through the endoscope can collect tissue samples or remove minor abnormalities, such as polyps.

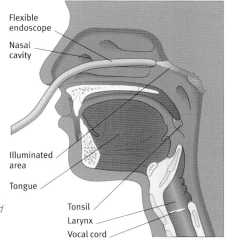

Flexible endoscope

Nasal cavity

Illuminated area

Tongue

Tonsil

Larynx

Vocal cord

VIEW

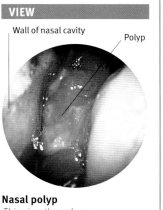

Wall of nasal cavity

Polyp

Nasal polyp
This view through an endoscope shows a polyp in the nasal cavity.

What can I do?

If you have other symptoms, such as daytime sleepiness or lack of concentration, you should consult your doctor in case you have sleep apnoea. Otherwise, the following self-help measures may bring relief. You may be able to prevent snoring by making it uncomfortable to sleep on your back, perhaps by sewing a small object, such as a tennis ball, into the back of your night clothes. If you are overweight, it will help to lose weight. You should also give up smoking, reduce alcohol consumption, and avoid taking sedatives or drinking alcohol before going to bed.

Sleep apnoea

Repeated temporary interruption of breathing during sleep

 Most common in children and in adults between the ages of 40 and 60

 More common in males

 Being overweight, drinking alcohol, and smoking are risk factors

 Genetics is not a significant factor

In sleep apnoea, breathing stops during sleep for at least 10 seconds at least five times an hour. Mild sleep apnoea causes few symptoms, but severe sleep apnoea may lead to low oxygen levels, which can cause serious symptoms. Sleep apnoea is more common in people who smoke, drink alcohol, or are overweight. It may occur at high altitudes.

What are the types?

Sleep apnoea can be divided into two types: obstructive sleep apnoea (OSA), which is common and due to blockage of the airway, and central sleep apnoea, which is rare and caused by a problem with the nerves that control breathing. In some cases, a mixture of both types of sleep apnoea occurs.

Obstructive sleep apnoea This condition mainly affects men aged between 40 and 60. OSA occurs when the air passages in the upper respiratory tract become obstructed during sleep. Most commonly, obstruction is caused by the soft tissue of the pharynx relaxing and blocking the flow of air. The obstruction prevents breathing until the low levels of oxygen in the blood cause a person to respond by waking up and taking a deep, snorting breath. Being overweight (particularly around the neck area) or having a large tongue or a small mouth can also cause or contribute to the obstruction. In children, enlarged tonsils (*see* **Tonsillitis**, p.546) or enlarged adenoids (p.546) are the most common causes of obstruction that can lead to OSA.

Central sleep apnoea In this rare type of sleep apnoea, the region of the brain and the nerves that regulate breathing do not function normally, and this causes breathing to be impaired. Causes of central sleep apnoea include brain damage following a head injury (p.322) or a stroke (p.329).

What are the symptoms?

The symptoms of OSA develop gradually, and it may be a partner or another member of your family who first notices your disturbed sleep. Central sleep apnoea may develop suddenly, depending on the cause. Symptoms of both types may include:

- Restless, unrefreshing sleep.
- Daytime sleepiness.
- Poor memory and concentration.
- Headache in the morning.
- Loud snoring (p.291).
- Change in personality.
- In men, erectile dysfunction (p.494).
- Frequent passing of urine at night.

In severe cases, daytime sleepiness may result in accidents, such as when driving. Taking sleeping drugs (p.591) and drinking alcohol may aggravate the symptoms. Left untreated, complications may develop, such as an irregular heartbeat (*see* **Arrhythmias**, p.249) and pulmonary hypertension (p.309). There is also an increased risk of high blood pressure developing (*see* **Hypertension**, p.242). Severe sleep apnoea may eventually be life-threatening.

How is it diagnosed?

If your doctor suspects that you have sleep apnoea, he or she will examine your nose and throat to look for an obvious cause of obstruction to your breathing. You may also have an endoscopy of the nose and throat (p.291). To confirm the diagnosis and assess the severity of sleep apnoea, you may be asked to undergo sleep studies (right).

What is the treatment?

If you have mild OSA, you should avoid sleeping drugs and alcohol. If you are overweight, losing weight often helps. You should also try to sleep on your side or elevate the head of the bed, which may relieve the symptoms. If it is caused by high altitudes, sleep apnoea should disappear when you acclimatize or return to lower altitudes.

▶ TEST

Sleep studies

Sleep studies monitor the changes in body processes during a period of normal sleep. Variables that are usually monitored during sleep include oxygen levels in the blood, brain activity, heart rate, blood pressure, airflow in the respiratory passages, and movement of the chest wall and the abdomen. If you undergo testing in a sleep laboratory, you may need to stay overnight.

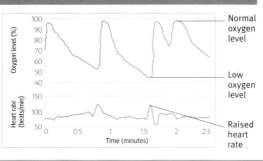

Monitor   Control panel

Electrode

Oximeter
This monitors oxygen levels

In the sleep laboratory
You will be attached to instruments that will continuously monitor various body functions while you are sleeping.

RESULTS

Trace indicating sleep apnoea
A trace of a 2.5 minute period of sleep shows oxygen levels falling each time breathing temporarily stops, indicating sleep apnoea. The heart rate rises in response to the lower oxygen levels.

Oxygen level (%)

Heart rate (beats/min)

Time (minutes)

Normal oxygen level

Low oxygen level

Raised heart rate

The first choice of treatment for OSA is usually positive pressure ventilation (below), in which air is steadily pumped through a mask. The increased air pressure keeps the airways open so that breathing is easier. The treatment is easy to use, but some people may find the mask uncomfortable and difficult to tolerate. If positive pressure ventilation is not effective, surgery to reduce the size of the soft palate or base of the tongue may be considered. If OSA is caused by enlarged tonsils or adenoids, surgery may be necessary to remove them (*see* **Tonsillectomy and adenoidectomy**, p.546).

Treatment for OSA is usually successful. Central sleep apnoea is more difficult to treat because, in most cases, the underlying causes are less likely to be reversible.

▶ TREATMENT

Positive pressure ventilation

During positive pressure ventilation, a steady supply of air is pumped to the nose during sleep through a tube and mask. The high pressure of the pumped air keeps the upper airways open. Positive pressure ventilation may be used to treat people with sleep apnoea, in which breathing repeatedly ceases for short periods of time during sleep. The treatment needs to be carried out every night during sleep, and it can be given easily at home.

Wearing the mask
A compressor supplies a flow of air at high pressure to the nose through a tube and mask. The mask is held in place by straps around the back of the head above and below the ears.

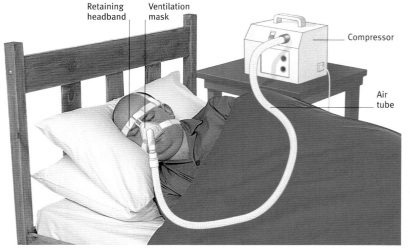

Retaining headband   Ventilation mask

Compressor

Air tube

Pharyngitis and tonsillitis

Inflammation of the pharynx (throat) and/or the tonsils

 Pharyngitis more common in adults; tonsillitis more common in children

 Smoking and drinking alcohol are risk factors

 Gender, genetics, and lifestyle are not significant factors

Pharyngitis and tonsillitis are common disorders, which are often described as a sore throat. The pharynx connects the back of the mouth and nose to the larynx (voice box) and the oesophagus. The tonsils lie at the top of the pharynx. Tonsillitis (p.546) is much more common in children because they have large tonsils, which shrink substantially as children get older. Adults tend to get pharyngitis. However, pharyngitis and tonsillitis can occur together in adults and children.

What are the causes?
Pharyngitis and tonsillitis are usually the result of a viral infection, such as a common cold (p.164) or infectious mononucleosis (p.166). Other causes include bacterial infections, such as with streptococcal bacteria, and fungal infections, such as candidiasis (p.177). Smoking and drinking alcohol may lead to pharyngitis in adults.

What are the symptoms?
Pharyngitis and tonsillitis have similar symptoms that tend to become worse over about 12 hours. They may include:
■ Sore throat.
■ Difficulty in swallowing.
■ Pain in the ear, which may be worse on swallowing.
■ Enlarged and tender lymph nodes in the neck.
Pharyngitis and tonsillitis may also be associated with a fever and feeling unwell, especially if the conditions are caused by a bacterial infection.

Are there complications?
In severe cases, the pharynx and/or the tonsils may become so swollen that difficulties with breathing develop. Occasionally, an abscess forms next to a tonsil, a condition

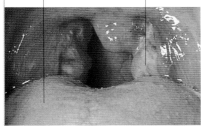
Tonsillitis
The tonsils shown here have become inflamed and covered with a white coating, a condition known as tonsillitis.

Tongue | Inflamed tonsil

Soothing a sore throat
A sore throat may be caused by pharyngitis, tonsillitis, or both. The following measures may help to relieve the discomfort:
■ Drink plenty of fluids, especially warm (not hot) or cold drinks.
■ Eat ice cream or suck ice lollies or ice cubes.
■ Gargle with warm salt water.
■ Take painkillers (p.589), such as paracetamol, at the recommended dose.
■ Suck throat lozenges containing a local anaesthetic (these are only suitable for adults).
■ Install a humidifier or place bowls of water near radiators to keep the air moist.

known as a peritonsillar abscess. Rarely, if pharyngitis and/or tonsillitis is caused by a streptococcal infection, the kidney disorder glomerulonephritis (p.446) may develop some weeks later.

What might be done?
There are self-help measures that you can take to ease a sore throat (*see* **Soothing a sore throat**, above). Both pharyngitis and tonsillitis normally clear up with these measures after a few days. However, if the pain is severe or has not improved after about 48 hours, or if you have difficulty breathing or swallowing, seek medical advice.

Your doctor may take a blood sample to test for infectious mononucleosis. If the doctor suspects that you have a bacterial infection, you may be given antibiotics (p.572). A peritonsillar abscess may be treated with intravenous antibiotics. It may also need to be drained under general or local anaesthesia. In some circumstances, it may be necessary to remove the tonsils, especially if a person has had repeated attacks of tonsillitis or a peritonsillar abscess.

Laryngitis

Inflammation of the larynx (voice box), usually caused by infection and producing hoarseness

 Smoking is a risk factor; drinking alcohol aggravates the condition

 Age, gender, and genetics are not significant factors

Laryngitis is inflammation of the larynx, which lies between the throat and the trachea (windpipe) and contains the vocal cords. The condition may be acute, lasting for only a few days, or be chronic and persist for months. It is rarely serious but can cause breathing difficulties in children (*see* **Croup**, p.545).

Acute laryngitis is usually caused by a viral infection, such as a common cold (p.164), but it may occur after straining the voice. Chronic laryngitis may be caused by smoking and long-term overuse of the

---

voice, which may damage the larynx. Drinking alcohol, particularly spirits, may aggravate laryngitis.

What are the symptoms?
The symptoms of laryngitis usually develop over a period of 12–24 hours and vary depending on the underlying cause. Symptoms may include:
■ Hoarseness.
■ Gradual loss of the voice.
■ Pain in the throat, especially when using the voice.
Sometimes, laryngitis is associated with vocal cord nodules (p.293).

What can I do?
Acute laryngitis that is caused by a viral infection usually clears up without treatment. There is no specific treatment for chronic laryngitis. For both forms of the condition, resting your voice can help to relieve pain and to avoid further damage to the vocal cords.

Steam inhalations (p.291) may also help to relieve symptoms. To prevent a recurrence of chronic laryngitis, you should try not to overuse your voice. If you smoke, you should try to stop completely, and, if you drink heavily, you should reduce your intake of alcohol.

Since hoarseness can be a symptom of cancer of the larynx (p.294), you should consult your doctor if a voice change persists for more than 2 weeks. He or she will probably arrange for you to go to hospital for mirror laryngoscopy (p.294) or endoscopic laryngoscopy (examination of the larynx with a viewing instrument).

Vocal cord nodules

Small, noncancerous lumps on the vocal cords, causing hoarseness

 More common in boys and adult females

 Excessive use of the voice is a risk factor

 Age and genetics are not significant factors

Constant strain on the voice sometimes leads to the formation of small, greyish-white nodules on the vocal cords of the larynx (voice box). Vocal cord nodules are noncancerous. The size of the nodules ranges from that of a pinhead to a grape seed. They sometimes cause scarring of the vocal cords.

The condition is common in people who tend to overuse their voices over a long period of time. For example, singers and teachers may be affected by vocal cord nodules. Drinking alcohol and smoking aggravate the symptoms. Nodules sometimes occur in persistently noisy children, especially boys who shout a lot.

The symptoms include increasing hoarseness, which develops suddenly or gradually, and rapid voice loss. You should consult a doctor if symptoms last more than 2 weeks because some types of cancer of the larynx (p.294) have similar symptoms.

What might be done?
Your doctor will probably arrange for you to go to hospital for mirror laryngoscopy (p.294) or endoscopic laryngoscopy (examination of the larynx with a viewing instrument) and possibly for a biopsy, in which a sample of tissue is removed using an endoscope (*see* **Endoscopy of the nose and throat**, p.291). If the nodules are small, you may be taught how to avoid straining your voice by a speech therapist (p.621). The nodules may then shrink or gradually disappear. Your doctor may suggest that you have larger nodules removed surgically. Sometimes the condition recurs.

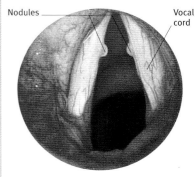
Nodules | Vocal cord

Vocal cord nodules
This view of the larynx (voice box) through an endoscope shows the vocal cords. A nodule can be seen on each vocal cord.

Cancer of the nasopharynx

A cancerous growth in the nasopharynx, the passage connecting the back of the nose to the throat

 Most common between the ages of 50 and 60

 More common in people from China or with Chinese ancestry

 Smoking, alcohol abuse, eating foods containing certain chemicals, and inhaling some dusts are risk factors

 Gender is not a significant factor

Cancer of the nasopharynx is a rare condition in which a tumour originates in the nasopharynx, the passage connecting the nasal cavity to the throat. This type of cancer occurs most frequently in people from China or with Chinese ancestry. The precise reason for this is unknown, but it may involve genetic factors or certain chemicals present in foods such as salted fish and fermented dishes. Other factors that may increase the risk of nasopharyngeal cancer include smoking or using snuff, alcohol abuse, and exposure to the Epstein–Barr virus (a common virus that can cause infectious mononucleosis, p.166). If cancer of the nasopharynx is diagnosed early, it is usually easily treated. However, if the cancer is not diagnosed at an early stage, it may spread to the lymph nodes of the neck and to other parts of the body and in some cases can be fatal.

What are the symptoms?

Initially, cancer of the nasopharynx may not cause symptoms and may not be noticed until the tumour spreads to a lymph node, causing a painless swelling in the neck. If symptoms do develop, they may include:

- Facial pain and swelling.
- Earache and loss of hearing.
- Loss of sense of smell.
- Repeated nosebleeds.
- Blocked or runny nose, usually affecting one nostril only.
- Discomfort on swallowing.
- Repeated sinusitis (p.290).

Left untreated, the cancer may spread, causing your voice to change or one side of your face to become paralysed.

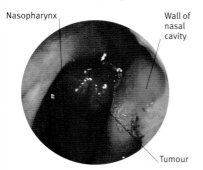

Cancer of the nasopharynx
This view through an endoscope shows a tumour in the nasopharynx, the passage connecting the nasal cavity and throat.

What might be done?

You may have endoscopy of the nose and throat (p.291) If a tumour is found, you may have a biopsy, in which a sample of tissue is removed from the growth and examined for signs of cancer. You may have CT scanning (p.132) or MRI (p.133) to assess the size of the tumour and to see if the cancer has spread.

If cancer is diagnosed early, a cure is possible. The usual treatment is radiotherapy (p.158), although if the lymph nodes in the neck are affected, surgery may be required. Both procedures may also be used to relieve symptoms. The outlook depends on how far the cancer has advanced, but overall, about 50 per cent of people survive for more than 5 years after diagnosis.

Cancer of the larynx

Cancer of the larynx (voice box), often causing persistent hoarseness

 Most common after the age of 50

 Four times more common in males

 Smoking and alcohol abuse are risk factors

 Genetics is not a significant factor

Cancer of the larynx is rare in the UK, accounting for only about 1 in every 100 cases of cancer. It usually occurs after the age of 50

▶ TEST

Mirror laryngoscopy

Also known as indirect laryngoscopy, mirror laryngoscopy involves viewing the larynx by shining a light on to a mirror held at the back of the palate. It may be used to detect disorders of the larynx, although laryngoscopy using an endoscope (viewing tube) is more common (p.291). Mirror laryngoscopy may be performed under local anaesthesia; if so, you should not eat or drink until the anaesthetic has worn off to avoid inhaling food or fluids.

Viewing the larynx
After spraying your throat with a local anaesthetic, the doctor places an angled mirror at the back of the palate. This enables the doctor to examine the larynx and vocal cords for abnormalities.

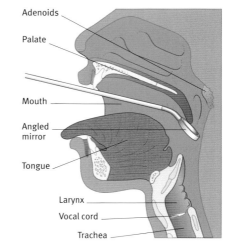

Adenoids
Palate
Mouth
Angled mirror
Tongue
Larynx
Vocal cord
Trachea

VIEW

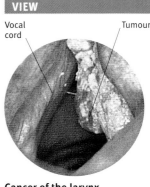

Vocal cord
Tumour

Cancer of the larynx
In this view of the larynx, one vocal cord is normal and the other vocal cord has a cancerous tumour.

---

and is four times more common in men than women. In about 6 in 10 cases, cancer develops on the vocal cords; in the remainder, it begins above or below the cords. If the cancer is on the cords, symptoms develop early, allowing prompt diagnosis and treatment. If cancer develops elsewhere in the larynx, it is more likely to be fatal.

The cause of laryngeal cancer is not known, but it is commonly associated with smoking and alcohol abuse. Without treatment, it may spread to lymph nodes in the neck and eventually to other areas.

What are the symptoms?

If a tumour develops on the vocal cords, the first noticeable symptom is hoarseness. If the tumour is not detected, it may spread above and below the vocal cords, causing symptoms such as:

- Loud breathing.
- Difficulty in breathing.
- Difficult and painful swallowing.

These symptoms may also occur if cancer develops above or below the vocal cords, although often these tumours do not produce symptoms at first. Tumours developing anywhere in the larynx may spread to lymph nodes in the neck, causing them to become enlarged.

How is it diagnosed?

Your doctor will examine your throat and, if cancer is suspected, will refer you for endoscopy of the larynx (examination of the larynx with a viewing instrument, p.291). In this procedure, which is carried out under anaesthesia, a tissue sample may also be removed. If the lymph nodes in the neck are enlarged, fine needle aspiration may be performed, in which a tissue sample is taken from a lymph node using a needle attached to a syringe. You may also have CT scanning (p.132) or MRI (p.133) to see how far the cancer has spread.

What is the treatment?

Treatment will depend on how far the cancer has spread. You may be offered radiotherapy (p.158), and you will possibly be given sur-

---

gery. If surgery to remove the entire larynx is necessary, you will need a permanent laryngectomy, in which a hole (stoma) is made in the windpipe (trachea) to maintain an airway for breathing. You may need a similar procedure called a tracheostomy temporarily while you are undergoing radiotherapy, but it can be reversed when treatment is completed.

If the larynx has to be removed, normal speech will no longer be possible. However, several techniques have been developed that allow speech without a larynx. A speech therapist (*see* **Speech therapy**, p.621) may teach you to speak using your oesophagus,

---

or a small device known as a tracheo-oesophageal valve may be fitted to help you to speak. Alternatively, you may be taught to speak using a hand-held electromechanical device that generates sounds.

In more than 9 in 10 cases in which the tumour develops on the vocal cords and is detected and treated early, treatment is successful. The chances of a cure are reduced if the cancer originates elsewhere in the larynx because symptoms appear later and the cancer may have already spread. In these cases, treatment may be given only to relieve symptoms, and survival rates are much lower.

Lung disorders

The lower part of the respiratory system consists of the trachea, which divides into the two main bronchi and then into smaller air passages, and the lungs. The lungs can be damaged by many factors, such as inhaled smoke and dust, infections, and allergies. The resulting disorders vary in severity from mild conditions, such as a cough, to life-threatening illnesses, such as lung cancer.

This section starts with two common symptoms, cough and hiccups. More serious disorders of the airways are discussed next, including asthma, a common long-term disorder in developed countries.

Many common lung diseases, such as pneumonia and tuberculosis, are caused by infections. After discussion of these disorders, articles follow on disorders of the pleura. Occupational lung diseases are then covered.

The next article discusses primary lung cancer, one of the most common types of cancer in the world and the most likely to prove fatal. Lung cancer is almost always caused by smoking. The final articles cover acute, potentially life-threatening lung disorders, such as acute respiratory distress syndrome.

Lung diseases specific to children are dealt with elsewhere (*see* **Infancy and childhood**, pp.524–565).

✚ KEY ANATOMY

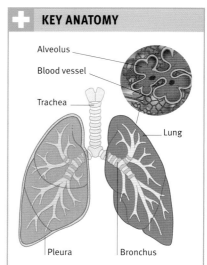

Alveolus
Blood vessel
Trachea
Lung
Pleura
Bronchus

For more information about the structure and function of the lungs, *see* pp.294–310.

Cough

A reflex response to irritation or infection of the respiratory tract

 More common in smokers

 Age, gender, and genetics are not significant factors

A cough is a protective reflex action that helps to clear irritants or blockages from the airways. If sputum is produced, the cough is termed productive; if no sputum is produced, the cough is called dry.

Most coughs are due to short-term irritation of the respiratory tract and generally disappear spontaneously. In other cases, coughing may be a sign of a serious disorder of the lungs that requires medical treatment.

What are the causes?

Many coughs are caused by irritation of the upper airways (the throat and trachea), either by inhaled particles or by mucus dripping from the back of the nose. Coughing is also often caused by inflammation of the upper airways, usually as a result of a viral infection such as influenza (p.164) or the common cold (p.164). Less commonly, a small foreign object, for example a peanut, is inhaled and causes violent coughing. Gastro-oesophageal reflux disease (p.403), a disorder in which acidic fluid from the stomach is regurgitated into the oesophagus, may result in a persistent cough.

More severe coughing may indicate damage to the lungs caused by inflammation associated with infections such as pneumonia (p.299), which is usually caused by bacterial infection, and acute bronchitis (p.297). In asthma (right), the airways in the lungs become narrowed and inflamed, producing a cough that is often worse at night or following exercise. The lungs may also be damaged by smoking, which provokes a characteristic "smoker's cough". Such a cough may indicate the development of chronic obstructive pulmonary disease (p.297). A smoker's cough is frequently much worse in the morning before the chest has been cleared of mucus that has accumulated overnight. Smoking-induced damage to the cilia (tiny hairs) that line the airways interferes with the normal process by which the lungs are cleared of excess mucus.

If a long-term smoker's cough suddenly becomes more intense or occurs more frequently than usual, this change may indicate the development of primary lung cancer (p.308) and requires immediate medical investigation.

A cough may also develop as a side effect of ACE inhibitor drugs (p.582), which are used in the treatment of high blood pressure and heart disease.

What can I do?

The majority of coughs clear up after a few days without requiring treatment. However, you should consult your doctor as soon as possible if you develop a cough that persists for more than about 2 weeks. You should also seek medical advice if the cough is severe or painful, produces bloody or discoloured sputum, or is accompanied by symptoms such as chest pain or shortness of breath.

You may be able to relieve a mild cough with an over-the-counter remedy (*see* **Cough remedies**, p.588). For example, some coughs may be relieved by taking a cough suppressant, which works by inhibiting the cough reflex. However, cough suppressants should not be used to treat a productive cough because coughing is the body's natural mechanism for clearing excess mucus from the lungs. Steam inhalation (p.291) may help to loosen the mucus.

What might the doctor do?

Your doctor may be able to diagnose the cause by listening to your cough and examining your chest. Sometimes, chest X-rays (p.300) or lung function tests (p.298) are necessary to confirm the diagnosis. Drugs can relieve a cough, but the cause may require specific treatment. For example, antibiotics (p.572) may be used to treat bacterial infection.

Hiccups

A sudden and involuntary intake of air, producing an unmistakable sound

 Age, gender, genetics, and lifestyle are not significant factors

Almost everyone has occasional attacks of hiccups. Usually, they last for only a few minutes and are no cause for concern. When you have hiccups, the muscles you use in order to breathe in, primarily the diaphragm, contract suddenly, causing a sharp intake of breath. This is interrupted almost immediately by an involuntary closure of the throat, which causes the characteristic sound of a hiccup. Hiccups occur even before birth; babies hiccup inside the uterus.

What are the causes?

In most cases, there is no obvious cause for hiccups. If they are persistent, hiccups may be due to physical irritation of the diaphragm or the nerves that supply it. Such irritation may be caused by a gastrointestinal problem, such as abnormal stretching of the stomach as a result of an obstruction, or by an accumulation of fluid under the diaphragm. In rare cases, hiccups are a symptom of a severe imbalance in body chemistry caused by disorders such as kidney failure (p.450) or liver failure (p.411).

What might be done?

There are a vast number of popular home remedies for hiccups, such as holding your breath or drinking a glass of water rapidly. If your hiccups are persistent, your doctor may prescribe a drug that relaxes your diaphragm, such as chlorpromazine (*see* **Antipsychotic drugs**, p.592).

Asthma

Intermittent narrowing of the airways, causing shortness of breath and wheezing

 Can occur at any age, but more common in children than adults

 More common in male children and adult females

 Sometimes runs in families

 Exposure to common allergens, including house dust mites, pollens, and pet fur, are risk factors

People with asthma have attacks of wheezing and shortness of breath that vary in severity from day to day and from month to month. Some people have only occasional mild attacks, while others may experience severe disabling symptoms on most days. Most people have symptoms that fall somewhere between these two extremes, but, when their asthma attacks occur, they tend to be unpredictable in length and severity. Severe attacks of asthma are potentially life-threatening if they are not given immediate medical treatment.

Although asthma can begin at any age, most adults with the condition developed it as children. More boys than girls are affected but, in adults, asthma is more common in women. The problems associated with asthma and its management are different in children. For this reason, there is a separate article on asthma in children (p.544) in the section on childhood disorders.

How common is it?

The UK has one of the highest rates of asthma in the world, although the reasons for this are unclear. About 5.4 million people in the UK are being treated for asthma, of whom about 4.3 million are adults (about 1 in 12 of all adults) and 1.1 million are children (about 1 in 11 of all children). It is the most common long-term medical problem affecting children in the UK.

What are the causes?

During an asthma attack, the muscle in the walls of the bronchi (airways) contracts, causing narrowing. The linings of the airways also become swollen and inflamed, producing excess mucus that can block the smaller airways.

In some people, an allergic response triggers the airway changes. This allergic type of asthma tends to occur in childhood, and may develop in association with eczema or certain other allergic conditions, such as hay fever (*see* **Allergic rhinitis**, p.283). Susceptibility to these conditions frequently runs in families and may be inherited.

Some substances, called allergens, are known as trigger attacks of allergic asthma. They include pollen, house dust mites, mould, and dander and saliva from furry animals, such as cats and dogs. Rarely, certain foods, such as milk, eggs, nuts, and wheat, provoke an allergic asthmatic reaction. Some people who have asthma are sensitive to aspirin or other anti-inflammatory drugs (such as ibuprofen) and taking them may trigger an attack.

When asthma starts in adulthood, there are usually no identifiable allergic triggers. The first attack is often brought on by a respiratory infection.

Factors that can provoke attacks in a person with asthma include cold air, exercise, smoke, and occasionally emotional factors such as stress and anxiety. Although industrial pollution and exhaust emissions from motor vehicles do not normally cause asthma, they do appear to worsen symptoms in people who already have the disorder. Pollution in the atmosphere may also trigger asthma in susceptible people.

In some cases, a substance that is inhaled regularly in the work environment can cause a previously healthy person to develop occupational asthma, one of the few occupational lung diseases (p.305) that is still increasing in incidence. If you develop wheezing and shortness of breath that improve when you are not in your work environment, you may have this disorder.

There are more than 200 substances found in the workplace that are known to triggers symptoms of asthma, including isocyanates (used in spray-painting, for example); dust from flour, grain, wood, and from insects and other animals; glues; resins; and latex. However, occupational asthma can be difficult to diagnose because a person may be regularly exposed to a particular trigger substance for weeks, months, or even years before the symptoms begin to appear.

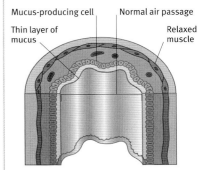

NORMAL AIRWAY

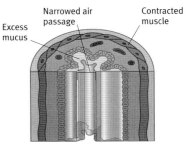

CONSTRICTED AIRWAY

The effect of asthma on the airways
Normally, air flows freely through the airways. In an asthma attack, the muscles of the bronchi walls contract, and excess mucus collects, restricting the flow of air.

What are the symptoms?

The symptoms of asthma may develop gradually and may not be noticed until a trigger provokes the first severe attack. For example, exposure to an allergen or a respiratory tract infection may cause the following symptoms:

- Wheezing.
- Painless tightening in the chest.
- Shortness of breath.
- Difficulty exhaling.
- Dry, persistent cough.
- Feelings of panic.
- Sweating.

These symptoms often become considerably worse at night and in the early hours of the morning.

Some people find that they develop mild wheezing during a common cold or a chest infection, but usually this does not indicate asthma. The main feature that distinguishes asthma from other respiratory conditions is its variability.

If asthma becomes severe, the following symptoms may develop:

- Wheezing that is almost inaudible because so little air flows through the airways.
- Inability to complete a sentence due to shortness of breath.
- Blue lips, tongue, fingers, and toes due to lack of oxygen.
- Exhaustion, confusion, and coma.

If you are with someone who is having a severe attack of asthma or your own symptoms continue to worsen, you need to call an ambulance.

How is it diagnosed?

If you have had breathing problems recently but are free of symptoms when you consult the doctor, he or she will ask you to describe your symptoms and will examine you. Your doctor may also arrange for you to have various tests, such as spirometry, to measure how efficiently your lungs work (see **Lung function tests**, p.298). As part of these tests, your doctor may ask you to exercise for a few minutes in an attempt to induce a mild attack of asthma. Less commonly, the doctor will measure how irritable your airways are by getting you to breathe in a small dose of a test chemical. If you do have an asthma attack as a result of these tests, you will be given medication to relieve it.

You may also be given a peak flow meter to take home and asked to record measurements over a period of weeks. A peak flow meter is a small device that measures the speed at which you exhale air. Your doctor or a nurse will show you how to use the device and how to record measurements (see **Monitoring your asthma**, below). You may also be asked to record your symptoms to help the doctor make a diagnosis.

If you have a severe attack of shortness of breath, you may be treated and sent to hospital for assessment. Once you are admitted to hospital, the oxygen level in your blood will be assessed (see **Measuring blood gases**, p.306), and you may have a chest X-ray (p.300) to rule out other serious lung disorders, such as a pneumothorax (p.303).

If you are diagnosed with asthma, your doctor may suggest that you have further tests at a later date to check for allergies to substances that are known to trigger attacks. If the timing and occurrence of your symptoms suggests that you have occupational asthma, your doctor will ask about substances used in your workplace to try to identify a specific trigger for your asthma.

What is the treatment?

Some people with asthma do not need treatment if they manage to avoid the factors that trigger their symptoms (see **Living with asthma**, opposite page). However, there are so many triggers that it is very difficult to avoid them all, and for this reason treatment is often necessary.

Today, asthma attacks can usually be treated with short-acting drugs. In addition, long-term maintenance treatment can prevent asthma attacks developing. The current approach to asthma treatment is to give you the knowledge and confidence to be able to manage the condition yourself on a day-to-day basis, in partnership with your doctor. The most important aspects of controlling your asthma effectively are the careful planning of drug treatment and regular monitoring of your condition.

The aim of all drug treatment is to eliminate symptoms and reduce the frequency and severity of asthma attacks so that visits to an accident and emergency department are no longer needed. Severe, potentially fatal attacks rarely develop without warning. Recognizing a serious change in your condition and taking prompt action by adjusting your treatment or contacting your doctor are essential to prevent an attack occurring.

Types of drugs The drugs that are used to treat asthma fall into two distinct categories: quick-relief drugs (relievers), which are used to relieve an attack of wheezing; and preventer drugs, which help to prevent attacks occurring. Most relievers are bronchodilators. There are several different types of bronchodilator, all of which relax the muscles that narrow the airways and treat breathing problems as they occur. Relievers are usually effective within a few minutes if they are inhaled, but their effect lasts for only a few hours. They should be used as soon as symptoms develop or, if recommended by your doctor, before you start to exercise.

Most preventers of asthma are corticosteroid drugs (see **Corticosteroids for respiratory disease**, p.588), which slow the production of mucus, reduce inflammation in the airways, and make the airways less likely to narrow when they are exposed to a trigger substance. Non-steroidal preventers, such as sodium cromoglicate and leukotriene antagonist drugs (see **Antiallergy drugs**, p.585), are sometimes used to reduce the allergic response and to prevent narrowing of the airways. This type of treatment must be used on a daily basis and can take several days to become effective.

Both relievers and preventers are usually inhaled from a special device called a metered-dose inhaler, which delivers a fixed dose of the drug. Your doctor or another healthcare professional will show you how to use an inhaler. For acute asthma attacks, some people find drugs are most effective when inhaled using a spacer attached to the inhaler or through a device called a nebulizer. This device produces a fine mist of drugs to be inhaled through a mouthpiece or face mask (see **Taking inhaled asthma drugs**, opposite page). Spacers are also useful if you find it difficult to coordinate releasing the drug and inhaling. Children may need to use spacers.

People with long-term severe asthma may occasionally be given additional preventers in the form of low-dose oral corticosteroids rather than just inhaled drugs. Oral corticosteroids may also be given to relieve severe attacks.

Day-to-day management Adults who have asthma are encouraged to take as much responsibility as possible for managing their condition. Asthma may vary in severity from day to day or over longer periods. For this reason, you and your doctor will probably develop an asthma management plan which helps you to assess your symptoms and make adjustments to your treatment accordingly. The key to controlling asthma is regular monitoring of symptoms and self-assessment using a symptom diary and a peak flow meter, which determines the rate at which you are able to exhale.

As you follow your management plan, your asthma treatment will move up a level, down a level, or stay the same, depending on your most recent symptoms and peak flow readings. A different level of treatment may involve altering a drug dosage; taking the medicine in another way, such as orally instead of by inhaling; taking a different drug; and/or using the treatment more or less frequently. If one level of treatment is not controlling your asthma, you move up to the next level.

If you are an adult newly diagnosed with asthma, treatment may start with a reliever drug only. Preventers may be added gradually if you find that you are using relievers more than a few times a week. Your doctor will closely monitor your progress over a period of time to determine whether your treatment plan needs to be changed. If you use your peak flow meter to monitor your asthma every day, you will get an early warning sign of worsening of your condition and can adapt your treatment in accordance with the prescribed plan. Discuss your treatment plan with your doctor and ensure that you understand it. Your plan should include specific advice on what to do if you experience a severe attack of asthma.

Emergency treatment If you have a sudden, severe attack of asthma, you should use your reliever inhaler as instructed by your doctor. If this treatment does not appear to be working, call for an ambulance immediately. If you have been given a reserve supply of corticosteroids as part of

---

▶ **TEST**

Monitoring your asthma

The best way to monitor your asthma is with a peak flow meter, which is used every morning and evening to measure the maximum rate at which you can exhale in litres per minute. The reading indicates whether your airways are narrowed. Plotted on a chart, your peak flow results show how effectively your asthma is being controlled. You can then adjust your treatment, following advice given to you previously by your doctor.

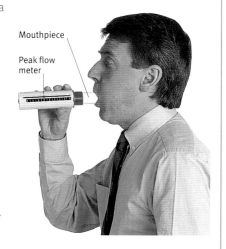

Mouthpiece

Peak flow meter

Using a peak flow meter
You should take a full breath in, seal your lips around the mouthpiece, and exhale as hard as you can. The pointer on the side of the meter shows your peak flow result.

RESULTS

Charting your peak flow
This chart shows twice-daily peak flow readings with marked variations between the morning and evening readings. These variations indicate that the asthma is poorly controlled.

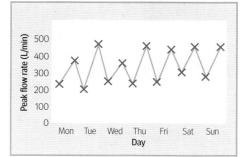

Taking inhaled asthma drugs

Drugs to prevent or treat asthma are often inhaled. Inhaled drugs reach the lungs quickly and have few side effects because only a small amount of drug enters the circulation. A metered-dose inhaler delivers a precise dose when the inhaler is pressed. A spacer can be used to hold the dose before it is inhaled. For treatment of a severe asthma attack, a nebulizer, which enables the delivery of large drug doses, may be used. Different devices are available for children (see **Giving inhaled drugs to children**, p.544).

Metered-dose inhaler

Drug suspended inside spacer

Metered-dose inhaler

Mouthpiece

SPACER

Using an inhaler
Place the inhaler in front of the lips or in the mouth. Press the inhaler while breathing in deeply at the same time. Hold your breath for 10 seconds, then breathe out. Spacers allow the drug to be inhaled over several breaths.

Using a nebulizer
A nebulizer creates a fine mist of drugs by forcing compressed air or oxygen through a liquid dose of the drug. The drug in mist form is then inhaled, through either a mouthpiece or a face mask.

Mouthpiece

Drug chamber
The drug is dissolved in 3–5 ml of fluid

Tube
This delivers compressed air

Compressor

your treatment plan, take them as advised by your doctor. You should try to stay calm and sit in a comfortable position. Place your hands on your knees to help to support your back; do not lie down. Try to slow down the rate of your breathing to prevent yourself from becoming exhausted.

In hospital, you will probably be given oxygen and corticosteroids and also bronchodilators at a high dose, either through a nebulizer or using a spacer. On the rare occasions when emergency drug treatment is not immediately effective, mechanical ventilation to force oxygen-enriched air into the lungs may be needed.

Living with asthma

Without doubt, the single most important aspect of controlling your asthma is the careful and planned use of drug treatments. However, there are several things that you can do to reduce your risk of an attack and to decrease the severity of your symptoms:

- Do not smoke and try to avoid polluted or smoky atmospheres.
- Take regular exercise to improve your stamina. Swimming is a particularly beneficial form of exercise. Avoid exercising outside when it is cold because this may provoke an attack.
- Avoid substances that are likely to provoke an allergic response; do not keep furry animals as pets if you are allergic to them.
- Always carry a reliever inhaler, and be sure that you take medication with you on holiday.
- If your attacks are triggered by stress, try to practise relaxation exercises (p.32).

What is the prognosis?

The majority of children and adults with asthma are able to lead normal lives if they receive medical advice for their condition and then follow their treatment plans. Asthma that begins during childhood disappears by the age of 20 in at least half of all cases.

Generally, the outlook is excellent for adults who have asthma but are otherwise healthy as long as there is careful monitoring of their condition.

In spite of this encouraging outlook, about 1,170 people in the UK died from severe asthma attacks in 2011. In most cases, the cause of death is a delay in recognizing the severity of an asthma attack and consequently a delay in getting to hospital.

Acute bronchitis

Short-term inflammation of the airways, most often due to a viral infection

 More common in adults

 Smoking and air pollution are risk factors

 Gender and genetics are not significant factors

In otherwise healthy adults, acute bronchitis may develop as a complication of respiratory infection. It is a recurrent problem for people with chronic obstructive pulmonary disease (right), who often have several episodes each winter. In acute bronchitis, the lining of the bronchi (the main airways of the lungs), becomes inflamed, often due to infection. The inflammation produces a large amount of mucus, which is usually coughed up as sputum. In adults who are otherwise well, acute bronchitis does not usually cause permanent damage, but in older people or those who have a heart or lung disorder, infection may spread further into the lungs, causing pneumonia (p.299).

Acute bronchitis is often caused by a viral infection, such as a common cold (p.164) that has spread from the nose, throat, or sinuses. Smokers, people who have an existing lung disorder, or those who are exposed to high levels of air pollution are more prone to attacks.

What are the symptoms?

The symptoms of acute bronchitis usually develop quickly over 24–48 hours and may include the following:

- Irritating, persistent cough that produces clear sputum.
- Central chest pain on coughing.
- Tightness of the chest and wheezing.
- Mild fever.

If you have a long-term heart or lung disease and develop the above symptoms, or if you cough up discoloured sputum, indicating a secondary infection, contact your doctor promptly. If you have a reserve supply of antibiotics, take them as instructed by your doctor.

What might be done?

In a person who is otherwise in good health, acute bronchitis caused by a viral infection usually clears up within a few days. Taking an over-the-counter painkiller (p.589), such as paracetamol, may help to bring down your temperature. If you smoke, give up immediately.

If your doctor suspects that you have developed a secondary bacterial infection, he or she will probably prescribe antibiotics (p.572). You should make a full recovery within 2 weeks of starting treatment. If acute bronchitis persists, your doctor may arrange for you to have additional investigations, such as a chest X-ray (p.300), to look for an underlying lung disorder.

Chronic obstructive pulmonary disease

Progressive damage to the lungs, usually caused by smoking, resulting in wheezing and shortness of breath

 More common over the age of 40

 Twice as common in males

 Rarely, due to an abnormal gene inherited from both parents

 Smoking especially, and air pollution are risk factors

In chronic obstructive pulmonary disease (COPD), the airways and tissues of the lungs gradually become damaged over time, causing increasing shortness of breath. Eventually, some people with COPD become so short of breath that they are seriously disabled and unable to carry out even simple daily activities. COPD is twice as common in men and is almost always caused by smoking.

People with COPD usually have two separate lung conditions, chronic bronchitis and emphysema. Either one may be dominant. In chronic bronchitis, the bronchi (airways) become inflamed, congested, and narrowed, and this obstructs the flow of air through them. In emphysema, the alveoli (air sacs) in the lungs become enlarged and damaged, making them less efficient in transferring oxygen from the lungs to the blood. The damage to the lungs is usually irreversible, although coughing and sputum production may lessen after a person gives up smoking. In the UK, about 900,000 people have been diagnosed with COPD and it is estimated that about 2 million people have undiagnosed COPD. It is also a leading cause of death in the UK.

What are the causes?

The main cause of both chronic bronchitis and emphysema, and hence of COPD, is smoking. Atmospheric pollution also contributes to the condition. For this reason, COPD is more common in industrialized areas where there is a high percentage of smokers in the population. Occupational exposure to dust, noxious gases, or other lung irritants can worsen existing COPD.

In chronic bronchitis, the linings of the airways of the lungs respond to smoke irritation by becoming thickened, narrowing the passages that carry air into and out of the lungs. Mucus glands in the bronchial linings multiply so that more mucus is produced, and the normal mechanism for clearing the airways and coughing up excess mucus as sputum is impaired. As the disease progresses, retained mucus in the airways easily becomes infected, which may lead to further damage. Repeated infections eventually cause the linings of the airways to become permanently thickened and scarred.

In emphysema, tobacco smoke and other airborne pollutants damage the air sacs. The sacs lose their elasticity, and the lungs become distended. Eventually, the air sacs tear and merge, reducing their total surface area, and air becomes trapped in the dilated sacs. As a result, the amount of oxygen that enters the blood with each breath is reduced. Rarely, the principal cause of emphysema is an inherited condition known as alpha₁-antitrypsin deficiency (opposite page). In such cases, damage occurs whether or not the person smokes, but smoking accelerates the disease.

What are the symptoms?
The symptoms of COPD may take many years to develop. When they do appear, symptoms often occur in this order:

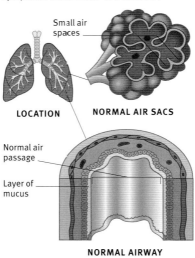

LOCATION NORMAL AIR SACS

Small air spaces

Normal air passage

Layer of mucus

NORMAL AIRWAY
NORMAL LUNG

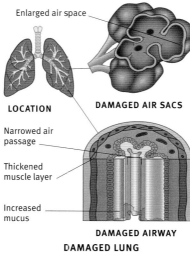

LOCATION DAMAGED AIR SACS

Enlarged air space

Narrowed air passage

Thickened muscle layer

Increased mucus

DAMAGED AIRWAY
DAMAGED LUNG
Damage to the lungs from COPD
In chronic obstructive pulmonary disease, the lungs are damaged in two ways. The air sacs of the lungs become stretched and coalesce, reducing the area over which oxygen is absorbed, and the air passages narrow due to thickened walls and increased mucus.

- Coughing in the morning that produces sputum.
- Coughing throughout the day.
- Increasing production of sputum.
- Frequent chest infections, especially in the winter months, producing yellow or green sputum.

- Wheezing, especially after coughing.
- Shortness of breath on mild exertion, becoming progressively worse so that eventually breathlessness occurs even when at rest.

Cold weather and infections such as influenza (p.164) cause symptoms to worsen.

Some people with emphysema develop a barrel-shaped chest as their lungs become distended. Respiratory failure (p.310) may develop, in which lack of oxygen causes the lips, tongue, fingers, and toes to turn blue. In addition, there may be ankle swelling due to reduced kidney function and chronic heart

---

▶ **TEST**

Lung function tests

Two tests are used to detect airflow problems in the lungs: spirometry, which measures how quickly the lungs fill and empty, and the lung volume test, which shows how much air the lungs can hold. These tests distinguish between disorders that narrow the airways and those that cause lung shrinkage. Gas transfer tests (not shown) use a small amount of inhaled carbon monoxide to determine how fast a gas is absorbed from the lungs into the blood.

Spirometry
A spirometer is used to measure the volume of air (in litres) that you can inhale and exhale over a period of time. The results show whether the airways are narrowed as a result of lung disorders such as asthma. Spirometry can also be used to monitor the effectiveness of certain treatments for lung disorders, such as bronchodilator drugs, which widen the airways.

Using the spirometer
You will be asked to inhale and exhale fully through a mouthpiece several times. The volume of air inhaled and exhaled is displayed on the monitor.

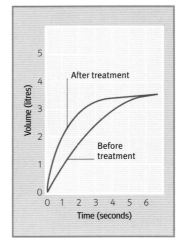

Monitor Nose clip

Spirometer

RESULTS

After treatment

Before treatment

Volume (litres)

Time (seconds)

Spirometry graph
This graph shows the effect of drug treatment to widen the air passages in a person with asthma. The volume of air that is exhaled in 1 second rises from about 1 litre to 2 litres soon after the drugs have been taken.

Lung volume test
This test measures the volume of air (in litres) that can be taken in with a full breath and the volume of air that remains in the lungs when the breath is fully exhaled. The lung volume test is used to help diagnose disorders such as chronic obstructive pulmonary disease that affect the volume of air retained by the lungs after breathing out.

RESULTS

Normal breathing

Full inhalation

Volume (litres)

Volume remaining in the lungs

Full exhalation

Time (seconds)

Lung volume graph
This shows the amount of air exhaled and inhaled by normally functioning lungs.

During the test
You will be asked to sit in an airtight booth and breathe in and out through a tube as fully as you can. The volume of air you can inhale and exhale is displayed as a graph on a monitor.

Technician

Airtight booth Mouthpiece Nose clip

Monitor

Printer

failure (p.247). Some people with severe airway narrowing compensate by working hard at breathing and manage to keep their oxygen levels within a normal range when they are at rest. They tend to have a rosy flush to the skin and may be thin because of the amount of energy they expend on breathing and because they find it difficult to eat and breathe at the same time. Other people with severe COPD can only manage shallow, ineffective breathing and consequently carbon dioxide builds up in the blood and oxygen levels fall. These people tend to have a blue complexion and tissue swelling in the feet and legs. Their condition is often compounded by heart failure.

How is it diagnosed?

If you have a history of smoking, the doctor may suspect COPD from your symptoms and a physical examination. He or she may arrange for you to have lung function tests (opposite) to assess the extent of lung damage. You may also have a chest X-ray (p.300) or CT scan (p.132). Part of the assessment of lung function may involve taking blood samples to check the levels of oxygen and carbon dioxide (see **Measuring blood gases**, p.306).

If members of your family have developed COPD before the age of 60, you may need a blood test to check the levels of the enzyme alpha₁-antitrypsin to look for a deficiency. Your doctor may take a sample of sputum to check for infection, and you may also have electrocardiography (see **ECG**, p.243) or echocardiography (p.255) to see if your heart is working unusually hard to pump blood through the lungs.

Chronic asthma (p.295) can produce similar symptoms to those of COPD. If your doctor suspects that you have asthma, you may be prescribed corticosteroid drugs (see **Corticosteroids for respiratory disease**, p.588). If your symptoms improve dramatically, this suggests that you may have asthma rather than COPD.

What can I do?

If you develop COPD and you smoke, giving up permanently is the only act on that can slow the progression of COPD. Simply cutting down on your smoking will have little or no effect on the progression of the disorder. Your environment should be kept as free as possible from smoke, pollution, dust, dampness, and cold. If you are overweight, losing the excess weight may help to alleviate breathlessness. Your doctor may suggest that you attend a pulmonary rehabilitation programme. Run by healthcare professionals, this is a programme of exercise and education that typically includes advice about lung health and coping with breathlessness, individually tailored physical exercises and breathing exercises, nutritional advice, and psychological and social support.

How might the doctor treat it?

The damage caused by COPD is largely irreversible but there are treatments that may ease the symptoms. You doctor may pre-scribe an inhaler containing a bronchodilator drug (p.588) to open up the airways of the lungs. If the bronchodilator drug does not relieve symptoms adequately, your doctor may suggest an inhaled corticosteroid drug (p.600) in addition to the bronchodilator. For people with severe COPD, it may be recommended that the drugs are taken via a nebulizer (which converts the drugs to a fine mist that is inhaled through a face mask or mouthpiece) rather than by an inhaler.

Some people may be offered continuous home oxygen therapy (p.310) to relieve shortness of breath. However, this must be used continuously for at least 15 hours each day to help prevent heart failure and improve life expectancy.

If you have swollen ankles, your doctor may prescribe diuretics (p.583) to reduce the build-up of fluid. Antibiotics (p.572) may be prescribed if a chest infection develops. You should be immunized against influenza, and you may also be given a vaccine to protect against *Streptococcus pneumoniae*. Both these infections are likely to be serious in people with COPD.

In rare cases of very severe COPD in which the lungs are distended, surgery may be suggested. A procedure called lung volume reduction surgery involves removing damaged areas of lung to allow the remaining areas to inflate and deflate more easily and increase oxygen in the blood. As a last resort for a very small minority of patients who are terminally ill with COPD, a lung transplant may be a possibility.

What is the prognosis?

If your COPD is mild and has been diagnosed at an early stage, you may be able to avoid severe, progressive lung damage by giving up smoking at once. However, most people with COPD do not realize they have the condition until it is well advanced. These people may need to retire from work early and may become housebound by shortness of breath. Fewer than 1 in 20 people with COPD survives for more than 10 years after diagnosis.

Alpha₁-antitrypsin deficiency

An inherited disorder that can result in damage to the lungs and liver

 Present from birth, but effects usually appear after the age of 40

 Due to a genetic abnormality on chromosome 14

 Smoking and drinking alcohol may hasten onset of symptoms

 Gender is not a significant factor

The enzyme alpha₁-antitrypsin prevents other enzymes in the body from destroying tissues, mainly those in the lungs and liver. People with alpha₁-antitrypsin deficiency lack this protective enzyme due to an abnormality in a gene on chromosome 14 (called the A1AT gene) that regulates production of the enzyme. The abnormal A1AT gene is usually inherited in an autosomal recessive pattern, which means that a person must inherit one copy of the abnormal gene from each parent to develop the condition (see **Gene disorders**, p.151). However, there are many variants of the A1AT gene and there are therefore variations in the severity of the condition.

In severe cases, alpha₁-antitrypsin deficiency causes jaundice in newborn babies (see **Neonatal jaundice**, p.531). However, the effects of the disorder most often appear after the age of 40 and include damage to the air sacs (alveoli) in the lungs (see **Chronic obstructive pulmonary disease**, p.297). Liver cirrhosis (p.410) may also develop.

What might be done?

The diagnosis is made by measuring levels of the enzyme in the blood, and a blood test should establish if you have the genetic abnormality. Other family members may also need to be tested. If you are planning to start a family, you may wish to consult your doctor about having genetic counselling (p.151).

At present, no specific treatment for alpha₁-antitrypsin deficiency is available, but trials of enzyme replacement therapy are in progress. Your doctor may prescribe inhaled bronchodilator drugs (p.588) to assist your breathing. People with severe lung or liver disease may be helped by an organ transplant. You should not smoke or drink alcohol if you have alpha₁-antitrypsin deficiency because these activities may cause lung and liver disease to worsen.

Pneumonia

Inflammation of the alveoli (air sacs) of the lungs, usually resulting from infection

 Most common in infants, children, and elderly people

 Smoking, alcohol abuse, and malnutrition are risk factors

 Gender and genetics are not significant factors

In pneumonia, some of the alveoli (air sacs) in the lungs become inflamed and fill with white blood cells and secretions. As a result, it is more difficult for oxygen to pass across the walls of the alveoli into the bloodstream. Usually, only part of one lung is affected, but, in some severe cases, pneumonia affects both lungs and can be life-threatening.

The cause of the inflammation is usually a bacterial infection, but other organisms, including viruses, protozoa, and fungi, may also cause pneumonia. Less commonly, inhaling certain substances, such as chemicals or vomit, causes inflammation, which may lead to a serious condition called acute respiratory distress syndrome (p.309).

In the UK, pneumonia affects about 1 in 1,000 adults each year, and most people with the disorder recover completely. However, it can still be fatal, particularly in vulnerable groups such as the elderly, infants, and those with another underlying illness. Some forms of pneumonia are becoming more difficult to treat due to the increasing resistance to antibiotics of some of the organisms responsible for the disease. For this reason, pneumonia is one of the most common fatal infections acquired in hospital.

Infants, elderly people, and people who are already seriously ill or have a long-term disease, such as diabetes mellitus (p.437), are at the greatest risk of developing pneumonia. Other people more likely to develop pneumonia are those who have lowered immunity as a result of a serious disease such as AIDS (see **HIV infection and AIDS**, p.169). Impaired immunity can also occur during treatment with immunosuppressant drugs (p.585) or chemotherapy (p.157). People who smoke, abuse alcohol, or who are malnourished are also at increased risk of pneumonia.

What are the causes?

Most cases of pneumonia in adults are caused by infection with a bacterium, most commonly *Streptococcus pneumoniae*. This type of pneumonia (sometimes called pneumococcal pneumonia) may develop as a complication of a viral infection in the upper respiratory tract, such as a common cold (p.164). Other common causes of bacterial pneumonia in healthy adults include infection with the bacteria *Haemophilus influenzae* and *Mycoplasma pneumoniae*.

The bacterium known as *Legionella pneumophila* causes a form of pneumonia called Legionnaires' disease, which can be spread through air-conditioning systems. Legionnaires' disease may also lead to liver and kidney disorders.

Pneumonia caused by the bacterium *Staphylococcus aureus* usually affects people who are already in hospital with another illness, particularly very young children and the elderly. This type of pneumonia can also develop as a serious complication of influenza (p.164). Other causes of pneumonia that are acquired in hospital include infection with klebsiella and pseudomonas bacteria. Viral causes of pneumonia include the organisms that are responsible for influenza and chickenpox (p.165).

In some cases, pneumonia is due to other organisms, such as fungi and protozoa. These infections tend to be rare and mild when they occur in otherwise healthy adults but are more common and potentially more serious in those with reduced immunity. For example, *Pneumocystis jirovecii* may live harmlessly in healthy lungs but can cause severe pneumonia in people who have AIDS (see **Pneumocystis infection**, p.177).

A rare type of pneumonia, known as aspiration pneumonia, may be caused by the accidental inhalation of vomit. Aspiration pneumonia is most likely to occur in people who have no cough reflex, often because they are unconscious after consuming an excessive amount of alcohol, taking a drug overdose, or sustaining a head injury (p.322).

What are the symptoms?
Bacterial pneumonia usually has a rapid onset, and severe symptoms generally develop within a few hours. You may experience the following symptoms:
■ Cough that may produce bloody or rust-coloured sputum.
■ Chest pain that becomes worse when you inhale.
■ Shortness of breath at rest.
■ High fever, delirium, or confusion.

When pneumonia is caused by organisms other than bacteria, it produces less specific symptoms that may develop gradually. You may feel generally unwell for several days and develop a fever, and you may lose your appetite. Coughing and shortness of breath may be the only respiratory symptoms.

The symptoms associated with all types of pneumonia are often less obvious in infants, children, and elderly people. Infants may initially vomit and can develop a high fever that may cause a convulsion. Elderly people may have no respiratory symptoms but often become progressively confused.

Are there complications?
Inflammation may spread from the lungs to the pleura (the membrane that separates the lungs from the chest wall), causing pleurisy (p.301). Fluid may accumulate between the two pleura (see **Pleural effusion**, p.302), compressing the underlying lung and making breathing difficult.

In severe cases, the microorganism that initially caused the infection may enter the bloodstream, leading to blood poisoning (see **Septicaemia**, p.171). In some vulnerable

people, such as young children, elderly people, or those with a weakened immune system, the inflammation caused by pneumonia may spread widely into the lung tissue and result in respiratory failure (p.310), which is a life-threatening condition.

How is it diagnosed?
If your doctor suspects pneumonia, the diagnosis may be confirmed by a chest X-ray (below), which will show the extent of infection in the lung. A sample of sputum may be collected and tested to identify the organism that has caused the infection. The doctor may also arrange for you to have blood tests to help to reach a precise diagnosis.

What is the treatment?
If you are otherwise healthy and have a mild form of pneumonia, you can probably be treated at home. Painkillers (p.589) should help to reduce fever and chest pain. If a bacterial infection is the cause of the pneumonia, your doctor will treat it with antibiotics (p.572). If pneumonia is caused by a fungal infection, antifungal drugs (p.574) may be prescribed. No drug treatment is usually needed for mild viral pneumonia.

Hospital treatment will probably be needed in severe cases of pneumonia and also for infants, children, elderly people, and people whose immune systems are suppressed. In all these cases, drug treatment is essentially the same as for people treated at home. Severe pneumonia caused by a viral infection, such as infection by the varicella zoster virus that causes chickenpox, may be treated with oral or intravenous aciclovir (see **Antiviral drugs**, p.573).

If the oxygen levels in your blood are low or if you are short of breath, you will be given oxygen through a face mask. Less commonly, mechanical ventilation in an intensive therapy unit (p.618) may be

required. You may have chest physiotherapy (p.620) regularly while you are in hospital to help to loosen excess mucus in the airways so that it can be coughed up as sputum.

What is the prognosis?
Young people who are in good health are generally able to recover from most types of pneumonia within 2–3 weeks, and there is no permanent damage to the lung tissue. Recovery from bacterial pneumonia usually begins within a few hours of starting treatment with antibiotics. However, some severe types of pneumonia, such as Legionnaires' disease, may be fatal, especially in people whose immune systems are weakened.

Can it be prevented?
Vaccination against pneumococcus (which is part of the routine childhood immunization programme) and influenza can help to prevent pneumonia, as can stopping smoking. Good personal hygiene can help to prevent spreading the causative organism.

Tuberculosis

A bacterial infection that most often affects the lungs but may also affect many other parts of the body

 Most common in children and in adults over the age of 60

 Overcrowded conditions and malnutrition are risk factors

 Gender and genetics are not significant factors

Tuberculosis (TB) is a slow-developing bacterial infection that usually begins in the lungs but can spread to many other parts of the body. TB can now be treated very effectively using oral antibiotics (see

Antituberculous drugs, p.573), but, left untreated, it may cause long-term ill health and can be fatal.

Worldwide, TB causes more deaths among adults than any other bacterial infection. The disease is still common in developing countries, especially in Asia. In developed countries, the number of cases steadily decreased during most of the 20th century due to improved health care, diet, and housing. However, since 1985 there has been a worldwide increase in the number of cases of TB. In the UK, TB is a notifiable disease, and about 7,890 cases were reported in 2013. This rise in TB is associated with an increase in travel and the spread of strains of TB bacteria that are resistant to antibiotics. Another factor is the emergence of HIV infection and AIDS (p.169), which lowers resistance to infection.

What is the cause?
The bacterium *Mycobacterium tuberculosis* causes most cases of TB and is usually transmitted in airborne droplets produced when an infected person coughs. Although many people are infected with the bacterium at some point in their lives, only a small proportion develops TB.

When the bacteria are inhaled, an initial minor infection develops in the lungs. The outcome of this initial lung infection will depend on the strength of a person's immune system. In many healthy people, the infection does not progress. However, some TB bacteria lie dormant in the lungs, and the disease may be reactivated years later if a person's immunity is reduced.

In some cases, the bacteria enter the bloodstream and spread to other sites in the body. Rarely, the infection does not begin in the lungs but in another part of the body. For example, TB may affect the gastrointestinal tract if a person drinks unpasteurized milk from a cow infected with TB.

Who is at risk?
People with reduced immunity are more likely to develop TB. This includes people who are infected with HIV, those who have diabetes mellitus (p.437), and those who are taking immunosuppressant drugs (p.585). Others at risk of TB include people with long-term lung disease; those who are on dialysis due to kidney failure; those living in overcrowded conditions with poor sanitation; and people who have a poor diet. Generally, elderly people and children are more susceptible.

What are the symptoms?
During the initial stages of the infection, many people have no symptoms. However, some people may experience:
■ Cough, which may be dry.
■ Generally feeling unwell.
■ Enlarged lymph nodes, especially in the neck.

If the disease progresses, further symptoms usually appear over 2–6 weeks, but progression may be more rapid. Later symptoms may include:

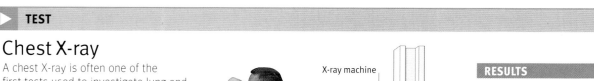

▶ **TEST**

Chest X-ray

A chest X-ray is often one of the first tests used to investigate lung and heart conditions because it is painless, quick, and safe. To create the image, X-rays are passed through your chest on to a detector. Dense tissues, such as the bones, absorb X-rays and appear white; soft tissues appear grey; and air appears black. Damaged or abnormal lung tissue or excess fluid in the chest shows up as a white area because it does not contain air as it should. Chest X-rays are usually taken from behind, although side views may also be required.

Having a chest X-ray
You will be asked to raise your arms to move your shoulder blades away from your lungs and to take a deep breath. While the X-ray is being taken, you must remain still to prevent the image from blurring.

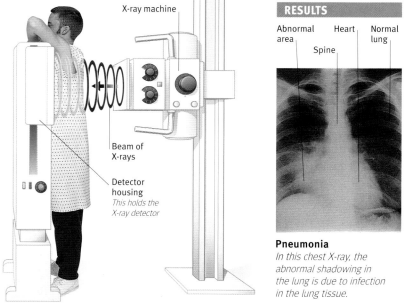

X-ray machine

Beam of X-rays

Detector housing
This holds the X-ray detector

RESULTS

Abnormal area   Heart   Normal lung

Spine

Pneumonia
In this chest X-ray, the abnormal shadowing in the lung is due to infection in the lung tissue.

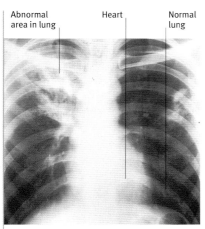

Chest X-ray in tuberculosis
This X-ray image shows an abnormal area at the top of one of the lungs due to an infection with tuberculosis.

Abnormal area in lung | Heart | Normal lung

- Persistent cough, which may produce greenish or yellowish sputum that is sometimes blood-streaked.
- Chest pain when inhaling deeply.
- Shortness of breath.
- Fever.
- Poor appetite and weight loss.
- Excessive sweating at night.
- Tiredness.

Untreated TB that begins in the lungs can spread directly to the tissue covering the heart (*see* **Pericarditis**, p.258). The infection may also be carried in the blood to the brain (*see* **Meningitis**, p.325), the bones, the kidneys, and many other parts of the body.

The onset of TB in areas of the body other than the lungs is very slow, and symptoms are not specific, making the condition difficult to diagnose.

How is it diagnosed?
Your doctor may suspect TB from your symptoms and a physical examination. He or she may also arrange for you to have a chest X-ray (opposite page) and possibly CT scanning (p.132) to look for evidence of lung damage.

If you are coughing up sputum, a sample will be sent to the laboratory so that it can be examined for bacteria and tested for sensitivity to particular drugs. In the meantime, you will be treated with a combination of antituberculous drugs.

Sometimes, a bronchoscopy (p.308) may be necessary to obtain lung tissue samples for examination. In addition, if your doctor suspects that you may have infection in a part of the body other than the lungs, such as in the lymph nodes, a sample of tissue may be taken from the area to look for TB.

If you have recently been in close contact with someone with TB bacteria in his or her sputum, you need to be screened. A chest X-ray may be carried out to look for signs of infection, along with a blood test (known as an interferon gamma release assay, or IGRA). If the blood test is positive, this indicates that you have either active or latent TB.

What is the treatment?
If you have TB, you will probably be treated at home unless you are very ill. You will be prescribed a combination of antituberculous drugs. Drug treatment is usually for at least 6 months if you have active TB, or for 3 months if you have latent TB. Using a combination of drugs helps to prevent the development of resistance to antibiotics. The drugs used depend on the antibiotic sensitivity of the bacteria and whether the infection has spread to other areas of the body. TB affecting areas that drugs do not penetrate easily, such as the bones, generally needs treatment for a longer period.

It is important to complete the full course of antituberculous drugs to help prevent the development of drug resistance. Since it is easy to forget to take the drugs, some people need help with their treatment using directly observed therapy, in which they attend a health centre to be given the drugs under medical supervision. While you are undergoing treatment for TB, you will probably need to have regular chest X-rays and blood tests to make sure that the infection is responding to treatment and to detect side effects of the drugs.

Can it be prevented?
The BCG vaccine against TB is recommended for particular at-risk groups, including newborns and infants in areas where there is a high rate of TB; new immigrants from countries where there is a high rate of TB; healthcare workers who are likely to have contact with TB patients; and those intending to live in a country with a high rate of TB. Those who are recommended for immunization will generally first be given a skin test to check whether they have been previously immunized, have had previous contact with TB, or have active TB infection. If the test is positive, BCG immunization is not given.

What is the prognosis?
Most people make a full recovery from TB if antituberculous medication is taken regularly as directed. However, in people who have a type of TB that is resistant to two or more drugs, in those whose immunity is severely weakened, or in people with widespread TB, the disease may be fatal.

Pertussis

A bacterial infection, also called whooping cough, that causes bouts of coughing

 Can occur at any age but more common under the age of 5

 Gender, genetics, and lifestyle are not significant factors

Pertussis is a distressing and extremely infectious disease that is caused by the *Bordetella pertussis* bacterium, which infects and inflames the trachea (windpipe) and the bronchi (airways) in the lungs. The

bacteria are transmitted in the airborne droplets that are produced when infected people cough and sneeze. Pertussis brings about violent fits of coughing that often end in a characteristic, high-pitched "whoop" when the affected person inhales.

Pertussis is most serious in children under the age of 12 months, when the disease can be life-threatening. Before the introduction of a reliable vaccine, pertussis was responsible for a considerable proportion of childhood deaths in the UK.

What are the symptoms?
The first symptoms usually appear 2–3 weeks after infection. They are mild and resemble those of a common cold, typically a dry cough, runny nose, and sneezing. During this initial stage, lasting about 7–14 days, the disease is highly infectious. Following this period, symptoms worsen and may include:
- Attacks of coughing followed by a sharp intake of breath that may produce a whooping sound. Coughing bouts are often much worse at night.
- Production of large amounts of sputum during coughing fits.
- Vomiting, which is caused by severe, repeated fits of coughing.

Episodes of prolonged coughing may cause small blood vessels to burst, resulting in a rash of small, flat, red spots, especially around the face, hairline, and eyes. Nosebleeds may also occur if vessels in the nose burst.

Complications of pertussis include pneumonia (p.299) and bronchiectasis (p.303), in which the airways become abnormally widened. Infants may stop breathing temporarily after a severe coughing spasm, which may result in a lack of oxygen that may cause seizures and brain damage.

What might be done?
The doctor will usually be able to diagnose pertussis from the symptoms. In some cases it may be necessary to confirm the diagnosis by taking a throat swab and culturing it to check for the causative bacterium or by taking a blood sample to check for antibodies to the bacterium.

The treatment of pertussis varies according to the age of the person affected and the stage of the disease.

Babies and children under 5 years old may sometimes be treated at home but often need treatment in hospital because the infection is more serious for this age group. There, they may be given antibiotics intravenously, and may also be given intravenous fluids. If they are having breathing difficulties, they may also be given corticosteroid drugs (p.600), and oxygen therapy.

Older children and adults can usually be treated at home. If the infection is diagnosed in its early stages, your doctor will probably prescribe antibiotics. The drugs will stop the person from being infectious after he or she has been taking them for 5 days; without antibiotics, the person may still be infectious until 3 weeks after the

coughing bouts started. If pertussis is not diagnosed until the later stages, antibiotics will probably not be prescribed because the bacterium is no longer in the body and the person is no longer infectious. If treated at home, the person should get plenty of rest, keep warm, drink plenty of fluids, and stay away from others until he or she is no longer infectious. To prevent the infection from spreading, antibiotics may also be prescribed for people who have been in close contact with an infected person.

The symptoms of pertussis usually improve within 4–10 weeks if there are no complications, but a dry cough may persist for months.

Can it be prevented?
The pertussis vaccine is part of the routine childhood immunization programme in the UK. It is given as part of the diphtheria, pertussis, tetanus, polio, and *Haemophilus influenzae* type b combined vaccine at 2, 3, and 4 months old. A booster dose is given as part of the diphtheria, pertussis, tetanus, and polio combined vaccine before starting school, at between 3 years 4 months and 5 years of age. Your child should receive the full course of immunization.

Pertussis is most dangerous in infants, including those too young to be immunized. Older siblings and parents may infect younger children. It is therefore important to maintain a high level of immunity to protect infants. Reactions to the vaccine are rare; the disease itself, which can cause brain damage and death, presents a far greater risk than any possible risk from the vaccine.

Pleurisy

Inflammation of the pleura, the two-layered membrane separating the lungs from the chest wall

 Age, gender, genetics, and lifestyle as risk factors depend on the cause

Normally, when people breathe, the two layers of the pleura (the membrane that separates the lungs from the chest wall) slide over each other, allowing the lungs to inflate and deflate smoothly. In pleurisy, inflammation of the pleura prevents the layers from moving over each other easily, and they grate as they rub against each other, causing sharp, severe chest pain when inhaling.

What are the causes?
Pleurisy may be caused by a viral illness, such as influenza (p.164), which affects the pleura itself. However, the disorder is often a reaction to damage to the lung just beneath the pleura. This lung damage may be due to pneumonia (p.299) or pulmonary embolism (p.302), in which the blood supply to part of the lung is blocked by a blood clot. The pleura can also be affected by primary lung cancer (p.307). Occasionally, an autoimmune disorder, such as rheumatoid arthritis (p.222) or systemic lupus

erythematosus (p.281), in which the immune system attacks healthy tissues, affects the pleura and leads to pleurisy.

What are the symptoms?

If an infection or a pulmonary embolism is the cause of the inflammation, the symptoms usually develop rapidly over 24 hours. In other cases, the symptoms occur gradually. They may include:

- Sharp chest pain that causes you to catch your breath on inhaling.
- Difficulty in breathing.

The pain is often restricted to the side of the chest affected by the underlying inflamed pleura. In some cases, fluid accumulates between the layers of the pleura (*see* **Pleural effusion**, below). This condition may actually lessen the pain because it eases the movements of the pleural layers over each other.

What might be done?

If you suspect that you have pleurisy, you should consult your doctor within 24 hours. He or she may be able to hear the layers of the pleura rubbing against each other when listening to your chest with a stethoscope. You may need a chest X-ray (p.300) to check for a problem in the underlying lung or for the presence of a pleural effusion.

You may be prescribed nonsteroidal anti-inflammatory drugs (p.578) to relieve the pain and inflammation. You may also find that holding the affected side while coughing helps to relieve the discomfort. In addition, you will probably need treatment for the underlying condition that is causing the pleurisy. For example, if a lung infection is the cause, you may be prescribed a course of antibiotics (p.572). If you have a pulmonary embolism, you will probably be given anticoagulant drugs (*see* **Drugs that prevent blood clotting**, p.584). In the majority of affected people, the condition clears up within 7–10 days of starting treatment.

Pleural effusion

An accumulation of fluid between the layers of the pleura, the membrane that separates the lungs from the chest wall

 Age, gender, genetics, and lifestyle as risk factors depend on the cause

A pleural effusion occurs when fluid accumulates between the layers of the pleura, the two-layered membrane separating the lungs from the chest wall. As fluid accumulates, the lung underneath becomes compressed, gradually causing shortness of breath. In some cases, the amount of fluid accumulated may be as much as 2–3 litres (4–6 pints).

What are the causes?

In some cases of pleural effusion, the pleura itself is inflamed and produces fluid (*see* **Pleurisy**, p.301). The inflammation may be

▶ TEST

Radionuclide lung scanning

Radionuclide lung scanning may occasionally be used to diagnose pulmonary embolism. It involves two scans performed simultaneously: one to assess blood flow through the lungs and the other, which is called a ventilation scan, to assess airflow.

A diagnosis can be made by comparing the ventilation scan and the blood flow scan because many lung disorders disrupt the flow of both blood and air in a specific area, whereas a pulmonary embolism disrupts only blood flow. The procedure takes about 20 minutes.

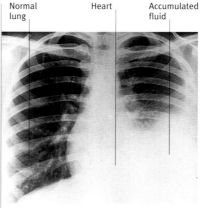

Syringe
This is used to inject radioactive material into the blood

Gamma camera
The gamma camera records radioactive emissions inside the body

Mask
Radioactive gas is inhaled

Monitor
The scan image builds up on the screen

During the procedure
A radioactive material is injected into a vein, and you inhale a radioactive gas. Scans may be taken from various angles using a gamma camera.

RESULTS

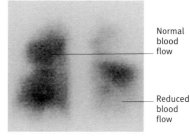

Gas in left lung

Gas in right lung

VENTILATION SCAN

Normal blood flow

Reduced blood flow

BLOOD FLOW SCAN

Comparison of air and blood flow
The ventilation scan above indicates normal airflow, but radioactivity is reduced in several areas on the blood flow scan. This result is characteristic of pulmonary embolism, in which only blood flow in a lung is affected.

---

due to a lung infection, such as pneumonia (p.299) or tuberculosis (p.300), or to other disorders that affect the lung, such as lung cancer (*see* **Primary lung cancer**, p.307) or cancer that has spread to the pleura from elsewhere in the body, for example from the breast, ovary, or bowel. Less often, the cause may be an autoimmune disorder, such as systemic lupus erythematosus (p.281), in which the immune system attacks the body's own tissues.

In most cases, the pleura itself is not the cause of the effusion. Instead, fluid leaks into the space between the pleural layers as a result of a serious underlying disorder, such as heart failure (*see* **Acute heart failure** and **Chronic heart failure**, pp.247–248), or kidney disease. In these cases, a pleural effusion is often associated with a build-up of fluid elsewhere in the body, such as in the ankles or abdomen.

A pleural effusion that produces little fluid may not cause symptoms. In severe cases, a large amount of fluid between the pleural layers compresses the lungs and may result in shortness of breath.

What might be done?

Your doctor may be able to detect a pleural effusion while examining your chest. You may also have a chest X-ray (p.300) to confirm the diagnosis and to assess the severity of the effusion. In order to identify the underlying cause, your doctor may

Normal lung   Heart   Accumulated fluid

Pleural effusion
In this X-ray, the left lung (on the right of the image) is partly obscured by the accumulated fluid of a pleural effusion.

take a sample of fluid by inserting a needle through the chest wall under local anaesthesia. A sample of the pleura may also be removed. The sample is examined under a microscope to look for evidence of infection or cancer. A sample of blood may be taken for testing to exclude other problems, such as kidney disorders.

Shortness of breath due to a severe pleural effusion may be relieved by removing some of the fluid through a tube inserted into the chest and between the two pleura under local anaesthesia. Your doctor may prescribe antibiotics (p.572) if a bacterial

infection is the cause of the effusion. Diuretic drugs (p.583) may be given to reduce the volume of fluid in the body. A pleural effusion that is associated with lung cancer may also be treated by draining the fluid through a tube.

In some people, particularly those who have lung cancer, pleural effusion may recur. If an effusion does recur, a chemical can be injected between the two layers of the pleura to make them stick together and prevent further recurrences.

Pulmonary embolism

Obstruction of the blood flow to the lungs by one or more blood clots

 Rare in children

 More common in females

 Sometimes runs in families

 Smoking, using oral contraceptives or HRT, and long periods of immobility are risk factors

In pulmonary embolism, a piece of a blood clot (embolus) becomes lodged in an artery in the lungs and partly or completely blocks blood flow in the affected area. Usually, the clot has broken off from a larger clot in the veins of the legs or the pelvic region (*see*

Deep vein thrombosis, p.263) and travelled to the lungs in the bloodstream. Pulmonary embolism may be mild if the blocked artery is small, but blockage of a major artery may suddenly cause severe symptoms and can be fatal. Rarely, small clots can block numerous small arteries in the lungs over months or years, and symptoms may not appear for some time. This condition is called recurrent pulmonary embolism.

Pulmonary embolism is most likely to occur in people who have developed deep vein thrombosis as a result of a period of immobility, such as that following childbirth or surgery (especially repair of fractures or pelvic surgery) or, rarely, during a long journey. A tendency to develop blood clots (see Hypercoagulability, p.275) increases the risk of deep vein thrombosis, as does smoking and using combined oral contraceptives or hormone replacement therapy.

What are the symptoms?
The symptoms depend on the extent of blockage to the flow of blood. Massive pulmonary embolism, in which a large blood clot blocks a major pulmonary artery, may cause sudden death. Single small clots may not cause symptoms. In most cases, however, symptoms develop over a few minutes and may include:
- Shortness of breath.
- Sharp chest pain that may be worse when inhaling.
- Coughing up blood.
- Feeling faint.
- Palpitations.

In some cases of recurrent pulmonary embolism, shortness of breath that worsens over months is the only symptom. Eventually, so many vessels may become blocked that pressure in the pulmonary arteries is increased (see Pulmonary hypertension, p.309) and chronic heart failure (p.247) may then develop.

How is it diagnosed?
If your doctor suspects that you have a pulmonary embolism, you may be admitted to hospital as an emergency. You will be given tests to measure the levels of oxygen and carbon dioxide in your blood (see Measuring blood gases, p.306). You will also have a chest X-ray (p.300) to exclude other lung conditions, and the blood flow in the veins of your legs may be measured using Doppler ultrasound scanning (p.259). You may also have a special blood test (the D-dimer test) to check if there has been significant clot formation and breakdown in the body; a contrast CT scan (p.132) to image the blood vessels in the lungs and pinpoint the exact location of blockages; and, in some cases, a radionuclide lung scan (opposite page). You may also have a blood test to check if you have a clotting disorder.

What is the treatment?
Treatment depends on the severity of the blockage. You may have a continuous intravenous infusion or injections of heparin, an anticoagulant drug that acts immediately to prevent the existing clots from enlarging and new clots from developing (see Drugs that prevent blood clotting, p.584). At the same time, you may be started on an oral anticoagulant drug, such as warfarin, which also prevents further clotting by thinning the blood but takes a few days to become effective. Anticoagulant drug treatment may last for 3 months if pulmonary embolism followed a single period of immobility. If the embolism is due to a long-term condition, such as hypercoagulability, you may need drug treatment indefinitely. If you have been prescribed warfarin, you will have regular blood tests to check your blood clotting, and the drug dosage altered as necessary.

In severe cases, thrombolytic drugs (p.584) may be used to dissolve the clot. If the main artery supplying the lungs is affected, life-saving emergency surgery may be necessary to remove the clot. If clots recur despite anticoagulant drug therapy, or if anticoagulants are not suitable, you may need to have a procedure in which a filter to trap blood clots is placed in the main vein that leads from the lower half of the body to the heart.

What is the prognosis?
Massive pulmonary embolism is fatal in about 1 in 3 cases. However, if you survive the first few days, you are likely to make a full recovery. People who have recurrent pulmonary embolism may remain short of breath.

If you have already had pulmonary embolism, you have a higher than average risk of further episodes and should avoid periods of prolonged immobility, such as sitting down continually during a long journey. You may need to have preventive treatment, such as heparin injections, after any surgery that involves prolonged immobility.

Bronchiectasis

Abnormal widening of the larger airways in the lungs (bronchi), causing a persistent cough with large amounts of sputum

 May begin in childhood but may not become apparent until after the age of 40

 In some cases, the underlying cause is inherited

 Gender and lifestyle are not significant factors

In bronchiectasis, the larger branches of the airways in the lungs (the bronchi) become abnormally wide, and their lining is damaged. Bronchiectasis usually starts in childhood as a result of a lung infection, but the symptoms of the disorder may not appear until after the age of 40. The main symptoms are a persistent cough that produces large amounts of sputum and shortness of breath that becomes progressively more severe. The disorder was once fairly common, but it is now rare in the developed world due to the greatly reduced incidence of childhood lung infections.

What are the causes?
Childhood infections such as whooping cough (see Pertussis, p.301) and measles (p.167) were once very common causes of bronchiectasis. Today, the main cause is repeated bacterial infections of the lungs in people with the inherited condition cystic fibrosis (p.535), in which the mucus produced by the lining of the airways is thicker than normal and tends to collect in the lungs. The repeated infections damage the bronchi, which become distorted so that small pockets form in the tissue. Stagnant mucus then builds up in the pockets, where it may become infected. When the condition is confined to just one area of the lung it may be caused by a blockage in one of the bronchi, which may be due to an inhaled object or a tumour.

What are the symptoms?
The symptoms of bronchiectasis gradually worsen over a period of several months or years and may include:
- A persistent cough that often produces very large quantities of dark green or yellow sputum. The cough is often worse when lying down.
- Coughing up blood.
- Bad breath.
- Wheezing and shortness of breath.
- Recurrent chest infections.
- Enlarged fingertips with abnormal fingernails, known as clubbing (see Nail abnormalities, p.209).

Eventually, an affected person will also experience the effects of long-term infection, such as weight loss and anaemia (p.271). Bronchiectasis may affect an increasing number of bronchi, causing extensive damage to a large area of the lung tissue. Rarely, it may lead to respiratory failure (p.310).

How is it diagnosed?
Your doctor may suspect that you have bronchiectasis from the large amount of sputum that you cough up. Your sputum may be tested in order to identify an infection, and you may also have a chest X-ray (p.300) and lung function tests (p.298). A high-resolution CT scan (p.132), which provides a very detailed and clear image of the bronchi, may be used to confirm the diagnosis.

What might be done?
If you have bronchiectasis, you should not smoke, and you should avoid smoky atmospheres and dust.

There are several exercises that can help remove mucus from the lungs, which can help to improve breathlessness and coughing. Your doctor can refer you to a physiotherapist to teach you these techniques. They should not be performed without having had proper instruction as they could cause lung damage if carried out incorrectly. A common exercise is called active cycle breathing therapy (ACBT), which involves a period of breathing normally, followed by several slow, deep breaths, then breathing out suddenly and forcefully through your open mouth. Another technique is postural drainage. There are different variations of this technique, but typically you lie on a flat surface with your head and chest hanging over the edge so that the mucus can drain into your windpipe. A relative or friend then uses their hands to vibrate certain areas of your back while you cough and "huff" to clear the mucus. Keeping the lungs as clear of mucus as possible reduces the risk of infections that may cause further lung damage. It is also important to ensure you have had the pneumococcal vaccine to protect against pneumonia and to have the annual influenza vaccine.

Your doctor may prescribe inhaled bronchodilator drugs (p.588) or corticosteroid drugs (see Corticosteroids for respiratory disease, p.588) to help you to breathe more easily. If an infection develops, it will be treated with antibiotics (p.572). In severe cases, continuous antibiotic treatment to prevent infections may be required and a lung transplant may be considered.

Pneumothorax

Presence of air between the layers of the pleura, the two-layered membrane that separates the lungs from the chest wall

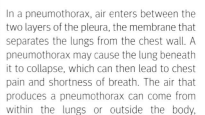

 Most common in young people

Much more common in males

Sometimes runs in families

Lifestyle is not a significant factor

In a pneumothorax, air enters between the two layers of the pleura, the membrane that separates the lungs from the chest wall. A pneumothorax may cause the lung beneath it to collapse, which can then lead to chest pain and shortness of breath. The air that produces a pneumothorax can come from within the lungs or outside the body, depending on the cause. The condition often affects only one side of the chest.

The amount of air between the layers of the pleura may be small, and in such cases breathing is not severely affected. However, a large pneumothorax may cause severe shortness of breath. In a tension pneumothorax, air that enters between the layers of the pleura cannot get back out and causes the pressure inside the pleural layers to rise. This condition also causes severe shortness of breath and can be fatal. It requires immediate medical treatment.

What are the causes?
In most cases, the cause of a pneumothorax is the spontaneous rupture of an abnormally dilated alveolus (air sac), known as a bulla, on the surface of the lung. Most bullae are present from birth. Rupture of a bulla is often caused by vigorous exercise but can

sometimes occur at rest. A pneumothorax due to the rupture of a bulla occurs most frequently in tall, thin young men.

A pneumothorax may develop as a complication of lung disorders such as asthma (p.295) and chronic obstructive pulmonary disease (p.297). Repeated pneumothoraces may be associated with Marfan's syndrome (p.534), a rare inherited disorder that affects connective tissue and results in abnormalities of the bones, heart, and eyes.

Other possible causes of a pneumothorax include a penetrating chest wound that allows air to enter between the layers of the pleura from outside the body, fractured ribs that tear the lung beneath them, or surgical procedures performed on the chest.

What are the symptoms?

Symptoms of a pneumothorax usually develop rapidly and may include:

■ Chest pain, which may be felt as sudden and sharp or may cause only slight discomfort.
■ Shortness of breath or a sudden worsening of pre-existing shortness of breath in someone with a long-term respiratory disorder.
■ Tightness across the chest.

In a tension pneumothorax, there is severe pain and shortness of breath. The high pressure caused by a tension pneumothorax prevents blood from returning to the heart from the lungs, which in turn causes low blood pressure, fainting, and shock (p.248).

What might be done?

If your doctor suspects that you have a pneumothorax, a chest X-ray (p.300) will be carried out to confirm the diagnosis. A small pneumothorax usually disappears by itself over the course of a few days as the leak that created it heals and the air is gradually absorbed by the body. If the pneumothorax is larger or you have an underlying lung disorder such as asthma, you may need hospital treatment. The doctor will either withdraw some air with a needle or insert a drainage tube through the chest wall under local anaesthesia to enable air to escape (see **Chest drain**, above right).

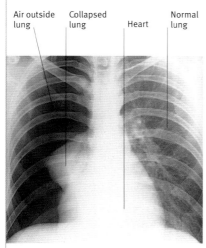

Pneumothorax
This X-ray image shows a large volume of air trapped inside one side of the chest, causing the lung beneath it to collapse.

▶ TREATMENT

Chest drain

A chest drain is used to treat a pneumothorax, in which air enters between the layers of the pleura (the membrane that separates the lungs from the chest wall). It may also be needed following chest surgery. A tube is inserted between the layers of the pleura, allowing air to escape. The tube may be connected to a pump that extracts the air. A chest drain must remain in place until the lung heals, which often takes several days.

Insertion of a chest drain
A local anaesthetic is applied to the skin and an incision made in the chest wall. A drainage tube, often with a one-way valve to control airflow, is then inserted.

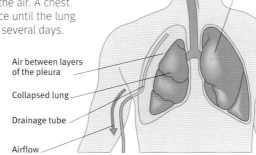

Normal lung

Air between layers of the pleura

Collapsed lung

Drainage tube

Airflow

A tension pneumothorax is a medical emergency. It is treated by inserting a large, hollow needle directly into the affected side of the chest to allow air to escape. This procedure provides immediate relief of symptoms.

If an air leak persists or returns, a technique known as pleurodesis may be used to prevent further lung collapse. This procedure introduces a chemical irritant (usually talc) between the two layers of the pleura to make them stick together. However, pleurodesis is not always successful and, rarely, surgery may be required to repair the damaged area.

With appropriate treatment, most people with a pneumothorax recover completely. However, in 1 in 5 cases the condition recurs, usually within a year.

Pulmonary fibrosis

Scarring of the lung tissue, mainly affecting the air sacs, resulting in shortness of breath

 Usually occurs over the age of 40 but is most common over the age of 60

 More common in males

 Genetics is not a significant factor

Scarring and hardening of the walls of the alveoli (air sacs) in the lungs is called pulmonary fibrosis. As a result of this condition, it is difficult for oxygen to pass into the bloodstream, and the level of oxygen in the blood falls. Because the alveoli lose their elasticity, shortness of breath also develops.

Usually, pulmonary fibrosis is a long-term disorder, developing over months or years. The condition most commonly occurs in people over the age of 60 and is more common in men.

What are the causes?

Pulmonary fibrosis may be caused by a wide variety of factors, including damage from previous lung infections; exposure to certain mineral dusts, such as asbestos (see **Asbestos-related diseases**, p.306), or coal dust (see **Coalworkers' pneumoconisis**, opposite page); autoimmune diseases (in which the immune system attacks the body's own tissues), such as rheumatoid arthritis (p.222) or systemic lupus erythematosus (p.281); radiotherapy (p.158) of the organs in the chest; and certain medications, such as amiodarone (sometimes used to treat heart rhythm problems). However, in most cases no cause can be identified, and the condition is then known as idiopathic pulmonary fibrosis (IPF).

What are the symptoms?

Typically, symptoms worsen gradually over months or years. They may include:

■ Shortness of breath.
■ Persistent, dry cough.
■ Recurrent chest infections.
■ Loss of appetite and weight loss.
■ Thickening of the tissue at the base of the fingernails and toenails (clubbing).

As the condition progresses, breathing becomes increasingly difficult, especially on exertion, and cyanosis may occur (blueness of the skin and mucous membranes due to a poor supply of oxygenated blood).

How is it diagnosed?

Your doctor may suspect that you have pulmonary fibrosis from your symptoms and medical history and from listening to your chest with a stethoscope. You may have a chest X-ray (p.300) or CT scanning (p.132) to look for scarred lung tissue. Your doctor may also arrange for you to have a blood test to check the levels of oxygen and carbon dioxide in your blood (see **Measuring blood gases**, p.306) and lung function tests (p.298). You may also have broncho-

---

scopy (p.308), in which a flexible viewing tube is passed into the lungs to examine the lung tissue; during the procedure, a small sample of lung cells may be taken for analysis. In some cases, keyhole surgery may be used to remove a larger sample of lung tissue for analysis.

What is the treatment?

If the underlying cause can be identified, treatment is usually primarily aimed at that. For idiopathic pulmonary fibrosis, treatment is aimed at relieving symptoms and slowing progression of the disease. It typically involves general measures, such as stopping smoking; ensuring that you have had the pneumococcal vaccine to protect against pneumonia, and also have the annual influenza vaccine; trying to avoid people with respiratory infections, such as colds and influenza; eating a healthy diet; and pulmonary rehabilitation (see **Chronic obstructive pulmonary disease**, p.299). In more severe cases, home oxygen therapy (p.310) may be needed. In some cases, medication may also be recommended, although it is not suitable in every case. Drugs that may be used include pirfenidone and nintedanib, which may slow down progression of the disease. If all these treatments are ineffective and the condition is severe and worsening, a lung transplant may be recommended.

What is the prognosis?

The outlook depends on the underlying cause and can vary greatly. If the pulmonary fibrosis is mild and the underlying cause can be treated successfully, it may stabilize or even improve. With idiopathic pulmonary fibrosis, where the underlying cause is not known, some people respond well to treatment and stay comparatively free of symptoms for several years. However, often other serious conditions develop, such as respiratory failure (p.310), pulmonary hypertension (p.309), or chronic heart failure (p.247), and the average survival time after diagnosis is only about 3 years.

Sarcoidosis

Inflammation of tissue in one or many parts of the body, most often affecting the lungs, lymph nodes, skin, and eyes

 Most common in young adults

 More common in females

 Sometimes runs in families

 Lifestyle is not a significant factor

In sarcoidosis, areas of inflammation develop in one or more parts of the body, frequently in the lungs. In some cases, only a single type of tissue is affected; in others, the condition affects several different organs. Sarcoidosis is thought to be caused by an abnormal, exaggerated response of the immune system. The trigger for this response is not fully understood, but it is thought that an infection may be involved.

Sarcoidosis may not produce symptoms. If symptoms do develop, they either appear suddenly over a period of a few days (acute sarcoidosis) or progress slowly over several years (chronic sarcoidosis). There is no cure, but symptoms disappear spontaneously in many cases. The condition, particularly in its acute form, is more common in women than in men. Sarcoidosis sometimes runs in families.

What are the symptoms?
Some people who have sarcoidosis never develop symptoms. However, those who have acute sarcoidosis may experience the following symptoms:
- Cough.
- Fever and excessive sweating at night.
- Weight loss.
- Tiredness.
- Pain in the joints.
- Painful red lesions on the shins (*see* **Erythema nodosum**, p.202).

People with chronic sarcoidosis may not experience symptoms initially, but they may gradually develop:
- Increasing shortness of breath.
- Cough.

Both acute and chronic sarcoidosis may cause redness of the eyes, blurred vision (*see* **Uveitis**, p.357), skin lesions on the nose and face, and swelling of the lymph nodes. There may also be high levels of calcium in the blood and/or urine, which may cause nausea and constipation and eventually lead to kidney damage.

How is it diagnosed?
If there are no symptoms, chronic sarcoidosis is usually discovered only after a chest X-ray (p.300) has been taken for another reason. Sarcoidosis may also be diagnosed by an X-ray taken to investigate symptoms such as coughing and shortness of breath. The X-ray usually shows swollen lymph nodes in the chest or shadows on the lungs. Sarcoidosis may also be diagnosed by the presence of skin lesions and confirmed by an examination of affected tissue from a skin sample or from a sample of tissue taken from the lung or airways. You may also have lung function tests (p.298) and blood tests to measure your calcium levels.

What is the treatment?
There is no cure for sarcoidosis, but your symptoms may be relieved by using corticosteroids (*see* **Corticosteroids for respiratory disease**, p.588). These drugs are usually effective, although you may need low-dose treatment for several years if you have chronic sarcoidosis. Corticosteroids (p.600) may be used for serious complications such as uveitis. You may need regular blood tests, chest X-rays, and lung function tests to monitor your response to treatment.

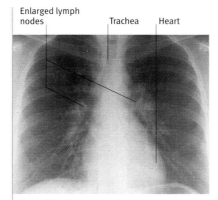

Enlarged lymph nodes   Trachea   Heart

Sarcoidosis
This chest X-ray shows enlarged lymph nodes due to sarcoidosis, a disorder causing inflammation of various body tissues.

What is the prognosis?
In most people with sarcoidosis, most commonly those with acute sarcoidosis, the disorder clears up spontaneously within about 3 years. Sarcoidosis is progressive in only a minority of people with the disorder. Rarely, it may be fatal.

Occupational lung diseases

A variety of disorders caused by inhaling damaging dusts or gases at work

 More common over the age of 40

 More common in males due to increased risk of occupational exposure

 Smoking causes some disorders to progress more quickly

 Genetics is not a significant factor

In developed countries, the number of cases of most occupational lung diseases is decreasing. This is partly due to the improved measures now used to protect workers, such as masks and protective clothing. In addition, regulations are in place that limit the maximum exposure levels for inhaled substances. A decline in the number of workers in industries such as mining in developed countries has also led to a reduction in occupational lung diseases. However, the diseases are still common in developing countries where workers are less likely to have adequate protection.

Occupational lung diseases are initiated by the body's reaction to small solid particles or gases that are breathed into the lungs while a person is in the workplace. The nature of the lung disorder depends on the type and amount of particles that are inhaled.

What are the types?
Occupational lung diseases associated with mineral dusts include coalworkers' pneumoconiosis (right), silicosis (p.306), and asbestosis (*see* **Asbestos-related diseases**, p.306). In the most severe cases, these disorders can result in irreversible scarring of lung tissue. Asbestos can also cause thickening of the pleura (the two-layered membrane that separates the lungs from the chest wall) and mesothelioma, a form of cancer that affects the pleura. Silicosis and coalworkers' pneumoconiosis are rare in developed countries. However, the incidence of mesothelioma is still increasing because it takes many years for symptoms to develop. Workers who have been exposed to asbestos before the introduction of safer working practices are still at risk of developing the disease at a later date.

Exposure to certain biological dusts, spores, and chemicals may induce allergic reactions, causing inflammation of the alvoli (air sacs) inside the lungs (*see* **Extrinsic allergic alveolitis**, p.307) or asthma (p.295). Although occupational asthma has probably been occurring for centuries, doctors have only relatively recently begun to recognize the extent of the disorder. The number of cases of occupational asthma has fallen in recent years but it remains a major health concern.

What might be done?
If you have respiratory symptoms, such as shortness of breath or a persistent cough, you should consult your doctor. Tell the doctor if your past or current occupation has involved working with dust or other irritants that could be causing your symptoms. He or she may arrange for you to have a chest X-ray (p.300) and lung function tests (p.298) to look for evidence of lung damage.

If your doctor suspects that you have occupational asthma, he or she will need to identify a trigger substance and confirm its presence in your workplace.

It is vital that you have no further contact with the substance that is causing your symptoms. If you are not able to do this, you will have to consider changing your occupation to prevent a deterioration in your condition. Avoiding these triggers should help to relieve symptoms. Otherwise, treatment is the same as for other forms of asthma.

Coalworkers' pneumoconiosis

Scarring of the lung tissue caused by long-term exposure to coal dust, also known as black lung

 More common over the age of 40

 More common in males due to increased risk of occupational exposure

 Caused by exposure to coal dust; smoking aggravates the disease

 Genetics is not a significant factor

Coalworkers' pneumoconiosis is a serious lung disorder caused by inhaling coal dust. The dust causes a gradual build-up of scar tissue in the lungs over many years, which leads to progressive and disabling shortness of breath. The severity of the condition depends on the degree to which a person has been exposed to coal dust. Pneumoconiosis was once a common disease in coalmining areas. However, the decline of the coal industry and improved safety practices have made it increasingly rare in developed countries.

What are the causes?
In pneumoconiosis, minute particles of coal dust are inhaled into the lungs, where they reach the alveoli (air sacs). Over many years of exposure, the dust causes irritation of the lung tissue. This form of the disorder is known as simple pneumoconiosis. Continuing exposure to the dust results in a serious complication known as progressive massive fibrosis (PMF). In this condition, lung tissue becomes heavily scarred. The disorder is likely to be worse if the coal dust contains a high level of silica (*see* **Silicosis**, p.306). Smoking causes the condition to progress more rapidly.

What are the symptoms?
Although the condition does not initially produce symptoms, the following symptoms of simple pneumoconiosis and PMF may develop over time:
- Coughing up black sputum.
- Shortness of breath on exertion that becomes progressively worse.

People with simple pneumoconiosis or PMF are also more susceptible to many other lung disorders, including chronic bronchitis (*see* **Chronic obstructive pulmonary disease**, p.297) and tuberculosis (p.300). Coalworkers who also have rheumatoid arthritis (p.222) may develop Caplan's syndrome, in which inflamed nodules form in the lungs.

As simple pneumoconiosis or PMF progresses, breathing difficulties may become so severe that respiratory failure (p.310) develops.

How is it diagnosed?
Your doctor will probably base the diagnosis on your occupational history and symptoms. He or she may arrange for a chest X-ray (p.300) and lung function tests (p.298) to confirm the diagnosis and assess existing damage to the lungs. You will probably also have tests that measure the levels of oxygen and carbon dioxide in your blood (*see* **Measuring blood gases**, p.306). These tests show how effectively oxygen from your lungs is reaching the bloodstream.

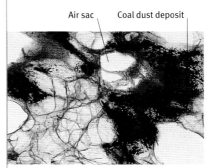

Air sac   Coal dust deposit

Coalworkers' pneumoconiosis
This magnified view of lung tissue shows black deposits of coal dust in and around the alveoli (air sacs). Eventually, the coal dust deposits cause scarring of lung tissue.

What is the treatment?

You should not smoke and should avoid further exposure to coal dust as far as possible. If you have simple pneumoconiosis and are no longer exposed to the dust, no treatment is necessary because the disease will not progress. If you have PMF, the symptoms may get worse even after exposure to the dust has stopped. Although there is no complete cure for PMF, your doctor may prescribe bronchodilator drugs (p.588) and oxygen therapy (see **Home oxygen therapy**, p.310) to help to relieve your symptoms. You may also need to have chest physiotherapy (p.620) regularly to help to remove mucus from the airways, and a friend or member of the family may be taught how to do this.

Can it be prevented?

In most developed countries, there are regulations governing the coalmining industry that require adequate ventilation in the workplace and other safety measures. Appropriate face masks and equipment to control dust may also be needed for people who work underground. Workers exposed to coal dust should have a chest X-ray every few years to detect the presence of simple pneumoconiosis before PMF develops.

Silicosis

Scarring of the lung tissue caused by inhaling dust containing silica

 More common over the age of 40

 More common in males due to increased risk of occupational exposure

 Caused by exposure to silica dust; smoking aggravates the disease

 Genetics is not a significant factor

Once common in developed countries, silicosis is a disorder that leads to irreversible lung damage. It tends to affect people who work with sandstone, granite, slate, and coal, as well as foundry workers, potters, and sandblasters. The number of new cases of silicosis diagnosed each year in the UK is now less than 100, due to safer working practices.

Most people with silicosis have the long-term form of the disease, which usually develops following 20–30 years of exposure to silica dust. The acute form of silicosis, which tends to develop suddenly after only a few months' exposure to a high level of silica dust, can lead to death in less than a year.

Unlike most other dust particles that are breathed into the lungs, silica dust causes a strong inflammatory response in lung tissue. Over time, the inflammation causes thickening and scarring, and the lungs become less efficient in supplying oxygen to the blood. Symptoms of silicosis may be more severe and the condition may progress more rapidly in people who smoke.

What are the symptoms?

The symptoms of chronic and acute silicosis are the same but develop over different time periods. They include:
- Coughing up sputum.
- Shortness of breath on exertion.
- Tightness of the chest.

A complication of both forms of silicosis is an increased susceptibility to tuberculosis (p.300). Even without further exposure to silica dust, silicosis may progress and may eventually lead to respiratory failure (p.310).

What might be done?

You should tell your doctor if your past or current work has involved handling materials that produce silica dust. He or she will probably arrange for a chest X-ray (p.300) and for lung function tests (p.298) to assess the level of damage to the lungs. There is no treatment for silicosis, but avoiding further exposure to the dust may slow the progress of the disease. If you have silicosis, you should not smoke, and, if you cannot avoid exposure to silica dust at work, your doctor may advise you to change your job. If you have severe silicosis, you may be given home oxygen therapy (p.310) to ease your breathing.

Can it be prevented?

If you think that you are at risk of silicosis, you should discuss the matter with your doctor and your employer. It is very important that you and your employer take immediate measures to reduce the amount of silica dust that you inhale. Appropriate ventilation, dust-control facilities, face masks, and showers should all be used.

Asbestos-related diseases

Serious lung disorders that develop as a result of inhaling asbestos fibres many years earlier

 Rare under the age of 40; more common with increasing age

 More common in males due to increased risk of occupational exposure

 Caused by exposure to asbestos in the workplace or at home

 Genetics is not a significant factor

Asbestos is a fibrous mineral that can cause serious lung damage if inhaled. Inhaling even very small numbers of asbestos fibres can lead to problems decades later, but those with the heaviest exposure are at greatest risk. The damage caused by inhaling asbestos fibres is irreversible, and preventing exposure to the dust is very important. The families of people who are exposed to asbestos at work may also be at risk of developing asbestos-related diseases because fibres from the workplace may be brought into the home on clothing.

In the UK, asbestos is now used only for a limited number of specialist applications. However, it was previously used extensively in building and so it is still found in many older buildings. There are now strict guidelines governing working with and disposing of asbestos to minimize the risk of exposure. However, the number of people with asbestos-related diseases is continuing to rise because there is a time lag of up to about 50 years between first exposure to asbestos and the development of lung disease.

What is the cause?

Asbestos fibres are needle-shaped. They are drawn into the lungs when inhaled, where they can penetrate the lung tissue. The fibres then trigger a reaction from white blood cells in the lungs, which try to engulf the fibres. However, the fibres usually destroy the blood cells, and inflammation and eventual scarring of the lung tissue may follow.

Asbestos fibres are divided into three main types: white, blue, and brown. All three types are dangerous and can cause asbestos-related diseases.

What are the types?

The inhalation of asbestos fibres can result in three different types of disease: asbestosis; diffuse pleural thickening, in which the pleura (the membrane that separates the lungs from the chest wall) becomes abnormally thickened; and mesothelioma, a cancerous tumour of the pleura. Often, more than one type of asbestos-related disease occurs simultaneously in one person.

Asbestosis In this condition, widespread fine scarring occurs in the lung tissue. The disease may progress even when exposure to asbestos is discontinued. Asbestosis tends to develop among people who have been heavily exposed to asbestos, such as asbestos miners, people who work in asbestos factories, and workers who regularly handle insulation materials that contain asbestos.

The period of time between first exposure to asbestos and development of symptoms is usually at least 20 years and is often longer. The main symptom is shortness of breath on exertion, which may eventually become disabling. Other symptoms include a dry cough, an abnormal shape to the fingernails known as clubbing (see **Nail abnormalities**, p.209), and a bluish tinge to the complexion. Some people with asbestosis develop primary lung cancer (opposite page).

Diffuse pleural thickening Pleural thickening may develop after only a brief exposure to asbestos. Usually, the condition produces no obvious symptoms and is detected only if a chest X-ray (p.300) is performed for another reason. However, in some cases, pleural thickening is severe and widespread, and the ability of the lungs to expand is restricted, causing shortness of breath.

Mesothelioma This disorder is a cancerous tumour of the pleura or less often of the peritoneum (the thin membrane that lines the abdominal cavity). Mesotheliomas most commonly result from working with blue or brown asbestos. It may take

---

▶ **TEST**

Measuring blood gases

Measuring the levels of oxygen and carbon dioxide in the blood helps in the diagnosis and monitoring of many lung disorders. To measure these gases, a blood sample is taken from an artery, usually in the wrist. This test also measures blood acidity (pH), which may be abnormal in conditions such as diabetes mellitus and in some forms of poisoning. Oxygen levels in the blood can also be measured continuously using a pulse oximeter, which detects changes in the amount of light that blood absorbs.

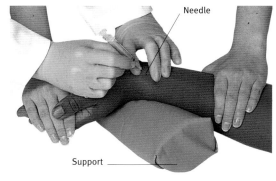

Needle

Support

Taking blood
To obtain a blood sample, the skin is cleaned and a local anaesthetic may be given before the blood is withdrawn from an artery with a needle and syringe. The procedure may be uncomfortable, but it is quick. Pressure must be applied for a few minutes afterwards to prevent bleeding.

Pulse oximeter
A machine called a pulse oximeter shines a light through the soft tissues of the finger or earlobe to measure oxygen levels in the blood painlessly.

Pulse oximeter

Cable to monitor

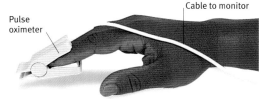

30–50 years from the initial exposure for symptoms to first appear. Mesotheliomas that affect the pleura usually cause chest pain and shortness of breath. In the peritoneum, they may cause an intestinal obstruction (p.419), resulting in symptoms such as abdominal pain and vomiting.

Are there complications?
People with asbestos-related diseases are particularly susceptible to developing primary lung cancer (right). People who smoke and who also have an asbestos-related disease are considered 75–100 times more likely to develop lung cancer than people with neither factor. Asbestos-related diseases may also increase a person's susceptibility to other serious lung conditions, including tuberculosis (p.300) and chronic obstructive pulmonary disease (p.297).

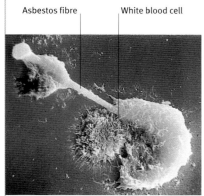

Asbestos fibre   White blood cell

Asbestos fibre in the lungs
Fibres of asbestos inhaled into the lungs are engulfed by white blood cells, as shown above, but destroy the cells. The result is scarring of the lungs called asbestosis.

How is it diagnosed?
If your doctor suspects that you have an asbestos-related disease, he or she will ask you about your current occupation and work history. Asbestos-related disease is usually diagnosed using a chest X-ray (p.300) to look for signs of thickening of the pleura. Your doctor may also listen to your chest for abnormal sounds and may arrange for lung function tests (p.298) to assess the extent of your breathing problems. A sample of sputum from the lungs may be examined for evidence of asbestos fibres. If a mesothelioma is suspected, CT scanning (p.132) or MRI (p.133) may be performed. To confirm the diagnosis of mesothelioma, a sample of tissue may be taken from the pleura under local anaesthesia to check for cancerous cells.

What is the treatment?
No treatment can reverse the progress of an asbestos-related disease. However, further exposure to asbestos may cause the condition to worsen more rapidly and should therefore be avoided. If you have asbestosis, you may be given oxygen (*see* **Home oxygen therapy**, p.310) to relieve shortness of breath. Diffuse pleural thickening requires no specific treatment because the

condition rarely causes severe symptoms. Mesothelioma may be treated with chemotherapy (p.157), and radiotherapy (p.158) may be given to help relieve pain.

Can it be prevented?
The only way to prevent asbestos-related diseases is to minimize your exposure to asbestos. In the UK, restrictions on the use of asbestos were first introduced in the 1970s, although it was not comprehensively banned until 1999 (except for a small number of special applications). Most cases of asbestos-related diseases now being diagnosed are the result of working practices before the ban. If you are carrying out repair work on a house that was constructed before 2000, you should check for the presence of asbestos. If you find asbestos, you should seek professional advice.

What is the prognosis?
About 4 in 10 people with asbestosis or diffuse pleural thickening will eventually die of lung cancer, and smoking should be avoided to lower this risk. Only a few people with asbestos-related mesothelioma survive for longer than 2 years after the diagnosis.

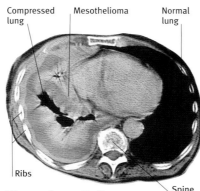

Compressed lung   Mesothelioma   Normal lung

Ribs   Spine

CT scan of mesothelioma
The lung seen on the left is encased in a mesothelioma, a cancerous tumour, which consists of a mass of thickened pleura.

Extrinsic allergic alveolitis

An allergic reaction to inhaled dusts or chemicals, causing cough and fever

 More common in adults

 More common in males due to increased risk of occupational exposure

 Exposure to certain organic dusts and chemicals is a risk factor

 Genetics is not a significant factor

In some people, inhaling certain dusts or chemicals containing organic substances, such as proteins and fungal spores, triggers an allergic reaction that causes inflammation of lung tissue and shortness of breath. This condition is called extrinsic allergic alveolitis (also known as hypersensitivity pneumonitis).

The dusts, fungal spores, and chemicals that cause it may be found in the workplace and can affect people in a variety of different occupations.

What are the causes?
Many substances in the workplace can trigger the allergic response that results in extrinsic allergic alveolitis. There are several forms of the disorder, which tend to be named according to the occupation that typically causes them. For example, in farmer's lung, the allergic reaction is triggered by fungal spores from mouldy hay. If particles from bird droppings are the cause, the disorder is known as bird fanciers' lung. Other substances that can trigger extrinsic allergic alveolitis include cheese mould, coffee dust, mushroom soil, and certain chemicals that are used in manufacturing products such as insulation and packing materials. Certain microorganisms that may be in air-conditioning systems and humidifiers can also trigger the disorder.

The allergic reaction causes inflammation of the alveoli (air sacs) and small airways in the lungs. The walls of the alveoli thicken, reducing their efficiency in transferring oxygen to the blood, and the airways narrow. Not everyone who is exposed to these dusts and chemicals will develop an allergic reaction if they inhale them. However, some people are particularly susceptible to allergies, and, in such people, exposure to these substances provokes a sudden acute attack. If exposure to the trigger substance continues after the allergy has become established, some people may go on to develop a long-term form of the disorder, which may cause permanent damage to the lungs.

What are the symptoms?
The symptoms of an acute attack of extrinsic allergic alveolitis have a rapid onset and are similar to those of influenza. They usually develop 4–8 hours after initial exposure and may include:
■ Fever and chills.
■ Coughing and wheezing.
■ Tightness in the chest and, in some people, shortness of breath.
If exposure to the substance stops, these symptoms usually begin to clear up spontaneously within 12–24 hours and often disappear completely within 48 hours. If there is further exposure to the substance, sudden attacks are eventually followed by continuous symptoms.

In long-standing (chronic) extrinsic allergic alveolitis, symptoms develop over time and include:
■ Coughing that may become progressively worse over time.
■ Progressive shortness of breath.
■ Loss of appetite and weight loss.
In chronic extrinsic allergic alveolitis, symptoms may continue even after exposure to the substance has stopped. If exposure to the substance continues, progressive lung damage may eventually lead to respiratory failure (p.310).

What might be done?
Your work or hobbies may alert your doctor to the diagnosis, which can be confirmed by blood tests to look for antibodies against the substance causing the allergic reaction. Your doctor may also arrange for a chest X-ray (p.300) and lung function tests (p.298) to look for evidence of lung damage.

If you have a severe, sudden attack of extrinsic allergic alveolitis, you may be given corticosteroids (*see* **Corticosteroids for respiratory disease**, p.588) to help to reduce inflammation in the lungs and bronchodilator drugs (p.588) to help to widen the airways. If the lung damage is severe, you may also be given oxygen (*see* **Home oxygen therapy**, p.310). In most acute attacks, the symptoms clear up once exposure to the dust has stopped. In long-term cases, continued treatment that includes corticosteroids may be necessary even after exposure to the trigger has ended.

Can it be prevented?
If you become sensitive to substances in your workplace, you should wear a protective mask. Employers should store materials safely and ensure that air conditioners are serviced regularly. You may consider changing your lifestyle or finding alternative employment to prevent the allergy from becoming persistent.

Primary lung cancer

A cancerous tumour that develops in the tissue of the lungs

 Most common in older people; most cases diagnosed in the over-70s

 More common in males

 Smoking and certain occupations are risk factors

 Genetics is not a significant factor

Primary lung cancer, in which a tumour originates in lung tissue, is the second most common type of cancer in the UK (after breast cancer) and the leading cause of death due to cancer. In men, it is the second most commonly diagnosed form of cancer (after prostate cancer). In women, it is also the second most common cancer (after breast cancer). Lung cancer is more common in men. It is rare in people under about 40 and becomes increasingly common with age. It is most commonly diagnosed in people over 70. In the UK, there were about 44,500 new cases in 2012.

Smoking is by far the most important cause of lung cancer, and the prevalence of smoking is closely related to the incidence of the disease. In the UK, the levels of both smoking and lung cancer rose sharply in the first half of the 20th century. Smoking among men reached a peak around 1950, when more than 80 per cent of men smoked, and has since declined to about 22 per cent in 2013. In women, the number of smokers reached a high of 45 per cent in 1966 and has since declined to about 17 per cent in 2013. However, because lung cancer can take many years to develop, the effects of smoking can take 20 or 30 years to appear. Among men, the incidence of lung cancer peaked in the 1970s and has declined steadily since then. In contrast, in women, the incidence of lung cancer has increased steadily since the 1970s.

The more cigarettes you smoke, the sooner you may develop cancer. For example, if you smoke 20 cigarettes a day, you may develop lung cancer after 20 years, but if you smoke 40 a day, you may develop the disease after only 10 years.

What are the types?
The type of cancer that develops depends on the type of cell in the lungs that becomes cancerous. Most lung cancers fall into one of four types squamous cell carcinoma, adenocarcinoma, large cell carcinoma, and small cell carcinoma. Squamous cell carcinoma, adenocarcinoma, and large cell carcinoma are sometimes collectively known as non-small-cell carcinoma.

Each type of cancer has a different growth pattern and response to treatment. In general terms, small cell carcinoma is the most highly malignant (cancerous) type; this type of cancer tends to grow rapidly and spread very quickly throughout the body. Non-small-cell carcinomas tend to grow more slowly (although large cell carcinoma may grow quite quickly) and may not spread beyond the lungs until later in the disease.

Lung metastases (opposite page) are cancers that have spread to the lung from a tumour elsewhere in the body. The lungs are a common site for metastases because all circulating blood (which can carry cancer cells) passes through them.

What are the causes?
Smoking is the cause of lung cancer in approximately 90 per cent of cases. The more you smoke, the greater the risk of developing lung cancer. It is also more likely to develop in people who start smoking at a young age. For people who have never smoked, the risk of developing lung cancer is small, but it increases slightly for anyone who is exposed to other people's tobacco smoke (passive smoking) on a regular basis.

Working with particular substances, such as radioactive materials, asbestos (*see* **Asbestos-related diseases**, p.306), chromium, and nickel, may lead to an increased risk of lung cancer, especially when the exposure is combined with smoking. Exposure to radon, a radioactive gas that is released slowly from granite rock, also leads to a slightly increased risk for people who live in areas that have a lot of granite. Living in an environment with a high level of air pollution may be a factor in some cases of lung cancer, but it is far less important as a cause than smoking. Other risk factors for lung cancer include a family history of the disease in a first-degree relative (parent or sibling);

previous treatment for cancer, especially in smokers who have had radiotherapy to the chest and have continued to smoke; and reduced immunity, for example, due to HIV/AIDS or immunosuppressant drugs.

What are the symptoms?
The symptoms of lung cancer depend on how far advanced the tumour is, but initial symptoms may include:
- A new, persistent cough or change in a long-standing cough, sometimes with blood-streaked sputum.
- Chest pain, which may be a dull ache, or a sharp pain that is worse on inhaling.
- Shortness of breath.
- Wheezing if the tumour is positioned so that it blocks an airway.
- Abnormal curvature of the fingernails, known as clubbing (*see* **Nail abnormalities**, p.209).

Some lung cancers do not produce any symptoms until they are advanced, when they may cause shortness of breath.

Are there complications?
In some cases, pneumonia (p.299) may develop in an area of the lung if an airway is blocked by a tumour. This may be the first indication of lung cancer. A tumour may also cause fluid to accumulate between the layers of the pleura, the thin membrane that separates the lungs from the wall of the chest (*see* **Pleural effusion**, p.302), which may lead to increased shortness of breath. Later, as the disease progresses, loss of appetite followed by weight loss and weakness may develop. A tumour at the top of the lung may affect the nerves that supply the arm, making the arm painful and weak. Small cell carcinomas may

You should consult your doctor as soon as possible if you develop a new cough that is persistent, experience a change in a long-term cough, or develop any of the other symptoms associated with lung cancer listed above.

produce chemicals that mimic different hormones in the body and upset body chemistry as a result.

In addition, there may be symptoms from tumours that have spread from the lungs to other parts of the body. For example, headaches may result from cancer that has spread to the brain.

How is it diagnosed?
A chest X-ray (p.300) is often one of the first investigations used when a person has a lung problem. A tumour is usually visible as a shadow on the X-ray. A CT scan (p.132) of the chest may also help to identify a possible tumour.

Samples of sputum may be taken to look for cancerous cells. Your doctor may also examine your airways using either bronchoscopy (left) or endobronchial ultrasound. The latter procedure is similar to bronchoscopy but uses a viewing instrument with an ultrasound probe on the tip; this enables the airways and interior of the chest to be imaged clearly and biopsy tissue samples to be taken under ultrasound guidance. If a tumour is found during either of these procedures, a biopsy sample of the tumour will be removed and examined under a microscope. If the tumour is cancerous, tests may be carried out to determine whether cancerous cells have spread to other parts of the body. In addition to blood tests, PET–CT scanning (a combined PET scan, p.137, and CT scan, p.132) and MRI (p.133) of the brain, chest, and abdomen may be carried out to assess the extent of cancer spread.

What is the treatment?
Treatment of lung cancer depends on the type of cancer and whether it has spread to other parts of the body.

For non-small-cell carcinomas that have not spread outside one lung, surgery is usually the first option. This may involve removal of a small section of the lung, removal of one or more lobes of the lung, or, occasionally, removal of an entire lung. Surgery may be followed by chemotherapy (p.157) to destroy any remaining cancer cells. If the cancer has not spread but surgery is not possible, radiotherapy (p.158), possibly combined with chemotherapy, may be used. In some cases, biological therapy (medication that modifies the activity of the immune system) to inhibit the growth of cancer cells may be used instead of or after chemotherapy. If the cancer has spread too far for surgery to be an option, treatment is usually with chemotherapy and/or radiotherapy.

If small cell carcinoma is detected at an early stage, it may be possible to remove the tumour surgically. However, in most cases the cancer has spread beyond the lungs by the time it is diagnosed and surgery is not a feasible option. In these cases, treatment is usually treated with chemotherapy, either by itself or combined with radiotherapy.

▶ **TEST AND TREATMENT**

Bronchoscopy

Bronchoscopy may be used to diagnose or treat lung disorders. A rigid or flexible tube called a bronchoscope is used to view the bronchi (airways). The rigid type is passed through the mouth into the lungs under general anaesthesia. The flexible type is passed into the lungs through the nose or mouth, which are first numbed by a local anaesthetic. Instruments to take tissue samples and perform laser surgery can be introduced through the tube.

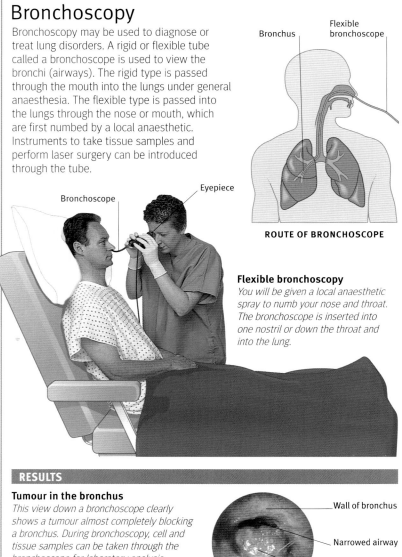

Bronchus — Flexible bronchoscope

Eyepiece

Bronchoscope

ROUTE OF BRONCHOSCOPE

Flexible bronchoscopy
You will be given a local anaesthetic spray to numb your nose and throat. The bronchoscope is inserted into one nostril or down the throat and into the lung.

RESULTS

Tumour in the bronchus
This view down a bronchoscope clearly shows a tumour almost completely blocking a bronchus. During bronchoscopy, cell and tissue samples can be taken through the bronchoscope for laboratory analysis.

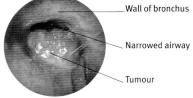

Wall of bronchus

Narrowed airway

Tumour

Other treatment options that may sometimes be possible for some early-stage tumours include radiofrequency ablation or photodynamic therapy. Radiofrequency ablation involves guiding a thin needle to the tumour then sending radio waves through the needle; the radio waves produce heat, which destroys the tumour cells. Photodynamic therapy involves administering a medication that makes cells sensitive to light. Strong light (often a laser) is directed on to the tumour which, being sensitive to light, is destroyed.

As well as treatment for the cancer, you may also be given treatment to control symptoms or relieve a blockage if a tumour is obstructing an airway. This may involve radiofrequency ablation, photodynamic therapy, cryotherapy (freezing the tumour), or insertion of a stent (rigid tube) to keep the airway open.

Lung cancer
In this colour-enhanced chest X-ray, a large cancerous tumour can be seen in one lung. The other lung is normal.

Labels: Normal lung | Heart | Cancerous tumour

What is the prognosis?
The outlook is best for people whose cancer is detected early. When lung cancer is diagnosed at its earliest stage, more than a third of people survive for 5 years or more after diagnosis. However, taking into account all cases, the outlook is less good: overall, about 1 in 10 people diagnosed with lung cancer survives for 5 years or more after diagnosis, and only about 1 in 20 survives for 10 years or more.

Can it be prevented?
Lung cancer is closely linked to smoking. People who stop smoking greatly improve their chances of avoiding lung cancer, and long-term ex-smokers have only a slightly greater risk of developing lung cancer than nonsmokers.

Lung metastases

Cancerous tumours in lung tissue that have spread from another part of the body

 Most common between the ages of 50 and 70

 More common in females

 Genetics and lifestyle as risk factors depend on the cause

Lung metastases, also known as secondary lung cancer, are tumours that have spread to the lungs from other parts of the body. Lung tissue is a very common site for metastases because all circulating blood passes through the lungs, allowing cancerous cells to be carried into lung tissue from other parts of the body. The primary (original) cancers that spread most often to the lungs include cancers of the breast, colon, prostate gland, and kidney.

Secondary lung cancers may not cause symptoms. However, if many secondary tumours have formed in the lung, you may feel short of breath. You may also develop a cough, which can produce blood if a tumour is blocking an airway.

What might be done?
If cancer has already been diagnosed elsewhere in your body, your doctor may arrange for you to have a chest X-ray (p.300) to check whether the cancer has spread to your lungs. If the site of the original cancer has not been confirmed, further tests may be carried out to locate it. For example, women will probably have a breast X-ray (*see* **Mammography**, p.487) to look for evidence of a breast tumour.

Treatment is aimed at destroying the primary cancer. Chemotherapy (p.157), radiotherapy (p.158), or hormonal treatment (*see* **Anticancer drugs**, p.586) may be used, depending on the type and extent of the primary tumour. To some extent, the overall outlook depends on the type of primary cancer. However, by the time lung metastases have been detected, there are usually several tumours, and treatment is difficult.

Pulmonary hypertension

Abnormally high pressure in the blood vessels supplying the lungs

 More common over the age of 40

 Lifestyle as a risk factor depends on the cause

 Gender and genetics are not significant factors

Blood is normally pumped through the lungs by the heart at a lower pressure than blood is pumped around the rest of the body. In pulmonary hypertension, the pressure of the blood in the arteries supplying the lungs is abnormally high. Consequently, the right side of the heart, which pumps the blood through the lungs, must contract much more vigorously than normal to maintain an adequate flow of blood through the arteries of the lungs. This causes enlargement of the muscle wall on the right side of the heart.

What are the causes?
There are various lung and heart conditions that may result in pulmonary hypertension. For example, in chronic obstructive pulmonary disease (p.297), resistance to blood flow in the lungs is caused by destruction of lung tissue. In diseases that cause extensive scarring of the tissue in the lungs, such as pulmonary fibrosis (p.304), blood vessels in the lungs are destroyed, making blood flow more difficult. Blood clots in the lungs (*see* **Pulmonary embolism**, p.302) may obstruct the flow of blood and lead to pulmonary hypertension. Narrowing of the mitral valve in the heart prevents blood from leaving the lungs, causing back pressure (*see* **Mitral stenosis**, p.255) and pulmonary hypertension.

In some forms of congenital heart disease (p.542), the heart pumps more blood than is normal into the lungs, and as a result the pressure rises.

Rarely, sleep apnoea (p.292) leads to pulmonary hypertension. Occasionally, there is no obvious cause for the condition, and it is then known as primary pulmonary hypertension.

What are the symptoms?
Many people who develop pulmonary hypertension already have symptoms of a long-term heart or lung disorder. The additional symptoms associated with pulmonary hypertension may include:
- Shortness of breath that tends to become worse on exertion.
- Tiredness.

As the disease progresses, shortness of breath becomes increasingly severe until it may occur at rest. Eventually, the right side of the heart, which pumps blood through the lungs, may fail, leading to tissue oedema (swelling caused by fluid build-up), especially around the ankles.

What might be done?
If you have an existing long-term heart or lung disorder and your symptoms suddenly become worse, your doctor may suspect that you are developing pulmonary hypertension. He or she may arrange for a chest X-ray (p.300) to look for enlarged arteries. An echocardiogram (*see* **Echocardiography**, p.255) and an electrocardiogram (*see* **ECG**, p.243) may be carried out to look for signs of heart disease, and lung function tests (p.298) are useful to assess the extent of lung damage. If the diagnosis is still unclear, a procedure called right heart catheterization may be used. This involves passing a tube through a vein in the arm or leg into the right side of the heart to measure blood pressure there.

If you have already developed pulmonary hypertension, treatment will first be directed at the underlying cause if one is found. Your doctor may advise long-term home oxygen therapy (p.310) if you have low oxygen levels due to a disorder such as chronic obstructive pulmonary disease. Drugs that prevent blood clotting (p.584) may be prescribed if the blood vessels in the lungs have become blocked by clots. You may also be prescribed drugs to dilate blood vessels in the lungs and lower the pressure in them. If heart failure has developed, you may be given diuretic drugs (p.583) to reduce excess fluid.

What is the prognosis?
If the underlying cause of pulmonary hypertension is identified and can be treated successfully, it is possible that the condition may improve. However, in most cases, pulmonary hypertension becomes progressively worse.

In primary pulmonary hypertension and cases in which the underlying cause is untreatable, the disorder may progress to chronic heart failure (p.247), which may be life threatening. For this reason, if you have pulmonary hypertension, are under the age of 55, and are otherwise in good health, you may be considered for a heart and lung transplant.

Acute respiratory distress syndrome

Inflammatory response of the lungs to severe disease or injury

Age, gender, genetics, and lifestyle are not significant factors

Acute respiratory distress syndrome (ARDS) is a serious lung disorder that develops suddenly as a result of severe damage either to the lungs or elsewhere in the body. In ARDS, the tiny blood vessels (capillaries) in the lungs leak fluid into the alveoli (air sacs), reducing the amount of oxygen that reaches the blood and preventing the lungs from expanding fully. This in turn can lead to the failure of other vital organs, including the kidneys and liver. ARDS is a life-threatening disorder that requires emergency medical treatment.

What are the causes?
ARDS can develop after any serious illness or injury. A third of cases result from widespread bacterial infection of the blood (*see* **Septicaemia**, p.171). In other cases, major trauma such as multiple fractures, crushed internal organs, or severe burns are the cause. Less commonly, ARDS results from pneumonia (p.299), obstetric emergencies, inhaling vomit, or an overdose of an

opioid drug such as heroin. How these conditions and emergencies cause leakage in the lungs remains unclear.

What are the symptoms?
The symptoms of ARDS usually begin 24–48 hours after the injury or onset of the disease that brings about the condition and may include the following:
- Severe shortness of breath.
- Wheezing.
- Mottled blue skin.
- Confusion or unconsciousness.

These symptoms develop in addition to those related to the underlying disorder that has caused the lung damage. As well as being a possible cause of ARDS, pneumonia may develop as a complication. Other complications, such as acute kidney injury (p.450), may also occur.

What might be done?
A doctor will probably suspect ARDS if a person who is already seriously ill develops sudden, unexpected breathing difficulties. The diagnosis can often be confirmed by a chest X-ray (p.300), which is used to look for evidence of fluid in the alveoli, and analysis of the oxygen levels in the blood (see **Measuring blood gases**, p.306).

People with ARDS are usually treated in an intensive therapy unit (p.618). High concentrations of oxygen are given using artificial ventilation in order to increase the amount of oxygen that passes from the lungs into the blood. Diuretic drugs (p.583) may be given to reduce the amount of fluid in the lungs. The underlying cause and any complications are treated, and the condition of major organs is monitored.

What is the prognosis?
Only 1 in 2 people who develop ARDS survive. In those who recover, symptoms usually improve over 7–10 days. There is often little or no permanent damage to the lungs, and the majority of people who do make a recovery experience no further problems.

Respiratory failure

Abnormally low levels of oxygen in the blood, resulting from lung damage

 Age, gender, genetics, and lifestyle are not significant factors

Respiratory failure occurs if the amount of oxygen that enters the bloodstream from the lungs is greatly reduced, leading to severe shortness of breath and eventually to profound confusion or unconsciousness. Simultaneously, there may be an excess of carbon dioxide in the blood. Respiratory failure is a life-threatening condition that should be treated promptly to prevent damage to other organs, such as the heart, which need an adequate supply of oxygen to maintain their function.

What are the causes?
There are two broad groups of conditions that lead to respiratory failure. In the first group, there is no difficulty in moving air into and out of the lungs, but less oxygen than normal is transferred to the blood as a result of damage to the alveoli (air sacs) in the lungs. The most common causes of this type are long-term lung disorders such as pulmonary fibrosis (p.304). Less commonly, the alveoli may become filled with fluid, as occurs in acute respiratory distress syndrome (p.309). In this case, the levels of oxygen in the blood are low, but levels of carbon dioxide are usually normal.

The second group of conditions consists of ventilation disorders, in which a person cannot move sufficient air into and out of the lungs. A ventilation disorder may develop suddenly after a stroke (p.329) or an injury to the area of the brain that controls breathing. A drug overdose (see **Drug overdose and accidental ingestion**, p.185) or injury to the chest wall may also reduce breathing. In addition, breathing difficulties may result from disorders, such as chronic obstructive pulmonary disease (p.297), and myasthenia gravis (p.339), in which the muscles involved in breathing become progressively weakened. Ventilation problems usually lead to low levels of oxygen and high levels of carbon dioxide in the blood.

What are the symptoms?
Disorders that involve damage to the alveoli are usually long-term conditions, and symptoms develop gradually. In ventilation disorders, symptoms of respiratory failure may develop either suddenly or gradually over a period of time, depending on the cause.

The symptoms of respiratory failure are mainly due to low levels of oxygen in the blood and may include:
- Shortness of breath.
- A bluish tinge to the lips and tongue, a condition known as cyanosis.
- Anxiety.
- Agitation.
- Confusion.
- Sweating.

In addition to the symptoms listed above, ventilation disorders may cause other symptoms, such as headache and drowsiness, due to the high concentration of carbon dioxide in the blood.

What might be done?
Respiratory failure can usually be diagnosed from the symptoms, and its severity can be assessed by measuring the levels of oxygen and carbon dioxide in blood (see **Measuring blood gases**, p.306). If the cause is not obvious, you may need further tests.

Respiratory failure due to permanent damage to the alveoli cannot be treated except with a lung transplant. However, symptoms may be relieved by long-term home oxygen therapy (below), which needs to be used continuously for at least 15 hours a day to prevent chronic heart failure (p.247).

If you develop respiratory failure caused by a ventilation disorder, you may need help from a ventilator to breathe. This is usually performed in hospital at first, but, if long-term ventilation is required, it may be possible to continue the treatment at home.

If respiratory failure occurs suddenly due to a ventilation disorder, recovery is possible if the underlying cause can be treated successfully. Cases of gradual respiratory failure are less likely to show significant improvement, but the symptoms can be controlled effectively with long-term oxygen therapy.

▶ **TREATMENT**

Home oxygen therapy

Oxygen therapy can be used at home to relieve symptoms of many lung disorders that lead to low blood oxygen levels. You can use either oxygen cylinders or an oxygen concentrator. In people with chronic respiratory failure, the treatment improves symptoms and can delay the development of complications and prolong life if used for at least 15 hours a day. Smaller, portable oxygen cylinders can be used when outside, enabling you to move around freely while receiving extra oxygen.

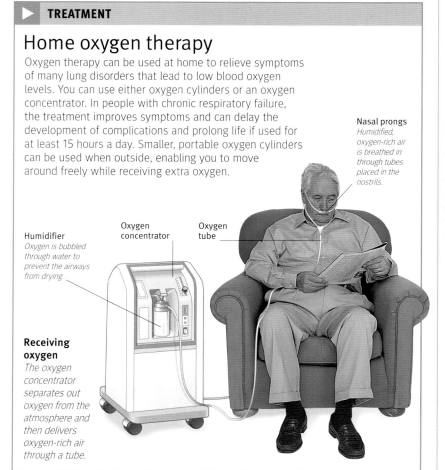

Nasal prongs
Humidified, oxygen-rich air is breathed in through tubes placed in the nostrils.

Oxygen tube

Oxygen concentrator

Humidifier
Oxygen is bubbled through water to prevent the airways from drying

Receiving oxygen
The oxygen concentrator separates out oxygen from the atmosphere and then delivers oxygen-rich air through a tube.

Nervous system and mental function

The nervous system is the most complex system in the body and regulates hundreds of activities simultaneously. It is the source of our consciousness, intelligence, and creativity and allows us to communicate and experience emotions. It also monitors and controls almost all bodily processes, ranging from automatic functions of which we are largely unconscious, such as breathing and blinking, to complex activities that involve thought and learning, such as playing a musical instrument and riding a bicycle.

THE NERVOUS SYSTEM has two parts: the central nervous system (CNS), which consists of the brain and spinal cord; and the peripheral nervous system (PNS), which is made up of all the nerves that emerge from the CNS and branch throughout the body. Nerve signals are processed and coordinated by the CNS, while the PNS transmits nerve signals to and from the CNS and other parts of the body.

The nervous system has immediate control over our voluntary actions, such as walking, and our automatic body functions, such as salivation. The longer-term control of automatic body activities, such as maintaining normal blood pressure and temperature, is aided by some of the hormones produced by the endocrine system.

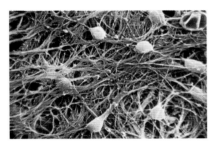

Nerve fibres
Brain tissue consists of networks of nerve fibres along which electrical signals travel.

How the nervous system works

Most of the activity of the nervous system is carried out by cells called neurons. Each neuron typically has a long projection known as a nerve fibre (axon), which relays information in the form of electrical signals. When a signal reaches the end of a nerve fibre, it is carried in chemical form to the next neuron or to another kind of cell. In the PNS, nerve fibres form bundles called nerves, and these carry messages

concerning the outside world and the inside of the body. For example, information about sound is detected by sensory receptors in the ear and converted into nerve impulses. These signals travel along nerve fibres towards the brain. In response to these nerve impulses, the CNS then transmits signals to the motor nerves in the PNS, which communicate with glands, organs, or muscles to produce an appropriate response to the original stimuli. The CNS also receives a constant stream of data concerning the inner organs and bodily functions, such as blood pressure and body temperature, from other sensory organs throughout the body. This information is monitored continuously and elicits appropriate responses, often without any input from the conscious mind.

Complex activities

Many complex activities and functions, including creativity and logic, involve conscious thought. However, some activities that require the coordination of several physical tasks are regulated unconsciously. For example, your first attempts to ride a bicycle require a conscious effort but when you have learned and memorized the necessary skills you can cycle without conscious thought. However, you still remain conscious of sensory stimuli, such as sight and sound, that aid navigation.

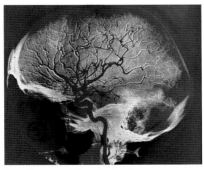

Arteries supplying the brain
Four arteries branch at the base of the brain to supply it with about one-fifth of the body's total supply of blood.

✚ FUNCTION

Nervous system organization

The nervous system is divided into two parts: the central nervous system (CNS), which regulates bodily activity; and the peripheral nervous system (PNS), which transmits signals between the body and the CNS. The PNS is divided into nerves that control voluntary actions or transmit sensations, and nerves that regulate internal functions.

Nerve links between brain and body
Nerve fibres leave the brain and enter the spinal cord to form a thick bundle of nerves. Individual nerves then emerge from the spinal cord and branch out through the body, supplying every tissue.

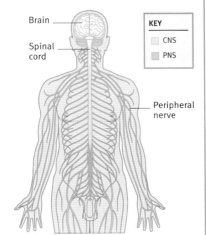

Brain
Spinal cord
Peripheral nerve

KEY
☐ CNS
☐ PNS

✚ **STRUCTURE**

Nervous system

The brain and spinal cord form the central nervous system and are protected by the bones of the skull and the vertebral column. Inside these hard outer coverings, further protection is provided by three membranes called the meninges and a clear liquid known as cerebrospinal fluid. The cranial nerves emerge directly from the brain, and the spinal nerves from the spinal cord. Together, these form the peripheral nerves that branch to every part of the body.

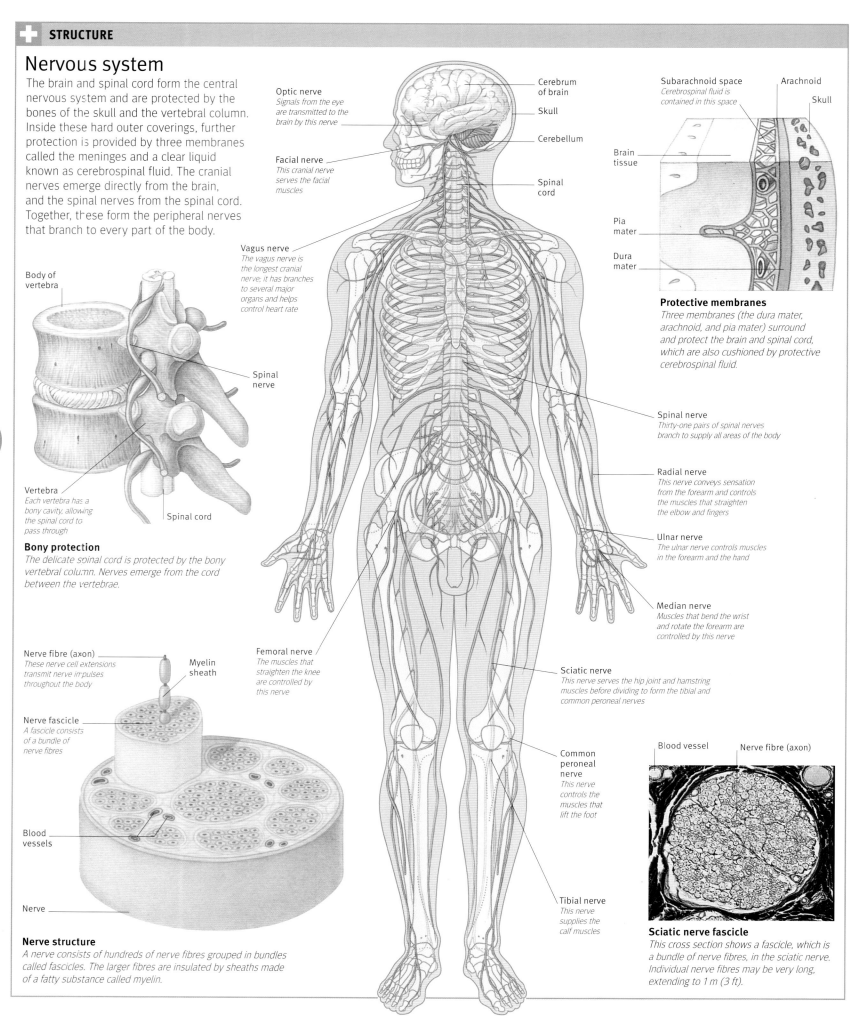

Optic nerve
Signals from the eye are transmitted to the brain by this nerve

Facial nerve
This cranial nerve serves the facial muscles

Vagus nerve
The vagus nerve is the longest cranial nerve; it has branches to several major organs and helps control heart rate

Cerebrum of brain

Skull

Cerebellum

Spinal cord

Body of vertebra

Spinal nerve

Vertebra
Each vertebra has a bony cavity, allowing the spinal cord to pass through

Spinal cord

Bony protection
The delicate spinal cord is protected by the bony vertebral column. Nerves emerge from the cord between the vertebrae.

Nerve fibre (axon)
These nerve cell extensions transmit nerve impulses throughout the body

Myelin sheath

Nerve fascicle
A fascicle consists of a bundle of nerve fibres

Blood vessels

Nerve

Nerve structure
A nerve consists of hundreds of nerve fibres grouped in bundles called fascicles. The larger fibres are insulated by sheaths made of a fatty substance called myelin.

Femoral nerve
The muscles that straighten the knee are controlled by this nerve

Common peroneal nerve
This nerve controls the muscles that lift the foot

Tibial nerve
This nerve supplies the calf muscles

Subarachnoid space
Cerebrospinal fluid is contained in this space

Arachnoid

Skull

Brain tissue

Pia mater

Dura mater

Protective membranes
Three membranes (the dura mater, arachnoid, and pia mater) surround and protect the brain and spinal cord, which are also cushioned by protective cerebrospinal fluid.

Spinal nerve
Thirty-one pairs of spinal nerves branch to supply all areas of the body

Radial nerve
This nerve conveys sensation from the forearm and controls the muscles that straighten the elbow and fingers

Ulnar nerve
The ulnar nerve controls muscles in the forearm and the hand

Median nerve
Muscles that bend the wrist and rotate the forearm are controlled by this nerve

Sciatic nerve
This nerve serves the hip joint and hamstring muscles before dividing to form the tibial and common peroneal nerves

Blood vessel

Nerve fibre (axon)

Sciatic nerve fascicle
This cross section shows a fascicle, which is a bundle of nerve fibres, in the sciatic nerve. Individual nerve fibres may be very long, extending to 1 m (3 ft).

Brain, spinal cord, and nerves

The brain contains more than 100 billion neurons and weighs about 1.4 kg (3 lb). The brain and spinal cord contain two main types of tissue: grey matter, which originates and processes nerve impulses; and white matter, which transmits them. The largest structure in the brain is the cerebrum, which is divided into two halves or hemispheres. Other structures include the cerebellum, the brain stem, and a central region that includes the thalamus and hypothalamus. The spinal cord is an extension of the brain stem and continues downwards from the base of the skull.

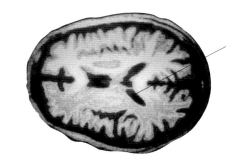

Lateral ventricles
The left and right lateral ventricles appear X-shaped when viewed in cross section

MRI scan of the brain
Protective cerebrospinal fluid is made in four ventricles, or cavities, in the brain. This section of the brain shows the lateral ventricles.

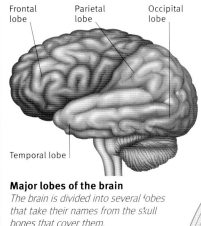

Frontal lobe
Parietal lobe
Occipital lobe

Temporal lobe

Major lobes of the brain
The brain is divided into several lobes that take their names from the skull bones that cover them.

Cerebrum
The cerebrum consists of grey and white matter. It is the largest part of the brain and links to every part of the body

Skull

Meninges
Surrounding the brain and the spinal cord are three protective membranes called the meninges

Cerebral cortex
This outer layer of the cerebrum governs higher brain functions, including thought. It receives and processes sensations and initiates movement

Subarachnoid space
This region contains cerebrospinal fluid, which protects the brain and spinal cord as it circulates around them before draining back into the venous sinuses

Arachnoid granulation
Cerebrospinal fluid is absorbed from here into the blood

Venous sinus
This is one of several major blood vessels that drain blood away from the brain

Corpus callosum
This large bundle of about 300 million nerve fibres connects the two cerebral hemispheres

Hypothalamus
The hypothalamus controls the endocrine system. It regulates sleep, sexual function, body temperature, and water content

Grey matter
Grey matter consists mainly of neuron cell bodies, from which nerve impulses originate

Choroid plexus
This area is involved in producing cerebrospinal fluid

Thalamus
Sensory nerve impulses pass through the thalamus on their way to the cerebral cortex

Pituitary
This gland regulates other glands throughout the body

Basal ganglia
These islands of grey matter help to coordinate movement

White matter
White matter consists largely of nerve fibres; its main role is to transmit nerve impulses

Brain stem
The main motor pathways cross over in the brain stem to the opposite sides of the spinal cord

Cerebellum
This area is involved in balance and the control of muscle movement

Midbrain

Pons

Medulla

Brain stem
The brain stem relays nerve impulses between the spinal cord and the brain; it controls vital functions such as heart rate and breathing

Brain tissue
The outer layer of the brain, the cerebral cortex, is made of grey matter. Beneath are white matter and islands of grey matter.

Cerebellum

Spinal cord
Nerve impulses sent between the brain and the peripheral nerves travel along nerve fibres that run through tracts (pathways) in the spinal cord

Brain, spinal cord, and nerves (continued)

Cranial nerves

Twelve pairs of cranial nerves emerge directly from the underside of the brain. Most of these nerves supply the head, face, neck, and shoulders. Certain organs in the chest and abdomen, including the heart, lungs, and much of the digestive system, are supplied by the vagus nerve.

Trigeminal nerve
Sensations from the face are relayed by this nerve, which also controls muscles used in chewing

Vestibulocochlear nerve
Fibres in this nerve carry information about sound and balance from the ear

Glossopharyngeal and hypoglossal nerves
These nerves carry information about taste in addition to controlling movements of the tongue

Cranial nerve functions
The cranial nerves contain sensory and/or motor fibres, which control various conscious and unconscious functions.

Spinal accessory nerve
This nerve controls some movements of the head and shoulder muscles

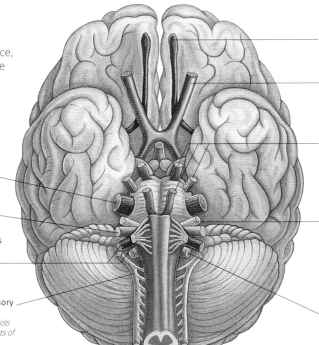

Olfactory nerve
This nerve relays information about smell from the nose

Optic nerve
This nerve transmits information about visual images

Oculomotor, trochlear, and abducent nerves
These nerves supply muscles that move the eyes

Facial nerve
This nerve transmits information from the taste buds and controls facial expression

Vagus nerve
This nerve performs many roles, such as regulation of heart rate and speech

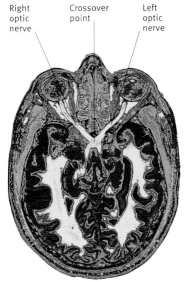

Right optic nerve   Crossover point   Left optic nerve

MRI scan of optic nerves
The optic nerves from the left and the right eyes merge and then diverge in the centre of the brain so that each cerebral hemisphere receives data from both eyes.

Spinal nerves

Thirty-one pairs of spinal nerves emerge from the spinal cord and extend through the protective, bony spinal column. These nerves divide to supply all parts of the trunk and the limbs. Before reaching the limbs, bundles of nerves converge to form braid-like plexuses, called the brachial and lumbar plexuses, which then branch further along.

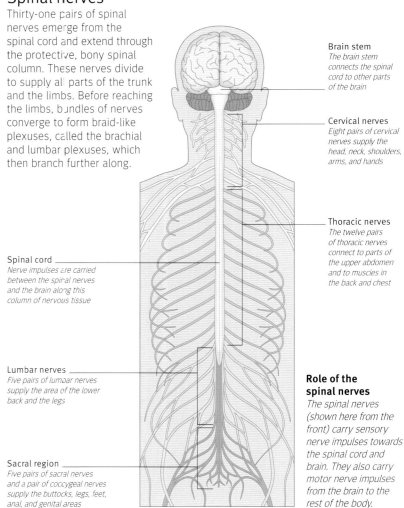

Spinal cord
Nerve impulses are carried between the spinal nerves and the brain along this column of nervous tissue

Lumbar nerves
Five pairs of lumbar nerves supply the area of the lower back and the legs

Sacral region
Five pairs of sacral nerves and a pair of coccygeal nerves supply the buttocks, legs, feet, anal, and genital areas

Brain stem
The brain stem connects the spinal cord to other parts of the brain

Cervical nerves
Eight pairs of cervical nerves supply the head, neck, shoulders, arms, and hands

Thoracic nerves
The twelve pairs of thoracic nerves connect to parts of the upper abdomen and to muscles in the back and chest

Role of the spinal nerves
The spinal nerves (shown here from the front) carry sensory nerve impulses towards the spinal cord and brain. They also carry motor nerve impulses from the brain to the rest of the body.

Structure of the spinal cord

The spinal cord has a core of grey matter containing nerve cell bodies, dendrites, and supporting cells. Surrounding the grey matter is white matter containing columns of nerve fibres that carry signals to and from the brain along the length of the spinal cord.

Sensory nerve root
These sensory fibres carry data about sensations and enter the rear of the cord

Motor nerve root
These motor nerve fibres control movement and leave the front of the spinal cord

Grey matter

White matter

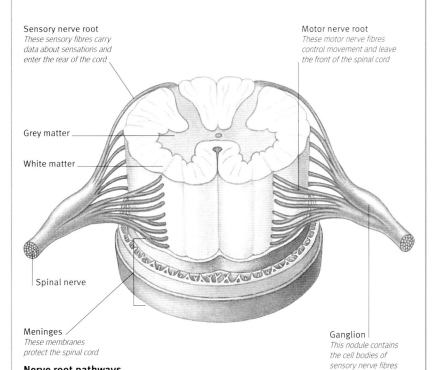

Spinal nerve

Meninges
These membranes protect the spinal cord

Ganglion
This nodule contains the cell bodies of sensory nerve fibres

Nerve root pathways
Each spinal nerve has motor and sensory nerve roots. The sensory nerve roots enter the back of the spinal cord to join fibres that lead to the brain. Nerve fibres carrying signals from the brain join motor nerve roots leaving the front of the cord.

Nerve cells

Neurons are nerve cells that originate, process, transmit, and receive nerve impulses. They are connected to other neurons or to cells in muscles, organs, or glands. Nerve impulses travel electrically along the neuron and are transmitted by chemical messengers (neurotransmitters) to the next neuron across a tiny gap, called a synapse, between the neuron and the adjacent cell, which is known as the target cell. In addition to neurons, the nervous system contains large numbers of other types of cell, called neuroglia, which protect, nourish, and support neurons.

Neural connection
This magnified image shows two neurons. The nerve fibre of one neuron links to the cell body of the other.

Cell body of
neuron

Nerve fibre
(axon)

Neurons

In addition to features common to all cells, such as a nucleus, neurons have specialized projections, known as nerve fibres (axons), that carry nerve signals. Neurons in the brain form densely packed clusters. Neurons in the spinal cord and around the body form long communication tracts.

Nerve fibre (axon)
Nerve fibres may link to the cell bodies or the dendrites of other neurons or to other cells

Node of Ranvier
These gaps in the myelin sheath help the conduction of nerve impulses

Myelin sheath
Some fibres have this fatty coating, which speeds up nerve impulse transmission

Dendrite
A neuron may have up to 200 of these short, branching projections

Synapse
This gap separates a fibre's end bulb from an adjacent cell body or a dendrite

Synaptic end bulb
This swelling at the end of the nerve fibre holds chemicals that are able to travel across the synapse

Neuron structure
A typical neuron has one or two long nerve fibres and many dendrites. Nerve fibres carry signals away from a neuron's cell body, and dendrites carry signals toward it.

Nucleus

Neuron
cell body

Conduction of nerve signals

Nerve impulses travel along neurons in the form of electrical signals. These signals cross the synapses (tiny gaps) between one neuron and the next in chemical form before being transmitted again in electrical form. Signals are also chemically transmitted to other target cells, such as those in muscles, which make appropriate responses.

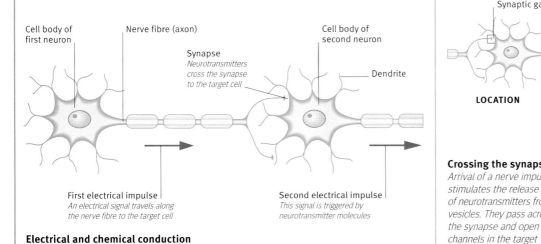

Cell body of
first neuron

Nerve fibre (axon)

Synapse
Neurotransmitters cross the synapse to the target cell

Cell body of
second neuron

Dendrite

First electrical impulse
An electrical signal travels along the nerve fibre to the target cell

Second electrical impulse
This signal is triggered by neurotransmitter molecules

Electrical and chemical conduction
When an electrical signal arrives at the end of a nerve fibre, it triggers the release of neurotransmitter molecules, which transmit the signal in chemical form to the next cell.

How neurotransmitters work

More than 50 neurotransmitters have been identified. Their task is to carry nerve impulses across the synapse (a tiny gap) between neurons and target cells. Neurotransmitters either stimulate or inhibit electrical impulses in target cells.

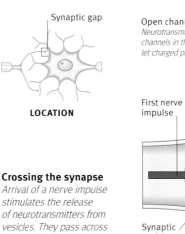

Synaptic gap

LOCATION

Crossing the synapse
Arrival of a nerve impulse stimulates the release of neurotransmitters from vesicles. They pass across the synapse and open channels in the target cell. Charged particles can then enter and trigger a second impulse.

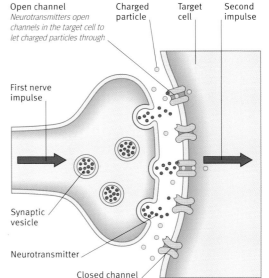

Open channel
Neurotransmitters open channels in the target cell to let charged particles through

Charged
particle

Target
cell

Second
impulse

First nerve
impulse

Synaptic
vesicle

Neurotransmitter

Closed channel

Sensory receptors

Sensory receptors respond to stimuli and transmit data about them to the brain. In the skin, receptors detect touch, pressure, vibration, temperature, and pain. Elsewhere in the body, more specialized receptors detect light (*see* **How the eye works**, p.353), sound (*see* **The mechanism of hearing**, p.372), smell, and taste. Internal receptors called proprioceptors sense body position and the location of body parts in relation to each other.

Touch

Touch receptors are found all over the body. The most common are free nerve endings, which sense pain, pressure, and temperature in addition to touch. Other touch receptors include Merkel's discs and Meissner's corpuscles, which detect light touch, and Pacinian corpuscles, which sense deep pressure and vibration.

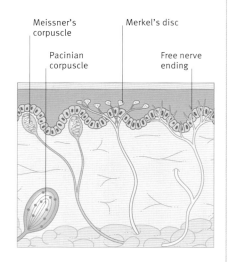

Meissner's corpuscle

Merkel's disc

Pacinian corpuscle

Free nerve ending

Receptors in the skin
Merkel's discs and Meissner's and Pacinian corpuscles end in a capsule. Free nerve endings are uncovered.

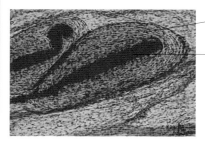

Capsule of layered membranes

Nerve ending

Pacinian corpuscle
This receptor consists of a nerve ending surrounded by layered membranes. Pacinian corpuscles are found in the palms, soles, genitals, and nipples.

Smell

Olfactory receptors in the roof of the nasal cavity are stimulated by odours. Nerve impulses from these receptors travel to the olfactory bulb (the end of the olfactory nerve) and then to the olfactory centres in the brain. Our sense of smell is thousands of times more sensitive than our sense of taste, and we can detect more than 10,000 odours.

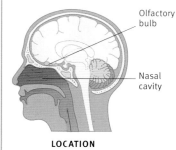

Olfactory bulb

Nasal cavity

LOCATION

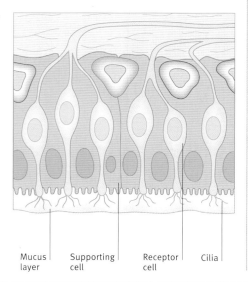

Olfactory receptors
When odour molecules enter the nose, they stimulate the cilia (tiny hairs) attached to receptor cells, causing nerve impulses to pass to the olfactory bulb and then to the brain.

Mucus layer

Supporting cell

Receptor cell

Cilia

Taste

There are about 10,000 taste buds on the upper surface of the tongue. Each bud contains about 25 sensory receptor cells, on which tiny taste hairs are exposed to drink and food dissolved in saliva. Buds sense the five basic tastes: bitter, sour, salty, sweet, and umami (a savoury, meaty taste). A combination of odours and these basic tastes produce more subtle tastes.

Taste bud structure
Substances in the mouth come into contact with taste hairs on the tongue. These tiny hairs generate nerve impulses that travel along nerve fibres to a specialized area of the brain.

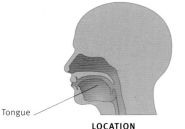

Tongue

LOCATION

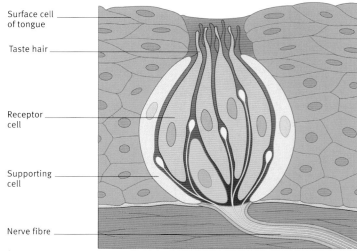

Surface cell of tongue

Taste hair

Receptor cell

Supporting cell

Nerve fibre

Proprioceptors

Proprioceptors are types of internal sensory receptors that monitor the degree of stretch of muscles and tendons around the body. This information gives us our sense of balance and our awareness of the position of various parts of the body in relation to each other.

Muscle

LOCATION

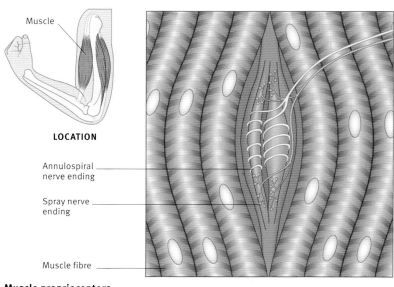

Annulospiral nerve ending

Spray nerve ending

Muscle fibre

Muscle proprioceptors
Two types of muscle proprioceptor are annulospiral sensory endings, which wind around the muscle fibres, and spray endings, which lie on top of the fibres.

✚ **FUNCTION**

Voluntary and involuntary responses

The responses of the nervous system to stimuli may be voluntary or involuntary. Voluntary responses are mainly under conscious control, but some voluntary movements, such as walking, require less conscious attention. There are two types of involuntary response, autonomic and reflex. Autonomic responses regulate the body's internal environment. Reflexes mainly affect those muscles that are normally under voluntary control.

Voluntary responses

All voluntary activities involve the brain, which sends out the motor impulses that control movement. These motor signals are initiated by thought and most also involve a response to sensory stimuli. For example, people use sight and sense of position to help them coordinate the action of walking.

Voluntary pathways
The sensory impulses that trigger voluntary responses are dealt with in many parts of the brain.

Cerebral cortex
The cortex processes sensory data and sends impulses to the muscles

Cerebellum
The cerebellum monitors sensory data on body position, fine-tuning motor nerve impulses from the cerebral cortex to coordinate movement

Sensory nerve impulse

Motor nerve impulse

Spinal cord

Basal ganglia
These masses of grey matter help to control coordinated movements, such as walking

Nerve–muscle junction
At this junction, a nerve fibre transmits signals to produce a response from muscle fibres.

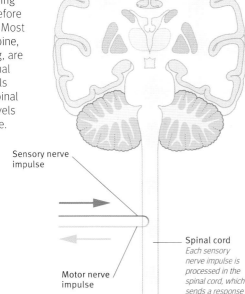

Nerve fibre

Muscle fibre

Autonomic responses

The autonomic nervous system controls the body's internal environment without conscious intervention and helps to regulate vital functions, such as blood pressure. The two types of autonomic nerves, sympathetic and parasympathetic, have opposing effects but balance each other most of the time. At certain times, such as during stress or exercise, one system dominates.

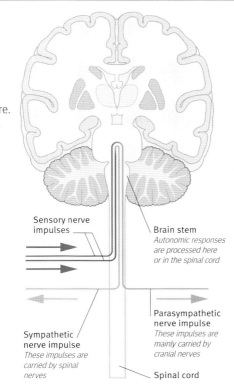

Sensory nerve impulses

Brain stem
Autonomic responses are processed here or in the spinal cord

Autonomic pathways
Information collected by internal receptors travels along sensory nerves to the spinal cord and the brain stem for processing. Sympathetic and parasympathetic response signals have separate pathways.

Parasympathetic nerve impulse
These impulses are mainly carried by cranial nerves

Sympathetic nerve impulse
These impulses are carried by spinal nerves

Spinal cord

Divisions of the autonomic system

Organ Affected	Sympathetic response	Parasympathetic response
Eyes	Pupils dilate	Pupils constrict
Lungs	Bronchial tubes dilate	Bronchial tubes constrict
Heart	Rate and strength of heartbeat increase	Rate and strength of heartbeat decrease
Stomach	Enzymes decrease	Enzymes increase
Liver	Releases glucose	Stores glucose

Two types of responses
Sympathetic and parasympathetic nerves each produce different responses in a particular organ. The sympathetic responses prepare the body to cope at times of stress. Parasympathetic responses help conserve or restore energy.

Reflexes

A reflex is an involuntary response to a stimulus, such as withdrawing your hand from a hot surface before you become aware of the heat. Most reflexes are processed in the spine, although some, such as blinking, are processed in the brain. In a spinal reflex, the stimulus signal travels along a sensory nerve to the spinal cord, and a response signal travels back by means of a motor nerve.

Sensory nerve impulse

Spinal cord
Each sensory nerve impulse is processed in the spinal cord, which sends a response signal directly to the correct muscle

Motor nerve impulse

Spinal reflex pathway
Spinal reflexes involve the simplest nerve pathways: the sensory and motor neurons are directly linked together in the spinal cord.

Information processing

Different types of sensory information are processed in different parts of the nervous system, which sends out appropriate response signals. Complex information, such as data about music and emotion, is processed in the cerebral cortex, which is known as the "higher" part of the brain. Some specialized functions, such as the interpretation of language, are processed mainly in one side of the brain, the "dominant hemisphere". The left hemisphere is dominant in more than 9 out of 10 people.

Processing higher functions

Neuroscientists can now pinpoint those parts of the brain's cortex that process nerve impulses concerned with higher human functions, such as intellect and memory. Areas of the cortex that are mainly concerned with detecting nerve impulses are known as primary areas; the parts that are concerned with analysing impulses are known as association areas.

Language interpretation in the brain
The coloured areas in this PET scan show the regions of the brain that are most active while interpreting language. There is more activity in the left dominant hemisphere than in the right hemisphere.

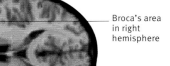

Broca's area in right hemisphere

Wernicke's area in left hemisphere

Broca's area in left hemisphere

Primary sensory cortex
This area receives data about sensations in skin, muscles, joints, and organs

Motor cortex
The motor cortex sends signals to muscles to cause voluntary movements

Premotor cortex
This part of the cortex coordinates complex movement sequences, such as piano playing

Prefrontal cortex
The prefrontal cortex deals with various aspects of behaviour and personality

Sensory association cortex
Data about sensations are analysed here

Broca's area
This area is vital for the formation of speech

Primary auditory cortex
This area detects discrete qualities of sound, such as pitch and volume

Visual association cortex
Images are formed once visual data have been analysed here

Primary visual cortex
This part of the cortex receives nerve impulses from the eye

The brain map
Different areas of the cortex have specific functions. Many areas of the cortex are involved in complex functions such as learning.

Auditory association cortex
This area analyses data about sound. Data about individual sounds are combined, so that words or melodies can be recognized

Wernicke's area
This area interprets spoken and written language

Movement and touch

Each side of the brain has its own motor and sensory cortices, which control movement and sense touch in the opposite side of the body. Movement signals are processed by a particular region at the top of the cerebrum in the motor cortex. An adjacent area, known as the sensory cortex, processes touch signals. Movements that involve great complexity or body parts that are extremely sensitive to touch are allocated a larger proportion of motor or sensory cortex. In general, those parts of the body capable of complex movement are also highly sensitive to touch.

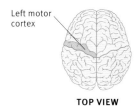

Left motor cortex

Motor map of the brain
Areas of the body that require great skill and precision of movement, such as the hands, are allocated relatively large areas of the motor cortex.

TOP VIEW

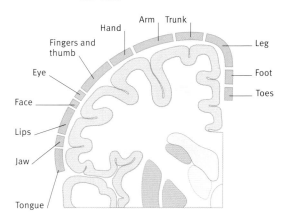

Hand · Arm · Trunk

Fingers and thumb

Eye

Face

Lips

Jaw

Tongue

Leg

Foot

Toes

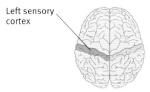

Left sensory cortex

Touch map of the brain
Very sensitive areas of the body, such as the fingers, lips, and genitals have disproportionately large areas of the sensory cortex allocated to them.

TOP VIEW

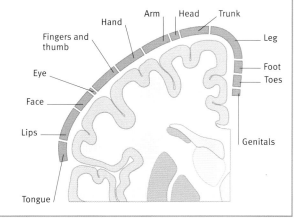

Hand · Arm · Head · Trunk

Fingers and thumb

Eye

Face

Lips

Tongue

Leg

Foot

Toes

Genitals

General nervous system disorders

The nervous system is composed of the brain and spinal cord, together known as the central nervous system, and a vast array of peripheral nerves that transmit information to and from these central structures. The nervous system may be damaged by infection, injury, vascular problems, inflammation, and degeneration. However, the causes of many general nervous system disorders are not fully understood.

The first article deals with pain, which is a common symptom of many disorders. A description of the pain often helps in the diagnosis of a disorder. Effective painkillers and treatments such as transcutaneous electrical nerve stimulation (TENS) mean that prolonged, severe pain can be effectively treated and/or controlled.

The different types of headache are discussed next. Tension headaches cause discomfort and pain to millions of people every year, often due to stress or tension. Migraine is also relatively common, while cluster headaches are a severe but less common type of headache that occur in a characteristic pattern. A headache can be a sign of an underlying disorder, and persistent or severe headaches associated with other symptoms, such as vomiting, should be assessed by a doctor without delay.

The final article in this section discusses chronic fatigue syndrome, a complex and debilitating condition.

Headaches and migraine in children are covered elsewhere (*see* **Infancy and childhood**, pp.524–565).

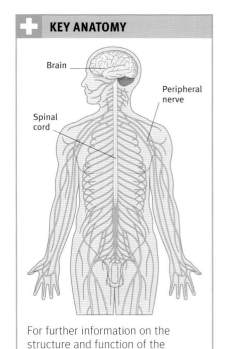

KEY ANATOMY

Brain

Peripheral nerve

Spinal cord

For further information on the structure and function of the nervous system, *see* pp.311–318.

Pain

An unpleasant sensation often felt as a result of tissue disease or damage

 Age, gender, genetics, and lifestyle are not significant factors

Pain is the body's response to an injury or a disease that results in tissue damage. Pain usually functions as a protective warning mechanism that helps to prevent further damage, although chronic (long-term) pain often seems to serve no useful function. Everyone has experienced pain, but its type and severity depend to some extent on the cause. For example, pain that results from a sports injury may be less severe than that of a similar injury caused by a violent assault. Mood and personality also affect the way we perceive pain. For example, fear or anxiety can make pain worse, while relaxation may help to relieve it to a certain extent.

The brain and spinal cord produce their own painkillers, known as endorphins, in response to pain. Endorphins are natural chemicals that are closely related to morphine and act as highly effective pain relievers for short periods but are less effective for chronic pain.

Most forms of pain can now be controlled as a result of improvements in treatment, and it is uncommon for someone to have to live with persistent pain.

What are the causes?

When tissue is damaged – for example, by trauma, infection, or a problem with its blood supply – specialized nerve endings called pain receptors are stimulated. Electrical signals travel along the nerves and through the spinal cord to the brain, which interprets them as pain. While this is happening, the damaged tissues release chemicals known as prostaglandins, which cause inflammation and swelling. The prostaglandins further stimulate the pain receptors. The skin and other sensitive parts of the body, such as the tongue and the eyes, have a large number of pain receptors and are therefore very sensitive to painful stimuli. The internal organs of the body have fewer pain receptors and so are generally less sensitive to most types of injury.

What are the types?

Although each individual may describe the character or the site of pain in a different way, there are some types of pain that usually result from specific problems. For example, throbbing pain is often due to increased blood flow, either as a result of widening of the blood vessels or because of an increase in blood flow through injured tissues. Severe, shooting pains, such as sciatica (p.338), can be caused by pressure or irritation of the nerve at the point where it emerges from the spinal cord. Colicky pain is caused by intermittent stretching and contraction of muscles in the walls of the intestines, or in other parts of the body such as the bile ducts, which lead from the liver to the intestine.

The location of the pain usually acts as a good guide to its source. However, in some cases, overlapping nerve pathways can result in a confused message, causing pain to be felt in a different area of the body from the site where it originates. This type of pain, known as referred pain, occurs when the nerves carrying the sensation of pain merge with other nerves before they reach the brain. For example, hip problems may be felt as knee pain, while problems with a tooth may be felt as earache. Heart problems can cause pain across the chest, into the neck, and in one or both arms. Pain due to problems in the intestines tends to be felt in the centre of the abdomen and is felt locally only when the abdominal wall is affected, as in the late stages of appendicitis (p.420).

Sudden (acute), severe pain may be associated with other symptoms, such as pale skin, sweating, nausea or vomiting, rapid pulse, and dilated pupils, and may even result in fainting. Prolonged periods of severe pain that continue for weeks or months may lead to depression (p.343), loss of weight as a result of decreased appetite, and disturbed sleep (*see* **Insomnia**, p.343).

What might be done?

If you experience severe or recurrent unexplained pain you should see your doctor, who may be able to establish the cause of pain after a physical examination. Further investigations, including blood tests and imaging tests such as ultrasound scanning (p.135), may be necessary if there is no obvious cause.

Since it is difficult to measure the severity of pain, your doctor may ask how the pain affects your sleep and your ability to cope with daily activities. You may also be asked to describe the severity of the pain on a scale of 1 to 10, using 1 for slight discomfort and 10 for almost unbearable pain.

The most effective remedy for pain is treatment of the underlying cause, if possible. However, pain relief is also important until treatment of the cause takes effect. There are many different ways to relieve pain, including drugs and physical methods. The form of pain relief chosen depends on the cause and type of pain you experience.

Since pain, especially persistent pain, is influenced by other factors, such as personality and levels of stress, treatment has to be tailored to the individual.

Drug treatment Virtually all short-lived pain and much long-term pain can be relieved by painkillers (p.589). When pain is caused partly by local prostaglandin release, treatment with a nonsteroidal anti-inflammatory drug (p.578) such as ibuprofen often works well because these drugs limit the release of prostaglandins.

Opioid drugs, such as morphine and codeine, act directly on the part of the brain that perceives pain and are usually highly effective. Opioid drugs may be needed to relieve intense pain, such as that following surgery, and the severe pain associated with some cancers (*see* **Pain relief for cancer**, p.159). The risk of addiction to these drugs is small when they are used for short periods, and dependence is not a cause for concern when they are used in caring for a terminally ill person.

In addition to painkillers, a number of other drugs are prescribed for certain types of pain. These include local anaesthetics (p.590) and drugs that affect the transmission of nerve impulses, such as antidepressant drugs

▶ TREATMENT

Pain relief using TENS

Transcutaneous electrical nerve stimulation (TENS) is sometimes useful for relieving severe, persistent pain, such as back pain. In TENS, electrical impulses are relayed from an impulse generator to electrodes placed on the skin in the area of the pain. After about 30 minutes, pain may be significantly reduced. Relief may last for several hours. TENS can be used while pursuing normal activities.

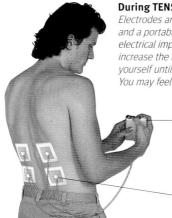

During TENS
Electrodes are placed on the skin, and a portable device generates electrical impulses. You can increase the level of stimulation yourself until the pain is relieved. You may feel a tingling sensation.

Impulse generator
This battery-operated device can be clipped on to a belt

Electrode
The electrodes can be left on the skin between treatments

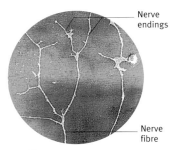

Nerve endings

Nerve fibre

Nerve endings
Branching nerve endings, as shown here, may respond to tissue damage by sending electrical signals to the brain. These signals are then interpreted as pain.

(p.592) and anticonvulsant drugs (p.590). Pain that is caused by muscle tension may be relieved by small doses of antidepressants. Anticonvulsant drugs are often used to treat pain associated with neuropathies, such as trigeminal neuralgia (p.338).

Physical treatment A wide range of nondrug therapies is available to help to relieve pain, including gentle massage and the use of hot or cold compresses. These treatments both alter blood flow through damaged tissues and stimulate other nerve endings, blocking pain.

Acupuncture may be helpful for some types of pain and may be used to relieve pain after surgical operations or for persistent pain that does not respond to other types of treatment.

If your pain is due to damaged ligaments or muscles, your doctor may offer ultrasound treatment, in which sound waves produce vibrations in the tissues and generate heat. Transcutaneous electrical nerve stimulation (*see* **Pain relief using TENS**, p.319) uses electric impulses to reduce pain and is sometimes used for lower back pain (p.225) or during labour.

What is the prognosis?
Almost all pain can be relieved to some degree, even if the underlying cause of the pain cannot be definitively treated. However, persistent pain is often more difficult to control than acute pain.

entire head. The type of pain varies; it may be sharp and sudden or dull and constant. Sometimes, other symptoms, such as nausea, occur at the same time.

What are the causes?
There are many possible causes of headache that determine the site and nature of the pain. About 3 in 4 of all headaches are caused by tension in the scalp or neck muscles. Tension headaches (below) tend to recur frequently and cause moderate pain that affects both sides of the head. Other types of headache, including migraine (below right) and cluster headaches (p.321), have a variety of possible causes. Headache can also result from prolonged use of painkillers (p.589).

Very few headaches have a serious underlying cause (*see* **Symptom chart: Headache**, p.50), but those that do require urgent medical attention. For example, a severe headache may be a sign of meningitis (p.325), a condition in which the membranes covering the brain and spinal cord become inflamed; encephalitis (p.326), in which the brain tissue is inflamed; or subarachnoid haemorrhage (p.330), in which there is sudden bleeding between the membranes covering the brain. In an elderly person, a headache with tenderness of the scalp or temple may be due to giant cell arteritis (p.282), an inflammation of the blood vessels in the head.

If your headache is severe, lasts more than 24 hours, or is accompanied by other symptoms, such as abnormal sensitivity to light, vomiting, or a rash, you should seek medical advice without delay.

What might be done?
You will be physically examined by your doctor. If it appears that an underlying disorder is causing your headache, you may have tests, such as CT scanning (p.132) or MRI (p.133) of your brain, or a lumbar puncture (p.326).

Treatment depends on the cause of the headache. A tension headache will usually clear up with rest and painkillers. Cluster headaches and migraine headaches can be treated with a specific drug, such as a triptan drug (*see* **Antimigraine drugs**, p.590).

persistent headaches that last for days or weeks. Recurrent tension headaches often affect people with depression (p.343) or those who are under continuous stress. Tension headaches are often made worse by noise and hot, stuffy environments. This type of headache occurs most commonly in women over the age of 20.

What are the symptoms?
Symptoms often begin late in the morning or in the early afternoon and may persist for several hours. They include:
■ Pain that is usually constant and is felt above the eyes or more generally over the head.
■ Feeling of pressure behind the eyes.
■ Tightening of neck muscles.
■ Feeling of tightness around the head.
People who have persistent headaches often find it difficult to sleep (*see* **Insomnia**, p.343) and may also feel depleted of energy.

What can I do?
Taking an over-the-counter painkiller (p.589) may help to relieve a tension headache. However, prolonged use of painkillers may cause headaches. Other self-help measures include gentle massage and applying heat to the neck and forehead to relieve tension. If you have a severe headache that lasts for more than 24 hours, does not respond to self-help measures, or is associated with symptoms such as vomiting or blurred vision, consult your doctor immediately.

What might the doctor do?
Your doctor will ask about the severity and frequency of your headaches and may look for signs of stress or depression. A diagnosis of tension headache is often clear from the symptoms, but you may need further tests, such as MRI (p.133) or CT scanning (p.132) of the brain, to check for an underlying cause.

Your doctor may recommend ways of dealing with stress, such as yoga or relaxation exercises (p.32). If you have depression, you may be prescribed antidepressants (p.592). Once stress or depression has been relieved, tension headaches usually clear up, but they may recur in the future.

attack before the age of 30. First attacks can occur in children as young as 2 years old (*see* **Migraine in children**, p.549) but their onset is rare in people over the age of 50. Migraine headaches recur at varying intervals. Some people have attacks several times a month; others have fewer than one a year. Most people find that migraine attacks occur less frequently and become less severe as they get older.

There are two major types of migraine: migraine with aura and migraine without aura. Aura is the term used for a group of symptoms, including visual disturbances, that develops before the onset of the main headache. Migraine with aura accounts for about 1 in 5 of all migraine cases. Some people have attacks of both types of migraine.

What are the causes?
The underlying cause of migraine is not clear but it is thought that it may be due to abnormal activity in the brainstem and changes in the levels of certain neurotransmitters (chemicals in the brain), which then affect other parts of the brain and cause changes in the brain's blood vessels.

About 8 in 10 people who suffer from migraine have a close relative with the disorder. Stress (p.31) and depression (p.343) may be trigger factors, as may the relief of stress, such as relaxing after a difficult day. Other potential triggers include missed meals, lack of or too much sleep, dehydration, and certain foods or drinks, such as cheese, chocolate, and red wine. Many women find that their migraines tend to occur around the time of menstruation.

What are the symptoms?
Migraine headaches, either with or without aura, are sometimes preceded by a group of symptoms that are collectively known as a prodrome. These prodrome symptoms tend to appear about an hour before the main symptoms begin. The prodrome often includes:
■ Anxiety or mood changes.
■ Altered sense of taste and smell.
■ Either an excess or a lack of energy.
■ Yawning.
People who have a migraine with aura experience a number of further symptoms before the migraine, including:
■ Visual disturbances, such as blurred vision and bright flashes.
■ Pins and needles, numbness, or a sensation of weakness on the face or on one side of the body.
The main symptoms, common to both types of migraine, then develop. These symptoms include:
■ Headache that is severe, throbbing, made worse by movement, and usually felt on one side of the head, over one eye, or around one temple.
■ Nausea or vomiting.
■ Abnormal sensitivity to bright light, loud noises, or certain smells.
A migraine may last for anything from a few hours to a few days but eventually clears up. After a migraine, you may feel tired and unable to concentrate.

Headache

Pain in the head of variable severity due to a variety of causes

 More common over the age of 20

 More common in females

 Stress is a risk factor

 Genetics is not generally a significant factor, although migraine sometimes runs in families

In the UK, 8 in 10 people have at least one headache each year. The majority of headaches last for only a few hours, but some persist for weeks. The pain may occur in only one part of the head, such as above the eyes, or it may be spread across the

---

Tension headaches

Moderate or severe pain, affecting one or more areas around the head, often as a result of stress

 More common over the age of 20

 More common in females

 Stress is a risk factor

 Genetics is not a significant factor

Tension headaches are often the result of stress (p.31) or bad posture, which causes tightening of the muscles in the neck and scalp. The headaches usually last only a few hours, although some people have

---

Migraine

A severe headache often associated with visual disturbances and nausea or vomiting

 First attack usually occurs by the age of 30; incidence decreases with age

 More common in females

 Sometimes runs in families

 Various things may trigger an attack, including stress, certain foods, too little or too much sleep, and dehydration.

Each year about 1 in 10 people in the UK has a migraine. Migraine is more common in women, and people usually have their first

Preventing a migraine

Many factors are known to trigger a migraine. You need to identify the ones that affect you. Avoiding these factors may reduce the frequency and severity of attacks.

- Keep a diary for a few weeks to help to pinpoint trigger factors.
- Avoid any food that brings on an attack. Common dietary triggers of migraine include red wine, chocolate, and cheese (especially matured cheese).
- Eat regularly, because missing a meal may trigger an attack.
- Drink plenty of water.
- Follow a regular sleep pattern if possible, because changing it may trigger an attack.
- If stress is a trigger, try relaxation exercises (p.32).

What might be done?

Your doctor will usually be able to diagnose a migraine from your symptoms. Rarely, tests such as MRI (p.133) or CT scanning (p.132) of the brain may be carried out to rule out more serious causes such as a brain tumour (p.327).

There is no cure for migraine but it is often possible to alleviate symptoms with medication or to reduce the likelihood of further attacks. For example, painkillers (p.589) or nonsteroidal anti-inflammatory drugs (p.578) may reduce pain. They are generally most effective if taken at the first signs of an attack. If these drugs are not effective, your doctor may prescribe an antimigraine drug (p.590) such as a triptan, which, if taken in the early stages of an attack, may help to prevent the attack from progressing. If you experience nausea or vomiting, antiemetic drugs (p.595) may help.

Self-help measures may help to prevent further migraines (see **Preventing a migraine**, above). If you have severe or frequent attacks, your doctor may prescribe a drug such as propranolol (see **Beta-blockers**, p.581) or the anticonvulsants topiramate or sodium valproate to take every day to prevent attacks.

Cluster headaches

Severe short-lived headaches that recur over a few days

 Rare under the age of 30

 More common in males

 Smoking and drinking alcohol are risk factors

 Genetics is not a significant factor

Cluster headaches are brief episodes of often excruciating pain experienced in one part of the head. They occur in a characteristic pattern, usually between one and four times a day, and there may be gaps of months or years between each group of headaches. However, a few people have persistent cluster headaches that occur at regular intervals with very few remission periods between attacks. Like migraines (opposite page), cluster headaches are likely to be related to an increase in blood flow as a result of widening of the blood vessels in the brain. These headaches affect about 1 in 1,000 people in the UK and tend to be more common in men. Smoking and drinking alcohol increase the risk.

What are the symptoms?

Cluster headaches often develop early in the morning. The major symptoms, which appear suddenly and affect one side of the head or face, include:

- Severe pain around one eye or temple.
- Watering and redness of the eye.
- Drooping of the eyelid.
- Stuffiness in the nostril or, sometimes, a runny nose on one side.

Individual episodes of pain may last from a few minutes to about 3 hours. The average attack lasts 15–30 minutes. If you have a sudden, severe headache for the first time or if you have symptoms that are different from those of previous headaches, you should consult your doctor at once.

What might be done?

Treatment for cluster headache comprises treatments for acute attacks and treatments aimed at preventing the headaches. For acute attacks, oxygen inhaled through a mask may bring relief. Alternatively, a triptan drug (see **Antimigraine drugs**, p.590), administered by injection or nasal spray, may be effective.

To prevent attacks, your doctor may prescribe verapamil, a calcium channel blocker (p.582), or corticosteroids (p.600). These should be gradually reduced in dose, as advised by your doctor, as the headaches disappear. If attacks are particularly severe and debilitating, lithium (see **Mood-stabilizing drugs**, p.593) may be prescribed.

If you are prone to cluster headaches, you should not smoke or drink even small amounts of alcohol.

Cluster headaches may continue for the rest of your life, but you may have prolonged periods of remission.

Chronic fatigue syndrome

Prolonged fatigue and a wide range of other symptoms, lasting at least 6 months

 Most common between the ages of 25 and 45

 More common in females

 Genetics and lifestyle are not significant factors

Chronic fatigue syndrome is a complex illness that produces extreme fatigue over a prolonged period. The condition has also been called post-viral fatigue syndrome, myalgic encephalomyelitis (ME), or chronic fatigue and immune dysfunction syndrome. The condition can be extremely debilitating and may continue for months or years.

Since the symptoms are so variable, chronic fatigue syndrome is often unrecognized or misdiagnosed. This makes it difficult to estimate the number of people affected, but it is thought to be about 250,000 in the UK. The condition is most often seen in women aged between 25 and 45, but it can affect children or adults of any age and people from all ethnic groups.

What are the causes?

The cause of chronic fatigue syndrome is unknown, although it is believed that several different factors are likely to be involved. In some cases, chronic fatigue syndrome develops after recovery from a viral infection or after an emotional trauma, such as bereavement. In other cases, there is no specific preceding illness or life event. Sometimes, chronic fatigue syndrome is associated with depression (p.343), although it is unclear whether depression is a result of the condition or a cause of it.

What are the symptoms?

Although the number and severity of symptoms may vary, the major symptoms of chronic fatigue syndrome are:

- Persistent, extreme tiredness.
- Impairment of short-term memory or concentration.
- Sore throat.
- Tender lymph nodes.
- Muscle and joint pain without swelling or redness.
- Difficulty sleeping, unrefreshing sleep, or insomnia.
- Headaches.
- Prolonged muscle fatigue and feeling ill after even mild exertion.

Coping with chronic fatigue syndrome

If you develop chronic fatigue syndrome, you are likely to have fluctuating energy levels. You will need to be flexible and adjust your lifestyle to help you to live with the condition. The following self-help measures may be useful:

- Try to divide the day into sessions of rest and work.
- Graded exercise may be useful. Try to set yourself a progressive increase in activity week by week.
- Set realistic goals for yourself.
- Make dietary changes: in particular, reduce your intake of alcohol and cut out drinks containing caffeine.
- Try to reduce stress (see **Relaxation exercises**, p.32).
- Join a support group so that you do not feel isolated.

Many people who have chronic fatigue syndrome also develop symptoms of depression, such as loss of interest in their work and leisure activities, or of anxiety (see **Anxiety disorders**, p.341). Conditions involving an allergic reaction, such as eczema (p.193) and asthma (p.295), may become worse in people who have chronic fatigue syndrome.

How is it diagnosed?

Your doctor may suspect chronic fatigue syndrome if you have had prolonged fatigue for more than 4 months (or 3 months in a child) with no obvious cause and you also have at least four of the other symptoms listed above. However, since persistent tiredness is a symptom of many other disorders, including an underactive thyroid gland or adrenal glands (see **Hypothyroidism**, p.432, and **Addison's disease**, p.436) and anaemia (p.271), your doctor will try to exclude other causes first.

Your doctor will probably perform a general physical examination, and he or she may ask you questions to find out if you have psychological problems, such as depression. Blood tests may also be arranged. If no underlying cause is identified, a diagnosis of chronic fatigue syndrome will be made if your symptoms meet the criteria. Since there is no specific diagnostic test for chronic fatigue syndrome, confirmation of the disorder can take some time.

What is the treatment?

Although there is no specific treatment for chronic fatigue syndrome, there are a number of self-help measures that may help you to cope with the condition (see **Coping with chronic fatigue syndrome**, left). Your doctor may give you drugs to help to relieve some of your symptoms. For example, headaches and muscle and joint pain may be relieved by painkillers (p.589) or nonsteroidal anti-inflammatory drugs (p.578); the anticonvulsant drug pregabalin may also sometimes be prescribed to treat muscle or joint pain. Antidepressant drugs (p.592) may produce an improvement in your condition even if you have not developed symptoms of depression. You may find cognitive–behavioural therapy (p.623) beneficial. A course of physiotherapy (p.620) will help to build up your stamina. Your doctor may suggest counselling (p.624) to help you to cope with your illness, and joining a support group may also be helpful.

What is the prognosis?

Chronic fatigue syndrome is a long-term disorder, but there may be periods of relief from some symptoms. Many people find symptoms are worst in the first 1–2 years. In more than half of all cases, the condition clears up after several years.

Disorders of the brain and spinal cord

The brain and spinal cord process all incoming information from different sense organs throughout the body and coordinate appropriate responses. Both the brain and the spinal cord are connected to other parts of the body by the peripheral nerves. The brain and spinal cord are protected by overlying membranes as well as by the skull and the flexible, bony vertebral column.

The first articles in this section cover head injuries and different states of unconsciousness, such as coma. Spinal injuries, often caused by whiplash in road accidents, are described next.

Disorders associated with abnormal brain function, such as epilepsy and narcolepsy, which causes an irresistible tendency to sleep are then discussed. The next articles focus on infectious disorders affecting the brain, such as meningitis, in which the membranes surrounding the brain and spinal cord are inflamed, and viral encephalitis, in which the brain becomes inflamed. Cancerous and noncancerous brain tumours are then described.

Different types of stroke and brain haemorrhages, all of which may affect speech, mobility, or mental ability, are discussed next. The final articles in this section deal with degenerative disorders, such as types of dementia and motor neuron disease.

General disorders that affect the brain, such as headache, are discussed elsewhere (*see* **General nervous system disorders**, pp.319–321).

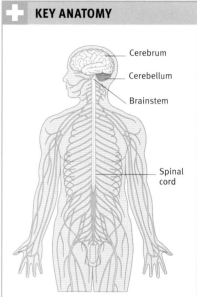

KEY ANATOMY

Cerebrum
Cerebellum
Brainstem
Spinal cord

For more information on the structure and function of the brain and spinal cord, *see* pp.311–318.

Head injuries

Damage to the scalp, skull, or brain that can vary in severity from minor to life-threatening

 More common under the age of 35

 More common in males

 Drinking alcohol and certain sports are risk factors

 Genetics is not a significant factor

Many people sustain a head injury at some time in their lives, but most are minor and have no long-term consequences. For example, from time to time most children fall over and bump their heads. However, head injuries can be serious and they are a major cause of death in young men. Approximately 700,000 people attended hospital emergency departments in England in 2011/2012 as a result of a head injury. Falls, assaults, and road traffic accidents are the most common causes.

The severity of a head injury should not be judged simply by appearance because serious brain damage can occur with no sign of damage to the scalp or skull.

What are the types?

Head injuries vary in severity and can involve damage to the scalp, skull, or brain, or a combination of all three. In some head injuries, the eyes may also be damaged (*see* **Eye injuries**, p.363).

Scalp injuries alone are usually minor and have no long-term harmful consequences. However, a small cut to the scalp may result in profuse bleeding because many of the blood vessels are close to the skin surface. As a result, the injury often appears worse than it is.

Fractures of the skull may result from a blow to the head. There may be no bleeding from the scalp, but fractures are sometimes associated with bleeding inside the skull or damage to the brain.

The brain can be damaged directly or indirectly. Direct damage usually occurs in conjunction with a skull fracture or after a penetrating injury, such as a stab wound. Indirect damage tends to occur as a result of a hard blow to the head that does not damage the skull. For example, if the head is struck on one side, the brain can be bruised as it is shaken violently within the skull. The brain may also be damaged by pressure inside the skull caused by a build-up of fluid in the brain after an injury. Bleeding between the membranes that cover the brain (*see* **Subdural haemorrhage**, p.330) may also cause dangerous compression of brain tissue.

What are the symptoms?

Initial symptoms often develop soon after a head injury and, in minor cases, usually include a mild headache and a lump, bruise, or cut on the scalp. However, an injured person may appear well at first, and then symptoms that can be indications of a more serious head injury develop hours or even days later. These symptoms include:

- Blurred or double vision.
- Headache accompanied by nausea and vomiting.
- Slurred speech.
- Vomiting.
- Blood or clear fluid leaking from the nose or ears.
- Confusion or drowsiness.
- Loss of consciousness.

In severe cases, the person may be persistently unconscious (*see* **Coma**, p.323). Sometimes, a very serious head injury is immediately fatal.

If you have a severe headache or a cut that requires stitches or if additional symptoms develop, you must go to hospital or get medical help at once.

A very young child who is unable to describe his or her symptoms should be watched closely after a head injury. If the child vomits or becomes distressed or drowsy, you should seek medical attention immediately. A head injury that causes loss of consciousness should be assessed in hospital without delay.

Are there complications?

Following a head injury, a few people develop long-term problems that continue for several months or more. These problems include frequent headaches, dizziness, poor concentration, and loss of balance. Persistent ringing in the ears (*see* **Tinnitus**, p.378) may also develop. People such as boxers who sustain repeated head injuries may eventually develop parkinsonism (*see* **Parkinson's disease and parkinsonism**, p.333).

If a head injury results in an open wound, bacteria can enter the skull and cause an infection (*see* **Brain abscess**, p.327). Rarely, brain damage may affect speech, movement, or mental ability. Some injuries may result in recurrent seizures (*see* **Epilepsy**, p.324).

What can I do?

If you have sustained a blow to the head but have not lost consciousness and have only a mild headache, it is safe to take paracetamol (*see* **Painkillers**, p.589) to relieve the pain. However, painkillers such as aspirin and other nonsteroidal anti-inflammatory drugs (p.578) should not be taken because they may make bleeding worse.

If you are with someone who has a head injury, you should try to control bleeding by pressing a clean pad firmly over the wound. If the person has lost consciousness, however briefly, or if you are concerned about the severity of the injury, you should seek medical advice immediately.

What might the doctor do?

Your doctor will examine you and, if necessary, will arrange for you to have tests at a hospital. These may include X-rays (p.131) to look for a fracture and MRI (p.133) or CT scanning (p.132) to look for swelling or bleeding. You may also need to be admitted to hospital overnight for observation.

If you have a minor injury, your doctor may advise you to rest at home. However, you must seek medical attention if further symptoms develop. A person with a severe head injury is usually admitted to an intensive therapy unit (p.618), where continuous monitoring can be carried out. If there is swelling of the brain, corticosteroids (p.600) may be given. Antibiotics (p.572) are given if there is a risk of infection. Surgery may be needed to relieve pressure on the brain caused by a build-up of fluid or from the skull pressing on it. You may also need surgery to remove a blood clot.

If brain damage has affected speech or movement, speech therapy (p.621), physiotherapy (p.620), and occupational therapy (p.621) may be required.

What is the prognosis?

Most people with a minor head injury recover completely within a few days. The outcome of a serious head injury is often difficult to predict. About 1 in 2 people survives such an injury, although recovery may take up to 2 years, and some impairment, such as speech problems, may remain. In the most severe cases of head injury, there may be paralysis, coma, persistent loss of consciousness (*see* **Persistent vegetative state**, p.323), or death.

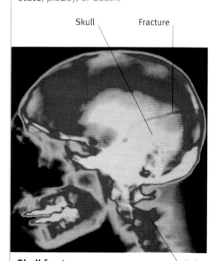

Skull   Fracture
Spine

Skull fracture
This colour-enhanced X-ray shows a long horizontal line in the skull, which is a fracture caused by a head injury.

Coma

A state of unconsciousness in which a person's responses to stimuli are absent or reduced

 Age, gender, genetics, and lifestyle are not significant factors

Coma is an unconscious state in which a person does not respond to outside stimuli such as sound, light, or touch. There are varying depths of coma. In less severe forms, a person may still respond to certain stimuli, move his or her eyes, cough, and murmur occasionally. A person who is deeply comatose does not make any movements or respond to any form of stimulation.

In the past, being in a state of coma was usually fatal within a short time. Nowadays, recovery is possible because vital functions, such as breathing, can be sustained with life-support machines (*see* **Intensive therapy unit**, p.618).

In severe cases of coma, some people lose all automatic functions irreversibly (*see* **Brain death**, right). Other people still retain these basic functions but are otherwise unresponsive. This condition is called a persistent vegetative state (right).

What are the causes?

A state of coma is caused by damage to the brain. Although such damage is often treatable, very severe damage may be irreversible and is sometimes fatal.

A serious head injury (opposite page) or a disorder that prevents blood flow to the brain, such as a stroke (p.329) or cardiac arrest (p.252), may damage enough brain tissue to result in a state of coma. Other causes of coma include infections that affect the brain, such as meningitis (p.325) and viral encephalitis (p.326).

Excessively high or low levels of certain substances in the blood may result in a state of coma. For example, a person with diabetes mellitus (p.437) may become comatose if his or her blood glucose (sugar) level rises or falls excessively. In such circumstances, it is usually possible to reverse the condition with appropriate treatment. A state of coma may also be caused by a drug overdose (*see* **Drug overdose and accidental ingestion**, p.185) or by drinking an excessive amount of alcohol or be associated with kidney or liver failure.

How is it diagnosed?

A person who is unconscious on admission to hospital will be examined for evidence of injury and to assess nervous system function. Family members and friends will be asked about possible causes. Coma is diagnosed when a person is persistently unconscious. The depth of coma is assessed against a standard scale (such as the Glasgow Coma Scale) by measuring the person's response to stimuli such as pain. For example, the doctor may rub the sternum

(breastbone) or press hard at the base of a nail bed. Blood tests are used to look for an underlying cause, such as a drug overdose, high levels of alcohol, or abnormal levels of glucose. Imaging tests, such as MRI (p.133) or CT scanning (p.132), may be carried out to look for brain damage.

If meningitis is suspected, a lumbar puncture (p.326) may be performed. In this test, a sample of fluid from around the spinal cord is taken and tested for evidence of an infection.

What is the treatment?

A person who is comatose is likely to need care in an intensive therapy unit, and mechanical ventilation may be necessary if breathing is impaired. If possible, underlying causes are treated immediately. For example, antibiotics (p.572) are given for an infection. The level of consciousness is assessed at regular intervals. Monitoring the pressure inside the skull may also be necessary because a state of coma may be associated with raised pressure. If the pressure rises, drugs can be given to reduce it.

What is the prognosis?

If brain damage is minor or reversible, a person may come out of a state of coma and make a full recovery. However, sometimes it is difficult for doctors to predict the likelihood of a complete recovery. Deep coma caused by severe head trauma often leads to long-term neurological problems. Problems may include muscle weakness or changes in behaviour for which long-term treatments such as physiotherapy (p.620) or occupational therapy (p.621) may be needed. If the damage to the brain is severe and irreversible, particularly if the brainstem has been affected, the person is unlikely to recover, and death may be the eventual outcome.

Persistent vegetative state

A long-term state of unconsciousness caused by damage to the brain

 Age, gender, genetics, and lifestyle are not significant factors

If large areas of both sides of the brain or the brainstem are damaged, coma (left) may result. In persistent vegetative state, the parts of the brain that control higher mental functions, such as thought, are damaged. However, the areas that control vital automatic functions, such as heart rate and breathing, are intact. Although the affected person is physically and mentally unresponsive to noise, light, and other stimuli, he or she can breathe without any assistance. Random movements of the head or limbs may occur.

People in a persistent vegetative state appear to have normal sleep patterns, with their eyes closing and opening as if

sleeping and waking. However, they do not appear to feel physical sensations, such as pain, or experience emotional distress. Since areas of the brain that control breathing and other vital functions are intact, a person in a persistent vegetative state can remain alive for months or even years, provided appropriate medical treatment is given.

The most common cause of the condition is a severe head injury (opposite page). It can also be caused by an infection of the brain, such as viral encephalitis (p.326), or by oxygen deprivation of the brain as a result of near-drowning or cardiac arrest (p.252).

What might be done?

The diagnosis of persistent vegetative state is made if a person who is unconscious fails to respond to stimulation or to communicate, but vital functions, such as breathing, are maintained. There is no evidence that the mind of the person is functioning consciously.

There is no treatment for persistent vegetative state. However, general supportive measures and nursing care will ensure that an affected person is kept as comfortable as possible. A person in a persistent vegetative state can live for several years, but recovery is unlikely.

Brain death

Irreversible cessation of the functions of the brain and brainstem

 Age, gender, genetics, and lifestyle are not significant factors

When a person does not respond to external stimuli because of brain damage, he or she is in a state of coma (left). In some cases, damage may affect the whole brain, including the brainstem. This part of the brain controls many of the body's vital automatic functions, such as heart rate and breathing. If the brainstem is severely damaged, such as after a head injury (opposite page), these vital functions may be affected; if this damage is irreversible, the person may be certified as brain dead.

A person who is brain dead is unable to respond to any stimuli and cannot breathe independently. Without a life-support machine (*see* **Intensive therapy unit**, p.618), death occurs within a few minutes and, even with life support, death occurs within a few days.

What might be done?

If doctors believe that brain death has occurred, a series of tests is carried out by two experienced medical consultants to confirm the diagnosis. These tests check the person's response to stimuli and the functions that are controlled by the brainstem. They include testing the ability to breathe independently without a life-support machine.

A diagnosis of brain death is made only if doctors confirm that brain and brainstem functions have been lost, and that the cause has been identified but cannot be reversed, in spite of everything possible having been done.

Someone with brain death will not survive for more than a few days, even with care in an intensive therapy unit. Full medical support, including mechanical ventilation, will continue while relatives are given counselling. Doctors will discuss the situation fully with the family, and involve family members as much as possible in the decision of when to switch off the life-support machine.

Depending on the age and previous health of the person and the cause of death, relatives may be asked about their wishes regarding organ donation.

Spinal injuries

Damage to the back or neck that may involve the spinal cord

 More common under the age of 30

 More common in males

 Drinking and driving and certain sports are risk factors

 Genetics is not a significant factor

Injuries to the neck and back are most commonly caused by traffic accidents. The areas most often damaged are the muscles of the back and neck, the bones of the spine (vertebrae), and the ligaments that hold the bones together.

Injuries to the spine may also damage the spinal cord, which lies in a narrow canal in the vertebrae and carries all the major nerve pathways connecting the limbs and trunk to and from the brain. Damage to the spinal cord may cause numbness and weakness in part of the body. If damage is severe, it can result in paralysis, which may be permanent and even life-threatening. Spinal injuries occur more commonly in young men, often as a result of risk-taking behaviour or playing contact sports.

What are the types?

The most common type of spinal injury is whiplash, in which the ligaments and muscles of the neck are damaged. The spinal cord is not usually affected by this type of injury. Whiplash is caused by sudden, extreme bending of the spine when the neck is "whipped" back, usually as the result of a road accident.

A spinal injury may dislocate or fracture one or more of the vertebrae. The vertebrae may be damaged by an impact, such as being hit by a car, or by compression, usually due to a fall from a considerable height. The spinal cord may be damaged by dislocated or broken vertebrae or by a penetrating injury.

What are the symptoms?

Symptoms of a spinal injury depend on the type and severity of the damage and on which part is injured. A whiplash injury may lead to one or more of the following symptoms:

- Headache.
- Neck pain and stiffness.
- Swelling of the affected area.
- Shoulder pain.

Displacement or damage to vertebrae, including compression of a disc, may cause pain and inflammation. If there is damage to the spinal cord, symptoms occur in other parts of the body. These symptoms may include:

- Loss of sensation.
- Weakness
- Inability to move the affected part.
- Problems with control of the bladder and bowels.
- Difficulty in breathing.

The areas of the body that are affected by symptoms depend on which part of the spinal cord has been damaged. The higher up the spinal cord the damage has occurred, the more parts of the body will be affected. For example, damage to the mid-chest area of the spine may cause weakness and numbness in the legs but will not affect the arms. If the spinal cord is severely damaged in the neck area, there may be total paralysis of all four limbs (quadriplegia), the trunk, and the muscles that control breathing, and death may result.

Anyone who has a suspected neck or spinal injury must not be moved without medical supervision because any movement may damage the spinal cord. Emergency medical help must be sought at once.

How are they diagnosed?

Once the injured person is in hospital, a full neurological assessment will be performed. This will include measuring the person's responses to different kinds of stimuli, which helps to assess whether the spinal cord has been damaged. If there is damage, CT scanning (p.132) or MRI (p.133) may be used to determine its nature and extent. If a fracture of the vertebrae is suspected, X-rays (p.131) of the spine may be taken.

What is the treatment?

If there is ligament and muscle damage, but the vertebrae are undamaged and unlikely to become displaced, bed rest and regular monitoring will probably be the only measures that are needed. Nonsteroidal anti-inflammatory drugs (p.578) may be used to relieve pain and swelling of tissues, and physiotherapy (p.620) may be required to strengthen the damaged muscles. If the injury has caused vertebrae to become displaced or damaged, the affected bones will need to be stabilized. Surgery may be carried out to realign damaged vertebrae and prevent possible damage to the spinal cord. People who have irreversible damage to the spinal cord may be paralysed. Sometimes, early treatment with drugs

reduces inflammation and limits the extent of the damage. Long-term physiotherapy is necessary to maintain muscle strength.

What is the prognosis?

Recovery from a spinal injury involving only muscles and ligaments is likely to take 4–6 weeks. Fractures usually heal in 6–8 weeks. If the spine is stable and there is no damage to the spinal cord, the person usually makes a complete recovery. When paralysis occurs, a long period of rehabilitation is needed. If there is no improvement after 6 months, the paralysis is likely to be permanent.

Epilepsy

A disorder of brain function causing recurrent seizures

 Usually develops in children and young adults

 Some types run in families

 Gender and lifestyle are not significant factors

In a person who has epilepsy, recurrent seizures or brief episodes of altered consciousness are caused by abnormal electrical activity in the brain. Epilepsy is a common disorder, affecting nearly 1 in 100 people in the UK.

The condition usually develops in childhood but may gradually disappear. However, elderly people are also at risk of developing epilepsy because they are more likely to have conditions that can cause it, such as stroke (p.329).

Many people with epilepsy lead normal lives. However, people who have recurrent seizures may have to limit certain aspects of their lifestyle, such as driving.

What are the causes?

In about a third of people with epilepsy, the underlying cause is not clear, although a genetic factor may be involved. In other cases, recurrent seizures may be the result of disease or damage to the brain, which may have various causes, including infections such as meningitis (opposite page), a stroke, a brain tumour (p.327), a severe head injury (p.322), a birth injury, or prolonged febrile convulsions as a baby.

In people with epilepsy, seizures may be triggered by lack of sleep or missing a meal, drinking excessive alcohol, and visual effects such as flashing lights and flickering television and computer screens.

A single seizure is not labelled as epilepsy. For example, high fever in a child can result in a single febrile convulsion (p.550). People who abuse alcohol over a long period may have a seizure, either while drinking heavily or during withdrawal from alcohol (*see* **Alcohol dependence**, p.350). Very low blood glucose levels, which can occur as a result of treatment for diabetes mellitus (p.437), can also trigger a seizure, as can low blood calcium levels.

▶ TEST

EEG

Electroencephalography (EEG) may be used to help diagnose conditions, such as epilepsy, that are associated with abnormal electrical activity in the brain. Electrodes are attached to a person's scalp, and recordings are made of brain activity with the eyes open and closed. A strobe light may be switched on for short periods to see if brain activity changes. The procedure takes approximately 20–30 minutes and is painless.

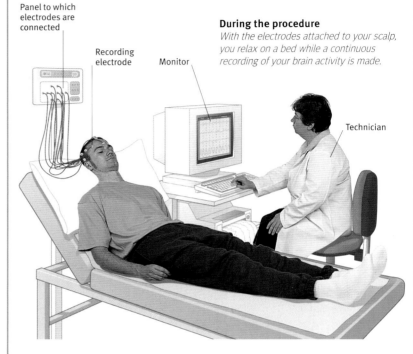

Panel to which electrodes are connected

Recording electrode

Monitor

Technician

During the procedure
With the electrodes attached to your scalp, you relax on a bed while a continuous recording of your brain activity is made.

RESULTS

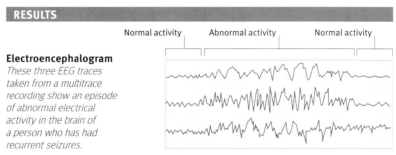

Normal activity | Abnormal activity | Normal activity

Electroencephalogram
These three EEG traces taken from a multitrace recording show an episode of abnormal electrical activity in the brain of a person who has had recurrent seizures.

What are the types?

Epileptic seizures may be generalized or partial, depending on how much of the brain is affected by abnormal electrical activity. During a generalized seizure, all areas of the brain are affected at the same time, whereas during a partial seizure only one part of the brain is affected. There are two main types of generalized seizure: tonic–clonic seizures and absence seizures. There are also two main types of partial seizure: simple partial seizures and complex partial seizures. Both simple partial and complex partial seizures can become generalized tonic–clonic seizures.

Tonic–clonic seizures This type of seizure may be preceded by a warning of an attack, known as an aura. This aura lasts for a few seconds and gives people an opportunity to sit or lie down before they lose consciousness and fall. Auras may consist of a sensation of fear, unease, or an unusual taste. During the first 30 seconds of a seizure, the body stiffens and breathing may become irregular or stop briefly. This stage is followed by several minutes of uncontrolled movement of the limbs and trunk. After the seizure, consciousness is regained, breathing returns to normal, and the muscles relax. Relaxation of the muscles in the bladder can cause incontinence. The person may be confused and disoriented for a few hours afterwards and may develop a headache. After a tonic–clonic seizure, the person affected usually has no memory of what has happened.

Status epilepticus is a serious condition in which a person has repeated tonic–clonic seizures without regaining consciousness in between. The condition can be life-threatening, and medical attention should be sought urgently.

Absence seizures Formerly known as petit mal seizures, they mainly affect children, although they may continue into adolescence and, rarely, may also affect adults. During an attack, the child loses touch with his or her surroundings and seems to be daydreaming because his or her eyes remain open and staring. Each attack lasts for between 5 and 30 seconds, and the child is usually unaware afterwards that anything was wrong. Since the seizures are almost never associated with abnormal movements or the child falling down, they may not be noticed. However, frequent attacks can affect schoolwork.

Simple partial seizures During a simple partial seizure, the affected person remains conscious. The head and the eyes may turn to one side, the hand, arm, and one side of the face may twitch, or the person may feel a tingling sensation in some of these areas. Temporary weakness or paralysis of one side of the body may follow an attack. The person may also have strange sensations, such as odd smells, sounds, and tastes.

Complex partial seizures Before this type of seizure, an affected person may experience odd tastes or smells or have a feeling of having already experienced what is happening (déjà vu). A brief dream-like state follows during which the person may be uncommunicative. During the attack, there may be smacking of the lips, grimacing and fidgeting. Afterwards, the person may not remember what has happened. Sometimes, a generalized seizure occurs as a progression of the complex partial seizure.

SELF-HELP

Living with epilepsy

If you have recently been diagnosed as having epilepsy, the following points may be helpful:

- Avoid anything that has previously triggered or may trigger a seizure, such as flashing lights.
- Learn relaxation exercises (p.32) to help you cope with stress, which may trigger seizures.
- Eat and sleep at regular times.
- Avoid drinking too much alcohol.
- Check with your doctor before taking medications that may interact with anticonvulsant drugs.
- Make sure that you have someone with you if you are swimming or playing water sports.
- Wear protective headgear when participating in contact sports.
- Before applying for a driving licence, talk to your doctor and contact the Driver and Vehicle Licensing Agency for regulations.
- Consult an adviser before choosing a career because some types of employment may not be suitable.
- Seek advice from your doctor if you plan to become pregnant.

How is it diagnosed?

You should consult a doctor if you lose consciousness for an unknown reason or if someone witnesses you having a seizure. If your child has a seizure, you should also seek medical advice immediately. It is helpful if you can obtain full details of your seizure from a witness so that you are able to give the doctor a reliable account of what happened. The doctor may arrange tests to look for an underlying cause of the seizure, such as a brain tumour or an infection such as meningitis. If no cause is found or if you have recurrent seizures, you may have an EEG (opposite page) to look for abnormal electrical activity in the brain. An EEG also helps to diagnose the particular type of epilepsy because some forms produce a distinctive pattern of electrical activity. Your doctor may also arrange for CT scanning (p.132) or MRI (p.133) of the brain to look for structural abnormalities that may be causing epilepsy.

How might the doctor treat it?

If only one seizure has occurred, treatment may not be needed. However, an underlying problem, such as poor control of diabetes, may need to be treated. If you have had recurrent seizures, you will probably be treated with anticonvulsant drugs (p.590). Usually, the dose of the drugs is gradually increased until the seizures are controlled. Occasionally, a second anticonvulsant is needed.

You will probably have regular blood tests to monitor drug levels. If you have no seizures for 2–3 years, it may be possible to reduce the drug treatment or even stop it, depending on a number of factors including the results of the EEG tests and the brain scan. However, any changes in dosage must be carried out under medical supervision. Up to 4 in 5 people who stop taking anticonvulsant drugs have seizures again within 2 years. If drugs do not control the seizures and a small area of brain tissue is found to be their cause, it may be removed surgically.

People with status epilepticus need to be admitted to hospital immediately, where they will be given intravenous drugs to control the seizures.

What can I do?

If you have epilepsy, you should avoid anything that triggers an attack, such as stress or lack of sleep (see **Living with epilepsy**, left). You should carry identification that will alert others to your condition in case you have a seizure.

If you witness someone having an epileptic seizure, you can help by turning the person onto his or her side and protecting him or her from self-injury. If the seizure lasts for more than 5 minutes, you should call an ambulance and stay with the person until it arrives.

What is the prognosis?

About 1 in 3 people who have a single seizure will have another one within 2 years.

The risk of recurrent seizures is highest in the first few weeks after an attack. However, the outlook for most people with epilepsy is good: with medication, more than 7 in 10 people go into long-term remission within 10 years.

Narcolepsy

An extreme tendency to fall asleep during normal waking hours

 Usually develops between the ages of 15 and 30

 Sometimes runs in families

 Gender and lifestyle are not significant factors

People with narcolepsy fall asleep at any time of the day, often when carrying out a monotonous task. Sleep may also occur at inappropriate times, such as while eating. Affected people can be awakened easily but may fall asleep again soon afterwards.

Some people with narcolepsy have vivid hallucinations just before falling asleep. Others find that they are unable to move while they are falling asleep or waking up (sleep paralysis). About 3 in 4 people with narcolepsy also have cataplexy, in which there is a temporary loss of strength in the limbs that causes the person to fall to the ground. Cataplexy is sometimes triggered by an emotional response, such as fear or laughter.

Narcolepsy is due to low levels of the hormone hypocretin (also called orexin) in the brain. This hormone is produced by cells in the hypothalamus and helps to regulate wakefulness and sleep. In people with narcolepsy, the cells that produce hypocretin are damaged, although it is not known why this damage occurs. Narcolepsy usually first appears between the ages of 15 and 30, although its onset sometimes occurs during childhood or middle age.

What might be done?

Your doctor will probably diagnose narcolepsy from your symptoms. EEG (opposite page) may also be used to record the electrical activity of your brain while you sleep. To confirm the diagnosis, you may also be given polysomnography, which involves an overnight stay in hospital where video monitoring, EEG, and measurement of other body activities are used to assess your sleep pattern.

You should take regular, short naps during the day and keep busy while awake. Your doctor may prescribe stimulant drugs (p.593) to help you to keep awake. Certain tricyclic antidepressant drugs (p.592) are useful in treating people with cataplexy. If you have been diagnosed with narcolepsy, you must contact the Driver and Vehicle Licensing Agency before driving or applying for a driving licence. Narcolepsy is usually lifelong, although in some cases there is a spontaneous improvement over time.

Meningitis

Inflammation of the meninges, the membranes that cover the brain and spinal cord, due to an infection

 Age and lifestyle as risk factors depend on the cause

 Gender and genetics are not significant factors

In meningitis, the meninges, the membranes that cover the brain and spinal cord, are inflamed. The disease is most often caused by a viral or bacterial infection. The viral form of meningitis is the more common and is usually not as severe as bacterial meningitis. The bacterial form is rarer but can be life-threatening. Although both forms of meningitis can occur at any age, bacterial meningitis occurs predominantly in children and young people between the ages of about 15 and 25 (see **Meningitis in children**, p.549), and viral meningitis is most common in young adults. In rare cases, meningitis may be caused by a fungal infection. This type predominates in people with AIDS (see **HIV infection and AIDS**, p.169) and in those with other disorders that impair the immune system, such as leukaemia.

What are the causes?

Many different viruses can result in meningitis. Among the most common are enteroviruses, such as the coxsackie virus, which can cause sore throats or diarrhoea, and, more rarely, the virus that causes mumps (p.167). Viral meningitis tends to occur in small outbreaks, most commonly in summer.

Bacterial meningitis most commonly occurs as a result of infection of the meninges with the bacterium *Neisseria meningitidis* (meningococcus) in an otherwise healthy child or teenager. This bacterium is the cause of meningococcal meningitis and has several types, including types A, B, C, W, and Y. Type B is the most common in the UK. Although many people carry *Neisseria meningitidis* bacteria in the back of the throat, only a fraction develop meningitis. Other bacteria that can cause the disease include *Haemophilus influenzae* type b (Hib) and *Streptococcus pneumoniae*, both of which can also cause infections in the lungs and the throat.

Less often, bacterial meningitis is a complication of an infection that has already developed elsewhere in the body. For example, the bacterium that causes tuberculosis (p.300) can spread from the lungs to the meninges.

Bacterial meningitis usually occurs as single cases only. However, there may be small outbreaks, especially in institutions such as schools and colleges. This form of meningitis is most common during the winter.

People who have a weakened immune system as a result of an existing illness or a particular treatment, such as people with HIV infection or those having chemotherapy (p.587), are at increased risk of all types of meningitis.

▶ **TEST**

Lumbar puncture

A lumbar puncture is usually performed to look for evidence of meningitis or other nervous system disorders, such as multiple sclerosis. The procedure is carried out under local anaesthesia and takes about 15 minutes. During the procedure, the pressure of the cerebrospinal fluid is checked, and a sample is taken for analysis. To help prevent a headache after the procedure, you should remain lying down flat for about an hour and drink plenty of fluids, including caffeine-containing ones such as tea and coffee.

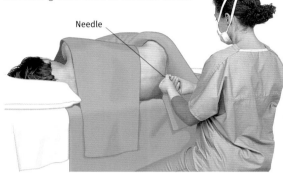

Cerebro-spinal fluid — Spinal cord — Needle — Vertebra

CROSS SECTION

During the procedure
A hollow needle is inserted between two vertebrae near the base of the spine and into the cerebrospinal fluid. A small sample of the fluid is removed for analysis.

RESULTS

Evidence of meningitis
This magnified view of a sample of cerebrospinal fluid shows several meningococcal bacteria, which confirm meningitis. The large numbers of white blood cells are a response to the infection.

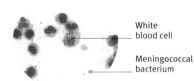

White blood cell — Meningococcal bacterium

What are the symptoms?
Initially, meningitis may produce vague flu-like symptoms, such as mild fever and aches and pains. More pronounced symptoms may then develop. Symptoms are the most severe in bacterial meningitis and may develop rapidly, often within a few hours.

The symptoms of viral meningitis may take only hours to develop, while in fungal and tuberculosis meningitis, symptoms develop slowly and may take several days to become pronounced. In adults, the main symptoms of meningitis may include the following:
- Severe headache.
- Fever.
- Stiff neck.
- Dislike of bright light.

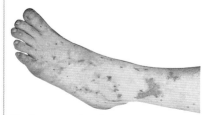

Meningococcal rash
In meningococcal meningitis, dark red or purple spots may appear that develop into blotches. The rash does not fade when pressed and viewed under a glass.

- Nausea and vomiting.
- In meningococcal meningitis, a rash of flat, reddish-purple lesions, varying in size from pinheads to large patches, that do not fade when pressed (see **Checking a red rash**, p.57).

Unless prompt treatment is given, bacterial meningitis may lead to seizures, drowsiness, and coma (p.323). In some cases, pus collects (see **Brain abscess**, p.327), which results in compression of nearby tissue.

What might be done?
If meningitis is suspected, immediate medical attention and admission to hospital is necessary. Intravenous antibiotics (p.572) are started immediately. A sample of fluid from around the spinal cord is then taken and tested for evidence of infection (see **Lumbar puncture**, above). In some cases, CT scanning (p.132) or MRI (p.133) of the brain may also be carried out before the lumbar puncture is performed.

If bacterial meningitis is confirmed by the lumbar puncture test, antibiotics are continued for at least a week. If meningitis is found to be caused by tuberculosis bacteria, antituberculous drugs (p.573) will be given. In cases of bacterial meningitis, continuous monitoring in an intensive therapy unit (p.618) is often needed. Intravenous fluids,

anticonvulsant drugs (p.590), and drugs to reduce inflammation in the brain, such as corticosteroids (p.600), may be given.

There is no specific treatment for viral meningitis. If bacterial meningitis has been excluded by tests, people with viral meningitis are usually allowed to go home. They may be given drugs to relieve symptoms, such as painkillers (p.589) for headaches. Fungal meningitis is treated with intravenous antifungal drugs (p.574) in hospital.

What is the prognosis?
Recovery from viral meningitis is usually complete within 1–2 weeks. It may take weeks or months to make a complete recovery from bacterial meningitis. Occasionally, there may be long-term problems, such as impaired hearing or memory impairment due to damage to a part of the brain. About 1 in 10 people with bacterial meningitis dies despite treatment. Deaths most commonly occur in infants and elderly people.

Can it be prevented?
People in close contact with someone with meningococcal meningitis are usually given antibiotics. This treatment kills any meningococcal bacteria that may be present in the back of the throat and prevents their spread to other people. In the UK, the routine vaccination schedule includes immunization against *Haemophilus influenza* type b (Hib) and meningococcus types B, C, and A, C, W, and Y. People travelling to high-risk areas, such as parts of Africa, might be advised to be immunized against several types of meningitis (types A, C, W, and Y; see **Travel immunizations**, p.35), even if they had already been immunized as a child.

Viral encephalitis

Inflammation of the brain as a result of a viral infection

ⓘ Age, gender, genetics, and lifestyle are not significant factors

Viral encephalitis is a rare condition in which the brain becomes inflamed as a result of a viral infection. Often, the meninges, the membranes surrounding the brain and spinal cord, are also affected. Viral encephalitis varies in severity. An attack can be so mild that it causes almost no symptoms and is barely noticeable. However, occasionally it is serious and potentially life-threatening.

What are the causes?
Many different viruses can cause viral encephalitis. Mild cases are sometimes the result of infectious mononucleosis (p.166). In addition, viral encephalitis still occurs as a complication of some childhood infections, such as measles (p.167) and mumps (p.167), although routine immunization (p.13) has made these disorders much less common.

The most common cause of life-threatening viral encephalitis is the herpes simplex virus (see **Herpes simplex infections**, p.166).

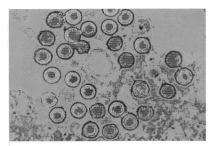

Herpes simplex virus
This highly magnified view shows the herpes simplex virus, the most common cause of life-threatening viral encephalitis.

In tropical countries, viral encephalitis can be caused by mosquito- and tick-borne infections, such as yellow fever (p.169).

In the past, the disorder was frequently caused by infection with the polio virus. However, this disease is now rare in developed countries as a result of routine immunization.

What are the symptoms?
Mild cases of viral encephalitis usually develop gradually over several days and may cause only a slight fever and mild headache. However, in severe cases, the symptoms usually develop quickly over 24–72 hours and may include:
- High fever.
- Intense headache.
- Nausea and vomiting.
- Problems with speech, such as slurring of words.
- Weakness or paralysis in one or more parts of the body.
- Confusion.

If the membranes that surround the brain become inflamed (see **Meningitis**, p.325), other symptoms such as a stiff neck and intolerance of bright light may develop. The person affected may have seizures. In some cases, there is drowsiness, which may progress to a gradual loss of consciousness and coma (p.323).

How is it diagnosed?
If viral encephalitis is suspected, you will be admitted to hospital. Your doctor may arrange for a blood test to look for signs of viral infection. You may also have CT scanning (p.132) or MRI (p.133) to look for areas of brain swelling caused by inflammation and to exclude other possible reasons for the symptoms, such as a brain abscess (p.327). A sample of the fluid surrounding the brain and spinal cord may be taken (see **Lumbar puncture**, above, left) to look for evidence of infection. You may have an EEG (p.324) to look for abnormal electrical activity in the brain. Rarely, a brain biopsy is performed, in which a sample of tissue is taken from the brain under general anaesthesia and then examined to confirm the diagnosis.

What is the treatment?
Viral encephalitis that is caused by the herpes simplex virus can be treated with intravenous doses of aciclovir (see **Antiviral drugs**, p.573) and possibly also with

corticosteroids (p.600) to reduce inflammation of the brain. In severe cases, intravenous aciclovir may be given, even if the cause has not been identified. Anticonvulsant drugs (p.590) may be prescribed if seizures develop. Severely affected people may need to be treated in an intensive therapy unit (p.618).

What is the prognosis?

It is often difficult to predict the outcome of viral encephalitis. People who have mild encephalitis usually make a full recovery over several weeks, but occasional headaches may occur for a few months. However, in severe cases, the condition may be fatal. Encephalitis caused by the herpes simplex virus often produces long-term effects, such as memory problems. In children, herpes simplex viral encephalitis may cause learning difficulties. The effects of this type of viral encephalitis can usually be minimized if treatment is begun early.

Brain abscess

A pus-filled swelling in the brain caused by bacterial or fungal infection

 More common in males

 Intravenous drug abuse is a risk factor

 Age and genetics are not significant factors

Brain abscesses are collections of pus. They are rare and, if left untreated, can be life-threatening. Pus may collect to form a single abscess or may form several abscesses in different parts of the brain. Brain tissue around the abscess or abscesses becomes compressed, and the brain itself may swell, increasing pressure inside the skull.

People who have impaired immunity, including those with HIV infection (*see* **HIV infection and AIDS**, p.169) and those having chemotherapy (p.587), are more likely to develop a brain abscess. The risk of a brain abscess is also higher in intravenous drug users than in other people because reused needles may be contaminated with infectious microorganisms. Men are twice as likely as women to develop a brain abscess.

What are the causes?

Most brain abscesses are caused by a bacterial infection that has spread to the brain from an infection in nearby tissues in the skull. For example, the infection may spread from a dental abscess (p.385) or from an infection in the sinuses (*see* **Sinusitis**, p.290). If the skull is penetrated (*see* **Head injuries**, p.322), bacteria may enter the brain and cause infection. Bacterial infection can also be carried in the bloodstream to the brain from an infection in another part of the body, such as the lungs (*see* **Pneumonia**, p.299) or the heart (*see*

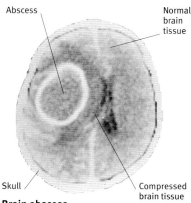

Abscess · Normal brain tissue
Skull · Compressed brain tissue

Brain abscess
This CT scan shows a large brain abscess caused by bacterial infection compressing and displacing brain tissue.

Infective endocarditis, p.256). In a few cases, the source of the infection cannot be found. Occasionally, a brain abscess may be the result of a fungal infection or, particularly in people with HIV/AIDS, of the protozoal infection toxoplasmosis (p.176).

What are the symptoms?

The symptoms of a brain abscess may develop in a few days or gradually over a few weeks. They may include:
- Headache.
- Fever.
- Nausea and vomiting.
- Stiff neck.
- Seizures.

Other symptoms, including speech and vision problems or weakness of one or more limbs, may develop depending on which part of the brain is affected. Without treatment, consciousness may be impaired and may lead to coma (p.323).

What might be done?

If your doctor suspects a brain abscess, you will be admitted to hospital immediately. The diagnosis can be confirmed by MRI (p.133) or CT scanning (p.132) of the head. You may have blood tests to identify the infecting organism and X-rays (p.131) to look for its source.

Brain abscesses caused by bacterial infections are treated with high doses of antibiotics (p.572), given intravenously at first and then orally for about 6 weeks. If the abscess is large or causing considerable brain swelling, a small hole may be drilled through the skull under general anaesthesia to allow pus to drain. The pus is then analysed to identify the infecting organism. You may have corticosteroids (p.600) to control swelling of the brain. Anticonvulsant drugs (p.590) may be prescribed to reduce the risk of seizures. In severe cases, mechanical ventilation in an intensive therapy unit (p.618) may be needed.

What is the prognosis?

Up to 8 in 10 people recover from a brain abscess if treatment is begun early. However, some have persistent problems, such as seizures, slurred speech, or weakness of a limb.

Brain tumours

Abnormal growths developing in brain tissue or the coverings of the brain

 Most common between the ages of 60 and 70. Some types occur only in children

 More common in males

 Genetics and lifestyle are not significant factors

Brain tumours may be cancerous or noncancerous. Unlike most tumours in other parts of the body, cancerous and noncancerous brain tumours can be equally serious. The seriousness of a tumour depends on its location, size, and rate of growth. Both types of tumour can compress nearby tissue, causing pressure to build up inside the skull.

Tumours that first develop in brain tissues are called primary tumours. They can arise from various types of brain cell, including the brain's support cells (tumours of which are called gliomas) and cells in the meninges (meningiomas). Gliomas are often cancerous, but most meningiomas are noncancerous. Primary brain tumours are slightly more common in men and usually develop between the ages of 60 and 70. Some types only affect children (*see* **Brain and spinal cord tumours in children**, p.550). Pituitary tumours (p.430) are those that arise in the pituitary gland, at the base of the brain.

Secondary brain tumours (metastases) are more common than primary tumours. They are always cancerous, having developed from cells that have been carried in the blood from cancerous tumours in areas such as the breast or the lungs. Several metastases may develop in the brain simultaneously.

What are the symptoms?

Symptoms usually occur when a primary tumour or metastasis compresses part of the brain or raises the pressure inside the skull. They may include:

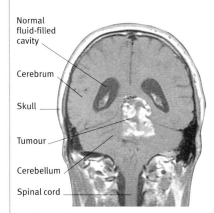

Normal fluid-filled cavity
Cerebrum
Skull
Tumour
Cerebellum
Spinal cord

Brain tumour
This MRI scan shows a brain tumour in the cerebellum, the part of the brain that helps to maintain posture and control movement. Balance and coordination are affected when the cerebellum is damaged.

- Headache that is usually more severe in the morning and is worsened by coughing or bending over.
- Nausea and vomiting.
- Blurred vision.

Other symptoms tend to be related to whichever area of the brain is affected by the tumour and may include:
- Slurred speech.
- Unsteadiness.
- Double vision.
- Difficulty in reading and writing.
- Change of personality.
- Numbness and weakness of the limbs on one side of the body.

A tumour may also cause seizures (*see* **Epilepsy**, p.324). Sometimes, a tumour blocks the flow of the cerebrospinal fluid, which circulates in and around the brain and spinal cord. As a result, the pressure inside the ventricles (the fluid-filled spaces inside the brain) increases and causes further compression of brain tissue. Left untreated, drowsiness can develop, which may eventually progress to coma (p.323) and death.

How are they diagnosed?

If your doctor suspects a brain tumour, he or she will refer you to hospital for immediate assessment by a neurologist. You will have CT scanning (p.132) or MRI (p.133) of the brain to look for a tumour and check its location and size. If these tests suggest that a brain tumour has spread from a cancer elsewhere in the body, you may need to have other tests, such as chest X-rays (p.300), mammography (p.487), or a PET scan (p.137) to check for other tumours elsewhere. You may also need to have a brain biopsy, in which a sample of the tumour is removed surgically under general anaesthesia. The sample is then examined in a laboratory to find the type of cell from which the tumour has arisen.

What is the treatment?

Treatment for brain tumours depends on whether there is one tumour or several, the precise location of the tumour, and the type of cell affected. Primary brain tumours may be treated surgically. The aim of surgery is to remove the entire tumour, or as much of it as possible, with minimal damage to the surrounding brain tissue. Surgery will probably not be an option for tumours located deep within the brain tissue. Radiotherapy (p.158) may be used in addition to surgical treatment, or as an alternative to it, for both cancerous and noncancerous primary tumours. Chemotherapy (p.587) may also be an option for certain types of primary tumours. Small meningiomas may not be treated if they are not causing problems; in such cases, regular monitoring is carried out to ensure that, if any problems do develop, they are detected and treated early.

As brain metastases are often multiple, surgery is not usually an option. However, in cases where there is a single metastasis, surgical removal may be successful. Multiple tumours are usually treated with radiotherapy or, less commonly, with chemotherapy.

Other treatments may be necessary to treat the effects of brain tumours. For example, the drug dexamethasone (*see* **Corticosteroids**, p.600) may be given to reduce the pressure inside the skull, and anticonvulsant drugs (p.590) may also be prescribed to prevent or treat seizures. If a tumour blocks the flow of cerebrospinal fluid in the brain and fluid builds up in the ventricles, a small tube may be inserted through the skull to bypass the blockage.

You may also benefit from treatments for the physical effects of the tumour, such as physiotherapy (p.620) to help with mobility problems or speech therapy (p.621) for speech problems.

What is the prognosis?

The outlook for primary brain tumours varies considerably, depending on their location, size, rate of growth, type of cell they affect, and whether they can be surgically removed or respond well to other treatments. The outlook is usually better for a noncancerous tumour that grows slowly; for example, overall about 8 in 10 people with a slow-growing, noncancerous meningioma survive for at least 5 years after diagnosis. In contrast, for the most aggressive type of glioma, the average life expectancy of adults after diagnosis is less than a year, and overall only about 6 in 100 adults survive for more than 5 years. In general, the outlook for children tends to be better than for adults.

For people with secondary brain tumours (metastases) the overall outlook is poor. Most people do not live longer than 6 months, although in rare cases a person with a single metastatic tumour may be cured.

Transient ischaemic attacks

Episodes of temporary loss of function in one area of the brain due to a reduced blood supply, commonly called "mini strokes"

 More common over the age of 45

 More common in males

 Sometimes runs in families

 Smoking and an unhealthy diet are risk factors

In a transient ischaemic attack (TIA), part of the brain suddenly and briefly fails to function properly because it is temporarily deprived of oxygen by blockage of its arterial blood supply. Commonly known as "mini strokes", transient ischaemic attacks can last for anything from a few seconds to a few hours and have no after-effects. If the symptoms persist for longer than 24 hours, the attack is classified as a stroke (opposite page).

Transient ischaemic attacks are more common in those aged 45 or older and affect about three times more men than women.

It is important that a transient ischaemic attack is not ignored because there is a strong possibility that it may be followed by a stroke. Without treatment, about 1 in 3 people who has an attack goes on to have a stroke later on.

What are the causes?

Two conditions can lead to blockage of an artery supplying the brain. A blood clot, called a thrombus, may develop in an artery, or a fragment from a blood clot, called an embolus, may detach itself from elsewhere in the body and travel in the blood to block an artery (*see* **Thrombosis and embolism**, p.259).

A thrombus usually forms in blood vessels affected by atherosclerosis (p.241), in which fatty deposits build up on vessel walls. People at increased risk of atherosclerosis include smokers and those who have an unhealthy diet. People who have an inherited tendency towards high levels of fat (*see* **Inherited hyperlipidaemias**, p.440) or people with diabetes mellitus (p.437) are at risk. High blood pressure (*see* **Hypertension**, p.242) increases the risk of atherosclerosis.

The emboli that cause transient ischaemic attacks usually originate in the heart, the aorta (the main artery of the body), or the carotid or vertebral arteries in the neck. Blood clots are more likely to form in the heart if it has been damaged by a heart attack (*see* **Myocardial infarction**, p.245), if the heartbeat is irregular (*see* **Atrial fibrillation**, p.250), or if the heart valves are damaged or have been replaced (*see* **Heart valve disorders**, p.253). Sickle-cell disease (p.272) can also increase the risk of transient ischaemic attacks because the abnormally shaped red blood cells tend to clump together and block blood vessels.

What are the symptoms?

The symptoms of a transient ischaemic attack usually develop suddenly and are often short-lived. Symptoms vary, depending on which part of the brain is affected, and may include the following:

- Drooping of one side of the face.
- Loss of vision in one eye or blurred vision in both.
- Slurred speech.
- Difficulty in finding the right words.
- Problems understanding what other people are saying.
- Numbness or pins and needles on one side of the body.
- Weakness or paralysis on one side of the body, affecting one or both limbs.
- Feeling of unsteadiness and general loss of balance.

Although the symptoms of transient ischaemic attacks disappear within a few hours, attacks tend to recur. People may have a number of attacks in one day or over several days. Sometimes, several years may elapse between attacks.

Transient ischaemic attacks themselves cause no permanent after-effects but people who have them are at increased risk of stroke and it is therefore important to seek urgent medical help.

Carotid Doppler scanning

Carotid Doppler scanning uses ultrasound to look at the flow of blood through blood vessels in the neck. The procedure is generally used to investigate disorders such as transient ischaemic attacks or stroke.

Ultrasound waves from a transducer produce a picture of the blood flow, which can reveal narrowing of the carotid blood vessels in the neck. The procedure takes about 20 minutes and is painless and safe.

Having a scan
The technician applies a gel to the skin before slowly and gently moving a Doppler transducer over the neck in the area of the carotid arteries. During the procedure, the technician views images of the arteries displayed on a monitor.

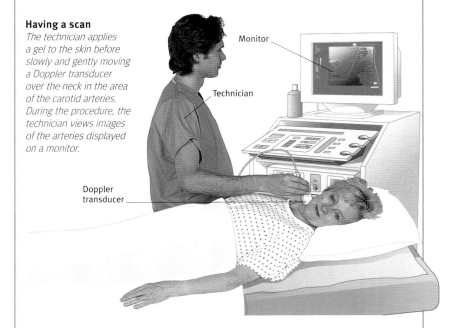

Monitor

Technician

Doppler transducer

RESULTS

Carotid Doppler scan
This ultrasound image shows the blood flow through a branched carotid artery. After the blood passes through a narrowed section of the artery, the flow becomes disrupted.

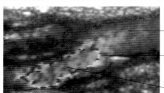

Normal blood flow

Narrowed area

Turbulent blood flow

How are they diagnosed?

Your doctor will carry out a physical examination, which will include checking your blood pressure, heart rhythm, and neurological function. He or she may arrange for CT scanning (p.132) or MRI (p.133) of your brain to look for other causes of your symptoms. You might also have ultrasound scanning of the arteries in your neck (*see* **Carotid Doppler scanning**, above) to look for narrowing. If these arteries are significantly narrowed, further imaging tests will be carried out to assess the severity of the narrowing. For example, you may have MRA (magnetic resonance angiography, a form of MRI) or cerebral angiography (opposite page).

Tests to look for the source of the blood clots include echocardiography (p.255), which is used to look at the structure of your heart and the movement of its valves. Your heart rate may also be monitored for up to about a week to look for irregularities in your heart rhythm (*see* **Ambulatory ECG**, p.249).

You may have blood tests to look for other factors that increase the risk of having a transient ischaemic attack, such as diabetes mellitus and hyperlipidaemias. Blood tests may also be used to check for blood disorders that increase the risk of a clot forming.

What is the treatment?

Once a transient ischaemic attack has been diagnosed, the aim of treatment is to reduce your risk of having a stroke in the future. You will be advised to eat a healthy diet (p.16) and, if you smoke, you should stop. If you have diabetes mellitus, you should make sure your blood glucose levels are well controlled. Your doctor will prescribe appropriate drugs to treat high blood pressure (*see* **Antihypertensive drugs**, p.580) or an irregular heartbeat (*see* **Antiarrhythmic drugs**, p.580) if you have either of these conditions.

Treatment after a transient ischaemic attack can be as simple as taking half an aspirin daily to help to prevent blood clots from forming inside blood vessels. Other drugs that help to prevent blood clotting (p.584), such as warfarin, may be prescribed if emboli originate from clots that have formed in the heart.

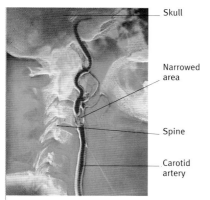

Narrowed carotid artery
This coloured X-ray shows a narrowed area in the carotid artery, which supplies blood to the brain. This narrowing may result in transient ischaemic attacks.

- Skull
- Narrowed area
- Spine
- Carotid artery

If your doctor finds that the arteries in your neck are severely narrowed, he or she may suggest that you have a surgical procedure called a carotid endarterectomy to clear fatty deposits from the narrowed arteries. If this procedure is not suitable, it may be recommended that you have carotid artery stenting instead. In this procedure, a catheter (thin tube) is used to insert a short, rigid tube (stent) at the site of narrowing in the affected artery or arteries. Both procedures improve the blood supply to the brain.

What is the prognosis?
Transient ischaemic attacks may occur intermittently over a long period or they may stop spontaneously. However, if you have had a transient ischaemic attack, you are at high risk of having a stroke in future, and the more frequently you have transient ischaemic attacks, the higher your risk. You can reduce your risk of further attacks or a stroke by lifestyle changes, such as giving up smoking and eating a healthy diet.

Stroke

Damage to part of the brain caused by an interruption in its blood supply, sometimes called a brain attack

 More common with increasing age; about 3 in 4 strokes occur in those over 65

 More common in males

 Smoking and an unhealthy diet are risk factors

 Genetics as risk factor depends on the cause

If the blood supply to part of the brain is interrupted, the affected region no longer functions normally. This condition is called a stroke, although it is often described as a "brain attack" to highlight the need for urgent medical attention. A stroke may be due to either a blockage or bleeding from one of the arteries supplying the brain.

There is usually little or no warning of a stroke. Immediate admission to hospital for assessment and treatment is essential if there is to be a chance of preventing permanent brain damage. The after effects of a stroke vary depending on the location and extent of the brain tissue affected. They range from mild, temporary symptoms, such as blurred vision, to lifelong disability or death.

If the symptoms disappear within 24 hours, the condition is known as a transient ischaemic attack (opposite page), which is a warning sign of a possible future stroke.

How common is it?
Each year, about 150,000 people in the UK have a stroke. The condition is more common in men and in older people. The risk of having a stroke roughly doubles every decade after the age of 55, and about 3 in 4 strokes occur in those over 65. Although the number of deaths from stroke has fallen over the last 50 years, it is still one of the leading causes of death in the UK, accounting for about 1 in 14 of all deaths.

What are the causes?
About 80 per cent of all strokes are due to blockage of an artery supplying the brain; these are known as ischaemic strokes. This type of stroke occurs as a result of cerebral thrombosis or cerebral embolism. In cerebral thrombosis, a blood clot forms in an artery in the brain. In cerebral embolism, a fragment of a blood clot that has formed in another part of the body, such as the heart or the main arteries of the neck, travels in the blood and lodges in an artery supplying the brain.

The remaining 20 per cent of strokes are due to bleeding from an artery supplying the brain (cerebral haemorrhage); these are known as haemorrhagic strokes. Cerebral haemorrhage occurs when an artery supplying the brain ruptures, causing blood to leak out into the surrounding tissue.

The blood clots that lead to cerebral thrombosis and cerebral embolism are more likely to form in an artery that has been damaged by atherosclerosis (p.241), a condition in which fatty deposits build

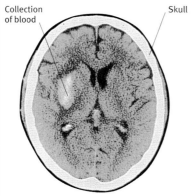

Cerebral haemorrhage
Bleeding into the brain tissue, as shown in this CT brain scan, is known as a cerebral haemorrhage and is one cause of stroke.

- Collection of blood
- Skull

▶ TEST

Cerebral angiography

Cerebral angiography uses X-rays to look for abnormalities of the vertebral or carotid arteries, which supply blood to the brain. It may be used to investigate transient ischaemic attacks and stroke. Under local anaesthesia, a thin, flexible tube called a catheter is inserted into an artery, usually at the groin or elbow, and guided to an artery in the neck. A dye that shows up on X-rays is then injected through it. The outline of blood flow through the arteries is then seen on the X-ray (angiogram).

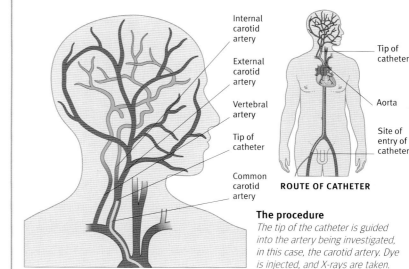

- Internal carotid artery
- External carotid artery
- Vertebral artery
- Tip of catheter
- Common carotid artery
- Tip of catheter
- Aorta
- Site of entry of catheter

ROUTE OF CATHETER

The procedure
The tip of the catheter is guided into the artery being investigated, in this case, the carotid artery. Dye is injected, and X-rays are taken.

RESULTS

Angiogram
This colour-enhanced contrast X-ray, called an angiogram, shows the internal carotid artery, a main artery supplying the brain, branching into many smaller blood vessels. In this angiogram, the artery is normal.

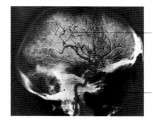

- Cerebral blood vessels
- Internal carotid artery

up in artery walls. Factors that increase the risk of atherosclerosis developing are high blood pressure (*see* **Hypertension**, p.242), an unhealthy diet, smoking, diabetes mellitus (p.437), and high levels of lipids in the blood (*see* **Inherited hyperlipidaemias**, p.440).

Cerebral embolism may be a complication of heart rhythm disorders (*see* **Arrhythmias**, p.249), heart valve disorders (p.253), and recent myocardial infarction (p.245), all of which can cause blood clots to form in the heart. The risk of cerebral embolism, thrombosis, or haemorrhage is increased by high blood pressure. Sickle-cell disease (p.272), an abnormality of the red blood cells, also increases the risk of cerebral thrombosis because the abnormal blood cells tend to clump together and block the blood vessels. Less commonly, thrombosis occurs as a result of the cerebral arteries becoming narrowed due to inflammation of the arteries, a condition known as vasculitis. This inflammation may, in turn, be due to various underlying conditions, such as the autoimmune disorder polyarteritis nodosa (p.283).

What are the symptoms?
In most people the symptoms develop rapidly over a matter of seconds or minutes. The exact symptoms depend on the area of the brain affected. The symptoms may include:
- Facial weakness, which may cause drooping of the face, mouth, or eye on one side, drooling, and the inability to smile.
- Arm weakness or numbness, causing the inability to raise both arms and keep them raised.
- Speech problems, such as slurred speech.
- Weakness, numbness, or paralysis on one side of the body.
- Clumsiness.
- Visual disturbances, such as loss of part of the field of vision or loss of vision in one eye.
- Difficulty in finding words and in understanding what others are saying.
- Difficulty swallowing.
- Headache.

If the stroke is severe, areas of the brain that control breathing and blood pressure may be affected or the person may lose consciousness or even lapse into a coma (p.323). in these circumstances, the outcome may be fatal.

How is it diagnosed?
If you suspect that a person has had a stroke, get emergency medical help.

Imaging of the brain, such as CT scanning (p.132) or MRI (p.133), will be used to find out whether the stroke was caused by bleeding or a blockage in a vessel. Cerebral angiography (p.329), MRA (magnetic resonance angiography, a form of MRI), or carotid Doppler scanning (p.328) may be performed to help identify narrowed arteries that can be corrected by surgery. Further tests may be carried out to look for the source of an embolus. These tests may include echocardiography (p.255) to assess the heart valves and heart monitoring (see ECG, p.243) to check the heart rhythm.

What is the treatment?
The initial treatment following a stroke is close monitoring and nursing care to protect the person's airways during recovery. If scanning reveals a clot in a blood vessel, immediate treatment with a thrombolytic drug (p.584) to dissolve the clot will be given. This treatment may improve the outcome and is now used routinely. However, the drug increases the risk of bleeding within the brain and must be given within a few hours of the onset of symptoms.

Long-term treatment to reduce the risk of further strokes will depend on the cause of the stroke. If the cause was a cerebral embolism, you may be given drugs such as aspirin, clopidogrel, or warfarin, which act on clotting factors in the blood to reduce the risk of further clots (see Drugs that prevent blood clotting, p.584). If a narrowed artery has been identified, it may be widened surgically.

After a cerebral haemorrhage, treatment may be focused on the underlying cause, although in a few cases it may first be necessary to perform emergency surgery to remove blood from the brain and repair ruptured blood vessels. Long-term treatment may include antihypertensive drugs (p.580) to lower blood pressure and a statin (see Lipid-lowering drugs, p.603) to reduce blood cholesterol levels. If the stroke is the result of inflammation of the arteries, corticosteroids (p.600) may be given. Depression is quite common after a stroke and may need treatment.

In all cases of stroke, rehabilitative therapies, such as physiotherapy (p.620), occupational therapy (p.621), and speech therapy (p.621) are essential. Lifestyle changes, such as eating a healthy diet and giving up smoking, can reduce the risk of another stroke.

What is the prognosis?
The outlook after a stroke is often difficult to predict at first and depends to some extent on the cause. Stroke is fatal in about 1 in 4 cases. Many of those who survive are left with long-term problems, and about half are left with a disability that is severe enough to significantly affect everyday activities.

Subarachnoid haemorrhage

Bleeding into the space between the two inner membranes covering the brain

 Most common between the ages of 40 and 60

 Sometimes runs in families

 Smoking and excessive alcohol consumption are risk factors

 Gender is not a significant factor

A subarachnoid haemorrhage occurs when an artery near the brain ruptures spontaneously and leaks blood into the subarachnoid space, the area between the middle and innermost of the three membranes that cover the brain. When this happens, the immediate symptom is an intensely painful headache.

Subarachnoid haemorrhage is rare, affecting about 6–12 in 100,000 people in the UK each year. It sometimes runs in families, although no single causative gene has been identified, and is most common in middle-aged people. When the condition does occur, it is life-threatening and needs emergency medical attention.

What are the causes?
About 8 in 10 subarachnoid haemorrhages are caused by the rupture of a berry aneurysm, an abnormal swelling in an artery often found at a Y-shaped junction in the arteries that supply the brain. Berry aneurysms are thought to be present at birth, and there may be one or several. Some do not rupture. However, if rupture does occur, it is usually between the ages of 40 and 60.

A further 1 in 10 subarachnoid haemorrhages are the result of a rupture of a knot of arteries and veins on the surface of the brain. The defect, known as an arteriovenous malformation, is present from birth, but haemorrhages do not occur until between the ages of about 20 and 40. The cause of 1 in 10 subarachnoid haemorrhages is unknown.

In people who are at risk, subarachnoid haemorrhage may be triggered by intense exertion. The disorder is more likely to occur in people who have high blood pressure (see Hypertension, p.242), smoke, and drink excessive amounts of alcohol.

What are the symptoms?
The onset of symptoms is usually sudden and without warning. Typical symptoms may include the following:
- Sudden, agonizing headache.
- Nausea and vomiting.

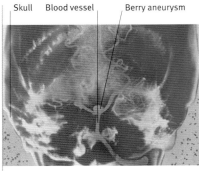

Skull   Blood vessel   Berry aneurysm

Berry aneurysm
This contrast X-ray shows a small swelling called a berry aneurysm at the base of the brain. Rupture of an aneurysm can result in a subarachnoid haemorrhage.

- Stiff neck.
- Dislike of bright light.
- Irritability.

In a few minutes, these may lead to:
- Confusion and drowsiness.
- Seizures.
- Loss of consciousness.

The body may react to the haemorrhage by constricting the arteries in the brain. As a result, the supply of oxygen to the brain is further reduced, and this may cause a stroke (p.329), possibly resulting in muscle weakness or paralysis.

What might be done?
If a subarachnoid haemorrhage is suspected, the affected person should be admitted to hospital immediately. CT scanning (p.132) is carried out to identify the location and extent of bleeding. If the CT scan shows no bleeding, a lumbar puncture (p.326) will be performed to look for signs of bleeding into the fluid surrounding the brain and spinal cord. If a subarachnoid haemorrhage is confirmed, MRI (p.133) or cerebral angiography (p.329) may also be performed to look at the blood vessels of the brain.

Once tests have confirmed a subarachnoid haemorrhage, drugs called calcium channel blockers (p.582) are usually given to reduce the risk of a stroke.

If the tests have shown that one or more berry aneurysms are present, they may be treated by endovascular embolization or surgery. In endovascular embolization, a catheter (thin tube) is passed into an artery in the groin and up to the aneurysm. Special coils, glue, or plastic particles are then passed inside the catheter to seal off the aneurysm. Alternatively, conventional surgery may be used to apply clips to the affected artery to prevent it from bleeding again.

If damage to the brain has caused persistent symptoms, such as muscle weakness as a result of a stroke, physiotherapy (p.620) and/or occupational therapy (p.621) may be arranged.

What is the prognosis?
Nearly half of all people with a subarachnoid haemorrhage die before they reach hospital. Of those people admitted to hospital, about half are treated successfully, but the remainder have another subarachnoid haemorrhage. If there is no further haemorrhage within the next 6 months or if treatment is successful, further bleeding is unlikely. However, everybody who has had a subarachnoid haemorrhage should avoid smoking and excessive drinking and, if necessary, take measures to reduce high blood pressure.

Subdural haemorrhage

Bleeding inside the skull between the two outer membranes that surround the brain

 One type is more common in elderly people

 Contact sports and excessive alcohol consumption are risk factors

 Gender and genetics are not significant factors

In a subdural haemorrhage, a vein in the subdural space is torn due to a head injury. The subdural space lies between the two outer membranes of the three membranes that surround the brain. Subsequent bleeding into the subdural space causes a blood clot, known as a haematoma, to form. As the blood clot enlarges, it compresses the surrounding brain tissue, causing symptoms such as headache and confusion.

A subdural haemorrhage is a potentially life-threatening condition that requires prompt medical treatment. It is one of the most common causes of death from contact sports such as boxing.

What are the types?
After a head injury, bleeding may occur within minutes (acute subdural haemorrhage) or blood may build up slowly over a period of days or even weeks (chronic subdural haemorrhage).

An acute subdural haemorrhage may follow a severe blow to the head, the type of injury sustained in a road accident or while playing contact sports. Bleeding occurs immediately, and the blood clot enlarges quickly.

A chronic subdural haemorrhage can result from an apparently trivial head injury, especially in the elderly. Bleeding is slow, and it may be several months before the blood clot begins to cause symptoms. Chronic subdural haemorrhage often affects people who have frequent falls and therefore occurs more commonly in elderly people or in people who drink excessive amounts of alcohol. Disorders or treatments that impair blood clotting, such as treatment with drugs that prevent blood clotting (p.584), also increase the risk of chronic subdural haemorrhage.

What are the symptoms?
Symptoms may develop at any time between a few hours and a few months

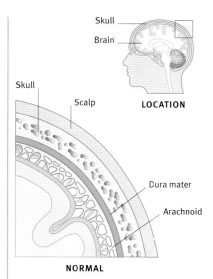

Skull
Brain

LOCATION

Skull
Scalp

Dura mater

Arachnoid

NORMAL

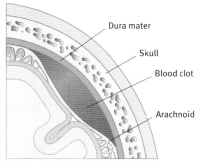

Dura mater

Skull

Blood clot

Arachnoid

SUBDURAL HAEMORRHAGE

Subdural haemorrhage
Bleeding (haemorrhage) between two of the membranes that cover the brain, the dura mater and the arachnoid, leads to the formation of a blood clot.

after the head injury, depending on whether the subdural haemorrhage is acute or chronic. In both types, symptoms are variable and often fluctuate in severity. The symptoms of acute subdural haemorrhage may include:
■ Drowsiness.
■ Confusion.
■ Coma.
The symptoms of a chronic subdural haemorrhage may include:
■ Headaches.
■ Gradually developing confusion and drowsiness.
■ Progressive weakness and unsteadiness.
If any of the symptoms of acute or chronic subdural haemorrhage develop, seek medical attention immediately.

What might be done?
If your doctor suspects that you have a subdural haemorrhage, he or she will arrange for CT scanning (p.132) or MRI (p.133) of your brain to look for a clot. If the condition is confirmed, a surgical procedure in which blood is drained through small holes made in the skull (called burr holes) will probably be necessary.

If a chronic subdural haemorrhage is small and produces few symptoms, the affected person may be monitored with regular scans, and the clot may clear without the need for surgery.

In all cases, the prognosis is determined by the size and location of the clot. Many people recover rapidly, but some residual symptoms, such as weakness, may persist. If the haemorrhage has affected a large area of brain, the condition may be fatal.

Dementia

A deterioration in mental function due to disorders affecting the brain

 More common over the age of 65

 Sometimes runs in families

 Lifestyle as a risk factor depends on the cause

Gender is not a significant factor

Dementia is a combination of problems associated with deterioration of the brain and mental functioning, including memory loss, problems with language, understanding, and judgement, and general intellectual decline. The affected person may not realize that there is anything wrong, but his or her condition is usually distressing for close friends and family. Poor memory alone is not a sign of dementia because some memory impairment is a natural part of aging. Dementia is relatively common in elderly people, with an estimated 1 in 14 people in the UK over the age of 65 affected to some degree. Although dementia is usually progressive and cannot be treated, in a few cases the underlying cause is treatable. An elderly person with severe depression (p.343) may seem to have dementia because the conditions have similar features, such as forgetfulness.

What are the causes?
The underlying abnormality in dementia is a decline in the number of brain cells, resulting in shrinkage of brain tissue. Alzheimer's disease (right), which occurs mainly in people over 65 and may occasionally run in families, is the most common cause of dementia. In multi-infarct dementia (p.332) – also known as vascular dementia – blood flow in small vessels of the brain is blocked by clots. Interruption to the brain's blood supply due to a stroke (p.329) may also sometimes result in dementia. In Lewy body dementia, small, spherical structures (Lewy bodies) accumulate inside the brain, leading to death of nerve cells and loss of brain tissue. In frontotemporal dementia, symptoms are due to damage to the brain's frontal and temporal lobes (at the front and sides of the brain, respectively). This type of dementia is a significant cause of dementia in those under 65. Its cause is not known, although it often runs in families, suggesting a genetic factor. Less common causes of dementia include other brain disorders such as Huntington's disease (p.333) and

Creutzfeldt–Jakob disease (p.334). People with Parkinson's disease (p.333) may also eventually develop dementia but it is thought that the Parkinson's disease alone is not responsible for the dementia.

Dementia may also occur in young people. For example, people with AIDS (*see* **HIV infection and AIDS**, p.169) may eventually develop AIDS-related dementia. Long-term abusers of alcohol are at risk of dementia because of direct damage to the brain tissue and because their poor diet often leads to vitamin B$_1$ deficiency. Severe vitamin B$_1$ deficiency can cause the brain disorder Wernicke–Korsakoff syndrome (p.332). In pernicicus anaemia (*see* **Megaloblastic anaemia**, p.272), there is a deficiency of vitamin B$_{12}$ due to impaired absorption in the digestive tract. A severe deficiency of this vitamin can result in dementia. Dementia may also be associated with repeated head injuries (p.322). Rarely, underactivity of the thyroid gland (*see* **Hypothyroidism**, p.432) may cause symptoms that resemble dementia.

What are the symptoms?
The symptoms may develop gradually over a few months or years, depending on the cause. They may include:
■ Impairment of short-term memory.
■ Gradual loss of intellect, affecting reasoning and understanding.
■ Difficulty engaging in conversations.
■ Reduced vocabulary.
■ Emotional outbursts.
■ Personality changes.
■ Wandering and restlessness.

SELF-HELP

Caring for someone with dementia
If you are taking care of someone with dementia, you need to balance his or her needs with your own. In the early stages, it is important to allow the person to remain as independent and active as possible. As the disorder progresses, there are several measures you can take which help to compensate for the person's failing memory, loss of judgment, and unpredictable behaviour:

■ Put up a bulletin board with a list of things that need to be done during each day.
■ If wandering is a problem, persuade the person to wear a badge with your contact details and phone number on it.
■ Place notes around the house that help the person to remember to turn off appliances.
■ Consider installing bath aids to make washing easier.
■ Try to be patient. It is common for people with dementia to have frequent mood changes.
■ Give yourself a break whenever you can by finding someone who can help for a few hours.
■ Join a carers' support group and investigate day centres and respite care options.

■ Neglect of personal hygiene.
■ Urinary incontinence.
In the early stages of the disorder, a person is prone to becoming anxious (*see* **Anxiety disorders**, p.341) or depressed due to awareness of the memory loss. As the dementia gets worse, the person may become more dependent on others.

What might be done?
The doctor may arrange for the person to have tests to look for the underlying cause and to exclude other disorders. If a treatable underlying cause is found, treatment of that cause may improve or even cure the dementia. However, such cases are rare and the treatment of dementia is based on management of the symptoms and, if possible, slowing the progression of the condition. For example, depression may be treated with antidepressants (p.592), and drugs called acetylcholinesterase inhibitors may slow the progression of Alzheimer's disease.

A person who has dementia usually needs support at home and may eventually need full-time care in a nursing home. Carers may also need support (*see* **Caring for someone with dementia**, left, and **Home care**, p.618).

Alzheimer's disease

A progressive deterioration in mental function due to degeneration of brain tissue

 More common over the age of 65

 More common in females

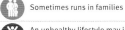 Sometimes runs in families

 An unhealthy lifestyle may increase the risk of developing the condition

It is normal to become mildly forgetful with increasing age, but severe impairment of short-term memory may be a sign of Alzheimer's disease. In this disorder, brain cells degenerate and deposits of an abnormal protein (known as amyloid plaques or tau tangles) build up in the brain. As a result of these changes, the brain tissue shrinks and there is a progressive loss of mental abilities, known as dementia (left).

Alzheimer's disease is the most common cause of dementia, affecting about 520,000 people in the UK. It mainly affects those over 65 and becomes more common with increasing age; an estimated 1 in 6 people over the age of 80 is affected. However, it can also affect younger people, and in the UK about 1 in 20 cases of Alzheimer's disease occurs in those under 65. Alzheimer's disease is also more common in women; the reason for this is not known, but it is not entirely due to women living, on average, longer than men. Various medical conditions increase the risk of developing Alzheimer's disease, including diabetes, high blood pressure, cardiovascular disease, and stroke. Therefore, lifestyle factors that increase the risk of developing such condition, notably smoking, excessive alcohol use, insufficient exercise, and an unhealthy diet, also increase the risk of developing Alzheimer's disease.

Although various risk factors for developing Alzheimer's disease have been identified, the underlying cause of the condition is not known in the majority of cases. In a few cases, the disease runs in families and a number of genes have been identified that are associated with development of the disease. For example, a gene known as APOE, which is on chromosome 19, is associated with Alzheimer's disease that develops in older people (late-onset Alzheimer's disease). Various other genes linked with Alzheimer's disease have also been identified but all of them are rare and, overall, they are thought to be involved in fewer than 1 in 1,000 cases. People with Down's syndrome (p.533) who live into their 50s or beyond are also at increased risk of developing Alzheimer's disease.

What are the symptoms?

The first symptom of Alzheimer's disease is usually forgetfulness. The normal deterioration of memory that occurs in old age becomes much more severe and begins to affect intellectual ability. Memory loss is eventually accompanied by other symptoms, which may include:

- Poor concentration.
- Difficulty in understanding written and spoken language.
- Difficulty with simple arithmetical tasks, such as calculating change.
- Wandering and getting lost, even in familiar surroundings.

In the early stages of the disease, people are usually aware that they have become more forgetful. This may lead to depression (p.343) and anxiety (see Anxiety disorders, p.341) Over a longer period, the existing symptoms may get worse and additional symptoms may develop. These may include:

- Slow movements and unsteadiness when walking.
- Rapid mood swings from happiness to tearfulness.
- Personality changes, aggression, and feelings of persecution.

Sometimes people find it difficult to sleep (see Insomnia, p.343) and become restless at night. After several years, most people with the disease cannot look after themselves and need full-time care.

How is it diagnosed?

There is no single test that can be used to diagnose Alzheimer's disease. The doctor will discuss the symptoms with the affected person and his or her family. Tests may be arranged to exclude other possible causes of dementia. For example, blood tests may be carried out to check

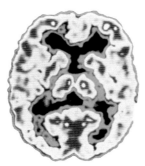

NORMAL BRAIN

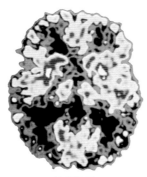

**BRAIN IN
ALZHEIMER'S DISEASE**

Effect of Alzheimer's disease

PET scans show a pattern of large, bright areas of high activity and small, dark areas of low activity in a normal brain compared to patchy activity in the brain of a person with Alzheimer's disease.

for vitamin B deficiencies, and a lumbar puncture (p.326) may be performed to check for possible infection. CT scanning (p.132) or MRI (p.133) may be carried out to exclude other brain disorders, such as multi-infarct dementia (right), subdural haemorrhage (p.330), or a brain tumour (p.327). If the results of CT or MRI scanning are uncertain, PET scanning (p.137) may also sometimes be performed. An assessment of mental functioning, which may include tests of memory and writing, may be used to determine the severity of the dementia.

What is the treatment?

There is no cure for Alzheimer's disease, but acetylcholinesterase inhibitor drugs may slow the loss of mental function in some cases. Some of the symptoms that are sometimes associated with Alzheimer's disease, such as depression and sleeping problems, can be relieved by antidepressant drugs (p.592). A person who is agitated may be given a sedative drug to calm him or her down.

Eventually, full-time care may be necessary, either at home (see Home care, p.618), and Caring for someone with dementia, (p.331) or in a nursing home. Caring for a person who has Alzheimer's disease is often stressful, and carers need practical and emotional support, especially if the affected person starts to become hostile and aggressive. Support groups can help a person to cope with caring for an elderly relative with the disease.

Alzheimer's disease is associated with a reduced life expectancy but its progress in individual cases is often unpredictable. However, many people with the condition survive for up to about 10 years from the time of diagnosis.

Multi-infarct dementia

A deterioration in mental function due to blood clots in small blood vessels in the brain that cause tissue damage

 More common over the age of 60

 More common in males

 Smoking and an unhealthy diet are risk factors

Genetics is not a significant factor

Multi-infarct dementia, also known as vascular dementia, occurs when blood flow in the small blood vessels supplying the brain is obstructed by blood clots. Each of these clots prevents oxygen from reaching a small part of the brain, and this causes tissue death (infarcts) in the affected parts. Infarcts occur in a number of distinct episodes. People who have multiple small infarcts are at increased risk of a major stroke (p.329), which can be life-threatening.

The risk of multi-infarct dementia is increased by atherosclerosis (p.241), in which fatty deposits build up in the artery walls, causing them to become narrowed and increasing the risk of clots forming. The risk of atherosclerosis is increased if a person has high blood pressure (see Hypertension, p.242). Lifestyle factors, such as eating an unhealthy diet and smoking, can also contribute to the development of atherosclerosis. Multi-infarct dementia is more common in men and is more likely to occur in people over the age of 60.

What are the symptoms?

Symptoms of multi-infarct dementia vary from one individual to another because they depend on the part of the brain affected. Unlike other types of dementia, which progress steadily, multi-infarct dementia gets abruptly worse following each separate episode. Symptoms are similar to those of other forms of dementia and include:

- Poor memory, particularly when trying to recall recent events.
- Difficulty in making decisions.
- Problems with simple, routine tasks, such as getting dressed.
- Tendency to wander and get lost in familiar surroundings.

It is common for a person with multi-infarct dementia to develop depression (p.343) and have episodes of agitation. There may be other symptoms, depending on which part of the brain is affected. These may include partial loss of sight; slow, sometimes slurred, speech; and difficulty walking.

What might be done?

Diagnosis of multi-infarct dementia is usually possible from the symptoms, although various tests, such as blood tests, may also be carried out to rule out other types of dementia. The doctor may arrange for CT scanning (p.132) or MRI (p.133) of the brain to look for evidence of multiple small infarcts.

Although the dementia itself cannot be cured, treatment can help to prevent further infarcts that would make the condition worse. A person with multi-infarct dementia should eat a healthy diet (p.16) and take regular exercise. Smokers should stop smoking immediately. Antihypertensive drugs (p.580), which help to control raised blood pressure, and a daily dose of aspirin, which reduces the risk of blood clots, may be prescribed.

Weakness and loss of movement can be treated with physiotherapy (p.620), and speech therapy (p.621) can help to alleviate speech problems. Antidepressants (p.592) and counselling (p.624) may be used to treat depression.

What is the prognosis?

Many people with multi-infarct dementia find that their symptoms improve for short periods of time but later become worse again. Early recognition of the condition and treatment of risk factors, such as high blood pressure, may prevent further progression of the disorder and increasing disability and reduce the risk of a future, potentially fatal stroke.

Wernicke–Korsakoff syndrome

A brain disorder caused by severe vitamin B₁ deficiency, usually the result of long-term alcohol abuse

 More common over the age of 45

 More common in males

 Long-term alcohol abuse is a risk factor

 Genetics is not a significant factor

Wernicke–Korsakoff syndrome is a rare disorder of the brain, causing dementia, abnormal eye movements, and an abnormal gait. The condition develops rapidly and is due to a severe deficiency of vitamin B₁. It is a medical emergency. If untreated, coma (p.323) and death may occur. About 2 in 10 individuals with the disorder die within 5 days. Vitamin B₁ deficiency is usually caused by many years of severe alcohol abuse, but rarely it may be due to extreme malnutrition or starvation. Wernicke–Korsakoff syndrome is most common in people over the age of 45 and affects more men than women.

What are the symptoms?

Symptoms may start gradually or suddenly, sometimes after heavy drinking, and are easily mistaken for drunkenness. They include the following:

- Abnormal movements of the eyes, which often result in double vision.
- Unsteadiness when walking.
- Confusion and restlessness.

Unless the individual is given urgent treatment, he or she will develop severe memory loss, become drowsy, go into a coma, and eventually die.

What might be done?

A person with Wernicke–Korsakoff syndrome needs immediate hospital treatment with high-dose vitamin B₁. After treatment, many of the symptoms may be reversed within days, but memory loss may persist. If untreated, the disorder is fatal.

Huntington's disease

An inherited brain disorder that causes personality changes, involuntary movements, and dementia

 More common over the age of 30

 Due to an abnormal gene inherited from one parent

 Gender and lifestyle are not significant factors

Huntington's disease is an inherited disorder that causes degeneration of a particular part of the brain. Also known as Huntington's chorea, the condition causes jerky, involuntary movements, clumsiness, and progressive dementia. Huntington's disease is rare, affecting only about 6,000 people in the UK. The symptoms commonly develop between the ages of 30 and 50.

Huntington's disease is caused by an abnormal dominant gene. To develop the disease, a person only has to inherit the abnormal gene from one parent (*see* **Gene disorders**, p.151). People who have the gene have a 1 in 2 chance of passing it on to each of their children. Because symptoms do not develop until later in life, an abnormal gene may be passed on to children before the affected parent becomes aware that he or she has the disease. A genetic test may be offered to adults to find out if an individual has the abnormal gene.

What are the symptoms?

Symptoms develop gradually over a period of months or years. Initially, they may include the following:

- Jerks and spasms of the face, arms, and trunk.
- Clumsiness.
- Mood swings, including outbursts of aggressive, antisocial behaviour.
- Poor memory, especially for events that have occurred recently.

As the disease progresses, further symptoms of dementia, such as losing the ability to think rationally, may develop. There may be difficulty in speaking and swallowing,

and problems with urinary incontinence (p.454). Anxiety and depression (p.343) may also occur.

What might be done?

Unless the condition has already been diagnosed in a family, it may not be recognized during its early stages. Usually, a member of the affected person's family first realizes that there is a problem. The affected person may be suspicious of others and refuse help. Diagnosis is usually made from the symptoms and possibly an MRI scan (p.133) of the brain, which may show distinctive patterns of abnormality. A genetic test may be carried out to confirm the diagnosis.

There is no cure for Huntington's disease, but drugs may relieve certain symptoms. For example, antipsychotic drugs (p.592) help to control jerks and spasms. Speech therapy (p.621) and occupational therapy (p.621) are used to help an affected person to lead as normal a life as possible. However, care in a nursing home may be necessary if the person is unable to live at home or when carers need a period of respite.

Members of the family may decide to have a blood test to determine whether they have the abnormal gene themselves. These tests are performed after genetic counselling because the results are likely to have a bearing on whether or not they decide to have children.

Huntington's disease has a slow progression; a person may live for 15–20 years after the onset of symptoms.

Parkinson's disease and parkinsonism

A progressive brain disorder causing shaking and problems with movement

 More common over the age of 60

 More common in males

 Sometimes runs in families

 Lifestyle is not a significant factor

Parkinson's disease results from degeneration of cells in a part of the brain called the substantia nigra. These cells project into the basal ganglia, which controls the smoothness of muscle movements. Normally, the cells in the substantia nigra produce a neurotransmitter (a chemical that transmits nerve impulses) called dopamine, which acts with acetylcholine, another neurotransmitter, to fine-tune muscle control. In Parkinson's disease, the level of dopamine relative to acetylcholine is reduced, with the result that control of the muscles is impaired. About 1 in 500 people in the UK has Parkinson's disease. The disorder tends to occur after the age of 60 and is more common in men. Although the cause is not

known, Parkinson's disease occasionally runs in families and genetic factors may be involved in some cases.

Parkinsonism is the term used for symptoms of Parkinson's disease when they are due to another underlying disorder (such as multiple strokes) or certain drugs. Repeated head injuries (p.322) may cause parkinsonism, as may some antipsychotic drugs (p.592) used to treat severe psychiatric illness.

What are the symptoms?

The main symptoms of Parkinson's disease develop gradually over months or even years. Parkinsonism may have a gradual or sudden onset depending on the cause. Symptoms include:

- Tremor of one hand, arm, or leg, usually when resting, that later occurs on both sides.
- Muscle stiffness, making it difficult to start moving.
- Slowness of movement.
- Shuffling walk with loss of arm swing.
- Expressionless or mask-like face.
- Stooped posture.

As the disease progresses, stiffness, immobility, and constant trembling of the hands may make some daily tasks difficult. Various other symptoms may also develop, including urinary problems; sexual dysfunction; slow, hesitant, speech; loss of the sense of smell; sleeping problems; nerve pain; dizziness; excessive sweating and/or salivation; and swallowing difficulty. Many people with the disorder develop depression (p.343). An estimated 30 per cent of people with Parkinson's disease eventually develop dementia (p.331) but the dementia tends to develop in older people and is not thought to be solely due to the Parkinson's disease.

How is it diagnosed?

Since Parkinson's disease begins gradually, it is often not possible to diagnose the condition at first. Your doctor will examine you and arrange tests such as CT scanning (p.132) or MRI (p.133) to exclude other possible causes. If a specific underlying disorder is found, you will be diagnosed as having parkinsonism rather than Parkinson's disease.

How might the doctor treat it?

There is no specific cure for Parkinson's disease, but drugs, physical treatments, and, more rarely, surgery can relieve symptoms. If you have parkinsonism due to medications, your doctor may change your drugs. Symptoms then usually disappear within 8 weeks. If the symptoms persist, you may need to be treated with anti-parkinsonism drugs.

Drug treatment In the early stages of Parkinson's disease when symptoms are mild, treatment may not be necessary because drugs cannot change the progression of the disease. Later on, drugs are used to relieve symptoms and reduce disability by correcting chemical imbalances

in the brain, either by boosting dopamine levels or by blocking some of the effects of acetylcholine or a combination of both.

An anticholinergic drug such as trihexyphenidyl (benhexol) is often given initially to reduce shaking and stiffness. Anticholinergic drugs can be effective for several years but they may cause side effects such as dry mouth, blurred vision, and difficulty in passing urine. They may also cause confusion and are therefore rarely used for elderly people.

The main treatments for Parkinson's disease are dopamine agonists and levodopa. Dopamine agonists, such as ropinirole, pramipexole, and rotigotine, mimic the action of dopamine in the brain and help to control the main symptoms of the disease, such as tremor and mobility problems. Levodopa is converted into dopamine in the body and thereby increases dopamine levels in the brain. It is given in combination with an enzyme inhibitor (such as benserazide in the preparation co-beneldopa, or carbidopa in co-careldopa) to increase the amount of dopamine reaching the brain.

Levodopa preparations are generally more effective than dopamine agonists at controlling symptoms. However, they tend to work less well over time and the dose needs to be gradually increased. In addition, after several years of treatment (typically 5–7 years), levodopa preparations often produce side effects such as involuntary movements and an "on–off" effect (in which you suddenly switch from being able to move to being immobile). Consequently, young people are prescribed dopamine agonists first, and levodopa preparations are added later as the disease progresses.

Although many drugs are available for treating Parkinson's disease, none reverses its progress. However, drug treatment may give sustained relief of the major symptoms.

Physical treatment The doctor may arrange for physiotherapy (p.620) to help with mobility problems or speech therapy (p.621) for speech and swallowing problems. If you are finding it difficult to cope at home, an occupational therapist (p.621) may be able to suggest practical changes to help you move around.

Surgical treatment For people who are otherwise in good health, surgery may be recommended if the symptoms cannot be controlled by drugs. Known as deep brain stimulation, the most common surgical procedure involves implanting a device that sends electrical impulses into the affected area of the brain to control symptoms. Rarely, surgery to destroy a part of the brain tissue responsible for the tremor may be recommended instead.

What can I do?

It is important to pay attention to your general health. Taking a walk each day and doing simple exercises will help you to maintain mobility. Emotional and practical help from family, friends, and support groups is also important.

Many hospitals have a specialist Parkinson's disease nurse who can provide information and support.

What is the prognosis?
The course of the Parkinson's disease is variable, but drugs can be effective in treating the symptoms and improving the quality of life. People can lead active lives for many years after being diagnosed. However, most people with the disorder need daily help eventually, and their symptoms may be increasingly hard to control with drugs.

Creutzfeldt–Jakob disease

A rare, progressive, degenerative disease of the brain tissue due to an abnormal infectious protein

 More common over the age of 50

 Sometimes runs in families

 Lifestyle as a risk factor depends on the cause

 Gender is not a significant factor

Creutzfeldt–Jacob disease (CJD) is an extremely rare condition in which brain tissue is progressively destroyed by an unusual infectious agent. The disorder leads to a general decline in all areas of mental and physical ability and ultimately to death. CJD affects about one person in a million each year worldwide.

What is the cause?
CJD is caused by an abnormal type of protein known as a prion, which replicates in the brain and causes brain damage. There are four main types of CJD. One type, called sporadic CJD, mainly affects middle-aged or elderly people. No underlying cause for the accumulation of prions in the brain has been found for this form of CJD.

Another type of the condition is iatrogenic CJD, which is associated with contamination during surgical or medical treatment, such as brain surgery or treatment with products derived from human tissue. Before the use of synthetic growth hormone, human growth hormone was one source of infection.

Familial CJD is a very rare condition in which a genetic mutation causes prions to form in the brain. In the mid 1990s, a new variant of CJD (known as vCJD) was discovered in the UK. By the end of 2014, 177 people had been diagnosed with vCJD, of whom all had died. This variant was linked with eating contaminated meat from cattle with a disease called bovine spongiform encephalopathy (BSE). Since the link between vCJD and BSE was confirmed, strict controls have been introduced in the UK to prevent BSE from entering the human food chain.

What are the symptoms?
It is thought that CJD is present for 2–15 years before symptoms begin to develop gradually. They may include:
- Depression.
- Poor memory.
- Unsteadiness and poor coordination.

Other symptoms develop as the condition progresses and include:
- Sudden muscle contractions.
- Seizures.
- Weakness or paralysis on one side of the body.
- Progressive dementia.
- Impaired vision.

In the later stages of CJD, a person may be unable to move and talk.

What might be done?
CJD is usually diagnosed from a person's symptoms because no specific test is yet available. Anyone suspected of having CJD will have extensive tests, such as MRI (p.133) and lumbar puncture (p.326), and EEG (p.324) to look for characteristic changes in electrical activity in the brain. A brain or tonsil biopsy, in which a small piece of tissue is surgically removed for examination, may be performed.

There is no cure for CJD and no treatment to slow progression of the disease, although medication can relieve some of the symptoms. For example, depression may be treated with antidepressant drugs (p.592) and muscle contractions may be controlled with muscle relaxant drugs (p.579). However, as CJD progresses, the person will need considerable nursing care. This may be difficult to provide at home, so hospice care may be the best option. Eventually, CJD is fatal, usually within about 3 years.

Motor neuron disease

Progressive degeneration of the nerves in the brain and spinal cord that control muscular activity

 More common over the age of 40

 More common in males

 Sometimes runs in familiesv

 Lifestyle is not a significant factor

Motor neuron disease is rare, with about 2 people in every 100,000 developing the disease each year in the UK. In the disease, also known as amyotrophic lateral sclerosis, degeneration of the nerves involved in muscular activity results in progressive wasting of the muscles and weakness. There are several types of motor neuron disease. Some affect mainly the spinal nerves, while other types also affect the brain. The condition is not painful and does not affect bowel or bladder function or the senses, such as sight.

The cause of motor neuron disease is unknown in the vast majority of cases. In about 1 in 20 cases, genetic factors are involved and the disease runs in the family. Motor neuron disease is more common in men than in women and usually develops after the age of 40.

What are the symptoms?
Initially, weakness and wasting develop over a few months and usually affect the muscles of the hands, arms, or legs. Other early symptoms may include:
- Twitching movements in the muscles.
- Stiffness and muscle cramps.
- Sometimes, slurred speech, hoarseness, and difficulty swallowing.

As the disease progresses, other symptoms may include:
- Dragging one foot or a tendency to stumble when walking.
- Difficulty in climbing stairs or getting up from low chairs.

An affected person may have mood swings and may become anxious and depressed. If the muscles involved in breathing and swallowing are affected, small particles of food may enter the lungs and cause recurrent chest infections and possibly pneumonia (p.299). The head may fall forwards because the muscles in the neck are too weak to support it. Eventually, weakness of the muscles that control respiration may cause difficulty in breathing. In very rare cases, dementia (p.331) may develop in the later stages of the disease.

How is it diagnosed?
There is no specific test to diagnose motor neuron disease. However, electromyography (*see* **Nerve and muscle electrical tests**, p.337) may be carried out to detect a change in electrical activity in the muscles. To exclude other possible causes of the symptoms, such as a tumour or cervical spondylosis (p.222), additional tests may be carried out, such as a lumbar puncture (p.326) and MRI (p.133) or CT scanning (p.132) of the brain and neck.

What is the treatment?
At present, no treatment can significantly slow down the progression of motor neuron disease, although a drug called riluzole may have a small effect. Treatment for symptoms may include antidepressants (p.592) to relieve depression and antibiotics (p.572) to treat chest infections. If the person is having difficulty in swallowing, a gastrostomy may be created surgically. Known as a PEG or percutaneous gastrostomy, this is an opening through which a permanent feeding tube is inserted directly into the stomach.

Usually, a team of specialists provide support and care for an affected person and members of the family. Counselling (p.624) may be offered to both. The person affected by the disease may have physiotherapy (p.620) to keep joints and muscles supple and may be given aids to help with activities such as eating and walking (*see* **Occupational therapy**, p.621). A speech therapist (*see* **Speech therapy**, p.621) can supply communication aids to help with speech difficulties and advise on swallowing problems. Joining a self-help group is often helpful to the person with motor neuron disease and his or her family.

The outlook for motor neuron disease is variable, with approximately 2 in 10 affected people alive 5 years after diagnosis. About 1 in 10 affected people survives more than 10 years.

Multiple sclerosis

A progressive disease of nerves in the brain and spinal cord causing weakness and problems with sensation and vision

 Usually develops between the ages of 20 and 40

 More common in females

 Sometimes runs in families

 Stress and heat may aggravate symptoms

Multiple sclerosis (MS) is the most common nervous system disorder affecting young adults. In this condition, nerves in the brain and spinal cord are progressively damaged, causing a wide range of symptoms that affect sensation, movement, body functions, and balance. Specific symptoms may relate to the particular areas that are damaged and vary in severity between individuals. For example, damage to the optic nerve may cause blurred vision. If nerve fibres in the spinal cord are affected, it may cause weakness and heaviness in the legs or arms. Damage to nerves in the brain stem, the area of the brain that connects to the spinal cord, may affect balance.

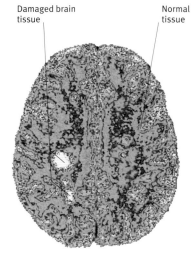

Damaged brain tissue · Normal tissue

Damage due to multiple sclerosis
This MRI scan of the brain of a person with multiple sclerosis shows damaged brain tissue caused by the destruction of the sheaths that surround nerve fibres.

▶ TEST

Visual evoked responses

A visual evoked response test measures the function of the optic nerve, the nerve that transmits messages from the eye to the brain. The test is most often used in the diagnosis of multiple sclerosis and can detect abnormalities even if visual symptoms are not apparent. The test records brain activity in response to a visual stimulus to find out the speed at which messages from the eye reach the brain. The test takes 20–30 minutes.

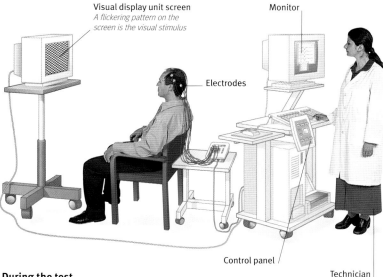

Visual display unit screen
A flickering pattern on the screen is the visual stimulus

Monitor

Electrodes

Control panel

Technician

During the test
Electrodes are attached to your scalp, and one eye is covered. You are asked to focus on a fixed dot of light while the checkered pattern flickers on the screen.

RESULTS

Visual evoked responses
This normal tracing shows electrical activity in an area of the brain as it receives messages from the eye. The first spike on the trace shows the moment of visual stimulus. The time taken for the signal to reach the brain is measured.

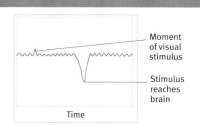

Moment of visual stimulus

Stimulus reaches brain

Time

In many people with MS, symptoms occur intermittently and there may be long periods of remission. However, some people have chronic (long-term) symptoms that gradually get worse.

In the UK, about 100,000 people are affected by MS. People who have a close relative with MS are more likely to develop the disorder. The condition is much more common in the northern hemisphere, which suggests that environmental factors also play a part. MS is more common in females and the disorder is more likely to develop between early adulthood and middle age.

What are the causes?

MS is an autoimmune disorder, in which the body's immune system attacks its own tissues, in this case those of the central nervous system. Many nerves in the brain and spinal cord are covered by a protective insulating sheath of material called myelin. In MS, small areas of myelin are damaged, leaving holes in the sheath, a process known as demyelination. Once the myelin sheath has been damaged, impulses cannot be conducted normally along nerves to and from the brain and spinal cord. At first, the damage may be limited to only one nerve, but myelin covering other nerves may become damaged over time. Eventually, damaged patches of myelin insulation are replaced by scar tissue.

It is thought that MS may be triggered by external factors such as a viral infection during childhood in genetically susceptible individuals.

What are the types?

There are two main types of MS: relapsing–remitting and progressive MS. In relapsing–remitting MS, the most common type, symptoms typically last for days or weeks (relapse) and then clear up for months or even years (remission). In a few cases of relapsing–remitting MS, the symptoms are very mild and may not cause significant disability even after as long as 20 years; this type is known as benign relapsing–remitting MS. However, whatever the type of relapsing–remitting MS, eventually some symptoms may persist between attacks.

About 1 in 10 people with MS have a type known as primary progressive MS, in which there is a gradual worsening of the symptoms from the start, with no remissions. Many people who initially have relapsing–remitting MS go on to develop secondary progressive MS, in which there is a progressive increase in symptoms with few, if any, remissions.

What are the symptoms?

The type, severity, and progression of symptoms vary considerably from person to person. In the initial stages, symptoms may occur singly, then, as the disease progresses, in combination. They may include:

■ Blurred vision, usually affecting only one eye.
■ Numbness or tingling in any part of the body.
■ Fatigue, which may be persistent.
■ Problems with coordination and balance, such as an unsteady gait.
■ Slurred speech.

Stress and heat sometimes make symptoms worse. Depression is common. Some people with muscle weakness develop painful muscle spasms. Spinal cord damage can lead to urinary incontinence (p.454), and men may have increasing difficulty in achieving an erection (*see* **Erectile dysfunction**, p.494). Eventually, damage to myelin covering nerves in the spinal cord may cause partial paralysis, and an affected person may need a wheelchair.

How is it diagnosed?

There is no single test to diagnose MS, and a diagnosis is only made once other possible causes of the symptoms have been excluded. Your doctor will take your medical history and examine you. If you have visual problems, you may be referred to an ophthalmologist, who will assess the optic nerve, which is commonly affected in the early stages of the disorder (*see* **Optic neuritis**, p.362). Your doctor may arrange for tests to find out how quickly your brain receives messages when particular nerves are stimulated. The most common test measures damage to the visual pathways (*see* **Visual evoked responses**, above left). You may also have a brain scan, such as an MRI scan (p.133), to look for demyelination.

Your doctor may arrange for a lumbar puncture (p.326), in which a sample of the fluid around the spinal cord is removed for analysis. Abnormalities in this fluid may confirm the diagnosis.

What is the treatment?

There is no cure for MS, but if you have relapsing–remitting MS, disease-modifying drugs will probably be prescribed to help reduce the number and severity of relapses; they may also help to slow the progression of the disease. There are several medications available, and the one you are prescribed will depend on your particular case. However, some of the more commonly used disease-modifying drugs include interferon beta (*see* **Interferon drugs**, p.586), glatiramer, teriflunomide, dimethyl fumarate, and fingolimod. Your doctor may also prescribe corticosteroid drugs (p.600) to shorten the duration of a relapse. At present, there is no treatment to halt the progression of progressive MS.

Many of the more common symptoms that occur in all types of MS can be relieved by drugs. For example, your doctor may treat muscle spasms with a muscle relaxant (p.579) and incontinence can often be improved by drugs (*see* **Drugs that affect bladder control**, p.606). Problems in getting an erection may be helped by a drug such as sildenafil. If you have mobility problems, your doctor may arrange for you to have physiotherapy (p.620), and occupational therapy (p.621) may make day-to-day activities easier.

Many people with MS believe that cannabis relieves symptoms such as muscle stiffness and pain, and there is experimental evidence to support that belief. However, cannabis has no approved medicinal use, cannot be prescribed by doctors, and its use is illegal.

What can I do?

If you are diagnosed with MS, you and your family will need time and possibly counselling (p.624) to come to terms with the disorder. You should minimize stress in your life and avoid exposure to high temperatures if heat makes your symptoms worse. Regular, gentle exercise will help to keep your muscles strong without overstraining them. Many hospitals have a specialist MS nurse, who can provide support and information.

What is the prognosis?

The progression of MS is extremely variable, but people who are older when the disease first develops tend to fare less well. About 7 in 10 people with MS have active lives with long periods of remission between relapses. However, some people, particularly those with progressive MS, become increasingly disabled. Half of all people with MS are still leading active lives 10 years after diagnosis, and the average lifespan from diagnosis is 25–30 years.

Peripheral nervous system disorders

The peripheral nervous system is composed of nerves that branch from the brain and spinal cord and then divide repeatedly to supply every part of the body. The nerves transmit information necessary for sensation, muscle stimulation, and the regulation of unconscious functions. Disorders of these nerves may be painful, cause loss of sensation, or lead to paralysis.

This section starts with an overview of peripheral neuropathies, in which one or more peripheral nerves are damaged. Peripheral neuropathies are relatively common and have many causes, including injuries, infection, nutritional deficiencies, and disorders such as diabetes mellitus. Diabetic neuropathy, the most common cause of peripheral nerve damage, is covered next. This is followed by an article on nutritional neuropathies, in which deficiency of essential nutrients in the diet, especially the vitamin B complex, causes the nerve damage.

The next articles cover disorders such as sciatica, carpal tunnel syndrome, and facial palsy, all of which may be caused by compression of a nerve. Rarer disorders that affect peripheral nerves are covered next. Such disorders include myasthenia gravis, in which the immune system affects the body's ability to transmit impulses from the nerves to muscles, and Guillain–Barré syndrome, which is the result of an abnormal response of the immune system after an infection. The final article covers nervous tics, which are often caused by stress.

KEY ANATOMY

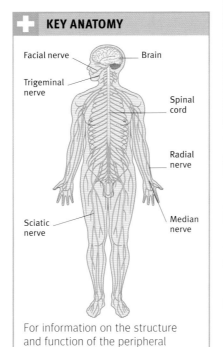

Facial nerve
Brain
Trigeminal nerve
Spinal cord
Radial nerve
Sciatic nerve
Median nerve

For information on the structure and function of the peripheral nervous system, *see* pp.311–318.

Peripheral neuropathies

Disorders of one or more of the nerves outside the brain and spinal cord, known as the peripheral nerves

 Age, gender, genetics, and lifestyle as risk factors depend on the cause

Disorders of the peripheral nerves, the nerves that branch from the brain and spinal cord to the rest of the body, are called neuropathies. Depending on the nerves affected, peripheral neuropathies may affect sensation, movement, or automatic functions, such as bladder control. Rarely, a peripheral neuropathy may be life-threatening.

What are the causes?

In developed countries, the most common cause of damage to the peripheral nerves is diabetes mellitus (*see* **Diabetic neuropathy**, right). Vitamin B complex deficiencies and some nutritional disorders may also result in nerve damage (*see* **Nutritional neuropathies**, opposite page). In the deve-

loped world, nutritional neuropathy is often the result of a poor diet in people who abuse alcohol. Drinking too much alcohol may also damage peripheral nerves directly.

Damage to a single nerve may occur as a result of an injury (*see* **Peripheral nerve injuries**, p.339) or because of compression. For example, in carpal tunnel syndrome (p.338), the median nerve, which supplies part of the hand, is compressed at the wrist.

Neuropathy may also be associated with an infection, such as leprosy (*see* **Hansen's disease**, p.173) or HIV infection (*see* **HIV infection and AIDS**, p.169). Guillain–Barré syndrome (p.340), a neuropathy that is rapidly progressive, is caused by an abnormal immune response that sometimes occurs after an infection.

Autoimmune disorders such as systemic lupus erythematosus (p.281), in which the immune system attacks the body's tissues, may cause nerve damage. Occasionally, a disorder such as polyarteritis nodosa (p.283) may damage nerves by causing inflammation of the blood vessels that supply them. Neuropathy may also result from certain cancers, particularly primary lung cancer (p.307), breast cancer (p.486), and

lymphoma (p.279). Occasionally, neuropathy is caused by amyloidosis (p.441), in which an abnormal protein is deposited in the body.

Some drugs, such as isoniazid (*see* **Antituberculous drugs**, p.573), may cause nerve damage, as may exposure to certain toxic substances, such as lead. In some cases, the cause is unknown.

What are the types?

Peripheral neuropathies may affect the nerves that transmit sensory information (sensory nerves), the nerves that stimulate the muscles (motor nerves), and/or the nerves that control automatic functions (autonomic nerves).

Sensory nerve neuropathies These neuropathies usually start in the extremities (commonly the feet first, then the hands), then progress up the limbs. The symptoms may include tingling, pain, and numbness in the affected area. If the fingertips are numb, everyday tasks may become difficult. This type of neuropathy is most often caused by diabetes mellitus, nutritional disorders, or drugs.

Motor nerve neuropathies If the motor nerves are damaged, the muscles they supply become weak, and wasting occurs eventually. In severe cases, mobility may become restricted, and, very rarely, breathing may have to be assisted by mechanical ventilation (*see* **Intensive therapy unit**, p.618). Lead poisoning may result in a neuropathy that affects the motor nerves only.

Autonomic nerve neuropathies A neuropathy that is affecting one or more autonomic nerves may result in constipation (p.398), fainting due to low blood pressure (*see* **Hypotension**, p.248), diarrhoea (p.397), urinary incontinence (p.454), or erectile dysfunction (p.494). This type of neuropathy is often caused by longstanding diabetes mellitus.

What might be done?

Your doctor may be able to tell which nerves are affected from your symptoms and an examination. If the cause of your neuropathy is not clear, he or she will probably arrange for blood tests to look for evidence of an underlying disorder, such as diabetes, nutritional deficiencies, or an autoimmune disorder. If there is evidence of compression of a nerve root, you may also have CT scanning (p.132) or MRI (p.133) to assess the severity and extent of nerve damage. Special tests to assess the function of the nerves (*see* **Nerve and muscle electrical tests**, opposite page) may also be carried out.

The treatment of a peripheral neuropathy depends on the cause and the type of nerve affected. For example, careful control of diabetes mellitus may keep diabetic neuropathy from worsening, and vitamin B complex injections (*see* **Vitamins**, p.598) may help a nutritional neuropathy. If motor nerves are affected, you may have physiotherapy (p.620) to help to maintain muscle tone. Wearing a foot splint may assist walking. Sometimes, the underlying cause can be treated, but longstanding nerve damage may be irreversible.

Diabetic neuropathy

Damage to one or more of the peripheral nerves caused by diabetes mellitus

 More common over the age of 40

 Diabetes mellitus sometimes runs in families

 Poor control of diabetes mellitus and smoking are risk factors

 Gender is not a significant factor

In diabetic neuropathy, one or more of the peripheral nerves that branch from the brain and spinal cord to the rest of the body are damaged as a result of diabetes mellitus (p.437). Diabetic neuropathy is the most common cause of peripheral neuropathy. If diabetes is poorly controlled, it results in high levels of glucose in the blood that damage the peripheral nerves directly and the blood vessels that supply them (*see* **Diabetic vascular disease**, p.260). Good control of diabetes reduces this risk.

Neuropathy may affect as many as half of people with diabetes, although not all of them develop significant symptoms.

People with diabetes mellitus who smoke increase the risk of damaging the blood vessels that supply the nerves.

What are the symptoms?

The symptoms of diabetic neuropathy usually develop slowly over a number of years. Rarely, they develop rapidly over days or weeks. Symptoms vary depending on which nerves are involved, but the feet are frequently affected. Less commonly, diabetic neuropathy may affect the larger nerves, mainly in the thighs. Symptoms may include:

■ Pins and needles.
■ Numbness.
■ Hypersensitivity.
■ Sharp, stabbing pains, which may disrupt sleep.
■ Discomfort or pain when walking (like walking on pebbles).

If sensation is lost, a minor injury to the foot, such as rubbing by badly fitting shoes, may not be noticed. Slow healing due to poor blood supply may lead to infection.

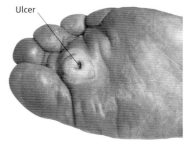

Ulcer

Foot ulcer
If nerves are damaged as a result of diabetic neuropathy, a painless ulcer, such as shown here on the sole, may develop.

▶ **TEST**

Nerve and muscle electrical tests

Nerve and muscle electrical tests consist of nerve conduction studies and electromyography (EMG). Nerve conduction studies are used to assess how well a nerve is conducting electrical impulses. They are often followed by EMG to see whether symptoms, such as weakness, are due to a disorder of the muscle or the nerve supplying it. Both tests are usually done on an outpatient basis. Each takes about 15 minutes and may cause some discomfort.

Nerve conduction studies

Nerve conduction studies are carried out to assess nerve damage in disorders such as peripheral neuropathies. A nerve is stimulated by an electrical impulse, and the response to the stimulus and the speed at which this response travels along the nerve indicates whether the nerve is damaged and the nature and extent of the damage.

Monitor
The results are displayed here as a trace

Control panel

Technician

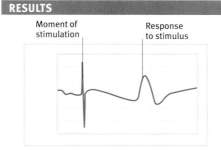

Stimulator

Recording electrode

During the procedure
A probe is held against the skin to stimulate the nerve to be tested. The signal that is produced by the nerve is picked up by a recording electrode placed further along the nerve on the skin.

RESULTS

Moment of stimulation

Response to stimulus

Nerve conduction trace
This trace shows a normal electrical impulse through a nerve. The nerve is stimulated, and the speed at which the impulse travels through the nerve is measured.

Electromyography

EMG is used to differentiate between nerve and muscle disorders and to diagnose disorders such as muscular dystrophy. A fine needle is used to record the electrical activity of a muscle at rest and when contracting. The results are recorded on a trace.

Recording needle

Ground electrode

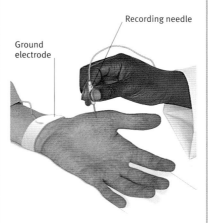

During the procedure
A needle placed in or on the muscle records electrical activity at rest and when you contract the muscle. A ground electrode eliminates background electrical activity.

RESULTS

Resting muscle

Muscle contraction

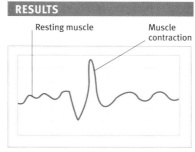

EMG trace
This trace shows normal patterns of electrical activity in a muscle at rest and when contracting.

If left untreated, ulcers may develop (*see* **Leg ulcer**, p.203) and, in severe cases, gangrene (p.262) occurs.

Eventually, diabetic neuropathy may also affect the autonomic nerves that regulate automatic body functions such as blood pressure control and digestion. Damage to these nerves causes symptoms such as dizziness when standing (*see* **Hypotension**, p.248), diarrhoea (p.397), and erectile dysfunction (p.494).

What might be done?

Careful control of diabetes reduces the risk of developing diabetic neuropathy. However, if you develop symptoms of nerve damage, you should consult your doctor. He or she will probably be able to diagnose the condition from your symptoms. However, nerve conduction tests may need to be carried out in hospital to confirm which nerves are affected and to assess the severity of the damage (*see* **Nerve and muscle electrical tests**, above).

The goal of treatment of diabetic neuropathy is to prevent further nerve damage and the development of complications. Your doctor will help you to monitor your blood sugar level carefully and advise you about good foot care (*see* **Living with diabetes**, p.438). For example, you should check your feet regularly for cuts or abrasions, particularly if you have been wearing new shoes. You should avoid wearing open-toed sandals or walking barefoot. If you smoke, you should try to give up.

To relieve pain, particularly at night, medications such as pregabalin or gabapentin (*see* **Anticonvulsant drugs,** p590), duloxetine, or amitriptyline (*see* **Antidepressant drugs,** p.592) may be prescribed.

What is the prognosis?

Good control of blood glucose levels in diabetes mellitus not only reduces the risk of developing diabetic neuropathy but may also halt further progression of the disease. However, in most cases, nerve damage is irreversible.

Nutritional neuropathies

Damage to peripheral nerves caused by nutritional deficiency

 Poor diet and excessive alcohol consumption are risk factors

 Age, gender, and genetics are not significant factors

In nutritional neuropathies, the peripheral nerves, which branch from the brain and spinal cord, are damaged by deficiencies of essential nutrients, particularly those of the vitamin B complex (*see* **Nutritional deficiencies**, p.399).

Worldwide, nutritional neuropathies are generally caused by malnutrition. In developed countries, such neuropathies are more commonly associated with excessive alcohol consumption. People who drink heavily often also have a poor diet, which can cause a vitamin B_1 deficiency. In addition, alcohol may directly damage the peripheral nerves. A person who has been drinking heavily for 10 years or more has a greatly increased risk of developing a nutritional neuropathy.

Nutritional deficiencies may occur in people with eating disorders, such as anorexia nervosa (p.348). People with long-term conditions that affect absorption of nutrients from the intestines (*see* **Malabsorption**, p.415) may also develop nutritional deficiencies.

What are the symptoms?

Nutritional neuropathies usually first affect the tips of the fingers and the toes. The symptoms appear gradually over several months or years and slowly progress up the limbs to the trunk. Symptoms may include:
■ Loss of sensation.
■ Pins and needles.
■ Pain in the feet and/or the hands.
Walking may be clumsy as a result of the loss of sensation in the feet and legs. If the motor nerves (nerves that stimulate the muscles) are affected, muscle weakness and wasting may develop and further affect the ability to walk.

What might be done?

Your doctor will examine you by checking your reflexes and your ability to feel sensation such as a pin prick. He or she may arrange for blood tests to look for a vitamin deficiency or for evidence of liver damage caused by excessive alcohol consumption. Your doctor may also arrange for tests that measure the extent of the nerve damage (*see* **Nerve and muscle electrical tests**, left).

Nutritional neuropathies are treated by replacing the missing nutrients. This is done either by giving a course of oral supplements or, in some cases, by injections (*see* **Vitamins**, p.598). Your doctor may also prescribe anticonvulsant drugs (p.590)

or antidepressants (p.592) to help to control the symptoms. You may also be prescribed painkillers (p.589) to relieve any discomfort.

Nerve damage is usually irreversible, but with treatment the progression of the disease can usually be halted.

Trigeminal neuralgia

Severe pain on one side of the face due to compression, inflammation, or damage to the trigeminal nerve

 More common over the age of 50

 More common in males

 Genetics as a risk factor depends on the cause

 Lifestyle is not a significant factor

The trigeminal nerve transmits sensation from parts of the face to the brain and controls some of the muscles that are involved in chewing. Damage to this nerve causes repeated bursts of sharp, stabbing pain, known as trigeminal neuralgia, in the lip, gum, or cheek on one side of the face. Attacks of trigeminal neuralgia may last for a few seconds or several minutes and may become more frequent over time. In severe cases, the pain may be so intense that the affected person is unable to do anything during the attack. Afterwards, the pain usually disappears completely. An attack may occur spontaneously or may be triggered by certain facial movements, such as chewing, or by touching a trigger spot on the face. Attacks rarely occur during the night.

Trigeminal neuralgia is most common in men over the age of 50. In most cases, it is due to compression of a nerve by a blood vessel in the skull. Rarely, it may be due to a tumour pressing on a nerve. However, in people under 50, the symptoms may be an early sign of multiple sclerosis (p.334).

What might be done?
There are no specific tests to diagnose trigeminal neuralgia. Your doctor will examine you to rule out any other causes of facial pain, such as toothache or sinusitis (p.290). He or she may also arrange for you to have MRI (p.133) to look for the presence of a tumour.

Your doctor may prescribe painkillers (p.589), such as paracetamol or ibuprofen. However, if the pain persists, your doctor may prescribe anticonvulsant drugs (p.590), such as carbamazepine, gabapentin, or lamotrigine, or certain antidepressants (p.592), all of which have been shown to be effective in treating trigeminal neuralgia. Unlike painkillers, which are taken only when the pain is present, both anticonvulsant and antidepressant drugs need to be taken every day to prevent attacks.

If a tumour is found, surgery may be necessary to remove it. Surgery may also be used to separate the trigeminal nerve from a blood vessel if the vessel is compressing the nerve. Rarely, people who have persistent, severe pain that does not respond to drugs are offered treatment to numb the affected side of the face. For example, pain can be alleviated by using a heated probe to destroy the nerve. Trigeminal neuralgia will not recur after treatment to numb the face, but you will need to take care when consuming hot food or drinks because of the lack of sensation in your face.

Attacks of neuralgia may stop spontaneously, become more frequent, or persist unchanged for months or years. However, symptoms usually improve significantly with treatment.

Sciatica

Pain in the buttock and down the back of the leg, occurring when the sciatic nerve or its roots are compressed or damaged

 Age, gender, and lifestyle as risk factors depend on the cause

 Genetics is not a significant factor

Sciatica is a form of nerve pain that may be felt anywhere along the course of one of the sciatic nerves, the two largest nerves in the body and the main nerve in each leg. The sciatic nerves are formed from nerve roots in the lower part of the spinal cord. They run from the base of the spine down the backs of the thighs to above the knees, where they divide into branches that supply the front and back of the leg and foot. The pain of sciatica is caused by compression of or damage to the sciatic nerve, usually where it leaves the spinal cord. Many people have at least one episode of sciatica during their lives. Often, only one leg is affected. In most cases, the pain disappears gradually over about 1–2 weeks, but it may recur.

What are the causes?
The most common cause of sciatica is a prolapsed or herniated disc (p.227) in the spinal column that presses on a spinal nerve root. In older people, sciatica may be caused by changes in the spine as a result of various conditions, such as osteoarthritis (p.221). Women may develop sciatica during the last months of pregnancy because of posture changes that cause increased pressure on the sciatic nerve (*see* **Common complaints of normal pregnancy**, p.506). Muscle spasm and sitting in an awkward position for long periods of time are relatively common causes of brief episodes of sciatica in all age groups. Rarely, a tumour on the spinal cord may press on the sciatic nerve roots and cause sciatica.

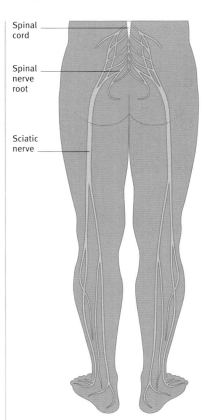

Spinal cord
Spinal nerve root
Sciatic nerve

The sciatic nerves
Each sciatic nerve is formed from nerve roots in the spinal cord and runs down the leg to the foot. Sciatic pain may occur anywhere along the sciatic nerve and its branches.

What are the symptoms?
The symptoms can be mild or severe, with spasmodic or persistent pain in the affected leg. Symptoms may include:
■ Pain that is made worse by movement or by coughing.
■ Tingling or numbness.
■ Muscle weakness.
If sciatica is severe, you may have difficulty in lifting the foot on the affected side, and you may be unable to stand upright. Some people have difficulty in walking.

What might be done?
The doctor will examine you and test your leg reflexes, muscle strength, and sensation. You will probably be advised to continue your normal activities as much as possible but stop any activity that makes the pain worse. If the pain is severe, you may be prescribed painkillers (p.589); you may also be advised to rest in bed for a short period (prolonged bed rest may make the pain worse). If symptoms persist or if you have muscle weakness, you may have tests, such as MRI (p.133) of the spine, to look for changes in the bones or a prolapsed disc.

Sciatica as a result of pregnancy will usually disappear after childbirth. Pain caused by muscle spasm or sitting awkwardly also tends to clear up without treatment. Occasionally, the condition can be helped by regular physiotherapy (p.620) or exercise. However, sciatica can recur. In some cases, surgery may be necessary to relieve pressure on the nerve, especially if there is weakness of the leg or foot muscles.

Carpal tunnel syndrome

Tingling and pain in the hand and forearm due to a compressed nerve at the wrist

 Most common between the ages of 40 and 60

 More common in females

 Work that involves repetitive hand movements is a risk factor

 Genetics is usually not a significant factor. Rarely, may run in families

The carpal tunnel is the narrow space formed by the bones of the wrist (carpal bones) and the strong ligament that lies over them. In carpal tunnel syndrome, the median nerve, which controls some hand muscles and conveys sensation from nerve endings in part of the hand, is compressed where it passes through the tunnel. This compression causes painful tingling in the hand, wrist, and forearm. Carpal tunnel syndrome is a common disorder, especially in women aged 40–60, and often affects both hands.

What are the causes?
In some cases, the underlying cause of nerve compression is not known. In others, it occurs because the soft tissues within the carpal tunnel swell, compressing the median nerve at the wrist. Such swelling may be due to diabetes mellitus (p.437), or it may occur during pregnancy. The carpal tunnel may also be narrowed by a joint disorder, such as rheumatoid arthritis (p.222), or by a wrist fracture. The syndrome is associated with work that involves repetitive hand movements, such as typing, which can result in inflammation of the tendons in the wrist (*see* **Tendinitis and tenosynovitis**, p.231). Rarely, carpal tunnel syndrome may occur as a feature of a generalized nerve disorder which may run in families.

What are the symptoms?
Symptoms mainly affect specific areas of the hand, such as the thumb, the first and middle fingers, the inner side of the ring finger, and the palm of the hand. Initially, symptoms may include:
■ Burning and tingling in the hand.
■ Pain in the wrist and up the forearm.
As the condition worsens, other symptoms may gradually appear including:
■ Numbness of the hand.
■ Weakened grip.
■ Wasting of some hand muscles, particularly at the base of the thumb.
Symptoms are typically worse at night. Shaking the affected arm may temporarily relieve symptoms, but the numbness may become persistent if left untreated.

What might be done?
Your doctor may suspect carpal tunnel syndrome from your symptoms. He or she will examine your wrists and hands. Nerve

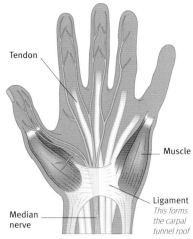

Tendon

Muscle

Median nerve

Ligament
This forms the carpal tunnel roof

Carpal tunnel
The carpal tunnel is formed by the bones of the wrist and the ligament over them. Compression of the median nerve in the tunnel causes carpal tunnel syndrome.

conduction studies (*see* **Nerve and muscle electrical tests**, p.337) may be carried out to confirm the diagnosis. If pregnancy is the cause of carpal tunnel syndrome, the symptoms usually disappear after childbirth. In other cases, treating the cause, if it can be identified, usually relieves symptoms.

The symptoms of carpal tunnel syndrome may be relieved temporarily by nonsteroidal anti-inflammatory drugs (p.578) or by wearing a wrist splint, particularly at night. In certain cases, a corticosteroid injection (*see* **Locally acting corticosteroids**, p.578) under or around the ligament may reduce swelling. If symptoms persist or recur, you may have surgery to release pressure on the nerve. After surgery, there are usually no further symptoms.

Facial palsy

Weakness or paralysis of the facial muscles on one side of the face due to damage to one of the facial nerves

 Age, gender, genetics, and lifestyle are not significant factors

The facial nerve controls the muscles of expression and emotion in the face and carries taste sensations from the front of the tongue to the brain. In facial palsy, one of the two facial nerves is damaged, compressed, or inflamed, and this results in weakness of the facial muscles, causing the eyelid and corner of the mouth to droop on one side of the face. People with facial palsy are often concerned that they have had a stroke (p.329), but this is unlikely if only the face is affected because a stroke is usually also associated with muscle weakness in other parts of the body, such as the limbs. Facial palsy is usually temporary, but a full recovery may take several months.

What are the causes?

The most common form of facial palsy is Bell's palsy, which in most cases is thought to arise as a result of infection with the herpes simplex virus, the virus that causes cold sores (p.205). In other types of facial palsy, causes of facial nerve damage include the viral infection shingles (*see* **Herpes zoster**, p.166) and the bacterial infection Lyme disease (p.174). In addition, the facial nerve sometimes becomes inflamed as a result of a middle-ear infection (*see* **Otitis media**, p.374). In rare cases, the facial nerve may be compressed by a tumour called an acoustic neuroma (p.380). Facial palsy can also result from injury or from damage to the nerve from a tumour of the parotid salivary gland (p.403).

What are the symptoms?

In some cases, such as in Bell's palsy, the symptoms of facial palsy appear suddenly over about 24 hours. In other cases, including facial palsy caused by an acoustic neuroma, symptoms may develop slowly. The symptoms include:

- Partial or complete paralysis of the muscles on one side of the face.
- Pain behind the ear on the affected side of the face.
- Drooping of the corner of the mouth, sometimes associated with drooling.
- Inability to close the eyelid on the affected side and watering of the eye.
- Impairment of taste.

If facial palsy is very severe, you may have difficulty in speaking and eating, and, occasionally, sounds may seem unnaturally loud in the ear on the affected side. If the eyelid cannot be closed, the eye may become infected, leading to ulceration of the cornea, the transparent front part of the eye. In facial palsy due to shingles, you will also have a rash of crusting blisters on your ear.

How is it diagnosed?

Your doctor will probably be able to diagnose facial palsy from your symptoms alone. A rapid onset over about 24 hours suggests Bell's palsy. Symptoms that develop more slowly usually indicate another cause.

If your doctor suspects a tumour may be compressing the facial nerve, he or she may arrange for you to have CT scanning (p.132)

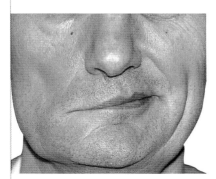

Facial palsy
Facial palsy caused by nerve damage has affected the muscles on the right side of this man's face, causing a lopsided smile.

or MRI (p.133). Nerve and muscle electrical tests (p.337) may also be arranged to assess nerve damage. If you live in a part of the UK where Lyme disease is common, you may have a blood test to look for evidence of this disorder.

What might be done?

If your symptoms have appeared in the last 48 hours, your doctor may prescribe corticosteroids (p.600) for up to 2 weeks to reduce inflammation of the nerve, and an antiviral drug (p. 573) such as aciclovir. He or she may also recommend that you take painkillers (p.589). To prevent damage to the cornea, you may be given artificial tears (*see* **Drugs acting on the eye**, p.594), and you will probably be advised to tape the affected eye shut when you go to sleep.

Bell's palsy usually clears up without further treatment. For other types of facial palsy, the underlying cause will be treated, if possible. For example, if it is due to shingles, aciclovir or another antiviral drug will be prescribed. To be effective, treatment with aciclovir should begin as soon as the rash appears. If you have an acoustic neuroma, it will be removed surgically to relieve compression of the facial nerve.

If muscle paralysis persists, surgery may be used to graft nerve tissue or reroute another nerve to the face. Facial exercises or massage may help to maintain tone (*see* **Physiotherapy**, p.620).

What is the prognosis?

With appropriate treatment, facial palsy usually improves within about 2 weeks. However, a full recovery may take up to about 12 months. Some people are left with residual weakness.

Peripheral nerve injuries

Damage to a nerve outside the brain or spinal cord as a result of physical injury

 Age, gender, genetics, and lifestyle are not significant factors

Any of the peripheral nerves, which connect the brain and the spinal cord to the rest of the body, may be damaged by physical injury. This damage may cause weakness and loss of sensation in the part of the body that the nerve supplies. A peripheral nerve may be partially or completely severed, or it may be compressed. Damage may not be permanent because peripheral nerves can regenerate if they are not completely cut.

What are the symptoms?

The part of the body affected depends on which peripheral nerve is damaged. Symptoms usually include:

- Tingling and numbness.
- Muscle weakness or paralysis.
- Eventually, muscle wasting.

The severity of the symptoms depends on whether the nerve is damaged or completely severed.

What might be done?

Your doctor will check for loss of sensation, test your reflexes, and assess the strength of your muscles. You may also have nerve and muscle electrical tests (p.337), in which the function of the affected nerve is tested to assess how severely it has been damaged.

Treatment is often unnecessary if a peripheral nerve is only compressed or partially severed. After a few weeks, nerve and muscle tests may be repeated to see if there has been an improvement in your condition. If the nerve is totally severed, it cannot regenerate by itself, and you may be offered microsurgery (p.613) to try to repair it. After the operation, you may have physiotherapy (p.620) to help to regain lost muscle strength and coordination. However, even with the most skilled surgery, full recovery may not be possible, and you may continue to have symptoms.

Myasthenia gravis

An autoimmune disorder causing fluctuating weakness of the muscles, especially of the eyes, face, throat, and limbs

 Most common between the ages of 20 and 40 in females and 50 and 70 in males

 More common in females

 Stress may aggravate the symptoms

 Genetics is not a significant factor

Myasthenia gravis is a rare autoimmune disorder in which the immune system produces abnormal antibodies that block the receptors in muscles that receive nerve impulses. As a result, the affected muscles fail to respond or respond only weakly to nerve impulses. The muscles of the face, throat, and those that control eye and eyelid movements are most often affected, causing speech problems, double vision, and drooping eyelids. However, other muscles may be affected, including those in the arms and legs and, rarely, the respiratory muscles.

Myasthenia gravis is a long-term condition that varies in severity. It is more common in women, especially in those aged 20 to 40 years. In men, the disorder tends to occur between the ages of 50 and 70. In the UK, it affects about 1 in 10,000 people.

What are the causes?

In some people, myasthenia gravis is associated with a thymoma, a tumour of the thymus gland (a gland that forms part of the immune system and is located behind the upper part of the breastbone). Myasthenia

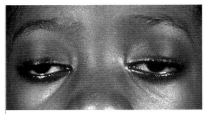

Myasthenia gravis
The rare immune disorder myasthenia gravis has affected the muscles controlling the eyelids, causing them to droop.

gravis may also be associated with other autoimmune disorders, such as the joint disorder rheumatoid arthritis (p.222) and pernicious anaemia, a type of megaloblastic anaemia (p.272). Certain drugs, such as penicillamine (*see* **Antirheumatic drugs**, p.579) may worsen the symptoms of myasthenia gravis.

What are the symptoms?

The symptoms of myasthenia gravis usually develop gradually over several weeks or months and tend to fluctuate. In some cases, symptoms appear suddenly. Symptoms may include:

■ Drooping eyelids.
■ Double vision.
■ Slurred speech.
■ Difficulty chewing and swallowing.
■ Weakness in the arm and leg muscles.

Symptoms usually improve with rest but worsen when the affected muscles are used. Symptoms may also be made worse by stress and, in women, by menstruation. Rarely, if respiratory muscles are weakened, life-threatening breathing difficulties may develop.

About 1 in 7 babies born to mothers with myasthenia gravis develops symptoms immediately after birth, but these usually disappear over a few weeks.

How is it diagnosed?

Your doctor may suspect myasthenia gravis from your symptoms. To confirm the diagnosis, you will probably have a blood test to look for the antibodies that block the receptors in muscles. In some cases, you may also be given an injection that increases the levels of neurotransmitters, the chemicals responsible for conveying nerve impulses from nerves to muscle receptors. If there is a rapid but only temporary improvement in muscle strength, you probably have myasthenia gravis. You may also have electromyography (*see* **Nerve and muscle electrical tests**, p.337) to look for muscle weakness by measuring electrical activity. CT scanning (p.132) of the chest may also be carried out to look for a thymoma.

What is the treatment?

Your doctor may prescribe drugs that raise the levels of neurotransmitters. If your symptoms are mild, this treatment may control them sufficiently. If your symptoms are persistent, you may be prescribed oral corticosteroids (p.600) or other immunosuppressant drugs (p.585), such as azathioprine, to reduce antibody production.

Treatment with oral corticosteroids may be started in hospital because the drugs may have an adverse effect initially, and symptoms may become worse.

In severe cases, regular plasmapheresis may be necessary. In this procedure, plasma (the fluid part of the blood) is taken from the body, treated to remove the abnormal antibodies, and replaced. Alternatively, intravenous immunoglobulin therapy may be used, which involves infusing into a vein large numbers of normal antibodies. If breathing becomes difficult, mechanical ventilation may be needed (*see* **Intensive therapy unit**, p.618).

If a tumour of the thymus is found, surgery will be performed to remove the thymus gland. Some people under the age of 45 with severe symptoms but no thymoma may also benefit from surgical removal of the thymus gland.

People with myasthenia gravis should avoid extremes of temperature, infections, stress, and becoming overtired, all of which intensify muscle weakness.

What is the prognosis?

About 8 in 10 people with myasthenia gravis can be cured or their symptoms substantially improved with treatment. In a few people, the symptoms disappear spontaneously after about a year. Rarely, if the respiratory muscles are involved, the disorder may be fatal.

Guillain–Barré syndrome

A disorder in which damage to the peripheral nerves results in weakness that spreads upwards from the legs

 Age, gender, genetics, and lifestyle are not significant factors

Guillain–Barré syndrome is a rare and potentially life-threatening disorder that causes progressive loss of feeling and weakness that can rapidly lead to paralysis. The condition is the result of an abnormal immune response that develops 2–4 weeks after certain infections. In most cases, the infection is viral, for example, the common cold, influenza, or cytomegalovirus infection (p.167), but sometimes the triggering infection may be bacterial, such as with *Campylobacter* bacteria (*see* **Food poisoning**, p.398).

In Guillain–Barré syndrome, antibodies produced in response to an infection attack the peripheral nerves, causing the nerves to become inflamed. Initially, the legs are affected, followed by the trunk, arms, and head. The condition is often mild, but, if severe, Guillain–Barré may cause difficulty in swallowing and breathing. In such circumstances, the affected person may need to have artificial feeding and mechanical ventilation. Each year, about 1,200 people in the UK are affected by the syndrome.

What are the symptoms?

The symptoms may develop in a few days or weeks and include:

■ Weakness in the legs, which may spread up the trunk and to the arms.
■ Numbness and tingling of the limbs.

Usually, no further symptoms develop, but, in severe cases, symptoms become progressively worse and include:

■ Blurred or double vision.
■ Paralysis of the limbs.
■ Difficulty in speaking and swallowing.

If the muscles of the ribcage and diaphragm are affected, serious breathing difficulties may develop.

How is it diagnosed?

Your doctor will probably diagnose Guillain–Barré syndrome from your symptoms. However, you may have tests to confirm the diagnosis, including nerve conduction studies (*see* **Nerve and muscle electrical tests**, p.337). You may also have a lumbar puncture (p.326), in which a sample of fluid from around the spinal cord is removed under local anaesthesia for analysis.

What is the treatment?

During the early stages of Guillain–Barré syndrome you will be admitted to hospital, where you will probably be given intravenous infusions of immunoglobulin. An alternative treatment is plasmapheresis, in which plasma (the fluid part of the blood) is withdrawn, treated to remove abnormal antibodies, and replaced. If you have difficulty swallowing, you may be given fluids intravenously or through a tube. If you develop breathing difficulties, mechanical ventilation may be necessary (*see* **Intensive therapy unit**, p.618). While you are recovering, you may have physiotherapy (p.620) to help to maintain muscle tone.

What is the prognosis?

About 75 per cent of people with Guillain–Barré syndrome make a full recovery. Mild symptoms usually disappear in a few weeks, but severe symptoms may persist for months. About 20 per cent of people are left with some disability, such as residual numbness or weakness. In about 5 per cent of cases, the syndrome is fatal.

Nervous tics

Involuntary repeated contraction of one or more muscles

 More common in children

 More common in males

 Stress is a risk factor

 Genetics as a risk factor depends on the cause

Nervous tics occur when a muscle or a group of muscles controlled by peripheral nerves contracts repeatedly and involuntarily.

The condition most often affects the facial muscles, but sudden, uncontrolled movements of the limbs and sounds such as grunts and throat clearing can also occur. Typical nervous tics include repetitive blinking, mouth twitching, and shrugging. Tics are common, recurrent, and painless. However, they may result in self-consciousness and teasing by others. Nervous tics usually develop during childhood and occur more commonly in boys than girls.

Often, the cause is unknown, but tics may be associated with stress because they tend to occur when children are tired or upset. In Tourette's syndrome (p.348), a rare neurological disorder that occurs more frequently in boys, there may be involuntary movements of the head, arms, and legs and repetitive shouts, noises, grimaces, and spoken obscenities.

What are the symptoms?

A tic usually lasts only a fraction of a second. The muscle contraction may occur repeatedly and may cause:

■ Rapid, uncontrolled blinking.
■ Twitching of the muscles around the mouth.
■ Shrugging of the shoulders or jerking movements of the neck.
■ Involuntary contractions of the diaphragm, causing grunting or hiccups.

Nervous tics may be suppressed for a short period, but, in doing this, people often become more tense. When children are absorbed in an activity or asleep, tics usually disappear.

What might be done?

You should consult your doctor if you or your child has persistent nervous tics. Often, no treatment is necessary. In other cases, your doctor may suggest one or more psychological therapies (pp.622–624) to help to relieve stress. If symptoms are severe, your doctor may prescribe an antianxiety drug (p.591) for short periods of time. In some cases, tics produced by Tourette's syndrome can be controlled by medication.

Nervous tics, particularly those that occur in children, will usually disappear within about a year of the disorder first developing. However, in a few children, nervous tics tend to persist and continue in adulthood. Tourette's syndrome is a long-term condition for many people, although symptoms often diminish over time; in some cases, symptoms eventually disappear completely.

Mental health disorders

Few people hesitate to seek treatment for a physical illness, but many find it hard to accept that they may have a mental health problem. However, disorders such as depression, anxiety, and problems with alcohol and other drugs are common, increasingly understood, and treatable. No one needs to be embarrassed about a mental illness or feel that he or she must deal with it alone.

This section begins with anxiety disorders, which are among the most common mental health problems in the UK. Feeling worried is a natural reaction to problems and stress. However, persistent anxiety, often with no obvious cause, needs treatment to prevent it from becoming a long-term problem. Phobias, excessive fears of anything from spiders to confined spaces, can dominate many areas of a person's life. Other anxiety-related illnesses include post-traumatic stress disorder, a response to events such as serious accidents and natural disasters, and obsessive–compulsive disorder, in which uncontrollable thoughts – obsessions – cause anxiety, leading to urges to perform certain acts – compulsions – to relieve the anxiety.

Insomnia, a symptom of many mental illnesses, particularly anxiety and depression, is covered next. Depression, a very common disorder that affects an

estimated 1 in 3 people at some time in their lives, is described in the article that follows. It requires prompt treatment to relieve symptoms and prevent persistent feeling of despair, and possibly even suicide. The next article cover bipolar affective disorder, in which mood alternates between extreme highs and lows.

The common factor in the next group of disorders, which includes Munchausen's syndrome, somatization, and hypochondriasis, is the relationship between the mind and physical symptoms. Schizophrenia, a severe mental illness that may cause disturbed emotions and disordered thinking, delusional disorders, personality disorders, and Tourette's syndrome are also discussed.

The final articles deal with the eating disorders anorexia nervosa and bulimia, alcohol and drug dependence, and compulsive gambling.

Anxiety disorders

Intense apprehension that may or may not have an obvious cause

 Some types more common in females

 Some types run in families

 Stress is a risk factor

 Age as a risk factor depends on the type

Temporary feelings of nervousness or worry in stressful situations are natural and appropriate. However, when anxiety becomes a general response to many ordinary situations and causes problems in coping with normal everyday life, it is considered a disorder.

Anxiety disorders occur in a number of different forms. The most common is generalized anxiety disorder, characterized by excessive, persistent anxiety that is difficult to control. Another type of anxiety disorder is panic disorder, in which there are recurrent panic attacks of intense anxiety and alarming physical symptoms. These attacks occur unpredictably, usually have no obvious cause, and generate fear of further attacks. Panic attacks may also feature in generalized anxiety disorder. In another type of anxiety disorder known as phobia, severe anxiety is provoked by an irrational fear of a situation, activity, creature, or object (*see* **Phobias**, right).

Generalized anxiety disorder affects about 2–4 per cent of people every year in the UK. The condition usually begins in early adulthood and affects more women than men. Sometimes, anxiety disorders exist alongside other mental health disorders, such as depression (p.343) or schizophrenia (p.346).

What are the causes?
An increased susceptibility to anxiety disorders may be inherited or may be due to experiences in childhood. For example, poor bonding between a parent and child and abrupt separation of a child from a parent have been shown to play a part in some anxiety disorders. Generalized anxiety disorder may develop after a stressful life event, such as the death of a close relative. However, frequently the anxiety has no identifiable cause. Similarly, panic disorder often develops for no obvious reason.

What are the symptoms?
People with generalized anxiety disorder and panic disorder experience both physical and psychological symptoms. However, in generalized anxiety disorder, the psychological symptoms tend to be persistent while physical symptoms are intermittent. During panic attacks, psychological and physical symptoms develop together suddenly and unpredictably. The psychological symptoms of generalized anxiety disorder include:
- A sense of foreboding with no obvious reason or cause.
- Being on edge and unable to relax.
- Impaired concentration.

► **SELF-HELP**

Coping with a panic attack

Rapid breathing in a panic attack reduces carbon dioxide levels in the blood and may cause tingling in the fingers. You can control these symptoms by breathing through the mouth into a paper bag. By doing this, you rebreathe air with more carbon dioxide and restore the body's levels to normal.

Paper bag
The paper bag should be held tightly to the mouth

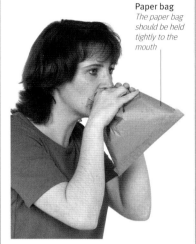

Rebreathing from a bag
Breathe in and out slowly into a paper bag about 10 times and then breathe normally for 15 seconds. Continue until you no longer need to breathe rapidly.

- Repetitive worrying thoughts.
- Disturbed sleep (*see* **Insomnia**, p.343) and, sometimes, nightmares.

In addition, you may have symptoms of depression, such as early waking or a general sense of hopelessness. Physical symptoms of the disorder, which occur intermittently, include:
- Headache.
- Abdominal cramps, sometimes with diarrhoea, and vomiting.
- Frequent passing of urine.
- Sweating, flushing, and tremor.
- A feeling of something being stuck in the throat.

Psychological and physical symptoms of panic attacks include the following:
- Shortness of breath.
- Sweating, trembling, and nausea.
- Palpitations (awareness of an abnormally rapid heartbeat).
- Dizziness and fainting.
- Fear of choking or that death may be imminent.
- A sense of unreality and fears about loss of sanity.

Many of these symptoms can be misinterpreted as signs of a serious physical illness, and this may increase your level of anxiety. Over time, fear of having a panic attack in public may lead you to avoid situations such as eating out in restaurants or being in crowds.

What might be done?
You may be able to reduce your anxiety levels yourself using methods such as relaxation exercises (p.32). If you are unable to deal with or identify a specific cause for your anxiety, you should consult your doctor. It is important to see a doctor as soon as possible after a first panic attack to prevent repeated attacks developing. There are several measures you can try to help to control an attack, such as breathing into a bag (*see* **Coping with a panic attack**, left). For any anxiety disorder, your doctor may suggest counselling (p.624) to help you to manage stress. You may also be offered cognitive–behavioural therapy (p.623) or behaviour therapy (p.622) to help you control anxiety. A self-help group may also be useful.

Your doctor may also prescribe various medications to help control symptoms. For example, antidepressants (p.592) may be useful in relieving the symptoms of anxiety and panic attacks whether or not depression is also present. If you are under particular stress, your doctor may prescribe a benzodiazepine drug (*see* **Antianxiety drugs**, p.591), but these drugs are usually prescribed for only a short time because of the danger of dependence. You may be prescribed beta-blocker drugs (p.581) to treat the physical symptoms of anxiety.

In most cases, the earlier anxiety disorders are treated, the quicker their effects can be reduced. Without treatment, an anxiety disorder may develop into a lifelong condition.

Phobias

Persistent and irrational fears of, and a compelling desire to avoid, particular objects, activities, or situations

 Most commonly develop from late childhood to early adulthood

 Gender and genetics as risk factors depend on the type

 Lifestyle is not a significant factor

Many people have particular fears, such as a fear of dogs or heights, that are upsetting occasionally but do not disrupt their everyday activities. A phobia is a fear or anxiety that has been carried to extremes. A person with a phobia has such a compelling desire to avoid contact with a feared object or situation that it interferes with normal life.

Being exposed to the subject of the phobia causes a panic reaction of severe anxiety, sweating, and a rapid heartbeat. A person with a phobia is aware that this intense fear is excessive or unreasonable but still feels anxiety that is alleviated only by avoiding the feared object or situation. This may disrupt routines and limit the person's capacity to take part in new experiences. About 1 in 10 people in the UK has a phobia. Phobias usually develop in late childhood, adolescence, or early adult life.

What are the types?

Phobias take many different forms, but they can be broadly divided into two types: simple and complex phobias.

Simple phobias Phobias specific to a single object, situation, or activity, such as a fear of spiders, heights, or air travel, are called simple phobias. For example, claustrophobia, a fear of enclosed spaces, is a simple phobia. A fear of blood is a common simple phobia that affects more men than women.

Complex phobias More complicated phobias that have a number of component fears are described as complex phobias. Agoraphobia is an example of a complex phobia that involves multiple anxieties. These fears may include being "looked at" when outdoors or being trapped in a public area with no exit to safety. The kind of situations that provoke agoraphobic anxiety include using public transport and lifts, and visiting crowded shops. Tactics to avoid these situations may disrupt work and social life, so that a person with severe agoraphobia may eventually become unable to leave the house. Agoraphobia occasionally develops in middle age and is more common in women.

Social phobias are also classified as complex phobias. People with a social phobia have an overwhelming fear of embarrassing themselves or of being humiliated in front of other people in social situations, such as when they are eating or speaking in public.

What are the causes?

Often, there is no reasonable explanation for the phobia, but occasionally a simple phobia can be traced to an earlier experience. For example, being trapped temporarily in a confined enclosed space during childhood may lead to claustrophobia in later life. Simple phobias appear to run in families, but this is thought to be because children "learn" rather than inherit their fear from a family member with a similar phobia.

The causes of complex phobias, such as agoraphobia and social phobia, are unclear, but they may develop from a tendency to be anxious. Agoraphobia sometimes develops after an unexplained panic attack. Some people recall a stressful situation as the trigger for their symptoms and then become conditioned to be anxious in similar circumstances. Most social phobias also begin with a sudden episode of intense anxiety in a social situation, which then becomes the main focus of the phobia.

What are the symptoms?

Exposure to or simply thinking about the object, creature, or situation that generates the phobia leads to intense anxiety accompanied by:

- Dizziness and feeling faint.
- Palpitations (awareness of an abnormally rapid heartbeat).
- Sweating and trembling.
- Nausea.
- Shortness of breath.

A factor that is common to every phobia is avoidance. Activities may become limited because of fear of unexpectedly encountering the subject of the phobia, and this may lead to depression (opposite page). Persistent anxiety and panic attacks (see **Anxiety disorders**, p.341) may develop. Sometimes, a person with a phobia attempts to relieve fear by drinking too much alcohol or abusing drugs.

What might be done?

If you have a phobia that interferes with your life, you should seek treatment. Many simple phobias can be treated effectively using a form of behaviour therapy (p.622), such as desensitization (see **Desensitization therapy**, p.623). During treatment, a therapist gives support while you are safely and gradually exposed to the object or situation that you fear. Inevitably, you will experience some anxiety, but exposure is always kept within bearable limits. In addition, you may be prescribed antidepressant drugs (p.592) as some are useful in the treatment of certain complex phobias.

Members of your family may be given guidance on how to help you cope with your phobic behaviour. You may benefit from contacting a self-help group.

What is the prognosis?

A simple phobia often resolves itself as a person gets older. However, complex phobias, such as social phobias and agoraphobia, tend to persist unless they are treated. More than 9 in 10 people with agoraphobia are treated successfully with desensitization therapy.

Post-traumatic stress disorder

A prolonged emotional response to an extreme personal experience

 Children and elderly people are at increased risk

 Women are at increased risk

 Genetics and lifestyle are not significant factors

Post-traumatic stress disorder (PTSD) occurs when a person is involved in a stressful event that triggers persistent intense emotions for some time afterwards. Experiencing an event in which life and personal safety are perceived to be at risk or simply witnessing a traumatic event is often enough to trigger the disorder. The kind of events that result in PTSD include natural disasters, accidents, and being assaulted.

About 1 in 10 people experiences PTSD. Children, elderly people, and women are more susceptible, as are people who have a history of anxiety or obsessional disorders.

▶ TREATMENT

EMDR

Eye movement desensitization and reprocessing – commonly known simply as EMDR – is a type of psychotherapy that was developed to treat the anxiety associated with post-traumatic stress disorder and other anxiety disorders, although it may also sometimes be used in the treatment of other mental health problems, such as depression. EMDR involves rhythmically moving your eyes – by tracking the therapist's back-and-forth finger movements, for example – while simultaneously recalling the anxiety-provoking event or trauma. In addition to moving your eyes from side to side, other forms of bilateral stimulation may also be used, such as sounds. The aim of the therapy is to break the link between your memories and anxiety symptoms.

What are the symptoms?

The symptoms of PTSD occur soon after the event or develop weeks, months, or, rarely, years later. They may include:

- Involuntary thoughts about and repeated reliving of the experience.
- Daytime flashbacks of the event.
- Panic attacks with symptoms such as shortness of breath and fainting.
- Avoidance of reminders of the event and refusal to discuss it.
- Sleep disturbance and nightmares.
- Poor concentration and irritability.

People with PTSD often feel emotionally "numb", detached from events, and estranged from family and friends. After a while, they may lose interest in their normal everyday activities. Other psychological disorders, such as anxiety (p.341) and depression (opposite page), may coexist with PTSD. Occasionally, the disorder leads to alcohol or drug abuse.

What might be done?

The doctor will assess the severity of symptoms and ask about the person's past mental health. Cognitive–behavioural therapy (p.623) has been found to be helpful, as has EMDR (eye movement desensitization and reprocessing). Support for the individual and family members is often an important part of treatment. Drugs such as antidepressants (p.592) may also be used. Although this approach often produces an improvement within about 8 weeks, drugs may need to be taken for at least a year. Often, most of the symptoms of PTSD disappear after a few months of treatment, but some symptoms may persist for years. Once a person has experienced PTSD, there is an increased likelihood of it recurring following another stressful event.

Obsessive–compulsive disorder

Uncontrollable thoughts that are often accompanied by irresistible urges to carry out acts or rituals to relieve anxiety

 Usually develops in adolescence

 Sometimes runs in families

 Stress is a risk factor

 Gender is not a significant factor

A person with obsessive–compulsive disorder (OCD) feels dominated by unwanted thoughts that enter the mind repeatedly. Obsessive thoughts are frequently accompanied by a form of compulsive ritual, in which a behaviour or action, such as checking that keys are still in a pocket, is repeated again and again. The affected person does not want to perform these actions but feels driven to do so to relieve the associated anxiety. Thoughts may be concerns about hygiene, personal safety, or security of possessions. Alternatively, there may be violent and obscene thoughts that are completely out of character. Examples of common compulsions include handwashing, checking that windows and doors are locked, and arranging objects on a desk in precise patterns. Carrying out the ritual brings short-lived relief, but, in severe cases, the ritual is performed hundreds of times a day and interferes with work and social life.

About 1 in 100 people in the UK has obsessive–compulsive disorder, which sometimes runs in families. Stressful life events may trigger the condition.

What are the symptoms?

An obsession or compulsion can focus on any object, event, or idea. The most common symptoms include:

- Intrusive, senseless thoughts or mental images.
- Repeated attempts to resist thoughts.
- Repetitive behaviour in the attempt to relieve anxiety.

The person may be aware that the behaviour is irrational and be distressed by it but cannot control these symptoms.

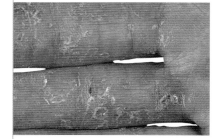

Effects of compulsive handwashing
Repeated handwashing by a person with obsessive–compulsive disorder has made the skin of the hands raw and chapped.

▶ **TEST**

Psychological assessment

To help diagnose a mental health disorder, your doctor may arrange for you to have a psychological assessment. You will be asked a series of questions to establish the nature of your problem and its effects on your life. Areas of discussion include your family, your history, how life was before you became ill, and any factors that might have triggered the mental health problem, such as a bereavement.

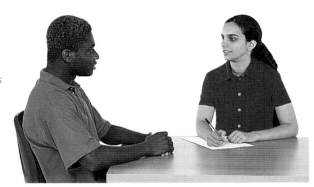

Having an assessment
Although questions are intimate and personal, they are part of a standard assessment procedure. The doctor usually records answers on a checklist.

What might be done?

Your doctor will probably be able to diagnose obsessive–compulsive disorder from your symptoms. To help reduce the severity of your symptoms, your doctor may suggest treatment with a form of psychotherapy, such as cognitive–behavioural therapy (p.623). He or she may prescribe an antidepressant drug (p.592) because drugs combined with psychotherapy usually offer the best chance of success. Initially, therapy may make your anxiety, thoughts, and compulsion to perform rituals worse, but, given time, it may help you to feel more in control of your thoughts as well as your compulsive urges.

As part of your treatment, you may want to involve a family member or friend to encourage you. You should also try to identify stress factors that may contribute to your condition and seek ways to reduce them. Many people find joining a self-help group is beneficial.

More than 7 in 10 people begin to improve within a year of starting treatment. Other people have a long-term illness that fluctuates in severity.

Insomnia

A regular inability to fall asleep or stay asleep, leading to excessive tiredness

 More common in elderly people

 More common in females

 Stress and a high intake of caffeine or alcohol are risk factors

 Genetics is not a significant factor

At some point in their lives, about 1 in 3 people has regular difficulty in sleeping, known as insomnia. Problems include difficulty in falling asleep, and waking during the night and being unable to get back to sleep. Insomnia is distressing and may lead to excessive tiredness, a general inability to cope, and a greater risk of accidents. Sleep problems are more common in women and in elderly people of both sexes.

Sleeping difficulties most commonly start when a person is worried or anxious. A high intake of caffeine or alcohol during the day may also lead to sleeplessness. Often, not sleeping properly then becomes persistent because good sleep habits are lost. Insomnia may be caused by an illness with symptoms that cause problems at night, such as asthma (p.295), the metabolic disorder hyperthyroidism (p.432), or other sleep disorders such as sleep apnoea (p.292). Insomnia is often associated with mental health problems such as depression (right) and anxiety disorders (p.341).

What might be done?

Your doctor will first treat any physical and mental problems that may be causing your insomnia. For example, if you are depressed, an antidepressant drug (p.592) may be prescribed. If there is no obvious cause, your doctor may arrange for you to be assessed during sleep at a sleep clinic. Tests often show that many people sleep more hours than they think they do but wake frequently. Reassurance that you are getting sufficient sleep may be all you need.

Your doctor may suggest changes to your lifestyle, such as exercising or reducing caffeinated drinks (*see* **Sleep**, p.31). You may be advised to avoid taking daytime naps because they reduce the need for sleep at night. Rarely, the doctor may prescribe sleeping drugs (p.591) for a few days to help to restore a normal sleep pattern. These drugs should not be taken for a longer time because of the risk of dependence.

Depression

Feelings of sadness, often accompanied by loss of interest in life and reduced energy

 More common from the late 30s onwards

 More common in females

 Sometimes runs in families

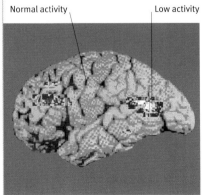 Social isolation is a risk factor

Sadness is an expected reaction to adversity or personal misfortune and may last for a considerable time. Depression exists when feelings of unhappiness intensify and daily life becomes difficult. Depression is one of the most common mental health disorders in the UK. It affects about 1 in 5 people at some time in life, most commonly from the late 30s onwards. Women are twice as likely to have depression as men. In some cases, the disorder lifts spontaneously after days or weeks, but other people may need professional help and support. In severe cases, hospital admission may be necessary to protect a person from neglect or self-harm.

Depression is often accompanied by symptoms of anxiety (*see* **Anxiety disorders**, p.341). For example, there may be a

Normal activity   Low activity

BRAIN OF NORMAL PERSON

Normal activity   Low activity

BRAIN OF DEPRESSED PERSON

Reduced brain activity in depression
These images show large areas of low activity in the brain of a depressed person compared with small areas of low activity in the brain of a normal person.

persistent sense of foreboding and repetitive, worrying thoughts. People with depression may also misuse alcohol or other drugs.

What are the causes?

Depression may develop when a person has to face one or more stressful life events. The trigger is often some form of loss, such as the breakdown of a close relationship or a bereavement.

A traumatic experience in childhood, such as abuse or the death of a parent, may increase susceptibility to depression later on. A tendency towards the disorder may also run in families.

Several physical illnesses may cause depression. These include some infections, such as infectious mononucleosis (p.166); neurological disorders, such as Parkinson's disease (p.333); and hormonal disorders, such as Cushing's syndrome (p.435). Hormonal changes at the menopause or after childbirth may also trigger the disorder (*see* **Depression after childbirth**, p.521).

A number of mental health disorders may lead to depression. They include phobias (p.341), the eating disorder anorexia nervosa (p.348), alcohol dependence (p.350), and drug dependence (p.349). Some people feel generally low and become depressed only during the winter months, a condition known as seasonal affective disorder. Depression can also be a side effect of certain drugs, such as oral contraceptives and beta-blockers (p.581). However, often depression has no identifiable cause.

What are the symptoms?

A typical sign of depression is a feeling of sadness, even misery, that is worse in the morning and lasts for most of the day. Other common symptoms include:

- Loss of interest in and enjoyment of work and leisure activities.
- Diminished energy levels.
- Poor concentration.
- Reduced self-esteem.
- Feelings of guilt.
- Tearfulness.
- Inability to make decisions.
- Early waking and inability to resume sleep (*see* **Insomnia**, left) or an excessive need to sleep.
- Loss of hope for the future.
- Recurrent thoughts of death.
- Weight loss or increase in weight.
- Decreased sex drive (p.494).

In an elderly person, other symptoms may occur, including confusion, forgetfulness, and personality changes, that may be mistakenly attributed to dementia (p.331). Neglect of personal hygiene and diet in an elderly person may also be an indication of underlying depression. Sometimes, depressive illness manifests itself as a physical symptom, such as tiredness (*see* **Somatization**, p.346), or may cause associated physical problems, such as constipation or headache.

Recovering from depression

There are a number of strategies that help you to rebuild your self-confidence and regain control of your life while you are recovering from depression. Try to plan your day so that any potentially difficult tasks become easier to deal with, and practice relaxation techniques on a regular basis. You might like to try some of the following ideas:

- Make a list of things that you have to do each day, beginning with the most important.
- Tackle one task at a time, and reflect on what you have achieved when each is done.
- Set aside a few minutes each day to relax by breathing deeply or stretching (*see* **Relaxation exercises**, p.32).
- Exercise regularly to help to reduce feelings of stress (*see* **The benefits of exercise**, p.20).
- Eat a healthy diet (p.17).
- Take up a pastime or hobby that distracts you from worries.
- Join a support group where you can meet other people who have had similar experiences.

Severely depressed people may see or hear things that are not there. Irrational delusions may also occur. For instance, a depressed person may become convinced that his or her partner is having a sexual relationship with someone else.

Depression may also alternate with periods of euphoria in a person who has manic depression (*see* **Bipolar affective disorder**, right).

Are there complications?
Rarely, if the condition is not treated, a depressive stupor may develop, in which speech and movement are greatly reduced. Left untreated, depression can delay recovery from a physical illness and intensify pain whatever the cause, which then increases the depression. A person who is severely depressed may contemplate or attempt suicide (*see* **Attempted suicide and suicide**, right).

What might be done?
If your depression is mild, your symptoms may disappear spontaneously if you are given sympathy and support from those close to you.

However, if you do need help for depression, it can almost always be treated effectively, and you should not put off seeing your doctor if you continue to feel low. He or she may examine you and arrange for blood tests to make sure that your low energy levels and mood are not caused by a physical illness. You may be asked to have a psychological assessment (p.343) in case there are other mental health problems that may be causing or contributing to your depression.

If depression is diagnosed, you may be treated with drugs, a psychological therapy such as cognitive–behavioural therapy (p.623), or therapy and drugs. Rarely, severe cases are treated with electroconvulsive therapy.

Drug treatments The doctor usually prescribes a course of antidepressant drugs (p.592). There are several different types, and your doctor will choose the one most suitable for your needs. Although some have undesirable side effects, other side effects may be useful. For example, an antidepressant drug that is mildly sedating may relieve a sleeping problem. Your mood usually improves after you have been taking an antidepressant for 2–4 weeks, although some symptoms may improve more quickly. If your depression shows little improvement after a month or if you have troublesome side effects from your treatment, your doctor may adjust the dosage or prescribe an alternative drug. Once your depression has lifted, you should continue taking antidepressants for as long as your doctor suggests. Treatment usually lasts for at least 6 months, but the length of time depends on the severity of the depressive symptoms and whether you have ever had any previous episodes of depression. Depression may recur if antidepressant drugs are stopped too soon.

Psychological treatments Support from your doctor or other health professionals is essential while you are depressed. Your doctor may refer you to a therapist for treatments such as cognitive–behavioural therapy (p.623) to help you to change negative patterns of thinking or psychoanalytic-based psychotherapy (p.622) to look into the reasons for your depression. Counselling (p.624), either on an individual basis or as part of a group, may help you to identify your feelings and make sense of them.

Electroconvulsive therapy In rare cases, treatment with electroconvulsive therapy (ECT) is given for severe depression. In this procedure, which is carried out under general anaesthesia, an electrical stimulus that causes a brief seizure in the brain is given by placing two electrodes on the head. Between 6 and 12 treatments may be given over a period of about 1 month. ECT is particularly useful for treating depression that is accompanied by delusions. After treatment, antidepressants are given for at least a few months to prevent relapse.

What is the prognosis?
Antidepressants are effective in treating about 3 in 4 people with depression. When drug treatments and psychological therapy are used in combination, the symptoms of depression can often be relieved completely in 2–3 months. Of the small number of people who are treated with ECT, about 9 in 10 make a successful recovery. However, for some people, depression can last for years or recur with no obvious trigger.

Attempted suicide and suicide

An attempt to end one's life that may have a nonfatal or fatal outcome

 More young people attempt suicide, but more elderly people die from an attempt

 More females attempt suicide, but more males die from an attempt

 Family history of suicide or attempted suicide may increase the risk

Social isolation and living in urban areas are risk factors

Most people who attempt suicide are in their teens or are elderly. Among those who attempt suicide, some are certain that they wish to die while others use the attempt to signal their desperation rather than end their lives. More than half of all suicides and suicide attempts involve a drug overdose (*see* **Drug overdose and accidental ingestion**, p.185), most commonly of a painkiller (p.589) such as paracetamol.

The suicide rate in the UK in 2013 was about 19 per 100,000 for men and 5 per 100,000 for women. About 6,230 deaths were attributed to suicide in 2013, but the exact number of suicides is unknown because some are recorded as deaths from other causes. It is estimated that more than 140,000 people each year attempt suicide, and women are about three times more likely than men to make a suicide attempt. However, men are four times more likely to die as a result of a suicide attempt because they use methods, such as hanging, that have a greater potential to kill.

What are the causes?
The majority of suicides in people of all ages are associated with an underlying mental health disorder. About half of all suicide attempts are a consequence of depression (p.343) or bipolar affective disorder (right).

Teenage suicide attempts are often impulsive and may follow family quarrels or the breakup of a relationship. These attempts rarely indicate a wish to die, but a fatal dose of tablets may be taken by mistake. Suicide in elderly people is often the result of depression caused by bereavement and loneliness. Incurable physical illnesses lead to an estimated 1 in 5 suicides of people over the age of 65.

Other mental health disorders associated with suicide are schizophrenia (p.346), drug dependence (p.349), and alcohol dependence (p.350).

What might be done?
If suicide has been attempted, admission to hospital is usually necessary for assessment and treatment. In the case of an overdose, as much of the ingested substance as possible is removed from the body to prevent it from being absorbed. If the substance is

identifiable, an antidote will be given if there is one available. Any physical effects of an attempted suicide, such as cuts to the wrists, are treated appropriately.

Treatment for underlying psychiatric problems is particularly important to prevent future suicide attempts. Drugs such as antidepressants (p.592) may be prescribed, and a form of psychotherapy or counselling (*see* **Psychological therapies**, pp.622–624) may be recommended. Any problems that may have precipitated the suicide attempt will be identified and, if possible, help offered to resolve them. After a first attempt, there is an increased risk of future ones.

Can it be prevented?
Some people talk about their wish to kill themselves before they attempt suicide, and these threats should be taken seriously. Family and friends should try to remove any available means and seek professional help urgently. If there is a high risk of suicide, it may be necessary to admit the person to hospital, with, or possibly without, his or her consent.

After a suicide attempt, treatment for any underlying mental health problems and family support and vigilance may prevent further attempts. However, a person who has a strong desire to die may try to prevent discovery during an attempt and is more likely to choose a method that will prove fatal.

Bipolar affective disorder

A disorder in which mood fluctuates between extremes of highs and lows

 Usually develops in the early 20s

 Often runs in families

 Life events may trigger episodes

 Gender is not a significant factor

About 1 in 100 people in the UK has bipolar affective disorder, also known as manic depression. In this disorder, episodes of elation and abnormally high activity levels (mania) tend to alternate with episodes of low mood and abnormally low energy levels (depression). More than half of all people with bipolar affective disorder have repeated episodes. The factors that trigger manic and depressive episodes are not generally known, although episodes are sometimes brought on in response to a major life event, such as a marital breakup or bereavement. Bipolar affective disorder usually develops in the early 20s and can run in families, but exactly how it is inherited is not known.

What are the symptoms?
Symptoms of mania and depression tend to alternate, each episode lasting an unpredictable length of time. Between periods of mania

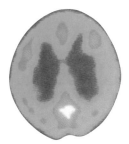

BRAIN IN NORMAL PERIODS

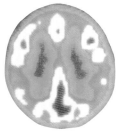

BRAIN IN MANIC PHASE

Increased brain activity in bipolar affective disorder
These PET scans of the brain of a person with bipolar affective disorder show high levels of activity during a manic episode.

and depression, mood and behaviour are generally normal. However, occasionally, a manic phase may be followed immediately by depression. Sometimes, either depression or mania predominates to the extent that there is little evidence of a pattern of changing moods. Occasionally, symptoms of depression and mania occur in the same period. The symptoms of a manic episode may include:

■ Elated, expansive, or sometimes irritable mood.
■ Inflated self-esteem, which may lead to delusions of great wealth, accomplishment, creativity, and power.
■ Increased energy levels and decreased need for sleep.
■ Distraction and poor concentration.
■ Loss of social inhibitions.
■ Unrestrained sexual behaviour.
■ Spending excessive sums of money on luxuries and holidays.

Speech may be difficult to follow because the person tends to speak rapidly and change topic frequently. At times, he or she may be aggressive or violent and may neglect diet and personal hygiene.

During an episode of depression, the main symptoms include:

■ Feeling generally low.
■ Loss of interest and enjoyment.
■ Diminished energy level.
■ Reduced self-esteem.
■ Loss of hope for the future.

While severely depressed, a person affected by the disorder may not care whether he or she lives or dies. About 1 in 10 people with bipolar disorder eventually attempts suicide (*see* **Attempted suicide and suicide**, opposite page).

In severe cases of bipolar affective disorder, delusions of power during manic episodes may be made worse by hallucinations.

When manic, the person may hear imaginary voices praising his or her qualities; in the depressive phase, these voices may describe the person's failures. In such cases, the disorder may resemble schizophrenia (p.346).

What might be done?
During a manic phase, people usually lack insight into their condition and may not be aware that they are ill. Often, a person's erratic behaviour is first noticed by a relative or friend, who seeks professional advice. A diagnosis of bipolar affective disorder is based on the full range of the person's symptoms, and treatment will depend on whether the person is in a manic or a depressive phase. For the depressive phase, antidepressants (p.592) are used, but their effects have to be monitored to ensure that they do not precipitate a manic phase. During the first days or weeks of a manic phase, symptoms may be controlled initially by antipsychotic drugs (p.592). During both phases, treatment with a mood-stabilizing drug (p.593), such as lithium, may be started for longer-term symptom control. Some people may need to be admitted to hospital for assessment and treatment during a manic phase or a severe depressive phase. They may feel creative and energetic when manic and may be reluctant to accept long-term medication because it makes them feel "flat".

Most people make a recovery from manic–depressive episodes, but recurrences are common. For this reason, initial treatments for depression and mania may be augmented with lithium, which has to be taken continuously to prevent relapse. If lithium is not fully effective, other drugs, such as certain anticonvulsants (p.590), may be given. In severe cases, in which drugs have no effect, electroconvulsive therapy (ECT) may be used to relieve symptoms by inducing a brief seizure in the brain under a general anaesthetic.

Once symptoms are under control, the person will need regular checkups to look for signs of mood changes. A form of psychotherapy (*see* **Psychological therapies**, pp.622–624) may help the person develop an insight into their disorder and reduce stress factors in his or her life that may contribute to it

Mental problems due to physical illness

One or more psychological conditions resulting from a physical illness

 Unsettled domestic or financial circumstances are risk factors

 Age, gender, and genetics are not significant factors

Changes in mental state are a common response to a physical illness. A serious physical illness may cause anxiety (*see* **Anxiety disorders**, p.341), depression

(p.343), anger, or denial of the problem. Usually, reactions are transient and disappear when the person adjusts to the change in his or her physical condition. However, illnesses that may be fatal or long-term disorders that involve lengthy treatment or continued disability may cause persistent mood problems. People who have had previous psychiatric disorders are more at risk, as are people who are under additional stress, such as from an unstable home life or financial problems, or those who find it hard to deal with adversity.

Mood problems are sometimes a recognized symptom of a physical illness. For example, anxiety is a symptom of the hormonal disorder hyperthyroidism (p.432), and depression is associated with strokes (p.329), multiple sclerosis (p.334), and also Parkinson's disease (*see* **Parkinson's disease and parkinsonism**, p.333).

What are the symptoms?
The psychological symptoms that may result from a physical illness include:

■ Feelings of anxiety, ranging from mild apprehension to fear and panic.
■ Depressive symptoms, such as a sense of hopelessness and worthlessness.
■ Irritability and anger.

In extreme cases, there may be social withdrawal and drug or alcohol abuse.

What might be done?
If your doctor thinks you are at risk of developing a psychological problem as a result of illness, you will be offered support and counselling (p.624) to help you adjust. If there are signs that you are avoiding coming to terms with an illness, your doctor will encourage you to ask questions and talk about possible anxieties. Home and work problems may be discussed, and your doctor will want to know if you have a history of depression or anxiety disorders.

A person who has developed psychological problems as a result of illness may not be aware of the fact, and a family member or friend may first contact the doctor on his or her behalf. The doctor may prescribe antidepressant drugs (p.592). Less commonly, an antianxiety drug (p.591) may be given for a short time. The person may be referred to a psychologist, who will encourage a problem-solving approach to illness that concentrates on seeking solutions rather than focusing on difficulties.

The outlook for a mental problem resulting from physical illness depends on how well the person develops an ability to cope with the demands of his or her illness. Given continued support, most people are able to recognize and deal with mood problems, which gradually diminish as a result.

Munchausen's syndrome

A condition in which medical care is sought repeatedly for nonexistent or self-induced symptoms

 Usually begins in early adulthood

 More common in males

 Working in a health-related profession is a risk factor

 Genetics is not a significant factor

Munchausen's syndrome is a rare condition in which a person claims to have symptoms of illness, such as abdominal pain, blackouts, or fever, and may repeatedly seek treatment from a number of hospitals. This unexplained desire to assume the role of a patient is seen as an attempt to escape from everyday life and be cared for and protected.

The syndrome usually develops in early adulthood and is more common in men. Those affected tend to have some knowledge of symptoms and hospital procedures, which may have been acquired through working in a health-related profession. For this reason, their bogus claims to illness may be taken seriously until test results prove negative or exploratory surgery is carried out. People with the disorder tend to conceal personal details or give extraordinary accounts of their circumstances. If challenged, they may accuse doctors of incompetence and leave the hospital.

In factitious disorder, a variant of Munchausen's syndrome, a person aggravates an existing condition or causes deliberate self-injury. The disorder occurs

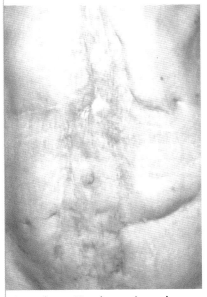

Scars due to Munchausen's syndrome
The numerous scars on the abdomen of this person with Munchausen's syndrome are the result of multiple operations to investigate fictitious symptoms.

most often in health professionals. In another related condition, Munchausen's syndrome by proxy, a parent, often the mother, repeatedly claims her child is ill and in need of treatment.

What are the symptoms?

Munchausen's syndrome and factitious disorder have similar typical patterns of behaviour, which may include:
- Dramatic presentation of symptoms and their history.
- Histrionic and argumentative behaviour towards medical staff.
- Wide knowledge of medical terms and medical procedures.

There may be evidence of multiple surgical operations, such as a number of scars on the abdomen. An affected person may demand strong painkillers, possibly because he or she has an addiction. In Munchausen's syndrome by proxy, the parent may fake physical signs of illness in a child and give a false description of symptoms. The child may be repeatedly admitted to hospital for unnecessary tests or treatment.

What might be done?

Treatment is difficult because as soon as staff begin to suspect that a person is feigning symptoms, he or she may leave the hospital to avoid being discovered. Munchausen's syndrome may be identified only with hindsight.

It is often difficult to treat Munchausen's syndrome and related conditions because deception is a characteristic of the disorders. The doctor may try to prevent further unnecessary treatments and tests by building a calm and supportive relationship with the person. In cases of Munchausen's syndrome by proxy, a social worker should be alerted in case a child needs to be placed in care.

Somatization

The expression of psychological problems as physical symptoms

 Usually develops in adolescence or early adulthood

 More common in females

 Stress is a risk factor

Genetics is not a significant factor

Somatization describes a process in which a psychological problem manifests itself as a physical symptom or a range of physical symptoms. Although occasionally bizarre, these symptoms are not fabricated and may be frightening if they are interpreted as signs of a progressive or potentially fatal disease. The condition is related to hypochondriasis (right), a condition in which there are constant, unfounded worries that minor

symptoms are caused by a serious underlying disorder. However, in somatization, psychological problems generate actual physical changes, which cause debilitating symptoms.

People with somatization may make repeated visits to their doctor to ask for investigations into their symptoms and treatment. When test results are normal, and reassurance is given that there is no underlying physical illness, an affected person feels no relief and may consult other doctors to find a physical cause for the symptoms. In extreme cases of somatization, life is continually disrupted by numerous follow-up medical appointments, and health is placed at risk by invasive tests and investigations.

Several psychiatric illnesses may be associated with somatization, including anxiety disorders (p.341) and depression (p.343). Some people may be unable to express their emotions and may use somatic symptoms and complaints to express their emotional state. Somatization usually develops in adolescence or early in adult life and may become a lifelong problem. It is more common in women and is associated with stress.

What are the symptoms?

A person who has a somatization disorder may have a long history of varying physical symptoms that fluctuate in severity and have no identifiable medical cause. Symptoms that sometimes have psychological causes include:
- Headaches.
- Chest pain, often accompanied by shortness of breath and palpitations.
- Abdominal pain and nausea.
- Tiredness.
- Itching of the skin.
- Partial weakness of a limb.
- Difficulty in swallowing.

In addition, there may be psychological symptoms of anxiety, depression, and substance abuse. Severely affected people may attempt suicide (*see* **Attempted suicide and suicide**, p.344).

What might be done?

The doctor will first carry out a physical examination and may arrange for blood and urine tests to exclude a physical illness. Medical records will give a picture of past symptoms and investigations.

Treating somatization is often difficult because the affected person may be convinced there is a physical illness in spite of normal test results. The doctor may prescribe treatment for symptoms, such as painkillers (p.589) for headaches, but will try to avoid further tests and investigations by offering reassurance that physical symptoms are taken seriously and explaining how they may be caused by psychological problems.

The doctor may recommend a psychological assessment (p.343) to look for an underlying mental health disorder, but this

may be resisted by the person. Cognitive–behavioural therapy (p.623) and behaviour therapy (p.622) can be particularly helpful for some people.

If depression is causing somatization, it may be treated with antidepressant drugs (p.592) and a form of psychological therapy (pp.622–624).

Hypochondriasis

A morbid preoccupation with one's state of health

 Most common between the ages of 20 and 30

 Long-term illness in childhood, close contact with people who are seriously ill, and stress are risk factors

 Gender and genetics are not significant factors

People who suffer from hypochondriasis are constantly anxious about their health and interpret all symptoms, no matter how minor, as indications of serious illness. They may be concerned about a combination of symptoms or a single symptom, such as a headache.

Inevitably, the disorder leads to frequent visits to the doctor to have tests. Even when the results are negative, people affected by hypochondriasis remain convinced that they are seriously ill. They may reject the doctor's findings and react with strong feelings of frustration and hostility. Frequently, their anxiety about illness causes problems with relationships, work, and social life.

Somatization (left) is a related condition in which psychological problems are expressed as physical symptoms.

Hypochondriasis is most common between the ages of 20 and 30 and may be a complication of other psychological disorders, such as depression (p.343) or anxiety (*see* **Anxiety disorders**, p.341). Often, the cause is unknown, but people who were very ill in childhood or who have prolonged contact with someone with a long-term illness are more susceptible. Stress increases the risk of the disorder developing.

What might be done?

The doctor will first look for and treat any underlying psychological disorders. For example, he or she may prescribe antidepressant drugs (p.592) for depression. The doctor will avoid unnecessary tests by reassuring the person that he or she does not have a serious illness and will explain normal body reactions if the person is mistaking responses, such as rapid heartbeats during exercise, for signs of serious illness. In some people, cognitive–behavioural therapy (p.623) and behaviour therapy (p.622) can be helpful.

Schizophrenia

A serious mental disorder in which there are disturbed emotions, disorganized thinking, and an inability to function socially

 Usually develops in males aged 15–25 and females aged 25–35

 Sometimes runs in families

 Stressful life events are risk factors

 Gender is not a significant factor

Schizophrenia is a severe and disruptive mental illness that occurs in all cultures and affects about 1 in 100 people worldwide. Although the term is sometimes used mistakenly to refer to a split personality, schizophrenia is actually an impairment of a person's sense of reality that leads to irrational behaviour and disturbed emotional reactions. People with schizophrenia may hear voices, and this may contribute to their bizarre behaviour. In addition, they are often unable to function at work and sometimes have difficulty maintaining relationships with other people. Without proper support and treatment, people with schizophrenia are likely to neglect or harm themselves. About 1 in 10 people with the condition commits suicide (*see* **Attempted suicide and suicide**, p.344).

What are the causes?

No single cause of schizophrenia has been identified, but genetic factors are known to play a major part. A person who is closely related to someone with schizophrenia has a significantly increased risk of developing the disorder. In addition, a stressful life event, such as a serious illness or a bereavement, may trigger the disorder in a person who is susceptible. Evidence also points to abnormalities in brain structure, such as enlarged fluid-filled cavities that suggest loss of brain tissue.

What are the symptoms?

Schizophrenia tends to develop in men during their teens or early 20s, but the onset in women may be 10–20 years later. The condition usually develops gradually, with the person losing energy and personal motivation and becoming increasingly withdrawn over a period of months or years. In other cases, the illness is more sudden and may be a response to an episode of stress. Some people have clear-cut episodes of illness and recover completely in between. In other cases, the disorder is more or less continuous. Symptoms may include:
- Hearing hallucinatory voices.
- Having irrational beliefs, in particular that thoughts and actions are being controlled by an outside force.
- Delusions of persecution or a conviction that trivial objects and events have deep significance.

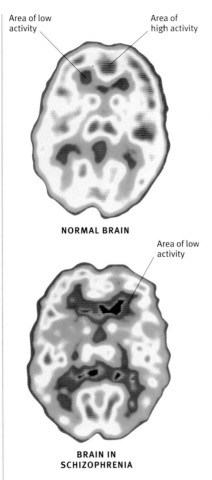

Area of low activity

Area of high activity

NORMAL BRAIN

Area of low activity

BRAIN IN SCHIZOPHRENIA

Brain activity in schizophrenia
PET scans show a distinctive pattern of large areas of low activity in the brain of a person with schizophrenia when compared with the brain of an unaffected person.

- Expression of inappropriate emotions, such as laughing at bad news.
- Rambling speech with rapid switching from one topic to another.
- Impaired concentration.
- Disordered thoughts.
- Agitation and restlessness.

A person with schizophrenia may be depressed, lethargic, and socially withdrawn. He or she may begin to neglect personal care and become increasingly isolated. In some cases, alcohol or drug abuse may occur.

How is it diagnosed?
If you are concerned that a close friend or family member may be suffering from schizophrenia, you should contact a doctor. Normally, the doctor will carry out a detailed assessment of the person's symptoms to look for evidence of a profound break with reality suggestive of a diagnosis of schizophrenia. He or she will also carry out a full physical examination, and blood or urine tests may be arranged to exclude other possible causes of abnormal behaviour, such as alcohol or drug abuse. The doctor may arrange for imaging of the brain by CT scanning (p.132) or MRI (p.133) to exclude an underlying physical disorder, such as a brain tumour (p.327).

What is the treatment?
If schizophrenia is suspected, it may be necessary to admit the person to hospital for further assessment and to begin treatment. Antipsychotic drugs (p.592) are prescribed to help to calm the affected person and control symptoms such as hallucinations and delusions. Up to 6 weeks of treatment may be needed to reduce the more obvious symptoms of schizophrenia. Some drugs may cause serious side effects, such as tremors, and doses may have to be reduced or other drugs prescribed to minimize these effects. Treatment with adjusted doses of drugs usually continues after symptoms have subsided.

After assessment and treatment, people with schizophrenia are usually sent home, but it is essential that they have support and a calm and unthreatening home environment. People who have schizophrenia need to be protected from stressful situations because anxiety may trigger symptoms. They also need frequent, regular contact with community mental health service workers, who will supervise their progress and wellbeing.

Counselling (p.624) may be offered both to the person with schizophrenia and to family members. People close to the affected person should watch for signs of relapse and indications that the person is sinking into a general state of apathy and self-neglect.

What is the prognosis?
For most affected people, schizophrenia is a long-term illness. However, about 1 in 5 of those affected have one sudden episode from which they recover and lead a normal life. The majority have a number of episodes of severe symptoms that may require hospital stays, interspersed with periods of recovery. Drugs have improved the outlook for people with schizophrenia, but adequate community care and support is essential to prevent relapse. The outlook is worse for people who develop schizophrenia gradually while they are young.

Delusional disorders

The development of one or more persistent delusions of persecution or jealousy

 More common over the age of 40

 More common in females

 Stress may be a risk factor

 Genetics is not a significant factor

Delusional disorders are rare, affecting only about 3 in 10,000 people worldwide. The main characteristic of these disorders is an irrational belief or set of beliefs that is not associated with other symptoms or caused by another mental illness, such as schizophrenia (opposite page). These beliefs or delusions persist in spite

of all rational arguments and evidence to the contrary. However, apart from behaviour related to the delusion, the person appears well, and work and relationships may not be affected.

There are several types of delusion, the most common of which is persecutory. People with this type of delusion believe they are being hounded or that somebody is trying to harm them. Extreme jealousy, in which a person has the unreasonable belief that his or her partner is unfaithful, is a common form.

Major life events, such as moving to another country, and long-term stress factors, such as poverty, may contribute to the development of delusions. A person who has a paranoid personality (*see* **Personality disorders**, below) is at an increased risk of delusions, as is a person who is alcohol dependent (p.350).

Delusional disorders usually develop insidiously, most often in middle age or late in life, and tend to occur more commonly in women than in men.

What might be done?
People with a delusional disorder are often suspicious or dismissive of others who are trying to help them. They may be reluctant to discuss their beliefs and unable to recognize that their delusions are irrational. Family members often seek medical advice on their behalf.

The doctor will look for additional symptoms in case delusions are being caused by another psychological illness, such as schizophrenia. The doctor will try to find out how firmly held or "fixed" the delusions are and whether the person is likely to act on them. If there is a risk of violence or self-harm, the person may need to be admitted to hospital, possibly without his or her consent.

Occasionally, an antipsychotic drug (p.592) is used to reduce the intensity of severe delusions. Counselling (p.624) may bring about a shift in perspective. Generally, delusional disorders tend to persist but without causing major disruption, although delusions of jealousy may pose a risk of violence to a partner.

Personality disorders

A group of disorders in which habitual patterns of thought and behaviour cause persistent life problems

 Develop in adolescence or early adulthood

 Gender, genetics, and lifestyle as risk factors depend on the type

People with personality disorders have ingrained patterns of thought and behaviour that prevent them from fitting in with society. Affected people often fail to see that their personality is causing distress to themselves or others. Although many

people have strong personalities, this is not the same as a personality disorder. People with personality disorders are inflexible and unable to adapt.

Personality disorders tend to develop in adolescence and early adulthood but may not be properly diagnosed until later in life. The cause of most of these disorders is unknown, although genetic influences and childhood experiences are thought to play a role in many cases.

What are the types?
Personality disorders are divided into three broad groups: emotional or erratic, eccentric or odd, and anxious or fearful. Each group has its own pattern of thought processes and behaviour, although they may often overlap.

Emotional or erratic This personality disorder further divides into four different types: antisocial, borderline, histrionic, and narcissistic.

An antisocial personality is typified by impulsive, destructive behaviour that often disregards the feelings and rights of others. A person with this disorder lacks a sense of guilt and cannot tolerate frustration. He or she will have problems with relationships and may often be in trouble with the law.

A person with a borderline personality has multiple abnormalities that may include an uncertainty about personal identity and an inability to form stable relationships. People with this disorder describe feelings of emptiness and may indulge in promiscuity, reckless spending, or substance abuse. They may self-harm or threaten suicide.

People with a histrionic personality have emotions that are exaggerated but shallow. They are self-centred, inconsiderate, and easily bored and constantly seek reassurance and approval.

People with a narcissistic personality believe themselves to be unique, special, and superior to others. They constantly seek attention and admiration and lack concern for the problems of others.

Eccentric or odd This group can be divided into three types of personality: paranoid, schizoid, and schizotypal.

A person with a paranoid personality tends to be mistrustful, jealous, and self-important. He or she readily interprets other people's actions as hostile and may feel continually rebuffed.

People who have a schizoid personality are emotionally cold and indifferent to others. They tend to be prone to fantasy and ill at ease in company. This disorder is not related to the mental illness schizophrenia (opposite page).

People with a schizotypal personality display eccentric and suspicious behaviour, often accompanied by odd ideas, such as a belief in magic or telepathy. They may have an unkempt appearance and vague, abstract speech patterns and may talk to themselves.

Anxious or fearful The four different types of personality that make up the anxious or fearful group of disorders are: avoidant, passive–aggressive, obsessive–compulsive, and dependent.

A person with an avoidant personality is timid, oversensitive to rejection, and cautious of new experiences and responsibilities. He or she is generally ill at ease in social situations.

People with a passive–aggressive personality react to any demands made on them by being stubborn and argumentative. They put off tasks at work and at home and may be deliberately inefficient and critical of people in authority.

An obsessive–compulsive personality is marked by a continual striving for perfection with limited regard for the feelings of other people. Generally, people with this disorder are inflexible, pedantic, and overly conscientious.

People with a dependent personality seem weak-willed and submissive. They appear helpless, lack self-reliance, and leave decisions to other people.

What might be done?

A person with a personality disorder is often aware that he or she does not fit in, but it may be a family member who contacts the doctor. The doctor will first assess the person's behaviour and how it affects others and then look for provoking factors. If drug or alcohol abuse is contributing to difficulties, part of the treatment plan will include advice on overcoming the problem.

People in whom relationship difficulties or low self-esteem are the main problems may benefit from a form of psychological therapy (pp.622–624). A few people with severe problems may have prolonged treatment in a special community where they can learn to deal with day-to-day experiences.

Generally, the manifestations of an abnormal personality tend to decrease in severity as people get older.

Tourette's syndrome

A neurological condition characterized by repetitive, involuntary physical or vocal tics

 Usually starts between the ages of 7 and 12

 More common in males

 Usually runs in families

 Lifestyle is not a significant factor

Also sometimes known by its full name, Gilles de la Tourette's syndrome, this condition is a comparatively rare neurological disorder in which the affected person makes involuntary movements and/or sounds. The precise number of people with Tourette's syndrome is not known but it has been estimated that as many as 1 in 100 people are affected by

the condition. It typically starts in childhood and affects more boys than girls. The cause of Tourette's syndrome is not known, although in most cases it runs in families so genetic factors may be involved, although no specific genetic abnormality has been identified.

What are the symptoms?

Characteristically, the symptoms of Tourette's syndrome start between the ages of about 7 to 12 and include:
- Repetitive, involuntary physical tics (called motor tics), such as facial twitches, blinking, mouth movements, and head and foot movements.
- Repetitive, involuntary vocal tics (called phonic tics), such as coughing, throat-clearing, snorting, and grunting.

In some cases, the affected person may repeatedly utter obscenities (known as coprolalia), copy what other people say (echolalia) or do (echopraxia), or say the same thing repeatedly (palilalia). He or she may also repeatedly make complex physical movements, such as bending, jumping, or touching or hitting things or people.

In general, the symptoms are made worse by stress or boredom but may be diminished or even temporarily disappear by concentrating on a task, relaxation, or engaging in a pleasurable activity.

Various other conditions may be associated with Tourette's syndrome, including obsessive–compulsive disorder (p.342), attention deficit hyperactivity disorder (p.554), depression (p.343), and self-harming behaviour.

What might be done?

Some people with mild symptoms learn to live with the disorder without treatment, although support from family and self-help groups can be beneficial in this process. However, most people with the disorder benefit from medication and/or psychological therapy, such as behaviour therapy (p.622). Depending on the individual, various drugs may be used, such as the antipsychotic drug haloperidol, which may reduce or even stop the tics. In addition to a therapist, a range of other specialists may also be involved in treatment, such as child psychologists and neurologists. In a few adults with Tourette's syndrome who have not responded to other treatments, brain surgery has been tried, but with only occasional benefit.

If the affected individual also has any associated conditions – for example, obsessive–compulsive disorder or attention deficit hyperactivity disorder – treatment for those conditions may also be given.

What is the prognosis?

Although Tourette's syndrome is a lifelong condition for many of those affected, more than half have only mild or moderate symptoms, and in most people the symptoms become less frequent and less serious over time. In some cases, the symptoms eventually disappear completely.

Anorexia nervosa

Extreme concern about body shape and weight that results in a long-term refusal to eat and severe loss of weight

 Usually develops in early adolescence

 More common in females

 Sometimes runs in families

Social and job-related pressure to be slim is a risk factor

People with anorexia nervosa tend to be obsessively preoccupied with their body shape and weight. Often they have a distorted body image and, against all evidence to the contrary, are convinced that they are fat, even when they are very thin. They deliberately lose weight by various means, including dieting, exercising excessively, vomiting, and using laxatives. They often go to great lengths to conceal these strategies and hide their weight loss from others.

The condition can cause changes in hormone levels that may affect growth during adolescence and menstruation in girls and women. In severe cases, the loss of weight may be life-threatening.

Anorexia nervosa occurs mainly in the developed world. It is most common in girls and young women, but it can affect people of all ages and in recent years has become more common in younger children and also in boys and men. Anorexia nervosa may run in families and may be associated with the binge-eating disorder bulimia (opposite page).

What are the causes?

Anorexia nervosa often develops following a normal weight-loss diet. In Western culture, the importance placed on having a slim body leads many people of normal size to diet unnecessarily, particularly if they lack self-confidence. Sometimes, the condition is triggered by stress (p.31) or depression (p.343).

Anorexia nervosa often affects young people who are under pressure to succeed in a family that overemphasizes achievement.

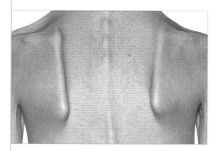

Wasting due to anorexia nervosa
The prominent shoulder blades and spine of this person with anorexia nervosa are signs of the extreme weight loss that is associated with the disorder.

In these circumstances, a teenager may feel driven to take control over an aspect of his or her life by refusing to eat. The condition has become an occupational hazard for people such as models, gymnasts, and ballet dancers, who are required to be extremely slim to succeed in their profession.

What are the symptoms?

Almost everyone attempts to lose some weight from time to time, and teenagers are usually especially anxious to be slim. However, normal dieting needs to be distinguished from anorexia nervosa, in which a person who is already of average or low weight follows a weight-loss diet for a prolonged period. Symptoms and behaviour patterns that may be apparent early in the disorder include:
- Refusal to eat, particularly foods that are high in calories.
- An obsessional interest in the subject of food.
- Preoccupation with body weight and body size.
- Weight loss that may be concealed by wearing baggy clothes.
- A conviction that one is overweight.
- Use of appetite suppressants and laxative drugs.
- Exercising excessively.

Depression may develop as a complication and lead to self-harm and suicide attempts (see **Attempted suicide and suicide**, p.344). Physical symptoms may appear gradually over weeks or months and become more obvious and extreme as the condition develops. They include:
- Extreme weight loss.
- Muscle wasting.
- Swollen ankles.
- Fine body hair on the trunk and limbs.
- In women, an absence of menstrual periods (see **Amenorrhoea**, p.471).

If anorexia nervosa develops before or around the onset of puberty, the development of adult sexual characteristics may be delayed or stop (see **Abnormal puberty in females**, p.474).

If there is a continued refusal to eat, extreme weight loss leads to complications such as chemical imbalances in the blood, nutritional deficiencies (p.399), loss of bone density (see **Osteoporosis**, p.217), infertility, chronic heart failure (p.247), and eventually death.

How is it diagnosed?

A person with anorexia nervosa is usually reluctant to admit that there is a problem. Often a concerned parent or friend consults the doctor first. The doctor will examine the affected person to assess the degree of weight loss and exclude other causes of weight loss, such as a digestive disorder or cancer. He or she will arrange for blood tests to see if an imbalance of chemicals in the blood has developed. The doctor will also look for an underlying or associated psychological disorder, such as depression.

What is the treatment?

Treatment is often difficult because of the person's refusal to acknowledge the illness. If the person's weight is very low or there is a risk of self-harm, he or she may be admitted to hospital. In less severe cases, treatment can be carried out at home under the doctor's supervision. Initially, the doctor sets a healthy weight target and monitors weight gain on a weekly basis. A dietitian will talk to the person about the importance of nutrition in general health and plan a healthy, balanced diet. In hospital, a person with anorexia nervosa is closely observed while eating habits are carefully monitored and modified until an agreed-upon weight has been achieved. At home, family members or a friend may be asked to closely monitor the person's diet.

People with anorexia nervosa are usually referred for psychological therapy. The doctor may suggest cognitive–behavioural therapy (p.623) to help an affected person develop a more realistic self-image or behaviour (p.622) to bring about changes in abnormal behaviour. Family therapy may be arranged if it appears that family problems are contributing to the disorder. Antidepressant drugs (p.592) may be given if there are symptoms of depression.

What is the prognosis?

About 1 in 5 people makes a complete recovery following treatment, but the same number remain severely ill. Even when a person has achieved his or her weight target, he or she needs continued professional support to maintain it.

For the remaining 3 in 5 people, the disorder persists but fluctuates in severity. Some people gain enough weight to recover but retain abnormal eating habits. Symptoms may also recur in response to stress. In some cases, bulimia develops up to 5 years after anorexia nervosa is first diagnosed.

About 1 in 20 people with anorexia nervosa dies from complications caused by malnutrition or commits suicide as a result of severe depression.

Bulimia

Episodes of binge-eating followed by strategies to avoid weight gain

 Usually develops in early adulthood

 More common in females

 Episodes can be brought on by stress

 Genetics is not a significant factor

People with bulimia (known medically as bulimia nervosa) worry excessively about their weight, body shape, and self-image. They typically binge on high-calorie food items, such as ice cream or chocolate, and then report a loss of control over their eating.

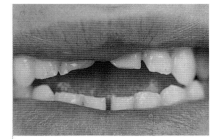

Effect of bulimia
Frequent self-induced vomiting leads to erosion of tooth enamel by stomach acid and eventually to the loss of front teeth.

After binge-eating, they use a number of methods to avoid weight gain, such as self-induced vomiting, using laxatives (p.597), and excessive exercising.

A person affected by bulimia is usually of average weight, and binge-eating and purging by vomiting and using laxatives are carried out secretly. He or she may have had anorexia nervosa (opposite page) in the past or may alternate between the two conditions. The disorder is more common in women and usually develops between the ages of 18 and 30. The person may have poor self-control and low self-esteem and may also indulge in substance abuse. Bouts of bulimia may be triggered by stress.

What are the symptoms?

Binge-eating followed by vomiting may occur once or several times a day. Over time, bulimia causes psychological and physical symptoms. The psychological symptoms include:

- A constant craving for food.
- Feelings of isolation as a result of eating alone and in secret.
- Guilt and disgust after binge-eating.

There may also be symptoms of depression (p.343) and anxiety (*see* **Anxiety disorders**, p.341). The physical symptoms caused by repeated episodes of binge-eating and vomiting include:

- Severe abdominal pain and swelling immediately following a binge.
- Physical weakness.
- Erosion of tooth enamel by stomach acids contained in vomit.
- Lesions on the knuckles from using fingers to induce vomiting.
- Bleeding from injuries to the lining of the oesophagus caused by vomiting.

Bulimia is unlike anorexia nervosa in that it rarely leads to severe weight loss. However, repeated excessive vomiting may cause dehydration and chemical imbalances in the blood. These imbalances sometimes lead to irregular heart rhythms (*see* **Arrhythmias**, p.249) that, very rarely, cause sudden death.

What might be done?

People with bulimia may be distressed by their behaviour and seek medical help themselves, or a family member or friend may encourage a person to see a doctor. The doctor will establish the severity of the illness by asking the person about his or her attitude to food. The doctor will look for signs of psychological problems, such as depression, anxiety, and substance abuse, and may arrange for blood tests to look for chemical imbalances in the blood.

The doctor may recommend a type of psychological therapy, such as cognitive–behavioural therapy (p.623), with a therapist who specializes in eating disorders. The goal of treatment is to boost self-esteem and help develop a rational approach to eating, while establishing a regular eating pattern. The doctor may prescribe antidepressant drugs (p.592) because they can be helpful even if a person with bulimia does not feel depressed.

What is the prognosis?

It is rare for bulimia to disappear spontaneously. In many cases, there is a risk of relapse weeks or even months after treatment is completed. However, in about 4 out of 5 cases, the frequency of binge-eating is reduced by therapy.

Drug dependence

Compulsive use of drugs, producing withdrawal symptoms when stopped

 Usually develops in adolescence

 More common in males

 Genetics may be a significant factor

 Stress, social factors, and peer pressure are risk factors

Drug dependence, or addiction, is the excessive and compulsive use of drugs for their effects on mental state. Often, increasing quantities of the drug are needed to produce the desired effect, and physical symptoms may develop if use stops or is delayed. Some drugs, such as LSD, do not cause this physical addiction but may cause psychological craving (*see* **Drugs and health**, p.26).

Drugs that may produce dependence include those obtained illegally, such as heroin and cocaine, and prescribed drugs, such as benzodiazepines (*see* **Sleeping drugs**, p.591) and opioid painkillers (p.589). Two common types of dependence are nicotine dependence (*see* **Tobacco and health**, p.25) and alcohol dependence (p.350). Nicotine dependence rarely affects work and social life, but alcohol dependence is often damaging. Drug addictions may lead to debt, loss of work, and breakdown in close relationships.

What are the causes?

Initially, drugs may be taken for the psychological "high" they produce and because they relieve symptoms such as anxiety (*see* **Anxiety disorders**, p.341) and insomnia (p.343). People who find it difficult to cope with stress may be more susceptible, as may people who have a parent who has abused drugs or alcohol. There is also some evidence that genetic factors may play a role in a person's susceptibility to drug dependence.

Dependence is more common in males than females, and peer pressure in adolescence and readily available illegal drugs make young people particularly vulnerable. The risk of dependence developing depends on which drug is taken. For example, heroin may cause dependence after only a few doses.

What are the symptoms?

There are different symptoms for each drug. However, certain areas of behaviour tend to be altered by most drugs that cause dependence. Symptoms of drug dependence often include:

- Mood changes.
- Changes in concentration levels.
- Altered energy levels.
- Faster or slower speech rate.
- Increased or decreased appetite.

Typically, withdrawal symptoms develop within 12 hours of last using or taking a drug. Effects range from mild to extremely severe and may include:

- Anxiety and restlessness.
- Overheating and sweating, alternating with chills and shivering.
- Confusion and hallucinations.
- Muscle aches and abdominal cramps.
- Diarrhoea and vomiting.
- Seizures.

Rarely, withdrawal from opioid drugs, such as heroin, may lead to coma (p.323). If drugs are injected, sharing needles may transmit diseases such as HIV infection (*see* **HIV infection and AIDS**, p.169) and hepatitis B and C (*see* **Acute hepatitis**, p.408). Drug dependence often leads to depression (p.343).

What might be done?

People who are dependent on drugs may not accept that they need help, and a member of their family or a friend may consult a doctor on their behalf. The doctor will ask which drugs are used and about the length and pattern of use.

Once a person has accepted that he or she needs treatment, withdrawal from the drug can begin. If the symptoms of withdrawal are likely to be severe or if there have been failed attempts in the past,

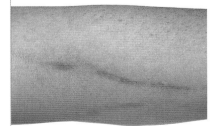

Needle tracks from drug injections
When a drug-dependent person repeatedly injects drugs, the veins can be damaged. In this picture, the damage is visible as needle tracks on the inside of the arm.

admission to hospital or a drug rehabilitation centre will be arranged. Otherwise, withdrawal may be closely supervised at home. Withdrawal symptoms are usually treated with substitute drugs that are less likely to cause dependence. For example, methadone may be used to replace or treat the symptoms of withdrawal from heroin. The doctor will offer support and specialized drug services for long-term counselling (p.624).

What is the prognosis?

Treatment of drug dependence is difficult and often unsuccessful. Sometimes there are several withdrawal attempts before dependence is overcome. Success is most likely if the person is strongly motivated and has good support from family, friends, and counselling services. Joining a support group also increases the chance of overcoming dependence.

Alcohol dependence

Compulsive regular consumption of alcohol, producing withdrawal symptoms when intake is stopped

 Most common between the ages of 20 and 40

 More common in males

Sometimes runs in families

 Stress and occupations that are associated with social drinking are risk factors

A person who is dependent on alcohol has an irresistible compulsion to drink, which takes priority over almost everything else in life. This craving for drink, coupled with withdrawal symptoms when drinking stops, is what separates alcohol dependence from alcohol abuse, a term used to describe regular drinking to excess (*see* Alcohol and health, p.24). About 5 million people in the UK abuse or are dependent on alcohol. Drinking problems are more common in men, particularly between the ages of 20 and 40. In addition to causing damage to the liver and brain, the need to drink to excess regularly is damaging to mental health and may destroy a person's family and social life and career.

What are the causes?

Alcohol dependence is often the result of a combination of factors. Sometimes,

alcohol dependence runs in families, partly as a result of children growing up in an environment of heavy drinking and partly because of an inherited predisposition. People who are shy, anxious, or have a social phobia (*see* Phobias, p.341) or depression (p.343) may rely heavily on alcohol. Working in an occupation that is associated with social drinking increases the risk of dependence. Stressful events may turn a moderate drinker into a heavy one.

What are the symptoms?

Alcohol dependence may develop after a number of years of moderate to heavy drinking. Symptoms may include:

- A compulsion to drink and loss of control over the amount consumed.
- Increased tolerance to the effects of alcohol, leading to greater consumption to achieve the desired effects.
- Withdrawal symptoms, such as nausea, sweating, and tremor, that start a few hours after the last drink.

In severe cases, withdrawal seizures develop after alcohol is stopped. After about 2 days without alcohol, delirium tremens may develop with symptoms of fever, shakes, seizures, disorientation, and hallucinations. Symptoms last for 3 to 4 days and are usually followed by a deep, prolonged sleep. In extreme cases, shock (p.248) occurs and may be fatal.

Are there complications?

Alcohol has direct effects on the body and may cause many diseases. Long-term alcohol dependence is the most common cause of severe liver disease (*see* Alcohol-related liver disease, p.409) and may damage the digestive system, causing peptic ulcers (p.406).

Heavy drinkers often have a poor diet, which may lead to a deficiency in vitamin B_1 (thiamine) that may eventually cause dementia (p.331). Rarely, severe thiamine deficiency leads to Wernicke–Korsakoff syndrome (p.332), a severe brain disorder that causes confusion and amnesia and may lead to coma. If excessive drinking continues for a prolonged period of time, damage to vital organs may be life-threatening.

Psychiatric problems associated with alcohol dependence include anxiety, depression, delusional disorders (p.347), and suicidal behaviour (*see* Attempted suicide and suicide, p.344). Generally, heavy drinkers tend to become self-centred and lack concern for family and friends.

How is it diagnosed?

Before the doctor can make a diagnosis, a person may need to be persuaded to seek help. The doctor will ask about the extent of the person's drinking and look for evidence of dependence. Blood tests to assess possible damage to the liver and other organs may be arranged.

What is the treatment?

Gradual reduction of alcohol intake or limiting alcohol consumption to social drinking is rarely possible. Instead, the person will be asked to stop drinking completely. In mild to moderate cases, withdrawal can take place at home, provided that adequate support is available. Antianxiety drugs (p.591), such as a benzodiazepine, may be prescribed for a short time to reduce agitation and other physical effects of withdrawal.

When heavy drinking is stopped suddenly, withdrawal seizures or delirium tremens may develop. The symptoms of delirium tremens are potentially life-threatening and require admission to hospital or a detoxification unit. Withdrawal symptoms are usually treated with antianxiety drugs.

Treatment for physical problems as a result of long-term alcohol dependence includes ulcer-healing drugs (p.596) for peptic ulcers and vitamin B_1 injections for a thiamine deficiency.

When the symptoms of withdrawal have been treated, the doctor may prescribe drugs that reduce cravings for alcohol or cause unpleasant reactions when it is consumed. Support is given to help prevent a relapse. Individual counselling (p.624) or group therapy (p.624) help people to address the problems that contribute to alcohol dependence.

What is the prognosis?

Accepting that there is a problem and receiving emotional support during the effort to give up drinking greatly improve a person's chance of recovery. Attending a self-help group, such as Alcoholics Anonymous, reduces the risk of relapse. However, after a long period of dependence, several attempts at detoxification may be needed before a person abstains from alcohol altogether.

In about 1 in 5 cases in which delirium tremens develops and is untreated, the condition proves fatal.

Compulsive gambling

Frequent gambling that dominates a person's life

 Usually develops by the age of 25

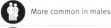 More common in males

 Exposure to gambling in adolescence is a risk factor

 Genetics is not a significant factor

In compulsive gambling or pathological gambling, a person has an intense urge to gamble that dominates his or her life. Compulsive gamblers continually increase their spending to achieve their desired intensity of excitement. They build up large debts and may lie, steal, and defraud to continue gambling. This behaviour continues regardless of its effects on family and social life and jeopardizes work and relationships.

Compulsive gambling is more common in men and usually develops before the age of 25. Growing up with a parent who gambles compulsively or who is dependent on alcohol has been shown to increase the risk. Adolescents who gamble are at an increased risk of developing a gambling problem. A person who gambles compulsively often appears optimistic and full of confidence. However, the disorder may be associated with mood disorders, such as anxiety (*see* Anxiety disorders, p.341) and depression (p.343), and with an antisocial personality disorder (p.347).

What might be done?

If a person is gambling excessively, a family member or friend may consult the doctor. The person will be assessed and treated for any underlying psychological disorders, such as anxiety or depression. Most self-help groups offer valuable support and encouragement, and a number of groups also give support to family and friends in their efforts to help a compulsive gambler.

Psychological therapies (pp.622–624) may be beneficial once the person has managed to refrain from gambling for a period of at least 3 months. Generally, therapy works best when a person has managed to gain some control over the compulsion to gamble.

Eyes and vision

The human eye is a remarkable organ, and our visual capabilities are among the most sophisticated of any living creature. We can judge speed and distance well enough to catch a fast-moving ball. Close up, we can see an incredible level of detail, allowing us to thread a needle or read small print. We can detect a vast range of colours, and, when we look rapidly from a close to a distant object or move from bright to dim light, our eyes automatically adjust. The eyes are protected by the eyelids and by tears, which flush out dirt and foreign matter.

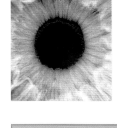

Detail of iris
The colour of the iris depends on the amount of pigment it contains.

FOR MOST HUMANS, vision dominates their conscious perception from the moment of birth. Working with but often overshadowing our other senses, vision supplies vast quantities of information about our surroundings and enables us to interact with our environment and the people within it.

The eye acts as a highly sophisticated biological video camera, focusing light from everything around us to form sharp images on a light-sensitive layer, the retina, at the back of the eye. Cells in the retina convert the images into electrical signals – nerve impulses – that travel along the optic nerve to the brain.

Visual perception depends not only on the eye but also on highly complex processing within the brain. In certain areas of the cortex (the outer layer of the brain), signals from both eyes are merged to provide three-dimensional vision. Also in the brain, signals from the eyes are combined with other information, such as memories and nerve impulses from other senses, to give meaning and structure to the visual world.

Forming an image
For us to see clearly, light rays entering the eye must be focused precisely on the retina. The first part of the eye to focus is the cornea, the transparent part of the front of the eye. The lens of the eye then fine-focuses the light rays by adjusting its focusing power automatically to create clear and sharp images of near and distant objects. The image formed on the retina is upside down, but the brain interprets the image so that we see the world the right way up.

When light falls on the retina, light-sensitive cells called rods and cones produce tiny electrical impulses in a pattern corresponding to the visual image. Each cone responds to one of the primary colours of light (red, green, or blue), and together these cells allow us to see a wide range of colours.

Our visual acuity (the level of detail we can see) is determined by the density of the light-sensitive cells in the retina. Compared with animals, our visual acuity is very good. However, birds of prey have a much higher density of both rods and cones, which gives them much greater visual acuity. For example, an eagle could spot an object at 5 km (3 miles) that we would struggle to see from a distance of 1 km (^{1}/2 mile).

The electrical impulses from all of the cells in the retina form the visual signal, which travels from the eye to the brain along the optic nerve. Impulses from both eyes are sent to a part at the back of the brain called the occipital, or visual, cortex. Here, the visual signals are integrated, giving a complete view of the visual field.

Protecting the eyes
The eyes are protected by the eyelids and by tears. The eyelids have the ability to close together to prevent harmful material from entering the eyes, while tears help to stop infection by washing away potentially dangerous materials that might damage the eye. Tears also contain a natural antiseptic.

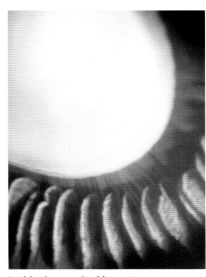

Inside the eye, looking out
This magnified view of the eye shows the delicate fibres that support the eye's elastic lens.

FUNCTION

The tear apparatus
Tears are produced by the lacrimal (tear) glands, which are situated above each eyeball. The glands continually secrete a small amount of salty fluid that is distributed over the surface of the eyes through the action of blinking and drain into the nose. Tears form a protective film that lubricates the eye and flushes out any dust and dirt. They also contain an antibacterial ingredient. Tear production increases when you cry or if the eye is irritated by a chemical or foreign particle.

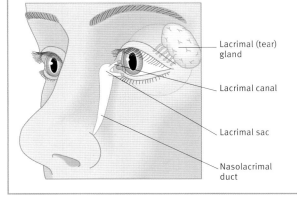

Lacrimal (tear) gland
Lacrimal canal
Lacrimal sac
Nasolacrimal duct

Drainage of tears
Tears drain away through the lacrimal canals into the lacrimal sac and then into the nose via the nasolacrimal duct.

✚ **STRUCTURE**

Structure of the eye

Each eyeball is roughly spherical, about 2.5 cm (1 in) in diameter, and lies in a protective bony socket in the skull. The eyeball has a tough outer coat called the sclera that maintains its shape. The choroid, which supplies the eye with nutrients, lies inside the sclera. The innermost layer, the retina, contains two types of light-sensitive cells: rods, which respond to dim light; and cones, which detect colour.

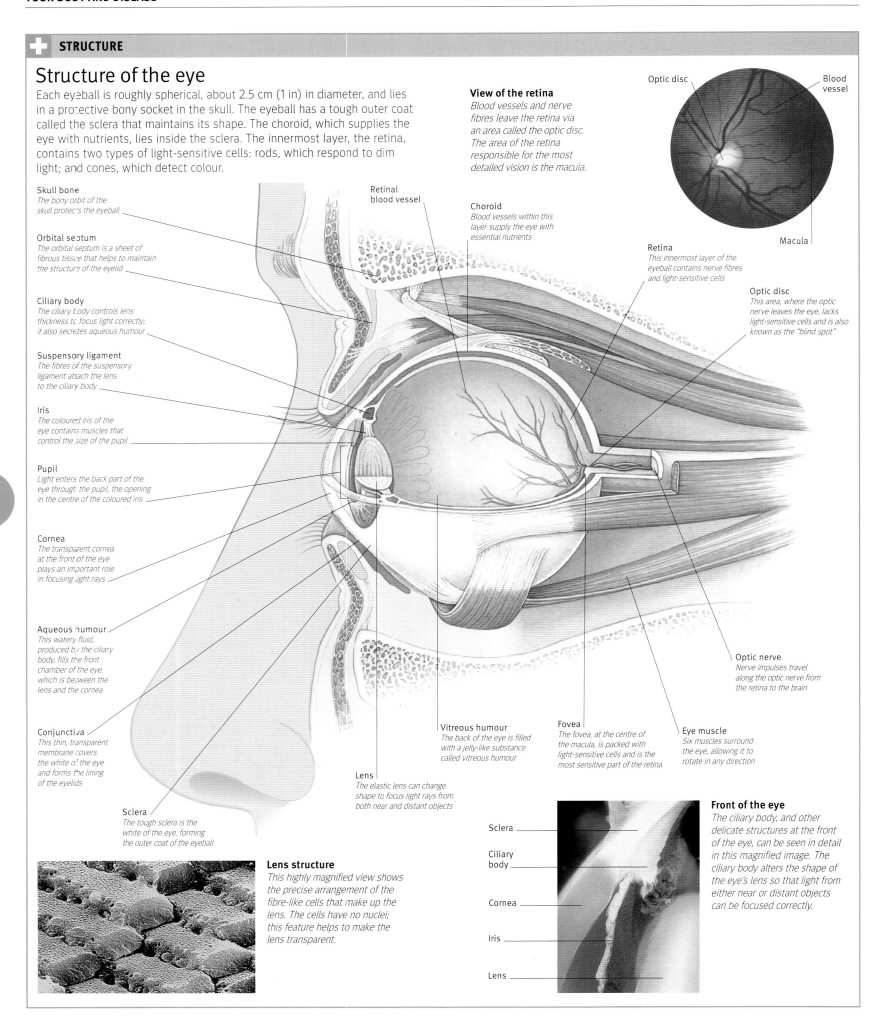

View of the retina
Blood vessels and nerve fibres leave the retina via an area called the optic disc. The area of the retina responsible for the most detailed vision is the macula.

Optic disc

Blood vessel

Macula

Skull bone
The bony orbit of the skull protects the eyeball

Orbital septum
The orbital septum is a sheet of fibrous tissue that helps to maintain the structure of the eyelid

Ciliary body
The ciliary body controls lens thickness to focus light correctly; it also secretes aqueous humour

Suspensory ligament
The fibres of the suspensory ligament attach the lens to the ciliary body

Iris
The coloured iris of the eye contains muscles that control the size of the pupil

Pupil
Light enters the back part of the eye through the pupil, the opening in the centre of the coloured iris

Cornea
The transparent cornea at the front of the eye plays an important role in focusing light rays

Aqueous humour
This watery fluid, produced by the ciliary body, fills the front chamber of the eye, which is between the lens and the cornea

Conjunctiva
This thin, transparent membrane covers the white of the eye and forms the lining of the eyelids

Sclera
The tough sclera is the white of the eye, forming the outer coat of the eyeball

Retinal blood vessel

Choroid
Blood vessels within this layer supply the eye with essential nutrients

Retina
This innermost layer of the eyeball contains nerve fibres and light-sensitive cells

Optic disc
This area, where the optic nerve leaves the eye, lacks light-sensitive cells and is also known as the "blind spot"

Optic nerve
Nerve impulses travel along the optic nerve from the retina to the brain

Vitreous humour
The back of the eye is filled with a jelly-like substance called vitreous humour

Fovea
The fovea, at the centre of the macula, is packed with light-sensitive cells and is the most sensitive part of the retina

Eye muscle
Six muscles surround the eye, allowing it to rotate in any direction

Lens
The elastic lens can change shape to focus light rays from both near and distant objects

Lens structure
This highly magnified view shows the precise arrangement of the fibre-like cells that make up the lens. The cells have no nuclei; this feature helps to make the lens transparent.

Sclera

Ciliary body

Cornea

Iris

Lens

Front of the eye
The ciliary body, and other delicate structures at the front of the eye, can be seen in detail in this magnified image. The ciliary body alters the shape of the eye's lens so that light from either near or distant objects can be focused correctly.

How the eye works

When you look at an object, light rays reflected from the object hit the transparent cornea at the front of your eye. The rays are partly focused and pass through the pupil, which enlarges or constricts depending on light conditions. The lens varies its focusing power for near and distant objects and fine-focuses the rays to create a sharp image on the fovea, the most responsive area of the light-sensitive retina at the back of the eye.

The mechanism of vision

Light rays focused by the cornea and lens produce an image on the retina that is upside down. Electrical signals from stimulated cells in the retina travel along the optic nerve to the brain, where the image is interpreted as being upright.

Action of the pupil

In dim conditions, the pupil widens (dilates) to allow the maximum amount of light to reach the light-sensitive retina. In bright light, the pupil constricts. Two sets of muscles in the coloured iris control these processes.

Changes in pupil size
To make the pupil constrict, the circular muscles contract; and to widen (dilate) it, the radial muscles contract.

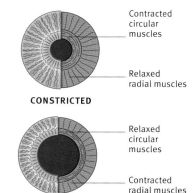

Contracted circular muscles
Relaxed radial muscles
CONSTRICTED

Relaxed circular muscles
Contracted radial muscles
DILATED

Blood vessel
Retinal arteries and veins supply nutrients and remove waste from the retina

Ciliary body
The muscles of the ciliary body control the shape and focusing power of the lens

Lens
The lens provides fine focusing of light rays

Cornea
Incoming light rays are initially refracted (bent) by the cornea

Object
Light reflected from an object travels in all directions. Some rays enter the eye

Pupil
Light rays enter the pupil to reach the retina

Iris
The ring of muscles in the iris controls the pupil's size to allow in more or less light

Retina
Light-sensitive cells (rods and cones) in the retina transform light into nerve signals

Macula
The macula, the area of the retina surrounding the fovea, is responsible for detailed vision

Fovea
The fovea contains the highest density of cells

Optic nerve
Fibres of the optic nerve carry impulses from the retina to the brain

Inverted image
The image on the retina is upside down

Light rays
Rays of light from the object cross in the eye and are focused on the retina

Accommodation

The eye adjusts for near and distant vision by changing the shape of its lens. This varies the extent to which incoming light is refracted (bent). To create a sharp image on the retina, light rays from near objects must be bent more than those from distant objects. This process is called accommodation.

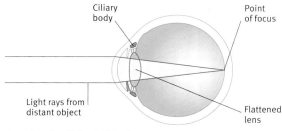

Ciliary body
Point of focus
Light rays from distant object
Flattened lens

Focusing for distant objects
When you look at an object in the distance, muscles in the ciliary body relax and the lens assumes a flatter shape.

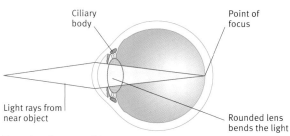

Ciliary body
Point of focus
Light rays from near object
Rounded lens bends the light

Focusing for near objects
When you look at a close object, muscles in the ciliary body contract, allowing the elastic lens to assume a more spherical shape.

How the eye works (continued)

Visual pathways

Electrical signals from each retina pass along the optic nerves, which meet at a junction called the optic chiasm. Here, half of the nerve fibres from the left eye cross to the right side and vice versa, and the fibres continue along the optic tracts to the brain. Information from the right half of each retina passes to the right visual cortex; information from the left half of each retina goes to the left visual cortex. The brain then integrates these messages into a complete visual picture.

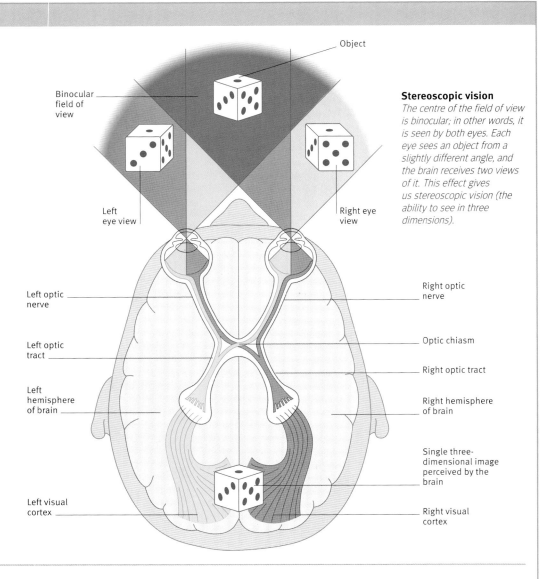

Stereoscopic vision
The centre of the field of view is binocular; in other words, it is seen by both eyes. Each eye sees an object from a slightly different angle, and the brain receives two views of it. This effect gives us stereoscopic vision (the ability to see in three dimensions).

Object

Binocular field of view

Left eye view

Right eye view

Left optic nerve

Left optic tract

Left hemisphere of brain

Left visual cortex

Right optic nerve

Optic chiasm

Right optic tract

Right hemisphere of brain

Single three-dimensional image perceived by the brain

Right visual cortex

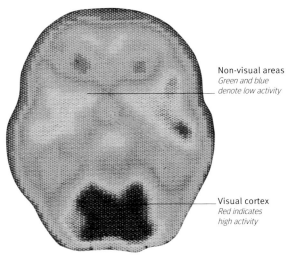

Non-visual areas
Green and blue denote low activity

Visual cortex
Red indicates high activity

Brain during visual stimulation
The visual cortex, which is located at the back of the brain, exhibits high activity compared with the rest of the brain when a detailed coloured picture is observed.

Rods and cones

There are two types of light-sensitive cells in the retina: rods and cones. Up to 120 million rods are distributed throughout the retina. Although rods are sensitive to all visible light, they contain only one type of pigment and cannot distinguish colours. They are therefore responsible mainly for night vision. In contrast, the 6.5 million cones provide detailed and colour vision. Every cone responds to red, green, or blue light, working only in bright light. They are most concentrated in the central part of the retina, the fovea.

LOCATION

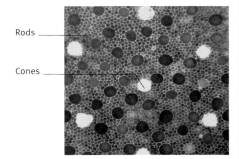

Rods

Cones

Rods and cones
This magnified view of the retina shows that rods greatly outnumber cones. Here, the cones are shown in two colours.

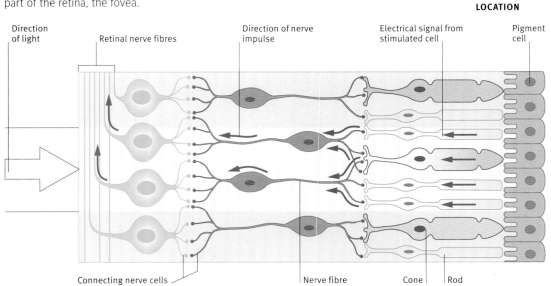

Direction of light

Retinal nerve fibres

Direction of nerve impulse

Electrical signal from stimulated cell

Pigment cell

Connecting nerve cells

Nerve fibre

Cone

Rod

How the retina responds to light
When light strikes the retina, the rods and cones produce electrical signals that trigger further impulses in the nerve cells to which they are connected. These signals travel along the optic nerve to the brain. Pigment cells behind the rods and cones absorb light and prevent reflection inside the eye.

Eye disorders

The eye is a complex organ made up of several highly specialized components. Many eye disorders do not threaten sight, but a few serious conditions may damage the eye's components and lead to loss of vision. Eye disorders are very common, but early diagnosis usually leads to successful treatment.

This section covers disorders caused by disease, structural abnormality, or injury to the eye. Conditions that involve the front covering of the eye (the conjunctiva and cornea) are described first, followed by disorders that affect the front chamber of the eye and the structures within it, including the iris and lens.

The next group of articles discusses disorders of the light-sensitive retina at the back of the eye and conditions affecting the optic nerve, which carries nerve signals from the retina to the brain. The final articles in this section cover conditions in which the eye is displaced or injured in some way. Impaired vision, whether occurring in healthy eyes or as a consequence of serious underlying causes, is described separately (*see* **Vision disorders**, pp.365–369), as are disorders of the eyelid and tear system (pp.363–365) and eye disorders that usually or only affect children. These include congenital blindness (p.555), cancer of the retina (*see* **Retinoblastoma**, p.556), and misalignment of the gaze of the eyes (*see* **Strabismus**, p.555).

Many major eye disorders that in the past would have ultimately progressed to blindness can now be treated successfully if detected early. For example, diabetic retinopathy is often now treated by laser surgery to prevent further sight loss. Regular eye examinations are therefore important, especially for people over the age of 40.

KEY ANATOMY

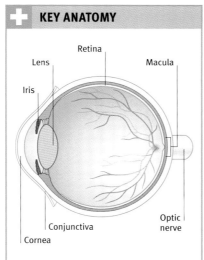

Retina
Lens
Macula
Iris
Optic nerve
Conjunctiva
Cornea

For more information on the structure and function of the eye, *see* pp.352–354.

Conjunctivitis

Inflammation of the conjunctiva, the membrane covering the white of the eye and the inside of the eyelids

 Wearing contact lenses and using cosmetics or eyedrops are risk factors

 Genetics as a risk factor depends on the type

 Age and gender are not significant factors

Conjunctivitis, also called pink eye, is a common condition in which the conjunctiva, the clear membrane covering the white of the eye and lining the eyelids, becomes inflamed. The affected eye becomes red and sore and may look alarming, but the condition is rarely serious. One or both of the eyes may be affected, and in some cases it begins in one eye then spreads to the other.

What are the causes?
Conjunctivitis may be caused by a bacterial or viral infection, or result from

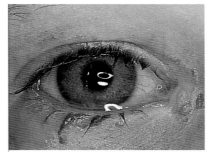
Conjunctivitis
This eye shows signs of conjunctivitis, including swollen eyelids, a discharge, and redness over the white of the eye.

an allergic reaction or irritation of the conjunctiva, for example by smoke, pollution, or ultraviolet light.

Bacterial conjunctivitis is common, and may be due to several types of bacteria. Viral conjunctivitis can occur in epidemics caused by one of the viruses that causes the common cold (p.164). One viral form of conjunctivitis, called herpes kerato-conjunctivitis, results from a herpes simplex infection (p.166). Conjunctivitis due to viruses or bacteria can be spread by hand-to-eye contact and is highly contagious.

Newborn babies sometimes develop conjunctivitis. This can happen if an infection is transmitted to the baby's eyes from the mother's vagina during the birth. This form of conjunctivitis is usually caused by the microorganisms responsible for certain sexually transmitted infections, including chlamydial infection (p.492), gonorrhoea (p.491), and genital herpes (p.493).

Allergic conjunctivitis is a common feature of hay fever and of allergy to dust, pollen, and other airborne substances (*see* **Allergic rhinitis**, p.283). The condition may also be triggered by chemicals found in eyedrops, cosmetics, or contact lens solutions. Allergic conjunctivitis often runs in families.

What are the symptoms?
The symptoms of conjunctivitis usually develop over a few hours and are often first experienced on waking. The symptoms generally include:
- Redness of the white of the eye.
- Gritty and uncomfortable sensation in the eye.
- Swelling and itching of the eyelids.
- Discharge that may be yellowish and thick or clear and watery.

The discharge may dry out during sleep and form crusts on the eyelashes and eyelid margins. As a result, the eyelids sometimes stick together on waking.

What can I do?
If you think you may have bacterial conjunctivitis, chloramphenicol drops and ointment are available over the counter to treat the condition in those over 2 years old. To avoid spreading infection, wash your hands after touching the eye and do not share towels or facecloths. Once conjunctivitis has cleared up, sight is rarely affected.

If you are susceptible to allergic conjunctivitis, avoid exposure to triggering substances. Antiallergy eyedrops can be used to ease the symptoms (*see* **Drugs acting on the eye**, p.594). If conjunctivitis does not clear up with self-help measures or if an eye becomes painful and red, you should consult your doctor.

What might the doctor do?
Your doctor will probably make a diagnosis from your symptoms. If infection is suspected, he or she may take a sample of the discharge to identify the cause.

Bacterial conjunctivitis is treated by applying antibiotic drops or ointment and the symptoms usually clear up within 48 hours. However, the treatment should be continued for as long as recommended by your doctor, even if there is improvement, to ensure the infection is eradicated.

Viral conjunctivitis caused by a herpes infection may be treated with eyedrops containing an antiviral drug (p.573). Although other types of viral conjunctivitis cannot be treated, their symptoms usually clear up within 2–3 weeks. Your doctor may prescribe eyedrops or oral antiallergy drugs if you have allergic conjunctivitis.

Subconjunctival haemorrhage

Bleeding between the white of the eye and the conjunctiva, the membrane covering the white of the eye and lining the eyelids

 Age, gender, genetics, and lifestyle as risk factors depend on the cause

Ruptured blood vessels in the conjunctiva, the clear membrane covering the white of the eye and lining the eyelids, cause bleeding under the membrane. The condition, called subconjunctival haemorrhage, is common because the blood vessels in the conjunctiva are easily damaged. The bleeding causes a red area over the white of the eye.

The condition may result from a minor eye injury (p.363), sneezing, coughing, or, rarely, a bleeding disorder (p.274). Most often, it is spontaneous, especially in elderly people. Although the haemorrhage looks dramatic, it is generally painless and usually clears up without treatment within 2–3 weeks. If the eye is painful or the redness persists, you should consult your doctor.

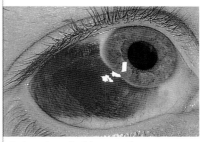
Subconjunctival haemorrhage
The red area on this eye is caused by bleeding under the conjunctiva, the outer membrane covering the white of the eye.

Corneal abrasion

A scratch on the surface of the cornea, the transparent front part of the eye

 Wearing contact lenses is a risk factor

 Age, gender, and genetics are not significant factors

The cornea, situated at the front of the eye, is susceptible to minor damage. For example, if it is scraped by the edge of a newspaper or by a foreign particle such as a speck of dirt, an injury known as a corneal abrasion may occur. People who wear soft contact lenses and rub their eyes excessively are particularly at risk of damage because tiny particles can become stuck behind a lens and scratch the surface of the cornea.

What are the symptoms?
The symptoms of a corneal abrasion usually occur suddenly. They include:

- Pain in the eye.
- Redness and watering of the eye.
- Blurred vision.
- Sensitivity to bright light.
- Frequent blinking.

A corneal abrasion is not usually serious. However, there is a risk that the abrasion may become infected and a corneal ulcer (below) may develop.

What might be done?
Painkillers (p.539) will relieve the discomfort of an abrasion, but you should consult your doctor or go to an accident and emergency department for treatment. The doctor will place drops containing fluorescein dye in your eyes and examine them with an instrument known as a slit lamp (see **Slit-lamp examination**, p.358). If an abrasion is highlighted by the dye, your doctor may recommend an eye patch and also prescribe antibiotic eyedrops to prevent infection and ulceration (see **Drugs acting on the eye**, p.594). A corneal abrasion usually heals within a few days.

Corneal ulcer

A deep erosion in the cornea, the transparent front part of the eye

 Wearing contact lenses is a risk factor

 Age, gender, and genetics are not significant factors

An eroded area in the cornea, the transparent outer part of the front of the eye, is known as a corneal ulcer. These ulcers can be very painful and, if left untreated, may cause scarring and lead to permanently impaired vision, blindness (p.369), or even loss of the eye. People who wear contact lenses are at increased risk of corneal ulcers.

What are the causes?
Corneal ulcers may be caused by an eye injury, an infection, or a combination of both. A relatively small injury, such as a corneal abrasion (p.355), can develop into a corneal ulcer if the damaged area becomes infected. A more severe injury, such as that caused by a caustic chemical, can produce an ulcer in the absence of infection. However, an ulcer that becomes infected may enlarge and penetrate more deeply into the cornea. Only rarely do infections cause corneal ulcers without prior injury. The most common of these infections are herpes zoster (p.166), known as shingles, and herpes simplex infections (p.166).

What are the symptoms?
If you have a corneal ulcer, you may experience the following symptoms:
- Intense pain in the eye.
- Redness and discharge from the eye.
- Blurred vision.
- Increased sensitivity to light.

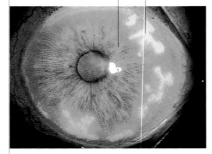
Normal area of the cornea   Ulcerated area

Corneal ulcer
Fluorescein eyedrops placed in this eye revealed an ulcerated cornea. These ulcers are due to a herpes simplex infection.

With an untreated infected ulcer, the infection may spread and permanently impair vision and cause damage to the eye itself. You should consult a doctor immediately if you develop a painful, red eye together with blurred vision.

What might be done?
The doctor may place fluorescein eyedrops in the affected eye and examine it under blue light with a slit lamp (see **Slit-lamp examination**, p.358). He or she may also take a swab to identify the cause. If the dye reveals an ulcer, you may be given antibiotic or antiviral eyedrops to treat the infection (see **Drugs acting on the eye**, p.594). Even severe ulcers usually clear up within 1–2 weeks of treatment, but they can leave scars that permanently affect vision.

Hyphaema

A pool of blood in the front chamber of the eye, behind the transparent cornea

 Participating in sports that may lead to a blow to the eye is a risk factor

 Age, gender, and genetics are not significant factors

A blow to the eye may rupture a blood vessel in the iris (the coloured part of the eye). The damaged blood vessel may bleed into the fluid-filled chamber between the lens and the cornea, the transparent front part of the eye, forming a pool of blood known as a hyphaema. Initially, the blood mixes with the clear fluid behind the cornea, resulting in severely blurred vision, but within a few hours the blood cells sink to the bottom of the chamber, which enables the vision to return to normal.

If you have an eye injury, you need to obtain prompt medical advice: consult your doctor immediately or go to hospital. Hyphaema blood usually disappears in less than a week. Restricting your activities may stop further bleeding. If bleeding recurs, the pressure in the eye can rise and cause acute glaucoma (p.358), a serious condition that needs urgent treatment.

Trachoma

A persistent eye infection that causes damage to the cornea, the transparent front part of the eye

 Particularly common in children

 Living in an area with limited water and poor hygiene is a risk factor

 Gender and genetics are not significant factors

Trachoma is a serious, persistent eye infection that causes permanent scarring of the cornea, the transparent front part of the eye. Although very rare in developed countries, trachoma is one of the world's main causes of blindness. It is responsible for visual impairment in more than 2 million people worldwide, of whom about 1.2 million are completely blind.

Trachoma is due to the bacterium *Chlamydia trachomatis*, which is spread to the eyes by direct contact with contaminated hands or by flies. Trachoma is common in poor parts of the world, particularly in hot, dry countries that have poor sanitation and limited water supplies. Overcrowding encourages the spread of the trachoma infection.

To avoid becoming infected in a high-risk area, you should wash your hands and face regularly and avoid touching your eyes with dirty fingers.

What are the symptoms?
Initially, trachoma causes inflammation of the conjunctiva, the membrane that covers the white of the eye and lines the eyelids (see **Conjunctivitis**, p.355). Later symptoms include:
- Thick discharge from the eye that is affected.
- Redness of the white of the eye.
- Gritty sensation in the eye.

Over time, repeated episodes of trachoma can cause scarring on the inside of the eyelids. The scars may pull the eyelids inwards and cause the eyelashes to rub against the delicate cornea (see **Entropion**, p.364). Left untreated, the condition can lead to blindness.

What is the treatment?
In the early stages, trachoma is treated with antibiotic eyedrops or ointment (see **Drugs acting on the eye**, p.594). If trachoma has caused the eyelids to turn inwards, an operation may be needed to prevent the eyelashes from rubbing against the cornea. If the cornea has become scarred, sight may be restored by an operation called a corneal graft, in which a cornea from a donor is used to replace the scarred one.

Keratoconus

Progressive change in the shape of the cornea, the transparent front part of the eye, causing blurred vision

 Usually develops around puberty

 Sometimes runs in families; more common in people of Asian descent

 Gender and lifestyle are not significant factors

In keratoconus, the central area of the transparent cornea that forms the front of the eye grows abnormally, becoming cone-shaped and thin. Also known as conical cornea, keratoconus is a rare condition that is sometimes inherited and is more common in people of Asian descent. It usually begins at puberty and may affect one or both eyes. As the shape of the cornea changes, astigmatism (p.366) develops and vision becomes blurred. As the distortion of the cornea progresses, symptoms worsen, in some cases quite rapidly.

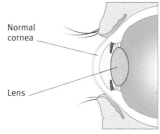
Normal cornea

Lens

NORMAL EYE

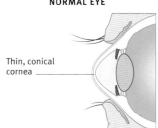
Thin, conical cornea

KERATOCONUS

Effects of keratoconus
The normal cornea has an even, spherical curvature. Keratoconus causes the cornea to grow abnormally, becoming thinner and bulging forwards in a conical shape.

What might be done?
A slit lamp may be used to examine your eyes (see **Slit-lamp examination**, p.358), and the shape of your corneas may be measured using a technique called corneal topography. If keratoconus is detected in its early stages, your vision can be corrected by glasses or hard contact lenses (see **Glasses and contact lenses**, p.366). However, if your vision has seriously deteriorated, your doctor may suggest a corneal graft, an operation in which the abnormal cornea is replaced with a healthy one from a donor. This operation will usually restore normal vision permanently.

Cataract

Clouding of the lens of the eye, causing loss of vision

 More common after the age of 75 but may be present from birth

 Sometimes due to a chromosome disorder

 Contact sports and frequent exposure to the sun are risk factors

 Gender is not a significant factor

If you have a cataract, the normally transparent lens of the eye is cloudy as a result of changes in protein fibres in the lens. The clouding affects the transmission and focusing of light entering the eye, reducing clarity of vision.

If cataracts are present from birth, total loss of vision (*see* **Congenital blindness**, p.555) may result. However, cataracts do not usually affect children or young adults. Most people over the age of 75 have some cataract formation, but visual loss is often minimal as only the outer edges of the lens are affected.

Cataracts usually develop in both eyes, but generally one eye is more severely affected. A cataract in the central part of the lens or one that affects the whole lens can cause loss of clarity and detail in vision. However, the affected eye will still be able to detect light and shade.

What are the causes?
All cataracts occur as a result of structural changes to protein fibres within the lens. These changes cause part or all of the lens to become cloudy.

Changes in the protein fibres are a normal part of aging, but cataracts that develop in young adults may be the result of an eye injury (p.363) or prolonged exposure to sunlight. They may also develop due to diabetes mellitus (p.437), uveitis (p.357), or long-term treatment with corticosteroids (p.600). Cataracts are common in people with the chromosome disorder Down's syndrome (p.533).

What are the symptoms?
Cataracts usually develop over a period of months or years. In most cases, they are painless and usually cause only visual symptoms, such as:

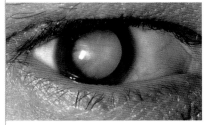

Severe cataract
This cataract, seen as a cloudy area behind the pupil, affects a large part of the lens. Cataracts cause visual impairment.

- Blurred or distorted vision.
- Star-shaped scattering of light from bright lights, particularly at night.
- Altered colour vision: objects appear reddish or yellow.
- In longsighted people, temporary improvement in near vision.

A severe cataract may make the pupil of the eye appear cloudy.

What might be done?
The doctor will examine your eyes with a slit lamp (*see* **Slit-lamp examination**, p.358) and an ophthalmoscope (*see* **Ophthalmoscopy**, p.360). If your vision is affected significantly, he or she may recommend that the cataract is removed surgically and an artificial lens put in the eye (*see* **Cataract surgery**, right). If there is no other reason for your visual deterioration, your sight should improve greatly after the operation. However, you may still need to wear glasses afterwards.

Scleritis

Inflammation of the sclera, the tough, white, outer covering of the eye

 More common in females

 May run in families if associated with rheumatoid arthritis

 Age and lifestyle are not significant factors

Scleritis is a rare, serious condition in which the sclera (the white outer coat of the eye) becomes inflamed. The condition is more common in women and is frequently associated with inflammatory disorders, such as rheumatoid arthritis (p.222). The main symptoms are severe pain in the eye, redness of the white of the eye, and excessive watering. If scleritis is linked with rheumatoid arthritis, you may experience repeated attacks. Rarely, severe cases of scleritis may cause perforation of the sclera and blindness (p.369) in the affected eye.

If you have any of these symptoms, contact your doctor immediately. Mild cases may need only anti-inflammatory eyedrops (*see* **Drugs acting on the eye**, p.594), but if rheumatoid arthritis is the cause, drug treatment for the arthritis can help both conditions.

▶ TREATMENT

Cataract surgery

A cataract is an opaque region in the lens of the eye causing loss of vision. During cataract surgery, the affected lens is removed and replaced with an artificial lens. The operation is usually performed under a local anaesthetic, and you will probably be able to go home the same day. In the technique shown here, the lens is first softened by an ultrasound probe. The softened tissue is extracted, and a new lens is inserted.

ARTIFICIAL LENS (ACTUAL SIZE)

LOCATION

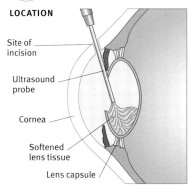
Site of incision
Ultrasound probe
Cornea
Softened lens tissue
Lens capsule

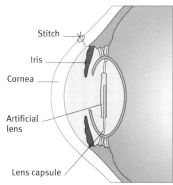
Stitch
Iris
Cornea
Artificial lens
Lens capsule

1 *An ultrasound probe is inserted into the lens through a small incision in the cornea. The probe softens the lens by emitting sound waves, and the softened tissue is then sucked out.*

2 *The back of the natural lens capsule is left in place, and an artificial lens is placed inside it. The incision in the cornea is either closed with surgical stitches or left to seal itself without stitching.*

Uveitis

Inflammation of any part of the uveal tract, which is a group of connected structures inside the eye

 Age, gender, genetics, and lifestyle as risk factors depend on the cause

The uveal tract consists of several connected structures: the iris (the coloured part of the eye); the ciliary body (a ring of muscle behind the iris); and the choroid (a layer of tissue that supports the light-sensitive retina). Inflammation of any part of the uveal tract is called uveitis. The condition may involve the iris and/or the ciliary body (anterior uveitis or iritis) or the choroid (posterior uveitis). If uveitis is not treated, vision can be seriously impaired.

What are the causes?
Uveitis is most commonly caused by an autoimmune disorder, in which the body attacks its own tissues, such as juvenile chronic arthritis (p.541). There may be links with some inflammatory disorders, such as sarcoidosis (p.304), ankylosing spondylitis (p.223), Crohn's disease (p.417), and ulcerative colitis (p.417). The condition may also occur with certain infectious diseases, including tuberculosis (p.300).

What are the symptoms?
Both anterior and posterior uveitis may affect only one eye. In anterior uveitis, the following symptoms may develop gradually over hours or days:
- Redness and watering of the eye.
- Sensitivity to bright light.
- Blurred vision.
- Aching in the eye.
- Small, irregularly shaped pupil.

Symptoms of posterior uveitis develop rapidly and include:
- Blurred vision.
- Spots or haziness in the visual field.

Consult your doctor at once if your eye becomes red and painful and if you develop blurred vision.

The main danger in anterior uveitis is that the inflamed iris may stick to the lens. This prevents normal drainage of fluid through the pupil and increases the pressure inside the eye (*see* **Acute glaucoma**, p.358). If this rise in pressure is not treated promptly, it can lead to blindness (p.369). The condition may also increase the risk of developing a cataract (left). Repeated attacks can lead to permanent damage to the iris and deterioration in vision.

Occasionally, parts of the retina may be damaged irreversibly by posterior uveitis, resulting in partial or total loss of vision in the affected eye.

What might be done?
If uveitis is suspected, you may have a slit-lamp examination (p.358) and ophthalmoscopy (p.360), which examines the inside of your eye. If this is your first attack of uveitis, you will probably have other diagnostic tests to establish the underlying cause.

▶ **TEST**

Slit-lamp examination

The slit lamp is used to examine structures at the front of the eye: the transparent cornea, which covers the front part of the eye; the coloured iris; the lens; and the front chamber, which lies between the cornea and the lens. The slit lamp produces a long, narrow beam of brilliant light that is focused onto the eye. Although the examination is painless, eye drops used to dilate the pupil may make your vision blurred for a few hours afterwards. Ophthalmologists may also sometimes use a slit lamp with a special lens placed in front of your eye to examine structures in the back of the eye, such as the retina.

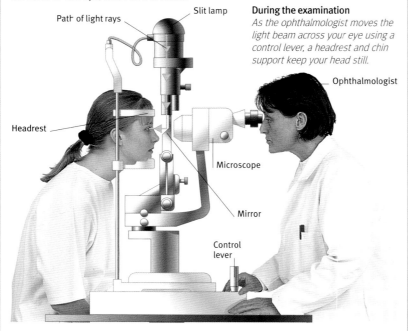

Path of light rays · Slit lamp

During the examination
As the ophthalmologist moves the light beam across your eye using a control lever, a headrest and chin support keep your head still.

Ophthalmologist

Headrest

Microscope

Mirror

Control lever

Your doctor may prescribe eyedrops to dilate the pupil and stop the iris from sticking to the lens, or corticosteroid eyedrops to reduce the inflammation (*see* **Drugs acting on the eye**, p.594). Treatment of uveitis is usually effective, but the condition tends to recur.

Glaucoma

Abnormally high pressure of the fluid inside the eye

 Rare under the age of 40; more common over the age of 60

 Some types run in families

 Gender and lifestyle are not significant factors

Fluid continually moves into and out of the eye to nourish its tissues and maintain its shape. In glaucoma, the flow of fluid out of the eye becomes blocked and pressure rises inside the eye. This high pressure may permanently damage nerve fibres in the light-sensitive retina and in the optic nerve, which carries nerve signals from the retina to the brain. Glaucoma becomes more common with age, and mainly affects people over the age of 60. If untreated, the condition may cause blindness (p.369).

What are the types?
There are two common types of glaucoma (acute and chronic) and two rarer types (secondary and congenital). Acute glaucoma (right) develops suddenly, causing rapid loss of vision and severe eye pain. In contrast, chronic glaucoma (opposite page) develops slowly and painlessly, often over many years. It may not cause noticeable symptoms until the eyes are badly damaged. Both types can run in families.

Secondary glaucoma occurs as a result of an underlying eye disorder, such as retinal vein occlusion (p.360) or uveitis (p.357), or from using certain drugs, such as corticosteroid eyedrops (*see* **Drugs acting on the eye**, p.594). Secondary glaucoma can result in blindness. Congenital glaucoma is due to a defect in the drainage apparatus of the eye. It is present from birth and can also result in blindness (*see* **Congenital blindness**, p.555).

Glaucoma is diagnosed by measuring pressure in the eye using an instrument called a tonometer (*see* **Tonometry**, right). Treatment should always be given immediately. Eyedrops are used first to reduce pressure in the eye (*see* **Drugs for glaucoma**, p.594). In some cases, surgery is necessary to increase drainage of fluid and prevent build-up of pressure in the eye (*see* **Laser iridotomy**, opposite page, and **Trabeculectomy**, opposite page). Correct treatment normally minimizes further vision loss.

Acute glaucoma

An abrupt blockage of the drainage system in the eye, causing a painful, rapid rise in fluid pressure

 Rare under the age of 40; more common over the age of 60

 More common in females

 Sometimes runs in families; more common in people of Asian descent

 Lifestyle is not a significant factor

Normally, the fluid that is secreted into the front of the eye to maintain the eye's shape and nourish the tissues drains away continuously. However, in acute (narrow-angle) glaucoma, the drainage system suddenly develops a blockage, and the fluid pressure inside the eye rises rapidly. Acute glaucoma is a medical emergency requiring prompt treatment. Left untreated, the eye can swiftly become damaged and a permanent reduction in vision can result.

What are the causes?
The fluid in the front part of the eye is produced continuously by a ring of tissue called the ciliary body, behind the eye's coloured iris. Normally the fluid flows out through the pupil and drains away through the trabecular meshwork, which surrounds the iris. This sieve-like meshwork is situated deep within the drainage angle, which is found between the outer rim of the iris and the edge of the cornea. In acute glaucoma, the iris bulges forwards and closes the drainage angle, trapping fluid within the eye. The pressure inside the eye rises as more fluid is secreted. As the pressure rises, it may damage the nerves in the light-sensitive retina and in the optic nerve, which carries nerve signals to the brain, causing impairment of vision.

Having a smaller eyeball than usual is a common cause of longsightedness (*see* **Hypermetropia**, p.366), and increases the risk of developing acute glaucoma. The disorder is more common in older people because the lens of the eye grows throughout life and may eventually press against the iris. Fluid builds up behind the iris, which bulges forwards and blocks the drainage angle.

Acute glaucoma can be triggered when dim light causes the pupil to widen. The iris thickens and the drainage angle can close. Acute glaucoma sometimes runs in families and is more common in women and in people of Asian descent.

What are the symptoms?
A full-blown attack of acute glaucoma may be preceded by mild attacks in the weeks before. Mild attacks usually take place in the evening. Symptoms include pain in the eyes and haloes appearing around lights; the symptoms are relieved by sleeping. If you have these symptoms,

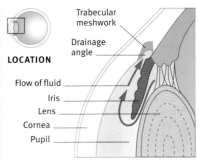

LOCATION

Trabecular meshwork

Drainage angle

Flow of fluid
Iris
Lens
Cornea
Pupil

NORMAL EYE

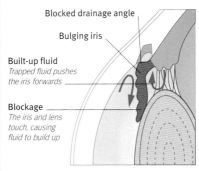

Blocked drainage angle

Bulging iris

Built-up fluid
Trapped fluid pushes the iris forwards

Blockage
The iris and lens touch, causing fluid to build up

ACUTE GLAUCOMA

Mechanism of acute glaucoma
Fluid normally flows out through the pupil and drains out of the meshwork deep within the drainage angle. If the iris and lens touch, fluid becomes trapped and the iris bulges forwards. This blocks the drainage angle, causing acute glaucoma.

▶ **TEST**

Tonometry

The eye condition glaucoma, in which the pressure inside the eye is elevated, can be detected using an instrument called a tonometer. Anaesthetic drops are put into your eye, then the tonometer is pressed gently against the cornea, the transparent front part of the eye, and the force needed to flatten the cornea is measured. The test takes only a few seconds and is painless. A simpler form of tonometry (called non-contact tonometry) may be carried out during a routine eye test. This involves having a puff of air directed at your eye. The pressure in your eye is then calculated on the basis of your eye's resistance to the puff of air.

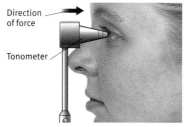

Direction of force

Tonometer

Contact tonometry
The tonometer is held against the cornea. As the internal pressure is measured, the pressure on your eye will increase slightly.

▶ TREATMENT

Laser iridotomy

This technique is used to treat acute glaucoma, in which pressure in the eye rises suddenly due to blockage in the outflow of fluid. The pressure is reduced using eyedrops, intravenous drugs, and, sometimes, oral drugs. Anaesthetic eyedrops are then put into the eye, and a thick contact lens is placed in front of it to focus a laser beam onto the iris. The laser cuts a small hole in the iris, releasing the fluid behind it. The iris flattens, opening the drainage angle and letting trapped fluid out. The hole remains in the eye with no ill effects.

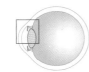
LOCATION

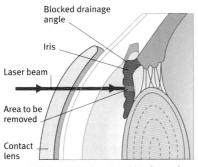

Blocked drainage angle
Iris
Laser beam
Area to be removed
Contact lens

1 *A thick contact lens is held in front of the eye, and a laser beam is focused through it onto the iris. The laser then cuts a small hole right through the iris.*

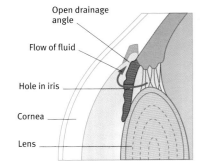

Open drainage angle
Flow of fluid
Hole in iris
Cornea
Lens

2 *Fluid trapped behind the iris flows through the hole. The iris returns to its normal shape, and the drainage angle opens, allowing the eye to drain normally.*

you should consult your doctor at once. Full-blown attacks develop suddenly. Symptoms include:
■ Rapid deterioration of vision.
■ Intense pain in the eye.
■ Redness and watering of the eye.
■ Sensitivity to bright light.
■ Haloes appearing around lights.
■ Nausea and vomiting.
If you develop a painful eye or your vision deteriorates suddenly, go to an accident and emergency department or consult your doctor immediately.

What might be done?

The pressure inside the eye is measured using a technique such as tonometry (opposite page). If acute glaucoma is detected, you will be given immediate drug treatment by intravenous injection, as eyedrops, and possibly also by mouth to reduce the pressure in the eye (*see* **Drugs for glaucoma**, p.594). Laser iridotomy (above) will probably be performed as soon as the pressure falls. In this technique, a laser is used to make a small hole in the iris so that fluid can be released. The unaffected eye may also be treated as a precaution.

After surgery, most people are symptom-free, but some loss of the outer edges of vision may remain. Long-term drug treatment or a second operation may be needed to prevent loss of sight.

Chronic glaucoma

A gradual, painless increase in the fluid pressure inside the eye

 Rare under the age of 40; more common over the age of 60

 Sometimes runs in families; more common in people of African descent

 Gender and lifestyle are not significant factors

Chronic glaucoma is also known as open-angle glaucoma. The condition causes a gradual deterioration of sight due to a progressive build-up of fluid pressure inside the eye (often over a period of years) causing nerve damage. There are often no symptoms until late in the disease, and loss of vision is permanent. The condition can lead to total blindness (p.369), but early treatment can prevent damage. Both eyes are usually affected, although the condition may be more severe in one eye.

What are the causes?

Fluid is continually secreted into the front of the eye to nourish the tissues and maintain the shape of the eye. Normally, this fluid drains away through the trabecular meshwork, a sieve-like structure at the back of the angle that is formed between the iris and the edge of the cornea (called the drainage angle).

However, in chronic glaucoma, a gradual blockage develops in the meshwork. Although the drainage angle remains open, fluid is prevented from draining normally, and the pressure in the eye gradually rises.

The increasing fluid pressure progressively damages the nerve fibres situated in the light-sensitive retina at the back of the eye and in the optic nerve, which carries nerve signals from the retina to the brain, causing loss of vision.

The underlying reason for the problem in the drainage system is not yet fully understood. Genetic factors may be involved and the condition sometimes runs in families. It is also more common in people of African descent. There is also an increased risk of developing chronic glaucoma if you are very shortsighted (*see* **Myopia**, p.365).

What are the symptoms?

Chronic glaucoma often has no symptoms until late in the disease, by which time it is probable that your vision has been permanently affected. During the later stages, the symptoms may include:
■ Bumping into objects because of loss of the outer edges of vision (peripheral vision).
■ Eventual blurring of objects that are straight ahead.
Always consult your doctor promptly if you notice a change in your vision. Because the risk of chronic glaucoma increases beyond middle age, everyone over the age of 40 should be tested for the condition every 2 years. If you are in a high-risk group, you should be tested regularly whatever your age.

How is it diagnosed?

Chronic glaucoma can often be detected at an early stage during a routine eye examination by an optometrist, who will refer you to an ophthalmologist for tests to confirm

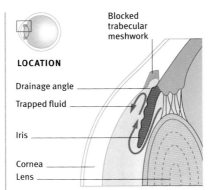

LOCATION

Blocked trabecular meshwork
Drainage angle
Trapped fluid
Iris
Cornea
Lens

Fluid flow in chronic glaucoma
Normally, fluid flows out of the eye through the meshwork around the iris. In chronic glaucoma, the meshwork is blocked, and pressure builds up.

the diagnosis. Ophthalmologists often use a technique known as tonometry (opposite page) to measure the pressure inside the eye. The retina will also be examined using ophthalmoscopy (p.360). This is a technique that will reveal damage to the optic nerve resulting from the high pressure. Your ophthalmologist will also perform a visual field test (p.369) to check for loss of peripheral vision.

What is the treatment?

If chronic glaucoma is diagnosed early, eyedrops to reduce the pressure in the eye will probably be prescribed (*see* **Drugs for glaucoma**, p.594). You will probably need to use these eyedrops for the rest of your life.

If the condition is advanced, or if eyedrops do not lower the pressure sufficiently, surgery may be needed to make a drainage channel in the white of the eye (*see* **Trabeculectomy**, below). In another surgical technique, called

▶ TREATMENT

Trabeculectomy

This surgical technique is used to treat chronic glaucoma, in which the pressure in the eye gradually rises due to a blockage of the trabecular meshwork, a sieve-like structure through which the fluid in the eye normally drains. Trabeculectomy may be carried out under a general or local anaesthetic and involves cutting out a section of the blocked meshwork so that fluid can flow out freely. Your doctor may advise you to wear an eye shield for a few days while the eye heals. You should also avoid strenuous activity for several weeks after the procedure.

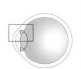

LOCATION

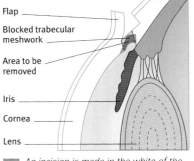

Flap
Blocked trabecular meshwork
Area to be removed
Iris
Cornea
Lens

1 *An incision is made in the white of the eye over the area where fluid normally drains away. The flap is pulled back to expose the trabecular meshwork, and a section of the blocked meshwork is cut out.*

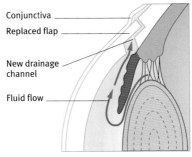

Conjunctiva
Replaced flap
New drainage channel
Fluid flow

2 *The flap in the white of the eye is replaced. Fluid can now drain around the edges of the flap and under the clear conjunctiva that covers the white of the eye. Pressure in the eye is then relieved.*

laser trabeculoplasty, a laser beam is used to increase flow through the trabecular meshwork, allowing fluid to drain away. In some cases, it may be necessary to continue using eyedrops after laser trabeculoplasty. If chronic glaucoma affects only one eye, the other will probably also need treatment eventually.

Floaters

Dark specks that appear to float and move in front of the eye

 More common with increasing age, especially after the age of about 40

 Gender, genetics, and lifestyle are not significant factors

It is quite common to see small specks, known as floaters, that appear to float in the field of vision. Although floaters seem to lie in front of the eyes, they are in fact fragments of tissue in the jelly-like vitreous humour that fills the back of the eye. These fragments cast shadows on the light-sensitive retina at the back of the eye. They move rapidly with any eye movement, but, when the eyes are still, they drift slowly.

The reason for most floaters is a pulling away of the vitreous humour from the retina. Floaters rarely affect vision, but you should consult your doctor immediately if they suddenly appear in large numbers or interfere with vision. A sudden increase in the number of floaters may indicate a serious eye disorder that requires urgent treatment, such as separation of the retina from its underlying tissue (*see* **Retinal detachment**, right), or a leakage of blood into the vitreous humour (*see* **Vitreous haemorrhage**, right).

Vitreous haemorrhage

Bleeding into the vitreous humour, the jelly-like substance that fills the back part of the eye, due to ruptured blood vessels

 Participating in sports that may lead to a blow to the eye is a risk factor

 Age, gender, and genetics are not significant factors

If blood vessels in the light-sensitive retina at the back of the eye rupture, blood from the ruptured vessels leaks into the jelly-like vitreous humour. This bleeding is known as a vitreous haemorrhage. The rupture may be due to a blow to the eye; a blocked vein in the retina (*see* **Retinal vein occlusion**, right); or the growth of abnormally fragile blood vessels in the retina because of other disorders, such as diabetic retinopathy (opposite page).

If the bleeding is minor, the only symptom may be the sudden appearance of large numbers of specks that seem to float in front of the eye (*see* **Floaters**, left). More severe bleeding can cause sudden loss of vision. Rarely, the blood in the vitreous humour clots, forming fibrous strands. Over a long period of time, new blood vessels may grow along these strands and pull on the retina, which may result in retinal detachment (right) and blindness (p.369).

You should call your doctor immediately if you have sudden loss of vision or if floaters appear in your eye in large numbers. He or she will examine the eye using ophthalmoscopy (below).

In mild cases of vitreous haemorrhage, floaters disappear within a few days. However, a large haemorrhage may take several weeks to clear, and, in severe cases, an operation may be needed to remove the affected vitreous humour and seal leaking blood vessels.

Retinal vein occlusion

Blockage of a vein in the light-sensitive retina at the back of the eye

 Increasingly common over the age of 50

 Gender, genetics, and lifestyle are not significant factors

Retinal vein occlusion (an obstructed vein in the eye's light-sensitive retina) is usually caused by a blood clot in the vein, preventing blood from draining away from the retina. This may cause the vein to burst, or the rising pressure may cause bleeding in the retina. Blockage of a small vein may not cause symptoms, but, if a large vein is affected, vision may deteriorate in a few hours.

Retinal vein occlusion affects mostly elderly people whose blood vessels are narrowed by atherosclerosis (p.241). It is also more common in people with glaucoma (p.358), high blood pressure (*see* **Hypertension**, p.242), or a disorder that makes blood clot easily (*see* **Hypercoagulability**, p.275).

The blockage of a small vein is often detected during a routine examination of the eye by ophthalmoscopy (left), but, if your vision deteriorates suddenly, see a doctor at once. In most cases, there is no treatment for the condition itself but treating the underlying cause may stop a recurrence. Small retinal vein occlusions may sometimes be treated by injections of drugs called anti-VEGF agents, which may restore vision in some people. You may also need retinal laser treatment to prevent or treat secondary glaucoma.

Retinal detachment

Separation of the light-sensitive retina at the back of the eye from the supporting tissues underneath

 More common over the age of 50

 Sometimes runs in families

 Participating in sports that may lead to a blow to the eye is a risk factor

 Gender is not a significant factor

The light-sensitive retina of the eye is normally attached to the underlying tissue, but in retinal detachment part of the retina peels away from this tissue. The

condition usually affects one eye only but, without rapid treatment, can cause partial or total blindness (p.369).

Retinal detachment usually begins with a small tear in the retina. Fluid is then able to pass through the hole and separates the retina from the supporting tissues underneath. Tears may be caused by disorders such as severe shortsightedness (*see* **Myopia**, p.365) or eye injuries. In some people, tears appear as a result of scarring after a vitreous haemorrhage (left). Retinal detachment sometimes runs in families.

What are the symptoms?
Retinal detachment is painless, but its visual symptoms may include:
■ Flashing lights in the corner of the eye.
■ Large numbers of tiny dark spots in the field of vision (*see* **Floaters**, left).
If a large area of the retina has become detached, you may experience a cloudy ring or a black area across your field of vision. If you experience any of these symptoms, you should go to an accident and emergency department or call your doctor immediately.

What might be done?
Retinal detachment is diagnosed by using a special head-mounted ophthalmoscope to examine the eye's internal structures. If only a small area of retina has detached, the tear may be sealed by laser treatment (p.613) or cryotherapy. However, if a large area has detached, surgery is necessary. If treated early, normal vision may be restored, but delayed treatment is less effective.

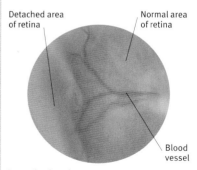
Detached area of retina
Normal area of retina
Blood vessel

Detached retina
In this view through an ophthalmoscope, the area of detached retina can be clearly distinguished from the normal area of retinal tissue seen on the right.

Retinopathy

Damage to the small blood vessels in the retina, the light-sensitive membrane at the back of the eye

 Age, gender, genetics, and lifestyle as risk factors depend on the cause

Some long-standing diseases can damage small blood vessels throughout the body. If the blood vessels in the retina (the light-sensitive membrane at the back of the eye) are affected, the damage is known as retinopathy. Retinal damage varies according to

---

▶ TEST

Ophthalmoscopy

In this technique, an instrument called an ophthalmoscope is used to examine the inside of the eye. You will be asked to focus on a distant object while the instrument directs a beam of light into your eye. Through the lenses in the ophthalmoscope, the ophthalmologist can examine the light-sensitive retina; the retinal blood vessels; the head of the optic nerve, which carries nerve signals from the eye to the brain; and the jelly-like vitreous humour, which fills the back of the eye. Ophthalmoscopy is painless, but if eyedrops are used to dilate the pupils, your vision may become temporarily blurred. Instead of an ophthalmoscope, a slit lamp (p.358) with a lens placed in front of your eye may sometimes be used to examine structures such as the retina.

Ophthalmoscope   Ophthalmologist

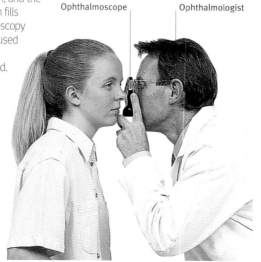
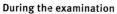

During the examination
The ophthalmologist looks through the lens of the ophthalmoscope to examine the structures inside the eye.

the underlying disorder but can include leakage of blood from damaged vessels, loss of blood flow to some areas, and abnormal development of new blood vessels. Retinopathy may cause loss of vision.

One of the most common causes of retinopathy is diabetes mellitus (*see* **Diabetic retinopathy**, below). The condition can also occur as a result of high blood pressure (*see* **Hypertension**, p.242), although vision is not usually affected in this case. Less frequently, retinopathy may be caused by AIDS (*see* **HIV infection and AIDS**, p.169), oxygen therapy in premature babies (*see* **Problems of the premature baby**, p.530), or by sickle-cell disease (p.272). Usually, only the underlying disease is treated. However, in diabetic retinopathy, laser treatment of the retina itself (*see* **Laser surgery for retinopathy**, right) can save vision.

Diabetic retinopathy

Damage to blood vessels in the retina, caused by diabetes mellitus

 Usually occurs in adults who have had diabetes mellitus for many years

 Sometimes runs in families

 Poor control of diabetes mellitus and smoking are risk factors

 Gender is not a significant factor

If you have diabetes mellitus (p.437), you have an increased risk of developing retinopathy. Diabetes mellitus can lead to abnormalities in small blood vessels anywhere in the body. If the damage affects vessels in the retina, the light-sensitive membrane at the back of the eye, diabetic retinopathy develops. The condition usually affects both eyes. At first, small blood vessels in the retina leak. Later, fragile new blood vessels may grow out into the jelly-like vitreous humour, a condition known as proliferative retinopathy. Loss of vision may result if retinopathy is left untreated, and blindness (p.369) may eventually follow.

The longer people have had diabetes and the less tightly the disorder is controlled, the greater the risk. Only a few people with type 1 diabetes mellitus develop retinopathy within the first 10 years after diabetes is diagnosed but, once retinopathy is established, it can progress rapidly. The condition may be present to some extent in type 2 diabetes mellitus by the time the diabetes has been recognized.

What are the symptoms?

Symptoms of diabetic retinopathy may not be noticeable until damage to the retina is severe, although there may be areas of blurred vision. As the disease progresses, vision may suddenly be lost in one eye due to rupture of one of the fragile new blood vessels in the retina (*see* **Vitreous haemorrhage**, opposite page) or the separation of the retina from the underlying tissue

(*see* **Retinal detachment**, opposite page). You should consult your doctor immediately if you experience sudden loss of vision.

Everybody over the age of 11 with diabetes should be registered with their local diabetic retinopathy centre, which arranges for every person to have regular photographs taken of their retina. These photographs are examined for signs of retinopathy so that it can be identified and treated as soon as possible. The photographs can also be used to detect diabetic maculopathy, in which fluid leaks into the centre of the retina, causing gradual impairment of central vision.

What might be done?

Established diabetic retinopathy can be identified by studying the retina with an instrument called an ophthalmoscope (*see* **Ophthalmoscopy**, opposite page). If your doctor suspects early retinopathy, he or she may arrange for fluorescein angiography (below), in which dye is injected into the circulatory system to show the retinal blood vessels in detail.

In some cases, your doctor may arrange for a diagnostic procedure called optical coherence tomography (OCT). This procedure, which is quick and painless, involves shining a light into the eye and then using the reflections from the back of the eye to produce a cross-sectional image of the retina, in an analogous way to how ultrasound scanning produces images using echoes.

If diabetic retinopathy is detected at an early stage, treatment may not be necessary, although your doctor will recommend regular monitoring. In later stages of the condition, laser surgery (*see* **Laser surgery**

for retinopathy, above) will probably be recommended, particularly if you have proliferative retinopathy. Any visual loss due to diabetic retinopathy that has already occurred is usually permanent but laser

surgery should prevent further loss of sight, although it may be necessary to have repeat treatments. If you have diabetic maculopathy, you may be given injections of an anti-vascular endothelial growth

▶ TREATMENT

Laser surgery for retinopathy

Laser surgery is used in the treatment of diabetic retinopathy to reduce abnormal blood vessels and prevent new ones from forming. Treatment is usually performed under a local anaesthetic, usually over several sessions. The laser makes tiny burns that destroy parts of the retina, which causes the abnormal blood vessels to regress and prevents new abnormal vessels from developing. Some vision may be lost, but blindness is prevented.

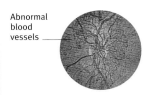

BEFORE SURGERY

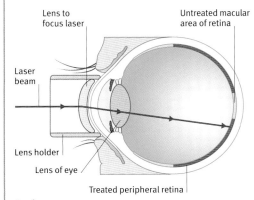

During surgery
A special lens held in front of your eye focuses the laser beam. Treatment is virtually painless, but you will see flashes of light as the laser strikes the retina.

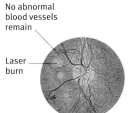

AFTER SURGERY

Results of laser treatment
Before laser surgery, new, abnormal blood vessels, which were formed on the surface of the light-sensitive retina, are visible. Following surgery, these abnormal blood vessels have regressed and the outer area of the retina appears much paler.

▶ TEST

Fluorescein angiography

This technique is used to study the blood vessels in the light-sensitive retina of the eye. A fluorescent dye (fluorescein) is injected into the circulatory system through one of the veins in the arm. As the dye passes through the retinal vessels, a series of photographs (fluorescein angiograms) is taken to define any underlying abnormalities. The ophthalmologist can then assess the extent of the damage. The test is painless, but your skin and urine may turn dark yellow until all the dye has been excreted.

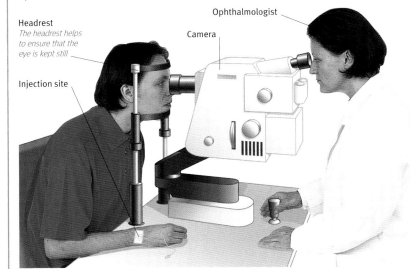

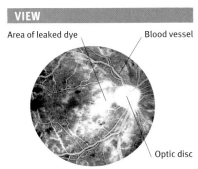

Leaking retinal blood vessels
This fluorescein angiogram shows an area of fluorescent dye that has leaked from damaged blood vessels into the retinal tissue.

During the test
The pupils are dilated with eyedrops, and fluorescein dye is injected into a vein in your arm. The dye then circulates in your bloodstream. When the dye reaches your eye and is moving through the retinal blood vessels, a series of photographs is taken.

(anti-VEGF) drug into your eye. This medication can reduce leakage of fluid and may allow the eye to heal itself to some extent.

Macular degeneration

Progressive damage to the macula, the area near the centre of the light-sensitive retina that is responsible for detailed vision

 Increasingly common with age, especially over the age of 70

 More common in females

 Sometimes runs in families

 Smoking and excessive exposure to sunlight are risk factors

Gradual deterioration of the macula, the most sensitive region of the light-sensitive retina at the back of the eye, is known as macular degeneration. The condition leads to progressive loss of central and detailed vision. Affected people become unable to read or to recognize faces. However, the edges of their vision (peripheral vision) remain clear. Usually both eyes are affected.

Macular degeneration is more common in females and sometimes runs in families. The condition usually develops after the age of 70, although there are some rare forms that affect younger people. The risk of developing macular degeneration is increased by excessive exposure to sunlight and smoking.

What are the types?

There are two main forms, but their causes are unknown. In dry macular degeneration, light-sensitive cells in the macula and cells in the supporting layer underneath die. In wet macular degeneration, fragile new blood vessels grow beneath the macula. As the blood vessels leak fluid or bleed, the light-sensitive cells in the macula are damaged.

What are the symptoms?

Macular degeneration causes progressive visual loss over several months. Symptoms may include:

- Difficulty in reading, watching television, and recognizing faces.
- Distortion of vision so that objects appear larger or smaller than normal, or straight lines appear wavy.

Wet macular degeneration may cause sudden loss of central vision due to rupture of an abnormal blood vessel. Without treatment, the damaged macula eventually becomes scarred, causing permanent visual impairment. Anybody who develops symptoms should consult their doctor promptly, particularly if they experience sudden distortion of vision.

What might be done?

Diagnosis is made by vision tests (p.367) and by ophthalmoscopy (p.360) of the retina.

If there is a possibility of wet macular degeneration, then fluorescein angiography (p.361) may be carried out to check for abnormal blood vessels.

Dry macular degeneration cannot be treated but there is limited evidence that large amounts of vitamins A, C, E, and the minerals zinc and copper may help to slow the progression of the disease. Smokers should also stop smoking.

The early stages of wet macular degeneration may be treated by a course of drugs called anti-vascular endothelial growth factor agents (anti-VEGF agents). These drugs inhibit the growth of new blood vessels under the macula and are given by injection into the eye. The drugs can be effective at preventing deterioration of vision and in a few cases may even restore some of the sight lost as a result of macular degeneration. However, not everybody regains some lost sight, and even in those that do, sight is not completely restored.

If sight becomes severely affected, aids such as magnifying glasses may help with tasks such as reading.

Retinitis pigmentosa

An inherited progressive degeneration in the retina, the light-sensitive membrane at the back of the eye

 Most commonly begins between the ages of 10 and 30.

 Slightly more common in males

 Due to an abnormal gene inherited from one or both parents

 Lifestyle is not a significant factor

Retinitis pigmentosa is a rare disorder in which the cells in the light-sensitive retina in the eye are progressively lost. Dark patches of pigment form on the retina, and vision deteriorates. The disorder is slightly more common in males and symptoms usually first appear between the age of 10 and 30, although they may sometimes appear earlier or not until middle age. Retinitis pigmentosa may be inherited in an autosomal dominant, autosomal recessive, or sex-linked manner (*see* **Gene disorders**, p.151), depending on the abnormal gene involved. Both eyes are affected equally, although there is a large variation in the severity of the condition from one person to another.

If you have retinitis pigmentosa, the first symptom you may notice is poor vision in dim light. Later, the outer edges of vision, known as peripheral vision, are lost, and sight deteriorates progressively inwards until only a small area of central vision remains (this is known as tunnel vision). Rarely, tunnel vision can cause blindness (p.369). Retinitis pigmentosa is diagnosed by examining the retina with an

ophthalmoscope (*see* **Ophthalmoscopy**, p.360). Although there is currently no treatment for retinitis pigmentosa, special glasses may help to widen the field of vision if you have tunnel vision. If you plan to have children, you may wish to have genetic counselling (p.151).

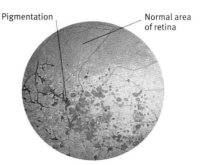

Pigmentation Normal area of retina

Retinitis pigmentosa
In this view through an ophthalmoscope, areas of pigmentation caused by retinitis pigmentosa are visible on part of the retina. The disorder leads to loss of vision.

Optic neuritis

Inflammation of the optic nerve, which carries signals from the light-sensitive retina to the brain

 Mainly affects young adults

 Three times more common in females

 Sometimes runs in families

 Lifestyle is not a significant factor

The optic nerve carries signals from the light-sensitive retina, found at the back of the eye, to the brain. Optic neuritis causes the nerve to become inflamed, resulting in pain and blurred vision. Usually, only one eye is affected.

Optic neuritis is most often caused by degeneration of the protective fatty sheath that surrounds the optic nerve fibres. This process, called demyelination, can be caused by a variety of conditions, including multiple sclerosis (p.334). Optic neuritis can also occur as a result of poisoning with chemicals, such as lead and methanol, or some viral infections, such as chickenpox (p.165). The condition can also occur for no obvious reason, most commonly in women in their late teens or twenties.

What are the symptoms?

Optic neuritis usually causes vision to deteriorate over hours or days. You may notice various symptoms, including:

- Loss of visual detail, making it difficult to read or to recognize faces.
- Loss of the central area of vision.
- Pain in the back of the eye that gets worse with eye movement.

If you experience a rapid deterioration in your vision, you should consult your doctor immediately.

What might be done?

Your doctor will use an ophthalmoscope (*see* **Ophthalmoscopy**, p.360) to examine your eye and may also carry out vision tests (p.367). The optic nerve and other parts of the nervous system may be tested for signs of multiple sclerosis (*see* **Visual evoked responses** p.335) because optic neuritis may be the first sign of this disorder.

If you have optic neuritis, you may be given oral corticosteroids (p.600) to relieve inflammation. Although vision often improves in 3–6 weeks, optic neuritis often recurs, and visual damage may be permanent. About half of all people who have optic neuritis develop multiple sclerosis within 5 years.

Papilloedema

Swelling of the optic disc, the area on the light-sensitive retina where the optic nerve enters the eye

 Age, gender, genetics, and lifestyle as risk factors depend on the cause

When the eye sends a signal to the brain, the signal travels along the optic nerve. The point on the light-sensitive retina where the optic nerve enters the eye is known as the optic disc, which can swell if pressure inside the skull increases. This condition is called papilloedema or optic disc oedema. There are several causes, including raised blood pressure (*see* **Hypertension**, p.242), head injuries (p.322), a brain tumour (p.327), or inflammation of the membranes that surround the brain (*see* **Meningitis**, p.325). The disorder itself does not cause pain, but the raised pressure of blood inside the head often causes headaches and vomiting.

Papilloedema is diagnosed with an instrument called an ophthalmoscope (*see* **Ophthalmoscopy**, p.360). MRI (p.133) or CT scanning (p.132) may be used to look for an underlying cause of the disorder. In the meantime, corticosteroids (p.600) may be given to reduce pressure in the skull and prevent lasting damage to the optic nerve.

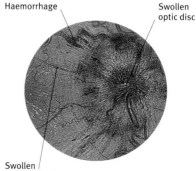

Haemorrhage Swollen optic disc

Swollen blood vessels

Papilloedema
This view through an ophthalmoscope shows a swollen optic disc (papilloedema) and distended retinal blood vessels caused by raised pressure inside the skull.

Exophthalmos

Bulging of one or both eyes, making them look abnormally prominent

 More common in females

 Age, genetics, and lifestyle are not significant factors

If the tissue in the eye socket swells, the eyeball can protrude, causing a staring appearance known as exophthalmos (also sometimes called proptosis). The condition usually affects both eyes and is more common in women. It is often linked with an overactive thyroid gland (*see* **Hyperthyroidism**, p.432). Less commonly, the cause may be bleeding or infection behind the eye, a tumour, or a cyst. In these cases, usually only one eye is affected.

Severe exophthalmos can result in blurred vision because of pressure on the eye. Abnormal eye movement may lead to a change in the position of the eye, which can result in double vision (p.368). Exophthalmos may keep the eyelids from closing properly, causing the front of the eye to dry out, increasing the risk of damage to the cornea.

What is the treatment?
Exophthalmos may be corrected by dealing with the underlying cause, such as by treating a bacterial infection with antibiotics (p.572). However, if the exophthalmos is due to hyperthyroidism, it often remains after the underlying condition has been treated.

If exophthalmos persists, you may need surgery to make more room for the eye by removing part of the socket.

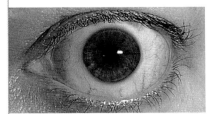

Exophthalmos
The staring appearance of this eye is due to swelling of tissues in the eye socket, making the eye bulge forwards (exophthalmos).

Eye injuries

Physical damage to the structures of the eye

 Certain occupations or sports are risk factors

 Age, gender, and genetics are not significant factors

The eyelid-closing reflex and the bony socket around the eye help to protect the eye from injuries. However, eye injuries are still common, and in some cases blindness may result if treatment is not given promptly.

The most common injury to the eye is a scratch on the transparent cornea caused by a foreign body in the eye (*see* **Corneal abrasion**, p.355). Minor injuries of this type rarely damage vision permanently unless an infection develops and remains untreated. However, penetrating injuries in which the eye is pierced by a tiny, fast-moving object, such as a metal chip from machinery, can lead to total loss of sight. Blunt injuries, such as those caused by a blow from a fist or ball, may also endanger vision. Injuries can also occur when using caustic chemicals or while looking directly at the sun.

Most eye injuries can be prevented by the use of protective eyewear when working with dangerous machines or chemicals or when participating in athletic activities. Never look directly at the sun, even while wearing sunglasses.

What are the symptoms?
The symptoms of eye injuries differ according to the type and severity of damage, but symptoms may include:
- Pain and watering of the eye.
- Inability to open the eye.
- Bleeding under the front surface of the eye (*see* **Subconjunctival haemorrhage**, p.355).
- Bruising and swelling of the skin around the eye.
- Reduced vision in the affected eye.

You should always seek prompt medical attention for any eye injury because all eye injuries are potentially serious. If the injury was caused by a blow to the eye, involves a penetrating foreign body, or results in reduced vision, hold a clean, dry cloth over the injured eye, making sure you do not touch or press on it. A chemical injury should be treated at once by washing the chemical out of the eye with copious amounts of water. Then go to the nearest accident and emergency department immediately.

What might be done?
Your doctor will probably assess the eye by ophthalmoscopy (p.360) and a slit-lamp examination (p.358). Ultrasound scanning (p.135) may also be used to look for a foreign body in the eye and assess the extent of the damage.

Most eye injuries can be treated under a local anaesthetic, although some will require surgery under a general anaesthetic. Many eye injuries heal completely with prompt treatment. Sometimes corneal injuries leave a scar, and, if the lens is damaged, part of it may become cloudy (*see* **Cataract**, p.357). Sunlight may cause permanent damage to the retina. Separation of the retina from its underlying layer (*see* **Retinal detachment**, p.360) may be due to a heavy blow and requires urgent treatment to prevent loss of sight. A serious eye injury can cause permanent blindness.

Eyelid and tear system disorders

Eyelids and tears work together to protect the eye against damage. The eyelids act as shutters, closing to stop material from entering the eyes. Tears keep the surface of the eyes moist and help to prevent infection. Disorders of the eyelids or tear system can damage the eyes, but most are easily treated if detected early.

The upper and lower eyelids provide essential protection for the eyes. If anything approaches the eye or face rapidly, the eyelids close together almost instantaneously as a reflex action. Furthermore, each eyelid has two or three rows of eyelashes, which help to prevent small particles from entering the eye.

Tears are another important part of the eyes' defences. They are made up of a salty fluid produced by the lacrimal (tear) glands, which are located above the upper eyelids. Tears lubricate the exposed surface of the eye and wash away potentially harmful materials, such as dust and chemicals. Tears also contain a natural antiseptic that helps to protect the eye against infection.

The initial articles in this section focus on conditions that affect the eyelids. These conditions include infections of the eyelid and disorders that alter the physical shape of the eyelids. The section then discusses disorders that affect the tear system, which include blockage of the tear drainage channels and problems with tear production. Disorders that affect the physical structures of the eye itself are covered elsewhere in the book (*see* **Eye disorders**, pp.355–363).

➕ KEY ANATOMY

For more information on the structure and function of the eye, *see* pp.351–354.

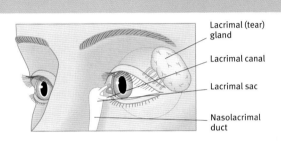

Lacrimal (tear) gland

Lacrimal canal

Lacrimal sac

Nasolacrimal duct

Stye

A painful, pus-filled swelling at the root of an eyelash due to a bacterial infection

 More common in children but can occur at any age

 Wearing contact lenses and using eye make-up may be risk factors

 Gender and genetics are not significant factors

An infection at the root of an eyelash may result in the formation of a pus-filled swelling called a stye. Most styes are caused by *Staphylococcus aureus*, a bacterium found on the skin of many healthy people. Adults are less likely than children to develop styes, but, if you use eye make-up or wear contact lenses, you may be at increased risk.

A stye begins as a red lump on the edge of the eyelid. Over about the next day, the eyelid becomes swollen and tender, and a yellow spot may form at the centre of the swelling.

What is the treatment?
Styes usually rupture, drain, and heal in a few days without treatment. You may be able to speed the process by placing a

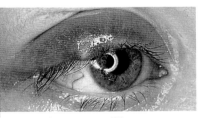

Stye on the upper eyelid
The swelling and redness of this eyelid are due to a stye, caused by a pus-producing infection at the root of an eyelash.

clean, warm, damp cloth on the stye for about 20 minutes four times a day. To avoid infecting other people or reinfecting yourself, always wash your hands after touching the infected eyelid and avoid sharing or reusing personal items such as towels or facecloths.

If a stye does not heal in a few days or if the swelling becomes worse, see your doctor. He or she may prescribe a topical antibiotic, which should be put directly on the stye and the skin surrounding it (*see* **Drugs acting on the eye**, p.594). However, if the stye persists, you may also need to take an oral antibiotic (p.572). The stye should clear up within 2–3 days of taking the antibiotic. Styes are unlikely to cause long-term damage, but they tend to recur in some people who are prone to them.

Blepharitis

Inflammation of the margin of the upper or lower eyelid or both

 Age, gender, genetics, and lifestyle are not significant factors

Blepharitis, in which the margin of one or both eyelids becomes inflamed, is often associated with the skin disorders seborrhoeic dermatitis (p.194) and rosacea (p.198). Blepharitis may also be due to a bacterial infection or an allergy to cosmetics.

If you have blepharitis, your eyelids will be swollen, red, and itchy. The margins of the eyelids may be covered with soft, greasy scales that dry into crusts, sticking the eyelashes together. In some cases, the roots of the eyelashes become infected, causing small ulcers or styes (p.363) to form.

What is the treatment?
You can relieve the symptoms by holding a clean, warm, damp cloth against the eyelid. The healing process may be helped by gently cleaning the eyelids twice a day with baby shampoo diluted half-and-half with water. If you have seborrhoeic dermatitis, treating it with a dandruff shampoo that contains an antifungal agent should also help the blepharitis. If the blepharitis recurs repeatedly, see your doctor, who may prescribe topical antibiotics (*see* Drugs acting on the eye, p.594) or a corticosteroid (p.600). The condition often clears up after 2 weeks of treatment, but it may recur. Allergic blepharitis usually improves on its own if you avoid contact with the trigger substance.

Chalazion

A swelling in the eyelid that may be painless

 Age, gender, genetics, and lifestyle are not significant factors

If an oil-secreting gland in the eyelid becomes blocked, the gland enlarges, creating a swelling called a chalazion. A chalazion may at first look like a stye (p.363), but, unlike a stye, it is not on the eyelid margin. Usually, the pain and redness associated with a chalazion disappear after a few days. However, if the swelling is large, it may cause long-term discomfort, and pressure on the front of the eye can interfere with vision.

What might be done?
If your doctor diagnoses a chalazion, he or she will probably wait for several weeks before arranging any treatment because it may disappear on its own. Meanwhile, if the chalazion is painful or irritating, holding a clean, warm, damp cloth against it may help.

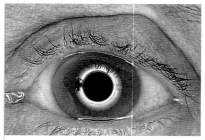

Chalazion
The swelling in the upper eyelid of this eye is a chalazion, caused by blockage of an oil-secreting gland.

A persistent chalazion can be treated by a simple operation in which a small cut is made in the inner surface of the eyelid and the contents of the swelling removed. The procedure is performed under local anaesthesia and is painless.

Ptosis

Abnormal drooping of one or both upper eyelids

 Age, gender, genetics, and lifestyle as risk factors depend on the cause

Drooping of the upper eyelid due to weakness of the muscle that raises it is called ptosis. The condition may be the result of a problem with the muscle or nerve that controls the eyelid. The sagging lid may partly or totally close the eye. One or both eyes may be affected.

Ptosis is occasionally present from birth. If a baby's eyelid droops and it covers the pupil, his or her vision may not develop normally (*see* Amblyopia, p.556) and early treatment is vital.

Ptosis in adults can occur as a part of the aging process, or it may be a symptom of myasthenia gravis (p.339), which causes progressive muscle weakness. If ptosis starts suddenly, it may be due to a brain tumour (p.327) or a defective blood vessel in the brain. If you develop ptosis, see your doctor to rule out a serious underlying disorder.

What is the treatment?
Ptosis in babies can be corrected by surgically tightening the eyelid muscle. If treatment is carried out early, the child's vision should develop normally.

In adults, surgery for ptosis should be carried out only after any possible significant underlying disorders have been ruled out. Surgery is very effective for ptosis caused by the aging process.

Entropion

Inward turning of the margin of the upper or lower eyelid or both

 More common in elderly people

 Gender, genetics, and lifestyle are not significant factors

In entropion, the eyelid turns inwards. The eyelashes rub against the cornea (the transparent front part of the eye) and the conjunctiva (which covers the white of the eye). Although the conjunctiva also lines the eyelids, this area is unaffected. Typical symptoms of the condition are pain in the eye area, watery eye (right) and irritation. Left untreated, the cornea may become damaged (*see* Corneal ulcer, p.356), leading to loss of vision.

In developed countries, entropion mainly affects elderly people because of the natural weakening of the muscles around the eyelids that takes place with increasing age. In developing countries, entropion affecting the upper eyelid most often follows bouts of the eye infection trachoma (p.356), which causes scar tissue to form on the inner surface of the eyelids. Eventually, this tissue may shrink, making the eyelids turn inwards.

A minor operation can be carried out to realign the eyelid. This procedure usually corrects the condition and prevents any further damage to the eye.

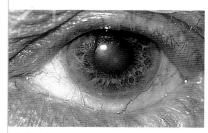

Entropion
This eye's lower lid has turned inwards, causing the eyelashes to rub against the eye. This condition is called entropion.

Ectropion

Outward turning of the margin of the lower eyelid

 More common in elderly people

 Gender, genetics, and lifestyle are not significant factors

If the edge of the lower eyelid turns outwards and the eyelid hangs away from the eye, the exposed inner surface of the lid becomes dry and sore. This condition is known as ectropion and may stop tears from entering the nasolacrimal duct, which runs from the eye to the nose, causing the eye to water continuously. Since the eyelids cannot close fully, the transparent cornea at the front part of the eye is constantly exposed and may become damaged (*see* Corneal ulcer, p.356) or repeatedly infected. The condition most often occurs in elderly people as a result of weakness of the lower eyelid that may occur with increasing age. Both eyes are usually affected. Ectropion may also be caused by contraction of a scar on the eyelid or cheek or by facial palsy (p.339), in which the muscles around the eye (and other facial muscles on the affected side) are paralysed. In these cases, only one eye is usually involved.

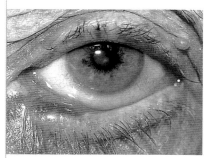

Ectropion
The lower eyelid of this eye has turned outwards (ectropion), exposing the inner surface and preventing drainage of tears.

What is the treatment?
If you think that you have ectropion, you should consult your doctor as soon as you can because treatment of the disorder is most successful when it is carried out early. Your doctor will probably recommend a straightforward surgical operation, performed under local anaesthesia, in which the skin and muscles around the eyelid are tightened. In severe cases, more complex plastic surgery (p.614) may be necessary.

Watery eye

Overflow of tears from the eye due to overproduction or poor drainage

 Most common in babies and elderly people

 Gender, genetics, and lifestyle are not significant factors

Watery eye may result from irritation of the eye by a foreign body such as a particle of dirt. Older people often have watery eye as a result of entropion (left), in which the eyelashes rub against the eye, or ectropion (left), in which tears do not drain away normally. The watering usually stops when the irritant is removed or the underlying condition is corrected. Watery eye may also occur as a result of a blocked nasolacrimal system (which drains tears), possibly caused by an infection of the eye.

Babies may have watery eyes because the nasolacrimal system is underdeveloped. Gently massaging between the corner of the eyelid and the nose may help. The condition usually corrects itself by the age of 6 months. Persistent blockages, at any age, must be treated by a doctor, who may clear the tear duct by inserting a fine probe.

Dacryocystitis

Painful swelling of the lacrimal (tear) sac, into which fluid drains from the surface of the eye

 Most common in babies and elderly people

 Gender, genetics, and lifestyle are not significant factors

Normally, tears from the eyes drain into the lacrimal sacs on either side of the nose. An infection of the lacrimal sacs is known as dacryocystitis. The condition is usually caused by a bacterial infection and most commonly results from a blockage in the nasolacrimal duct, which normally carries tears from the lacrimal sac to the nose. Nasolacrimal blockage is common in babies because the ducts are not fully developed until a year after birth. Elderly people may develop a blockage with no apparent cause, although it may be due to previous injury or inflammation.

Dacryocystitis usually starts with a red, watery eye. The area beside the nose just below the eye then becomes tender, red, and swollen. Pus may be discharged into the eye. Dacryocystitis usually affects only one eye at a time, but it can recur in either eye.

What might be done?

In adults, warm compresses and oral antibiotics (p.572) may help to clear the infection. If the problem continues, surgery may be required to bypass the blocked nasolacrimal duct. In babies, gentle massage of the lacrimal sac may help to relieve the condition. Antibiotics may also be given. In some cases, the blockage may be cleared by the insertion of a tiny probe.

Keratoconjunctivitis sicca

Persistent dryness of the eye due to insufficient production of tears, also known as dry eye

 Increasingly common over the age of 35

 More common in females

 Genetics and lifestyle are not significant factors

Insufficient tear production, known as keratoconjunctivitis sicca or dry eye, results from damage to the lacrimal (tear) glands. The condition causes eye irritation and often leads to eye infections (*see* **Conjunctivitis**, p.355). In severe cases, corneal ulcers (p.356) may develop. Dry eye affects more women than men and is more common over the age of 35. The condition may be linked to autoimmune disorders, such as Sjögren's syndrome (p.281), in which the body attacks its own tissues.

Your doctor will prescribe artificial tears to restore moisture to the eye. The tears may need to be used many times a day. The doctor may also investigate and treat an underlying cause. Sometimes, surgery may be performed to plug the channel through which the tears normally drain.

Xerophthalmia

Dryness of the eye due to a dietary deficiency of vitamin A

 More common in young children but can occur at any age

 Caused by a diet low in vitamin A

 Gender and genetics are not significant factors

Xerophthalmia, which occurs mainly in developing countries, means dryness of the eye. The condition is caused by a dietary deficiency of vitamin A (*see* **Nutritional deficiencies**, p.399).

Left untreated, xerophthalmia leads to chronic (long-term) infection and the transparent cornea at the front of the eye may soften and perforate. Infection may then spread inside the eye and blindness (p.369) may result. Artificial tears may relieve dryness, but the main treatment is vitamin A.

Vision disorders

Disorders of vision are very common; most people have a visual problem at some time in their lives. The most common disorders of vision are shortsightedness (myopia), longsightedness, (hypermetropia), and astigmatism, which are types of refractive (focusing) errors. Most refractive errors can be corrected by aids, such as glasses or contact lenses, or cured by surgical techniques.

The opening articles in this section discuss refractive errors and show how variations in the size and shape of the eye may lead to distortions of vision. Tests and treatments for refractive errors are also described. However, special tests for children's vision are covered separately (*see* **Vision tests in children**, p.555). Presbyopia, the deterioration of vision that occurs with aging, is covered next.

The following articles describe colour blindness, a condition that is more common in men, and serious visual problems, including double vision and partial or total blindness.

Disorders that affect the structure of the eye, including glaucoma, are covered elsewhere (*see* **Eye disorders**, pp.355–363), as are blindness at birth (*see* **Congenital blindness**, p.555) and two disorders that mainly affect children: crossed eyes (*see* **Strabismus**, p.555) and abnormal vision in an eye that is otherwise structurally normal (*see* **Amblyopia**, p.556).

KEY ANATOMY

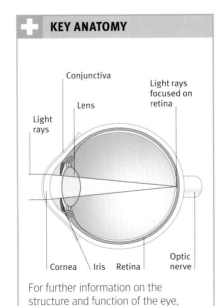

For further information on the structure and function of the eye, see pp.351–354.

Myopia

Inability to see distant objects clearly, commonly known as shortsightedness

 Usually becomes apparent around puberty

 Sometimes runs in families

 Gender and lifestyle are not significant factors

To enable us to see clearly, light rays need to be focused by the transparent cornea at the front of the eye and by the eye's lens so that they form a sharp image on the retina, the light-sensitive membrane at the back of the eye. In people who have myopia (shortsightedness), the eyeball is long relative to the combined focusing power of the cornea and the lens. Light rays from distant objects are therefore bent too much and are focused in front of the retina, resulting in blurred vision. Myopia is a very common condition that sometimes runs in families and can usually be corrected.

What are the symptoms?

The symptoms of myopia often become apparent around puberty, but the condition may begin to develop a few years before. The earlier myopia starts, the more severe it is likely to become. However, the condition usually stabilizes in early adulthood when growth stops. The main symptoms are:

- Increasing difficulty with distance vision.
- In children, deteriorating schoolwork as a result of not seeing clearly.

If you are severely myopic, you are more susceptible to eye disorders such as retinal detachment (p.360), chronic glaucoma (p.359), and macular degeneration (p.362). All of these disorders can badly damage eyesight. If you have problems with distance vision, you should visit your optometrist.

What might be done?

The optometrist will carry out vision tests (p.367) to check for myopia. Myopia can be corrected with concave-lensed glasses or, for older children and adults, contact lenses (*see* **Glasses and contact lenses**, p.366). In many cases, myopia can be treated effectively by surgery (*see* **Surgery for refractive errors**, p.368).

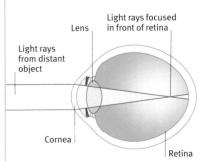

Myopia
In myopia, the eyeball is too long relative to the focusing power of the cornea and lens. Light from distant objects is focused in front of the retina and the image is blurred.

▶ **TREATMENT**

Glasses and contact lenses

Most refractive errors can be corrected by wearing glasses or, for older children and adults, contact lenses. Glasses are suitable for most refractive errors, are comfortable to wear, and do not cause complications. Contact lenses are also available for many refractive errors, but they are most effective for myopia (p.365) and hypermetropia (right). Nondisposable contact lenses require careful cleaning to reduce the chance of an infection of the transparent cornea over which they are placed.

How lenses work

Glasses and contact lenses correct refractive errors in the eye by altering the angle of light rays before the rays reach the surface of the cornea, the transparent front part of the eye. The cornea at the front of the eye and the lens can then focus the rays correctly on the retina. Concave lenses make the light rays diverge (bend apart) and convex lenses make the light rays converge (bend together).

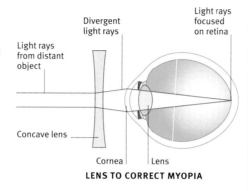

LENS TO CORRECT MYOPIA

Divergent light rays · Light rays from distant object · Light rays focused on retina · Concave lens · Cornea · Lens

Myopia and hypermetropia
Myopia is corrected by concave lenses, which make light rays diverge and focus on the retina, not in front of it. Hypermetropia requires a convex lens to make light rays converge, focusing them on the retina and not behind it.

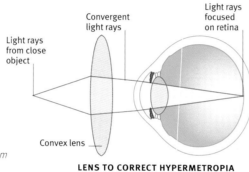

LENS TO CORRECT HYPERMETROPIA

Convergent light rays · Light rays focused on retina · Light rays from close object · Convex lens

Contact lenses

There are three main types of contact lenses: rigid, gas-permeable, and soft. Soft lenses are the most widely used and rigid the least. Some soft lenses are worn only once or for a few days. Nondisposable lenses should be disinfected daily unless worn for an extended period (not usually recommended). If an eye becomes red or painful, you should stop wearing your lenses and consult your optician immediately.

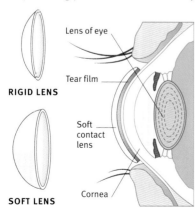

RIGID LENS
Lens of eye · Tear film

SOFT LENS
Soft contact lens · Cornea

Rigid and soft lenses
A contact lens floats on the tear film on the front of the eye. Soft lenses cover the whole cornea; rigid and gas-permeable lenses cover only the central part of the cornea.

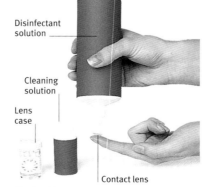

Disinfectant solution · Cleaning solution · Lens case · Contact lens

Contact lens care
Good lens hygiene prevents eye infections. Nondisposable lenses must be carefully cleaned before and after use and soaked overnight in disinfectant solution.

Hypermetropia

Inability to see close objects clearly, commonly known as longsightedness

 Most often detected at about the age of 5; may not cause problems until middle age

 Sometimes runs in families

 Gender and lifestyle are not significant factors

The transparent cornea and the lens act together to focus light rays and create a clear image on the light-sensitive retina at the back of the eye. Hypermetropia (longsightedness) occurs if the eyeball is short relative to the combined focusing power of the cornea and lens. When the image falls behind the retina, it causes blurred vision that is often worse when viewing near objects. Young people with hypermetropia often see distant objects very clearly because the lens is flexible and changes focus easily, but with age, focusing ability lessens and distant vision is also affected.

What are the symptoms?

Mild or moderate hypermetropia will probably not affect vision in young people because they can compensate by focusing the lens, but, the more severe the condition, the earlier in life symptoms may appear. Symptoms of severe hypermetropia, which may be apparent from infancy, can include:

- Lack of interest in small objects.
- Difficulty with reading or following picture stories.

If the eyes are not equally affected by hypermetropia, they may be unable to focus together on the same object. Without early treatment, young children may develop crossed eyes (*see* **Strabismus**, p.555) and may eventually lose vision in one eye (*see* **Amblyopia**, p.556). You should take your child to the doctor immediately if you notice any of the symptoms described here. If you have trouble seeing near objects clearly or have difficulty in reading or doing other close work, you should visit your optometrist for vision tests (opposite page). These problems may indicate that you have presbyopia (opposite page), which develops earlier in people with hypermetropia than in most people.

What might be done?

Your optometrist will check your visual acuity and the level of detail you can see, and then assess the severity of hypermetropia. Although the condition is sometimes detected in children during routine vision testing at school, all children who have a family history of severe hypermetropia should be tested before the age of 3 because early treatment is important.

Hypermetropia can be corrected with contact lenses or glasses that have convex lenses (*see* **Glasses and contact lenses**, left). The focusing power of the eye decreases gradually with age, and your prescription may need to be updated regularly. People who have hypermetropia may be helped by laser treatment that increases the focusing power of the cornea (*see* **Surgery for refractive errors**, p.368).

Hypermetropia does not cause complications, but people who have the condition are more prone to acute glaucoma (p.358), a condition that must be treated promptly. Regular tests for glaucoma (*see* **Common screening tests**, p.14) are therefore especially important.

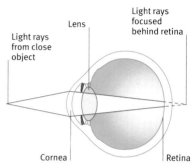

Hypermetropia
In hypermetropia, the eye is too short relative to the focusing power of the cornea and lens. Light rays are focused behind the retina and the image is blurred.

Light rays focused behind retina · Lens · Light rays from close object · Cornea · Retina

Astigmatism

Distorted vision caused by an uneven curvature of the transparent cornea at the front of the eye

 Sometimes runs in families

 Age, gender, and lifestyle are not significant factors

In people with astigmatism, the transparent cornea at the front of the eye is unevenly curved and refracts (bends) the light rays striking different parts of it to differing degrees. The lens of the eye is then unable to bring all the rays into focus on the light-sensitive retina at the back of the eye, and vision becomes blurred. Astigmatism can run in families and often occurs in combination with myopia (p.365) or hypermetropia (left).

What are the causes?

The most common form of astigmatism is present from birth and is due to a slight buckling of the cornea in both eyes. Instead of being round like a football, the cornea is shaped like a rugby ball, with a steep curvature in one direction and a shallow curvature in the other. This type may worsen slowly with age. Less often, astigmatism is due to an eye disorder such as keratoconus (p.356) or an eye injury that causes a corneal ulcer (p.356) to develop.

Vision tests

You should have your vision tested every 2 years, especially if you are over the age of 40. The most common tests assess the acuity (sharpness) of your distance vision and your ability to focus on near objects. The tests also show which corrective lenses, if any, you need. Additional tests for specific eye disorders, such as glaucoma (p.358), may be performed, depending on your age and medical history.

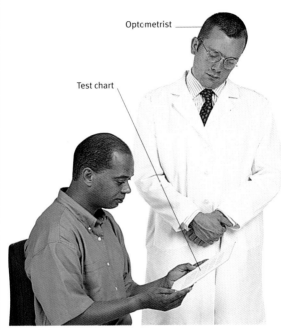

Optometrist

Test chart

Near-vision test
Wearing your usual glasses or contact lenses, if you use them, you will be asked to read very small print on a chart held at normal reading distance. This test checks your ability to focus on near objects.

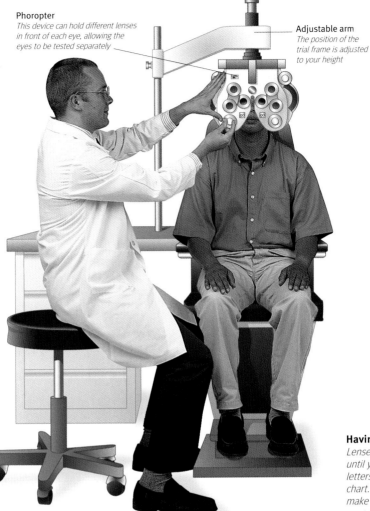

Phoropter
This device can hold different lenses in front of each eye, allowing the eyes to be tested separately

Adjustable arm
The position of the trial frame is adjusted to your height

Snellen chart
The acuity of your distance vision is tested separately for each eye. The test involves noting how far down a Snellen chart you can read letters of decreasing sizes.

Having a vision test
Lenses in the phoropter are changed until you can accurately read the letters near the bottom of the Snellen chart. This enables the optometrist to make the appropriate prescription for your corrective lenses.

What are the symptoms?

The majority of people have a slight degree of astigmatism. If you are only slightly affected, you probably will not notice much wrong with your vision. More severe astigmatism, however, may lead to significant visual problems.

Astigmatism can affect vision in a number of different ways. Symptoms may include the following:

■ Blurring of small print, causing difficulty in reading.

■ Inability to see both near and distant objects clearly.

If you are experiencing difficulty in seeing objects clearly at any distance, it is important to visit your optometrist as soon as possible to have a vision test (above).

What is the treatment?

In people with astigmatism, vision can usually be corrected by glasses that have special lenses that compensate for the unevenly shaped cornea. Rigid contact lenses are also effective because they smooth out the surface of the cornea. Conventional soft contact lenses mould to the shape of the cornea and can normally correct only mild astigmatism. However,

soft contact lenses known as toric lenses, which are specially designed to correct astigmatism, are also available.

In some people, astigmatism may be corrected permanently by laser treatment that alters the shape of the cornea. This procedure leaves only minimal scarring (see **Surgery for refractive errors**, p.368).

Presbyopia

Gradual age-associated loss of the eye's ability to focus on near objects

 Generally develops over the age of 40

 Gender, genetics, and lifestyle are not significant factors

After about the age of 40, almost everyone starts to notice increased difficulty in reading small print because of the development of presbyopia. A person with normal vision is able to see close objects clearly because the elastic lens of the eye changes shape, becoming thicker and more curved when

focusing on near objects. The thicker lens brings light rays from close objects into sharp focus on the light-sensitive retina at the back of the eye in a process known as accommodation. As we age, the lens becomes less elastic and the power of accommodation is reduced. Eventually, light rays from near objects can no longer be focused on the retina and the objects we see appear blurred.

What are the symptoms?

Since presbyopia develops very slowly, most people are unaware of the initial stages of this condition. However, the symptoms usually become noticeable between the ages of 40 and 50. Longsighted people (see **Hypermetropia**, opposite page) may have noticeable symptoms from an earlier age. Common symptoms of presbyopia include:

■ The need to hold newspapers and books at arm's length so that you can read them.

■ Increased difficulty in focusing on near objects in poor light.

■ If you are shortsighted (see **Myopia**, p.365), the need to take off your glasses to see near objects clearly.

If you develop any of these problems, consult your optometrist.

What is the treatment?

Presbyopia can be corrected by wearing glasses with convex (outward-curved) lenses, which bring light rays from near objects into focus on the retina. If you are longsighted, shortsighted, or have astigmatism (opposite page), you may be prescribed glasses with a different power in different parts of the lens. For example, bifocals have an upper lens to correct distance vision and a lower lens to correct presbyopia. Varifocal lenses that gradually alter the focusing power from top to bottom are also available. Presbyopia can sometimes be corrected with contact lenses, but glasses may still be necessary for reading.

Presbyopia tends to worsen with age, and you will probably need to have your lens prescription updated every few years. You should see your optometrist regularly in order to have vision tests. The condition eventually stabilizes at about the age of 60 by which time little natural focusing power is left. By this stage most of the focusing work is done by your glasses instead of the eye.

Double vision

Seeing two separate images of a single object instead of one

 Age, gender, genetics, and lifestyle as risk factors depend on the cause

People with double vision see two images of a single object. The images are separate but often clearly focused. This disorder can have a number of causes, and usually disappears when one eye is closed. You should consult your doctor immediately if you start to experience double vision because it may indicate that you have a serious underlying disorder.

What are the causes?

The most common cause of double vision is weakness or paralysis of one or more of the muscles that control the movements of one eye. The movement of the affected eye is impaired, causing crossed eyes (*see* Strabismus, p.555). Two different views of the same object are received by the visual system and the brain cannot combine them. Tilting or turning the head may briefly correct the problem. However, not all types of crossed eyes cause double vision.

Many serious conditions that affect the brain and nervous system may cause impaired eye movements, leading to double vision. Potential causes include multiple sclerosis (p.334), head injuries (p.322), brain tumours (p.327), and bulging of an artery inside the head due to a weakness in the vessel wall (called an aneurysm). In older people, impaired eye movement resulting in double vision may be linked with diabetes mellitus (p.437) and, rarely, with atherosclerosis (p.241) and high blood pressure (*see* Hypertension, p.242). Very rarely, double vision can also occur as a result of a tumour or blood clot behind one of the eyes, causing the movement of that eye to be affected.

How is it diagnosed?

Your doctor may ask you to shut one eye at a time to see whether the double vision disappears. He or she may also ask you to describe the double images, or ask if they appear side by side or one on top of the other or whether one of the images appears to be tilted. Your doctor will probably observe the movements of your eyes closely in order to establish whether any of the eye muscles are weak or paralysed. He or she may also carry out special vision tests to identify weak eye movement.

If double vision has come on suddenly, or if no obvious cause can be found, urgent CT scanning (p.132) or MRI (p.133) may be carried out to check for any abnormality in the eye sockets or brain that might be affecting the alignment of the eyes. You may also have a neurological examination.

▶ **TREATMENT**

Surgery for refractive errors

Some refractive errors can be corrected by surgery. The main techniques are corneal reshaping by laser in-situ keratomileusis (LASIK), laser epithelial keratomileusis (LASEK), or photorefractive keratectomy (PRK). In LASIK, a flap is created in the cornea, the middle layers of the cornea are reshaped by laser, and the corneal flap is replaced. LASEK is similar to LASIK but cuts less deeply into the cornea. In PRK, part of the front surface of the cornea is shaved away by laser. For some people with severe myopia, lens implant surgery may be a possible alternative to corneal reshaping. There are two main types of such treatment: phakic implant surgery and lens replacement. In the first, an artificial lens (phakic lens) is inserted into the eye through a small cut in the cornea but the natural lens is not removed. In the second, the natural lens is replaced with an artificial implant, in a procedure that is essentially the same as cataract surgery (p.357).

LOCATION

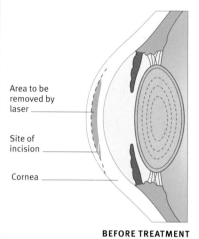

Area to be removed by laser

Site of incision

Cornea

BEFORE TREATMENT

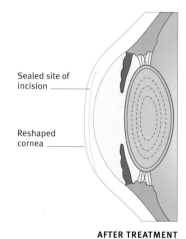

Sealed site of incision

Reshaped cornea

AFTER TREATMENT

LASIK treatment of myopia
After a flap has been created, a laser beam, guided by computer, removes part of the cornea. The flap is then replaced. The reshaped cornea is flatter, and light rays are focused to form a sharp image. The LASIK technique leaves very little scarring.

What is the treatment?

Treatment of double vision is aimed at the underlying cause. A serious disorder such as an aneurysm may need hospital treatment. Double vision due to diabetes mellitus usually disappears over time. If it does not, you may be advised to wear a patch over one eye to eliminate the second image. Surgery to adjust the eye muscles helps if double vision has been present for some time. In some cases, injection of botulinum toxin into an overactive eye muscle may relieve double vision by temporarily paralysing the muscle.

Visual field defects

Loss of part of the normal area of vision in one or both eyes

 Age, gender, genetics, and lifestyle as risk factors depend on the cause

Visual field defects take different forms, ranging from loss of areas at the outer edges of vision (peripheral vision) or small blind spots to loss of most of the area that you normally see (the visual field). If you notice a loss of vision, you should seek urgent medical advice because visual field defects sometimes indicate a serious underlying disorder. Regular vision tests (p.367) are important because visual field defects may develop slowly without being noticed.

What are the causes?

Visual field defects may be caused by damage to the light-sensitive retina at the back of the eye; the optic nerve, along which nerve signals are carried from the retina to the brain; or the parts of the brain involved with vision.

Several eye disorders cause characteristic patterns of visual field loss. For example, a gradual increase in fluid pressure in the eye (*see* Chronic glaucoma, p.359) can damage nerve fibres in the retina, which can cause loss of peripheral vision. If glaucoma is left untreated, only a narrow area of central vision will remain (known as tunnel vision). Inflammation of the optic nerve (*see* Optic neuritis, p.362) typically causes loss of central vision, and a pituitary tumour (p.430) often causes loss

of the outer half of the visual field in each eye. Brain damage due to a stroke (p.329) or tumour (*see* Brain tumour, p.327) may result in loss of the right or left half of the visual field in both eyes. Migraine (p.320) can cause temporary visual field defects.

What are the symptoms?

Visual field defects usually appear gradually and often remain unnoticed. In other cases, depending on the type of defect, symptoms may include:
- Bumping into objects on one side.
- Missing whole sections of text while you are reading.
- Being able to see only straight ahead (tunnel vision).

The majority of visual field defects can be detected during routine vision tests. However, you should see your doctor immediately if you notice a change in your normal field of vision.

What might be done?

Your doctor may carry out a visual field test (p.369) to assess the pattern and extent of the defect.

The treatment for the defect depends on the underlying cause. For example, if you have chronic glaucoma, you will be given drugs to reduce the pressure in the eye (*see* Drugs for glaucoma, p.594). Existing defects are usually permanent, but treatment of the underlying condition may prevent further deterioration. Many people who have a visual field defect become used to it, but it may affect their lifestyle or choice of occupation. For example, if you have tunnel vision, you should not drive.

Eyestrain

Temporary discomfort or aching in or around the eyes

 Age, gender, genetics, and lifestyle are not significant factors

Eyestrain is neither a medical term nor a diagnosis. In contrast to widespread belief, you cannot damage or strain your eyes by using them under difficult conditions, such as reading small print in poor light or wearing glasses of the wrong strength. Although aching and discomfort are commonly attributed to eyestrain, they are often headaches that are caused by tension or tiredness of the muscles around the eye as a result of frowning or squinting.

The symptoms normally attributed to eyestrain do not require treatment and normally disappear on their own but, if the problem worsens or persists, you should consult your doctor.

is caused by an eye disorder or by drugs, it may sometimes be possible to treat the underlying cause.

▶ **TEST**

Visual field test

Visual field testing (perimetry) is used to check the whole area that each eye can see (the visual field). The development of blank sections in the visual field may be caused by various underlying disorders (*see* **Visual field defects**, p.368). Many eye disorders cause characteristic visual field defects that can develop without being noticed. Testing allows early detection and treatment.

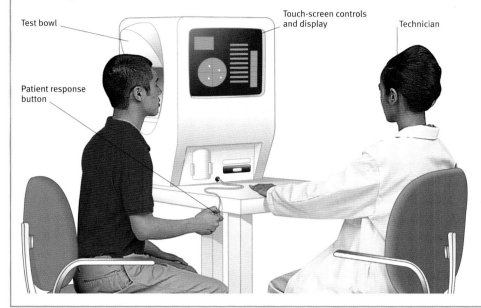

Test bowl

Touch-screen controls and display

Technician

Patient response button

RESULTS

Normal visual field perimeter

Centre of visual field

Grid lines on visual map

Area of visual loss

Visual field map
The blue area above represents the area of visual loss in the normal field of vision.

Visual field test
One eye is covered while you look at a central target inside the test bowl. When you see lights flashing in different parts of your visual field, you press a response button.

Colour blindness

Below-normal ability to distinguish between colours

 Usually present from birth

 More common in males

 Usually due to an abnormal gene inherited from the mother

 Lifestyle is not a significant factor

Colour blindness is the reduced ability to tell certain colours apart. It is due to a defect in the cones, the specialized cells in the light-sensitive retina at the back of the eye. There are three types of cone cell, each of which is sensitive to blue, green, or red light. If one or more type of cell is faulty, colour blindness results. The condition is usually inherited.

What are the types?
The most common type of colour blindness, red–green colour blindness, affects far more males than females, and may take one of two forms. In one form, people are unable to distinguish between pale reds, greens, oranges, and browns. The other form makes shades of red appear dull and indistinct. Red–green colour blindness is caused by an abnormal gene carried on the X chromosome. It mainly affects men because women have a second X chromosome that usually masks the effect of the gene (*see* **Gene disorders**, p.151). However, women may pass the abnormal gene to their children.

Another, much rarer, type of colour blindness makes it difficult to distinguish between blues and yellows. This form of the condition can be inherited, but because it is not linked to the X chromosome, it affects both females and males in equal numbers. Macular degeneration (p.362) and other eye disorders may cause colour blindness. The toxic effects of some drugs, including chloroquine (*see* **Antimalarial drugs**, p.574), may also cause colour blindness.

What might be done?
Colour blindness is usually noticed during routine vision testing in childhood (*see* **Vision tests in children**, p.555). It may also be detected during medical tests for jobs requiring normal colour vision, such as flying aeroplanes. The test checks your ability to see numbers in patterns of coloured dots.

Colour blindness is rarely a serious problem. Inherited forms of the condition are untreatable, but, if colour blindness

Blindness

Severe to total loss of vision that cannot be rectified by corrective lenses

 Age, gender, genetics, and lifestyle as risk factors depend on the cause

Complete or almost complete loss of sight, usually termed blindness, affects about 40 million people worldwide. Although most of those affected are in developing countries, about 360,000 people in the UK are registered as blind or partially sighted, and many more have some degree of visual impairment. The risk of becoming blind increases with age, but the condition can be present from birth (*see* **Congenital blindness**, p.555).

What are the causes?
Blindness may be caused by disorders of the eyes, the nerves that connect the eyes to the brain, or the areas of the brain that process visual information.

In developed countries, blindness is most often caused by a damaged retina due to macular degeneration (p.362) or diabetic retinopathy (p.361), raised fluid pressure in the eye due to glaucoma (p.358), or clouding of the lens due to cataracts (p.357). Cataracts are also a common cause in developing countries, together with the eye infection trachoma (p.356) and vitamin A deficiency (*see* **Xerophthalmia**, p.365).

What might be done?
Early diagnosis can help some underlying disorders that cause blindness to be treated to preserve vision. For example, if you have glaucoma, you will be given drugs to reduce the pressure in the eye (*see* **Drugs for glaucoma**, p.594).

If you are registered as blind or visually handicapped, you may be eligible for certain benefits and services. Visual aids, such as magnifying glasses, can make some daily tasks easier.

Ears, hearing, and balance

Our ears provide us with two vital but very different senses: hearing and balance. Sound detected by the ears provides essential information about our external surroundings and allows us to communicate in highly sophisticated ways, such as through speech and music. In addition, our ears contribute to our sense of balance, the largely unconscious understanding of the body's orientation in space that allows us to maintain an upright posture and move without falling over.

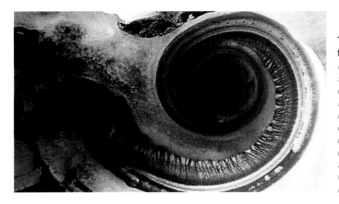

The cochlea in the inner ear
Resembling the shell of a snail, the cochlea is a coiled tubular structure in the inner part of the ear. The central duct of the cochlea contains the spiral organ of Corti, the receptor for hearing.

THE EAR CONTAINS separate organs of hearing and balance, which detect sound from the world around us and internal information about our posture and movement. Sensory structures inside our ears convert the different forms of information into nerve impulses, which travel along nerves to various parts of the brain where the information is analysed. Our ability to interpret sounds and use information about balance develops during infancy and childhood.

The qualities of sound
Sound is actually a vibration of the molecules in the air all around us. The pitch of a noise (how "high" or "low" it sounds) is determined by a property of sound waves called the frequency. Frequency is the number of vibrations per second and is measured in units called hertz (Hz). The higher the frequency, the higher the pitch.

The intensity or loudness of a sound depends on the power of the sound waves and is measured in units called decibels (dB). For every 10 dB increase in power, our ears hear double the loudness, so noises at 90 dB sound twice as loud as those at only 80 dB. Conversation is typically about 60 dB, and sound from nearby traffic is usually about 80 dB. Even brief exposure to noises over 120 dB can damage our hearing.

We all vary in the acuteness of our hearing (how loud a sound has to be for us to hear it) and in our ability to analyse complex sounds such as music. Young people can normally detect sounds with frequencies between about 20 Hz and 20,000 Hz, but our ability to hear high-frequency sounds tends to decline with age. Animals such as bats and dogs can hear sounds with frequencies much higher than the normal human range.

Balance and movement
The structures of the inner ear that are concerned with balance have two functions: awareness of the head's orientation (where it is in space) and detection of the head's rotation and movement in all directions. The brain combines information from the ears with that from position sensors in the muscles, tendons, and joints and visual information from the eyes. Taken together, this information enables us to move in many different ways without losing our balance.

✚ STRUCTURE

Connecting passageways

Although the ears may appear to be isolated structures, they are directly linked to the nose and throat. The visible part of the ear, the pinna, is connected to the ear canal, which ends at the eardrum. Beyond this membrane lies the middle ear, an air-filled space connected to the back of the nasal cavity and to the throat by a channel called the eustachian tube. This tube ensures that the air pressure is the same on both sides of the eardrum. The structures of the inner ear lie deep within the skull and contain the sensory organs for sound and balance.

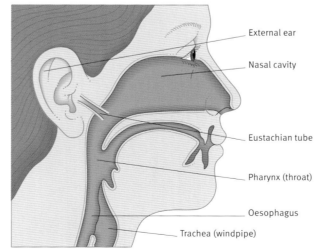

| External ear |
| Nasal cavity |
| Eustachian tube |
| Pharynx (throat) |
| Oesophagus |
| Trachea (windpipe) |

Link between the ear, nose, and throat
The eustachian tube connects the ear to the nasal cavity and throat and maintains equal air pressure on both sides of the eardrum.

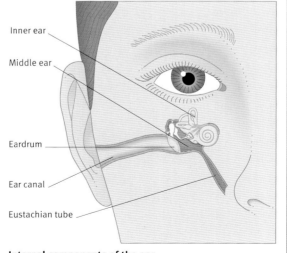

| Inner ear |
| Middle ear |
| Eardrum |
| Ear canal |
| Eustachian tube |

Internal components of the ear
The ear canal runs from the external ear to the middle and inner ear, which are situated inside the skull.

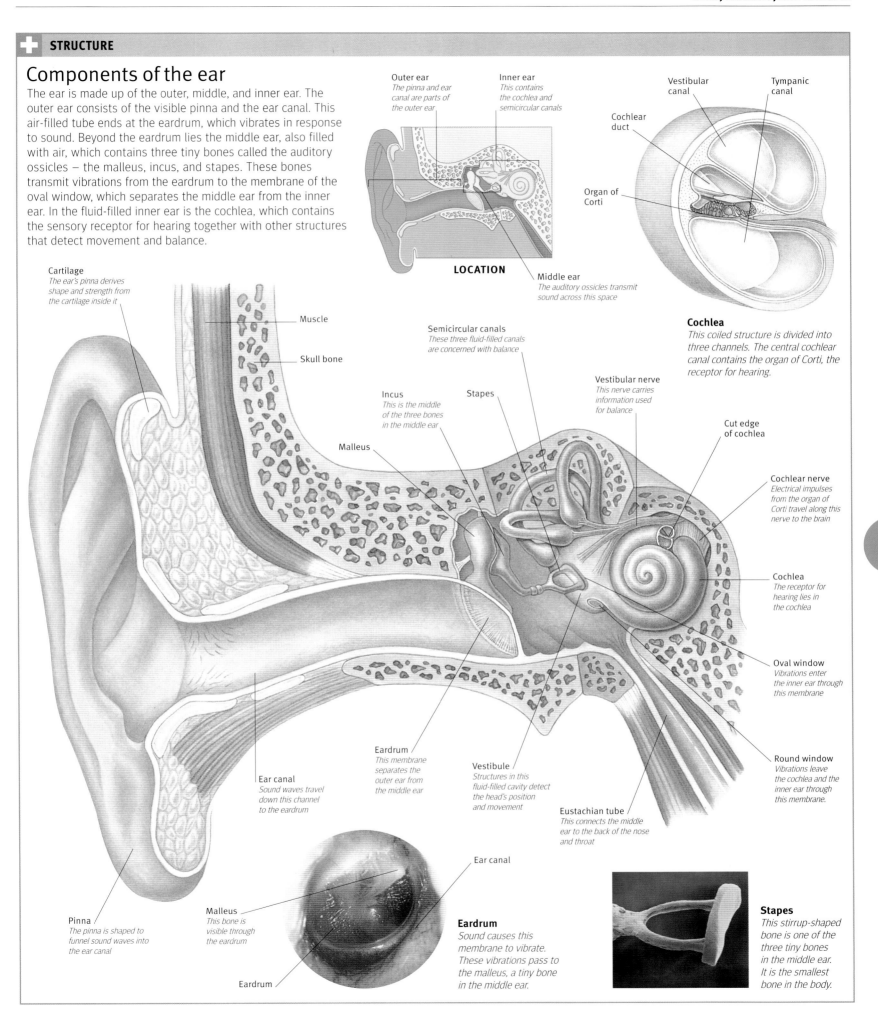

+ STRUCTURE

Components of the ear

The ear is made up of the outer, middle, and inner ear. The outer ear consists of the visible pinna and the ear canal. This air-filled tube ends at the eardrum, which vibrates in response to sound. Beyond the eardrum lies the middle ear, also filled with air, which contains three tiny bones called the auditory ossicles – the malleus, incus, and stapes. These bones transmit vibrations from the eardrum to the membrane of the oval window, which separates the middle ear from the inner ear. In the fluid-filled inner ear is the cochlea, which contains the sensory receptor for hearing together with other structures that detect movement and balance.

Outer ear
The pinna and ear canal are parts of the outer ear

Inner ear
This contains the cochlea and semicircular canals

Vestibular canal

Tympanic canal

Cochlear duct

Organ of Corti

LOCATION

Middle ear
The auditory ossicles transmit sound across this space

Cochlea
This coiled structure is divided into three channels. The central cochlear canal contains the organ of Corti, the receptor for hearing.

Cartilage
The ear's pinna derives shape and strength from the cartilage inside it

Muscle

Skull bone

Semicircular canals
These three fluid-filled canals are concerned with balance

Vestibular nerve
This nerve carries information used for balance

Cut edge of cochlea

Incus
This is the middle of the three bones in the middle ear

Stapes

Malleus

Cochlear nerve
Electrical impulses from the organ of Corti travel along this nerve to the brain

Cochlea
The receptor for hearing lies in the cochlea

Oval window
Vibrations enter the inner ear through this membrane

Eardrum
This membrane separates the outer ear from the middle ear

Vestibule
Structures in this fluid-filled cavity detect the head's position and movement

Ear canal
Sound waves travel down this channel to the eardrum

Eustachian tube
This connects the middle ear to the back of the nose and throat

Round window
Vibrations leave the cochlea and the inner ear through this membrane.

Pinna
The pinna is shaped to funnel sound waves into the ear canal

Malleus
This bone is visible through the eardrum

Ear canal

Eardrum

Eardrum
Sound causes this membrane to vibrate. These vibrations pass to the malleus, a tiny bone in the middle ear.

Stapes
This stirrup-shaped bone is one of the three tiny bones in the middle ear. It is the smallest bone in the body.

The mechanism of hearing

Our ability to hear depends on a complex series of events that occur in the ear. Sound waves in the air are transmitted as vibrations through a series of structures to the receptor for hearing, the organ of Corti in the inner ear. Inside the organ of Corti, these physical vibrations are detected by sensory hair cells, which respond by producing electrical signals. Nerves carry these signals to the brain, where they are interpreted. Sounds of different frequencies stimulate hair cells in different parts of the organ of Corti, allowing us to perceive the subtleties of sounds such as speech and music.

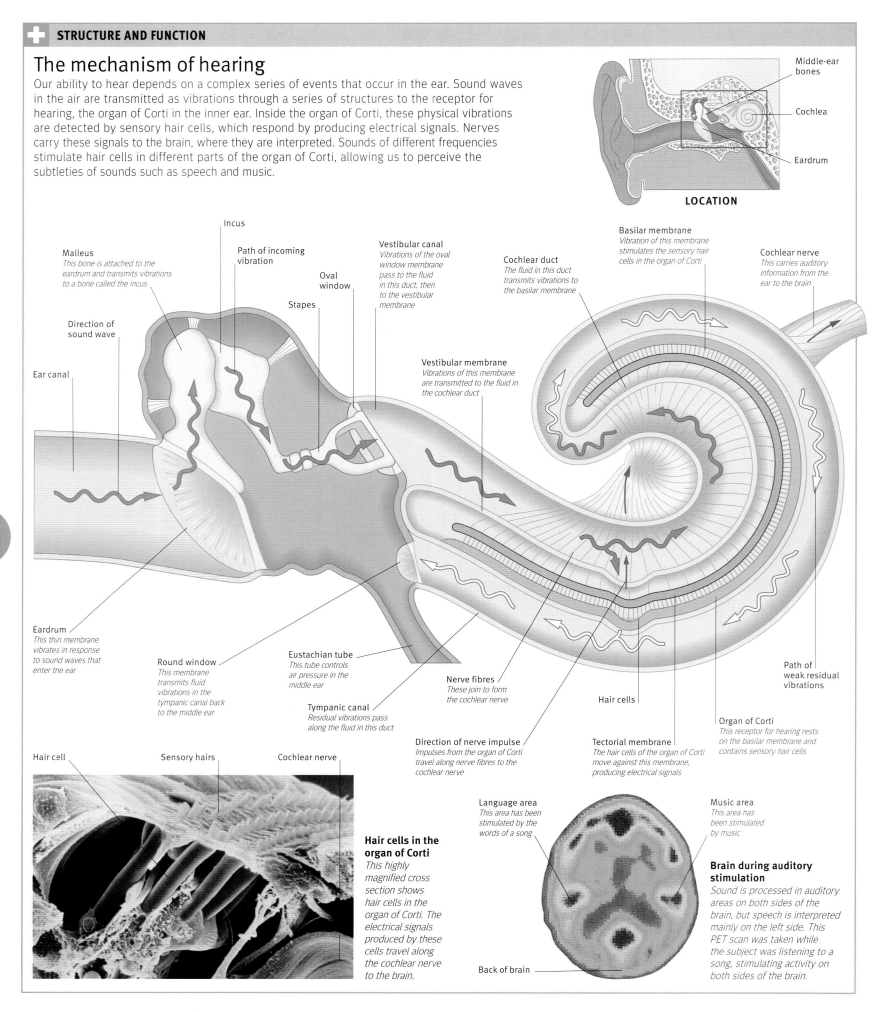

LOCATION

Middle-ear bones

Cochlea

Eardrum

Incus

Path of incoming vibration

Vestibular canal
Vibrations of the oval window membrane pass to the fluid in this duct, then to the vestibular membrane

Basilar membrane
Vibration of this membrane stimulates the sensory hair cells in the organ of Corti

Cochlear nerve
This carries auditory information from the ear to the brain

Cochlear duct
The fluid in this duct transmits vibrations to the basilar membrane

Malleus
This bone is attached to the eardrum and transmits vibrations to a bone called the incus

Oval window

Stapes

Direction of sound wave

Vestibular membrane
Vibrations of this membrane are transmitted to the fluid in the cochlear duct

Ear canal

Eardrum
This thin membrane vibrates in response to sound waves that enter the ear

Round window
This membrane transmits fluid vibrations in the tympanic canal back to the middle ear

Eustachian tube
This tube controls air pressure in the middle ear

Nerve fibres
These join to form the cochlear nerve

Hair cells

Path of weak residual vibrations

Tympanic canal
Residual vibrations pass along the fluid in this duct

Direction of nerve impulse
Impulses from the organ of Corti travel along nerve fibres to the cochlear nerve

Tectorial membrane
The hair cells of the organ of Corti move against this membrane, producing electrical signals

Organ of Corti
This receptor for hearing rests on the basilar membrane and contains sensory hair cells

Hair cell

Sensory hairs

Cochlear nerve

Hair cells in the organ of Corti
This highly magnified cross section shows hair cells in the organ of Corti. The electrical signals produced by these cells travel along the cochlear nerve to the brain.

Language area
This area has been stimulated by the words of a song

Music area
This area has been stimulated by music

Back of brain

Brain during auditory stimulation
Sound is processed in auditory areas on both sides of the brain, but speech is interpreted mainly on the left side. This PET scan was taken while the subject was listening to a song, stimulating activity on both sides of the brain.

+ STRUCTURE AND FUNCTION

The sense of balance

The ability to stand upright and move without falling over depends on our sense of balance. Structures in the inner ear, known as the vestibular apparatus, contribute to balance by detecting the position and movements of the head. The vestibular apparatus is composed of three semi-circular canals and the two-chambered vestibule.

The role of hair cells

The head's movements are detected by hair cells found in structures called cristae in the semicircular canals and in two structures called maculae in the vestibule.

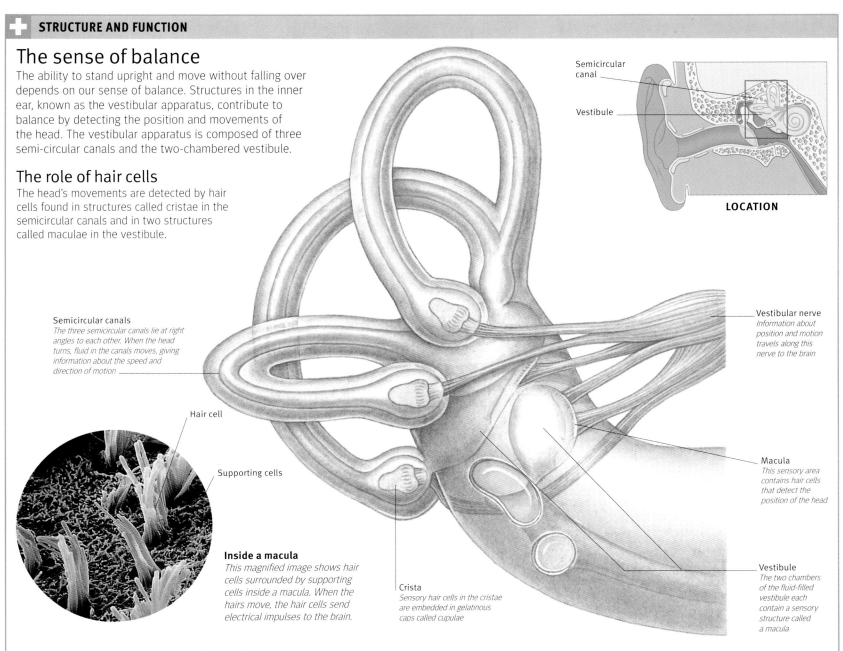

Semicircular canal

Vestibule

LOCATION

Semicircular canals
The three semicircular canals lie at right angles to each other. When the head turns, fluid in the canals moves, giving information about the speed and direction of motion

Hair cell

Supporting cells

Inside a macula
This magnified image shows hair cells surrounded by supporting cells inside a macula. When the hairs move, the hair cells send electrical impulses to the brain.

Crista
Sensory hair cells in the cristae are embedded in gelatinous caps called cupulae

Vestibular nerve
Information about position and motion travels along this nerve to the brain

Macula
This sensory area contains hair cells that detect the position of the head

Vestibule
The two chambers of the fluid-filled vestibule each contain a sensory structure called a macula

Linear movement and static position

The two maculae within the vestibule of the inner ear sense linear movements – for example, when travelling by car or using a lift – and the orientation of the head relative to gravity. Detecting the head's position in relation to gravity helps us, for example, to know instantly which way is up when we dive into deep water.

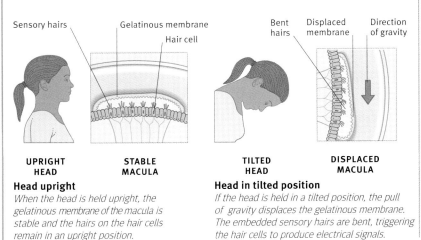

Sensory hairs   Gelatinous membrane   Bent hairs   Displaced membrane   Direction of gravity
Hair cell

UPRIGHT HEAD   **STABLE MACULA**   **TILTED HEAD**   **DISPLACED MACULA**

Head upright
When the head is held upright, the gelatinous membrane of the macula is stable and the hairs on the hair cells remain in an upright position.

Head in tilted position
If the head is held in a tilted position, the pull of gravity displaces the gelatinous membrane. The embedded sensory hairs are bent, triggering the hair cells to produce electrical signals.

Rotational movement

Rotational movements of the head are detected by the cristae in the fluid-filled semicircular canals. The three semicircular canals are at right angles to each other, so head rotation in any direction is detected by at least one canal. The information is used both to maintain balance and to keep vision stable when the head moves.

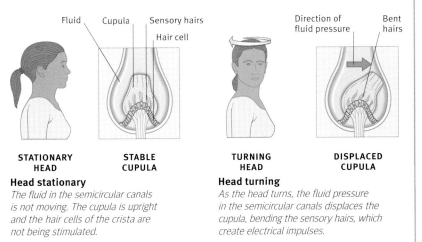

Fluid   Cupula   Sensory hairs   Direction of fluid pressure   Bent hairs
Hair cell

STATIONARY HEAD   **STABLE CUPULA**   **TURNING HEAD**   **DISPLACED CUPULA**

Head stationary
The fluid in the semicircular canals is not moving. The cupula is upright and the hair cells of the crista are not being stimulated.

Head turning
As the head turns, the fluid pressure in the semicircular canals displaces the cupula, bending the sensory hairs, which create electrical impulses.

Outer- and middle-ear disorders

The outer ear consists of the visible part, called the pinna, which is composed of skin and cartilage, and the ear canal, the channel that leads to the eardrum. Behind the eardrum is the air-filled middle ear, which contains three tiny, delicate bones. The middle ear is directly linked to the respiratory system by the eustachian tube, the passage connecting the ear to the nose and throat.

This section covers disorders of the visible parts of the ear and of the ear canal, followed by conditions that affect the eardrum and middle ear. Outer- and middle-ear disorders have a number of causes, including injury, infections, obstruction, damage from atmospheric pressure changes, and inherited disease. The symptoms of these disorders include irritation, discomfort, pain, and, in some cases, partial hearing loss.

Most outer- and middle-ear problems are more easily treatable than those affecting the inner ear and are less likely to lead to permanent loss of hearing. Most causes of hearing loss are covered elsewhere (*see* **Hearing and inner-ear disorders**, pp.376–380), as are disorders of the middle ear that particularly affect children (*see* **Acute otitis media in children**, p.557, and **Chronic secretory otitis media**, p.557).

KEY ANATOMY

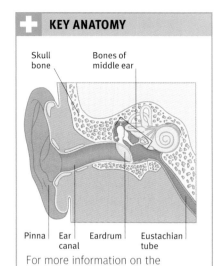

Skull bone | Bones of middle ear

Pinna | Ear canal | Eardrum | Eustachian tube

For more information on the structure and the function of the ear, *see* pp.370–373.

Outer-ear injury

Damage to the visible part of the ear, sometimes leading to deformity

 Playing contact sports is a risk factor

 Age, gender, and genetics are not significant factors

If the visible part of the outer ear is injured, blood may collect between the skin of the ear and its underlying cartilage, leading to pain and swelling. The collected blood (haematoma) may cut off the supply of blood to the cartilage, which may break down and be gradually replaced by scar tissue. Severe or repeated injury may result in a "cauliflower ear", a deformity that sometimes occurs in boxers and other athletes.

You can reduce the discomfort of an injured ear by applying an ice pack. If the ear is severely swollen, you should consult your doctor. He or she may drain a

haematoma under a local anaesthetic or apply a pressure bandage to reduce swelling. Plastic surgery may be necessary to correct a deformity.

When playing contact sports, make sure you wear headgear to protect your ears (*see* **Exercising safely**, p.22).

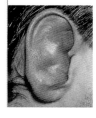

Outer-ear injury
The visible part of this ear is swollen and distorted due to a large collection of blood under the skin. The injury was caused by a blow to the ear.

Otitis externa

Inflammation of the ear canal, commonly known as "swimmer's ear"

 Swimming or wearing a hearing aid or earplugs are risk factors

 Age, gender, and genetics are not significant factors

In otitis externa, the ear canal becomes inflamed, usually because of bacterial, viral, or fungal infection. Otitis externa often develops after swimming because persistent moisture within the ear canal increases the risk of infection. The condition is also more common in people who work in a hot and humid environment or who wear a hearing aid or earplugs. Scratching the ear with a cotton swab or fingernail is another cause of otitis externa. Less commonly, the infection occurs as a reaction to chemicals such as those in eardrops or hair dye.

What are the symptoms?
The symptoms of otitis externa usually appear over 1–2 days and may include:
■ Itching and/or pain within the ear canal at the affected site.
■ Discharge of pus from the ear.
If pus blocks the canal, see your doctor rather than trying to remove it yourself.

What might be done?
Your doctor will examine your ear with an otoscope (*see* **Otoscopy**, below). If there is pus present, indicating infection, he or she may take a swab to identify the organism responsible. The ear canal may also be cleaned out using a suction device. Depending on the type of infection present, your doctor may prescribe eardrops that contain an antibiotic or antifungal and/or a corticosteroid (*see* **Drugs acting on the ear**, p.595). An oral painkiller (p.589) may also be given to relieve discomfort.

If you have a severe bacterial infection, your doctor may prescribe oral antibiotics (p.572). Most viral infections are treated solely with painkillers. However, if the condition is caused by the herpes virus, you may be prescribed an oral antiviral drug (p.573), sometimes with a corticosteroid (p.600). The disorder usually clears up in a few days.

Wax blockage

Blockage of the ear canal by earwax, often causing a feeling of fullness and irritation in the ear

 Age, gender, genetics, and lifestyle are not significant factors

Earwax, produced by glands in the ear canal, cleans and moistens the canal. Usually, wax is produced in small quantities and emerges naturally from the ear.

However, if the canal becomes blocked with wax, it causes a feeling of fullness and discomfort and sometimes hearing loss. A common cause of wax blockage is insertion of a cotton swab or finger into the canal in an attempt to remove the wax. This usually pushes the wax deeper into the canal. Excessive secretion of wax or narrow ear canals increase the likelihood of blockage.

Wax blockage can be treated with over-the-counter eardrops, which usually dissolve the earwax in about 4–10 days. If the ear remains blocked, you should consult your doctor. He or she will probably use a viewing instrument to inspect the ear canal (*see* **Otoscopy**, below) and may gently flush out the ear with warm water from a syringe to remove the wax. If flushing is ineffective, the wax may be removed with a suction device. Wax blockage sometimes recurs.

Otitis media

Inflammation of the middle ear, usually as a result of a bacterial or viral infection

 More common in children but can occur at any age

 Gender, genetics, and lifestyle are not significant factors

In otitis media, tissues lining the middle ear are inflamed, and pus and fluid accumulate in the middle ear, causing pain and partial hearing loss. The condition occurs when a viral infection, such as a common cold (p.164) or influenza (p.164), or a bacterial infection spreads from the throat to the middle ear. The infection may cause a ruptured eardrum (opposite page). Otitis media is common in children. This is because their eustachian tubes, which connect the ear to the back of the nose and throat and ventilate

▶ TEST

Otoscopy

The ear canal and eardrum can be examined directly by using an otoscope, a viewing instrument that illuminates and magnifies the inside of the ear. Otoscopy is used to diagnose disorders such as otitis media and ruptured eardrum.

Otoscope

VIEW

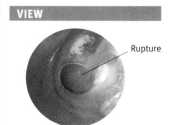

Rupture

Hole in eardrum
This eardrum has ruptured as a result of a long-standing bacterial infection of the middle ear.

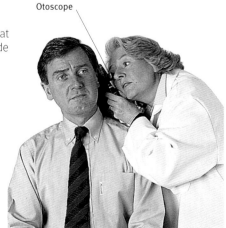

The examination
The doctor pulls the ear upwards and backwards to straighten the ear canal and then gently inserts the otoscope to look inside the ear.

the middle ear, are immature and easily blocked by large structures, such as adenoids (*see* **Acute otitis media in children**, p.557). Sometimes, a sticky fluid persistently collects in the middle ear, impairing hearing (*see* **Chronic secretory otitis media**, p.557).

What are the symptoms?
The symptoms of otitis media often develop over a few hours and include:
■ Pain in the ear, which may be severe.
■ Partial hearing loss.
■ Fever.
If the eardrum ruptures, there may be a bloodstained discharge from the ear and a decrease in pain. Untreated otitis media may become a chronic infection with a constant discharge of pus from the ear. Rarely, the infection results in a cholesteatoma, a collection of skin cells and debris, in the middle ear. This complication may damage the middle ear and rarely the inner ear, causing permanent loss of hearing.

What might be done?
Your doctor will examine your ear with an otoscope (*see* **Otoscopy**, opposite page) to check if your eardrum is inflamed and to see if there is pus in the middle ear. You may be prescribed oral antibiotics (p.572) and may be given painkillers (p.589). Decongestants (p.587) may also sometimes be prescribed. In most cases, the pain subsides in a few days, but mild hearing loss may sometimes persist for a week or two. If a cholesteatoma has developed, it is usually necessary for it to be removed by surgery.

Ruptured eardrum

A tear or hole in the membrane between the outer and middle ear

 Age and lifestyle as risk factors depend on the cause

 Gender and genetics are not significant factors

Rupture of the eardrum most commonly results from an acute bacterial infection of the middle ear (*see* **Otitis media**, opposite page). Pus or other fluid produced by the infection builds up inside the middle ear and eventually bursts through the eardrum. Less commonly, a rupture occurs when an object is poked into the ear. In some cases, the eardrum suddenly ruptures because there is an imbalance between the pressures inside the middle ear and the outer ear. Such a pressure imbalance in different parts of the ear may occur after a blow to the ear, an explosion, a head injury (p.322), or when flying or diving (*see* **Barotrauma**, p.375).

What are the symptoms?
The symptoms usually last for only a few hours and may include:
■ Sudden, sometimes intense pain in the affected ear.
■ Bloodstained discharge from the ear.
■ Partial hearing loss.

If you suspect that you have a ruptured eardrum, keep the affected ear dry and consult your doctor as soon as possible.

What might be done?
Your doctor may inspect your ear (*see* **Otoscopy**, opposite page). A ruptured eardrum usually heals within a month. Infection can be treated with antibiotics (p.572). Rarely, ruptures caused by an infection need to be repaired with a tissue graft.

Barotrauma

Damage or pain, mainly affecting the middle ear, caused by pressure changes

 Air travel and diving are risk factors

 Age, gender, and genetics are not significant factors

If the pressure on the outer side of the eardrum exceeds the pressure on the inner side, the middle ear may become damaged or painful, a condition called barotrauma. Changes in outside pressure are common when flying or diving and may cause pain or a feeling of fullness in the ears. If you swallow or hold your nose and exhale with your mouth closed, the eustachian tubes, which connect the ears to the nose and throat will usually open, allowing air into the middle ear and equalizing the pressure. If insufficient air enters the middle ear, barotrauma occurs. The condition is more likely if the eustachian tubes are blocked as a result of a cold or ear infection (*see* **Otitis media**, opposite page).

Small pressure changes may cause pain and temporary ringing or buzzing in the ears (*see* **Tinnitus**, p.378). An extreme pressure imbalance may lead to a ruptured eardrum (left), bleeding into the middle ear, or damage to the inner ear, which may result in hearing loss and vertigo (p.379).

If symptoms do not clear up in a few hours, see your doctor. If you have a cold or ear infection, avoid flying or diving. If you must fly, use a decongestant (p.587) beforehand to clear the eustachian tubes.

Otosclerosis

Abnormal growth of bone between the middle and inner ear, often leading to hearing loss

 Symptoms usually develop between the ages of 20 and 30

 Twice as common in females

 Often runs in families

 Lifestyle is not a significant factor

Otosclerosis is a condition in which bone begins to overgrow around the base of the stapes, the innermost of the three tiny bones in the middle ear. The stapes gradually becomes immobilized, preventing the transmission of sound vibrations to the inner ear and causing progressive loss of hearing. Usually both ears are affected, although not always equally. As the disease progresses, nerve damage may occur in the inner ear.

Otosclerosis affects about 1–2 in 100 people in the UK, and symptoms usually first appear between the ages of about 20 and 30. The disorder is twice as common in women as it is in men and may progress more quickly during pregnancy or after starting the contraceptive pill or hormone replacement therapy. In about 6 out of 10 people with otosclerosis, the condition runs in the family and is due to an inherited abnormal gene. In other cases, the underlying cause is unknown.

What are the symptoms?
The symptoms of otosclerosis develop gradually and may include:
■ Hearing loss in which sounds are muffled but may appear to be clearer if there is background noise.
■ Ringing or buzzing noises in the ears (*see* **Tinnitus**, p.378).
In severe cases, dizziness and imbalance (*see* **Vertigo**, p.379) may also develop.

What might be done?
Your doctor will probably be able to diagnose otosclerosis from hearing tests (p.377) and your family history.

If your hearing loss is mild, you may decide to wait until it becomes problematic before opting for treatment, which is either using a hearing aid (p.376) or surgery to replace the stapes (*see* **Stapedotomy**, below). Hearing aids are often very effective for moderate hearing loss but tend to be less effective when hearing loss is severe. Stapedotomy is usually successful in restoring hearing, but it carries the slight risk of further impairing hearing in the ear operated on. For this reason, it is usually recommended only when hearing loss is severe.

▶ TREATMENT

Stapedotomy
This operation is carried out to treat otosclerosis (above), a disorder in which the stapes bone in the middle ear becomes immobilized by bony overgrowth, causing hearing loss. Under local or general anaesthesia, parts of the stapes are removed and replaced by a prosthesis. Stapedotomy is usually successful, but there is a small risk that hearing may deteriorate further.

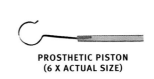
PROSTHETIC PISTON (6 X ACTUAL SIZE)

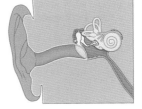
LOCATION

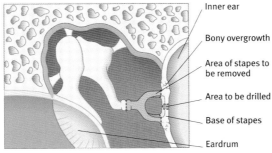

Inner ear
Bony overgrowth
Area of stapes to be removed
Area to be drilled
Base of stapes
Eardrum

Before surgery
The stapes has become immobilized due to bony overgrowth around its base, so that sound vibrations cannot travel to the inner ear. During the operation, the body of the stapes is removed and a hole is drilled or lasered in the bony area around the base.

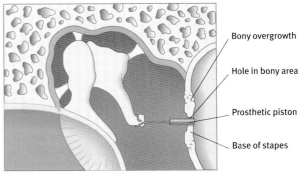

Bony overgrowth
Hole in bony area
Prosthetic piston
Base of stapes

After surgery
The body of the stapes is replaced by a prosthetic piston. The piston is able to move freely in and out of the hole in the bony area, transmitting vibrations to the inner ear.

Hearing and inner-ear disorders

Disorders of hearing are very common and, in severe cases, they may interfere with communication, causing significant disability. In some cases, hearing loss is due to a disorder of the ear canal or the middle ear, but inner-ear disorders can also cause hearing problems. The inner ear also contains the vestibular apparatus, which helps to maintain the sense of balance. Inner-ear disorders may therefore lead to other symptoms, such as dizziness.

This section starts by discussing all types of hearing loss from partial loss of hearing to total deafness. Hearing defects that are due to disorders of the inner ear, including noise-induced hearing loss and tinnitus (various sounds heard in one or both ears in the absence of an external source), are then covered in greater detail.

Problems in other parts of the ear that may cause hearing loss or deafness are covered elsewhere in the book (*see* **Outer- and middle-ear disorders**, pp.374–375), as is hearing loss or deafness that is present from birth (*see* **Congenital deafness**, p.556).

Inner-ear disorders do not only affect hearing; if the vestibular apparatus is disturbed, the sense of balance may be disrupted. Three common inner-ear disorders that affect balance – motion sickness, labyrinthitis, and Ménière's disease – are described in this section. All of these disorders may cause symptoms such as dizziness and nausea. Ménière's disease can also lead to hearing loss. The final article in this section discusses acoustic neuroma, a rare, noncancerous tumour affecting the vestibulocochlear nerve, which connects the inner ear to the brain.

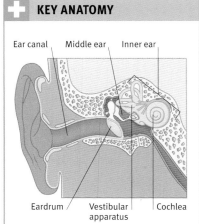

✚ KEY ANATOMY

Ear canal   Middle ear   Inner ear

Eardrum   Vestibular   Cochlea
apparatus

For further information on the structure and function of the ear, *see* pp.370–373.

Hearing loss

Partial or total loss of hearing in one or both ears

 Age, gender, genetics, and lifestyle as risk factors depend on the cause

Partial or total hearing impairment can severely restrict social interaction, leading to isolation and depression (p.343). Hearing loss may result from disease or injury, and most people experience deterioration of hearing with age (*see* **Presbyacusis**, right). Hearing defects may also be present from birth; about 2 in every 1,000 babies are born with some degree of hearing impairment (*see* **Congenital deafness**, p.556).

What are the types?

There are two types of hearing loss: conductive and sensorineural. Conductive hearing loss is caused by a failure of the outer or middle ear to transmit sound to the inner ear, and is often temporary. Sensorineural hearing loss is usually permanent, and may be caused by disorders of the cochlea (the part of the inner ear that detects sound), the vestibulocochlear nerve (which connects the inner ear to the brain), or parts of the brain involved with hearing.

Conductive hearing loss The most common cause of conductive hearing loss in children is chronic secretory otitis media (p.557), in which the middle ear fills with fluid following an infection. In adults, the condition is often due to blockage of the ear canal (*see* **Wax blockage**, p.374). It can also result from a ruptured eardrum (p.375), or sudden changes in air pressure (*see* **Barotrauma**, p.375). Rarely, the condition is due to otosclerosis (p.375), in which one of the tiny bones in the middle ear is immobilized and cannot transmit sound.

Sensorineural hearing loss This type of hearing loss is commonly due to deterioration of the cochlea with age and mostly affects people over 70. The condition may also result from damage to the cochlea by excessive noise (*see* **Noise-induced hearing loss**, p.378) or by the inner-ear disorder Ménière's disease (p.380). Rarely, hearing loss is caused by a tumour that affects part of the brain or the vestibulocochlear nerve (*see* **Acoustic neuroma**, p.380). Certain drugs, including antibiotics such as gentamicin and chemotherapeutic agents such as cisplatin, can be toxic to the inner ear, resulting in hearing loss.

What might be done?

Your doctor will examine your ear with a viewing instrument called an otoscope (*see* **Otoscopy**, p.374). Hearing tests (opposite page) may then be performed to establish the type and degree of hearing loss. If a tumour of the vestibulocochlear nerve is suspected, your doctor may arrange for an examination of the nerve using MRI (p.133).

If you have conductive hearing loss, treatment of the underlying cause may restore your hearing to near normal. Sensorineural hearing loss is often permanent, although a hearing aid (below) may be helpful. In cases of profound sensorineural deafness, a cochlear implant (p.378), in which electrodes are surgically implanted in the cochlea, may allow hearing of sounds such as speech.

Presbyacusis

Gradual loss of hearing that develops as a natural part of aging

More common over the age of 50

More common in males

Sometimes runs in families

Prior damage due to other middle- or inner-ear problems or to excessive noise exposure may increase the severity

Many people over the age of 50 notice that they find it hard to hear quiet or high-pitched sounds and conversation is sometimes difficult to understand, particularly when there is background noise, such as music. Over a period of years, sounds of all pitches may become increasingly difficult to hear. This progressive decline in hearing is known as presbyacusis and is a common feature of the normal process of aging.

Presbyacusis occurs in about 1 in 5 people aged 50–60, 1 in 3 people aged 60–70, and half of all people over 70. The condition is more common and severe in men and may run in families.

What are the causes?

The body's sensory receptor for hearing, located in the cochlea in the inner ear, is lined with sensory hair cells. Presbyacusis occurs when these sensory hair cells degenerate and die with age. The condition is occasionally more severe in people whose hearing has already been damaged by exposure to excessive levels of noise (*see* **Noise-induced hearing loss**, p.378) or by previous middle- or inner-ear problems, such as a perforated eardrum.

What are the symptoms?

The symptoms of presbyacusis develop gradually and may include:
- Loss of hearing, initially of high-pitched sounds and gradually of lower pitches.
- Difficulty in hearing speech, especially with noise in the background.
- Loss of sound clarity, so that even loud speech is difficult to understand.

▶ TREATMENT

Hearing aids

Hearing aids amplify sounds, improving hearing in people with most types of hearing loss. These devices have a tiny microphone, amplifier, and speaker, all powered by batteries. The range of sounds amplified by a hearing aid is tailored to the individual's pattern of hearing loss.

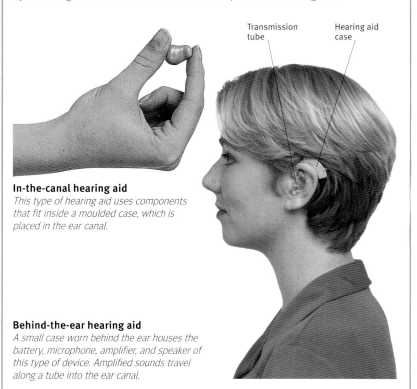

Transmission tube   Hearing aid case

In-the-canal hearing aid
This type of hearing aid uses components that fit inside a moulded case, which is placed in the ear canal.

Behind-the-ear hearing aid
A small case worn behind the ear houses the battery, microphone, amplifier, and speaker of this type of device. Amplified sounds travel along a tube into the ear canal.

▶ **TEST**

Hearing tests

Your doctor may recommend hearing tests if you have difficulty hearing speech or if you work in a noisy environment. He or she may perform preliminary tests in the surgery and may refer you to a hearing specialist for others. Some tests determine the type of hearing loss, while others assess how well you can hear sounds of varying frequency and volume. Babies are given a hearing screening test soon after birth; further hearing tests are carried out during childhood as part of routine developmental assessment and whenever hearing impairment is suspected (*see* **Hearing tests in children**, p.557).

Preliminary tests

A tuning fork is used to distinguish conductive hearing loss, resulting from a disorder of the outer or middle ear, from sensorineural loss, which is caused by a disorder of the inner ear or of the nerves that transmit hearing to the brain.

Vibrating tuning fork

Weber test
A vibrating tuning fork is held against your forehead. If you have conductive hearing loss, the sound will seem louder in the more affected ear. In sensorineural loss, it is louder in the less affected ear.

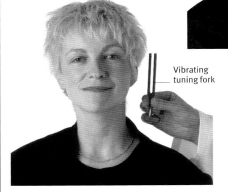

Vibrating tuning fork

Rinne test
A vibrating tuning fork is held near your ear and then against a bone behind the ear. If it sounds louder in the second position, you have conductive hearing loss. If it is louder in the first position, either the ear is healthy or the hearing loss is sensorineural.

Tympanometry

Detailed information about the movements of the eardrum and bones of the middle ear in response to sound can be obtained by tympanometry. The test is used to establish the cause of conductive hearing loss and is often used in children because it does not rely on responses from the person being tested.

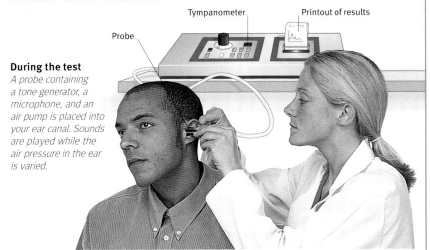

Tympanometer

Printout of results

Probe

During the test
A probe containing a tone generator, a microphone, and an air pump is placed into your ear canal. Sounds are played while the air pressure in the ear is varied.

Eardrum   Sound waves   Ear canal   Probe

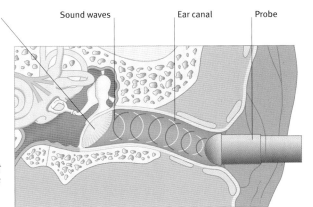

How the test works
The sounds bounce off the eardrum and are picked up by a microphone. The pattern of reflected sound varies at different air pressures and shows whether the eardrum is moving normally.

Audiometry

This test measures how loud a sound has to be for you to hear it. Sounds of varying frequency are transmitted to one ear at a time through headphones. For each frequency, the volume is increased until you hear it, and the results are recorded. The test is repeated with a speaker held against a bone behind the ear.

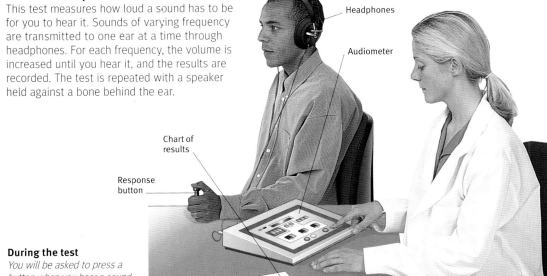

Headphones

Audiometer

Chart of results

Response button

During the test
You will be asked to press a button when you hear a sound in either ear. The softest sound that you can hear at each frequency will be recorded.

RESULTS

Left ear

Right ear

Hearing level (dB): -20, 0, 20, 40, 60, 80, 100

Frequency (hertz): 125, 250, 500, 1000, 2000, 4000, 8000

Audiometry trace
This trace is from a person with normal hearing in the left ear and sensorineural hearing loss in the right. At higher frequencies, the right ear can detect sound only if the sound level is much higher than normal.

Both ears are usually affected, although not always equally. The severity and progression of hearing loss vary from person to person. Severe hearing loss sometimes leads to feelings of isolation, loneliness, and depression (p.343).

What might be done?

Your doctor will examine your ears with a viewing instrument called an otoscope (*see* Otoscopy, p.374). He or she may also arrange for various hearing tests to determine the type and degree of hearing loss (*see* Hearing tests, p.377). There is no cure for presbyacusis. However, a hearing aid (p.376) may improve your ability to hear and communicate.

Noise-induced hearing loss

Hearing loss caused by prolonged or repeated exposure to excessive noise or by brief exposure to intensely loud noise

 A noisy workplace and using a portable music player are risk factors

 Age, gender, and genetics are not significant factors

Persistent or repeated exposure to loud noise or a single intensely loud sound can damage the delicate sensory hair cells that line the receptor for hearing within the inner ear. Temporary or permanent hearing loss may result.

Different individuals have different tolerances to noise and so it is impossible to establish absolute safe limits of noise exposure that apply to everybody. Furthermore, the risk of noise-induced hearing loss also depends on the length of time of exposure. However, in general, exposure to a sudden, extremely loud sound (above about 130 decibels) – an explosion, for example – can cause immediate and permanent hearing loss and may also lead to a ruptured eardrum (p.375). More commonly, noise-induced hearing loss results from prolonged and/or repeated exposure to lower levels of noise (between about 85 and 130 decibels).

A few simple steps, such as using earplugs, can reduce your risk of noise-induced hearing loss (*see* Protecting your hearing, opposite page).

What are the symptoms?

Exposure to very loud noises can cause immediate symptoms. These usually affect both ears and may include:

■ Loss of hearing, particularly of high-pitched sounds.
■ Ringing or buzzing sounds in the ears (*see* Tinnitus, right).
■ Pain in the ears following intensely loud noises.

Immediate symptoms of noise-induced hearing loss are almost always temporary, and hearing returns to normal after a few

RISK OF NOISE-INDUCED HEARING LOSS

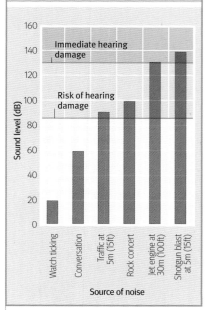

Noise levels and damage to hearing
The intensity of sound is measured in decibels (dB). A 10 dB increase doubles the loudness, so that 90 dB sounds twice as loud as 80 dB. Repeated and/or prolonged exposure to noise of about 85–130 dB may lead to hearing loss. Sounds louder than 130 dB can cause immediate hearing damage.

hours or days. However, permanent hearing loss may occur as a result of either a single, loud noise or repeated or prolonged exposure to excessive noise.

If your symptoms persist, or if you work in a noisy environment or regularly listen to loud music and notice a change in your hearing, you should consult your doctor.

What might be done?

Your doctor may perform hearing tests (p.377) and may arrange for further tests to assess the pattern of any hearing loss. Noise-induced hearing loss cannot be cured, although using a hearing aid (p.376) may make understanding conversation and communication easier.

Tinnitus

Sounds heard in one or both ears in the absence of external noise

 More common over the age of 60

 Previous exposure to excessive noise is a risk factor

 Gender and genetics are not significant factors

People with tinnitus hear sounds that originate within the ear itself. These sounds may include ringing, buzzing, whistling, roaring, or hissing noises in the ears. These sounds may vary in intensity and pulse in time with the heartbeat, but they are usually continuous.

▶ TREATMENT

Cochlear implants

A cochlear implant is used to treat profoundly deaf people who are not helped by hearing aids. The device consists of tiny electrodes surgically implanted in the cochlea deep in the inner ear and a receiver that is embedded in the skull just behind and above the ear. A microphone, sound processor, and transmitter are worn externally. A cochlear implant does not restore normal hearing, but it enables patterns of sound to be detected. Combined with lip-reading, it may enable speech to be understood.

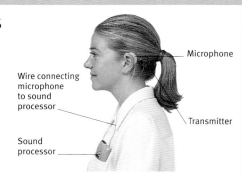

External components
The microphone detects sounds and converts them into electrical signals, which travel to the sound processor. Selected signals are relayed back to the transmitter behind the ear and then transmitted to the implanted components of the cochlear implant.

Inside the ear
Signals from the transmitter are detected by the implanted receiver and travel along a wire to the cochlea. Implanted electrodes are activated by the signals and stimulate the cochlear nerve to send impulses to the brain.

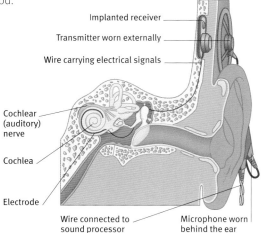

For some people, the episodes of tinnitus are brief, but for others it is a permanent condition.

In many cases, tinnitus is associated with hearing loss, and your risk of developing tinnitus is increased if you have previously been exposed to loud noises. The condition is more common in older people and affects approximately 3 in 10 people over the age of 60.

Most people with tinnitus are only aware of the sounds when they listen carefully, but for others the condition may be intrusive and lead to difficulties in concentrating or in getting to sleep (*see* Insomnia, p.343). In these cases, tinnitus may lead to depression (p.343) and anxiety disorders (p.341).

What are the causes?

Tinnitus may occur for no apparent reason, but it is often associated with certain ear disorders, such as Ménière's disease (p.380), presbyacusis (p.376), or noise-induced hearing loss (p.376).

In some cases, tinnitus can be the result of a deficiency of the blood pigment that carries oxygen (*see* Anaemia, p.271) or an overactive thyroid gland (*see* Hyperthyroidism, p.432). Other causes of tinnitus include head injuries (p.322) and

treatment with various drugs, such as aspirin (*see* Painkillers, p.589) and certain antibiotics (p.572). Tinnitus that affects one ear only may be a symptom of a tumour affecting the vestibulocochlear nerve, which carries information from the inner ear to the brain (*see* Acoustic neuroma, p.380).

If you develop tinnitus, particularly if it affects one ear only, you should consult your doctor.

What might be done?

Your doctor will examine your ear with a viewing instrument called an otoscope (*see* Otoscopy, p.374) and may arrange for hearing tests (p.377). He or she may also arrange for other tests to look for an underlying disorder. These tests may include a blood test for anaemia, as well as CT scanning (p.132) or MRI (p.133) to rule out a tumour.

If an underlying cause is found and successfully treated, the tinnitus may improve. If tinnitus persists, your doctor may recommend a device called a masker. This device, worn in or behind the ear like a hearing aid, produces sounds that distract you from the tinnitus. If tinnitus accompanies hearing loss, a hearing aid (p.376) may provide relief by increasing your awareness of background noise while masking the internal sounds. Many people with tinnitus find that background noise, such as playing music, reduces their awareness of the sounds in their ears.

If tinnitus is particularly distressing or leads to depression or anxiety, counselling (p.624), self-help groups, or relaxation exercises (p.32) may help.

Vertigo

A false sensation of movement often combined with nausea and vomiting

 Age, genetics, and lifestyle as risk factors depend on the cause

 Gender is not a significant factor

People with vertigo feel as if they or their surroundings are moving. These false sensations are often accompanied by a feeling of spinning and may be associated with nausea and, sometimes, severe vomiting. Vertigo may result from disturbance affecting the organs of balance in the inner ear (the vestibular apparatus), the nerve that connects the inner ear to the brain, or the areas of the brain concerned with balance. Rarely, it is a sign of a serious underlying condition and needs urgent medical attention.

Vertigo often develops suddenly and may last from a few seconds to several days, occurring either intermittently or constantly. The condition can be very distressing and, in severe cases, may make it impossible to walk or even to stand. In most cases, vertigo disappears on its own or following treatment of the underlying disorder.

What are the causes?

A common cause of vertigo is an infection of the vestibular apparatus (*see* **Labyrinthitis**, p.380). The infection usually begins as a viral infection of the respiratory tract, such as a common cold (p.164) or influenza (p.164) or, less frequently, a bacterial infection of the middle ear (*see* **Otitis media**, p.374). This type of vertigo usually starts suddenly and lasts for 1–2 weeks.

Recurrent vertigo combined with hearing loss and sounds in one or both ears (*see* **Tinnitus**, opposite page) may be due to the inner-ear disorder Ménière's disease (p.380). Vertigo may also be a side effect of certain antibiotics (p.572), due to excessive alcohol consumption, or be a symptom of food poisoning (p.393) or heatstroke (*see* **Heat exhaustion and heatstroke**, p.185).

Vertigo is sometimes caused by calcified material moving around in the inner ear and causing dizziness when the head is moved. This condition often improves over a few weeks or months.

Vertigo may occasionally be associated with arthritis in the neck (*see* **Cervical**

spondylosis, p.222), a disorder that mainly affects older people. In this condition, vertigo occurs when the head is turned or tilted, thereby compressing blood vessels that supply the parts of the brain involved with balance.

Rare causes of vertigo include a tumour affecting the nerve connecting the inner ear to the brain (*see* **Acoustic neuroma**, p.380), a stroke (p.329), a head injury (p.322), or multiple sclerosis (p.334). These serious conditions may also cause other symptoms, such as speech or vision problems or weakness in a limb. If vertigo is accompanied by symptoms of this type, you should seek immediate medical attention.

What can I do?

You may relieve vertigo by lying still and avoiding sudden movement. If you have been vomiting, take small sips of water every 10 minutes to avoid dehydration until the symptoms subside.

If the vertigo persists for more than a few minutes, or if it becomes recurrent, you should consult your doctor.

What might be done?

Your doctor may examine your ears, eye movements, and nervous system to look for a cause. Tests may include a caloric test, in which air at different temperatures is blown into the ear to check the function of the vestibular apparatus. A neck X-ray (p.131) may be done to look for cervical spondylosis. If you also have tinnitus, you may have CT scanning (p.132) or MRI (p.133) to rule out a tumour pressing on the brain.

Your doctor may recommend drugs to relieve the symptoms of vertigo (*see* **Antiemetic drugs**, p.595, and **Antihistamines**, p.585). If vertigo is a side effect of an antibiotic, you may be given an alternative drug. Other treatment will be aimed at the underlying cause. For example, vertigo caused by a bacterial infection of the vestibular apparatus may be treated with antibiotics.

In some cases your doctor may suggest special exercises to carry out once the acute vertigo has subsided. These exercises can help you to resume normal activities and can also help to prevent longer-term problems with balance from developing.

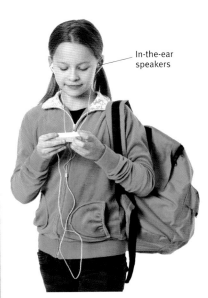

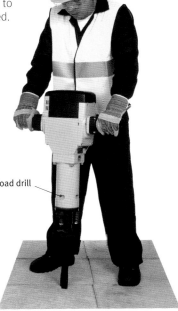

Ear protectors

In-the-ear speakers

Road drill

> **SELF-HELP**

Protecting your hearing

Excessive noise can damage the inner ear and lead to hearing loss. If possible, you should avoid exposure to loud noise. For example, do not listen to loud music, especially on a portable media player or similar device. If exposure is unavoidable in your work, always take steps to prevent hearing loss by using ear protectors or earplugs. You should also have regular tests to check that your hearing is not being damaged.

Using a portable media player
When listening to music on a portable media player, you should still be able to hear conversation.

Noise at work
If you are exposed to high noise levels at work, you should use appropriate ear protection to prevent noise-induced hearing loss.

Motion sickness

A range of symptoms, generally including nausea, caused by motion during travel by road, sea, or air

 Can occur at any age; most common in children aged 3–12

 Gender, genetics, and lifestyle are not significant factors

Most people experience some degree of motion sickness at some time in their lives. The condition is especially common in children. Motion sickness occurs when the brain receives messages from the organs of balance in the inner ear and from the eyes that conflict with one another. For example, when you travel in a car, the inner ear senses the motion, but, if you look at the interior of the car, the eyes may perceive it as stationary. The conflicting messages that the brain receives may lead to a feeling of nausea.

What are the symptoms?

In its mildest form, motion sickness may produce only a feeling of uneasiness. However, the initial symptoms of motion sickness usually include:

- Nausea.
- Headache and dizziness.
- Lethargy and tiredness.

If the motion continues after the onset of symptoms, the initial symptoms typically get worse and other symptoms, such as pale skin, excessive sweating, yawning, hyperventilation (abnormally deep or rapid breathing), and vomiting may occur. Poor ventilation in the vehicle may make the symptoms worse.

What can I do?

Before travelling, you should eat only small amounts and not drink alcohol. When travelling, you should try to sit in a cool, well-ventilated position and avoid reading or looking at nearby objects. Instead, try to look at the horizon or a distant object in the direction of travel. Drivers have to maintain their focus on the road ahead and so are usually unaffected by motion sickness.

There are many drugs, both over-the-counter and prescription, available to prevent or treat motion sickness (*see* **Antiemetic drugs**, p.595, and **Antihistamines**, p.585). To prevent symptoms, the medication should be taken before travelling, but, if you are driving, you should avoid certain drugs that may cause drowsiness. Many of these drugs can also increase the effects of alcohol.

Motion sickness remedies that are based on ginger may help to prevent nausea in some people. However, if you are taking any medication, you should check with your doctor or pharmacist before using ginger in case it interacts with the medication.

Labyrinthitis

Inflammation of the labyrinth of the inner ear, which contains the organs of balance and the receptor for hearing

 Age, gender, genetics, and lifestyle are not significant factors

The labyrinth of the inner ear consists of the vestibular apparatus, which is composed of the organs of balance, and the cochlea, which contains the receptor for hearing. Inflammation of the labyrinth, known as labyrinthitis, can therefore affect both balance and hearing. Labyrinthitis can be mild, but more often it is extremely unpleasant. The condition is not painful and rarely has serious consequences.

What are the causes?

The most common cause of labyrinthitis is a viral infection. Viral labyrinthitis may develop as a result of a viral infection of the upper respiratory tract, such as a common cold (p.164) or influenza (p.164). Less commonly, labyrinthitis is due to a bacterial infection, usually a complication of a middle-ear infection (*see* **Otitis media**, p.374) or, rarely, an infection elsewhere in the body.

What are the symptoms?

The symptoms of labyrinthitis usually develop rapidly and are most severe in the first 24 hours. They may include:

- Dizziness and a loss of balance (*see* **Vertigo**, p.379).
- Nausea and vomiting.
- Ringing and buzzing noises in the ears (*see* **Tinnitus**, p.378).

The symptoms may gradually decrease as the brain compensates for the disturbance to the vestibular apparatus, but you should consult your doctor immediately if you develop symptoms of labyrinthitis. Left untreated, bacterial infection of the labyrinth may cause severe damage to the cochlea, possibly leading to permanent hearing loss, or it may spread to the membranes covering the brain, causing meningitis (p.325).

What might be done?

Labyrinthitis can be diagnosed from your symptoms. Your doctor may prescribe an antiemetic drug (p.595) to ease the nausea. He or she may also advise you to lie in a darkened room with your eyes closed. Viral labyrinthitis often clears up without specific treatment, but, if you have bacterial labyrinthitis, your doctor will prescribe antibiotics (p.572). It may take several weeks to recover completely from labyrinthitis.

Ménière's disease

A disorder of the inner ear causing sudden episodes of severe dizziness, nausea, and hearing loss

 Most common between the ages of 20 and 60

 Sometimes runs in families

 A high-salt diet may increase the frequency of attacks

 Gender is not a significant factor

Ménière's disease is a rare disorder of unknown cause, although it may be related to excessive fluid pressure in the inner ear. The condition causes sudden attacks of distorted hearing and dizziness so severe that the affected person may fall to the ground.

Usually only one ear is affected, but both ears can become involved. The condition most commonly occurs in people aged between 20 and 60 years and sometimes runs in families. Ménière's disease may lead to permanent hearing loss.

What are the symptoms?

Attacks of Ménière's disease occur suddenly and may last from a few minutes to several days before gradually subsiding. The symptoms may include:

- Sudden, severe dizziness and loss of balance (*see* **Vertigo**, p.379).
- Nausea and vomiting.
- Abnormal, jerky eye movements.
- Ringing or buzzing noises in the affected ear (*see* **Tinnitus**, p.378).
- Loss of hearing, particularly of low-pitched sounds.
- Feeling of pressure or pain in the affected ear.

The length of time between attacks of Ménière's disease ranges from a few days to years. Tinnitus may be constant or may occur only during an attack. Between attacks, vertigo and nausea cease and hearing may improve. With repeated attacks, hearing often deteriorates progressively.

How is it diagnosed?

Your doctor may arrange for hearing tests (p.377) to assess your hearing loss. He or she may also arrange for a caloric test, in which air or water at different temperatures is introduced into the ears to check the functioning of the organs of balance. A tumour affecting the nerve that connects the ear to the brain (*see* **Acoustic neuroma**, right) may occasionally produce symptoms that resemble those of Ménière's disease. Your doctor may arrange for you to have tests such as CT scanning (p.132) or MRI (p.133) to rule out the possibility of a tumour.

What is the treatment?

You may be prescribed drugs to relieve nausea (*see* **Antiemetic drugs**, p.595). Your doctor may also recommend betahistine to

give further relief from nausea and vertigo and to reduce the frequency of the episodes. Sometimes, diuretic drugs (p.583) are used to help prevent further attacks.

There are steps you can take to help yourself if you have Ménière's disease. During an attack, lie still with your eyes closed and avoid noise, perhaps by wearing earplugs. Between attacks, try to avoid stress. Relaxation techniques may also be helpful.

For people who continue to have severe vertigo and whose hearing is already significantly impaired, one of various other options may be recommended. One course of action involves applying the antibiotic drug gentamicin to the middle ear. More invasive procedures include cutting the vestibular nerve (which carries information about position and motion to the brain) or surgically destroying the labyrinthine structure in the ear.

What is the prognosis?

The symptoms of Ménière's disease usually improve with medication. The frequency and severity of the episodes tend to decrease over a period of years. However, hearing usually becomes progressively worse with each successive attack, and permanent hearing loss may eventually result, although total deafness does not usually occur.

Acoustic neuroma

A noncancerous tumour affecting the vestibulocochlear (acoustic) nerve, which connects the ear to the brain

 Most common between the ages of 40 and 60

 One type runs in families

 Gender and lifestyle are not significant factors

An acoustic neuroma is a rare, noncancerous tumour affecting the vestibulocochlear (acoustic) nerve, which carries auditory and balance information from part of the inner ear to the brain. The tumour usually affects the vestibulocochlear nerve on one side of the head only, but it may affect both nerves.

The cause of acoustic neuroma is unknown but, if the tumour affects both acoustic nerves, it may be associated with neurofibromatosis (p.536), an inherited condition in which multiple tumours grow from the sheaths around nerves. Acoustic neuroma is most common between the ages of 40 and 60.

What are the symptoms?

An acoustic neuroma tends to grow slowly and may not cause any problems or symptoms when it is small. When symptoms do develop, they usually do so slowly and almost always affect only one ear. They may include:

- Progressive hearing loss.
- Ringing or buzzing noises in the ear (*see* **Tinnitus**, p.378).
- Headache and pain in the ear.
- Dizziness and a loss of balance (*see* **Vertigo**, p.379).

As an acoustic neuroma enlarges it may press on part of the brain, causing lack of coordination of body movements. The tumour may also compress the nerves that supply the face, causing weakness of the facial muscles (*see* **Facial palsy**, p.339) and pain. In such cases, an untreated neuroma may cause permanent nerve damage.

What might be done?

If you have symptoms of an acoustic neuroma, your doctor may arrange for imaging tests such as MRI (p.133) to look for a tumour and hearing tests (p.377) to check for hearing loss.

An acoustic neuroma that is small and is not causing troublesome symptoms may simply be monitored with MRI, because in many cases the tumour does not enlarge sufficiently to cause significant problems. Troublesome or larger tumours may be removed by surgery. This is often successful in eliminating many of the symptoms and, if the tumour is small, hearing may be restored in the affected ear. However, removal of a large tumour may damage the vestibulocochlear or facial nerves, which may result in permanent hearing loss in the affected ear and numbness, weakness, or paralysis of part of the face. Alternatively, it may be possible to treat the tumour using radiotherapy or by a technique called stereotactic radiosurgery (sometimes called a "gamma knife"), which delivers a very precise dose of radiotherapy to the tumour.

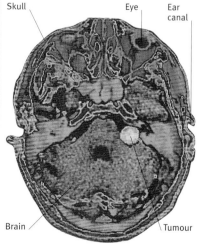

Acoustic neuroma
This MRI scan of the head shows an acoustic neuroma, a tumour of the nerve that connects the ear to the brain.

Teeth and gums

The primary function of teeth is to break down food ready for digestion. Teeth also help us to pronounce sounds clearly and give the face shape and definition. Each of us grows two sets of teeth in a lifetime, the second set gradually replacing the first during childhood. The gums help to keep the teeth firmly in the jaw and protect their roots from decay. Teeth and gums are vulnerable to the build-up of plaque (a sticky mixture of bacteria, saliva, and food particles), which causes decay and gum disease.

I N THE EARLY 20th century, it was common for people to have lost all of their secondary (adult) teeth by the age of 60 as a result of tooth decay and gum disease. Today, because of advances in dental health care, improvements in nutrition, and, in some areas, fluoridation of water, many people keep their secondary teeth for life.

The structure of the teeth

The part of the tooth that protrudes from the gum is called the crown; the part beneath the gumline is called the root. The crown is covered with a protective layer of enamel, the hardest substance in the body. Enamel is composed of rod-shaped calcium salt crystals and cannot renew itself. As a result, the enamel may eventually become worn down from abrasion, or it may be damaged by acid present in food and drinks or produced by bacteria in plaque in the presence of sugars from food and drink. If the enamel is damaged, a cavity is formed. This can be repaired with a dental filling.

Beneath the enamel layer lies the dentine, a hard ivory-like substance that surrounds the pulp cavity. This central cavity contains nerves and blood vessels that extend through tiny channels into the dentine, making the dentine sensitive to heat, cold, and pain.

About two-thirds of a tooth is made up of the root, buried below the gumline in a deep socket in the jaw. Each root is attached to the jawbone by a periodontal ligament, which cushions the root in its socket while the teeth are grinding down food.

Teeth have various shapes and sizes to enable them to hold, cut, tear, and chew food efficiently. For example, to enable teeth to grind down food effectively, the contoured chewing

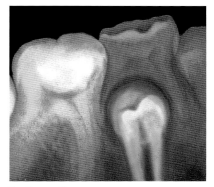

Tooth eruption
In this colour-enhanced X-ray of a child's lower jaw, a secondary tooth that has not yet erupted can be seen below a primary tooth.

surfaces of the upper and lower back teeth meet and are similar in shape. The actions of the teeth are controlled by the upper and lower jaws, which are able to clamp the teeth together with great force – up to 500 kg/sq. cm (7,000 lb/sq. in) – with the help of four powerful sets of muscles.

The role of the gums

The bone and periodontal ligaments that support the teeth in the jaw are covered by a layer of protective tissue known as the gums or gingiva. Healthy gums are pink or brown and firm. They form a tight seal around the neck of the tooth, preventing food particles and plaque from invading underlying tissues and the root of the tooth.

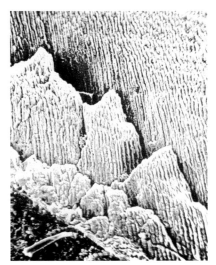

Tooth enamel
This magnified image of tooth enamel shows the many tiny, rod-shaped calcium crystals that lie at right angles to the surface of the tooth.

✚ STRUCTURE

Development of teeth

Our first set of 20 teeth appears between the ages of 6 months and 3 years. These teeth are known as primary, deciduous, or milk teeth. As the jaw grows, a set of 32 secondary (adult or permanent) teeth appears between the ages of 6 and 21. As the secondary teeth erupt, they displace the primary teeth, which usually fall out by the age of 13. In some cases, the third molars, also known as wisdom teeth, fail to develop or never erupt.

Patterns of eruption
The primary and secondary teeth usually erupt in a specific order (as indicated here by the numbers in brackets).

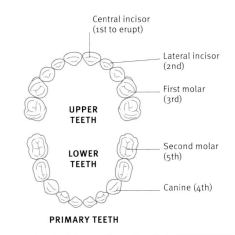

Central incisor (1st to erupt)
Lateral incisor (2nd)
First molar (3rd)
UPPER TEETH
Second molar (5th)
LOWER TEETH
Canine (4th)
PRIMARY TEETH

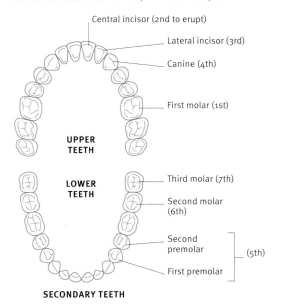

Central incisor (2nd to erupt)
Lateral incisor (3rd)
Canine (4th)
First molar (1st)
UPPER TEETH
LOWER TEETH
Third molar (7th)
Second molar (6th)
Second premolar (5th)
First premolar
SECONDARY TEETH

Teeth and gums

Teeth vary in shape and size but have an identical structure. Each tooth consists of a hard shell that surrounds a cavity of soft tissue, known as pulp. The crown (the exposed part of the shell) is coated in a tough layer of enamel, beneath which is a layer of a yellowish substance similar to ivory, called dentine. The dentine and pulp form long, pointed roots that extend into the jawbone and are covered by a layer of firm, fleshy tissue called the gums.

Temporo-mandibular (TM) joint

Molar

Mandible (lower jaw)

Maxilla (upper jaw)

Incisor

Canine

Premolar

SIDE VIEW OF THE JAWS AND TEETH

Crown
The crown is the part of the tooth exposed above the gumline

Neck
The part of the tooth that narrows slightly at the gumline is called the neck

Root
The root is the long pointed part of the tooth embedded in the jawbone; incisors and canines have one root, premolars one or two, and molars three or four

Incisor
The sharp chisel-like incisors, situated at the front of the mouth, cut and hold food.

Canine
Canines are longer and more pointed than incisors; they are used for tearing food.

Premolar
Premolars have two prominences (cusps) on their biting surfaces and are used for grinding food.

Molar
Molars, the largest teeth, are used for grinding. They have four or five cusps on their chewing surfaces.

Enamel
The crown is coated in enamel, an insensitive, nonliving substance

Dentine
Dentine is a tough, ivory-like material that connects with blood and nerves from the pulp tissue through microscopic tubules

Gum (gingiva)
This layer of protective tissue fits tightly around the base of the crown and covers the roots of the tooth

Pulp
At the centre of a tooth lies the soft pulp tissue, containing nerves and blood vessels

Periodontal ligament
This tissue joins the tooth to the jawbone and gums

Cementum
This layer of hard tissue covers the roots and anchors the fibres of the periodontal ligament

Jawbone
Deep sockets in the jawbone encase the roots of the tooth

Nerve
Nerves supply the periodontal ligament, pulp, gums, and jaw

Blood vessel
These blood vessels supply nutrients to the pulp tissue, bone, and gums

Using the jaws

The actions of biting and chewing require the lower jaw to move in all directions. This range of movement is made possible by the temporomandibular joint, a complex but exceptionally flexible type of hinge joint that attaches the lower jaw to the skull.

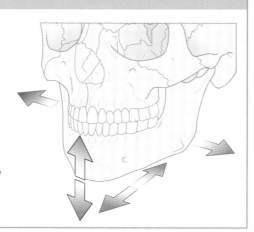

Moving the lower jaw
The lower jaw moves in six directions, side to side, up and down, and backwards and forwards. This mobility is essential for biting off and chewing food.

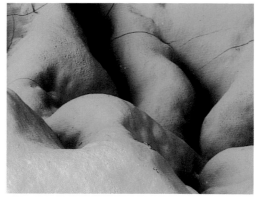

The upper surface of a molar
This magnified image shows the normal pits and fissures on the chewing surface of a molar tooth.

Disorders of the teeth

Teeth are necessary for chopping food into small pieces to make digestion easier. Each person has two sets of teeth: the primary teeth, which emerge in infancy, and the secondary teeth, which gradually replace the primary teeth in late childhood. Both sets are protected from damage and decay by a hard coating of enamel and by the gums, which cover the roots.

Good oral hygiene is essential because without regular brushing and flossing of the teeth and gums, tooth decay or gum disease may develop. Improved oral hygiene and the addition of fluoride to water in many parts of the world have made tooth decay far less common today than several decades ago.

The first articles in this section deal with tooth disorders that are usually caused by neglect of oral hygiene and consuming too much sugar, such as toothache and tooth decay. If left untreated, tooth decay may spread to the central parts of the teeth and cause pulpitis. Pus may eventually build up at the root of a tooth due to infection, resulting in a dental abscess. Poor oral hygiene can also cause teeth to become discoloured. Malocclusion caused by teeth that have grown unevenly or become overcrowded is covered next. Sometimes teeth are missing or are broken or lost due to injury. Problems of the temporomandibular joint are covered in the last article of this section. Teething (p.532) in babies is discussed in the children's section.

KEY ANATOMY

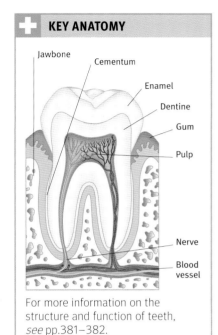

Jawbone · Cementum · Enamel · Dentine · Gum · Pulp · Nerve · Blood vessel

For more information on the structure and function of teeth, *see* pp.381–382.

Toothache

Pain or discomfort in one or more teeth or in the gums

 Poor oral hygiene and a diet high in sugar are risk factors

 Age, gender, and genetics are not significant factors

Pain in one or more teeth is usually a symptom of an underlying problem with the teeth or gums. Depending on the cause, the pain may range from a dull ache to a severe throbbing sensation. Toothache may last only a few minutes or it may be continuous.

What are the causes?
A sharp pain triggered by biting or consuming hot, cold, or sweet foods and drinks may be a symptom of the early stages of tooth decay (*see* Dental caries, p.384). A fractured tooth (p.387), receding gums (p.390), or advanced gum disease (*see* Periodontitis, p.389) may also result in toothache. A dull pain in the teeth while chewing may be due to inflammation of the gums (*see* Gingivitis, p.389) following a build-up of plaque (a deposit of food particles, saliva, and bacteria). Pain may also be caused by food trapped between the teeth.

A continuous, severe, throbbing pain is usually the result of advanced tooth decay (*see* Pulpitis, p.385), in which the pulp, the central part of the tooth containing the nerves and blood vessels, becomes inflamed. If the pain changes so that the tooth becomes tender to touch, it may be a sign that pulpitis has developed into a dental abscess (p.385) at the root, with infection and death of the pulp tissues. The infection may spread to surrounding tissues and be accompanied by facial swelling and, occasionally, fever. The lymph nodes in the neck may also become enlarged and tender.

Pain and tenderness at the back of the mouth may be due to emerging wisdom teeth. If the wisdom teeth only partially emerge (*see* Impacted teeth, p.386), the gum around the teeth can become inflamed or infected, which can be particularly painful.

In some cases, toothache occurs as a result of a disorder elsewhere in the body, such as sinusitis (p.290), an ear infection (*see* Otitis media, p.374), or a problem in the joint between the jaw and the skull (*see* Temporomandibular joint disorder, p.388).

What can I do?
If you have toothache, you should consult your dentist as soon as possible. If you have a fever and/or a swollen face in addition to toothache, you should see a dentist immediately.

▶ TEST

Dental checkup

To keep your teeth and gums healthy, you should have regular dental checkups. Your dentist will recommend how often you should have your teeth checked based on your risk of developing dental problems. This can range from 3–24 months. During a checkup, your dentist will examine your teeth for signs of decay and your gums for evidence of gum disease. If you have not been to the dentist for some time, you may have X-rays to look for evidence of decay between the back teeth and under existing fillings. Your dentist may also clean and polish your teeth and will advise you on good oral hygiene.

Looking at the teeth and gums
Your teeth and gums will be examined for signs of disease while you lie in a dental chair under a bright light. Your dentist will also check that all the teeth are present and aligned correctly and that teeth still emerging are not likely to become impacted.

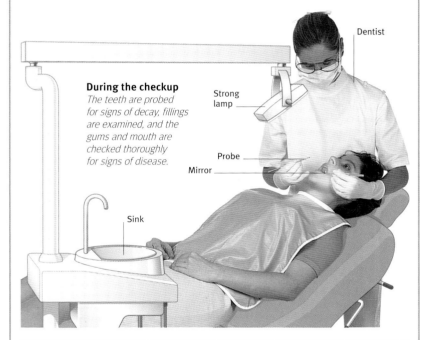

Dentist · **Strong lamp** · **Probe** · **Mirror** · **Sink**

During the checkup
The teeth are probed for signs of decay, fillings are examined, and the gums and mouth are checked thoroughly for signs of disease.

Bite-wing X-ray
A bite-wing X-ray is used to look for decay. The X-ray film is put in a holder, which is held between the teeth while the X-ray machine is placed near your cheek. An X-ray may be taken on both sides of the face.

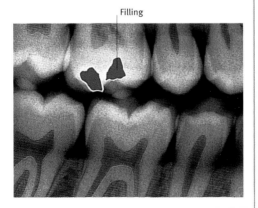

Filling

Bite-wing X-ray
This colour-enhanced X-ray shows two fillings in an upper molar tooth. No decay is present.

While you are waiting for an appointment to see your dentist, you can try using an over-the-counter painkiller (p.589), such as paracetamol, to help relieve the toothache. Rinsing out your mouth with warm salt water may also be helpful. However, the only permanent remedy for toothache is for the affected tooth to be treated by a dentist.

What might be done?
Your dentist will ask you about your symptoms and examine your teeth and gums. He or she may also take X-rays of your mouth to look for decay.

If toothache is caused by decay, your dentist will remove the decayed areas and may put in an ordinary filling to stop the pain and prevent further decay (*see* **Tooth filling**, opposite page). If tooth decay is acvanced and you have pulpitis or a dental abscess, you may need root canal treatment (p.386), in which the soft pulp tissues within the tooth are taken out. The cavity is sterilized to clear up the infection, and the root canals and decayed area are filled permanently. If you have gingivitis or periodontitis, your dentist will probably remove the plaque and tartar that is causing the inflammation by scaling your teeth. A tooth that is very badly damaged or decayed may need to be extracted. Likewise, painful, impacted wisdom teeth may need to be extracted. Your dentist may prescribe antibiotics (p.572) if there is an infection. If your toothache is due to a condition such as sinusitis or an ear infection, you may need to consult a doctor for the necessary treatment.

To prevent toothache, you should brush and floss your teeth and gums regularly and avoid sugary food and drinks (*see* **Caring for your teeth and gums**, below). You should also have regular dental checkups (p.383).

Dental caries

Progressive decay of one or more teeth, causing cavities to form

 More common under the age of 25

 Poor oral hygiene and a diet high in sugar are risk factors

 Gender and genetics are not significant factors

Gradual, progressive decay of a tooth is known as dental caries. This condition usually starts as a small cavity in the enamel (the hard, protective outer covering of a tooth). If left untreated, the decay eventually penetrates the outer layer of enamel and attacks the dentine, the softer material that makes up the bulk of a tooth. As the tooth decay progresses, the pulp (the living core of the tooth that contains the nerves and blood vessels) may be affected (*see* **Pulpitis**, opposite page). If the pulp is exposed to decay and becomes infected, it may die.

Most people develop dental caries at some time in their lives. In younger age groups, tooth decay most often occurs on the chewing surfaces of the teeth and on the smooth surfaces between adjacent teeth. In older people, tooth decay is more common at the gum margins where the teeth meet the gums.

In developed countries, the number of teeth lost as a result of dental caries has fallen considerably in recent years, particularly among children. This fall is partly due to the addition of fluoride to drinking water in some areas and to the widespread use of fluoride toothpaste, both of which help to harden the teeth, making them more resistant to decay.

What are the causes?
Tooth decay is usually caused by a build-up of plaque (a deposit of food particles, saliva, and bacteria) on the surface of the teeth. The bacteria in plaque break down the sugar in food to produce an acid that erodes the tooth enamel. If sugary foods are eaten often and the teeth are not cleaned regularly with fluoride toothpaste, a cavity is eventually likely to form.

The condition is especially common in children, adolescents, and young adults because they are more likely to have a diet high in sugar and fail to clean their teeth regularly. Babies or young children who drink milk or juice from a bottle frequently throughout the day or who sleep with a bottle of milk or juice in their mouth may also develop severe caries.

What are the symptoms?
There may be no signs of dental caries in the early stages, but the symptoms develop gradually as the decay progresses and may include:

- Toothache, which may be constant or sharp and stabbing and triggered by hot, cold, or sweet foods or drinks.
- Persistent, throbbing pain in the jaw and occasionally in the ear and face, which may be worse when chewing.
- Bad breath.

Pain in a tooth can take several forms. It may be persistent, recurrent, or set off by extremes of hot or cold or pressure on the tooth. You should see your dentist as soon as possible after the pain first appears and

---

▶ **SELF-HELP**

Caring for your teeth and gums

Daily care of your teeth is as important as having regular dental checkups. If you adopt a simple routine of regular brushing and flossing, you can prevent food particles and bacteria from building up on the surface of your teeth and reduce the risk of tooth decay and gum disease. If you cannot clean your teeth between meals, chewing sugar-free gum may help. You should avoid sugary foods and drinks, which contribute to tooth decay.

Brushing your teeth

Your teeth need brushing at least twice a day for 2 minutes and, if possible, after every meal. Use a small-headed, soft toothbrush and fluoride toothpaste. Check with your dentist how much fluoride your toothpaste should contain. Make sure that you clean all the surfaces of all your teeth, especially where they meet the gum. You should replace your toothbrush every 2–3 months.

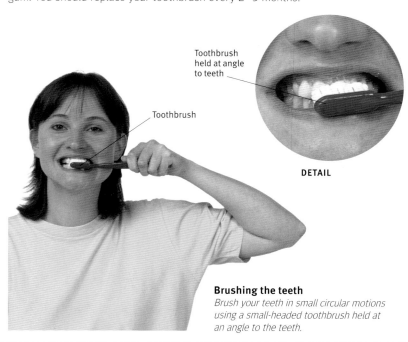

Toothbrush held at angle to teeth

Toothbrush

DETAIL

Brushing the teeth
Brush your teeth in small circular motions using a small-headed toothbrush held at an angle to the teeth.

Cleaning between teeth

Dental floss or dental tape is used to clean between the teeth and remove food particles and bacteria from areas between the teeth that cannot be reached easily with a toothbrush. Toothpicks and small interdental brushes may also be used. You should clean between each tooth in turn in a regular pattern so that no teeth are missed.

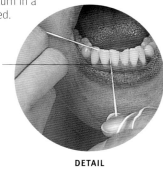

Floss curved around tooth

Dental floss

DETAIL

Flossing the teeth
Keeping the floss taut, guide it between the teeth. Gently scrape the side of the tooth away from the gum.

Food and drink

You should avoid consuming foods and drinks that have a high sugar content, such as desserts and colas, particularly if you cannot clean your teeth immediately. If you cannot brush soon after eating sugary foods, chew sugar-free gum.

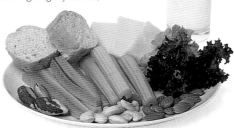

Sugarless snacks
Snacking on foods such as nuts, celery, carrots, and cheese is better for your teeth than eating sugary foods.

▶ **TREATMENT**

Tooth filling

Teeth are usually filled or restored because of tooth decay. Composite fillings are usually used in front teeth and are also often used in back teeth, although amalgam (a mixture of silver, tin, and mercury) is still sometimes used in back teeth. A local anaesthetic may be used to make the tooth and gum numb. The decayed area of tooth is drilled away and the hole is shaped to secure the filling; often, the hole is lined with a substance to protect the tooth pulp. The filling is then pushed into the hole as a soft paste. With composite fillings, a special curing light is used to harden the filling. Amalgam fillings harden naturally within a few hours.

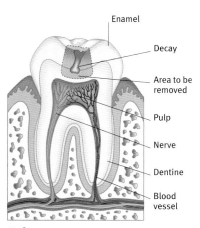

Before treatment
Tooth decay has penetrated the hard enamel covering of the tooth and invaded the dentine, the softer material that makes up the bulk of the tooth.

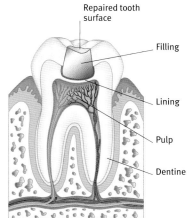

After treatment
The decayed area has been drilled out and the hole shaped to hold a filling. A protective lining has been inserted into the hole, which has then been filled.

make an immediate appointment if the pain ends abruptly because this may indicate that the nerves and blood vessels have died. Delaying a visit to your dentist may result in the spread of infection, and an abscess may eventually form (*see* **Dental abscess**, right).

What might be done?
Your dentist will examine your teeth with a probe and a mirror to look for areas of tooth decay. An X-ray may also be taken to look for decay that may be developing beneath the surface of the teeth (*see* **Dental checkup**, p.383).

If you have superficial dental caries restricted to the surface of the enamel, your dentist may only apply fluoride to the affected area and advise you to be more careful about oral hygiene.

If tooth decay has penetrated further into the enamel or if it has affected the dentine, your dentist will probably need to fill the affected tooth (*see* **Tooth filling**, above). An injection of a local anaesthetic is often used to numb the tooth and nearby gum to prevent you from feeling pain. When the area is numb, the decayed parts of the tooth are drilled out, and the cavity is cleaned and filled to prevent further decay. If you have pulpitis and the pulp cannot be saved, you may need to have root canal treatment (p.386).

Can it be prevented?
You can help to prevent caries by brushing and flossing your teeth and gums regularly (*see* **Caring for your teeth and gums**, opposite page) and by avoiding sugary foods and drinks. Your dentist can apply a fluoride varnish to your teeth, which can also help to prevent caries.

Pulpitis

Inflammation of the pulp, the living core of a tooth

 Poor oral hygiene and a diet high in sugar are risk factors

 Age, gender, and genetics are not significant factors

The soft centre (pulp) of a tooth contains the blood vessels and nerves. Inflammation of the pulp is called pulpitis. It may be caused by advanced tooth decay (*see* **Dental caries**, opposite page) that invades the pulp. Pulpitis may also develop if the pulp becomes exposed in a fractured tooth (p.387). Some people grind their teeth during sleep, which may inflame the pulp.

There are two varieties: reversible and irreversible. In reversible pulpitis, the decay has not affected the entire pulp, and the remaining tissue with its nerves and blood vessels can be saved. Without treatment, reversible pulpitis may eventually become irreversible, in which decay is so severe that the remaining pulp, nerves, and vessels die. Eventually, the tooth may become discoloured (*see* **Discoloured teeth**, p.386).

The main symptom of pulpitis is toothache. If it only occurs while eating or drinking, pulpitis is likely to be reversible. In irreversible pulpitis, pain tends to be more constant until the pulp dies. You may also notice pain if you tap the tooth. Left untreated, a dental abscess (below) may form.

What might be done?
Your dentist will examine your teeth and may take an X-ray to look for decay (*see* **Dental checkup**, p.383). To treat reversible pulpitis, he or she may remove the decayed area and fill the tooth to prevent further damage (*see* **Tooth filling**, left). If the pulpitis is irreversible, you will probably need root canal treatment (p.386), in which the pulp is removed and the root canals are filled.

Dental abscess

A pus-filled sac that develops in or around the root of a tooth

 Poor oral hygiene and a diet high in sugar are risk factors

 Age, gender, and genetics are not significant factors

An accumulation of pus in or around the root of a tooth is known as a dental abscess. An abscess usually develops as a complication of dental caries (opposite page), which gradually destroys the layer of enamel on the outside of the tooth and the inner dentine, allowing bacteria to invade the soft central core, or pulp, of the tooth (*see* **Pulpitis**, left). Eventually, a dental abscess may form. The pulp may also become infected if a tooth is damaged by a blow to the mouth (*see* **Fractured tooth**, p.387).

An abscess may also form as a result of certain types of gum disease (*see* **Periodontitis**, p.389). Periodontitis is usually caused by a build-up of dental plaque (a deposit including food particles, saliva, and bacteria) in a pocket that forms between a tooth and gum. An abscess can be extremely painful and may cause the tooth that is affected to loosen in its socket.

What are the symptoms?
The main symptoms of a dental abscess develop gradually and may include:
■ Severe pain on touching the affected tooth and on biting or chewing.
■ Loosening of the affected tooth.
■ Red, tender swelling of the gum over the root of the tooth.
■ Release of pus into the mouth.
If untreated, the infection may make a channel from the tooth to the surface of the gum (known as a sinus tract), and a painful swelling, known as a gumboil, may form. If the gumboil bursts, foul-tasting pus is released and the pain decreases. In some cases, the channel may persist, leading to a chronic (long-standing) abscess that discharges pus periodically.

If the infection spreads, the face may become swollen and painful, and a fever may also develop. If you suspect that you have a dental abscess, you should consult your dentist as soon as possible.

What can I do?
Taking painkillers (p.589), such as paracetamol, may help until you can see your dentist. Rinsing your mouth with warm salt water may also help to relieve the pain and encourage a gumboil to burst. If a gumboil does burst, you should wash away the pus thoroughly with more warm salt water.

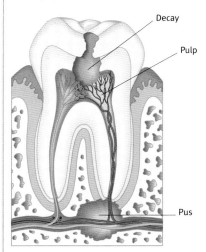

Dental abscess
Tooth decay and infection has spread through the tooth, and pus has gathered at the root of the tooth. If it is not treated, the tooth will have to be extracted.

What might the dentist do?
Your dentist will ask you about your symptoms and examine your teeth and gums. He or she may take an X-ray of your mouth to confirm the diagnosis (*see* **Dental checkup**, p.383).

If the abscess has been caused by decay, your dentist may try to save the tooth. Under a local anaesthetic, a hole is drilled through the top of the tooth to release the pus and relieve the pain. If there is a gumboil, a small cut may be made to drain the pus and the cavity is then cleaned with an antiseptic solution. You will probably also be given a course of antibiotics (p.572). Once the infection has cleared up, you will probably need root canal treatment (p.386). If it is not possible to save the tooth, it will be extracted.

To treat an abscess caused by gum disease, your dentist may use a scaler to scrape out the plaque from the pocket between the affected tooth and gum. The pocket is then washed out with an antiseptic solution. In a severe case, the affected tooth may need to be extracted.

What is the prognosis?
Treatment is usually successful, but a small area of infection may persist and further treatment may be required.

Discoloured teeth

Abnormal colouring of the teeth, which may be due to a number of factors

 More common with increasing age

 Poor oral hygiene, using tobacco, and drinking coffee and tea are risk factors

 Gender and genetics are not significant factors

Tooth colour varies among individuals, and secondary teeth are usually darker than primary teeth. Teeth also normally darken slightly with age. However, abnormal discoloration sometimes occurs because of changes within the teeth.

What are the causes?

A common cause of discoloration is the build-up of dental plaque (a deposit of food particles, saliva, and bacteria) on the surface of the teeth. Plaque-stained teeth are often yellowish-brown, but children's teeth may be black or even green. Regularly drinking tea and coffee and smoking or using chewing tobacco may also stain the surface of the teeth, as may some liquid medicines that contain iron.

Tooth discoloration may also be due to systemic (whole-body) factors, such as severe illness, while the teeth are developing. Some drugs, such as tetracycline (*see* **Antibiotics**, p.572), can cause a yellow discoloration of the teeth if given to young children while their

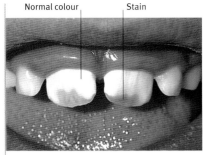

Normal colour | **Stain**

Discoloured teeth
The brown areas of discoloration on this child's two front teeth have been caused by excess amounts of fluoride. This condition is called fluorosis.

secondary teeth are developing; if given to a pregnant woman, her baby's teeth may be discoloured.

Fluorosis, in which the teeth develop a mottled colour, is due to an excess of natural fluoride in the water in some parts of the world. However, where fluoride is added to the water to reduce tooth decay, the concentration is too low to cause fluorosis. Fluorosis may also develop if children are given too high a dose of fluoride drops or pills.

A tooth may become darker than normal following irreversible pulpitis (*see* **Pulpitis**, p.385), when the soft centre, or the pulp, of the tooth dies. Root canal treatment (below) may cause a tooth to darken if the material used to fill the tooth is dark in colour.

What might be done?

Staining on the surface of the teeth is routinely removed by scaling and polishing of teeth by your dentist or oral hygienist. If

staining is severe, it may be possible to bleach the teeth. If a single tooth is discoloured as a result of a condition such as pulpitis or following root canal treatment, a porcelain or plastic veneer may be bonded to the front of the tooth, or alternatively the top of the tooth may be replaced by a crown (*see* **Crowns and replacement teeth**, p.388).

Most discoloration of teeth can be prevented by brushing and flossing the teeth and gums regularly (*see* **Caring for your teeth and gums**, p.384).

Impacted teeth

Failure of teeth to emerge completely from the gum and grow into their normal position, usually due to lack of room

 More common under the age of 25

 Gender, genetics, and lifestyle are not significant factors

Teeth usually become impacted when there is not enough room in the mouth for them to grow into their correct positions. Impacted teeth may sometimes remain entirely buried in the jawbone, producing few or no symptoms, or they may only partly erupt through the gum. Impaction may also occur if a tooth starts to grow in the wrong direction and pushes against other teeth or the jawbone.

Wisdom teeth are the most likely to become impacted, followed by the upper canines. The wisdom and upper canine teeth emerge at a later stage of life than other teeth, and often there is insufficient room in the mouth for them to erupt normally. Impacted teeth most frequently occur in adolescents and young adults when the teeth are still emerging.

Impacted teeth may cause pain and inflammation. A partly erupted tooth may be covered by a flap of gum under which plaque (a sticky deposit of food particles, saliva, and bacteria) accumulates, leading to inflammation of the gum and gradual decay of the tooth (*see* **Dental caries**, p.384).

Impacted wisdom teeth | **Molar tooth**

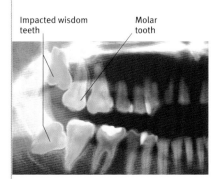

Impacted teeth
This colour-enhanced X-ray shows two wisdom teeth that have impacted on the roots of adjacent molars.

What might be done?

Your dentist will check at each visit (*see* **Dental checkup**, p.383) whether any emerging teeth are likely to become impacted. He or she may also take X-rays to look at unerupted teeth. One or more teeth may be extracted to allow room for other teeth to come through. You may also need orthodontic treatment (opposite page) to straighten the teeth.

Wisdom teeth that are impacted are not routinely removed unless they frequently become infected or are causing other problems. If canines are impacted, they may be fully exposed by removing gum tissue. An orthodontic device is then applied to guide the teeth into position.

Malocclusion

Unsatisfactory contact between the upper and lower teeth or misalignment of the teeth

 Most common between the ages of 6 and 14

 Often runs in families

 Poor oral hygiene and thumb sucking beyond the age of 6 are risk factors

 Gender is not a significant factor

Ideally, the upper front teeth should slightly overlap the lower front teeth and the molars should meet evenly. Most people have some teeth that are out of position but this is not usually a pressing problem unless appearance is adversely affected or biting and chewing are impaired.

Malocclusion may occur when the teeth are crooked because they are crowded and overlap each other or when the upper front teeth protrude too far in front of the lower front teeth. Less commonly, the lower teeth protrude in front of the upper front teeth. Sometimes, the back teeth prevent the front teeth from meeting properly, a condition known as an open bite.

What are the causes?

Malocclusion often runs in families and usually develops in childhood when the teeth and jaws are growing. The condition is usually caused by a discrepancy between the number and size of the teeth and the growth of the jaws. In children, protrusion of the front teeth may also be caused by thumb sucking beyond about the age of 6.

If the primary teeth are lost early (before about 9 or 10) because of decay (*see* **Dental caries**, p.384), the secondary molars already in position may move forwards to take up some of the space meant for the new premolar and canine teeth. The new teeth then become crowded and misaligned.

What are the symptoms?

From about the age of 6, the symptoms develop gradually and may include:
■ Out-of-line, crowded, or abnormally spaced teeth.

▶ **TREATMENT**

Root canal treatment

Sometimes, decay invades the pulp, the centre of the tooth, and root canal treatment may be performed. The pulp is removed, as well as the nerves and blood vessels, and an antiseptic solution is used to sterilize the cavity. If infection within the tooth is severe, a temporary filling may be inserted for a few days before the cavity is sterilized again. The root canals and the decayed area of the tooth are then filled.

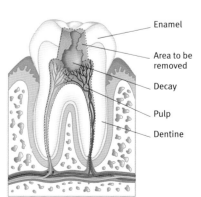

Before treatment
Tooth decay has penetrated the enamel and the dentine and has reached the pulp, the core of the tooth that contains the blood vessels and nerves.

Enamel
Area to be removed
Decay
Pulp
Dentine

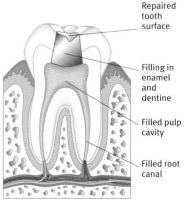

After treatment
The decayed area of the tooth and pulp have been removed, and the pulp cavity has been sterilized. The decayed area, pulp cavity, and root canals have been filled.

Repaired tooth surface
Filling in enamel and dentine
Filled pulp cavity
Filled root canal

- Excessive protrusion of the upper teeth in front of the lower, or a protruding lower jaw.
- Front teeth that do not meet.

Some children have mild symptoms, but these are often temporary and tend to result from a growth spurt.

Speech and chewing are affected in severe cases of malocclusion. An abnormal bite may be painful and may also affect the appearance, particularly the lower-jaw profile. Arthritis may develop in the temporomandibular joint (*see* **Temporomandibular joint disorder**, p.388) in rare cases.

What might be done?
The dentist will look for malocclusion as part of a dental checkup (p.383). If found, a specialist dentist called an orthodontist may take casts of the teeth to study the bite in detail. The orthodontist may also take X-rays, especially if some of the teeth have not erupted.

Treatment is usually necessary only if malocclusion is severe and is causing difficulties when eating and speaking or is affecting appearance. If the teeth are overcrowded, some of them may be extracted. If necessary, the teeth may then be aligned using an orthodontic appliance (*see* **Orthodontic treatment**, below). Surgical treatment for malocclusion is necessary only in rare cases.

It is best to treat malocclusion during childhood, when the teeth and jaw bones are still developing. However, if malocclusion is caused by a severe mismatch in the size of the jaws and teeth, surgery may be needed and treatment may be delayed until adulthood.

▶ **TREATMENT**

Orthodontic treatment

Orthodontics is the correction of crowded or unevenly spaced teeth. Orthodontic treatment is usually performed on older children and adolescents while their teeth are still developing, although adults can also benefit. Casts of the teeth are taken before an orthodontic appliance, or brace, is applied either to move or straighten the teeth gradually. In some cases, it is necessary to extract one or more teeth in order to make room for others. The treatment usually takes several months or years to complete and necessitates regular visits to the orthodontist for checkups.

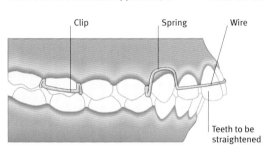

Clip Spring Wire

Teeth to be straightened

Removable appliances
Removable braces consist of a plastic plate, which fits into the roof of the mouth and clips into place. Springs and wires exert pressure on the teeth. To increase the amount of pressure, the brace may be connected to a headcap that is worn while sleeping.

Fixed appliances
Fixed braces consist of wires and springs carried by brackets that are fixed to the teeth with dental adhesive. These braces can exert greater pressure than removable appliances and produce more complex movements of the teeth.

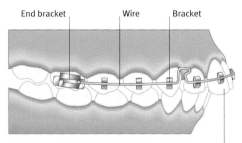

End bracket Wire Bracket

Teeth to be straightened

Orthodontic treatment
These two photographs show a set of teeth before and after orthodontic treatment. The irregular teeth have been brought into line by the treatment.

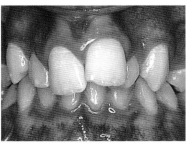

BEFORE TREATMENT

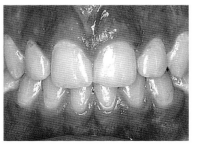

AFTER TREATMENT

Fractured tooth

A tooth that is cracked, chipped, or broken, often as a result of trauma

 More common under the age of 30

 More common in males

 Playing contact sports is a risk factor

Genetics is not a significant factor

A hard blow to the mouth is the most common cause of a fractured tooth. Young men are more likely to damage their teeth in this way because they are more likely to participate in contact sports. Protruding front teeth or teeth weakened by heavy filling are particularly susceptible to fracture.

The enamel, the hard outer covering of the crown, is most often damaged, but this does not usually produce any symptoms. Sensitivity to heat or cold and pain when biting may occur if the dentine beneath the enamel is affected. Pain and bleeding may indicate that the pulp, containing the nerves and blood vessels, has been damaged. You should consult your dentist within 24 hours if the damaged tooth feels sensitive or is bleeding because the pulp may become infected (*see* **Pulpitis**, p.385), and a dental abscess (p.385) may form at the root.

What might be done?
Treatment depends on the severity of the damage. Chipped enamel may only be treated for cosmetic reasons. A large fracture may be filled (*see* **Tooth filling**, p.385) or a crown may be fitted (*see* **Crowns and replacement teeth**, p.388). A tooth loosened by trauma and with an extensive fracture may be splinted to neighbouring teeth for 1–2 weeks. If the pulp is infected or has died, you may need root canal treatment (opposite page). Severely damaged teeth may have to be extracted.

Missing teeth

The lack of one or more secondary, or adult, teeth

 More common with increasing age

 More common in males

 In some cases, the cause is inherited

 Poor oral hygiene and playing contact sports are risk factors

Total absence of many or all of the secondary teeth is very rare. Failure of one or more teeth to develop is more common. Of all the teeth, the wisdom teeth are most likely to be absent, which may be an advantage as it reduces the risk of impaction (*see* **Impacted teeth**, opposite page). The emergence of some teeth may be delayed by the effects of chemotherapy (p.157) and radiotherapy (p.158) and in people with Down's syndrome (p.533) or those with certain other genetic conditions. A delay may also be due to impaction caused by overcrowding.

Teeth may be lost due to injury (*see* **Avulsed tooth**, below) or tooth decay caused by neglect of oral hygiene (*see* **Dental caries**, p.384). The risk of tooth loss is higher in men because they play more contact sports. If the secondary (adult) teeth are not present, adjacent teeth tend to grow into the remaining spaces, which may cause uneven teeth or malocclusion (opposite page).

What might be done?
The dentist will check a child's teeth during each checkup to make sure that all the teeth emerge. If one or more teeth are missing, he or she may take bite-wing X-rays to see if the teeth are absent or still in the jaw (*see* **Dental checkup**, p.383). If you lose a tooth, you should consult a dentist or go to an accident and emergency department at once.

Treatment depends on how many and which teeth are affected. If the teeth are held back or delayed by overcrowding, one or two teeth may be removed to make room for the others. A brace may be needed to move teeth into place or keep them locked in position until the missing teeth have emerged and have become established (*see* **Orthodontic treatment**, left). Teeth that have been lost can sometimes be reattached. If a tooth has failed to develop or one or more teeth have been lost, the missing tooth or teeth may be replaced (*see* **Crowns and replacement teeth**, p.388). Missing wisdom teeth are not replaced.

Avulsed tooth

A tooth that has been partly or completely knocked out of its socket as a result of a powerful impact to the jaw

 More common in children

 More common in males

 Playing contact sports is a risk factor

 Genetics is not a significant factor

Although teeth are commonly lost in childhood accidents, an avulsed tooth is really a problem only if a secondary (adult) tooth is lost because primary (baby) teeth are eventually replaced by secondary teeth. Avulsed teeth are much more common in men because they play more contact sports. The front teeth are most often involved. If you play contact sports, you can ask your dentist to make a plastic mouthguard to fit over your teeth and protect them.

▶ **TREATMENT**

Crowns and replacement teeth

If a tooth is damaged but the root and main body of the tooth are healthy, a crown can be used to restore the tooth. A crown is a tooth-shaped cap that covers the whole of the natural tooth. It reinforces and protects the tooth and can be coloured to match the surrounding teeth. If one or more teeth are missing, there are various types of artificial teeth that may be used to replace them. The type used depends on the number of teeth lost and the individual's oral health.

Crowns

Up to two or three visits to your dentist may be necessary for a crown to be fitted. White porcelain is usually used for crowns at the front of the mouth. Materials used for crowns at the back of the mouth include reinforced porcelain, composite, and various metal alloys.

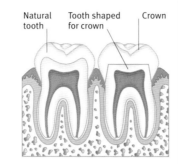

Fitting a crown
The tooth is shaped and an impression of it is taken. A temporary crown is made to fit over the shaped tooth while a permanent crown is made. The permanent crown is then cemented into place.

Replacement teeth

If one or more teeth have to be extracted, or if they are lost, they can be replaced by one of three different types of artificial teeth: a bridge, a dental implant, or dentures. Bridges and dental implants are permanent and fixed and are used to replace only one or two teeth at a time. Dentures can be removed and are used when many teeth need to be replaced.

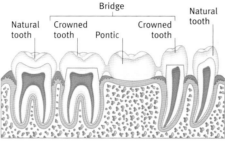

Bridge
A bridge is a permanent fixture used to replace one or two teeth. The teeth beside the gap (abutments) are crowned to support the artificial tooth (pontic).

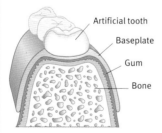

SECTION ACROSS FULL DENTURE

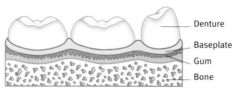

SECTION ALONG FULL DENTURE

Dentures
A denture can be removed and may replace any number of teeth. Full dentures stay in place by the baseplate resting on the gum ridges; partial dentures may be clasped to remaining natural teeth.

Implants
An implant is a permanent method of replacing a single tooth. A hole is drilled in the jaw at the site of the missing tooth, and an implant, usually titanium, is placed into the hole. The implant must heal for 4–6 months before an artificial tooth is attached to the top of the implant.

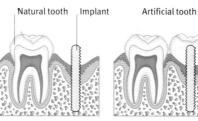

IMPLANT IN PLACE   **TOOTH IN PLACE**

If you have a tooth that is dislodged or knocked out, you should consult a dentist or visit an accident and emergency department immediately. If your tooth has been completely knocked out, you should avoid handling the root. If the tooth is very dirty, rinse it with milk or contact lens solution. Do not clean it with water or disinfectant, and do not let it dry out. The tooth should be pushed back firmly into the socket, and then you should bite on a clean handkerchief and see a dentist as soon as possible. If you cannot replace the tooth in its socket, you should ideally keep the tooth in your mouth (as long as there is no risk of swallowing it), where the saliva will protect it. Alternatively, put the tooth in a glass of milk or contact lens solution. In 9 out of 10 cases, a tooth will reattach itself to the jaw if it is replaced in the socket within 30 minutes of being knocked out.

What might be done?
The dentist will replace the tooth and splint it to other teeth to immobilize it for 10–14 days. Complete avulsion usually kills the pulp (containing nerves and blood vessels), in which case you may need root canal treatment (p.386) when the tooth has been replaced.

If you have lost a tooth and may have inhaled it, a chest X-ray (p.300) may be taken to ensure that the tooth is not lodged in your airways or lungs. A lost or damaged tooth may have to be replaced with an artificial tooth (*see* **Crowns and replacement teeth**, left).

Temporomandibular joint disorder

Problems in the joint between the jaw and skull, causing headaches or pain in the face

👥 Much more common in females

🧍 Stress may be a risk factor

🧍 Age and genetics are not significant factors

The temporomandibular joint connects the mandible (lower jawbone) to the part of the skull known as the temporal bone. The joint allows the lower jaw to move in all directions so that the teeth can be used to bite off and chew food efficiently. In temporomandibular joint disorder, the joint and the muscles and ligaments that control the joint do not work together properly, causing pain. The condition is three times more common in women than in men.

Temporomandibular joint disorder is most commonly caused by spasm of the chewing muscles, often as a result of clenching the jaw or grinding the teeth. Clenching the jaw and grinding the teeth may be increased by stress. A poor bite (*see* **Malocclusion**, p.386) places stress on the muscles and may also result in temporo-

---

mandibular joint disorder, as may an injury to the head, jaw, or neck that causes displacement of the joint. In rare cases, arthritis (p.220) is a cause of the condition.

What are the symptoms?
If you have temporomandibular joint disorder, you may notice one or more of the following symptoms:
■ Headaches.
■ Tenderness in the jaw muscles.
■ Aching pain in the face.
■ Severe pain near the ears.

In some cases, pain is caused by chewing or by opening the mouth too widely when yawning. There may be difficulty in opening the mouth, locking of the jaw, and clicking noises from the joint as the mouth is opened or closed.

What might be done?
Your dentist may take a panoramic X-ray of your mouth and jaws. He or she may also arrange for you to have special X-rays or an MRI (p.133) of the joint.

Treatment is aimed at eliminating muscle spasm and tension and relieving the pain. There are several self-help measures that you can take, including applying a warm, wet towel to the face, massaging the facial muscles, eating only soft foods, and using a device that fits over the teeth at night to prevent you from clenching or grinding your teeth. Taking a painkiller (p.589), such as paracetamol, may also help. If tension of the muscles used for chewing is severe, your doctor may prescribe a muscle relaxant drug (p.579). If stress is a major factor, you may find relaxation exercises (p.32) helpful.

If your bite needs to be adjusted, your dentist may recommend wearing a fixed or removable orthodontic appliance for a specified period of time (*see* **Orthodontic treatment**, p.387).

What is the prognosis?
In about 3 in 4 people, the symptoms improve within 3 months of treatment. However, in some cases, if symptoms do not improve, surgery may be needed to repair the temporomandibular joint.

Gum disorders

The gums form a layer of protective tissue that surrounds the base of each tooth and covers part of the jawbones. Healthy gum forms a tight seal around the crown of a tooth and protects the sensitive tissues below from bacterial invasion. If the gums are damaged, the teeth may become unsupported and loose. Most gum disorders can be prevented by good oral hygiene.

Most adults have some degree of gum disease which, if left untreated, may eventually lead to loss of teeth. Good oral hygiene is essential to help to prevent gum disorders. During regular dental checkups, most dentists and oral hygienists provide information on the correct way to brush and floss teeth and on general mouth care.

The first topics covered here are gum disorders such as gingivitis and periodontitis, which may be caused by poor oral hygiene. Inadequate teeth cleaning leads to a build-up of plaque (a deposit of food particles, saliva, and bacteria) on the surfaces of the teeth. If the plaque is not removed, it causes the gums to become inflamed. In more serious cases, the teeth may be affected and loosen or come out, either because the periodontal tissues are inflamed and detach from the teeth or because the gums recede, exposing the roots and leading to tooth decay. The final article in this section discusses a condition called dry socket, in which a tooth socket becomes inflamed after the tooth has been extracted.

KEY ANATOMY

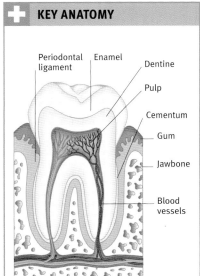

For more information on the structure and function of the gums, *see* pp.381–382.

Gingivitis

Inflammation of the gums, usually caused by poor oral hygiene

 More common in females

 Poor oral hygiene is a risk factor

 Age and genetics are not significant factors

Mild gingivitis, also known as gum disease, is very common and occurs in most adults at some time in their lives. Healthy gums are pink or brown and firm. In gingivitis, the gums become purple-red, soft, and shiny. They also bleed easily, especially when the teeth are brushed. The condition is usually caused by a build-up of plaque (a deposit of food particles, saliva, and bacteria) where the gums meets the base of the teeth. Once plaque has formed on the teeth, it can become hardened by taking up minerals from the saliva, and it is then known as calculus (tartar). This can only be removed by a dentist or hygienist.

Gingivitis can be made worse by taking certain drugs, such as phenytoin (*see* **Anticonvulsant drugs**, p.590), immuno-suppressants (p.585), and some antihypertensives (p.580). These drugs may cause overgrowth of the gums, making the removal of dental plaque difficult. Certain contraceptive drugs can also make symptoms worse. Pregnant women are more susceptible to gingivitis because of dramatic changes in hormone levels during pregnancy.

A rare but severe form of gingivitis is known as acute necrotizing ulcerative gingivitis (ANUG) or "trench mouth". ANUG usually occurs in teenagers and young adults. The condition sometimes develops from chronic gingivitis and is caused by an abnormal growth of the bacteria that normally exist harmlessly within the mouth. ANUG is more common in people who are under stress or run down and in people with AIDS (*see* **HIV infection and AIDS**, p.169).

What are the symptoms?
The symptoms of gingivitis develop gradually and usually include:
- Purple-red, soft, shiny, swollen gums.
- Gums that bleed easily when the teeth are brushed.

If gingivitis is not treated, the gums become inflamed and the fibres connecting the gum to the teeth are destroyed (*see* **Periodontitis**, right). This can leave a pocket between the gum and teeth in which more plaque and calculus accumulate, leading to further destruction. The inflammatory process can also destroy the bone supporting the teeth. The gums may recede and leave part of the tooth roots exposed. Eventually, one or more teeth may become loose and fall out.

Symptoms of ANUG usually develop over 1–2 days and may include:
- Bright red gums that are covered with a greyish deposit.
- Crater-like ulcers on the gums.
- Gums that bleed easily.
- Bad breath and a metallic taste in the mouth.
- Pain in the gums.

As ANUG progresses, the lymph glands in the neck may become enlarged, and a fever may develop.

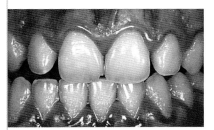

Gingivitis
In gingivitis, the gums become inflamed and soft due to a build-up of plaque on the teeth. The gums also bleed easily.

What is the treatment?
If you have gingivitis, your dentist will probably scale your teeth to remove the plaque and calculus (hardened plaque). The teeth are then polished. Regular follow-up visits may be needed to monitor the condition of your gums. Your dentist may also recommend that you use an antiseptic mouthwash to help prevent plaque from building up.

If you have ANUG, your dentist will clean carefully around all the teeth. He or she will also prescribe antibiotics (p.572) and an antiseptic mouthwash. Painkillers (p.589) may be prescribed. Once your teeth have been thoroughly scaled and cleaned, your gums should gradually return to normal.

You can prevent gingivitis by adopting good oral hygiene (*see* **Caring for your teeth and gums**, p.384).

Periodontitis

Inflammation of the tissues that support the teeth with loss of attachment between the teeth and gums

 More common over the age of 55

 In rare cases, the cause is inherited

 Poor oral hygiene and smoking are risk factors

 Gender is not a significant factor

Periodontitis affects many people over the age of 55 and is a major cause of tooth loss. In this condition, the gums become inflamed and the fibres that connect the gums to the teeth (the periodontal tissues) are destroyed. The teeth may become loose and may eventually fall out. The damage from periodontitis is irreversible, but further inflammation can be prevented with treatment and by improving oral hygiene (*see* **Caring for your teeth and gums**, p.384). There is evidence that if periodontal disease is left untreated, it may predispose to cardiovascular disease.

What are the causes?
The most common form of periodontitis is chronic adult periodontitis. This condition often develops as a complication of gingivitis (left), in which the gums are inflamed, usually due to poor oral hygiene and/or smoking. Periodontitis is also associated with certain disorders, such as diabetes mellitus (p.437). If toothbrushing is neglected, plaque (a deposit of food particles, saliva, and bacteria) and calculus (hardened plaque) build up on the teeth. As a result of this build-up, the gums become inflamed. The periodontal tissues also become inflamed and are gradually destroyed. This leaves pockets between the gums and teeth in which more plaque and calculus collect, which leads to further inflammation and tissue destruction. The inflammatory process can also result in the loss of bone supporting the teeth, and teeth may fall out.

Periapical periodontitis is another form of periodontitis and is caused by tooth decay (*see* **Dental caries**, p.384), usually due to poor oral hygiene. If tooth decay is left untreated, the hard enamel that covers the tooth and the dentine underneath will eventually be destroyed, allowing bacteria into the pulp (central part) of the tooth (*see* **Pulpitis**, p.385).

Some rare genetic forms of the disorder, such as juvenile periodontitis, occur in children or young adults and are particularly severe.

What are the symptoms?
In the early stages of periodontitis, there may be no symptoms. Symptoms of chronic periodontitis may include:
- Red, soft, shiny gums that bleed easily and may recede.
- Bad breath and an unpleasant taste.
- Toothache when hot, cold, or sweet foods or drinks are consumed.

In the late stages of chronic periodontitis, there may be loosening of the teeth.

The symptoms of periapical periodontitis may include:
- Toothache in a specific area, especially when biting.
- Loosening of a tooth.
- Swelling of the jaw.

In some cases, a dental abscess (p.385) forms. If any of these symptoms occur, consult your dentist promptly.

What might be done?
Your dentist will examine your teeth and gums and check the depth of the pockets between them using a special probe. He or she may also take dental X-rays

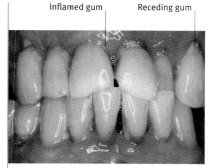

Inflamed gum   Receding gum

Periodontitis
*The gums and tissues securing the teeth
have become inflamed, and the gums have
receded, leaving the teeth unsupported.
The condition is known as periodontitis.*

(*see* **Dental checkup**, p.383) to check how
much of the bony support around the
teeth has been lost.

Chronic periodontitis is treated by removing plaque and calculus from the teeth in a
procedure known as scaling. In some cases,
a gingivectomy (surgical trimming of the
gums) may also be performed to reduce the
size of the pockets between the gums and
teeth. The diseased lining of the pockets
may be removed to allow healthy tissue to
attach itself to the teeth.

After surgery, you will probably be prescribed an antiseptic mouthwash, which you
should use regularly. If the periodontitis is
severe, your dentist may prescribe a course
of antibiotics (p.572), or an antibiotic paste
or pellet may be pushed into the deep pockets between the teeth and gums. Loose
teeth may be fixed to other teeth in order
to stabilize them.

Periapical periodontitis is treated by
removing the bacteria from the tooth and
carrying out root canal treatment (p.386).
A tooth that cannot be saved may need to
be extracted.

After treatment, your dentist will advise
that you brush and floss your teeth at least
twice a day to prevent further build-up of
plaque and calculus. If you smoke, giving up
will help to prevent further inflammation.

What is the prognosis?
If you have chronic periodontitis, better oral
hygiene and giving up smoking should help
to prevent the gums from receding further
and teeth becoming loose. It may also reduce
the risk of complications. Periapical periodontitis may need root canal treatment.
About 1 in 10 people with periodontitis has a
rapidly progressive form of the condition,
leading to loss of teeth around the age of 50.

Receding gums

*Withdrawal of the gums from
around the teeth, exposing part
of the roots*

 Usually develops after the age of 55

 Poor oral hygiene and abrasive
tooth-brushing are risk factors

 Gender and genetics are not
significant factors

Healthy gums form a tight seal around the
tooth where the crown of the tooth meets
the root. Receding of the gums is a result of
the supporting bone and gum around the
tooth being destroyed. When gum recession
is severe, there may not be enough bone
and soft tissue left to support the tooth.
Eventually, the tooth may become loose
and, in severe cases, may have to be
extracted by the dentist.

If the roots are exposed, the teeth may
be sensitive to hot, cold, or sweet substances. Since the roots are softer than the
enamel on the crown of the tooth, they are
also more susceptible to decay (*see*
Dental caries, p.384).

What are the causes?
Severely receding gums are usually a
symptom of periodontitis (p.389). This
disorder is usually a result of poor oral
hygiene, which results in a build-up of
plaque (a deposit of food particles, saliva,
and bacteria) and calculus (hardened
plaque) between the base of the teeth and
the gums.

The gums will eventually become
inflamed and recede, exposing the roots of
the teeth. Vigorous, abrasive toothbrushing
along the margins of the gums, particularly
in a horizontal direction with a hard toothbrush, may also cause the gums to recede.

What might be done?
If you have receding gums, improving your
oral hygiene (*see* **Caring for your teeth
and gums**, p.384) and giving up smoking
should prevent any further recession of
the gums.

Your dentist will probably use a procedure known as scaling to remove the
plaque and calculus from your teeth.
Scaling should help to prevent your gums
from receding further. He or she will also
advise you on your toothbrushing and
flossing techniques to avoid further

damage to the exposed roots. Your dentist
may suggest that you use a desensitizing
toothpaste or fluoride mouthwash, which
will also reduce the risk of decay. If your
teeth are very sensitive, the dentist may
treat them with a desensitizing varnish or
an adhesive filling material. Very rarely,
grafting procedures, which help to cover the
exposed surfaces of roots, are used. If
severely receding gums cause any teeth to
become loose, these loose teeth can sometimes be fixed to teeth that are more firmly
anchored in the jawbone.

Gingival hyperplasia

*Enlargement and swelling of the
gums due to various causes*

 Poor oral hygiene is a risk factor

 Age, gender, and genetics are not
significant factors

The gums most commonly enlarge and
swell, a condition known as gingival
hyperplasia, as a result of the gum disease
gingivitis (p.389). This condition is usually
the result of poor oral hygiene, which
allows plaque (a deposit of food particles,
saliva, and bacteria) and calculus (hardened plaque) to build up where the gums
meet the teeth. The gums become
inflamed and bleed easily, especially when
the teeth are brushed.

Gingival hyperplasia can also occur as
a side effect of certain drugs, such as
antihypertensives (p.580), anticonvulsants
(p.590), and some immunosuppressants
(p.585). The condition may occur during
pregnancy due to certain hormonal
changes. Less common causes of gingival
hyperplasia include acute leukaemia
(p.276) and scurvy, in which there is a
deficiency of vitamin C.

To treat gingival hyperplasia, your
dentist will probably scale your teeth
to remove the plaque and advise you
to brush and floss regularly (*see* **Caring
for your teeth and gums**, p.384). In
some cases, excess gum tissue may
be removed. If gingival hyperplasia is due
to drugs, alternatives will be given.
An underlying disorder, such as acute
leukaemia, will be treated if possible,
and the condition of your gums should
then improve. Gingival hyperplasia due to
pregnancy should clear up after the birth
as hormone levels return to normal.

Dry socket

*Inflammation of a tooth socket
that will not heal after extraction
of the tooth*

 Smoking and taking oral contraceptives
are risk factors

 Age, gender, and genetics are not
significant factors

After a tooth is extracted, the tooth socket
fills with blood. The blood clots and provides the framework for healing the
socket. If the clot is washed away for
some reason, such as by overvigorous
rinsing, or if the clot becomes infected,
the bony lining of the socket can become
inflamed, a condition that is known as "dry
socket" or post-extraction alveolitis. Dry
socket occurs after about 1 in 25 tooth
extractions and is more common following
a difficult extraction of a molar tooth from
the lower jaw. The condition occurs more
frequently in people who smoke and in
women taking oral contraceptives.

The symptoms of dry socket may include
a severe, throbbing pain that commonly
radiates to the ear 2–4 days after extraction of the tooth, a bad taste in the
mouth, and bad breath. The tooth socket
may only partly heal, and occasionally
small pieces of bone may come out of the
tooth socket.

What might be done?
Your dentist may prescribe antibiotics
(p.572) after extracting a tooth to help to
prevent the tooth socket from becoming
infected. If after a few days the socket is
not healing or you are still feeling pain,
make an appointment to see your dentist
as soon as possible. While waiting for an
appointment, you can relieve symptoms
with over-the-counter painkillers (p.589),
such as paracetamol.

To treat dry socket, your dentist
may initially wash out the tooth socket
with warm salt water or a dilute antiseptic
solution. He or she will then pack the
socket with antiseptic paste. This treatment is repeated every 2–3 days until
the tooth socket begins to heal. Your
dentist may also suggest that you use
hot saltwater mouthwashes at home to
help to reduce the inflammation. The
socket should start to heal within a few
days, and healing should be complete
within a few weeks.

Digestive system

The digestive system breaks down food into simple components that the body's cells can absorb and eliminates remaining waste. Food is propelled by muscular contractions through the digestive tract, the long tube that runs from the mouth to the anus. Digestion begins in the mouth, where saliva moistens and dissolves the food and the chewing action of the teeth and tongue breaks up large particles. The process of digestion is completed when nutrients (the useful parts of food) have been absorbed into the bloodstream and waste has passed out of the anus. The body uses nutrients for energy, growth, and tissue repair.

THE DIGESTIVE SYSTEM consists of a long, convoluted, muscular tube or tract, which extends from the mouth to the anus, and a number of other digestive organs. These associated organs include the salivary glands, liver, and pancreas. The digestive tract is made up of a series of hollow organs, which includes the stomach and the small and large intestines.

The functions of the digestive system are to ingest food, break it down, extract the useful components, or nutrients, and dispose of the remaining waste as faeces. Food can take many hours to pass through the tract. However, the oesophagus and stomach enable us to swallow a large amount of food quickly and digest it at leisure. In an average person's lifetime, the digestive system processes 30,000 kg (66,000 lb) of food. The digestive system can process a variety of diets, from a typical meat-based Western diet to a Japanese diet consisting mainly of rice and fish.

Food breakdown

Most food molecules are too large to pass through cell membranes and must be broken down before they can be absorbed. Organs of the digestive system secrete juices containing enzymes (proteins that speed up chemical reactions) and acids that help

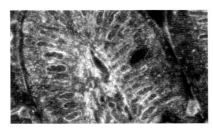

Villus
A villus is one of many, tiny, finger-like projections lining the small intestine.

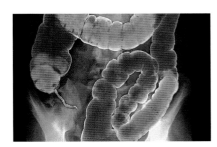

Colon
The colon, a looped tube about 1.3 m (4 ft) long, is the main component of the large intestine.

to convert large molecules into small, absorbable units. Chewing physically breaks down food into small particles, exposing a large surface area to the action of enzymes. In the stomach, food is churned with digestive juices to make chyme, a semi-liquid mixture.

Absorption

By the time food reaches the end of the small intestine, most large nutrient molecules have been broken down into smaller molecules. These are absorbed into the blood through tiny pores in the villi, the fronds that project from the intestinal wall. The blood carries nutrients to the liver, then to the body's cells. Indigestible matter passes into the large intestine, where some water is absorbed before the remainder is expelled from the anus as faeces.

Regulating digestion

The nervous and hormonal systems work together to ensure that digestive juices are secreted at the right time in different parts of the digestive tract. For example, when food enters the stomach or intestines, local glands release hormones that activate the production of digestive juices. These systems also control the action of the muscular walls of the digestive tract.

✚ PROCESS

Hunger and appetite

How much and how often we eat is determined by both hunger and appetite. When the body needs food or at times of day when it expects a routine meal, the nervous and hormonal systems cause the stomach to contract, resulting in hunger pangs. Appetite is a pleasurable sensation caused by the production of digestive juices in the mouth and stomach.

Stimulating hunger and appetite
Hunger is stimulated by the body's need for food or by the routine of meal times. The anticipation of food stimulates the appetite. Both sensations trigger a desire to eat.

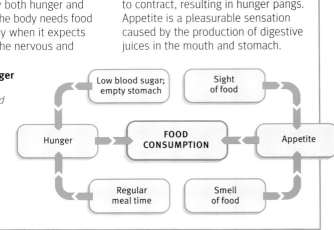

✚ **STRUCTURE AND FUNCTION**

The digestive system

The digestive system consists of the digestive tract and its associated organs. The digestive tract is a tube about 7 m (24 ft) long through which food passes while it is broken down. The tract consists of the mouth and pharynx (throat), oesophagus, stomach, the small and large intestines, and the anus. The associated digestive organs include three pairs of salivary glands, the liver, the pancreas, and the gallbladder.

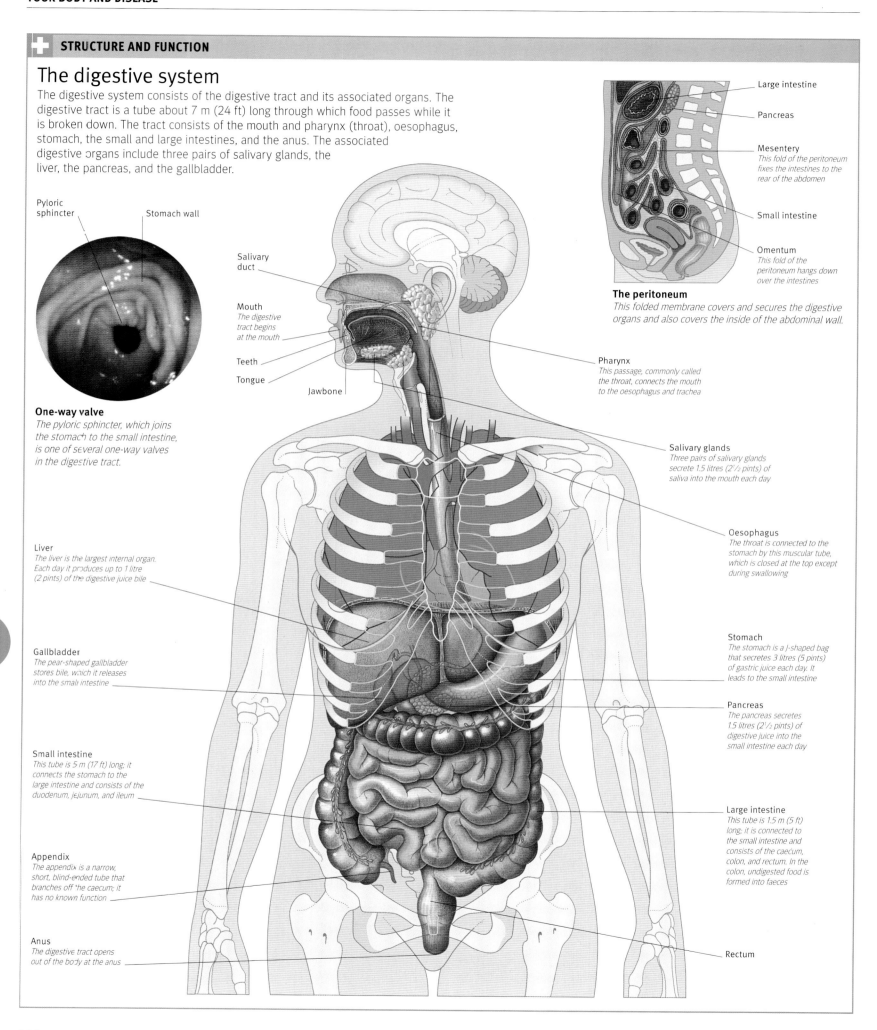

Pyloric sphincter

Stomach wall

One-way valve
The pyloric sphincter, which joins the stomach to the small intestine, is one of several one-way valves in the digestive tract.

Salivary duct

Mouth
The digestive tract begins at the mouth

Teeth

Tongue

Jawbone

Large intestine

Pancreas

Mesentery
This fold of the peritoneum fixes the intestines to the rear of the abdomen

Small intestine

Omentum
This fold of the peritoneum hangs down over the intestines

The peritoneum
This folded membrane covers and secures the digestive organs and also covers the inside of the abdominal wall.

Pharynx
This passage, commonly called the throat, connects the mouth to the oesophagus and trachea

Salivary glands
Three pairs of salivary glands secrete 1.5 litres (2½ pints) of saliva into the mouth each day

Liver
The liver is the largest internal organ. Each day it produces up to 1 litre (2 pints) of the digestive juice bile

Oesophagus
The throat is connected to the stomach by this muscular tube, which is closed at the top except during swallowing

Gallbladder
The pear-shaped gallbladder stores bile, which it releases into the small intestine

Stomach
The stomach is a J-shaped bag that secretes 3 litres (5 pints) of gastric juice each day. It leads to the small intestine

Pancreas
The pancreas secretes 1.5 litres (2½ pints) of digestive juice into the small intestine each day

Small intestine
This tube is 5 m (17 ft) long; it connects the stomach to the large intestine and consists of the duodenum, jejunum, and ileum

Appendix
The appendix is a narrow, short, blind-ended tube that branches off the caecum; it has no known function

Large intestine
This tube is 1.5 m (5 ft) long; it is connected to the small intestine and consists of the caecum, colon, and rectum. In the colon, undigested food is formed into faeces

Anus
The digestive tract opens out of the body at the anus

Rectum

+ STRUCTURE AND FUNCTION

The digestive tract

The digestive tract is a series of hollow organs – the mouth, oesophagus, stomach, small and large intestines, and anus – connected to form a long tube. The tract has muscular walls that rhythmically propel food along the tube (*see* **Peristalsis**, p.394), breaking it down and mixing it with digestive juices. Muscular activity is controlled by a network of nerves that covers the tract. Several muscular valves control the passage of food and prevent it from moving backwards.

Mouth

The tongue, teeth, and saliva work together to start digestion and aid swallowing. Teeth chop and grind food, increasing the surface area over which digestive enzymes in saliva can act. Saliva also softens food so that the tongue can mould it into a bolus, or ball, for swallowing.

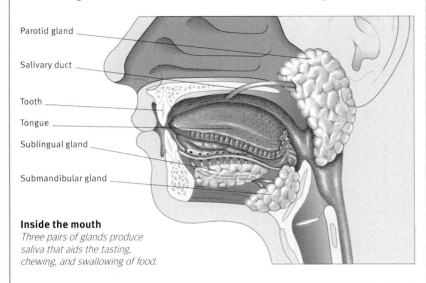

Parotid gland
Salivary duct
Tooth
Tongue
Sublingual gland
Submandibular gland

Inside the mouth
Three pairs of glands produce saliva that aids the tasting, chewing, and swallowing of food.

+ FUNCTION

Swallowing

Swallowing begins when you push a bolus (ball of food) towards the oesophagus with your tongue. This action triggers two involuntary events: the soft palate, the back of the roof of the mouth, closes off the nasal cavity, and the epiglottis, a flap of cartilage, tilts downwards to seal the trachea (windpipe).

1 *In their normal positions, the soft palate and the epiglottis allow air to pass from the nasal cavity into the trachea.*

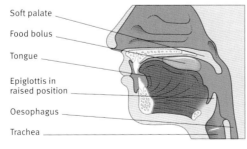

Soft palate
Food bolus
Tongue
Epiglottis in raised position
Oesophagus
Trachea

2 *While swallowing, the epiglottis tilts to seal the trachea, the soft palate lifts to close off the nasal cavity, and the bolus enters the oesophagus.*

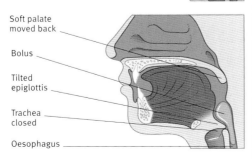

Soft palate moved back
Bolus
Tilted epiglottis
Trachea closed
Oesophagus

Oesophagus and stomach

The throat leads into the oesophagus, a muscular tube that propels food to the stomach. In the stomach, solid food spends up to 5 hours being churned to a pulp and mixed with gastric juice to form chyme before being squirted into the small intestine. Liquids pass from the mouth to the intestine in a matter of minutes.

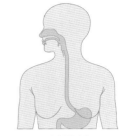

LOCATION

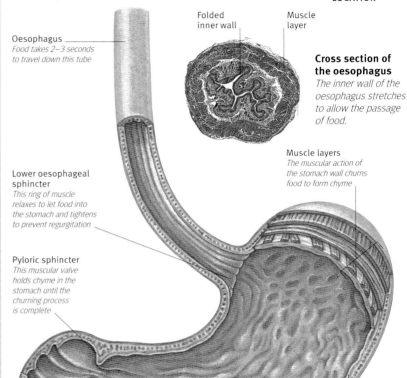

Oesophagus
Food takes 2–3 seconds to travel down this tube

Folded inner wall

Muscle layer

Cross section of the oesophagus
The inner wall of the oesophagus stretches to allow the passage of food.

Lower oesophageal sphincter
This ring of muscle relaxes to let food into the stomach and tightens to prevent regurgitation

Pyloric sphincter
This muscular valve holds chyme in the stomach until the churning process is complete

Muscle layers
The muscular action of the stomach wall churns food to form chyme

Mucosa

Submucosa

Duodenum

Rugae
An empty stomach is folded into creases, or rugae, that allow it to expand

Section of the stomach lining
The stomach is lined by mucosa, which secretes mucus to prevent the stomach from digesting itself.

Gastric pit
The bases of these pits contain gastric glands

Mucus-producing cell (goblet cell)

Gastric gland
Within each ruga, there are many gastric glands, which secrete acid and enzymes that make up gastric juice

Enzyme-producing cell

Acid-producing cell

✚ **STRUCTURE AND FUNCTION**

The digestive tract (continued)
Small and large intestines

At about 6.5 m (22 ft) in length, the intestines form the longest part
of the digestive tract. In the small intestine, which consists of the
duodenum, jejunum, and ileum, food mixes with digestive juices,
and nutrients and water are absorbed into the blood. In the large
intestine, which is divided into the caecum, colon, and rectum,
faeces are formed before passing out of the anus.

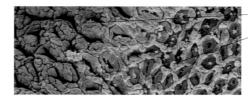

Lining of small intestine

Lining of large intestine

Intestinal junction
*The small intestine has a folded lining
to absorb nutrients; the lining of the
large intestine is flatter.*

Duodenum
*This tube mixes chyme with fluids
from the gallbladder and pancreas*

Colon
*The colonic walls absorb water from
faeces, and bacteria reduce the bulk
of the fibre that the faeces contain;
these processes can take up to 2 days*

Caecum
*This short pouch has a valve that
opens to receive chyme from the ileum*

Appendix

Jejunum
*The duodenum empties into this long
tube, which adds its own digestive juices*

Ileum
*The last part of the small intestine
has a rich supply of blood and lymph
to absorb nutrients*

Mucosa
*Absorption occurs in
tiny projections (villi)
lining this layer*

Submucosa
*This layer contains
nerves, blood vessels,
and lymph vessels*

Mesentery

Serosa
*The serosa is a thin
outer protective
membrane*

**Muscle
layers**

Muscle layers
*Faeces are mixed
up and propelled
by this layer of
muscle*

Mesentery
*Blood vessels and
nerves reach the
intestine through
this membrane*

Serosa

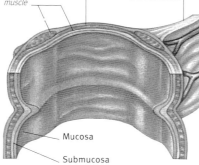

Mucosa

Submucosa

Cross section of the large intestine
*The large intestine wall is wider than the small
intestine and its inner layer lacks the finger-like
villi that project into the small intestine.*

Rectum
*When faeces enter the rectum, they
trigger an urge to defecate; the
urge can be overridden voluntarily*

Anus
*Faeces exit the digestive
tract through the anus; a ring
of muscle controls this action*

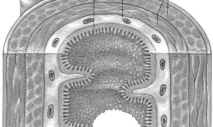

CROSS SECTION OF SMALL INTESTINE

✚ **FUNCTION**

Peristalsis

Food is propelled along the
digestive tract by a sequence
of muscular contractions called
peristalsis. The muscular wall
behind a piece of food squeezes
to push it forwards into the next
part of the tract, where the
muscle is relaxed. Other types
of muscular action churn food in
the stomach and form faeces
in the colon.

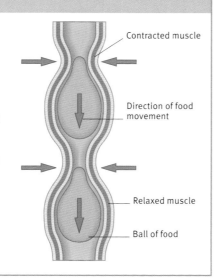

Contracted muscle

Direction of food
movement

Relaxed muscle

Ball of food

The peristaltic wave
*The muscular action of the digestive
tract moves food continuously in an
action known as a "peristaltic wave".*

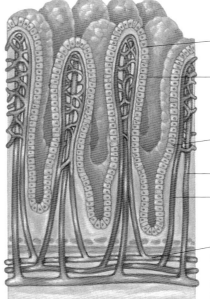

Enzyme-producing cell
*These cells line the villi
of the jejunum*

Villus
*Each villus is covered in hundreds
of projections called microvilli*

Mucus-producing cell

Lymph vessel
*These vessels transport the
products of fat digestion*

Artery

Vein
*Absorbed nutrients are
carried away by this vessel*

Villi of the small intestine
*The mucosa, the inner layer of the small
intestine, has millions of finger-like fronds
called villi covered in smaller fronds called
microvilli. These fronds provide a surface area
the size of a tennis court for nutrient absorption.*

**CROSS SECTION OF THE SMALL
INTESTINE LINING**

Liver, gallbladder, and pancreas

The liver, gallbladder, and pancreas all take part in the process of digestion by secreting digestive juices that break down food molecules. The liver produces a greenish digestive juice called bile, which is stored in the sac-like gallbladder. The pancreas produces a powerful digestive fluid known as pancreatic juice. When food enters the duodenum from the stomach, the duodenal lining releases hormones that stimulate the gallbladder and pancreas to release their juices.

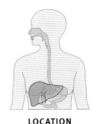

LOCATION

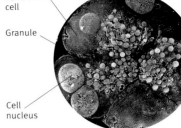

Pancreatic cell

Granule

Cell nucleus

Pancreatic enzymes
This magnified view shows granules that contain enzymes in pancreatic cells.

Wall of gallbladder
The heavily folded inner wall of the gallbladder can be seen in this highly magnified image.

Liver
The liver manufactures, stores, and breaks down substances as required by the body

Inferior vena cava
Blood that has been processed by the liver is carried to the heart by this vein

Hepatic veins
These veins drain blood from the liver

Oesophagus

Stomach

Gallbladder
This sac concentrates and stores bile, a digestive fluid made by the liver from waste products of the blood

Pancreas
The pancreas secretes enzymes and mucus that neutralize stomach acid

Central vein

Lobule

Pancreatic duct
This duct carries pancreatic juice into the duodenum

Hepatic artery
This artery carries oxygenated blood from the heart to the liver

Cross section of liver lobules
The liver consists of thousands of lobules, tiny blood-processing units each 1 mm (¹/₂₅ in) wide.

Cystic duct
This carries bile from the gallbladder to the common bile duct

Duodenum
When food enters this tube, the pancreas and gallbladder release digestive juices

Common bile duct
This carries bile from the liver and gallbladder to the duodenum

Portal vein
This vein carries nutrient-rich blood from the small intestine to the liver

Liver function

The liver is the body's chemical factory, converting molecules into simpler or more complex forms as the body requires. For example, nutrients are modified in the liver, then stored there or distributed throughout the body; toxins such as alcohol are broken down into less harmful substances. The liver also produces the digestive juice bile.

Lobule
Each lobule contains specialized cells that perform all of the liver's chemical functions

Central vein
Deoxygenated and processed blood from the lobule collects in this vein before returning to the heart

Branch of portal vein
Nutrient-filled blood from the small intestine enters each lobule through six small veins

Sinusoids
Blood is processed by hepatocytes as it passes along these channels to the centre of the lobule

Inside a liver lobule
Branches of the portal vein, hepatic artery, and bile duct surround each lobule. A central vein carries blood to the heart.

Branch of hepatic artery
Oxygenated blood from the heart reaches each lobule through six small arteries

Branch of bile duct
Bile made by liver cells flows into tiny channels that converge to form the common bile duct

✚ **PROCESS**

Chemical breakdown

Food consists mainly of water and the three main types of nutrients – protein, carbohydrate, and fat – that the body needs to survive. Before these nutrients can be used, their large molecules must be broken down in the digestive system into units small enough for the body to absorb. Absorption occurs in the small intestine (the duodenum, jejunum, and ileum) and the colon. Vitamins and minerals, which are also essential nutrients, consist of molecules tiny enough for the body to absorb without breaking them down first.

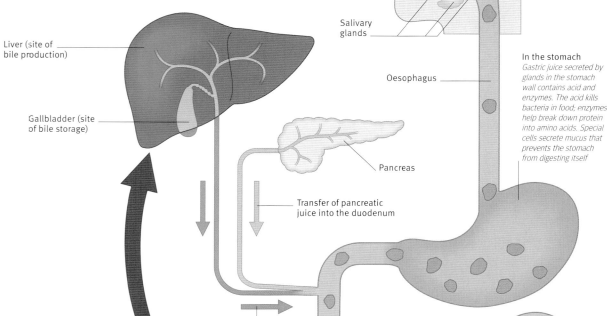

Liver (site of bile production)

Gallbladder (site of bile storage)

Salivary glands

Oesophagus

Pancreas

In the mouth
Enzymes in saliva begin to break down starch, a type of carbohydrate, into simple sugars

In the stomach
Gastric juice secreted by glands in the stomach wall contains acid and enzymes. The acid kills bacteria in food; enzymes help break down protein into amino acids. Special cells secrete mucus that prevents the stomach from digesting itself

Transfer of pancreatic juice into the duodenum

Transfer of bile into the duodenum

Nutrient transfer to liver
Absorbed nutrients flow in the bloodstream to the liver, where they are processed and either stored or distributed to other parts of the body. Some fats pass along lymph vessels before entering the bloodstream

In the duodenum
Bile breaks down fat particles into smaller droplets; pancreatic juice contains enzymes that convert fats into fatty acids and glycerol and sodium bicarbonate to neutralize stomach acid

In the jejunum
Pancreatic enzymes and enzymes produced by the jejunum wall complete the breakdown of carbohydrate, protein, and fat

In the ileum
The main function of the ileum is to absorb nutrients; bile is also absorbed here and returned to the liver through blood vessels

In the colon
The absorption of water from waste matter to form faeces, which consist mainly of fibre, is completed in the colon. Bacteria in the colon produce some vitamins that are then absorbed

In the rectum
Faeces formed in the colon collect in the rectum before being excreted

Anus

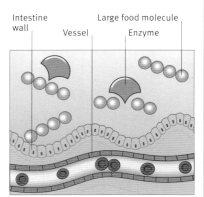

Indigestible fibre
This magnified view shows cells of fibre, an indigestible plant material that is a vital part of the diet. Fibre adds bulk to faeces and helps them to retain some water, making them easier to expel.

Digestive enzymes

Food molecules are too large to pass through the walls of the digestive tract into the blood and lymph vessels and must be broken down into smaller molecules. Digestive enzymes help to break down proteins into amino acids, fats into fatty acids and glycerol, and starch (a complex carbohydrate) into simple sugars.

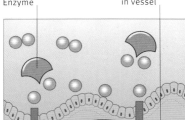

Intestine wall   **Large food molecule**
Vessel   **Enzyme**

1 *A particular enzyme combines with a large food molecule, such as a protein. The enzyme breaks down the large molecule into two or more smaller molecules.*

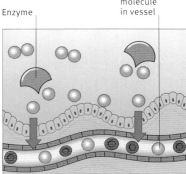

Enzyme   **Tiny food molecule in vessel**

2 *The tiny molecules separate from the enzyme and are able to pass through the wall of the digestive tract into the bloodstream. The enzyme molecule remains unchanged.*

General digestive and nutritional problems

Most common digestive problems cause short-term symptoms, such as indigestion, diarrhoea, and constipation. However, long-term symptoms affecting the digestive system may reflect a more serious underlying disorder.

The first part of this section looks at indigestion, the upper abdominal discomfort that most people feel at some time. Occasionally, as is described in the seconc article, discomfort may be more vague and persist without an identifiable cause, in which case it is known as nonulcer dyspepsia.

The next articles cover diarrhoea and constipation. These problems often clear up on their own. If they persist, you should seek medical advice because there may be an underlying disorder that needs treatment. Diarrhoea may be a result of gastroenterit s or food poisoning; both of these conditions can be potentially serious in elderly people and young children.

Bleeding from the digestive tract can indicate a serious disorder and is discussed n the next article. Now, most cases of digestive tract bleeding can be diagnosed and treated without the need for surgery.

The final articles look at nutritional deficiencies, which are rare in the UK, and obesity, which affects about a quarter of the UK's adult population.

KEY ANATOMY

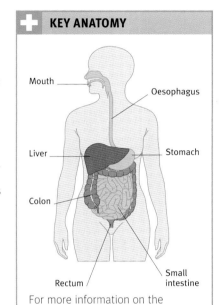

Mouth
Oesophagus
Liver
Stomach
Colon
Small intestine
Rectum

For more information on the structure and function of the digestive system, *see* pp.391–396.

Indigestion

Pain or discomfort in the upper abdomen, usually after eating, that may have a variety of causes

 More common in adults

 Stress, being overweight, smoking, and certain dietary habits are risk factors

 Gender and genetics are not significant factors

Most people have had a few episodes of upper abdominal discomfort related to eating, usually called indigestion. The condition is more common in adults. Smoking and being overweight increase the risk. Most cases are not serious.

Usually, indigestion follows a meal, especially one that includes rich, fatty, or heavily spiced food. Overeating, consuming too much alcohol or coffee, and eating too quickly can also cause discomfort, as can stress and drugs such as aspirin that irritate the digestive tract. If indigestion persists or becomes more severe, or if you start to vomit, lose your appetite, or lose weight, you should consult your doctor. These symptoms may be a sign of conditions such as gastro-oesophageal reflux disease (p.403), a peptic ulcer (p.406), or, in rare cases, stomach cancer (p.406).

Antacids (p.596) can usually relieve mild indigestion. There are also some self-help measures to avoid future attacks (*see* **Preventing indigestion**, above right).

Nonulcer dyspepsia

Pain or discomfort in the upper abdomen that is not associated with a structural abnormality

 More common in adults

 More common in males

 Stress, being overweight, smoking, and certain dietary habits are risk factors

 Genetics is not a significant factor

Nonulcer dyspepsia describes recurrent and persistent indigestion (left) that occurs without an identifiable anatomical cause or abnormality of the digestive tract. The condition is more common in adults, especially men, and may be made worse by stress, being overweight, smoking, and a diet high in rich, fatty foods.

The symptoms may include pain in the upper abdomen, often made worse by eating, and nausea, particularly in the morning. People who have nonulcer dyspepsia often

Preventing indigestion

To prevent or reduce the frequency of indigestion try the following:

- Eat small portions of food at regular intervals without rushing or overfilling your stomach.
- Avoid eating in the 3 hours before going to bed.
- Reduce or eliminate your intake of alcohol, coffee, and tea.
- Avoid rich, fatty foods.
- Keep a food diary to help identify foods that cause indigestion.
- Learn to overcome stress, which can often trigger episodes of indigestion (*see* **Relaxation exercises**, p.32).
- Try to lose excess weight and avoid tight-fitting clothing.
- If possible, avoid medicines that irritate the digestive tract, such as aspirin and other nonsteroidal anti-inflammatory drugs (p.578).

experience these symptoms several times a week. If you have such persistent symptoms, you should consult your doctor because they could be a sign of a more serious underlying disorder, such as a peptic ulcer (p.406) or, rarely, stomach cancer (p.406).

What might be done?

Your doctor will probably arrange for tests to exclude other disorders. For example, a faecal test may be carried out to check for infection of the stomach lining with the bacterium *H. pylori* (*see* **Helicobacter pylori infection**, p.405). In addition, upper digestive tract endoscopy (p.407) may be carried out to look for abnormalities in the digestive tract, and an ultrasound scan (p.135) may be done to check for gallstones (p.412). If no underlying disorder is found, you will be diagnosed with nonulcer dyspepsia.

There are measures that you can try to reduce the frequency or severity of symptoms (*see* **Preventing indigestion**, above). If these measures do not resolve the problem, your doctor may prescribe a drug to neutralize or reduce stomach acid production (*see* **Antacids**, p.596, and **Ulcer-healing drugs**, p.596). You may also be given drugs that help the stomach to empty more effectively (*see* **Antispasmodic drugs and motility stimulants**, p.598).

Diarrhoea

The passage of loose or watery stools and/or an increase in the frequency of bowel movements

 Poor food hygiene is a risk factor

 Age, gender, and genetics are not significant factors

Diarrhoea is the production of stools that are more watery, more frequent, or greater in volume than is normal for a particular

individual. Although it is not a disease in itself, diarrhoea may be a symptom of an underlying disorder.

In some cases, diarrhoea is accompanied by abdominal pain, bloating, loss of appetite, and vomiting. Severe diarrhoea can also lead to dehydration that may be life-threatening, particularly in babies (*see* **Vomiting and diarrhoea**, p.559) and elderly people.

Short bouts of diarrhoea, especially if they are associated with vomiting, are often due to gastroenteritis (p.398) or food poisoning (p.398). Diarrhoea that lasts more than 3–4 weeks usually indicates that there is an intestinal disorder and requires medical attention.

What are the causes?

Diarrhoea that starts abruptly in a person who is otherwise healthy is often caused by contaminated food or water and may last a few hours to 10 days. This sort of diarrhoea often occurs during travel in a developing country, where food hygiene and sanitation may be poor. Diarrhoea can also be caused by a viral infection that is spread by close personal contact. For example, infectious gastroenteritis is a common cause of diarrhoea in babies and young children.

People with reduced immunity, such as those with AIDS (*see* **HIV infection and AIDS**, p.169), are more susceptible to infectious gastroenteritis, which also tends to be more severe in these people. People taking drugs such as antibiotics (p.572) may develop sudden diarrhoea if the drugs disturb the normal balance of bacteria in the colon.

Persistent diarrhoea may result from long-standing inflammation of the intestine due to disorders such as ulcerative colitis (p.417) or Crohn's disease (p.417) or some conditions in which the small intestine is unable to absorb nutrients (*see* **Malabsorption**, p.415).

Preventing dehydration

For normal body functioning, the body's water and salt content must be kept at a constant level. During an attack of diarrhoea or vomiting, the body can become dehydrated due to loss of large amounts of fluids and salts. Babies, children, and elderly people are particularly vulnerable to dehydration, which can be reversed or prevented by following these simple measures:

- Drink plenty of fluids every 1–2 hours, while symptoms last. Choose fluids such as dilute orange juice, weak sweet tea, or rehydration solution, which is available over the counter as a powder that you reconstitute.
- Do not give children milk because it may perpetuate the diarrhoea. However, if a breast-feeding baby is affected, continue to breast-feed and give the baby additional fluids.
- Stay out of the sun and try to keep yourself cool in order to prevent further loss of body fluids in sweat.

Lactose intolerance (p.416), a disorder in which lactose (a natural sugar present in milk) cannot be broken down and absorbed, can also cause diarrhoea.

Infections with protozoal parasites, such as giardiasis (p.176) and amoebiasis (p.176), can cause persistent diarrhoea. Irritable bowel syndrome (p.415) may produce abnormal contractions of the intestine, which result in alternating episodes of diarrhoea and constipation.

What might be done?

In most cases, diarrhoea clears up after a day or two. Other symptoms that can accompany diarrhoea, such as headache, weakness, and lethargy, are most often caused by dehydration. The symptoms of dehydration disappear as soon as lost fluids and salts are replaced (see **Preventing dehydration**, p.397).

If your diarrhoea lasts longer than 3–4 days, you should consult your doctor, who may request a sample of faeces to look for evidence of infection. If the diarrhoea persists for more than 3–4 weeks or if there is blood in the faeces, your doctor will probably arrange for you to have investigations, such as blood tests, sigmoidoscopy, or colonoscopy (p.418).

Specific treatments given for diarrhoea depend on the underlying cause. If you need to relieve your diarrhoea quickly, your doctor may prescribe an antidiarrhoeal drug (p.597), such as loperamide. However, antidiarrhoeal drugs should be avoided if your diarrhoea is due to an infection because they may prolong the infection. Antibiotics are only needed to treat persistent diarrhoea that has a known bacterial cause.

Constipation

Difficult and infrequent passage of small, hard stools

 Most common in children and elderly people

 More common in females

 A low-fibre diet is a risk factor

 Genetics as a risk factor depends on the cause

If your stools are small and hard or if you have to strain to pass them, you are probably constipated. How frequently you pass stools is less important because healthy people have bowel movements at widely differing intervals. Usual intervals range from three times a day to three times a week. Most people tend to have a regular routine, and bowels usually function best if they are allowed to follow a consistent pattern.

Bouts of constipation are common and usually harmless, but occasionally they may indicate an underlying disorder. You should consult your doctor if you have recently developed constipation that is

Preventing constipation

There are some simple steps you can take to prevent or reduce the severity of constipation:

■ Increase your daily fibre intake. Fibre-rich foods include bran, wholemeal bread, cereals and wholegrains, fruit, leafy vegetables, beans, and dried peas.

■ Reduce your intake of highly refined and processed foods, such as cheese and white bread.

■ Increase your daily fluid intake, but avoid drinks containing caffeine or alcohol.

■ Do not use stimulant laxatives (p.597) persistently because the colon may eventually be unable to function without them.

■ Do not ignore the urge to defecate. The longer that faeces remain in the colon, the drier and harder they become.

■ Try to achieve a regular routine in which you go to the toilet at the same time of day.

severe or lasts more than 2 weeks, particularly if it first occurs after the age of 45 or if blood is present in the faeces. Persistent constipation may lead to faecal impaction, in which hard faeces remain in the rectum. Liquid faeces may leak around the partial obstruction, resulting in diarrhoea (p.397).

What are the causes?

A diet that is low in fibre and fluids is the most common cause of constipation. Drinking too much alcohol or drinks containing caffeine, which may lead to dehydration, can also make faeces hard and difficult to pass. Other factors that decrease the frequency of bowel movements are taking too little exercise and long periods of immobility. Several disorders, such as the metabolic disorder hypothyroidism (p.432) and depression (p.343), may also lead to constipation. In addition, the condition is associated with disorders of the large intestine, such as diverticular disease (p.420).

People recovering from abdominal surgery and people with anal disorders, such as haemorrhoids (p.422) or an anal fissure (p.423), may find it painful to defecate and then develop constipation. Certain drugs, including some antidepressants (p.592) and antacids (p.596) containing aluminium and calcium carbonate, may cause constipation.

Poor toilet training in infants (see **Constipation in children**, p.560) and increasing immobility in elderly people make constipation much more common in these age groups. For unknown reasons, it is more common in women.

What might be done?

If constipation is associated with your lifestyle, there are several measures you can take to relieve it and prevent recurrence (see **Preventing constipation**, above). If

constipation persists despite taking these self-help measures, you should consult your doctor, who will perform various tests to look for an underlying cause. He or she will probably first examine your abdomen and check your rectum by inserting a gloved finger. You may be asked to give a faecal sample, which will be examined for the presence of blood.

If a cause is not found, you may have your large intestine examined with a viewing instrument (see **Colonoscopy**, p.418) or have a CT scan (p.132) of your intestines to reveal abnormalities. If your doctor finds an underlying cause, its treatment should relieve constipation. Your doctor will prescribe an alternative drug if a particular drug is the cause of constipation.

You may have an enema, in which liquid is passed through a tube into the rectum to stimulate bowel movements. This treatment should be followed by a change in diet to include more fibre.

Constipation linked to a painful anal disorder may be relieved with a soothing ointment or suppositories.

Gastroenteritis

Inflammation of the lining of the stomach and intestines, usually due to infection

 Most common in babies and children but can occur at any age

 Poor food hygiene or unsanitary conditions are risk factors

Gender and genetics are not significant factors

Gastroenteritis usually starts suddenly, with symptoms of vomiting, diarrhoea (p.397), and fever. Outbreaks commonly occur within families and among people who are in close contact, such as schoolchildren. Most people recover from the disorder without problems, but gastroenteritis may be serious in elderly people and very young children (see **Vomiting and diarrhoea**, p.559) because there is a risk of dehydration. In developing countries, gastroenteritis is a common cause of death in these age groups.

What are the causes?

Gastroenteritis is usually due to a viral or bacterial infection that irritates the lining of the stomach and intestines. The infection may be acquired from contaminated food or water (see **Food poisoning**, right), or it may be spread among people who are in close contact, especially if hygiene is poor.

Viral gastroenteritis is often caused by rotaviruses or astroviruses, particularly in young children, and by noroviruses in older children and adults. Most people acquire immunity to these viruses by the time they are adults. Bacterial causes of gastroenteritis include salmonella, campylobacter, and *Escherichia coli*.

What are the symptoms?

The symptoms of gastroenteritis often develop rapidly over 1–2 hours and may vary in severity. They include:

■ Nausea and vomiting.
■ Cramping abdominal pain.
■ Fever, often with headache.
■ Diarrhoea.

In some people, vomiting or diarrhoea may lead to dehydration. Babies and elderly people are much more susceptible to the effects of dehydration, which are often difficult to recognize. Babies may become listless and cry feebly, and an elderly person may become confused. Consult your doctor promptly if you are not able to keep fluids down or have not passed urine for over 6 hours, especially if you have a long-term illness, such as diabetes mellitus (p.437) or kidney disease. Without appropriate treatment, dehydration may be life-threatening.

What might be done?

A mild attack of gastroenteritis usually clears up without treatment, but you should follow self-help measures and drink plenty of fluids every few hours (see **Preventing dehydration**, p.397). Over-the-counter antidiarrhoeal drugs (p.597) are useful if you need to relieve your symptoms quickly. However, these treatments are best avoided because they may prolong gastroenteritis by retaining the infective organism inside the gastrointestinal tract.

If your symptoms are severe or prolonged, you should consult your doctor. You may be asked to provide a sample of faeces, which will be tested for infection. Antibiotics (p.572) are rarely given unless a bacterial infection is identified. Severe dehydration requires emergency treatment in hospital to replace fluids and salts intravenously.

What is the prognosis?

Most people recover rapidly from gastroenteritis with no long-lasting effects. Occasionally, short-term damage to the intestine may reduce its ability to digest lactose, the natural sugar present in milk (see **Lactose intolerance**, p.416). This disorder occurs particularly in infants and often results in diarrhoea that can persist for days or weeks. In rare cases, gastroenteritis may trigger irritable bowel syndrome (p.415).

Food poisoning

Sudden illness caused by consuming food or drink contaminated by a toxin or infectious organism

 Poor food hygiene is a risk factor

 Age, gender, and genetics are not significant factors

Food poisoning is the term used to describe a sudden illness that is caused by consuming food or drink that may taste normal but is contaminated with a toxin or infectious organism.

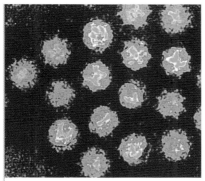

Norovirus
This magnified image shows particles of norovirus, which often contaminates shellfish and causes food poisoning.

The diagnosis of food poisoning is easily made if a group of people all develop the same symptoms, usually vomiting and diarrhoea, after they have consumed the same food or drink. The symptoms may start hours or days after consuming the food or drink.

Usually, the symptoms are confined to the gastrointestinal tract. However, some food poisoning may cause more widespread symptoms. For example, the *Clostridium botulinum* bacterium causes muscle weakness and paralysis (*see* **Botulism**, p.173), and listeriosis (p.172) may cause flu-like symptoms and lead to meningitis (p.325).

Food poisoning is very common, but it can usually be avoided by careful preparation, storage, and cooking of food (*see* **Food hygiene**, p.33).

What are the causes?
Most cases of food poisoning result from contamination of food or water by bacteria, viruses, or, less commonly, protozoal parasites. Poor food hygiene can enable microorganisms to multiply. In some cases of bacterial food poisoning, it is not the presence of the bacteria themselves that cause poisoning but the effect of toxins produced by the bacteria.

If infectious organisms are ingested with the food, they can multiply in the digestive tract. If the food poisoning is caused by bacterial toxins, they may be produced in the food before it is eaten.

Most types of food poisoning cause diarrhoea and/or vomiting, often with abdominal pain. The severity of symptoms, the speed at which they develop, and the duration of the illness depend on the cause of food poisoning.

Staphylococci bacteria A number of foods, such as poultry, eggs, pâté, and previously prepared sandwiches can be infected by staphylococci bacteria. These bacteria produce toxins that are ingested with food. The toxins usually produce diarrhoea and/or vomiting within 4 hours. In most cases, symptoms clear up within 24 hours.

Escherichia coli bacteria Certain types of *E. coli* can contaminate meat (commonly undercooked beef) and water and produce toxins of varying potency. Types of *E. coli* are usually responsible for causing traveller's

diarrhoea, which is usually mild. However, some types of *E. coli* (such as the strain called *E. coli* 0157) may cause a severe illness because they produce a potent type of toxin that can damage blood cells and lead to kidney failure (p.450).

Salmonella bacteria Up to half a million people develop the disease salmonellosis every year in the UK from eating eggs or poultry that are infected with salmonella bacteria. It typically causes symptoms such as vomiting, mild fever, and severe diarrhoea that may be bloodstained. The symptoms usually begin 12–72 hours after eating the contaminated food and last for 1–3 days.

Campylobacter bacteria These bacteria are the most common cause of food poisoning in the UK. They may contaminate meat and more rarely water or unpasteurized milk. Symptoms usually develop about 2–5 days after eating contaminated food and may include severe, watery diarrhoea. The diarrhoea may contain blood and/or mucus. In most cases, symptoms subside within 2–3 days, but bacteria may be present in faeces for up to 5 weeks after infection.

Other infections Viral infections can be contracted from contaminated food or water. Shellfish are a common source of infection, especially with noroviruses. Symptoms often start suddenly after contaminated food has been eaten, but recovery is usually rapid. Protozoal infections that may be contracted from contaminated food or water include cryptosporidiosis (p.176), amoebiasis (p.176), and giardiasis (p.176). Cryptosporidiosis may cause symptoms such as vomiting and loose, watery diarrhoea to develop about a week after contaminated substances have been consumed. Symptoms of amoebiasis may include watery, often bloody, diarrhoea persisting for several days or weeks. In giardiasis, there may be diarrhoea, bloating, and flatulence that often last more than a week.

Noninfectious causes In some cases, food poisoning may be caused by poisonous mushrooms or contamination of fruit or vegetables with high concentrations of pesticides. Symptoms may include vomiting and diarrhoea.

What might be done?
Usually, symptoms disappear without treatment. If your symptoms are mild, use self-help measures to prevent dehydration (*see* **Preventing dehydration**, p.397). If the symptoms are severe or last more than 3–4 days, consult your doctor. If an elderly person or child is affected, you should consult a doctor immediately. Keep a sample of any remaining food in addition to the faeces, which can be tested for the presence of infectious microorganisms. If the cause is noninfectious, such as poisonous mushrooms, you may need to be treated urgently to eliminate the poison from the body.

Treatment of food poisoning is usually aimed at preventing dehydration. In severe cases, fluids and salts may be administered intravenously in hospital. Antibiotics

(p.572) are given only if specific bacteria have been identified. People usually recover rapidly from a bout of food poisoning and rarely experience long-lasting consequences.

In rare cases, there is a risk of septicaemia (p.171) if bacteria spread into the bloodstream. Both dehydration and septicaemia can lead to shock (p.248), a condition that may be fatal. Infection with *E. coli* 0157 may also cause serious illness, which may occasionally be fatal.

Bleeding from the digestive tract

Loss of blood from the lining of the digestive tract, sometimes resulting in bloodstained faeces or vomit

 Age, gender, genetics, and lifestyle as risk factors depend on the cause

Bleeding can occur in any part of the digestive tract and should always be investigated because there may be a serious underlying cause. In some cases, only small amounts of blood are lost over a long period of time and go unnoticed. In other cases, severe, sudden bleeding from the digestive tract may result in blood being vomited or passed out of the anus in the faeces. You should seek medical help if you notice any bleeding.

What are the causes?
The causes of bleeding in the digestive tract include inflammation of or damage to the tract's lining and tumours.

Bleeding from the upper tract, which includes the oesophagus, stomach, and duodenum, may occur if stomach acid damages the lining. This is a common complication of gastro-oesophageal reflux disease (p.403) and peptic ulcers (p.406). Severe bleeding is sometimes due to enlargement of veins in the oesophagus, which may be a complication of chronic liver diseases (*see* **Portal hypertension and varices**, p.410).

Most cases of bleeding from the lower digestive tract, which includes the colon, rectum, and anus, are due to minor disorders, such as haemorrhoids (p.422) or anal fissure (p.423) caused by straining to defecate. However, bleeding may be a sign of colorectal cancer (p.421). Diverticular disease (p.420) and other disorders of the colon can also lead to the presence of blood in the faeces.

What are the symptoms?
The symptoms vary according to the site and severity of the bleeding. If it is mild, blood loss may go unnoticed, but it may eventually cause symptoms of iron-deficiency anaemia (p.271), such as pale skin and shortness of breath. Severe bleeding from the oesophagus, stomach, or duodenum may cause:

- Vomit containing bright red blood or resembling coffee grounds.
- Light-headedness.
- Black, tarry stools.

If there is a heavy loss of blood from the lower part of the tract, there will probably be visible blood in the stools. When there is severe blood loss from any part of the tract, shock (p.248) may develop. Shock causes symptoms that include fainting, sweating, and confusion and requires immediate hospital treatment.

What might be done?
Minor bleeding may be detected only during an investigation for anaemia or screening to detect colorectal cancer. If the bleeding is severe, you may need intravenous fluids and a blood transfusion (p.272) to replace lost blood. You will be examined to detect the location of the bleeding, usually by endoscopy through the mouth (*see* **Upper digestive tract endoscopy**, p.407) or anus (*see* **Colonoscopy**, p.418).

Treatment for bleeding depends on the underlying cause. For example, peptic ulcers are treated with antibiotics (p.572) and ulcer-healing drugs (p.596), but colorectal cancer requires surgery. It may be possible to stop the bleeding during endoscopy. If the cause of the bleeding is identified and treated early, treatment is usually successful.

Nutritional deficiencies

Deficiencies of one or more nutrients essential for normal body function

 More common in children

 Alcohol dependence and extreme dieting are risk factors

 Gender and genetics are not significant factors

Nutritional deficiencies occur when the body lacks essential elements that are obtained from food. In developing countries, such deficiencies are usually the result of poverty and insufficient food supplies. In the UK, nutritional deficiencies are due mainly to disorders that limit the body's intake or absorption of nutrients or to self-imposed dietary restrictions. Deficiencies may be noticed when nutritional needs increase, such as in growth spurts in childhood.

What are the types?
There are two main types of nutritional deficiency: a general deficiency of calories and all nutrients; and deficiency of specific nutrients. A general deficiency may be the result of poor eating because of severe illness or surgery. It may also be due to extreme dieting or deliberate starvation, as occurs in the eating disorder anorexia nervosa (p.348). Some people may neglect

their diet because of other psychological problems, such as alcohol dependence (p.350). A general deficiency of nutrients may also result from poor absorption of food in the small intestine (see **Malabsorption**, p.415). Symptoms of a general deficiency may include weight loss, muscle weakness, and tiredness.

Specific nutritional deficiencies may occur if people limit their diets because of certain beliefs. In some cases, malabsorption causes deficiency of a specific nutrient. For example, the bowel disorder Crohn's disease (p.417) can affect the last section of the small intestine, through which vitamin B$_{12}$ is absorbed. Specific nutritional deficiencies result in a variety of disorders. These include iron-deficiency anaemia (p.271) and the bone disorders osteomalacia and rickets (p.217), which are caused by a lack of calcium or vitamin D.

What might be done?

If your doctor suspects that you have a nutritional deficiency, he or she will weigh you and make a full assessment of your diet, possibly in consultation with a dietician. You may also have blood tests to look for anaemia and to measure levels of specific nutrients. Investigations, such as contrast X-rays (p.131) of the gastrointestinal tract, may be carried out to check for underlying disorders.

If the deficiency is severe, you will be admitted to hospital and given nutrients using a tube passed through the nose into the stomach or through a drip directly into the bloodstream.

If the deficiency is a result of a treatable physical problem, it should resolve with treatment. Changing your diet should resolve the problem if poor eating is the cause. Psychological problems will also require treatment. In some cases, such as Crohn's disease, long-term vitamin and mineral supplements (pp.598–600) may be required.

Obesity in adults

A condition in which an adult is severely overweight, usually due to overeating and too little exercise

 More common with increasing age

 Slightly more common in females

 Sometimes runs in families

 Overeating and a sedentary lifestyle are risk factors

Whether a person is a healthy weight, underweight, or overweight is assessed by using a measure called the body mass index (BMI). This provides an indication of the degree of fatness, although it is not a direct measure of body fat. A person's BMI is calculated by dividing his or her weight (in kilograms) by his or her height (in metres) squared. For most healthy adults, a BMI over 30 is classed as obese (see **Are you a healthy weight?**, p.19 and **Controlling your weight**, p.19). For children, the definition of obesity is different (see **Obesity in children**, p.552). About 1 in 4 adults in the UK is obese and the condition has become increasingly common in recent years, in children as well as adults.

Obesity can have an adverse effect on virtually any part of the body and can therefore lead to a wide variety of health problems. For example, back pain, painful hips and knees, and shortness of breath are common problems. It increases the risk of some serious disorders, such as coronary artery disease (p.243), stroke (p.329), high blood pressure (see **Hypertension**, p.242), type 2 diabetes mellitus (p.437), and certain cancers. Obesity may also lead to psychological problems, including depression (p.343).

What are the causes?

Obesity occurs when food taken into the body provides more energy than is used. The main causes are overeating and a sedentary lifestyle. Obesity may run in families as a result of learned eating habits in addition to inherited factors. In rare cases, it may be a symptom of a hormonal disorder, such as hypothyroidism (p.432). Some drugs, particularly corticosteroids (p.600), can lead to obesity. Occasionally, obesity may be due to an underlying psychological problem.

Are there complications?

Obesity increases the risk of various long-term problems. For example, obese people are more likely to have high blood cholesterol levels (see **Hypercholesterolaemia**, p.440). High cholesterol in turn increases the risk of atherosclerosis (p.241), in which fatty deposits build up on the inner linings of the arteries. Atherosclerosis may contribute to high blood pressure, coronary artery disease, and strokes. Arterial thrombosis and embolism (p.259), which is blockage of a blood vessel by a blood clot, occurs more frequently in obese people. Obese adults are at greater risk of gallstones (p.412) and are more likely to develop type 2 diabetes. Certain cancers, such as breast cancer (p.486), cancer of the uterus (p.479), and colon cancer (see **Colorectal cancer**, p.421) are also more common in obese people.

Excess weight puts strain on joints. Osteoarthritis (p.221), especially in the hips and knees, is common in obese people. Sleep apnoea (p.292), a respiratory disorder, is also linked to obesity.

What might be done?

Your doctor will probably measure your weight and height (to calculate your body mass index) and discuss your diet with you (see **A healthy diet**, p.16) as well as how much exercise you take (see **Exercise and health**, pp.20–23). Tests may be performed to measure blood sugar levels (to look for diabetes) and cholesterol levels. Rarely, you may have blood tests to check for a hormonal disorder.

Obesity is most commonly treated by a weight-reduction diet and increased exercise. Calorie intake per day is usually reduced to 500–1,000 calories less than the average requirement for a person of your age, sex, and height (see **Controlling your weight**, p.19). This type of eating plan is designed to produce slow, sustainable weight loss. The diet may be formulated by your doctor or a dietitian, although you may also choose to join a self-help group. Moderate, regular exercise is essential in losing weight. Changes in diet and lifestyle need to be maintained throughout life to maintain a healthy weight.

Drugs to aid weight loss are usually recommended only for people who are obese and who have not succeeded in losing weight through diet and exercise alone. These drugs may cause adverse side effects and should not be used long term; they should always be used in conjunction with diet and exercise. Orlistat (Xenical) inhibits fat absorption from the digestive tract. It may cause headaches, flatulence, the feeling of an urgent need to defecate, and an oily rectal discharge. Bulking agents, such as methyl cellulose, make you feel full but may cause bloating and flatulence.

Rarely, weight-loss surgery (known medically as bariatric surgery) is used to treat obesity, but usually only as a last resort because of the risk of serious complications. The most common forms of such surgery are gastric banding, gastric bypass, and sleeve gastrectomy They are usually carried out under general anaesthesia by endoscopic ("keyhole") surgery. In gastric banding, an inflatable band is placed around the top of the stomach to create a small pouch. When you eat, the pouch fills quickly, making you feel full sooner, and the band also slows the movement of food into the lower part of the stomach. The band is connected by a tube to an access port under the skin, allowing the tightness of the band to be adjusted. In a gastric bypass, surgical staples are used to create a small pouch at the top of the stomach. This pouch is then connected directly to the small intestine. As a result, food bypasses most of the stomach and the first part of the small intestine. After a gastric bypass, it takes less food to make you feel full, and you also get fewer calories from the food you eat. In a sleeve gastrectomy, a large part of the stomach is removed, leaving a banana-shaped stomach (the sleeve), which becomes your new stomach. As the new stomach is smaller, it takes less food to make you feel full. Unlike gastric banding or bypass, a sleeve gastrectomy cannot be reversed.

Disorders of the mouth, tongue, and oesophagus

Digestion begins in the mouth, where food is chewed by the teeth and mixed by the tongue with saliva secreted by the salivary glands. Swallowing forces the food into the oesophagus, where it progresses to the stomach by coordinated muscle contractions.

The first half of this section deals with disorders of the mouth and tongue. These conditions range from mouth ulcers, which are common and relatively mild, to the serious disease mouth cancer. Also included are disorders that involve inflammation, such as glossitis (inflammation of the tongue), and disorders that cause white patches in the mouth, such as leukoplakia.

Two disorders affecting the salivary glands are described next. Salivary gland stones are painful but can usually be removed successfully. The majority of salivary gland tumours are not cancerous, and their outlook is generally good, but they may recur.

The last part of the section covers disorders of the oesophagus, including gastro-oesophageal reflux disease, which is the most common, and cancer of the oesophagus.

For disorders specifically affecting the teeth and gums, see pp.381–390.

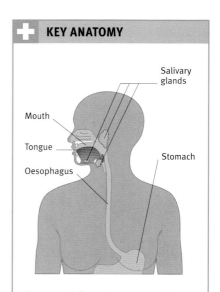

KEY ANATOMY

Salivary glands

Mouth

Tongue

Oesophagus

Stomach

For more information concerning the structure and function of the mouth, tongue, and oesophagus, see pp.391–396.

Mouth ulcers

Painful sores in the lining of the mouth, also called aphthous ulcers or canker sores

 Most common in adolescents and young adults

 Slightly more common in females

 Sometimes run in families

 Stress, illness, and poor general health are risk factors

Mouth ulcers are shallow, grey-white pits with a red border. They can cause pain, particularly when you are chewing spicy, hot, or acidic food. Mouth ulcers are extremely common and may occur singly or in clusters anywhere in the mouth. They may recur several times a year, but they usually disappear without treatment within 2 weeks.

The cause of mouth ulcers is not known, but the ulcers tend to occur in people who are run down or ill and before menstruation in women. Mouth ulcers are often stress-related. Injuries to the lining of the mouth caused by ill-fitting dentures, a roughened tooth, or careless toothbrushing can also result in the development of mouth ulcers.

Occasionally, recurrent mouth ulcers are due to anaemia (p.271), a deficiency of either vitamin B_{12} or folic acid, or an intestinal disorder such as Crohn's disease (p.417) or coeliac disease (p.416). In rare cases, they are due to the autoimmune disorder Behçet's syndrome (p.283).

Ulcers may also occur as a result of specific infections, such as herpes simplex infections (p.166). Rarely, an ulcer that enlarges slowly and does not heal may be mouth cancer (p.402).

Mouth ulcers usually heal without treatment. If you are prone to them, avoid possible irritants, such as spicy foods, and use an antiseptic or pain-relieving mouthwash. Over-the-counter treatments containing a corticosteroid to reduce inflammation or an anaesthetic are also available.

Consult a doctor or dentist about a mouth ulcer that does not heal within 3 weeks. He or she may carry out tests to look for an underlying cause.

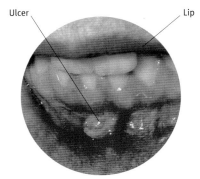

Mouth ulcer
The typical grey-white pit of a mouth ulcer has developed inside the lower lip of the mouth shown above.

Stomatitis

Inflammation of the lining of the mouth that may be mild or severe

 May occur at any age but most common in children and elderly people

 Poor oral hygiene, smoking, and a diet deficient in iron are risk factors

 Gender and genetics are not significant factors

Stomatitis is a general inflammation of the lining of the mouth including the tongue. The disorder is usually caused by an infection. If the inflammation affects the tongue, it is called glossitis (right); if it affects the gums, it is called gingivitis (p.389). Mouth ulcers (left) are another form of stomatitis. Whichever part of the mouth is affected, stomatitis is usually a short-lived condition and, although it may be painful, it does not usually cause serious problems.

What are the causes?

The most common causes of stomatitis are infections with viruses, bacteria, or fungi and eating a poor diet. Smoking may also cause the condition.

Viral stomatitis is mainly caused by the herpes simplex virus (*see* **Herpes simplex infections**, p.166) and the coxsackie virus. Viral stomatitis occurs most commonly in childhood.

Bacterial stomatitis, particularly gingivitis, usually results from neglected dental problems and poor oral hygiene, such as ineffective toothbrushing. Oral bacterial infections are also more likely when saliva production is reduced, such as in Sjögren's syndrome (p.281).

Stomatitis may also result from the fungal infection candidiasis (p.177), in which a fungus that is normally present in the mouth grows excessively and causes inflammation. Candidiasis occurs most commonly in infants, elderly people, those who wear dentures, and pregnant women. People with reduced immunity, such as those with diabetes mellitus (p.437) and people with AIDS (*see* **HIV infection and AIDS**, p.169), are also susceptible to candidiasis. The infection may also occur in people who are being treated with antibiotics (p.572) and in people who use inhaled corticosteroids to treat asthma (*see* **Corticosteroids for respiratory disease**, p.588) and fail to rinse their mouth thoroughly afterwards.

The most common deficiency that causes stomatitis is a shortage of iron, which also leads to anaemia (*see* **Iron-deficiency anaemia**, p.271). Deficiency of vitamin B_{12} or folic acid in the diet may also cause stomatitis.

What are the symptoms?

The symptoms of stomatitis may range from mild to severe and include:
- Sore mouth.
- Bad breath.
- In some cases, mouth ulcers.

In gingivitis, the gums may be sore and swollen and may bleed during toothbrushing. Chronic gingivitis and poor oral hygiene may lead to teeth loosening and eventually falling out.

What might be done?

If your doctor cannot make a diagnosis from your symptoms immediately, a swab may be taken from the affected area of the mouth and sent to a laboratory for testing. If stomatitis is due to infection, antibiotics or antifungal drugs (p.574) may be prescribed. Most viral infections clear up spontaneously, and treatment is usually aimed at relieving symptoms such as pain. Antiviral drugs (p.573) may also be prescribed.

To relieve the symptoms, you should keep your mouth clean by using saltwater mouthwashes regularly. If eating and drinking are particularly painful, your doctor may prescribe a painrelieving mouthwash or gel containing a local anaesthetic to apply to the inside of your mouth just before meals. If children are unable to drink, they may be admitted to hospital to be given fluids intravenously to rehydrate them.

Gingivitis can be prevented by good oral hygiene (*see* **Caring for your teeth and gums**, p.384). Once it has developed, more extensive treatment by your dentist or dental hygienist may be necessary to control the progression of the condition.

Glossitis

Inflammation of the tongue, making it smooth, red, and swollen

 Alcohol abuse and smoking are risk factors

 Age, gender, and genetics are not significant factors

Glossitis (inflammation of the tongue) is usually a temporary condition that heals quickly with treatment. The most common cause of glossitis is an injury to the tongue, which can be due to ill-fitting dentures, roughened teeth, or scalding liquids. Smoking, eating spicy foods, and excessive alcohol intake may cause mild irritation and inflame the tongue. Glossitis may also be the primary symptom of a fungal infection

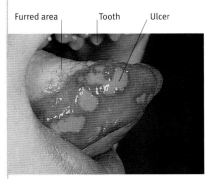
Furred area   Tooth   Ulcer

Glossitis
This tongue has inflammation (glossitis), along with thick furring and ulceration, as a result of herpes simplex infection.

such as candidiasis (p.177) or a viral infection such as herpes simplex infection (p.166). In some cases, the tongue becomes inflamed as a result of a deficiency of iron, vitamin B_{12}, or folic acid in the diet. Rarely, some people find that particular oral hygiene products, such as mouthwashes, breath fresheners, and toothpastes, cause an allergic reaction in the mouth, which leads to inflammation of the tongue.

What are the symptoms?

In many cases, the symptoms of glossitis develop gradually. With time, the tongue may become:
- Painful, swollen, and tender.
- Smooth and red.
- Furred.
- Dotted with multiple small ulcers.
- Cracked.

In cases of glossitis caused by damage from scalding liquids, a viral infection, or an allergic reaction, the symptoms often develop rapidly. Swallowing and speaking may become painful. Other symptoms may also be present in addition to a swollen tongue, depending on the cause. For example, you may have ulcers on your tongue if you have a herpes simplex infection, or if you have candidiasis, you may have sore patches that are creamy-yellow or white.

What might be done?

Your doctor may take swabs from the tongue to identify an infection. A blood sample may also be taken to look for mineral or vitamin deficiencies.

Whatever the cause, you can relieve the discomfort by rinsing your mouth with antiseptic or pain-relieving mouthwashes. It should also help if you stop smoking and avoid acidic and spicy foods that exacerbate the soreness. In many cases, the symptoms clear up without a cause being identified. However, if a clear diagnosis is made, specific treatment for the infection is usually effective. For example, if your condition is caused by candidiasis, your doctor may prescribe an antifungal drug (p.574), such as miconazole in an oral gel form.

Oral lichen planus

White patches in the mouth, sometimes associated with an itchy skin rash

 Most common between the ages of 30 and 60

 More common in females

 Genetics and lifestyle are not significant factors

Oral lichen planus is a rare condition in which small, white patches develop on the inside of the cheeks and sometimes elsewhere in the mouth. The patches often have a lacy pattern. In most people these white patches are painless, but sometimes they develop into persistent ulcers that can be very painful.

Oral lichen planus usually occurs in episodes that may last months or even years and frequently recurs after treatment. The condition occurs most often in people between the ages of 30 and 60 and affects more women than men. A few people who have oral lichen planus may also develop the general skin condition lichen planus (p.195), in which an itchy rash appears on the skin, most commonly on the wrists. In very rare cases, oral lichen planus may develop into mouth cancer (below right).

What are the causes?

Often no cause can be found, but oral lichen planus may be due to an abnormal immune response and may occur with other immune disorders, such as systemic lupus erythematosus (p.281). Oral lichen planus is sometimes due to an adverse reaction to amalgam tooth fillings or particular drugs, including gold-based antirheumatic drugs (p.579) and some of the drugs used to treat diabetes mellitus (p.437). Stress sometimes triggers the symptoms.

What might be done?

If you have white patches in your mouth that last longer than 3 weeks, you should consult your doctor or dentist. It may be possible to make a diagnosis from your symptoms, but to confirm the diagnosis and exclude other disorders, a sample of tissue from the affected area may be taken under local anaesthesia and examined microscopically.

If the symptoms are only mild, no treatment may be necessary. To avoid irritating the patches, you should avoid spicy or acidic foods and alcohol (including alcohol-containing mouthwashes). If the patches are painful, eat soft, bland foods, such as mashed potato; a topical corticosteroid in an oral paste may also be given to relieve pain. Oral lichen planus sometimes disappears spontaneously after several years.

Leukoplakia

Small, thickened, white patches on the lining of the mouth or tongue

	Nearly always occurs over the age of 40
	Twice as common in males
	Smoking, chewing tobacco, and alcohol abuse are risk factors
	Genetics is not a significant factor

In leukoplakia, thickened white patches develop on the lining of the mouth or on the tongue. The patches develop slowly and painlessly, starting most often on the sides of the tongue. Unlike the white patches in the mouth caused by oral thrush (see Candidiasis, p.177), leukoplakia patches cannot be scraped off. Sometimes, these patches may harden, causing the surface to crack.

What are the causes?

Occasionally, the condition is caused by repeated mild damage to one area of the mouth, such as by a roughened tooth, but often the cause is unknown. If there is no obvious cause, there is a small chance that the patch may become cancerous (see Mouth cancer, below). The risk of cancer is higher if the patch is on the floor of the mouth or is ulcerated. Leukoplakia is much more common in smokers and people who chew tobacco. The risk is increased further if people drink excessive alcohol. The disorder is twice as common in men as in women and nearly always occurs in those over 40.

A form of leukoplakia known as hairy leukoplakia affects people with reduced immunity, especially people with AIDS (see HIV infection and AIDS, p.169). White patches occur on the sides of the tongue and have a rough or corrugated surface. Hairy leukoplakia does not usually become cancerous.

Patch of leukoplakia   Tongue

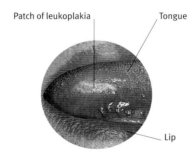

Lip

Leukoplakia
The thickened white patches of leukoplakia usually develop on the side of the tongue. The patches often harden and crack.

What might be done?

An obvious cause for the patches can be treated, and the patches may then disappear. If no cause is found or the condition persists, your doctor or dentist may take a tissue sample from your mouth to exclude mouth cancer. Persistent patches may be removed by surgery or laser treatment (p.613). Even with treatment, leukoplakia may recur and needs to be monitored regularly.

Mouth cancer

Cancerous tumour of the lips, tongue, or lining of the mouth

	Most common over the age of 60; rare under the age of 40
	Twice as common in males
	Smoking, chewing tobacco, alcohol abuse, and excessive exposure to sunlight are risk factors
	Genetics is not a significant factor

About half of all cancerous tumours of the mouth occur on either the tongue or the lower lip. The gums, inside of the cheeks, floor of the mouth, and palate are less commonly affected.

In developed countries, mouth cancer accounts for around 2 per cent of all new cases of cancer. In developing countries such as India, where people chew tobacco, betel leaves, and nuts, mouth cancer is much more common. Worldwide, the disease is twice as common in men as it is in women, although the incidence is increasing in women. Mouth cancer occurs most commonly in people over the age of 60 and is rare in those under the age of 40. The outlook for lip cancer is good. The outcome is generally poorer for other forms of mouth cancer but is improved with early diagnosis.

What are the causes?

Some people develop mouth cancer for no apparent reason. However, various risk factors increase the chance of developing mouth cancer. The main risk factors are tobacco use, either smoking or chewing tobacco; drinking large amounts of alcohol, particularly if combined with tobacco use; chewing betel leaves or nuts; infection with the human papillomavirus (HPV); and the presence of leukoplakia (left). Repeated, unprotected exposure to sunlight increases the risk of developing lip cancer. In addition, other factors that may increase the risk of mouth cancer include a poor diet and a suppressed immune system.

What are the symptoms?

If you have mouth cancer, you may experience the following symptoms:
- An ulcer or sore that fails to heal, occurring on the lining of the mouth or on the tongue.
- A white or red patch in your mouth or throat that does not clear up.
- Persistent pain or discomfort in the mouth.
- A swelling that develops anywhere inside the mouth or on the lips.
- Pain when swallowing.

Left untreated, mouth cancer usually spreads from the mouth to nearby tissues, the lymph nodes in the neck, and from there to other parts of the body.

How is it diagnosed?

Cancerous tumours in the mouth are often detected early by a dentist during a checkup. If your doctor suspects that a lump or nonhealing ulcer is a tumour, a small sample of tissue may be taken for

Tumour   Lip   Tongue

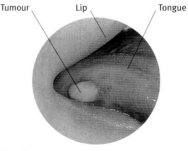

Mouth cancer
A cancerous tumour can be seen here in the form of a small, white lump that has developed on the right side of the tongue.

examination. If cancer is found, further tests will establish how far it has spread (see Staging cancer, p.157).

What is the treatment?

A small cancerous tumour that is discovered early may be removed surgically or by laser treatment (p.613). In about 8 in 10 people, surgery is successful and the cancer does not recur following removal of the tumour. If the tumour is large, it will be removed surgically, and plastic surgery (p.614) may be necessary to restore a more normal facial appearance. Following surgery, radiotherapy (p.158) may be carried out to ensure that all cancerous cells have been destroyed and the cancer does not recur. If the tumour has spread, chemotherapy may be used in conjunction with radiotherapy.

What is the prognosis?

Tumours that are found early and are in an accessible part of the mouth can usually be treated successfully. The outlook is best for lip cancer, which is the most accessible site. For cancers within the mouth, less than half of the affected people survive for 5 years.

Salivary gland stones

Stones that form in the ducts of the salivary glands

	More common over the age of 40
	Twice as common in males
	Genetics and lifestyle are not significant factors

There are three pairs of salivary glands in the mouth, and sometimes the salivary ducts (tubes through which saliva enters the mouth) become blocked by stones. The stones are composed of calcium salts and vary in size. They either partially or, rarely, completely block the duct. The salivary gland then becomes swollen and feels painful during eating because saliva cannot escape from the gland into the mouth. In most cases, no cause can be found. Stones are twice as common in men and occur most often in people over the age of 40.

What are the symptoms?

In most cases, the symptoms of salivary gland stones include:
- A visible swelling on the outside of the mouth or the sensation of a lump inside the mouth.
- Pain during or after a meal due to a build-up of saliva behind the stone.

A blocked salivary duct is liable to become infected, causing the swelling to become red and inflamed, with possible leakage of pus into the mouth.

What might be done?

To confirm the presence of a salivary gland stone, you may have imaging tests, such as X-rays (p.131), CT scanning (p.132), MRI (p.133), or ultrasound scanning (p.135). If the location is unclear, you may have a test called a sialogram, in which a dye is injected directly into the blocked duct and an X-ray of the area is taken. The doctor may be able to tease out the stone using a thin, blunt instrument. Alternatively, a procedure called sialendoscopy may be used. In this procedure, which is usually carried out under local anaesthesia, a thin endoscope (viewing tube) is inserted into the salivary duct and instruments are passed down the tube to remove the stone. Sometimes it may be necessary to remove a stone by surgery. Rarely, lithotripsy may be used in which ultrasound shock waves are used to break up the stone so that the fragments can be flushed out. Salivary gland stones may recur after treatment.

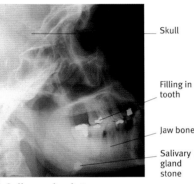

Salivary gland stone
In this X-ray, a salivary gland stone shows up as a white mass. The stone is blocking the duct of the gland beneath the jaw bone.

Skull

Filling in tooth

Jaw bone

Salivary gland stone

Salivary gland tumours

Noncancerous or cancerous tumours in the salivary glands

 More common over the age of 45

 Gender, genetics, and lifestyle are not significant factors

Tumours that affect the salivary glands are rare, particularly in people under the age of 45. Three-quarters of the tumours occur in one of the two parotid salivary glands that lie behind the angles of the jaw. Only about 1 in 5 salivary gland tumours is cancerous.

The symptoms of a salivary gland tumour depend on whether or not it is a cancerous tumour, but in all cases there is a lump that may be felt either protruding inside the mouth or on the face. Noncancerous tumours are usually painless, rubbery in consistency, and mobile when touched. These benign tumours usually grow slowly.

Cancerous tumours of the salivary gland usually grow quickly, feel hard, and are sometimes painful. The facial nerve, which passes through the gland, may be affected as the cancer develops, leading to paralysis of part of the face (*see* Facial palsy, p.339). If the tumour is left untreated, the cancer may spread to nearby lymph nodes in the neck and from there to other parts of the body, such as the chest and liver.

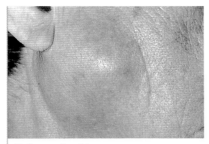

Salivary gland tumour
This swelling close to the ear and over the angle of the jawbone is caused by a noncancerous tumour of a salivary gland.

What is the treatment?
Treatment for a noncancerous tumour of the parotid gland is an operation to remove the affected part of the gland. This is a very delicate procedure and there is a risk that the facial nerve may be damaged. If damage does occur, the mouth may droop as a result. The nerve sometimes recovers, but in other cases the damage may be permanent.

If a tumour is cancerous, all of the affected gland is removed. If the tumour has spread to the lymph nodes in the neck, these nodes may also need to be removed. After surgery, it may be necessary to perform radiotherapy (p.158) to destroy remaining cancerous cells.

What is the prognosis?
Noncancerous tumours can usually be removed successfully but may sometimes recur. Rarely, a noncancerous tumour may become cancerous if it is not removed.

The outlook for people with cancerous tumours depends on which glands are affected and how far advanced the cancer is. For small parotid tumours treated early, before they have spread, approximately 8 in 10 people survive for at least 10 years after diagnosis. However, for advanced parotid tumours that have spread and affected the facial nerve, only about 1 in 10 people survives for more than 5 years. For cancerous tumours of the other salivary glands, the outlook is generally better.

Gastro-oesophageal reflux disease

Regurgitation of acidic stomach juices into the oesophagus, causing pain in the upper abdomen and chest

 Obesity, a high-fat diet, drinking too much coffee or alcohol, and smoking are risk factors

 Age, gender, and genetics are not significant factors

Commonly known as acid reflux, gastro-oesophageal reflux disease (GORD) is probably the most common cause of indigestion (p.397). The discomfort is due to acidic juices from the stomach flowing up into the oesophagus (the tube leading from the throat to the stomach). The lining of the oesophagus is not adequately protected against the harmful effects of stomach acid, which may cause inflammation and a burning pain known as heartburn.

Attacks of GORD are usually brief and relatively mild but if they are persistent, the lining of the oesophagus may be permanently damaged or scarred. In some cases, GORD causes bleeding from the digestive tract (p.393).

What are the causes?
The stomach contents are kept from entering the oesophagus by a double-action valve mechanism. One part of this mechanism is the muscular ring at the lower end of the oesophagus, called the lower oesophageal sphincter. The other part is the effect of the diaphragm muscle on the oesophagus as the tube passes through a narrow opening in the muscle, called the hiatus. These mechanisms provide an effective one-way valve.

GORD may develop as a result of several factors acting together to make the valve leak. These include poor muscle tone in the sphincter; increased abdominal pressure due to pregnancy; obesity; or a weakness in the hiatus that allows part of the stomach to slide into the chest (a hiatus hernia). Many people develop mild attacks of GORD after eating certain foods or drinks, especially pickles, fried or fatty meals, carbonated soft drinks, alcohol, or coffee. Smoking may also worsen symptoms.

What are the symptoms?
Some of the symptoms of GORD are most noticeable immediately after eating a large meal or when a person bends over. The main symptoms include:

■ Burning pain or discomfort in the chest behind the breastbone, known as heartburn.
■ Acidic taste in the mouth due to regurgitation of acidic fluid into the throat or mouth.
■ Persistent cough.

SELF-HELP

Managing gastro-oesophageal reflux disease
The following steps either relieve symptoms of gastro-oesophageal reflux disease (GORD) or prevent them from recurring:

■ Take antacids (p.596) to help neutralize stomach acids.
■ Avoid spicy, acidic, tomato-based foods and high-fat foods such as chocolate and cream.
■ Avoid alcohol, colas, and coffee.
■ Stop smoking.
■ Lose excess weight.
■ Eat smaller amounts of food to avoid overfilling the stomach and do not eat late at night.
■ After eating, do not exercise or lie down since both may lead to food being regurgitated.
■ Raise the head of your bed or sleep on extra pillows so that your head is higher than your feet during the night.

■ Belching.
■ Blood in the vomit or faeces.
GORD that persists for many years can cause scarring in the oesophagus, which may eventually cause a stricture (narrowing). A stricture can make swallowing difficult and may lead to weight loss. Long-term GORD can lead to a condition called Barrett's oesophagus, in which part of the oesophageal lining is replaced by the stomach lining. People with extensive Barrett's oesophagus are at increased risk of cancer of the oesophagus (p.404).

If you have recently developed pain in the centre of your chest that seems unrelated to eating or drinking, you should seek immediate medical help because the far more serious condition angina (p.244) is sometimes mistaken for the pain of severe heartburn.

What might be done?
Self-help measures can relieve many symptoms of GORD (*see* Managing gastro-oesophageal reflux disease, left). However, if your heartburn is persistent, consult your doctor.

The doctor may arrange for contrast X-rays to look for abnormalities in the oesophagus (*see* Barium swallow, p.404). You may also undergo endoscopy (p.138), in which a flexible viewing tube is used to examine the lining of the oesophagus. During this procedure, a small sample of tissue may be removed for examination under a microscope. Endoscopy is more sensitive than a barium swallow at detecting Barrett's oesophagus or inflammation or ulcers in the oesophagus.

If self-help measures do not relieve your symptoms, your doctor may prescribe a drug that reduces the stomach's acid production (*see* Ulcer-healing drugs, p.596). The rate at which the stomach is emptied may be increased by a drug such as metoclopramide (*see* Antispasmodic drugs and motility stimulants, p.598), making GORD less likely. Symptoms usually disappear with this treatment. If they do not, you may need an operation to return the stomach to its normal position and tighten the lower oesophageal sphincter. This may be carried out by laparoscopic surgery (*see* Laparoscopy, p.476), a type of endoscopic surgery (p.612).

Achalasia

Difficulty in swallowing due to a muscle disorder of the oesophagus

 Most common between the ages of 25 and 60; rare in childhood

 Gender, genetics, and lifestyle are not significant factors

In people with achalasia, the passage of food and drink into the stomach from the oesophagus is delayed or prevented. The problem is mainly caused by failure of the lower oesophageal sphincter (the ring of muscle at the lower end of the oesophagus) to relax normally and allow food to pass into the stomach during swallowing.

▶ **TEST**

Barium swallow

A barium swallow is a test used to visualize the oesophagus, the tube that connects the mouth to the stomach. The test can detect disorders or abnormalities of the oesophagus, such as narrowing or tumours. A barium solution is used because it shows up on X-rays, which are taken continuously to monitor the flow of the solution. The barium may cause temporary constipation.

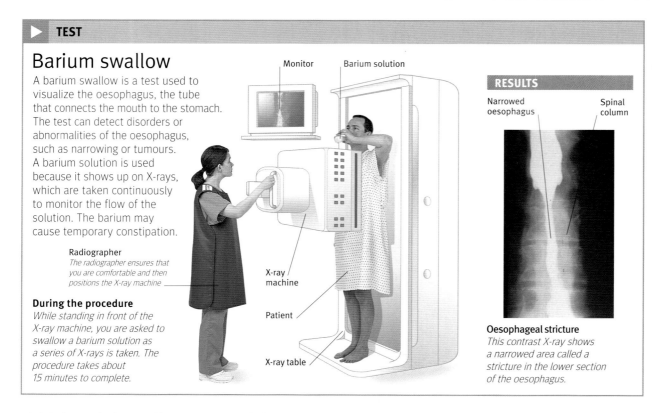

Radiographer
The radiographer ensures that you are comfortable and then positions the X-ray machine

During the procedure
While standing in front of the X-ray machine, you are asked to swallow a barium solution as a series of X-rays is taken. The procedure takes about 15 minutes to complete.

Labels: Monitor · Barium solution · X-ray machine · Patient · X-ray table

RESULTS

Labels: Narrowed oesophagus · Spinal column

Oesophageal stricture
This contrast X-ray shows a narrowed area called a stricture in the lower section of the oesophagus.

Achalasia may also be caused by poor muscle coordination in the oesophagus. The condition causes the lower part of the oesophagus to be progressively distorted and widened over months or years, and makes swallowing increasingly difficult. Achalasia most commonly occurs in people between the ages of 25 and 60.

What are the symptoms?
Symptoms of achalasia usually develop slowly and include the following:
■ Difficulty in swallowing.
■ Chest pain or a feeling of discomfort behind the breastbone, which may be related to eating.
■ Regurgitating undigested food during meals or some hours afterwards, especially at night.
■ Eventually, weight loss.
If achalasia is left untreated, there is a slightly increased risk of developing cancer of the oesophagus (right).

How is it diagnosed?
If your doctor suspects that you have achalasia, a chest X-ray (p.300) may be arranged to look for the typical widening and distortion of the oesophagus. The diagnosis may be apparent from a barium swallow (above). Your doctor may look down your oesophagus using a flexible viewing instrument called an endoscope (*see* **Endoscopy**, p.138) to confirm the diagnosis and eliminate other possible disorders, such as cancer of the oesophagus. Oesophageal manometry is considered the most reliable indicator of achalasia. In this procedure, a flexible tube is passed down the oesophagus in order to measure pressures. Normally, the procedure shows changing pressures as a result of the alternate contractions and relaxations of the oesophageal muscles. In

achalasia, these pressure changes are absent, and the overall pressure is high due to incomplete muscle relaxation.

What is the treatment?
Several different effective treatments are available for achalasia. The choice of treatment depends on your age and general health in addition to the severity and duration of your symptoms.

The simplest treatment is for your doctor to prescribe drugs called calcium channel blockers (p.582), which temporarily relax the lower oesophageal sphincter muscle. However, for longer-term relief, the treatment most often used is to pass a small balloon down to the oesophageal sphincter. Once the balloon is in place, it is inflated with either air or water to stretch the sphincter and is then removed. This procedure is successful in at least half of all people with the disorder. However, for a few people, it may have to be repeated over periods varying from 6 months to several years.

An alternative treatment is the injection of botulinum toxin into the sphincter. In small doses, the toxin paralyses the affected muscles, causing them to relax and allow food and liquids to pass. This effect typically lasts a little over a year and may need to be repeated.

If none of these methods is successful, laparoscopic surgery (p.476) may be performed using instruments passed through small incisions in the abdomen. Some of the muscle at the lower end of the oesophagus may be cut to allow food to pass into the stomach. In about 1 in 10 cases, this procedure leads to the stomach contents flowing back up the oesophagus, a condition that will also need treatment (*see* **Gastro-oesophageal reflux disease**, p.403).

Cancer of the oesophagus

Cancerous tumour in the tissue of the oesophagus

 Rare before the age of 60; thereafter, the risk increases with age

 About twice as common in males

 Smoking and alcohol abuse are risk factors

 Genetics is not a significant factor

In the UK, there are about 8,300 cases a year of oesophageal cancer. In certain other areas of the world, such as parts of East and Central Asia, the disease is much more common. In the UK, oesophageal cancer is about twice as common in men as in women and few cases are diagnosed in the under-60s. However, death rates from the cancer are relatively high because it is often present for some time before it begins to cause symptoms. As a result, the cancer has often spread by the time medical help is sought.

What are the causes?
The exact cause of oesophageal cancer is unknown, but factors known to increase the risk of developing it include smoking and excessive alcohol consumption. In East and Central Asia, diet may be at least partly responsible for the high rate of the cancer. People who have particular disorders of the oesophagus, such as gastro-oesophageal reflux disease (p.403) and Barrett's oesophagus (in which the lining of the stomach replaces part of the oesophageal lining), are at increased risk of developing oesophageal cancer. People who have long-term diseases

---

of the oesophagus may benefit from regular endoscopy (p.138) to look for early evidence of cancerous growths.

What are the symptoms?
Early in the disease, there are often no symptoms. They develop slowly over weeks or months as the oesophagus becomes obstructed and may include:
■ Difficulty swallowing solid foods.
■ Difficulty swallowing liquids as the oesophageal opening narrows further.
■ Regurgitation of recently eaten food.
■ Cough as a result of food that cannot be swallowed properly spilling into the lungs.
■ Loss of appetite and weight loss.
If the tumour spreads and involves the trachea, there may also be shortness of breath and coughing up blood.

If you have heartburn on most days for 3 weeks or more, or if you have any of the other symptoms listed above, you should consult your doctor so that the cause can be investigated.

How is it diagnosed?
Your doctor may arrange for a tissue sample to be taken during endoscopy, which involves passing a flexible viewing tube into the oesophagus (*see* **Upper digestive tract endoscopy**, p.407). A barium swallow (above, left) may be performed to detect an obstruction in the oesophagus. Once the diagnosis has been confirmed, tests such as CT scanning (p.132) may be carried out to determine if the tumour has spread. Tumour spread may also be investigated using endoscopic ultrasound, in which a special probe is passed down the oesophagus.

What is the treatment?
The treatment depends on whether the cancer is limited to the oesophagus or has spread. A localized cancer can be removed, but the operation is a major procedure and only a small proportion of affected people are diagnosed early enough to make surgery worthwhile. If surgery is performed, chemotherapy (p.157) or radiotherapy (p.158) may be given beforehand to maximize the chance of a cure.

If the cancer has spread or if general health is not good enough for surgery, treatment is given to ease symptoms. Insertion of a stent (a self-expanding tube) into the narrowed area of the oesophagus can relieve swallowing difficulties (*see* **Palliative surgery for cancer**, p.159). Treatment may also involve radiotherapy and chemotherapy.

About 40 per cent of people with oesophageal cancer survive for at least a year after diagnosis but only about 15 per cent survive for more than 5 years.

Disorders of the stomach and duodenum

The stomach and the duodenum (the first part of the intestine) are exposed to many potentially damaging substances, including acid produced by the stomach to aid food digestion, alcohol, and irritant foods such as spices. The stomach and duodenum have a natural defence mechanism that protects against damage, but sometimes this mechanism fails, leading to disease.

The first article in this section covers infection with the *Helicobacter pylori* bacterium, which was discovered in the early 1980s. It is now estimated that about half the world's population is infected with *H. pylori*. In most cases, there are no symptoms. However, *H. pylori* is known to be associated with the disorders of the stomach and duodenum discussed in this section: gastritis, which is inflammation of the lining of the stomach; peptic ulcer, which is an area of the stomach lining or the duodenum that has been eroded by acidic digestive juices; and stomach cancer. Both gastritis and peptic ulcer are common disorders of the digestive system that affect thousands of people in the UK every year. However, if either of these disorders occurs with *H. pylori* infection, it can usually be treated with drugs. The final article covers stomach cancer, which is now rare in many developed countries. General problems that may involve the stomach or another part of the upper digestive tract are covered elsewhere (*see* **Indigestion**, p.397; **Nonulcer dyspepsia**, p.397; and **Gastro-oesophageal reflux disease**, p.403).

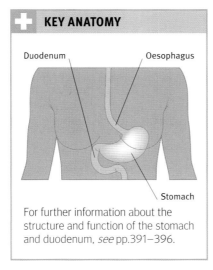

✚ KEY ANATOMY

Duodenum   Oesophagus

Stomach

For further information about the structure and function of the stomach and duodenum, *see* pp.391–396.

Helicobacter pylori infection

A common bacterial infection, which may lead to inflammation or ulceration in the upper digestive tract

 Often contracted in childhood, but symptoms usually develop in adulthood

 More common in males

 Living in overcrowded, unsanitary conditions is a risk factor

 Genetics is not a significant factor

The *Helicobacter pylori* bacterium is a common infection of the stomach and duodenum (first part of the small intestine), and is estimated to affect about half of the world's population. The infection is usually contracted during childhood and, in most cases, causes no symptoms, despite being associated with inflammation of the stomach lining (*see* **Gastritis**, right). However, in some people, *H. pylori* infection may lead to a peptic ulcer (p.406), in which an area of the lining of the stomach or the duodenum is eroded by the action of the acidic digestive juices.

The *H. pylori* bacterium can lead to peptic ulcers or gastritis when it damages the mucous layer of the stomach or duodenum. The mucus usually protects the lining of the stomach and the duodenum from acidic digestive juices, and the lining may become inflamed or eroded in areas where the mucous layer is damaged. Long-term infection with *H. pylori* may also increase the risk of developing stomach cancer (p.406).

The exact way in which *H. pylori* is transmitted is unknown. It is believed that the bacterium may be carried in faeces and saliva and is most readily passed on by close contact with others, especially among people living in overcrowded, unsanitary conditions. The infection is more common in males.

Stomach lining   Bacterium

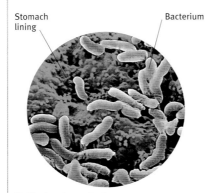

Helicobacter pylori
A number of Helicobacter pylori *bacteria can be seen in this magnified view of the mucous lining of the stomach.*

How is it diagnosed?

If you have discomfort or pain in the upper abdomen, your doctor may suspect that you have gastritis or a peptic ulcer. He or she may arrange for tests to check for *H. pylori* infection. The most common test is a faecal test for the presence of *H. pylori* proteins. Alternatively, you may be given a blood test to check for antibodies against *H. pylori*, or a breath test. The breath test involves first drinking a substance that is normally broken down by *H. pylori*. If the bacteria are present, the substance is changed into a chemical that can be detected with a breathalyser. You may also have an upper digestive tract endoscopy (p.407), in which the stomach or duodenum is examined with a flexible viewing tube. During the endoscopy procedure, a small piece of the lining may be taken for examination under a microscope.

What is the treatment?

Treatment for *H. pylori* is given only if the infection has led to a disorder such as gastritis or a peptic ulcer. Your doctor will prescribe a combination of antibiotics (p.572) to treat the *H. pylori* infection and other drugs to suppress the production of acid by the stomach (*see* **Ulcer-healing drugs**, p.596).

In about 9 in 10 cases, *H. pylori* infection can be successfully treated. The infection may recur in a small number of cases.

Gastritis

Inflammation of the stomach lining, which may be caused by irritation or infection

 More common over the age of 50; rare in children

 Sometimes runs in families

 Alcohol abuse and smoking are risk factors

 Gender is not a significant factor

Gastritis, which is inflammation of the stomach lining, is a common disorder. More than half of the population over the age of 50 have gastritis, although in some cases there are no symptoms. The disorder may be acute and have a sudden onset, but it is more frequently chronic, developing gradually over months or years. The symptoms commonly include discomfort in the upper abdomen. The inflammation may be complicated by bleeding from the stomach.

Some types of gastritis run in families. However, a major cause of chronic gastritis is *Helicobacter pylori* infection (left).

What are the causes?

Acute gastritis may occur when the stomach lining is damaged by drinking an excessive amount of alcohol or by taking aspirin or another nonsteroidal anti-inflammatory drug (p.578), such as ibuprofen. Acute gastritis can also develop after serious illness, such as blood poisoning (*see* **Septicaemia**, p.171).

Chronic gastritis is often caused by infection with *H. pylori* bacteria, which are found in the stomach lining of about half of the population. The bacterium damages the mucous layer that protects the stomach lining from digestive juices, allowing acid to attack the lining. Chronic gastritis may also occur in Crohn's disease (p.417), a disorder which may cause digestive tract inflammation. Long-term use of alcohol, tobacco, and nonsteroidal anti-inflammatory drugs (p.578), such as aspirin, may also lead to chronic gastritis.

One type of chronic gastritis, known as atrophic or autoimmune gastritis, is caused by an abnormal reaction of the immune system in which the body produces antibodies that attack the tissues of the stomach lining.

What are the symptoms?

Chronic gastritis often does not cause any symptoms, but it may gradually result in damage to the stomach lining that will eventually produce symptoms similar to those of acute gastritis. The onset of symptoms in acute gastritis is much faster and the symptoms are more severe. The symptoms of both types of gastritis may include:

- Discomfort or pain in the stomach area, often after eating.
- Nausea and vomiting.
- Loss of appetite.

Bleeding from the stomach lining may go unnoticed until it gives rise to iron-deficiency anaemia (p.271), which causes tiredness and pale skin. If the bleeding is severe, you may vomit blood or pass black, tarry stools (*see* **Bleeding from the digestive tract**, p.399).

Atrophic gastritis is usually painless, and the only symptoms may be those of pernicious anaemia due to a deficiency of vitamin B_{12}. Atrophic gastritis damages the stomach so that it cannot make intrinsic factor, a substance essential for the absorption of this vitamin. People with chronic gastritis, especially atrophic gastritis, also have an increased risk of developing stomach cancer (p.406).

What can I do?

The symptoms of mild gastritis can be treated with over-the-counter antacids (p.596), which neutralize the acid in the stomach. You may also find that your symptoms are relieved by eating small, regular meals, reducing your alcohol intake, and giving up smoking. If symptoms persist or are severe or if you are losing weight without apparent reason, you should consult your doctor.

What might be done?

Your doctor will ask you about your smoking, drinking, and dietary habits, and your use of medications. You may be given a faecal, blood, or breath test for *H. pylori* infection. You may also have a blood test for anaemia to see if there has been bleeding from the stomach lining. Your doctor may arrange for you to have endoscopy (*see* **Upper digestive tract endoscopy**, opposite page) to examine the stomach lining.

If *H. pylori* infection is confirmed, a combination of antibiotics (p.572) and ulcer-healing drugs (p.596) may be prescribed. If you have gastritis and need to take aspirin or another nonsteroidal anti-inflammatory drug for a period of time, you may also be advised to take a proton pump inhibitor drug, such as omeprazole. Proton pump inhibitors reduce the production of stomach acid and help to protect the stomach lining.

Gastritis usually improves if lifestyle changes, such as reducing intake of alcohol, are made. If chronic gastritis is caused by *H. pylori* infection, complete recovery usually follows treatment with antibiotics and ulcer-healing drugs. However, infection sometimes recurs, requiring further treatment.

Peptic ulcer

An eroded area of the tissue lining the stomach or the duodenum, the first part of the small intestine

 Stomach ulcers are more common over the age of 50; duodenal ulcers are most common between the ages of 20 and 60

 Peptic ulcers are more common in females

 Sometimes runs in families

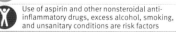 Use of aspirin and other nonsteroidal anti-inflammatory drugs, excess alcohol, smoking, and unsanitary conditions are risk factors

The lining of the stomach and duodenum normally has a barrier of mucus to protect it from the effects of acidic digestive juices. If this barrier is damaged, the acid may cause inflammation and erosion of the lining. The resulting eroded areas are known as peptic ulcers, of which there are two types: duodenal ulcers and gastric (stomach) ulcers. Duodenal ulcers are more common than gastric ulcers and usually occur in people aged 20 to 60. Gastric ulcers are more common in people over the age of 50. Peptic ulcers are common, and it is estimated that about 1 in 10 people in the UK develops an ulcer at some time.

What are the causes?

Peptic ulcers are most commonly associated with *Helicobacter pylori* infection (p.405). This bacterium is thought to be transmitted most easily in unsanitary living conditions and releases substances that reduce the effectiveness of the mucous layer. Acidic digestive juices are

then able to erode the protective lining of the stomach or the duodenum, thereby allowing peptic ulcers to develop.

Peptic ulcers may sometimes result from the long-term use of nonsteroidal anti-inflammatory drugs (p.578), such as ibuprofen or aspirin, that damage the lining of the stomach. Other factors that may lead to peptic ulcers include smoking and consumption of alcohol. In some people, there is a strong family history of peptic ulcers, suggesting that a genetic factor may be involved in their development. It used to be thought that stress could cause peptic ulcers but this is now no longer considered to be a significant causative factor.

What are the symptoms?

Many people with a peptic ulcer do not experience symptoms or dismiss their discomfort as indigestion (p.397). Those with persistent symptoms may notice:

- Pain or discomfort that is felt in the upper abdomen.
- Loss of appetite and weight loss.
- A feeling of fullness in the abdomen.
- Nausea and sometimes vomiting.

Pain is often present for several weeks and then disappears for months or even years. The pain from a duodenal ulcer can be worse before meals when the stomach is empty. This pain may be quickly relieved by eating but usually recurs a few hours afterwards. By contrast, pain caused by a gastric ulcer is often aggravated by food.

Are there complications?

The most common complication of a peptic ulcer is bleeding as the ulcer becomes deeper and erodes into nearby blood vessels (*see* **Bleeding from the digestive tract**, p.399). Minor bleeding from the digestive tract may cause no symptoms apart from those of iron-deficiency anaemia (p.271), such as pale skin, tiredness, and faintness. Bleeding from the digestive tract may lead to vomiting of blood. Alternatively, blood may pass through the digestive tract, resulting in black, tarry stools. In some cases, an ulcer perforates all the layers of the stomach or duodenum, allowing gastric juices to enter the abdomen and causing severe pain (*see* **Peritonitis**, p.421). Bleeding from the digestive tract and perforation of the stomach or the duodenum may be life-threatening and require immediate medical attention.

In rare cases, stomach ulcers may result in narrowing of the stomach outlet into the duodenum, which prevents the stomach from emptying fully. Symptoms may then include bloating after meals, vomiting undigested food hours after eating, and weight loss.

What might be done?

If your doctor suspects that you have a peptic ulcer, he or she may arrange an endoscopy (*see* **Upper digestive tract endoscopy**, opposite page) to view the stomach and duodenum. During endoscopy, a sample of the stomach lining may be taken to look for evidence of *H. pylori*

infection and exclude stomach cancer (below), which may cause similar symptoms. Your doctor may also arrange for a faecal, blood, or breath test to look for *H. pylori* infection, and blood tests to check for evidence of anaemia.

Treatment of a peptic ulcer is designed to heal the ulcer and to prevent it from recurring. You will be advised to make some lifestyle changes, such as giving up smoking and drinking less alcohol.

If *H. pylori* is found, a combination of antibiotics (p.572) and ulcer-healing drugs (p.596) will usually be prescribed. Ulcer-healing drugs are usually given to maximize the chance of healing even if tests for *H. pylori* prove negative.

If long-term treatment with aspirin or another nonsteroidal anti-inflammatory drug is the cause, your doctor may prescribe an alternative or an additional drug, such as omeprazole, to protect the lining of the stomach and duodenum.

A bleeding or perforated ulcer is an emergency requiring urgent admission to hospital. If bleeding is moderate, it can usually be stopped by injections of drugs. If blood loss is severe, a blood transfusion (p.272) may be necessary. Endoscopy will be used to view the stomach lining; during this procedure, bleeding blood vessels can be sealed off. If the bleeding continues or the ulcer is perforated, surgery is usually necessary.

With treatment, about 19 in 20 peptic ulcers disappear completely within a few months. However, an ulcer may recur if lifestyle changes are not made, if nonsteroidal anti-inflammatory drugs continue to be used, or if *H. pylori* is not eradicated or reinfection occurs.

Stomach cancer

A cancerous tumour in the lining of the stomach wall

 More common over the age of 55

 Twice as common in males

 More common in people with blood group A; sometimes runs in families

 Certain foods, smoking, and a high alcohol intake are risk factors

Worldwide, stomach cancer is one of the most common forms of cancer, accounting for about 7 per cent of all new cancer cases per year. It is a particular problem in Japan and China, possibly because of dietary factors. However, in most other countries the disease has become less common. In the UK the incidence has declined since the 1970s, and there are now about 7,000 new cases a year. Stomach cancer is rare before the age of 55 but the incidence then increases with age. It is about twice as common in males. It is also more common in people of blood group A and can run in families, suggesting a genetic factor.

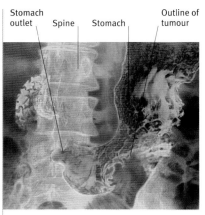

Stomach outlet   Spine   Stomach   Outline of tumour

Cancer in the lower stomach
In this X-ray, barium has been used to outline the stomach. The lining of the stomach has an irregular area where there is a large tumour.

In most cases, stomach cancer develops in the stomach lining. The cancer may spread rapidly to other parts of the body. Early diagnosis is rare because the symptoms are usually mild, and by the time people seek medical help, the cancer has often spread.

What are the causes?

The causes of stomach cancer are not fully understood, but there are a number of factors. Chronic gastritis due to infection with the *H. pylori* bacterium (*see* **Helicobacter pylori infection**, p.405) increases the risk of stomach cancer. Certain diets may increase the risk, such as a diet with a high intake of salt, pickled and smoked foods, and a low intake of fresh fruit and green vegetables. Smoking and a high alcohol intake are also risk factors.

What are the symptoms?

The early symptoms of stomach cancer are mild and vague, and many people ignore them. They may include:

- Discomfort in the upper abdomen.
- Pain in the stomach after eating.
- Loss of appetite and weight loss.
- Nausea and vomiting.

In many people, iron-deficiency anaemia (p.271) develops due to minor bleeding from the stomach lining. Later on, swelling may be felt in the upper abdomen.

How is it diagnosed?

Your doctor may arrange for you to have upper digestive tract endoscopy (opposite page), in which a flexible viewing tube is used to examine the lining of the stomach. Tissue samples from abnormal areas of the stomach lining are tested for the presence of cancerous cells. Rarely, you may also have a barium meal (*see* **Contrast X-rays**, p.132), in which a liquid barium mixture is swallowed to show the stomach clearly on an X-ray. The doctor may arrange blood tests for anaemia, which may show that there has been bleeding from the stomach lining.

If a diagnosis of stomach cancer is confirmed, further investigations, such as CT scanning (p.132) and blood tests, may be performed to check whether the cancer has spread to other organs (*see* **Staging cancer**,

Upper digestive tract endoscopy

This technique involves passing a flexible viewing tube through the mouth to examine the oesophagus, stomach, and duodenum (the first part of the small intestine) to look for disorders such as peptic ulcers. Diathermy (a heat treatment) or laser therapy can be performed or injections of drugs given to stop any bleeding.

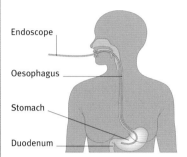

Endoscope
Oesophagus
Stomach
Duodenum

ROUTE OF ENDOSCOPE

During the procedure
You may have a local anaesthetic spray to numb the back of your throat and/or intravenous sedation. You then swallow the endoscope, through which the doctor views your upper digestive tract. The procedure usually takes about 15 minutes.

VIEW

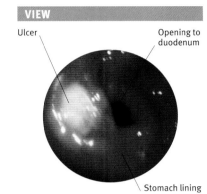

Ulcer
Opening to duodenum
Stomach lining

Gastric ulcer
In this view through an endoscope, a gastric ulcer is clearly visible in the mucous membrane lining the stomach. Close by is the opening from the stomach into the duodenum.

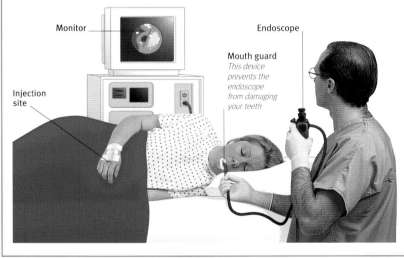

Monitor
Endoscope
Mouth guard
This device prevents the endoscope from damaging your teeth
Injection site

p.157). Endoscopic ultrasound, in which a probe is passed into the stomach to look for evidence of tumour spread, may also be performed.

What is the treatment?
The only effective treatment is early surgery to remove the tumour. However, in the majority of cases the cancer has already spread too widely to be operable. The operation involves the removal of part or all of the stomach. The surrounding lymph nodes are also removed since they are possible sites of cancer spread. In some cases in which the cancer has spread to other parts of the body, surgery may help to improve life expectancy. Surgery may also be carried out to relieve symptoms rather than attempt a cure; for example, if the cancer is obstructing the passage of food, a stent (tube) may be inserted to relieve the blockage. Chemotherapy (p.157) may also be used, either to slow the progress of the disease

and relieve symptoms if the cancer is not operable, or to reduce the risk of the cancer recurring after surgery. Radiotherapy is not commonly used to treat stomach cancer but may sometimes be used to shrink the tumour or help relieve symptoms. Strong painkillers (p.589) may also be given to relieve severe discomfort.

What is the prognosis?
If detected and treated early, stomach cancer has a good cure rate. Some countries in which stomach cancer is common, such as Japan, have efficient screening programmes to detect the cancer early, and in Japan about 90 per cent of people are alive 5 years after diagnosis. In the UK, stomach cancer tends to be diagnosed later and the survival rate is poorer. However, it has improved over the past 40 years, and now about 40 per cent of people survive for at least 1 year after diagnosis and 20 per cent survive for at least 5 years.

Disorders of the liver, gallbladder, and pancreas

One of the main functions of the liver and pancreas is to aid food digestion. The liver makes the digestive fluid bile, which is stored in the gallbladder. The pancreas makes digestive enzymes. These organs have other vital functions. The liver uses digestion products to make new substances such as proteins and fats, and the pancreas produces hormones that control the level of glucose in the blood.

The yellow discoloration of the skin and eyes known as jaundice is a sign of liver disease but also has other causes, which are discussed in the first article in this section. The next two articles cover hepatitis due to viral infection, which is the most common cause of liver disease worldwide, as well as other forms of hepatitis. Excessive alcohol consumption is the main cause of liver disease in Western countries; three articles deal with alcoholic liver disease and its complications – cirrhosis and portal hypertension and varices. Liver cancer is then described; the first type, which originates in the liver, is less common in Western countries than cancer that spreads from other organs to the liver (liver metastases). Liver failure, which may be fatal unless treated with liver transplantation, is also discussed.

Gallstones do not usually cause symptoms and may not need to be treated, as explained in the next articles,

but can lead to inflammation of the gallbladder, called cholecystitis. Articles on the inflammatory conditions, acute and chronic pancreatitis follow, and the final article covers pancreatic cancer, which is relatively uncommon in the UK.

✚ KEY ANATOMY

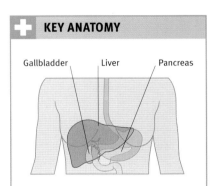

Gallbladder   Liver   Pancreas

For information on the structure and function of the liver, gallbladder, and pancreas, *see* pp.391–396.

Jaundice

Yellow discoloration of the skin and the whites of the eyes

👤 Age, gender, genetics, and lifestyle as risk factors depend on the cause

Jaundice, a yellow discoloration of the skin and the whites of the eyes, is a symptom of many disorders of the liver, gallbladder, or pancreas. It may also be caused by some blood disorders. Jaundice results from excessively high blood levels of the pigment bilirubin, a breakdown product of red blood cells. Bilirubin is processed by the liver and then excreted as a component of the digestive fluid bile.

Jaundice always requires investigation because the underlying disorder may be serious. A few days after birth, many babies develop a form of jaundice that is usually harmless and disappears quickly (*see* **Neonatal jaundice**, p.531).

What are the causes?
Levels of bilirubin in the blood can increase if the amount of bilirubin produced is too great for the liver to process. Damaged liver cells or obstruction of the bile ducts, which carry bile from the liver to the gallbladder

and small intestine, can also lead to high levels of bilirubin in the blood.

Excess red blood cell breakdown In a healthy person, red blood cells have a lifespan of about 120 days, after which they are removed from the blood and broken down by the spleen to produce bilirubin. The bilirubin then passes to the liver. If the number of red blood cells being broken down is above normal, the liver cannot process the large amounts of bilirubin produced. This condition is known as haemolytic jaundice and may be caused by disorders such as haemolytic anaemia (p.273), in which the lifespan of red blood cells is shorter than normal. It may be accompanied by other symptoms, such as tiredness.

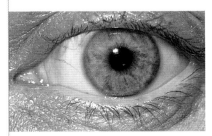

Jaundice
The skin and the white of the eye have become yellow. These symptoms, known as jaundice, can occur as a result of many disorders, including liver disease.

Liver cell damage If the liver cells are damaged, the liver is less able to process bilirubin. Possible causes of damage include infection (*see* **Acute hepatitis**, below, and **Chronic hepatitis**, opposite page), alcohol abuse (*see* **Alcohol-related liver disease**, opposite page), and an adverse reaction to some drugs. Jaundice that is due to liver cell damage is sometimes accompanied by nausea, vomiting, and abdominal pain and swelling.

Bile duct obstruction An obstruction in the bile ducts, the channels through which bile leaves the liver, may result in jaundice. Obstruction may be due to disorders such as pancreatic cancer (p.414) or gallstones (p.412). If bile ducts are blocked, bile builds up in the liver, and bilirubin is forced back into the blood. This type of jaundice may be accompanied by itching, dark-coloured urine, and paler than normal faeces.

What might be done?

Your doctor may arrange blood tests to assess liver function and to look for signs of excess red blood cell destruction, viral hepatitis, or other disorders affecting the liver. Ultrasound scanning (p.135) of your liver and gallbladder may be carried out, and sometimes also more detailed imaging techniques, such as CT scanning (p.132), MRI (p.133), ERCP (p.414), or endoscopic ultrasound (in which a viewing tube with an ultrasound probe attached is inserted into the body). A sample of liver tissue may also be taken and examined for underlying liver disease (*see* **Liver biopsy**, p.410).

If the underlying cause of jaundice can be treated, jaundice will disappear. If the cause is not curable, as in the case of advanced pancreatic cancer, treatment may be given to relieve symptoms associated with jaundice, such as itching.

Acute hepatitis

Sudden, short-term inflammation of the liver due to a variety of causes

 Lifestyle as a risk factor depends on the cause

 Age, gender, and genetics are not significant factors

Short-term inflammation of the liver is known as acute hepatitis. The condition has various causes and has a sudden onset. Most people with acute hepatitis recover within a month or two, but in some cases inflammation of the liver persists for many months or even years (*see* **Chronic hepatitis**, opposite page) or progresses to liver failure (p.411).

What are the causes?

Worldwide, the most common cause of acute hepatitis is infection with any one of the several types of hepatitis viruses. Until the late 1980s, there were only two known hepatitis viruses, hepatitis A and B. Additional hepatitis viruses have now been identified,

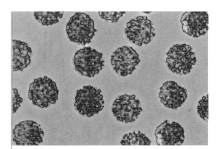

Hepatitis B viruses
This highly magnified image shows hepatitis B viruses. Infection with these viruses is one of the many causes of the acute hepatitis.

including hepatitis C, D, and E. Other hepatitis viruses are almost certainly yet to be discovered. The known viruses can all cause acute hepatitis, and they have many features in common, although the way in which they are transmitted and their long-term effects may differ. Infections with some types of bacteria, other nonhepatitis viruses, and some parasites can also lead to acute hepatitis. In addition, the condition may be caused by noninfectious agents, such as some drugs and toxins, including alcohol (*see* **Alcohol-related liver disease**, opposite page).

Hepatitis A virus The hepatitis A virus is common in southern and eastern Europe and some parts of Africa and Asia, but it is much less common in the UK. However, many cases are not reported because the virus often produces no symptoms or symptoms are so mild that the infection passes unrecognized. The virus can be detected in the urine and faeces of infected people, and it can be transmitted to other people in contaminated food or water.

Hepatitis B virus Worldwide, it is estimated that 240 million people are infected with the hepatitis B virus. In the UK, about 1 in 1,000 people is infected with the virus, and most of them are in high-risk groups, such as immigrants from countries in which there is a high prevalence of the infection, people who have been exposed to unscreened blood products, or intravenous drug users who have shared contaminated needles. The virus is spread by contact with an infected person's body fluids. Therefore it can be spread by sexual intercourse, for example, as well as by contaminated needles. In the UK, blood products are screened for hepatitis B and C, and so such products do not pose the threat of infection. In developing countries, hepatitis B infection is most commonly transmitted from mother to baby at birth. Before blood banks screened blood for the hepatitis B virus, blood transfusions were a source of infection, and a number of people with haemophilia (*see* **Haemophilia**, p.274) contracted hepatitis.

Hepatitis C virus An estimated 130–150 million people worldwide are infected with the hepatitis C virus. There is no accurate information on the number of people infected in the UK but the infection seems to be mainly in those who have been exposed to unscreened blood products (blood is now routinely screened for hepatitis B and C in the UK) or who have shared contaminated needles. There is also a small risk of mothers passing on the infection to their babies, usually at the time of birth. Sexual transmission between heterosexual partners is possible but uncommon, and there is concern about the possibility of sexual transmission between men who have sex with other men.

Hepatitis D virus Infection with hepatitis D occurs only in people who already have hepatitis B infection. It is spread by contact with infected body fluids.

Hepatitis E virus The hepatitis E virus is a rare cause of hepatitis in the UK. The virus is excreted in the faeces of infected people and infection can result from consuming contaminated water or food. The virus is also found in certain animals and can be acquired by eating undercooked meat, such as pork.

Other infectious causes Acute hepatitis may also be caused by other viral infections, such as cytomegalovirus (*see* **Cytomegalovirus infection**, p.167) and the Epstein–Barr virus, the cause of infectious mononucleosis (p.166). Some bacterial infections, such as leptospirosis (p.173) and typhoid (p.172), can cause acute hepatitis. Parasitic infections that may lead to acute hepatitis include infection with plasmodium organisms, the cause of malaria (p.175).

Noninfectious causes In developed countries, excessive alcohol intake is one of the most common causes of acute hepatitis. The disease can also be caused by other toxins, such as those found in poisonous fungi. Certain drugs, such as the anaesthetic gas halothane, some anticonvulsants (p.590), and an overdose of paracetamol (*see* **Painkillers**, p.589), may cause acute hepatitis. Occasionally, the condition occurs in pregnancy, although the cause is not fully understood.

What are the symptoms?

Some people infected with a hepatitis virus have no symptoms or symptoms are so mild that they are not recognized. In other cases, the disorder may be life-threatening. If hepatitis is due to a viral infection, the time from infection to the appearance of symptoms can vary from up to 6 weeks for hepatitis A to 6 months for hepatitis B. Some people who have no symptoms may become carriers of the virus. If symptoms do develop, they may initially include:

- Tiredness and a feeling of ill health.
- Poor appetite.
- Nausea and vomiting.
- Fever.
- Discomfort in the upper right side of the abdomen.

In some cases, several days after the initial symptoms develop, the whites of the eyes and the skin take on a yellow tinge, a condition known as jaundice (p.407). Often, the initial symptoms improve once jaundice appears. At this time, the faeces may become paler than usual, and widespread itching may be present. Acute hepatitis caused by the hepatitis B virus may also cause joint pains.

Severe acute hepatitis may result in liver failure, causing confusion, seizures, and sometimes coma (p.323). Liver failure is relatively common following an overdose of paracetamol but is less common with some types of hepatitis, such as those due to the hepatitis A virus. The hepatitis E virus rarely causes serious illness, although it can cause life-threatening severe acute hepatitis in women who are pregnant.

How is it diagnosed?

If your doctor suspects that you have hepatitis, he or she may arrange for you to have blood tests to evaluate your liver function and to look for possible causes of your symptoms. Blood tests will probably be repeated in order to help monitor your recovery. If the diagnosis is unclear, you may undergo ultrasound scanning (p.135) and may need to have a liver biopsy (p.410).

What is the treatment?

There is no specific treatment for most cases of acute hepatitis, and people are usually advised to rest. Consult your doctor before taking any medicines, such as painkillers, because there is a risk of side effects. If you have viral hepatitis, you will need to take precautions to prevent the spread of the disease, including practising safe sex (p.27).

You should avoid drinking alcohol during the illness and for a minimum of 3 months after you have recovered. However, if the cause was alcohol-related, you will be advised to give up drinking alcohol permanently.

What is the prognosis?

Most people with acute hepatitis feel better after 4–6 weeks and recover by 3 months. However, ongoing (chronic) infection occurs in about 60–80 per cent of those infected with hepatitis C and about 5 per cent of those infected with hepatitis B or hepatitis B and D. Very rarely, hepatitis E may cause chronic infection in those with impaired immunity. People with acute hepatitis caused by an infection other than the hepatitis viruses usually recover completely once the infection has cleared up. Recovery from acute hepatitis caused by excessive alcohol consumption, drugs, or other toxins depends on the extent of the resulting liver damage. The substance that caused acute hepatitis must be avoided in the future.

In the rare cases in which hepatitis progresses to severe liver failure, a liver transplant (p.412) may be necessary.

Can it be prevented?

Infection with hepatitis A and E may be prevented by maintaining good personal hygiene, such as always washing your hands thoroughly before handling food. The risk of infection with hepatitis B, C, and D can be reduced by practising safe sex and by not sharing needles or other objects that might be contaminated with infected body fluids. Those who have recovered from acute hepatitis A or B usually develop lifelong immunity to the respective viruses.

However, there are several different strains of the hepatitis C virus so further infections are possible.

Immunizations against the hepatitis A and B viruses are recommended for those at particular risk of infection, such as travellers (*see* **Travel immunizations**, p.35).

To avoid the transmission of hepatitis through blood transfusions, blood banks routinely screen all blood for the hepatitis B and hepatitis C viruses.

Chronic hepatitis

Inflammation of the liver, due to a variety of causes, that lasts more than 6 months

 Gender, genetics, and lifestyle as risk factors depend on the cause

 Age is not a significant factor

Chronic hepatitis is inflammation of the liver that lasts for at least 6 months. Sometimes, the condition persists for many years. Although chronic hepatitis is often mild with no symptoms, it can slowly damage the liver, causing cirrhosis (p.410), in which healthy liver tissue is replaced by fibrous scar tissue. Eventually, liver failure (p.411) may develop. People who are affected with chronic hepatitis and cirrhosis have a higher than normal risk of developing liver cancer (p.411).

What are the causes?
Chronic hepatitis can have a number of causes, including a viral infection, an autoimmune reaction in which the body's immune system attacks liver cells, certain drugs, alcohol abuse, and some metabolic disorders.

Some of the hepatitis viruses that cause acute hepatitis (opposite page) are more likely than others to cause persistent inflammation. The virus that most commonly causes chronic inflammation is the hepatitis C virus. Less commonly, the hepatitis B and D viruses are responsible. Some people may be unaware that they have had a previous episode of acute viral hepatitis until long-term symptoms of chronic hepatitis appear.

The underlying cause of autoimmune chronic hepatitis is still not known, but the condition is more common among women than it is in men.

Rarely, some drugs, such as isoniazid (*see* **Antituberculous drugs**, p.573) may cause chronic hepatitis. The condition can also result from regular excessive alcohol consumption (*see* **Alcohol-related liver disease**, right).

In addition, chronic hepatitis can be due to rare metabolic diseases in which liver inflammation is caused by excess amounts of certain minerals that accumulate in the body. For example, in the inherited disorder haemochromatosis (p.441) there are abnormally high levels of iron in the blood and tissues.

What are the symptoms?
In some cases, chronic hepatitis causes no symptoms. If symptoms do develop, they are usually mild but can vary in severity. They may include:
- Loss of appetite and weight loss.
- Tiredness.
- Yellowing of the skin and whites of the eyes (*see* **Jaundice**, p.407).
- Swelling of the abdomen.
- Abdominal discomfort.

If cirrhosis develops due to persistent inflammation, there may be increased blood pressure in the blood vessels that connect the digestive tract to the liver. This pressure may lead to bleeding into the digestive tract (*see* **Portal hypertension and varices**, p.410). In some cases, cirrhosis can result in liver failure, which may be fatal.

What might be done?
Your doctor will give you a physical examination and arrange for blood tests to evaluate your liver function and to look for causes of your symptoms. To confirm the diagnosis, he or she may use an imaging technique such as ultrasound scanning (p.135). A liver biopsy (p.410), in which a small piece of liver is taken for microscopic examination, may be used to determine the nature and severity of liver damage.

Chronic hepatitis caused by infection with the hepatitis B or C viruses may respond to treatment with antiviral drugs (p.573). For people with chronic hepatitis B infection, a course of injections of interferon (p.586) or a longer-term course of treatment with antiviral drugs such as tenofovir or entecavir may be recommended. For those with chronic hepatitis C, treatment with interferon and the oral antiviral drug ribavirin was the mainstay of therapy, but new combinations of oral antivirals (such as sofosbuvir, simeprevir, boceprevir, ledipasvir, ombitasvir, and paritaprevir) and ribavirin may be used in some cases and have proved very effective at eliminating the virus from the body.

People with chronic hepatitis caused by an autoimmune reaction are usually treated indefinitely with corticosteroids (p.600), which may be given in combination with other immunosuppressant drugs (p.585). If the liver has been damaged by a drug, it should recover slowly as long as the drug is stopped. If chronic hepatitis is due to a metabolic disorder, treatment of that underlying disorder may slow the progress of liver damage.

What is the prognosis?
The outlook depends on the cause of the hepatitis. Chronic viral hepatitis usually progresses slowly, and it may take decades before problems such as cirrhosis and liver failure develop. People with chronic hepatitis are at increased risk of developing liver cancer, particularly if hepatitis is due to infection with the hepatitis B or C virus.

Without treatment, approximately 1 in 2 people who have autoimmune chronic hepatitis develop liver failure after 5 years.

Hepatitis due to a metabolic disorder tends to get progressively worse, often ending in liver failure. In the case of liver failure, a liver transplant (p.412) may be considered.

Alcohol-related liver disease

Short-term or progressive liver damage due to excessive alcohol consumption

 More common over the age of 30

 More common in males

 Long-term excessive alcohol consumption is a risk factor

 Genetics is not a significant factor

The most common cause of severe long-term liver disease in developed countries is excessive alcohol consumption (*see* **Alcohol and health**, p.24, and **Alcohol dependence**, p.350). More men than women have alcohol-related liver disease because more men drink heavily. However, women are more susceptible to liver damage from alcohol because of differences in the way that men and women metabolize alcohol. The longer excessive alcohol consumption continues, the greater the likelihood of liver disease developing. Long-term alcohol-related liver disease increases the risk of liver cancer (p.411).

What are the types?
Alcohol may cause three types of liver disease: fatty liver, alcoholic hepatitis, and cirrhosis (p.410). Typically, these conditions occur in sequence, but this is not always the case. Over a period of several years, most heavy drinkers develop a fatty liver, in which fat globules develop within liver cells. If alcohol consumption continues, hepatitis (inflammation of the liver) develops. With continued drinking, cirrhosis develops. In this condition, liver cells that are damaged by alcohol are replaced by fibrous scar tissue. If cirrhosis has developed, liver damage is usually irreversible. It is not known why some heavy drinkers go on to develop hepatitis or cirrhosis while others do not.

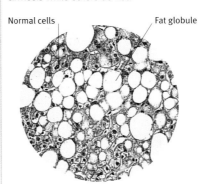

Normal cells | Fat globule

Fatty liver
Excessive alcohol consumption can damage the liver, causing fat globules to form in liver cells, as seen in this magnified view.

What are the symptoms?
In many cases, fatty liver does not cause symptoms and often remains undiagnosed. However, in about 1 in 3 affected people, the liver becomes enlarged, which may lead to discomfort in the right upper abdomen.

Alcoholic hepatitis may also produce no symptoms at first, but after about 10 years of heavy drinking in men and sooner in women, the first symptoms usually develop. These may include:
- Nausea and occasional vomiting.
- Discomfort in the upper right side of the abdomen.
- Weight loss.
- Fever.
- Yellowing of the skin and the whites of the eyes (*see* **Jaundice**, p.407).
- Swollen abdomen.

Cirrhosis often causes no symptoms for a number of years or only mild symptoms, including:
- Poor appetite and weight loss.
- Nausea.
- Muscle wasting.

In some cases, severe cirrhosis may lead to a serious condition in which there is bleeding into the digestive tract from abnormal blood vessels that develop in the wall of the oesophagus (*see* **Portal hypertension and varices**, p.410). Severe alcoholic hepatitis and cirrhosis can lead to liver failure (p.411), which may result in coma (p.323) and death.

How is it diagnosed?
A history of heavy alcohol consumption is essential for the diagnosis of alcohol-related liver disease. It is important that you are honest and tell your doctor exactly how much you drink.

Your doctor may arrange for blood tests to evaluate your liver function. You may also have a liver biopsy (p.410), a procedure in which a hollow needle is inserted into the liver to obtain a sample of liver tissue. The sample is then examined under a microscope to look for cell abnormalities.

What is the treatment?
People with alcohol-related liver disease must stop drinking permanently. Many people need professional help to achieve this. If drinking continues, the disease will probably progress and may be fatal. If drinking stops, the outlook is likely to improve.

Fatty liver often disappears after 3–6 months of abstinence from alcohol. Some people with alcoholic hepatitis who stop drinking recover completely. However, in most cases damage to the liver is irreversible, and the condition progresses to cirrhosis. Severe alcoholic cirrhosis can cause serious complications, which in some cases may be fatal. About half of all people who have cirrhosis die from liver failure within 5 years. More than 1 in 10 people who have cirrhosis go on to develop liver cancer. People who have alcohol-related liver disease but have no other serious health problems and have managed to stop drinking may be candidates for a liver transplant (p.412).

▶ **TEST**

Liver biopsy

In a liver biopsy, a sample of tissue is removed from the liver to diagnose a variety of disorders, including cirrhosis, hepatitis, and cancer. This procedure is performed in hospital under local anaesthesia and the sample is sent to a laboratory for microscopic examination. You will need to remain in bed for up to 6 hours afterwards, lying on your right side at first to prevent bleeding. The biopsy site may be tender for a few days.

During the procedure
A hollow needle is inserted into the liver through a small incision between the right lower ribs. A sample of tissue is collected. You will be asked to exhale and stay completely still until the needle is withdrawn.

Biopsy needle

Rib
Lung
Biopsy needle
Liver
Cartilage

DETAIL

RESULTS

Fibrous tissue

Normal cells

Cirrhosis
This magnified view of a sample of liver tissue shows normal liver cells surrounded by bands of fibrous scar tissue. Such an appearance is typical of the damage caused by cirrhosis.

Many of the symptoms and some of the complications of alcohol-related liver disease can be treated successfully. For example, swelling of the abdomen as a result of fluid accumulating in the abdominal cavity can be reduced by diuretic drugs (p.583) and by following a diet that is low in salt. Nausea and vomiting can frequently be relieved by antiemetic drugs (p.595).

Cirrhosis

Scarring of the liver, occurring in the late stages of various liver disorders

 More common over the age of 40

 More common in males

 In some cases, the underlying cause is inherited

 Long-term excessive alcohol consumption is a risk factor

In cirrhosis, normal liver tissue is destroyed and replaced by fibrous scar tissue. The condition may be caused by several different disorders, including viral infections and excessive alcohol consumption. The liver damage is usually irreversible and prevents the liver from functioning properly. Some people with cirrhosis may feel well for years despite having severe liver damage. However, with time they may develop complications, such as liver failure (opposite page) and liver cancer (opposite page).

Cirrhosis is more common in men than in women in the UK and accounts for about 4,000 deaths a year. Worldwide, cirrhosis resulted in about 1.2 million deaths in 2013.

What are the causes?

There are various causes of cirrhosis. Worldwide, the most common cause is infection with a hepatitis virus, particularly the hepatitis B and C viruses (*see* **Chronic hepatitis**, p.409). However, in developed countries, cirrhosis is most frequently caused by excessive alcohol consumption (*see* **Alcohol-related liver disease**, p.409).

Another cause of liver cirrhosis is the autoimmune disorder primary biliary cirrhosis, which is more common in women than in men. Bile, a liquid produced by the liver to aid digestion, normally leaves the liver through the bile ducts. In primary biliary cirrhosis, the bile ducts become inflamed, blocking the flow of bile from the liver. This causes bile to build up, damaging the liver tissue. Cirrhosis may also be caused by sclerosing cholangitis, a condition in which the bile ducts inside the liver become inflamed. The cause of this condition is not known, although it can be associated with the inflammatory bowel diseases ulcerative colitis (p.417) and Crohn's disease (p.417).

Cirrhosis may also develop after bile duct surgery or as a result of a blockage of the bile ducts by gallstones (p.412). In addition, certain inherited disorders may cause cirrhosis, for example haemochromatosis (p.441), in which excessive amounts of iron accumulate in the body.

What are the symptoms?

Often, cirrhosis produces no symptoms and is detected during a routine examination for another condition. If there are symptoms, they may include:

■ Poor appetite and weight loss.
■ Nausea.
■ Yellowing of the skin and the whites of the eyes (*see* **Jaundice**, p.407).

After some time, life-threatening complications may develop. For example, cirrhosis can lead to high blood pressure in veins in the oesophagus, which causes them to be fragile and to bleed easily (*see* **Portal hypertension and varices**, right). Malnutrition may also develop from being unable to absorb fats and certain vitamins. Eventually, cirrhosis can lead to liver cancer or liver failure. The symptoms of liver failure include a swollen, fluid-filled abdomen and visible spider-like blood vessels in the skin, known as spider naevi. A failing liver may also result in abnormal bleeding and easy bruising. This is as a result of reduced production of blood clotting factors in the liver.

What might be done?

If your doctor suspects that you have cirrhosis from your symptoms, he or she will take blood samples to assess liver function and look for hepatitis viruses. You may also have ultrasound scanning (p.135), CT scanning (p.132), or MRI (p.133) to assess the liver. To confirm the diagnosis, you may have a liver biopsy (above), in which a small sample of tissue is removed from your liver for microscopic examination.

Damage to the liver caused by cirrhosis is usually irreversible. However, if the underlying cause can be treated, further deterioration may be prevented. Whatever the cause of the cirrhosis, you should not drink alcohol. Nutritional deficiencies can be corrected by taking supplements and altering your diet. If the condition worsens but you are otherwise in good health, you may be suitable for a liver transplant (p.412).

What is the prognosis?

The outlook for cirrhosis is extremely variable and depends on the degree of liver damage, whether complications have developed, and whether further damage can be prevented. If the condition is mild, people may live for many years. About 9 in 10 people survive for more than a year after a liver transplant.

Portal hypertension and varices

Elevated pressure in the vein carrying blood to the liver, leading to distended veins, particularly in the oesophagus

 More common in adults, especially those over the age of 40

 More common in males

 Excessive alcohol consumption is a risk factor

Genetics is not a significant factor

In a liver damaged by disease, normal blood flow may become blocked. This obstruction leads to portal hypertension, in which the pressure is increased inside the portal vein, a large vein that carries blood from the digestive tract to the liver. The high pressure forces blood through other smaller veins in the digestive tract. These veins become distended and fragile (like varicose veins in the legs), and are known as varices.

In most cases, varices develop at the lower end of the oesophagus. They are prone to rupture, and heavy bleeding from them can be life-threatening. In some cases, varices develop in other areas of the body, such as in the skin over the abdomen and in the rectum.

Portal hypertension occurs mainly in adults and is more common in men. The condition is often associated with excessive consumption of alcohol (*see* **Alcohol and health**, p.24).

What are the causes?

In Western countries, about 8 in 10 cases of portal hypertension are associated with cirrhosis (left), which is often due to chronic hepatitis (p.409) or long-term alcohol abuse (*see* **Alcohol–related liver disease**, p.409). A blood clot blocking the portal vein, schistosomiasis (p.179), and in rare cases, congenital liver disorders may also cause portal hypertension.

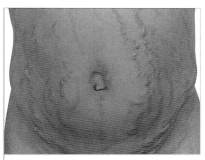

Effect of portal hypertension
Increased pressure in the portal vein, which carries blood from the digestive tract to the liver, can cause distended veins in the skin over the abdomen, as shown here.

What are the symptoms?

Portal hypertension is usually undetected until complications develop. If symptoms develop, they may include:

- Swollen abdomen due to accumulation of fluid (ascites).
- Visible swelling of the veins in the skin over the abdomen, sometimes around the navel.

In about 1 in 3 people with varices in the oesophagus, the veins eventually rupture. The bleeding is usually sudden and massive and leads to vomiting of blood and later passage of black, tarry faeces that contain partly digested blood (*see* **Bleeding from the digestive tract**, p.399). Loss of large volumes of blood can result in shock (p.248). If it is not treated immediately, shock may cause damage to internal organs and lead to disorders such as acute kidney injury (p.450) and liver failure (right). In some cases, the blood loss may be fatal.

What might be done?

Your doctor will check for signs of portal hypertension if you have chronic hepatitis. Ultrasound scanning (p.135) or CT scanning (p.132) may be done to detect enlarged veins, or endoscopy may be used to visualize them (*see* **Upper digestive tract endoscopy**, p.407).

Usually, once the disorder has developed, liver damage is irreversible, but beta-blockers (p.581) may be prescribed to lower pressure in the portal vein and decrease the risk of bleeding from varices.

Ruptured varices require urgent treatment in hospital with intravenous fluids and a blood transfusion (p.272), to replace lost blood. The source of internal bleeding will be investigated using endoscopy. If possible, the varices will be injected through the endoscope with a chemical that causes the vein to close and thus stops bleeding. Alternatively, bands may be placed around the varices during endoscopy. Drugs may also be given to help reduce bleeding.

If these steps do not stop the bleeding, a tube encircled by a deflated balloon may be passed through the mouth into the oesophagus. The balloon is inflated to compress the varices and left in place until bleeding stops. In some cases, a procedure is carried out to allow blood from the digestive tract to bypass the liver: X-rays may be used to direct

the insertion of a tube to connect the portal vein directly to the hepatic vein, through which blood normally leaves the liver.

What is the prognosis?

The outlook depends on whether or not varices develop and bleed and also on the severity of bleeding. About 7 in 10 people survive ruptured varices, but in over half of them bleeding will recur.

Liver cancer

A cancerous tumour that originates in the cells of the liver

 More common with increasing age

 Up to four times more common in males

 Excess alcohol consumption and intravenous drug abuse are risk factors

 Genetics is not a significant factor

Primary liver cancer is cancer of the liver tissue that originates within the liver itself. Tumours in the liver that originate elsewhere in the body are known as secondaries, or liver metastases (*see* right).

Worldwide, liver cancer is one of the more common forms of cancer, accounting for about 1 in 20 of all new cancer cases. However, in developed countries, the disease is less common, and most cases occur following long-standing cirrhosis (opposite page) due to long-term alcohol abuse.

In developing countries, liver cancer is closely linked with viral hepatitis, especially that due to the hepatitis B and C viruses (*see* **Chronic hepatitis**, p.409). People with haemochromatosis (p.441), a condition in which iron builds up in the liver, are also at high risk of developing liver cancer.

Another cause of liver cancer is contamination of food by carcinogens such as aflatoxin, a toxin produced by a fungus that grows on stored grain and peanuts. Occasionally, liver cancer results from infection with a form of liver fluke (a parasitic worm) common in the Far East or exposure to certain chemicals in the workplace.

What are the symptoms?

People with liver cancer may experience the following symptoms:

- Weight loss and fever.
- Pain in the upper right side of the abdomen.
- Yellowing of the skin and the whites of the eyes (*see* **Jaundice**, p.407).

As the disease progresses, the abdomen may become swollen because of an accumulation of fluid (ascites).

What might be done?

Your doctor may suspect liver cancer from your symptoms if you already have cirrhosis. You may have blood tests to look for signs of cancer and to assess liver function. Imaging tests, such as ultrasound scanning

(p.135) or MRI (p.133), may be performed to confirm the diagnosis. You may also have a liver biopsy (opposite page), in which a piece of tissue is removed and tested for cancer cells.

Treatment depends on various factors, such as your general health and the stage of the cancer. If the cancer is not too advanced, surgical removal of the tumour or a liver transplant (p.412) may be possible. In other cases, you may be given chemotherapy (p.157) or localized treatments to reduce the size of the tumour, such as chemoembolization, in which the blood supply to the tumour is blocked, causing it to shrink.

What is the prognosis?

Often the cancer is at an advanced stage by the time it is diagnosed and the outlook is poor; on average, about 10 per cent of people survive for 5 years or more after diagnosis. However, for those who are diagnosed early and are able to have a liver transplant, about 75 per cent survive for at least 5 years after treatment.

Liver metastases

Cancerous tumours in the liver that have spread from other parts of the body

 More common with increasing age

 Gender, genetics, and lifestyle are not significant factors

Metastases are cancerous tumours in the liver that originate from cancers elsewhere in the body, commonly those of the lung, breast, colon, pancreas, and stomach. Other types of cancer, such as leukaemia (p.276) and lymphoma (p.279), may also spread to the liver. Liver metastases form when cancerous cells separate from the original cancer, circulate in the blood, and settle in the liver, where they multiply. Several metastases of varying size may develop.

In developed countries, liver metastases occur more commonly than liver cancer (left). The disease is more common in elderly people.

What are the symptoms?

People may already have symptoms due to the original cancer, but sometimes this cancer is not apparent. The symptoms of liver metastases may be the only warning of illness. They include:

- Weight loss.
- Reduced appetite.
- Fever.
- Pain in the upper right side of the abdomen.
- Yellowing of the skin and the whites of the eyes (*see* **Jaundice**, p.407).

As the disease progresses, the abdomen may become swollen due to enlargement of the liver or fluid accumulation.

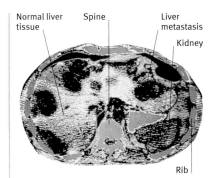

Liver metastases
The dark areas in the liver shown in this CT scan are metastases, which are cancerous tumours that have spread from a cancer elsewhere in the body.

What might be done?

Anyone who has cancer will have tests, such as ultrasound scanning (p.135), CT scanning (p.132), or MRI (p.133), to find out if the liver is affected. To confirm the diagnosis, a piece of liver tissue may be removed for microscopic examination (*see* **Liver biopsy**, opposite page).

Most treatment aims to maintain liver function and relieve symptoms. You may be offered painkillers (p.589) for pain and chemotherapy (p.157) or radiotherapy (p.158) to reduce the size of the metastases. Surgery may be considered if there is a solitary metastasis.

What is the prognosis?

The outlook is generally poor for most people with liver metastases because by this stage the cancer is usually advanced.

Liver failure

Severe impairment of liver function, occurring either suddenly or at the final stages of chronic liver disease

 Excessive alcohol consumption is a risk factor

 Age as a risk factor depends on the cause

 Gender and genetics are not significant factors

The liver performs many vital functions, such as the breakdown of toxins in the blood. Liver failure allows toxin levels to rise, affecting the brain and other organs. In acute liver failure, the liver may fail suddenly. In chronic liver failure, it may fail over months or years.

Acute liver failure may be due to a disorder such as acute viral hepatitis (*see* **Acute hepatitis**, p.408) or damage from drugs, such as an overdose of paracetamol. Chronic liver failure is usually due to an underlying disorder such as alcohol-related liver disease (p.409) or chronic hepatitis (p.409).

What are the symptoms?

The symptoms of acute liver failure can develop over several hours or days and are caused by the effect of toxins on the brain.

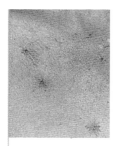

Spider naevi
In people with liver failure, numerous spider-like blood vessels known as spider naevi may appear on the skin, particularly in the chest area.

Symptoms of acute liver failure may include:
- Poor memory.
- Confusion and agitation.
- Drowsiness.

As acute liver failure progresses, other major organs, including the kidneys and the lungs, may gradually begin to fail. The condition may eventually lead to coma (p.323) and death.

Chronic liver failure may produce no symptoms for several months or even years. When the symptoms do begin to appear, they usually develop gradually and may include:
- Yellowing of the skin and whites of the eyes (*see* Jaundice, p.407).
- Itching.
- Easy bruising and bleeding.
- Swollen abdomen.
- Abnormally shaped fingernails.
- Numerous small, spider-like blood vessels in the skin, called spider naevi.
- Redness of the palms of the hands.
- Thickened tissue in the palms of the hands (*see* Dupuytren's contracture, p.231).
- In men, enlargement of the breasts and shrunken testes.

▶ **TREATMENT**

Liver transplant

This procedure involves the transfer of a healthy liver, usually from a recently deceased donor, into a person with liver disease. Sometimes, part of a liver is donated by a living donor. The donor and recipient must have the same blood type. After the transplant, the recipient is monitored in an intensive therapy unit for a few days and remains in hospital for up to 4 weeks. Most transplants are successful, but if the new liver fails, further transplants may be possible.

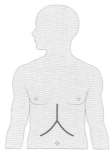

SITE OF INCISION

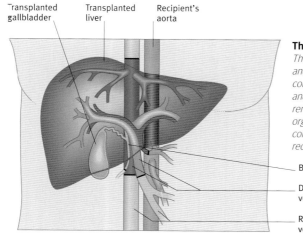

Transplanted gallbladder

Transplanted liver

Recipient's aorta

The procedure
The liver, gallbladder, and portions of the connected blood and bile vessels are removed. The donor organs and vessels are connected to the recipient's vessels.

Bile duct

Donor's blood vessels

Recipient's blood vessels

Bleeding into the digestive tract may occur from enlarged blood vessels that form in the wall of the oesophagus (*see* Portal hypertension and varices, p.410). Sometimes, chronic liver failure deteriorates suddenly and causes the symptoms of acute liver failure.

What might be done?
Liver failure that has deteriorated suddenly requires immediate hospital care, often in an intensive therapy unit (p.618). Antibiotics (p.572) may be given to reduce the numbers of intestinal bacteria. These bacteria produce toxins that accumulate in the blood and adversely affect the brain and other organs.

If you have chronic liver failure, your doctor will arrange for blood tests to determine the extent of damage to the liver. You may need to follow a diet that is low in protein to reduce the work of the liver and minimize the build-up of potentially damaging toxins. Your doctor may also advise you to reduce the salt in your diet and may prescribe diuretic drugs (p.583) to reduce swelling of the abdomen. You should stop drinking alcohol immediately and permanently. There is no treatment that can repair the damage that has already occurred to the liver.

What is the prognosis?
Most people who have severe liver failure need a liver transplant (below) to survive. Fewer than 1 in 10 people survive acute liver failure without a transplant. In those who do survive, the liver often recovers completely, provided that it was previously undamaged. In chronic liver failure, the outlook largely depends on the underlying cause. Many people with chronic liver failure lead normal lives for many years.

Gallstones

Stones of various sizes and content that form in the gallbladder

 More common over the age of 40; rare in childhood

 Twice as common in females

 Sometimes run in families; more common in people of Asian and white European origin

 Being overweight and eating a high-fat diet are risk factors

Gallstones occur in about 1 in 10 people over the age of 40, with twice as many women as men being affected. The stones usually occur in the gallbladder, and, in most cases, do not cause symptoms. Gallstones are formed from bile, a liquid that aids digestion and is produced by the liver and then stored in the gallbladder. Bile is made up mainly of the fatty substance cholesterol, pigments, and various salts. A change in the composition of bile may trigger stone formation. Most gallstones are a mixture of cholesterol, calcium salts, and pigments. In about 1 in 5 cases, stones consist of cholesterol only, and in about 1 in 20 cases, stones consist of pigment only. Often, there are many stones, and some can reach the size of a golf ball. Gallstones may run in families, and they are more common in people of Asian and white European origin, for reasons that are unclear.

What are the causes?
There is often no obvious cause for gallstones. However, cholesterol stones are more common in people who are very overweight (*see* Obesity in adults, p.400) and the risk of stones forming may also be greater than normal in people who have a high-fat diet.

Pigment stones may form if there is excessive destruction of red blood cells, as in the disorders haemolytic anaemia (p.273) and sickle-cell disease (p.272). Insufficient emptying of the gallbladder caused by narrowed bile ducts may also increase the risk of gallstones.

What are the symptoms?
Gallstones often cause no symptoms. However, symptoms may occur if one or more stones block the cystic duct (the exit tube from the gallbladder) or the common bile duct (the main bile duct from the liver to the duodenum). A stone that partially or completely blocks the flow of bile will cause attacks known as biliary colic, which cause symptoms that may include:
- Mild to severe upper abdominal pain.
- Nausea and vomiting.

Episodes are normally brief and typically occur following a fatty meal, which causes the gallbladder to contract.

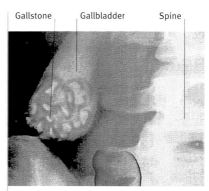

Gallstone   Gallbladder   Spine

Gallstones
A gallbladder full of gallstones is visible in this colour-enhanced X-ray. In some people, gallstones are detected only when an X-ray is taken for another purpose.

Are there complications?
Stones that remain lodged in the bile ducts block the drainage of bile. This can cause severe inflammation or infection of the gallbladder (*see* Cholecystitis, opposite page). Blocked bile ducts may also cause jaundice (p.407), in which the skin and whites of the eyes become yellow. In addition to jaundice, blockage of the common bile duct may cause inflammation of the pancreas (*see* Acute pancreatitis, opposite page).

How are they diagnosed?
Most people only become aware that they have gallstones by chance when an unrelated condition is being investigated. However, if your doctor suspects from your symptoms that you have gallstones, you may have blood tests to check your red blood cell count and cholesterol levels. You may also have imaging tests, such as ultrasound scanning (p.135). If a bile duct is found to be blocked, the exact position of the gallstones may be located using a special imaging procedure called ERCP (p.414), in which an endoscope (viewing tube) is used to inject a special dye into the bile ducts prior to X-rays being taken, or by an MRI scan (p.133).

What is the treatment?
Gallstones that do not cause symptoms need no treatment. If you have mild or infrequent symptoms, adopting a diet that is low in fat may prevent further discomfort. However, if your symptoms are persistent or become worse, you may have your gallbladder removed by conventional surgery or by minimal access surgery (*see* Having minimally invasive surgery, p.612). Removal of the gallbladder usually cures the problem. However, in very rare cases, the stones re-form in the bile duct and may need to be removed by open surgery or during ERCP. The absence of a gallbladder does not usually cause any health problems, and the bile simply drains continuously through a duct directly into the intestines.

Drugs are available that dissolve gallstones made of pure cholesterol, but it may take months or years for the stones to dissolve completely. Occasionally, you may be treated with ultrasonic shock waves (*see*

Lithotripsy, p.448), which shatter the stones into tiny pieces so that they pass painlessly into the small intestine and are excreted in the faeces. Use of drugs or ultrasonic shock waves avoids the need for surgery. However, because the gallbladder is still present there is an ongoing risk that further gallstones will form and so these therapies are rarely used.

Cholecystitis

Inflammation of the gallbladder, usually associated with gallstones blocking the flow of the digestive fluid bile

 More common over the age of 40; rare in childhood

 Twice as common in females

 Sometimes runs in families

 Being overweight and a high-fat diet are risk factors

Cholecystitis is inflammation of the gallbladder wall. It usually occurs when the outlet from the gallbladder, through which the digestive liquid bile is normally released, becomes blocked by a gallstone (opposite page). Bile becomes trapped in the gallbladder, causing inflammation of its walls. A bacterial infection may then develop in the stagnant bile. In rare cases, cholecystitis occurs when there are no gallstones present.

Anyone with gallstones is at risk of developing cholecystitis. Gallstones are more common in people over 40 and in women and sometimes run in families. Gallstones are associated with obesity (p.400), a high-fat diet, and blood disorders, such as sickle-cell disease (p.272).

What are the symptoms?

The symptoms of cholecystitis can vary in severity. They usually develop over a period of hours and may include:

- Constant pain in the right side of the abdomen, just below the ribcage.
- Pain in the right shoulder.
- Nausea and vomiting.
- Fever and chills.

Sometimes, jaundice (p.407), causing yellowing of the skin and the whites of the eyes, may develop. Symptoms often improve over a few days and disappear after about a week. However, in some cases symptoms become progressively worse and need urgent treatment.

Rarely, bacterial infection may cause the gallbladder to perforate. This allows irritant bile to leak into the abdomen, resulting in peritonitis (p.421), a serious condition in which the peritoneum (the membrane lining the wall of the abdomen) becomes inflamed. Cholecystitis may also be accompanied by acute pancreatitis (right), in which there is sudden inflammation of the pancreas.

What might be done?

Your doctor may suspect cholecystitis from your symptoms and after a physical examination. If so, he or she may arrange for you to have ultrasound scanning (p.135) or CT scanning (p.132) to confirm the diagnosis and to indicate the position of any gallstones.

What is the treatment?

If your symptoms are mild, you may be treated at home with antibiotics (p.572) and painkillers (p.589). If your symptoms are severe, you will need treatment in hospital with intravenous fluids, painkillers, and antibiotics. You may have a tube passed into your nose and down to your stomach to remove the contents by suction. This procedure stops digestive juices from entering the duodenum, which would cause the gallbladder to contract.

Although cholecystitis often subsides after treatment with antibiotics, surgery to remove the gallbladder is usually recommended to prevent the condition from recurring. Surgery is always necessary if complications arise, such as perforation of the gallbladder.

What is the prognosis?

Removal of the gallbladder, at the time cholecystitis occurs or some weeks later, prevents recurrences of the disorder. Absence of the gallbladder has no long-term ill effects on the digestive system.

Acute pancreatitis

Sudden inflammation of the pancreas due to damage from its own enzymes

 Almost exclusively affects adults

 Excessive alcohol consumption is a risk factor

 Gender and genetics are not significant factors

In acute pancreatitis, the pancreas suddenly becomes inflamed, causing severe abdominal pain. The condition is serious and can be life-threatening if left untreated. The main function of the pancreas is to secrete a fluid containing enzymes that aid digestion. In addition, the pancreas secretes the hormones insulin and glucagon, which control the level of sugar in the blood.

What are the causes?

Often, the cause of acute pancreatitis is unclear. If there is a cause, it may be a gallstone (opposite page) blocking the common bile duct (the duct that transports bile from the liver to the duodenum). The gallstone obstructs the flow of digestive juices from the pancreas so that enzymes in these juices leak into the pancreatic tissue and cause severe inflammation.

Excessive alcohol consumption over a long period can also cause the disorder. However, it is not fully understood how alcohol causes inflammation of the pancreas. Typically, an attack of acute pancreatitis occurs 12–24 hours after a heavy bout of drinking.

Certain drugs such as immunosuppressants (p.585) and thiazide diuretics (p.583) can cause pancreatitis. Less common causes include viral infection of the pancreas and high levels of fatty substances in the blood (*see* Inherited hyperlipidaemias, p.440).

What are the symptoms?

Acute pancreatitis causes a range of symptoms that occur suddenly and may be severe. These symptoms may include:

- Severe upper abdominal pain, often spreading to the back and made worse by movement.
- Nausea and vomiting.
- Bruised appearance of the skin around the abdomen.
- Fever.

In severe cases, inflammation affects the whole abdomen, making it rigid and increasing the pain (*see* Peritonitis, p.421). There is also a risk of shock (p.248), a potentially fatal condition in which blood pressure falls extremely low.

How is it diagnosed?

If your doctor suspects that you have acute pancreatitis, you will be admitted to hospital, where you may have blood tests to detect pancreatic enzymes that have leaked directly into the blood. You may need imaging tests, such as CT scanning (p.132), ultrasound scanning (p.135), or MRI (p.133), to look for a blockage of the common bile duct by gallstones. The imaging tests may also reveal enlargement of the pancreas due to inflammation.

What is the treatment?

If you have acute pancreatitis and the condition is severe, you may need continuous monitoring in an intensive therapy unit (p.618). Your stomach will be kept empty to prevent the pancreas from being stimulated to produce more enzymes. A tube will be passed through your nose into your stomach to remove its contents by suction, and you will be given fluids intravenously. If imaging tests have detected a

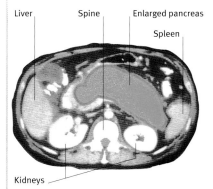

Liver | Spine | Enlarged pancreas
Spleen
Kidneys

Acute pancreatitis
The enlarged pancreas seen in this CT scan through the abdomen is due to the inflammatory disorder acute pancreatitis.

gallstone, ERCP (p.414) may be performed to locate the stone more precisely and remove it. In rare cases, damaged pancreatic tissue becomes infected and may need to be drained. If the pancreatitis was caused by gallstones, it may be advisable to have your gallbladder removed once you have recovered.

What is the prognosis?

Most people survive an attack of acute pancreatitis, but the gland may be damaged so that it is unable to produce adequate amounts of enzymes. You may then need to take enzyme supplements. Severe damage to the hormone-secreting areas of the pancreas may affect the production of insulin and lead to diabetes mellitus (p.437). Treatment with insulin will then be necessary to control your blood sugar levels. A single attack of acute pancreatitis may not cause permanent damage, and long-term treatment is needed only if the condition recurs. If your gallbladder is removed because of stones, there should be no long-term ill effects.

Chronic pancreatitis

Long-term inflammation of the pancreas, leading to progressive loss of function

 Most common between the ages of 35 and 45

 Excessive alcohol consumption is a risk factor

 Gender and genetics are not significant factors

Chronic pancreatitis is a progressive disorder in which the pancreas is persistently inflamed. One of the functions of the pancreas is to secrete a fluid containing digestive enzymes that is added to the intestinal contents. The pancreas also forms the hormones insulin and glucagon, which are released into the bloodstream to control blood sugar levels. In chronic pancreatitis, normal pancreatic tissue becomes damaged and is replaced by scar tissue, gradually impairing pancreatic function. The condition is usually painful and may lead to complications. Damage to the pancreas is usually irreversible.

What are the causes?

Most cases of chronic pancreatitis are due to long-term alcohol abuse. In most other cases, the causes are unknown. In a few cases, chronic pancreatitis may be associated with cystic fibrosis (p.535) or certain rare genetic conditions.

What are the symptoms?

Symptoms of chronic pancreatitis usually develop over several years and vary in severity depending on the extent of damage to the pancreas. Most people do not experience symptoms during the early stages, but, as the disease progresses, they may develop symptoms such as:

▶ **TEST**

ERCP

Endoscopic retrograde cholangiopancreatography (ERCP) is a procedure used to look for, and sometimes treat, blockages or other abnormalities in the bile ducts and pancreatic duct. Contrast dye is injected into the ducts using an endoscope passed through the mouth into the duodenum. The doctor's view down the endoscope can also be seen on a monitor. The flow of the dye is followed on X-ray images shown on a second monitor. ERCP is done in hospital under sedation and takes up to an hour.

Endoscope
Liver
Endoscope
Gallbladder
Duodenum
Stomach
Duodenum

ROUTE OF ENDOSCOPE

Common bile duct
Pancreatic duct
Pancreas

DETAIL

During the procedure
The endoscope is passed painlessly down the throat into the duodenum, and dye is injected into the ducts.

ERCP monitor | **X-ray monitor** | **X-ray beam**

X-ray machine | **Site of injection** | **Endoscope**

RESULTS

Endoscope
Common bile duct
Gallbladder

Contrast X-ray
The common bile duct and gallbladder, made visible by a dye injected through the endoscope, appear normal.

■ Persistent upper abdominal pain, often radiating to the back.
■ Nausea and vomiting.
■ Loss of appetite.
Complications result mainly from the reduced production of enzymes and hormones. A reduced level of pancreatic enzymes causes malabsorption (p.415), which may lead to greasy, bulky stools, vitamin deficiencies, and weight loss. Diabetes mellitus (p.437) may result if the production of insulin is reduced.

How is it diagnosed?
There is no simple test to diagnose chronic pancreatitis. Your doctor may arrange for X-rays (p.131), ultrasound scanning (p.135), or MRI (p.133) to look for calcium deposits in the pancreas, which are an indication that the pancreas has been inflamed. Other tests may include ERCP (above), in which a tube-like instrument called an endoscope is used to inject a contrast dye into the pancreatic duct to look for abnormalities. You may also have ultrasound scanning, which may be done through an endoscope, to look for gallstones. In addition, you may have blood tests to determine blood sugar levels.

What is the treatment?
Your doctor will probably advise you to avoid alcohol and fatty foods. You may need drugs to replace the hormones and enzymes that should be produced by the pancreas. Enzymes in tablet or powder form can be taken with each meal to aid digestion. Regular injections of insulin may also be necessary to control blood sugar levels and will probably be needed for life. If pain is severe, strong opiate painkillers (p.589) are given. In some cases, pain may be relieved by a nerve block. In this procedure, an injection is used to destroy the nerves that carry pain sensations from the pancreas to the spinal cord.

What is the prognosis?
The symptoms of chronic pancreatitis may recede over time, but in some cases the disorder worsens and symptoms become more severe. People who have chronic pancreatitis are more likely to develop pancreatic cancer (right).

Pancreatic cancer

A cancerous tumour of the pancreas that may cause no symptoms in its early stages

 More common over the age of 60

 Slightly more common in females

 Rarely, runs in families

 Smoking, a high-fat diet, and drinking alcohol to excess are risk factors

Pancreatic cancer is a relatively rare disorder; it is diagnosed in about 8,800 people every year in the UK. The disease mainly affects people over 60 and is slightly more common in women than in men. Pancreatic cancer is almost always fatal and is one of the 10 most common causes of death from cancer in the UK.

People with pancreatic cancer usually have few symptoms until the disorder reaches an advanced stage and often not

until it has spread to other parts of the body, typically to the lymph nodes in the abdomen and the liver.

Little is known about the causes of pancreatic cancer, but it has been linked with diet, in particular with fatty foods and high alcohol consumption. In a few cases, the cancer runs in a family, which indicates that a genetic factor may be involved in such cases. The risk of the disease is greater in people who smoke and in those with chronic pancreatitis (p.413).

What are the symptoms?
Symptoms often develop gradually over a few months and may include:
■ Pain in the upper abdomen that radiates to the back.
■ Loss of weight.
■ Reduced appetite.
Many pancreatic tumours cause obstruction of the bile ducts, through which the digestive liquid bile leaves the liver. Such blockage leads to jaundice (p.407), in which the skin and whites of the eyes turn yellow. Jaundice may be accompanied by itching, dark-coloured urine, and paler than normal faeces.

How is it diagnosed?
Imaging techniques, such as ultrasound scanning (p.135), CT scanning (p.132), or MRI (p.133), are normally used to diagnose pancreatic cancer. In addition, specialized imaging procedures such as ERCP (left) and ultrasound scanning through an endoscope may be used to look for abnormalities in the bile and pancreatic ducts. To confirm the diagnosis, a sample of pancreatic tissue may be taken for microscopic examination.

What is the treatment?
Surgery to remove part or all of the pancreas offers the only chance of cure. However, the cancer has usually spread by the time it is diagnosed. In such cases, the aim is to relieve symptoms and slow the progression of the disease. For example, if the bile duct is obstructed by a tumour, a tube or coil known as a stent may be inserted to keep the duct open. This procedure is usually carried out during ERCP and helps to reduce jaundice. Treatment such as chemotherapy (p.157) and radiotherapy (p.158) may be used to slow the progress of the disease.

Pain can often be relieved with painkillers (p.589). If the pain is severe, it may be treated by a nerve block, a procedure using an injection of a chemical to inactivate the nerves supplying the pancreas.

What is the prognosis?
In many cases, pancreatic cancer is not diagnosed until it has reached an advanced stage, at which time the outlook is poor. Most people survive for less than a year after diagnosis, and less than 5 per cent survive for more than 5 years. Even with surgery, only 7 to 25 per cent survive for more than 5 years.

Disorders of the intestines, rectum, and anus

The intestines, rectum, and anus are exposed to infectious agents and toxins in food, and disorders resulting from these factors are common. Disorders may also be linked to diet, but in many other cases the cause is unknown. Many problems cause changes in the consistency of faeces and in the frequency of bowel movements.

The first article in this section covers irritable bowel syndrome, an extremely common disorder affecting about 2 in 10 people. Disorders that affect the body's ability to absorb nutrients from food, such as malabsorption and lactose intolerance are described next. Two subsequent articles deal with the inflammatory bowel disorders Crohn's disease and ulcerative colitis. Digestive disorders that can affect the movement of the intestinal contents, such as hernias, are then discussed. The section also covers appendicitis and colorectal cancer, a common cause of death due to cancer in the UK. Disorders of the rectum and anus are described last.

Articles on diarrhoea (p.397) and constipation (p.398) can be found in the section that deals with general digestive and nutritional problems. Intestinal infections (*see* **Infections and infestations**, pp.160–180) and intestinal disorders in children (*see* **Infancy and childhood**, pp.524–565) are also covered elsewhere in the book.

KEY ANATOMY

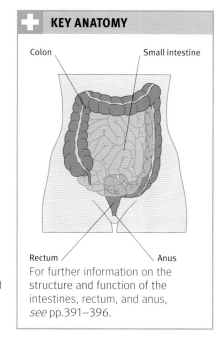

For further information on the structure and function of the intestines, rectum, and anus, *see* pp.391–396.

Irritable bowel syndrome

A combination of intermittent abdominal pain, constipation, and/or diarrhoea

 Most commonly develops between the ages of 20 and 30

 Twice as common in females

 Sometimes runs in families

 Stress and certain foods may make symptoms worse

Irritable bowel syndrome accounts for more referrals to gastroenterologists than any other disorder, although many affected people never consult a doctor. The condition most often develops in people between the ages of 20 and 30 and is twice as common in women as in men. As many as 2 in 10 people have symptoms of irritable bowel syndrome at some time in their lives. The symptoms, which include abdominal pain, constipation, and/or diarrhoea, tend to be intermittent but typically persist for many years. Although irritable bowel syndrome can be distressing, it does not lead to serious complications.

What are the causes?
The precise cause of irritable bowel syndrome is unknown. It may result from abnormal contractions of the muscles in the intestinal walls. An increased sensitivity to certain foods, such as fruit, sorbitol (an artificial sweetener), and fat, may also contribute. The disorder sometimes develops after a gastrointestinal infection (*see* **Gastroenteritis**, p.398). The problem can run in families, which suggests that genetic factors may be involved. Stress, anxiety, and depression can be associated with irritable bowel syndrome and may make symptoms worse.

What are the symptoms?
The symptoms are typically intermittent but usually recur for many years and often persist into old age. They vary widely among people and with each episode. The main symptoms include:
- Abdominal bloating combined with excessive quantities of wind.
- Abdominal pain, often on the lower left side, that may be relieved by defecation or passing wind.
- Diarrhoea, which may be most severe on waking and sometimes alternates with bouts of constipation that may produce "rabbit pellet" stools.
- Feeling that the bowel has not been emptied completely.
- Passage of mucus during defecation.
- Nausea and vomiting.
- Feeling of fullness and difficulty in finishing meals.

Many people have symptoms unrelated to the digestive tract, such as tiredness, headache, back pain, and an increased urge to pass urine. In women, sexual intercourse may be painful, and symptoms may be worse before menstrual periods.

You should consult your doctor if the symptoms are severe, persistent, or recurrent or if you have unexpectedly lost weight. If you are over 40 when the symptoms first develop, you should seek medical advice so that serious disorders with similar symptoms, such as colorectal cancer (p.421), can be ruled out.

How is it diagnosed?
There is no single test for irritable bowel syndrome and the diagnosis is made on the basis of your symptoms, medical history, and often tests to exclude other possible disorders. The type and number of tests used to investigate the disorder depend on your age.

If your symptoms suggest that you may have an inflammatory bowel disorder such as Crohn's disease (p.417) or if you are over the age of 40, your doctor will probably want to investigate your symptoms further. You may have a blood or faecal sample test to check for bowel inflammation. If the result is positive or if your doctor suspects a colorectal tumour, you will probably have a colonoscopy (p.418). You may also have tests to exclude food intolerance (p.416) and lactose intolerance (p.416), which cause symptoms similar to those of irritable bowel syndrome.

SELF-HELP

Living with irritable bowel syndrome

Some people learn to control the symptoms of irritable bowel syndrome by making dietary and lifestyle changes. The symptoms may improve if you follow a diet that is high in fibre and low in fat (*see* **Diet and health**, p.16). You may need to try several different approaches before finding one that helps you. Try the following:
- Keep a food diary. Try to eliminate any food or drink that seems to bring on an attack of irritable bowel syndrome.
- Avoid large meals; spicy, fried, fatty foods; and milk products.
- If constipation is a problem, try gradually increasing your fibre intake. If bloating and diarrhoea are particular problems, reduce your fibre intake.
- Cut out or reduce your intake of tea, coffee, milk, cola, and beer.
- Eat at regular times.
- Stop smoking.
- Try relaxation exercises (p.32) to alleviate stress, which is often a contributing factor.

What is the treatment?
Although the symptoms can be distressing, irritable bowel syndrome is not a serious condition. You should be able to control your symptoms with a combination of a change in diet and relaxation techniques (*see* **Living with irritable bowel syndrome**, below left). However, if symptoms are troublesome enough to interfere with daily routines, you should consult your doctor for advice on treatment. You may be given antispasmodic drugs to relax the contractions of the digestive tract and help to relieve abdominal pain (*see* **Antispasmodic drugs and motility stimulants**, p.598). Your doctor may also prescribe antidiarrhoeal drugs (p.597) to help to alleviate diarrhoea, especially if you have diarrhoea on waking. If you regularly have problems with constipation, bulk-forming agents (*see* **Laxatives**, p.597) may help.

If you have psychological symptoms such as anxiety or depression in addition to irritable bowel syndrome, your doctor may refer you to a therapist for advice on controlling them.

Irritable bowel syndrome tends to be a long-term disorder, often lasting into old age. However, attacks usually become less frequent and severe with time.

Malabsorption

Impaired absorption of nutrients from the small intestine

 Sometimes runs in families

 Age, gender, and lifestyle as risk factors depend on the cause

Malabsorption occurs when the small intestine cannot absorb nutrients from food passing through it. The disorder may cause various symptoms, including diarrhoea and weight loss. If malabsorption is left untreated, certain nutritional deficiencies (p.399) can develop, which may lead to further problems, such as anaemia (p.271) or nerve damage (*see* **Nutritional neuropathies**, p.337).

What are the causes?
Malabsorption is due to disorders that result in inadequate breakdown of food during digestion, damage to the lining of the small intestine, or impairment of motility, which is the ability of the muscular intestinal walls to contract.

In some cases, the small intestine cannot break down food because digestive enzymes or juices are missing or in short supply. For example, disorders affecting the pancreas, the organ that produces digestive juices, may prevent the breakdown of food. Such disorders include chronic pancreatitis (p.413) and cystic fibrosis (p.535). Sometimes, there is a problem in breaking down a specific nutrient. For example, people with lactose intolerance (opposite page) lack an enzyme in the intestine needed to break down the sugar lactose from milk.

Damage to the lining of the intestine may result from inflammation due to disorders such as coeliac disease (right) and Crohn's disease (opposite page) and certain infections, such as giardiasis (p.176). As a result, nutrients are unable to cross the lining and pass into the bloodstream. In the autoimmune disorder scleroderma (p.281), changes in the structure of the intestinal walls affect motility and lead to malabsorption of nutrients. Diabetes mellitus (p.437) may cause abnormal motility and malabsorption by damaging the nerves that supply the muscles in the intestinal walls.

What are the symptoms?
The most common symptoms of malabsorption include:
■ Bulky, pale, foul-smelling diarrhoea.
■ Flatulence and abdominal bloating.
■ Weight loss.
■ Abdominal pain with cramps.
■ Tiredness and weakness.
Left untreated, malabsorption can lead to deficiencies in vitamin B$_{12}$ and iron, which may result in anaemia, the symptoms of which include pale skin and shortness of breath. A deficiency of vitamin B$_{12}$ can also affect the spinal cord and peripheral nerves, causing numbness and tingling in the hands and feet.

How is it diagnosed?
Your doctor may arrange for a variety of blood tests to look for anaemia, vitamin deficiencies, and other signs of malabsorption. If the doctor suspects that your pancreas is damaged, he or she will probably arrange additional tests to assess its function. A test may be carried out to confirm the enzyme deficiency that causes lactose intolerance.

Further tests may be carried out to check for other disorders of the small intestine. You may have a blood test to look for the antibodies that are present in coeliac disease. A special X-ray in which barium is used to highlight the inside of the small intestine (see **Contrast X-rays**, p.132) or an MRI or CT scan may be carried out to look for damage to the digestive tract caused by Crohn's disease. You may also require an endoscopy (p.138) to obtain a sample of intestinal tissue for microscopic analysis.

What is the treatment?
If possible, the underlying cause of the malabsorption is treated. Coeliac disease can usually be treated with a special diet, and Crohn's disease usually responds to corticosteroids (p.600) or mesalazine (see **Aminosalicylate drugs**, p.596). If the cause of malabsorption is giardiasis, antiprotozoal drugs (p.574) will be prescribed. Specific nutritional deficiencies can be corrected by taking vitamin and mineral supplements (see **Vitamins**, p.598, and **Minerals**, p.599).

If you are severely malnourished, you may need treatment in hospital, where you will be given intravenous nutrients or special liquid food supplements.

Most disorders that lead to malabsorption can be treated effectively, and the majority of affected people recover fully from the condition.

Food intolerance

Symptoms that are related to eating a specific food

 Age, gender, genetics, and lifestyle are not significant factors

If you develop troublesome symptoms such as stomachache each time you eat a particular food, you may have food intolerance. The cause of food intolerance is usually unknown, although in some cases there is a definite abnormality, such as an enzyme deficiency (see **Lactose intolerance**, right). Food intolerance is different from a food allergy (p.284), in which the immune system reacts inappropriately to a specific food.

What are the symptoms?
The symptoms of food intolerance vary among individuals. Symptoms are usually related to a particular type of food, such as milk or wheat flour. They may occur within minutes or hours of eating and include the following:
■ Nausea and vomiting.
■ Abdominal pain.
■ Diarrhoea.
Some people develop other symptoms, such as aching muscles or headaches.

What might be done?
In most cases of food intolerance, the diagnosis is based on your symptoms. Tests may then be performed to exclude other possible conditions. In some cases, endoscopy (see **Upper digestive tract endoscopy**, p.407) may be carried out to examine the digestive tract with a flexible viewing tube and to look for evidence of an intestinal disorder such as coeliac disease (right). During the procedure, a small sample of tissue may be taken from the intestinal wall for examination under a microscope.

Often, the only way to diagnose food intolerance is by an exclusion diet, in which the suspect food is excluded from your diet for a period of time to see if there is an improvement in your symptoms. The food is later reintroduced, and you are monitored to see if your symptoms worsen. An exclusion diet, especially one for a child, should be undertaken only under the supervision of a doctor and a dietitian because restricted diets can cause vitamin and mineral deficiencies.

Once the cause of your intolerance has been identified, you should avoid eating foods that aggravate the problem. You will probably need to consult a dietitian, who will advise you on a diet that excludes the problem foods but still provides all the nutrients you need.

Lactose intolerance

An inability to digest lactose, the natural sugar found in milk

 Most commonly develops from adolescence onwards

 More common in certain ethnic groups

 Gender and lifestyle are not significant factors

A person who is lactose intolerant is unable to digest lactose, a natural sugar found in milk and dairy products. As a result, the lactose remains undigested in the intestines. In an affected person, even small amounts of lactose can cause abdominal pain and diarrhoea. Lactose intolerance usually develops in adolescence or adulthood, and only rarely affects babies. Worldwide, about 8 in 10 people of African, Native American, Asian, and Jewish origin develop an inability to digest lactose in the diet.

What are the causes?
Normally, the enzyme lactase breaks down lactose in the intestines to form the sugars glucose and galactose, which are easily absorbed through the intestinal wall. If this enzyme is absent, the unabsorbed lactose ferments in the large intestine and produces painful symptoms. Although high levels of lactase are present at birth, in many ethnic groups the levels can drop with increasing age, becoming very low by adolescence so that lactose can no longer be digested.

In children and babies, lactose intolerance sometimes develops temporarily following an attack of gastroenteritis (p.398) that causes short-term damage to the lining of the intestine.

What are the symptoms?
The symptoms of lactose intolerance usually develop a few hours after eating or drinking products containing milk. They may include the following:
■ Abdominal bloating and cramping.
■ Diarrhoea.
■ Vomiting.
The severity of the symptoms depends on the degree of lactase deficiency. One person may experience symptoms only after drinking several glasses of milk, but another may feel discomfort after consuming only a small amount of a dairy product.

What might be done?
Your doctor may be able to diagnose lactose intolerance from your symptoms. He or she will probably ask you to keep a diary of all the foods you eat and the symptoms that occur. You may then have a specialized test to confirm lactose intolerance. Alternatively, your doctor may ask you to eliminate all dairy products from your diet for a few days. If your symptoms improve but return when dairy products are reintroduced into your diet, the diagnosis of lactose intolerance is confirmed.

Lactose intolerance is usually permanent in adults. However, the symptoms can be completely relieved by eliminating lactose from the diet. In order to achieve this aim, it is important to remember that you should avoid all dairy products, such as milk, yogurt, cheese, cream, and butter. Milk products that have been specially treated by having the lactose broken down are available over the counter. In addition, your doctor may suggest that you take lactase supplements in the form of liquid or capsules. In babies whose lactose intolerance is caused by gastroenteritis, the condition usually improves over several days and milk can be continued during this period.

Coeliac disease

Malabsorption due to the intestine being damaged by a reaction to gluten, a protein found in many foods

 Typically occurs in the first year of life but can occur at any age

 More common in females

 Sometimes runs in families

 Lifestyle is not a significant factor

Coeliac disease, commonly called sprue, is a condition caused by the protein gluten, which is found in wheat, rye, barley, and to some extent in oats. In people with the disease, the lining of the small intestine is damaged so that food cannot be properly absorbed (see **Malabsorption**, p.415). The exact mechanism of damage is uncertain, but it seems to be due to an abnormal immune response in which antibodies against gluten are produced. The resulting malabsorption leads to a deficiency of many nutrients, including vitamins and minerals that are vital for good health. Coeliac disease can run in families, which suggests that genetic factors may be involved.

In the UK, coeliac disease affects about 1 in 100 people. The condition is very rare in Africa and Asia.

What are the symptoms?
In babies, the symptoms of coeliac disease first appear soon after cereals are introduced into the diet, usually at 3 or 4 months. In adults, the symptoms usually develop gradually and include:
■ Bulky, loose, foul-smelling faeces that look greasy.
■ Abdominal bloating and flatulence.
■ Weight loss.
■ Weakness and tiredness.
■ Sometimes, a persistent, itchy rash on the knees, buttocks, elbows, and shoulders (see **Blistering diseases**, p.194).
In babies and children, the following symptoms may also occur:
■ Diarrhoea.
■ Failure to grow or gain weight.
■ Muscle wasting, especially around the buttocks.

Vitamin and mineral deficiencies may lead to disorders such as iron-deficiency anaemia (p.271) and osteomalacia (*see* **Osteomalacia and rickets**, p.217), which is due to a lack of vitamin D and calcium. Untreated, coeliac disease may increase the risk of cancers, particularly cancer of the small intestine.

How is it diagnosed?

Your doctor may suspect coeliac disease from your symptoms, especially if you have the characteristic rash described above. A blood test for antibodies may help to confirm the diagnosis. The doctor may suspect the condition in a baby if symptoms developed soon after solid foods were introduced. However, in many cases, coeliac disease is discovered during investigations for other conditions.

Diagnosis involves removing a small sample of tissue from the lining of the small intestine. This procedure is performed using an endoscope inserted through the mouth (*see* **Upper digestive tract endoscopy**, p.407). When the tissue is examined under a microscope, the intestinal lining appears flattened. You may also have blood tests to look for evidence of anaemia.

What is the treatment?

Coeliac disease is treated by removing gluten from your diet. The recommended diet can be complicated, and it is advisable to see a dietitian for guidance. You should avoid foods that contain wheat, rye, and barley. Of the cereals, only rice, corn, and possibly oats are suitable. It is not advisable to eat mustard, pasta, salad dressing, and some margarines because they contain wheat or wheat extracts, and you should avoid drinking beer. Initially, you may also need to take supplements of vitamins (p.598) and minerals (p.599).

Removing gluten from the diet usually produces a substantial and rapid improvement, and eventually the symptoms may totally disappear. However, coeliac disease is a lifelong disorder and may reappear if gluten is reintroduced. Since coeliac disease sometimes runs in families, relatives of an affected person may be screened for the disorder by having a blood test to check for antibodies produced in the disease.

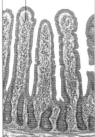
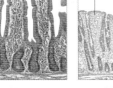

Projection	Flattened surface
NORMAL INTESTINE	**DISEASED INTESTINE**

Intestine in coeliac disease
These magnified sections of small intestine show the effects of coeliac disease. The finger-like projections that normally absorb nutrients are flattened in coeliac disease.

Crohn's disease

A lifelong inflammatory disease that can affect any part of the digestive tract

 Onset most common between the ages of 15 and 30

 Sometimes runs in families; more common in certain ethnic groups

 Smoking is a risk factor

 Gender is not a significant factor

Crohn's disease is a lifelong illness that usually begins in early adulthood and may cause serious ill health throughout life. Areas of the digestive tract become inflamed, causing a range of symptoms such as diarrhoea, abdominal pain, and weight loss. The disorder can occur in any part of the digestive tract from the mouth to the anus. However, the parts most frequently affected are the ileum (the last part of the small intestine) and the colon (the major part of the large intestine). Inflammation often occurs in more than one part of the digestive tract, with unaffected or mildly affected areas between the inflamed areas.

Crohn's disease is a relatively uncommon disorder in the UK, affecting about 115,000 people. In Europe and North America, the condition most commonly affects white people, especially those of Jewish origin, and the onset of symptoms usually occurs between the ages of 15 and 30. The symptoms of Crohn's disease tend to recur despite treatment, and the condition is lifelong.

The exact cause of Crohn's disease is unknown but it is thought that it may be due to an abnormal reaction of the immune system in the intestine. Genetic factors are likely to be involved in this abnormal reaction in at least some cases, because about 1 in 10 people with Crohn's disease has one or more relatives with the disease or another inflammatory bowel disorder. Environmental factors are also likely to be involved, especially smoking; smokers are three times more likely to develop the disease than are nonsmokers.

What are the symptoms?

The symptoms of Crohn's disease vary between individuals. The disorder usually recurs at intervals throughout life. Episodes may be severe, lasting weeks or several months, before settling down to periods when symptoms are mild or absent. The symptoms include:

- Diarrhoea.
- Abdominal pain.
- Fever.
- Weight loss.
- General feeling of ill health.

If the colon is affected, symptoms may also include the following:

- Diarrhoea, often containing blood.
- Rectal bleeding.

About 1 in 10 people also develops other disorders associated with Crohn's disease.

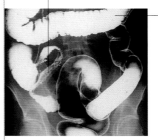

Inflamed small intestine — Normal colon

Crohn's disease
This contrast X-ray shows a normal colon and also shows a section of small intestine that has become inflamed and ulcerated as a result of Crohn's disease.

These other conditions may occur even in mild cases of Crohn's disease and include arthritis (*see* **Ankylosing spondylitis**, p.223), eye disorders (*see* **Uveitis**, p.357), kidney stones (p.447), gallstones (p.412), and a rash (*see* **Erythema nodosum**, p.202).

Are there complications?

Complications of Crohn's disease may include pus-filled cavities near the anus (*see* **Anal abscess**, p.423). These cavities can develop into abnormal passages between the anal canal and the skin around the anus, called anal fistulas.

Intestinal obstruction (p.419) caused by thickening of the intestinal walls is a fairly common complication of Crohn's disease. Damage to the small intestine may prevent the absorption of nutrients (*see* **Malabsorption**, p.415), and thus lead to anaemia (p.271) or vitamin deficiencies. Inflammation of the colon over a long period of time may also be associated with an increased risk of developing colorectal cancer (p.421).

How is it diagnosed?

If your doctor suspects that you have Crohn's disease, he or she may arrange for endoscopic examination of your upper bowel and of your lower bowel (*see* **Colonoscopy**, p.418). During these procedures, tissue is taken from affected areas for microscopic examination. You may also have a contrast X-ray (p.132) of the intestine, known as a small bowel enema study, or a CT (p.132) or MRI (p.133) scan to look for intestinal abnormalities.

Blood tests may be done to check for anaemia and to assess how severely the intestine is inflamed. If your doctor suspects that you have gallstones or kidney stones, you may have imaging tests such as ultrasound scanning (p.135).

What is the treatment?

Mild attacks can often be treated with antidiarrhoeal drugs (p.597) and painkillers (p.589). For an acute attack, your doctor may prescribe oral corticosteroids (p.600). As soon as symptoms subside, the dosage will be reduced to avoid the risk of side effects. If your symptoms are very severe, you may need hospital treatment with intravenous corticosteroids. In all cases, once the

corticosteroid dosage has been reduced, your doctor may recommend oral sulfasalazine or mesalazine (*see* **Aminosalicylate drugs**, p.596) to reduce the frequency of attacks. Immunosuppressant drugs (p.585), such as azathioprine, may also be used for this purpose. If your symptoms do not improve with corticosteroid treatment, you may be offered biological therapy. This involves injections or intravenous infusions of drugs (known as biologicals) that block a specific protein involved in inflammation of the intestinal wall.

You may need dietary supplements, such as extra protein and vitamins (p.598), to counteract malabsorption. During severe attacks, nutrients may have to be given intravenously.

Many people who have Crohn's disease need surgery at some stage. The procedure involves removing the diseased area of the intestine and rejoining the healthy ends (*see* **Colectomy**, p.421). However, surgery is not usually performed until it is absolutely necessary because further affected regions may develop in the remaining intestine.

What is the prognosis?

Crohn's disease is a lifelong disorder with symptoms that recur episodically. Most affected people learn to live reasonably normal lives, but 7 in 10 people eventually need surgery. Complications and repeated surgery can occasionally reduce life expectancy. Since the disorder may increase the risk of colorectal cancer, your doctor may advise regular checkups that include colonoscopy.

Ulcerative colitis

Lifelong, intermittent inflammation and ulceration of the rectum and colon

 Onset most common between the ages of 15 and 35

 Sometimes runs in families; more common in white people and in certain other ethnic groups

 More common in nonsmokers and ex-smokers

 Gender is not a significant factor

Ulcerative colitis is a lifelong, intermittent inflammatory disorder that most commonly develops in young adults. The disorder causes ulceration of the rectum and the colon (the major part of the large intestine). It may either affect the rectum alone (*see* **Proctitis**, p.422) or extend from the rectum further up the colon. In some cases, the disorder involves the entire colon.

Ulcerative colitis affects about 1 in 500 people in the UK. It occurs most frequently in white people, particularly those of Jewish descent, and is more common in nonsmokers and ex-smokers.

What is the cause?

The exact cause of ulcerative colitis is unknown. However, there is some evidence that genetic factors are involved, since

▶ **TEST AND TREATMENT**

Colonoscopy

In colonoscopy, a flexible tube called a colonoscope is used to view the colon to look for disorders such as polyps. The day before a colonoscopy, you will be given laxatives. You may also be given sedatives before the procedure, which takes 15–60 minutes and is usually painless. Instruments passed through the colonoscope can be used to take tissue samples or perform certain treatments. A similar viewing technique called sigmoidoscopy is used to examine the rectum and lower part of the colon.

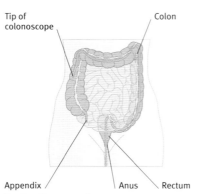

Tip of colonoscope · Colon · Appendix · Anus · Rectum

During the procedure
The colonoscope is passed through the anus and rectum into the colon. Once the tube is inside, you will not feel it moving.

VIEW

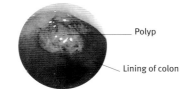

Polyp · Lining of colon

Intestinal polyp
An intestinal polyp attached to the wall of the colon can be seen in this view through a colonoscope. Small polyps can often be painlessly removed during the colonoscopy.

about 1 in 10 people with ulcerative colitis has a close relative who has the disease. There may also be a family history of intestinal diseases, such as Crohn's disease (p.417), and of allergic disorders, such as eczema (p.193).

What are the symptoms?
The symptoms of ulcerative colitis are often intermittent, and there may be several months or years in which there are few or no symptoms. In a mild episode, symptoms often develop over a few days and may include the following:
- Diarrhoea, sometimes with blood and mucus in the stool.
- Abdominal cramps.
- Tiredness.
- Loss of appetite.

In a severe attack, the symptoms may begin suddenly, developing over just a few hours. Symptoms may include:
- Severe bouts of diarrhoea, at least six times a day.
- Passage of blood and mucus from the anus.

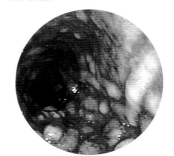

Ulcerative colitis
This endoscopic view of a colon affected by ulcerative colitis shows extensive ulceration of the intestinal lining.

- Pain and swelling in the abdomen.
- Fever.
- Weight loss.

People with ulcerative colitis often have other associated disorders. These include pain in the joints and in the spine (see **Arthritis**, p.220, and **Ankylosing spondylitis**, p.223), inflammation in the eye (see **Uveitis**, p.357), and the skin condition erythema nodosum (p.202).

Are there complications?
Rarely, a severe, sudden attack of ulcerative colitis may lead to toxic megacolon. In this condition, the inflamed colon becomes greatly distended. As a result, the wall of the colon can perforate, allowing intestinal contents containing bacteria to leak into the abdominal cavity. This leakage can cause peritonitis (p.421), a potentially fatal disorder.

People with ulcerative colitis are also at greater risk of developing colorectal cancer (p.421). The risk is increased further if the ulcerative colitis is extensive, severe, and of long duration.

How is it diagnosed?
If your symptoms are fairly mild, your doctor will probably ask you for a faecal sample, which will be tested to exclude the possibility of an infection. The definitive test for ulcerative colitis is direct examination of the colon with an endoscope. You may therefore have a colonoscopy (above), during which a small sample of tissue may be removed from the lining of the rectum or the colon for microscopic examination. You may also have blood tests to look for anaemia (p.271) and to assess the extent of inflammation of the colon.

What is the treatment?
Ulcerative colitis is usually treated with drugs, but surgery may be necessary if you are experiencing frequent severe attacks or if complications develop.

Drugs Your doctor may prescribe the anti-inflammatory drug mesalazine (see **Aminosalicylate drugs**, p.596) to prevent attacks of ulcerative colitis or treat mild episodes. If the inflammation is confined to the rectum or the lower part of the colon, your doctor may prescribe topical aminosalicylate drugs (in the form of suppositories or enemas) for you to self-administer. If the ulcerative colitis affects more of the colon, you will be given the drugs to take orally. In some cases, your doctor may prescribe both topical and oral aminosalicylates.

If you have sudden, severe attacks of the disorder, your doctor will probably prescribe corticosteroids (p.600). Long-term use of corticosteroids may cause various side effects, such as weight gain, a moon-shaped face, and thinning of the bones (see **Osteoporosis**, p.217). For this reason, the doctor will reduce the dose once your symptoms have started to subside and stop the treatment as soon as possible.

If these treatments are ineffective, your doctor may suggest immunosuppressant drugs, such as azathioprine. These drugs may produce potentially serious side effects and regular monitoring is required during treatment. If immunosuppressants are unsuitable or ineffective, biological medications, such as infliximab, adalimumab, or golimumab, may sometimes be used.

Surgery Surgical treatment is usually necessary for people who experience persistent symptoms despite treatment with drugs. It may also be recommended for people who have a sudden, severe attack that does not respond to medical treatment and that may lead to toxic megacolon. In addition, surgery may be advisable for people with an increased risk of colorectal cancer. Surgery usually involves the removal of the diseased colon and rectum (see **Colectomy**, p.421) and creation of a stoma, an artificial opening in the abdominal wall through which faeces can be expelled (see **Colostomy**, p.422). A newer procedure called a pouch operation is suitable for some people. In this procedure, part of the small intestine is used to create a pouch that connects the small intestine to the anus. This operation avoids the need for a stoma, but the pouch may become inflamed and the frequency of bowel movements often increases.

What is the prognosis?
Some people have only one attack of ulcerative colitis, but most have recurring episodes. About 1 in 5 people needs to have surgery. Colorectal cancer is the greatest long-term risk, and it eventually develops in about 1 in 6 people whose entire rectum and colon have been affected for 25 years or more. If you have long-standing, extensive ulcerative colitis but have not had surgery, you will need regular colonoscopy to detect early signs of colorectal cancer.

Polyps in the colon

Noncancerous growths in the large intestine that often do not produce symptoms

 More common over the age of 60, but some forms develop in childhood

 In some cases, the condition is due to an abnormal gene

 Gender and lifestyle are not significant factors

Polyps in the colon are very common in developed countries, where at least 1 in 3 people over the age of 60 may be affected. However, most people are unaware that they have polyps because they often do not cause symptoms.

Polyps are slow-developing growths that protrude inwards from the lining of the large intestine. Some are small and spherical and are attached directly to the intestinal wall; others are over 2.5 cm (1 in) long and attached to the wall by a stalk. Polyps can occur either singly or in groups. Growths larger than about 1 cm (½ in) in diameter have a higher risk than smaller polyps of becoming cancerous (see **Colorectal cancer**, p.421) and must be treated early.

What are the causes?
In most cases, the cause of the condition is not known. Rarely, polyps result from an inherited condition such as familial adenomatous polyposis (FAP). This condition, in which hundreds of polyps cover the lining of the large intestine, is due to an abnormal gene inherited in an autosomal dominant manner (see **Gene disorders**, p.151).

What are the symptoms?
In most cases, intestinal polyps do not cause symptoms. However, if symptoms do occur, they may include:
- Diarrhoea.
- Blood in the faeces or bleeding from the anus, sometimes with mucus.

In some cases, anaemia (p.271) develops due to blood loss, causing tiredness and shortness of breath. In rare cases, a polyp protrudes through the anus.

What might be done?
Polyps that do not cause symptoms may never be diagnosed. However, symptomless polyps can be detected by routine screening for colorectal cancer; they may also be found during investigations that are performed for other reasons. If you do have symptoms, your doctor may arrange for a colonoscopy (above left) to examine the lining of the intestine.

Most polyps can be removed painlessly during the colonoscopy, but occasionally surgery may be necessary to remove larger growths. Polyps that have been removed will be examined under a microscope to look for precancerous cells. If you are found to have precancerous polyps, you may need a colonoscopy every 3–5 years to check for new growths.

If you have FAP, the polyps will be too numerous to be removed individually. There is a high risk of colorectal cancer associated with FAP, and for this reason you will probably be advised to have your colon completely removed (see **Colectomy**, p.421). If you have a close relative who has FAP, you may be offered regular screening using colonoscopy (opposite page) so that any polyps that develop can be detected early. In some cases, testing for the abnormal gene that causes FAP may be carried out. If no polyps have developed by the time you reach the age of 40, they are unlikely to occur.

What is the prognosis?

Polyps can almost always be treated successfully, although they may recur and further treatment may be necessary. However, with treatment the condition can be controlled and the risk of colorectal cancer kept to a minimum.

Hernias

Protrusions of part of an organ, usually the intestine, through a weakened muscle

 Obesity and lifting heavy weights may be risk factors

 Age and gender as risk factors depend on the type

 Genetics is not a significant factor

Hernias, commonly called "ruptures", most often occur at sites in the abdomen where there is a weakness in the muscles. If pressure in the abdomen is increased due to activities such as lifting heavy weights, persistent coughing, or straining at defecation, the muscles of the abdomen become stretched at the weak point. A visible bulge can then develop, which may contain fatty tissue or part of the intestine. Abdominal hernias are frequently found in men who have manual jobs.

An abdominal hernia usually disappears when you lie flat, but sometimes a section of intestine becomes trapped inside the bulge. If the trapped portion of intestine

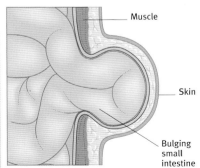

How a hernia develops
Part of the small intestine pushes through a weak area of muscle in the abdominal wall, causing a noticeable bulge to appear on the surface of the body.

becomes twisted, its blood supply may be cut off; this is known as a strangulated hernia. It causes worsening pain, nausea, and vomiting and is a medical emergency.

Hernias may occur in other areas. Hiatus hernias develop when part of the stomach protrudes into the chest cavity through a weak area in the diaphragm (the sheet of muscle that lies beneath the lungs and is involved in breathing,) and may be accompanied by gastro-oesophageal reflux disease (p.403).

What are the types?

Hernias are classified according to the site where they occur in the body. Some types occur more often in men; others are more frequently found in women.

Inguinal hernia This type of hernia occurs when a portion of the intestine pushes through into the inguinal canal, which is a

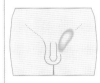

weak spot in the abdominal muscle wall. The hernia causes a visible bulge in the groin or scrotum. These hernias usually affect men, but sometimes occur in women.

Femoral hernia This type of hernia occurs in the part of the groin where the femoral vein and artery pass from the lower abdo-

men to the thigh. Women who are overweight or who have had several pregnancies are at increased risk of these hernias because their abdominal muscles are weakened.

Umbilical hernia Babies may be born with an umbilical hernia, which develops behind

the navel due to a weakness in the abdominal wall. Hernias that develop near the navel are known as paraumbilical hernias and are most common in women who are overweight or have had several pregnancies.

Other types of hernia Epigastric hernias develop in the midline between the navel and the breastbone and are three times more common in men. Incisional hernias may develop after abdominal surgery if there is weakness around the scar. Risk factors include being overweight and having several operations through the same incision.

What are the symptoms?

The symptoms of a non-strangulated hernia usually develop over a period of several weeks or months, although in some cases they may come on suddenly. They may include the following:
- A lump in the abdomen or groin; the lump may disappear when you lie down and reappear when you cough or strain to defecate.
- A dragging or aching sensation in the abdomen or groin.

It is essential to consult a doctor if you think you have a hernia, even if it is not causing pain, because surgery may be needed to prevent the hernia from becoming strangulated or from causing intestinal obstruction.

The symptoms of a strangulated hernia usually come on suddenly and may include:
- A steady pain that gradually gets worse.
- Nausea and vomiting.
- Swelling and redness around the hernia.
- Pain when the hernia is touched.
- Often, the hernia cannot be pushed back through the abdominal wall.

If you think you may have a strangulated hernia, you should get immediate medical help. A strangulated hernia is a medical emergency that requires urgent surgery to prevent the intestine from become gangrenous.

What might be done?

Your doctor may be able to feel a hernia by examining your abdomen or groin. Even small hernias eventually need to be repaired (see **Hernia repair**, below) because, if they are left untreated, they may become strangulated. A strangulated hernia requires immediate surgical repair. The type of operation depends largely on the size of the hernia and on your age and general health. Some procedures are done under local anaesthetic as day surgery and others under a general anaesthetic. Umbilical hernias in babies can usually be left untreated since they tend to disappear naturally by the age of 3–4 years. Surgery is usually effective. However, there is a risk that the hernia will recur in the same place or else-

where. You can help to prevent a recurrence by losing any excess weight, taking gentle exercise, and avoiding constipation.

Intestinal obstruction

Failure of partly digested material to move through the intestine due to a blockage or paralysis of the intestinal muscles

 Age, gender, genetics, and lifestyle as risk factors depend on the cause

In intestinal obstruction, a section of the intestine is partially or totally blocked (mechanical obstruction) or the intestinal walls stop contracting (functional obstruction). In both cases, the intestinal contents cannot move along the digestive tract normally. Left untreated, the condition can be life-threatening.

What are the causes?

Many disorders can cause mechanical obstruction. For example, the intestine may be blocked by a tumour inside it or by external pressure from a growth in another organ. Obstruction may also be due to narrowing of the intestine as a result of inflammation, as in Crohn's disease (p.417), or a strangulated hernia (see **Hernias**, left). After abdominal surgery, adhesions (scar tissue) can form between loops of intestine and cause an obstruction months or even years later.

▶ **TREATMENT**

Hernia repair

Repairing an inguinal hernia is a straightforward procedure, often performed as day surgery. Either a local or general anaesthetic can be used, depending on the location or size of the hernia and the health and age of the patient. The hernia may be repaired either by open surgery, in which a 5–7 cm (2–3 in) incision is made in the skin, or by endoscopic ("keyhole") surgery (p.612). Whichever technique is used, the contents of the hernia are repositioned and the overlying defect in the muscle is repaired. In most cases, the defect is repaired using a synthetic mesh, which significantly reduces the chance of the hernia recurring. After the operation, you will be encouraged to resume normal activities rapidly, although there may be some discomfort for several days; your surgeon will advise you when you can safely resume strenuous activities such as heavy lifting.

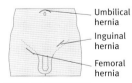

Umbilical hernia
Inguinal hernia
Femoral hernia

SITES OF INCISIONS

1 *An incision is made through the layers of skin and fat to uncover the hernia. The intestine is then repositioned inside the abdominal cavity.*

2 *A piece of synthetic mesh is then positioned either above or below the muscle (as here). The mesh is held in place with staples or stitches. Eventually, tissue grows through the mesh, creating an even stronger repair.*

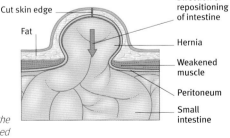

Cut skin edge
Fat
Direction of repositioning of intestine
Hernia
Weakened muscle
Peritoneum
Small intestine

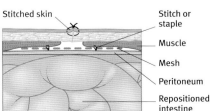

Stitched skin
Stitch or staple
Muscle
Mesh
Peritoneum
Repositioned intestine

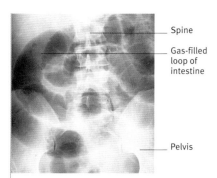

Intestinal obstruction
This abdominal X-ray shows enlarged loops of gas-filled intestine due to an obstruction in the colon.

Functional obstruction, in which the muscles of the intestine fail to contract properly, may be a complication of certain disorders, such as peritonitis (opposite page), or it may follow major surgery.

What are the symptoms?
The symptoms of intestinal obstruction may include:
- Vomiting fluid that may be greenish-yellow, or brown with a faecal odour.
- Severe constipation.
- Abdominal bloating.
- Pain, usually occurring in waves that may later become continuous.
- Total absence of flatulence.

Repeated vomiting may cause dehydration. The intestinal wall may tear due to increased pressure and leak its contents into the abdomen, causing peritonitis.

What might be done?
If an obstruction is suspected, you will be admitted to hospital immediately. You will have abdominal X-rays (p.131) and CT scanning (p.132) to confirm the diagnosis and help determine the nature and position of the obstruction. A tube may be inserted into your stomach to remove digestive juices and prevent vomiting. You will probably be given intravenous fluids to prevent further dehydration. Surgery is often needed to relieve an obstruction. If the cause is Crohn's disease or peritonitis, treating the inflammation may relieve the obstruction. If a blockage occurs after surgery, the intestinal wall usually starts to contract normally after a few days.

Diverticular disease

The presence of small pouches known as diverticula in the wall of the colon

 More common over the age of 50

 A low-fibre diet is a risk factor

 Gender and genetics are not significant factors

In diverticular disease, pea- or grape-sized pouches (diverticula) protrude from the wall of the large intestine, usually from the part of the colon closest to the rectum. The pouches form when parts of the wall of the intestine bulge outwards through weakened areas, often close to an artery. In many cases, the bulging of the intestinal wall is associated with persistent constipation (p.398) and occurs when the pressure inside the intestine increases as the person strains to defecate. Sometimes, one or more pouches become inflamed, a condition known as diverticulitis.

About 1 in 3 people between the ages of 50 and 60 has diverticular disease, and it becomes increasingly common after the age of 60. However, about three-quarters of affected people have no symptoms. The disease is strongly associated with a low-fibre diet, which can lead to constipation. The disease is very rare in developing countries, where fibre is a large part of the diet.

What are the symptoms?
Most people with diverticular disease are unaware of the condition because they have no symptoms. If symptoms are present, they may include:
- Episodes of abdominal pain, especially in the lower left abdomen, that are relieved by a bowel movement or a release of intestinal wind.
- Intermittent episodes of constipation and diarrhoea.
- Occasional bright red bleeding from the rectum, which may be painless.

Diverticular disease is sometimes difficult to distinguish from irritable bowel syndrome (p.415), which has similar symptoms. If diverticulitis develops, the symptoms may become worse and be accompanied by:
- Severe lower abdominal pain and tenderness in the abdomen.
- Fever.
- Nausea and vomiting.

If you notice any change in your bowel habits or you have rectal bleeding, you should consult your doctor immediately because these symptoms may indicate a more serious underlying disease, such as colorectal cancer (opposite page).

Are there complications?
If an inflamed diverticulum bursts, faeces and bacteria can spill into the abdominal cavity. As a result, an abscess may form next to the colon or peritonitis (opposite page), an inflammation of the membrane that lines the abdominal cavity, may develop. Peritonitis is a potentially life-threatening condition.

An abnormal channel called a fistula may develop between a diverticulum and the bladder, resulting in pain, a more frequent urge to pass urine, or recurrent bladder infections (see Cystitis, p.453). In some women, a fistula may develop between a diverticulum and the vagina, causing faecal material to be discharged through the vagina. An inflamed diverticulum may also cause intestinal obstruction (p.419).

How is it diagnosed?
If your doctor suspects that you have diverticular disease, he or she may arrange for you to have a CT scan (p.132) or, less com-

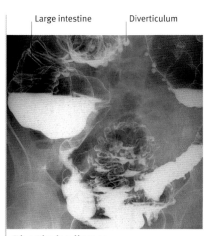
Large intestine   Diverticulum

Diverticular disease
In this special X-ray, a contrast dye shows small pouches (diverticula) protruding from the wall of the large intestine.

monly, a contrast X-ray (p.132) in which a barium enema is used to highlight the shape of the intestines. If your symptoms include rectal bleeding, a colonoscopy (p.418) may be carried out to examine the colon and exclude colorectal cancer. Sometimes, diverticular disease is found during an investigation for another disease.

If your symptoms develop suddenly, you may be admitted to hospital for investigative tests. You may have X-rays and a colonoscopy. In addition, CT scanning or ultrasound scanning (p.135) may be performed.

What is the treatment?
Often, a high-fibre diet with plenty of fluids is the only treatment needed for diverticular disease, together with antispasmodic drugs (*see* **Antispasmodic drugs and motility stimulants**, p.598) if you have abdominal pain.

If you develop severe diverticulitis, you will be admitted to hospital and given intravenous fluids and antibiotics (p.572) to treat bacterial infection. These measures produce improvements in most cases, and no further treatment is needed. However, surgery is sometimes necessary if you have severe rectal bleeding or if an abscess or a fistula develops. Anyone who has two or three attacks of diverticulitis within a few years may also need surgery. The most common operation is a partial colectomy (opposite page), in which the diseased part of the colon is removed and the healthy ends of the intestine are rejoined. At the same time, a temporary colostomy (p.422) may be performed.

What is the prognosis?
The outlook for diverticular disease is generally good. If a high-fibre diet is adopted early enough, the condition is unlikely to progress. Among people with diverticulitis, 2 in 3 have only one attack, but in other people it recurs and surgery may be needed. About 2 in 10 people who experience bleeding will have a recurrence within the next few months to a year unless the problem is treated surgically.

Appendicitis

Inflammation of the appendix, leading to severe abdominal pain

 More common under the age of 40, especially among adolescents

 Slightly more common in males

 A low-fibre diet is a risk factor

 Genetics is not a significant factor

Appendicitis is inflammation affecting the appendix, the small, blind-ended tube attached to the first section of the large intestine. The disorder is common, especially among adolescents, affecting about 40,000 people every year in England. Appendicitis is a common cause of sudden, severe pain in the abdomen, and removal of the appendix is one of the most commonly performed emergency operations. The disorder occurs most commonly in developed countries where the typical diet is low in fibre.

In most cases of appendicitis, no cause is detected, but in some instances the inflammation is the result of a blockage inside the appendix. Blockages sometimes occur when a lump of faecal material passes from the large intestine into the appendix and becomes lodged there. The closed end of the appendix beyond the obstruction then becomes infected with bacteria and inflamed.

What are the symptoms?
Symptoms differ from one person to another. The early symptoms usually develop over a few hours and include:
- Sudden onset of intermittent pain that is first felt in the upper abdomen or around the navel.
- Nausea, with or without vomiting.

Less often, there may be:
- Diarrhoea.
- Mild fever.
- Loss of appetite.
- Frequent passing of urine.

After a few hours, the pain shifts to the lower right abdomen. If treatment is delayed, the appendix may rupture, and intestinal matter containing a high concentration of bacteria can leak into the abdomen. The result may be peritonitis (opposite page), a potentially serious condition in which the membrane that lines the abdominal cavity becomes inflamed. If the appendix ruptures, the pain becomes widespread and severe.

What might be done?
Your doctor will first ask you about the development of your symptoms. He or she will then examine your abdomen and may also insert a gloved finger into the rectum to determine whether there is tenderness in the area around the appendix. You may also have a blood test to measure the white blood cell count. An elevated white cell count may be a sign of inflammation. If your doctor suspects that you have appendicitis, you will be

admited to hospital immediately, where imaging with ultrasound scanning (p.135) or CT scanning (p.132) may confirm the diagnosis.

The usual treatment is removal of the appendix by laparoscopic ("keyhole") surgery (*see* **Endoscopic surgery**, p.612) or by conventional open surgery. The operation is relatively simple and is performed under general anaesthesia. There are usually no long-term adverse effects following either type of operation.

Peritonitis

Inflammation of the peritoneum, the membranous lining of the abdomen

 More common in males

 Age, genetics, and lifestyle are not significant factors

Inflammation of the peritoneum, the membrane that surrounds the organs in the abdomen and lines the abdominal cavity, is called peritonitis. The condition is more common in men. It usually occurs as a complication of another abdominal disorder, such as appendicitis (opposite page). Severe peritonitis may be fatal if not treated rapidly.

What are the causes?
The most common cause of peritonitis is a bacterial infection that has spread from elsewhere in the abdomen. For example, bacteria from the intestine may escape into the abdominal cavity if the intestine is perforated. Possible causes of a perforation include a severe flare-up of a long-term inflammatory disorder, such as ulcerative colitis (p.417); intestinal obstruction (p.419); a wound such as a stab injury (p.184); or surgery.

A less common cause of peritonitis is irritation of the peritoneum. For example, stomach acid may leak into the abdominal cavity and cause irritation if a peptic ulcer (p.406) perforates the wall of the stomach

or the duodenum (the first part of the small intestine). Peritonitis may also develop if bile leaks out from an inflamed gallbladder (*see* **Cholecystitis**, p.413). Occasionally, the condition is caused by leakage of digestive enzymes into the abdominal cavity as a result of acute pancreatitis (p.413).

What are the symptoms?
The symptoms of peritonitis usually develop rapidly. They may include:
- Severe, constant abdominal pain.
- Fever.
- Abdominal swelling.
- Nausea and vomiting.

In severe cases, dehydration and shock (p.248) may also occur. Rarely, after an attack of peritonitis, adhesions may develop, in which bands of scar tissue grow between loops of intestine, causing the loops to stick together. Adhesions may cause abdominal pain months after the attack of peritonitis. Another complication may be intestinal obstruction.

If you believe that you may have peritonitis, you should seek medical attention without delay.

What might be done?
It is important that peritonitis is diagnosed and treated as soon as possible. If your doctor suspects that you have peritonitis, he or she will have you admitted to hospital immediately. In hospital, a doctor will examine your abdomen to check for pain or tenderness and you will have X-rays (p.131) or CT scans (p.132) of the abdomen. You may also have a laparoscopy (p.476), in which the abdominal cavity is examined for abnormalities.

If peritonitis is the result of a bacterial infection, you will be given antibiotics (p.572). You may also need intravenous fluids to treat dehydration and shock. Your doctor will treat the underlying cause of the peritonitis. For example, a perforated peptic ulcer will be repaired or a ruptured appendix removed.

If peritonitis is treated immediately, recovery is usually rapid and long-term problems, such as adhesions, are rare.

Colorectal cancer

A cancerous tumour of the lining of the colon or rectum

 Rare under the age of 40; becomes increasingly common over the age of 40

 Rectal cancer is more common in males; colon cancer is equally common in males and females

 In some cases, the condition is inherited

 A high-fat, low-fibre diet, high alcohol consumption, and obesity are risk factors

More commonly known as bowel cancer, colorectal cancer is one of the most common cancers in the UK and is the second leading cause of cancer death (after lung cancer). However, it can be detected early by screening people (*see* **Screening**, p.13, and **Colonoscopy**, p.418), and when it is detected early enough, it can be treated successfully by surgery.

Colorectal cancer is rare under 40 and most often occurs in people over 60. Rectal cancer tends to be more common in men, while colon cancer affects men and women equally. Cancer can occur anywhere in the colon or rectum, but most tumours develop in the lower third of the colon nearest the rectum.

What are the causes?
In less affluent countries, where people traditionally live on a high-fibre diet consisting mainly of cereals, fruit, and vegetables, colorectal cancer is rare. However, a typical Western diet, which tends to be high in meat and animal fats and low in fibre, seems to increase the risk of developing colorectal cancer. It is not known how fibre in the diet reduces the risk of the disorder. A possible explanation is that dietary fibre shortens the time that it takes for waste matter to pass through the intestines. As a result, potentially cancer-causing substances (carcinogens) in food are expelled from the body at a faster rate. Other lifestyle factors, such as high alcohol consumption, obesity, smoking, and lack of exercise, also increase the risk of developing colorectal cancer. The reasons for this increased risk are also unknown.

About 1 in 20 cases of colorectal cancer is hereditary. Most of these cases are caused by inheritance of an abnormal gene. Some genetic abnormalities increase the risk of developing a form of the cancer known as hereditary nonpolyposis colorectal cancer (HNPCC). Rarely, colorectal cancer may be caused by the inherited disorder familial adenomatous polyposis (FAP), in which polyps (growths of tissue) form inside the large intestine (*see* **Polyps in the colon**, p.418). In FAP, there is about a 9 in 10 chance that some of the polyps will become cancerous before the age of 40.

Inflammatory disorders affecting the large intestine, such as ulcerative colitis (p.417) or Crohn's disease (p.417), can also increase the risk of developing colorectal cancer if they are long-standing and most of the colon is affected.

What are the symptoms?
The symptoms of colorectal cancer vary depending on the site of the tumour. They may include the following:
- Changes in the frequency of bowel movements or in the general consistency of the faeces.
- Abdominal pain.
- Blood in the faeces.
- Rectal discomfort or a sensation of incomplete emptying of the rectum.
- Loss of appetite.

The symptoms of colorectal cancer may be mistaken for the symptoms of a less serious disorder, such as haemorrhoids (p.422). If there is heavy loss of blood from the rectum, iron-deficiency anaemia (p.271) may result. This condition produces symptoms such as pale skin, headaches, and tiredness. As the tumour grows bigger, it may eventually cause intestinal obstruction (p.419).

You should consult your doctor promptly if you notice blood in your faeces or an inexplicable change in your bowel habits (such as increased frequency, loose stools, or diarrhoea), especially if you are over 50. Left untreated, colorectal cancer will eventually spread via the bloodstream to the lymph nodes, liver, and other organs in the body.

How is it diagnosed?
Colorectal cancer may be diagnosed during screening before symptoms have developed. If you do have symptoms, your doctor may feel your abdomen to detect any swelling and carry out a rectal examination, in which a gloved finger is inserted into the rectum to feel for a tumour. A stool sample is tested for the presence of blood and a blood sample is tested for evidence of anaemia.

The rectum may be examined visually with a viewing instrument inserted through the anus. Your doctor may also arrange for a colonoscopy, in which a flexible viewing instrument is used to examine the entire colon. A biopsy, in which a sample of intestinal tissue is removed for microscopic examination, may be performed during the procedure. You may also have a "virtual colonoscopy", in which CT scans (p.132) are used to produce a three-dimensional image of your colon or rectum in order to identify abnormal areas. Alternatively, and less commonly, a contrast X-ray (p.132) with a barium enema may be used for the same purpose. If a cancerous tumour is detected, you will probably need to have CT scanning to see if the cancer has spread to the lymph nodes in the abdomen or to the liver or lungs. An MRI scan (p.133) may also sometimes be done to help plan surgical treatment.

In the UK, screening with the faecal occult blood (FOB) test is offered to older age groups and people at high risk. It checks for blood in the faeces, which may be an early sign of bowel cancer. You are sent a home-testing kit and you simply have to smear a series of faecal samples on to a specially treated card and then send off the card for analysis. If blood is detected in the samples (a positive result), further tests will be

Colectomy

A colectomy is an operation in which part or all of the large intestine (the colon and the rectum) is removed under general anaesthesia. It is usually performed to treat inflammatory conditions, such as Crohn's disease, or cancer of the colon. In most cases, the cut ends of the large intestine are rejoined once the diseased section has been removed, but sometimes a colostomy (p.422) is needed. You will have to stay in hospital for at least a week after the operation, depending on the extent of the surgery.

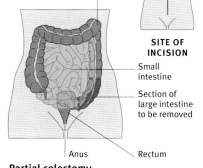

Colon

SITE OF INCISION

Small intestine

Section of large intestine to be removed

Anus   Rectum

Partial colectomy
During the procedure, the abnormal section of the colon is cut out, and the healthy ends of the remaining intestine are joined together. A colostomy is performed only in a minority of partial colectomies.

▶ **TREATMENT**

Colostomy

In a colostomy, part of the colon is cut and the edges are attached to the skin of the abdomen to form an artificial opening called a stoma. Faeces are expelled through the stoma into a disposable bag. A colostomy is performed following a colectomy (p.421) and may be either temporary or permanent. If part of the colon has been removed, a temporary colostomy may be carried out to allow the rejoined ends to heal without faeces passing through the site. A permanent colostomy is needed when the rectum and anus are removed with part of the colon.

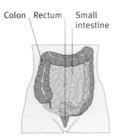

Colon Rectum Small intestine

LOCATION

Opening on skin surface Edge stitched to skin Healing colectomy site

Muscle

Loop of colon

Small intestine

Temporary colostomy
An incision is made in a loop of colon and the edges of the loop are stitched to the skin surface. When the colectomy site has healed, the incision in the colon is closed and the colon is then returned under the skin.

Opening on skin surface Edge stitched to skin

Skin

Muscle

Colon

Small intestine

Permanent colostomy
The cut end of the colon is passed through the abdominal wall. The edges are then stitched to the skin surface to create a permanent opening. Normal defecation is no longer possible.

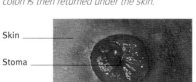

Skin

Stoma

Permanent stoma
An artificial opening (stoma) can be seen on the surface of the abdomen. Faeces discharged from the intestine are collected in a disposable bag fitted over the stoma.

needed. In England, an extra bowel screening test is offered to those at the age of 55. Known as bowel scope screening, this is a one-off procedure in which the inside of the lower bowel is inspected with an endoscope (a viewing instrument) to check for polyps (which might become cancerous) or other abnormalities. If any polyps are detected, they are usually removed immediately.

What is the treatment?
Treatment of colorectal cancer depends on the site of the tumour. In most cases of early cancer, the affected part of the intestine can be removed and the cut ends rejoined (*see* **Colectomy**, p.421). In a few cases, if most of the rectum has been removed, a permanent colostomy (above) may be necessary. In this procedure, an opening is created on the surface of the abdomen for the discharge of faeces. In some cases when the tumours are small and at an early stage, it may be possible to remove them by laparoscopic ("keyhole") surgery. If the cancer cannot be cured, treatment is aimed at relieving the symptoms. For example, surgery may be done to remove a tumour obstructing the bowel. If cancer has spread to other parts of the body, chemotherapy (p.157), radiotherapy (p.158), or both may be necessary to treat the disease. Chemotherapy and/or radiotherapy may also be used to shrink large tumours before surgery.

About 9 in 10 people treated at an early stage live at least 5 years. Surgical removal of affected tissue at a more advanced stage of the disease gives a 3 in 4 chance of living at least 5 years. If the cancer has spread, the outlook is less favourable.

Proctitis

Inflammation of the rectum, most often due to ulcerative colitis

 Rare in childhood

 Gender and lifestyle as risk factors depend on the cause

 Genetics is not a significant factor

In proctitis, the lining of the anus and the rectum becomes inflamed. The disorder most commonly develops as part of ulcerative colitis (p.417), a condition that can either be restricted to the rectum or be a more widespread disease that also affects the colon.

Proctitis may also result from an infection of the lining of the rectum. Unprotected anal sex increases the risk of contracting a sexually transmitted infection (STI). Because anal sex may also lead to proctitis by causing physical injury to the rectum, the disorder is more common in homosexual men. Other causes of proctitis include the gastrointestinal infection amoebic dysentery (*see* **Amoebiasis**, p.176) and radiotherapy (p.158) used to treat cancers close to the rectum, such as prostate cancer (p.464).

What are the symptoms?
In most cases, the symptoms of proctitis include the following:
- Blood, mucus, or pus in the faeces.
- Discomfort and pain in the anus and rectum that becomes more severe with a bowel movement.
- Diarrhoea or constipation.
- An increased urge to defecate.

Inflammation due to an STI may be accompanied by fever and pelvic pain. If the rectum is inflamed, there may also be an increased risk of acquiring or transmitting STIs, such as HIV infection through unprotected anal sex.

In some cases, proctitis is complicated by the presence of an anal fissure (opposite page) or an anal abscess (opposite page).

What might be done?
Your doctor may ask for a stool sample or take a rectal swab to look for infection. He or she may also examine your rectum by using a viewing instrument called a proctoscope. A small sample of rectal tissue may be taken for examination under a microscope.

Treatment of proctitis depends on the cause. However, pain and inflammation, whatever the cause, may be eased with painkillers (p.589) and drugs to soften the faeces (*see* **Laxatives**, p.597). If the cause is ulcerative colitis, mesalazine (*see* **Aminosalicylate drugs**, p.596) or corticosteroids (p.600) are generally used to reduce inflammation.

Antibiotics (p.572) are usually given to treat a bacterial STI. Topical corticosteroids (p.600) can be used to reduce rectal inflammation caused by injury. Avoiding anal intercourse will help to speed up the healing process. Antibiotics may be given to treat amoebic dysentery, while proctitis due to radiotherapy is often treated with corticosteroids. Treatment is usually successful.

Rectal prolapse

Protrusion of the lining of the rectum outside the anus

 Most common in young children and in elderly people

 More common in females

 A low-fibre diet is a risk factor

 Genetics is not a significant factor

Rectal prolapse is an uncommon condition in which the lining of the rectum protrudes through the anus. It is usually associated with a low-fibre diet and constipation (p.398). The condition is more common in females and in elderly people and may be a recurrent problem in people who have weak pelvic floor muscles. In addition, rectal prolapse may sometimes occur temporarily in very young children during toilet training.

What are the symptoms?
If you have a rectal prolapse, you may experience symptoms after straining to defecate. These include:
- Bleeding and discharge of mucus from the anus.
- Pain or discomfort on defecation.
- The sensation of a lump protruding from the anus.

If the prolapse is large, there may also be some faecal incontinence.

What might be done?
Your doctor may examine the prolapse with a gloved finger and gently push the rectum back into place. Further treatment is used to relieve the underlying cause, such as a high-fibre diet to relieve constipation. If the prolapse recurs and you have persistent constipation, your doctor may arrange for tests, such as colonoscopy (p.418) or contrast X-rays (p.132), to look for a possible underlying cause, such as colorectal cancer (p.421).

In children, rectal prolapse will usually disappear when measures are taken to prevent constipation. Elderly people may require surgery to fix the rectum in position permanently.

Haemorrhoids

Swollen veins inside the rectum and around the anus, also known as piles

 More common in adults

 More common in females during pregnancy and after childbirth

 Being overweight and a low-fibre diet are risk factors

 Genetics is not a significant factor

Haemorrhoids are a common problem that are estimated to affect up to half of all people at some time in their lives. In this disorder, veins in the soft tissues around the anus and inside the lower part of the rectum become swollen. Swellings around the anus are called external haemorrhoids, and those within the rectum are called internal haemorrhoids. Internal haemorrhoids that protrude outside the anus are called prolapsing haemorrhoids.

Haemorrhoids frequently cause bleeding, itching, and discomfort. However, these symptoms are usually intermittent, and the condition is not in itself serious.

What are the causes?
Haemorrhoids most often result from constipation, when a person strains to pass stools. Straining in this way increases the pressure inside the abdomen, which in turn causes blood vessels around the rectum to swell.

Constipation is often due to a low-fibre diet. Excess weight also exerts pressure on blood vessels and thus increases the risk of haemorrhoids. During pregnancy, the growing fetus has the same effect, frequently resulting in haemorrhoids.

What are the symptoms?

The symptoms of haemorrhoids commonly develop following constipation. Symptoms may include:

- Fresh blood on toilet paper or in the toilet after a bowel movement.
- Increasing discomfort on defecation.
- Discharge of mucus from the anus, sometimes leading to itching.
- Visible swellings around the anus.
- Feeling that the bowels have not been fully emptied.

A prolapsing haemorrhoid may protrude through the anus after a bowel movement and may then retract or can be pushed back inside with a finger. In some cases, a blood clot (thrombus) may form within a prolapsing haemorrhoid, causing severe pain and a visible, tender, blue, grape-sized swelling.

If you have bleeding from the anus, you should consult your doctor without delay, especially if you are over 40, since it may indicate a more serious disorder, such as colorectal cancer (p.421).

What might be done?

Your doctor will probably examine your rectum by inserting a gloved finger into it, and, if there has been bleeding that suggests a serious underlying disease, may arrange for colonoscopy (p.418).

Small haemorrhoids do not usually need treatment. Haemorrhoids due to pregnancy usually disappear soon after the birth. A high-fibre diet helps to prevent constipation, and laxatives (p.597) may help to ease defecation. Over-the-counter topical corticosteroids (p.600) and corticosteroid suppositories can reduce swelling and itching, and anaesthetic sprays may relieve pain. If these measures are not effective within a few days, you should consult your doctor, who may suggest surgery.

Small internal haemorrhoids may be treated by sclerotherapy, a procedure in which the affected area is injected with a solution that causes the veins to shrink. Alternatively, the doctor may place a band around the base of an internal haemorrhoid, causing the haemorrhoid to shrink and fall off (see Banding haemorrhoids, below).

Persistent, painful, bleeding haemorrhoids can be destroyed by electrical, laser, or infrared heat treatment or be removed surgically. Treatment is usually successful, but haemorrhoids may recur.

Anal abscess

An infected, pus-filled cavity in the anal or rectal area

 More common in males

 Anal sex is a risk factor

 Age and genetics are not significant factors

An anal abscess is a pus-filled cavity that develops when bacteria enter a mucus-secreting gland in the anus or rectum and multiply. The abscess may be deep within the rectum or close to the anus.

Inflammatory disorders of the colon, such as Crohn's disease (p.417), can be associated with anal abscesses. Anal sex also increases the risk.

You should consult a doctor if you have swelling or redness in the anal area or have a throbbing pain that worsens with defecation. If the infection spreads from the anal area, you may also have a fever and feel generally unwell.

An anal abscess is usually diagnosed by a physical examination. Treatment involves draining the abscess through an incision under local anaesthesia. Drainage of deep or large abscesses may need a general anaesthetic. You may be given oral antibiotics (p.572) and advised to soak the affected area in warm water three or four times a day. An abscess may take several weeks to heal.

Anal fissure

A tear in the lining of the anus that is usually a result of constipation

 A low-fibre diet is a risk factor

 Age, gender, and genetics are not significant factors

The most common cause of an anal fissure is the passage of a large, hard stool due to constipation (p.398). This type of stool can tear the anal lining so that subsequent defecation is extremely painful. You may also notice bright red blood on your faeces or the toilet paper.

An anal fissure can usually be diagnosed from a description of the symptoms, although in some cases the doctor may inspect the anal lining using a viewing instrument called a proctoscope.

Self-help measures to relieve constipation, such as using laxatives (p.597) and eating a high-fibre diet, may help the anal fissure to heal. In addition, a gel that relaxes the anal sphincter (the ring of muscle around the anus) or an anaesthetic gel may be helpful. In severe cases, surgery to stretch or cut the anal sphincter may be recommended.

Anal itching

Irritation in or, more commonly, around the anus

 Age, gender, and lifestyle as risk factors depend on the cause

 Genetics is not a significant factor

Anal itching (pruritus ani) is rarely a serious condition, although it may be embarrassing and hard to treat. Itching may be either localized around the anus or part of a generalized itching disorder (see Itching, p.196). It may be worse in older people because their skin is drier, less elastic, and more easily irritated.

Localized anal itching may be caused by poor personal hygiene, haemorrhoids (opposite page), or threadworm infestation (p.178). Generalized itching around the anal area may be a symptom of a skin disease, such as psoriasis (p.192) or eczema (p.193), or be due to an allergic reaction to a substance such as detergent or soap.

What might be done?

There are several measures you can take to relieve anal itching. It is important to keep the anal area clean by washing and drying carefully after a bowel movement. Avoid using soaps that irritate the skin, and try not to scratch because it will worsen the itching. A warm bath or shower before bed may soothe night-time itching. Loose underclothes made of natural fibres are less likely than synthetic materials to cause irritation. An over-the-counter cream containing a topical corticosteroid (p.600) may give relief. Itching that lasts for longer than 3 days should be assessed by a doctor.

Your doctor may examine your anus and arrange for tests to look for causes that require treatment. For example, haemorrhoids may need to be removed.

Anal cancer

Cancer of the anus or anal canal, which may cause pain and bleeding

 More common with increasing age

 More common in males

 Genetics and lifestyle are not significant factors

Cancer of the anus or the anal canal (the passage from the rectum to outside the body) is very rare. Although the cause is not known, there may be a link between anal cancer and human papillomaviruses, which cause genital warts (p.493) and are also associated with cancer of the cervix (p.481).

What are the symptoms?

The symptoms of anal cancer usually develop gradually and include:

- Bleeding from the anus.
- Itching or discomfort in the anal area.
- Frequent desire to defecate.
- A lump in or near the anus.

If you have any of these symptoms, you should consult your doctor to determine the cause. Left untreated, anal cancer may spread to nearby tissues and eventually to other parts of the body.

What might be done?

Your doctor will first examine the anus and then insert a gloved finger into the rectum to feel for lumps. Under local anaesthesia, your doctor may remove a sample of tissue from the anal canal for examination under a microscope.

If anal cancer is diagnosed, you will need further tests to detect whether the cancer has spread. These tests include blood tests and CT scanning (p.132) or MRI (p.133) of the abdomen and pelvis.

The usual treatment is chemotherapy (p.157) with radiotherapy (p.158). In about 2 in 3 people, this treatment causes the tumour to shrink so that surgery is not needed. In most people, treatment is curative. However, in rare cases, surgery is necessary to remove the anus and part of the rectum.

If the cancer has already spread to other parts of the body, the outlook is poor. However, surgery in combination with radiotherapy may relieve the symptoms and prolong life.

▶ **TREATMENT**

Banding haemorrhoids

Large or prolapsing haemorrhoids can be successfully treated by using a procedure called banding, in which a rubber band is placed around the base of the haemorrhoid. As a result, the haemorrhoid gradually shrinks over a period of several days and eventually drops off. Before the procedure, you may need a laxative to ensure that the rectum is empty. The procedure can be carried out in a doctor's surgery and is usually painless. The treated area may be sore for a few days afterwards.

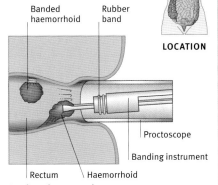

LOCATION

Banded haemorrhoid · Rubber band · Proctoscope · Banding instrument · Rectum · Haemorrhoid

During the procedure
Using a short tube called a proctoscope, the doctor first grasps the haemorrhoid with forceps and then attaches a rubber band around the base using a banding instrument.

Hormones and metabolism

The word hormone is derived from a Greek term meaning "to excite" or "to spur on". Hormones are chemical messengers that alter the activity of or "excite" targeted cells. They are produced in various specialized glands and cells throughout the body and are transported in the bloodstream to their specific sites of action. Hormones regulate many important body processes and functions, including growth, reproduction, and metabolism, the collective term for all the chemical reactions that occur in the body.

HORMONES ARE PRODUCED by a number of different glands and cells that are described collectively as the endocrine system. The major endocrine glands – the pituitary, thyroid, parathyroid, and adrenal glands and the pancreas, ovaries, and testes – are all primarily dedicated to the production of various hormones. However, other organs and tissues with functions of their own also produce hormones. For example, the main function of the kidneys is to filter the blood, but they also contain endocrine cells that secrete hormones.

Hormones are transported in the bloodstream to their target tissues, which may then be stimulated to produce other hormones in a chain reaction. For example, the pituitary gland produces thyroid-stimulating hormone (TSH), which travels to the thyroid gland where it stimulates the production of thyroid hormones.

Hormones also regulate the balance of certain substances in the blood. If there is too much or too little of a substance, a feedback mechanism restores the correct levels. The pituitary, a pea-sized gland situated at the base of the brain and regulated by a part of the brain called the hypothalamus, has overall control of most hormone production.

Some hormones work on cells throughout the body. For example, certain thyroid hormones influence metabolic rate. Others have specific target cells, such as the hormone vasopressin (also known as antidiuretic hormone, or ADH) which acts on specific cells in the kidneys to regulate urine concentration.

When we are under stress or excited, the two adrenal glands increase production of hormones that affect our blood pressure, circulation, and breathing, creating the heightened states that form part of our "fight or flight" response to danger.

In addition to short-term fluctuations, hormone levels can also change throughout life. For example, during puberty sex hormones rise sharply, and in women levels fall after the menopause.

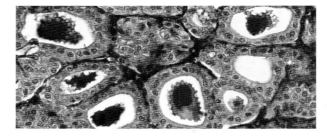

Thyroid gland tissue
This image shows hormone-secreting cells in the thyroid gland around bright red areas that are stores of hormones.

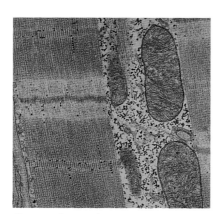

Glycogen in muscles
Glycogen stores, which break down into glucose to supply energy, appear as black dots in this view of muscle cells.

✚ **PROCESS**

Feedback mechanism

Hormone secretion is regulated by feedback mechanisms in order to maintain correct levels of substances in the blood. For example, a drop in the calcium level in the bloodstream stimulates an increase in the secretion of parathyroid hormone (PTH), which acts on various parts of the body to raise calcium levels. When calcium reaches the normal level, PTH secretion decreases.

Maintaining blood calcium levels
The parathyroid glands detect fluctuations in calcium levels in the blood and secrete appropriate amounts of parathyroid hormone (PTH) to correct them.

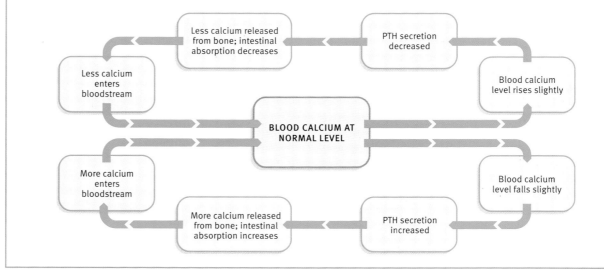

Less calcium released from bone; intestinal absorption decreases

PTH secretion decreased

Less calcium enters bloodstream

Blood calcium level rises slightly

BLOOD CALCIUM AT NORMAL LEVEL

More calcium enters bloodstream

Blood calcium level falls slightly

More calcium released from bone; intestinal absorption increases

PTH secretion increased

Hormone-secreting glands and cells

Most endocrine cells are grouped together in organs, such as the pituitary, thyroid, and adrenal glands, whose only purpose is to produce hormones. However, hormone-secreting cells are also present in many other tissues that have a different primary function. For example, the kidneys secrete hormones that stimulate red blood cell production, although their main role is to filter the blood. New chemical substances that act as hormones are still being discovered and their specific roles in the body clarified.

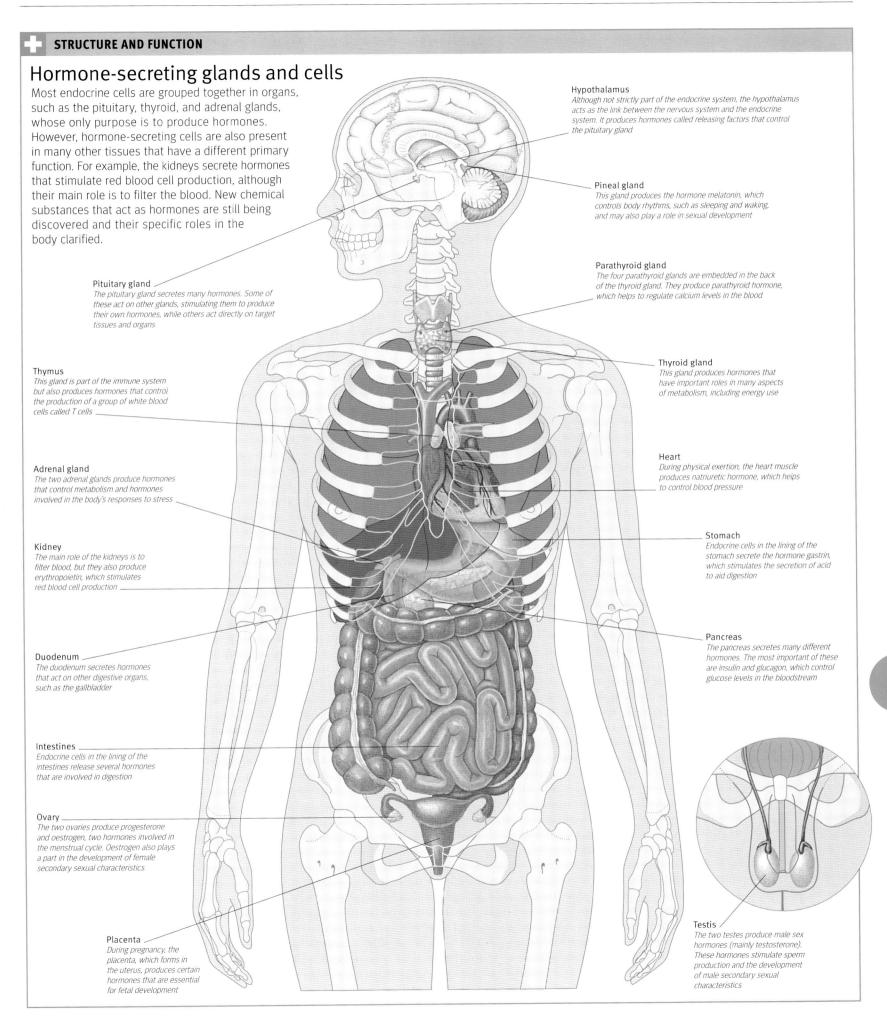

Hypothalamus
Although not strictly part of the endocrine system, the hypothalamus acts as the link between the nervous system and the endocrine system. It produces hormones called releasing factors that control the pituitary gland

Pineal gland
This gland produces the hormone melatonin, which controls body rhythms, such as sleeping and waking, and may also play a role in sexual development

Parathyroid gland
The four parathyroid glands are embedded in the back of the thyroid gland. They produce parathyroid hormone, which helps to regulate calcium levels in the blood

Thyroid gland
This gland produces hormones that have important roles in many aspects of metabolism, including energy use

Heart
During physical exertion, the heart muscle produces natriuretic hormone, which helps to control blood pressure

Stomach
Endocrine cells in the lining of the stomach secrete the hormone gastrin, which stimulates the secretion of acid to aid digestion

Pancreas
The pancreas secretes many different hormones. The most important of these are insulin and glucagon, which control glucose levels in the bloodstream

Testis
The two testes produce male sex hormones (mainly testosterone). These hormones stimulate sperm production and the development of male secondary sexual characteristics

Pituitary gland
The pituitary gland secretes many hormones. Some of these act on other glands, stimulating them to produce their own hormones, while others act directly on target tissues and organs

Thymus
This gland is part of the immune system but also produces hormones that control the production of a group of white blood cells called T cells

Adrenal gland
The two adrenal glands produce hormones that control metabolism and hormones involved in the body's responses to stress

Kidney
The main role of the kidneys is to filter blood, but they also produce erythropoietin, which stimulates red blood cell production

Duodenum
The duodenum secretes hormones that act on other digestive organs, such as the gallbladder

Intestines
Endocrine cells in the lining of the intestines release several hormones that are involved in digestion

Ovary
The two ovaries produce progesterone and oestrogen, two hormones involved in the menstrual cycle. Oestrogen also plays a part in the development of female secondary sexual characteristics

Placenta
During pregnancy, the placenta, which forms in the uterus, produces certain hormones that are essential for fetal development

Pituitary gland

The pituitary gland controls the activities of many other endocrine glands and hormone-producing cells around the body. The pituitary gland has two parts, the anterior and posterior lobes, which are under the control of a part of the brain known as the hypothalamus. The hypothalamus secretes releasing hormones that pass through the circulation to the pituitary's anterior lobe, where they trigger the production of hormones that control other glands. Nerve cells in the hypothalamus secrete two hormones (oxytocin and vasopressin, or ADH) that pass down nerve fibres to be stored in the posterior lobe of the pituitary until they are needed.

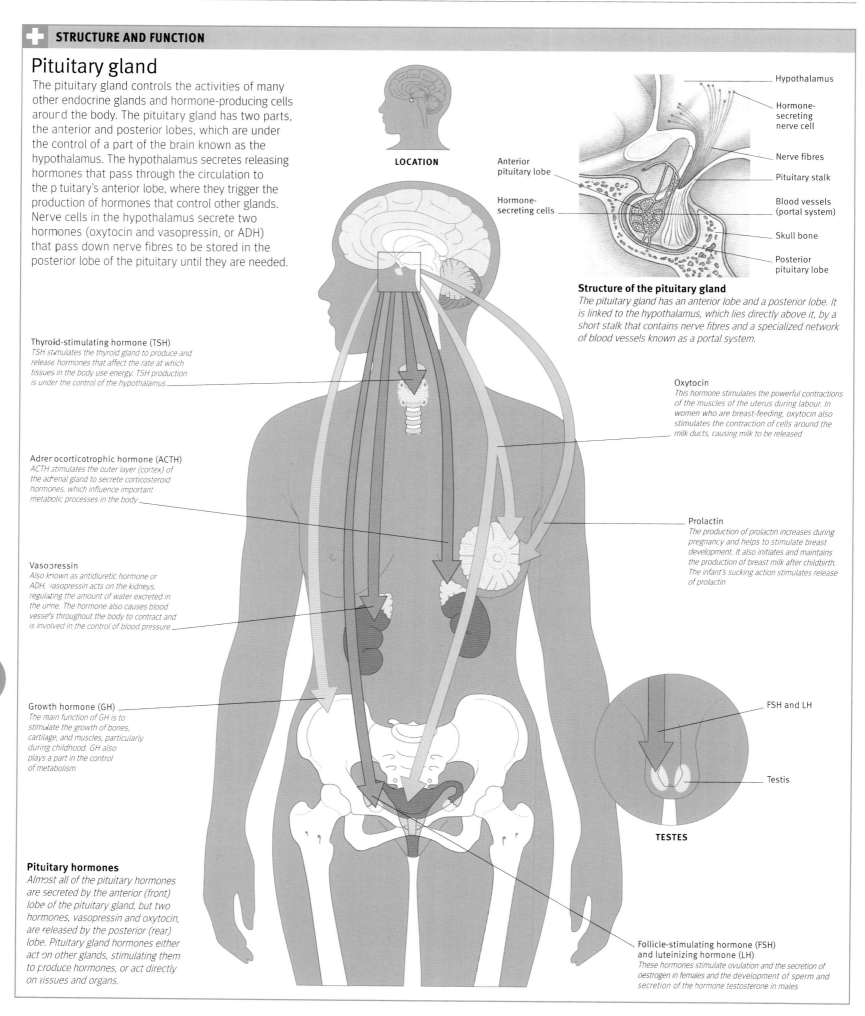

LOCATION

Structure of the pituitary gland
The pituitary gland has an anterior lobe and a posterior lobe. It is linked to the hypothalamus, which lies directly above it, by a short stalk that contains nerve fibres and a specialized network of blood vessels known as a portal system.

Labels for structure diagram:
- Hypothalamus
- Hormone-secreting nerve cell
- Nerve fibres
- Pituitary stalk
- Blood vessels (portal system)
- Skull bone
- Posterior pituitary lobe
- Anterior pituitary lobe
- Hormone-secreting cells

Thyroid-stimulating hormone (TSH)
TSH stimulates the thyroid gland to produce and release hormones that affect the rate at which tissues in the body use energy. TSH production is under the control of the hypothalamus.

Adrenocorticotrophic hormone (ACTH)
ACTH stimulates the outer layer (cortex) of the adrenal gland to secrete corticosteroid hormones, which influence important metabolic processes in the body.

Vasopressin
Also known as antidiuretic hormone or ADH, vasopressin acts on the kidneys, regulating the amount of water excreted in the urine. The hormone also causes blood vessels throughout the body to contract and is involved in the control of blood pressure.

Growth hormone (GH)
The main function of GH is to stimulate the growth of bones, cartilage, and muscles, particularly during childhood. GH also plays a part in the control of metabolism.

Oxytocin
This hormone stimulates the powerful contractions of the muscles of the uterus during labour. In women who are breast-feeding, oxytocin also stimulates the contraction of cells around the milk ducts, causing milk to be released.

Prolactin
The production of prolactin increases during pregnancy and helps to stimulate breast development. It also initiates and maintains the production of breast milk after childbirth. The infant's sucking action stimulates release of prolactin.

FSH and LH

Testis

TESTES

Pituitary hormones
Almost all of the pituitary hormones are secreted by the anterior (front) lobe of the pituitary gland, but two hormones, vasopressin and oxytocin, are released by the posterior (rear) lobe. Pituitary gland hormones either act on other glands, stimulating them to produce hormones, or act directly on tissues and organs.

Follicle-stimulating hormone (FSH) and luteinizing hormone (LH)
These hormones stimulate ovulation and the secretion of oestrogen in females and the development of sperm and secretion of the hormone testosterone in males.

Thyroid and parathyroid glands

The thyroid and parathyroid glands are situated close to each other in the front of the neck. The thyroid gland produces the hormone thyroxine (T_4) and its more active form, T_3, which act on body cells to regulate metabolism (the chemical reactions continually occurring in the body). Some thyroid cells secrete the hormone calcitonin, which lowers calcium in the blood. The parathyroid glands produce parathyroid hormone (PTH), the main regulator of calcium.

Parathyroid hormone (PTH)
If blood calcium is low, PTH secretion is increased. The hormone acts on the bones to release calcium into the blood, on the intestines to increase the absorption of calcium from food, and on the kidneys to prevent calcium loss in urine

T_4 and T_3
These hormones regulate the rate of many chemical processes in the body, including the use of energy

BODY CELLS

Calcitonin
This hormone inhibits calcium release from the bones if blood calcium levels are high

LOCATION

Thyroid cartilage

Thyroid gland

Parathyroid gland

Trachea (windpipe)

FRONT VIEW   **BACK VIEW**

Structure of the thyroid and parathyroid glands
The thyroid gland is wrapped around the front of the trachea. The four parathyroid glands are at the back of the thyroid gland.

Thyroid and parathyroid hormones
Iodine from the diet is used to make the hormones T_4 and T_3. These hormones are produced by the thyroid gland and regulate body metabolism. Parathyroid hormone (PTH) and, to a lesser extent, calcitonin regulate levels of calcium and phosphate.

Adrenal glands

Each adrenal gland has two parts. The cortex (outer layer) is controlled by the pituitary gland and produces several corticosteroid hormones, the most important of which affect metabolism and blood pressure. The cortex also secretes small amounts of male sex hormones (androgens). The medulla (core) influences the autonomic nervous system by releasing the hormones epinephrine (adrenaline) and norepinephrine (noradrenaline), which increase heart activity and blood flow in response to excitement or stress.

Epinephrine (adrenaline) and norepinephrine (noradrenaline)
These hormones trigger the "fight or flight" response. They increase heart rate and blood flow to the muscles

Cortisol
Cortisol helps the body to adapt to physical and emotional stress by boosting blood glucose levels

Aldosterone
This hormone acts on the kidneys to help regulate the excretion of salt to maintain blood pressure

Sex hormones
Adrenal androgens promote the development of secondary male sexual characteristics

BODY CELLS

Medulla

Cortex

Fat

Kidney

LOCATION

Structure of the adrenal gland
The adrenal glands rest on pads of fat above the kidneys. Each gland has an outer cortex, which makes up 90 per cent of its weight, and an inner medulla.

Adrenal hormones
The corticosteroid hormones cortisol and aldosterone and small amounts of male sex hormones are secreted by the cortex. The medulla secretes epinephrine (adrenaline) and norepinephrine (noradrenaline).

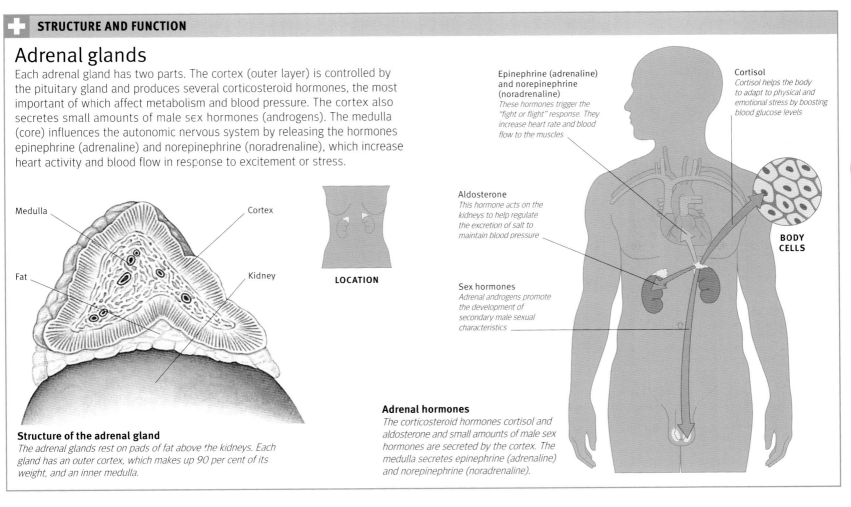

STRUCTURE AND FUNCTION

Pancreas

The pancreas has two main functions. It plays a major role in digestion, releasing enzymes that break down fat, starch, and proteins through the pancreatic ducts into the intestine. It also contains clusters of cells, called islets of Langerhans, that secrete hormones directly into the bloodstream. These cells secrete insulin and glucagon, two hormones that regulate glucose levels in the body, and other digestive hormones.

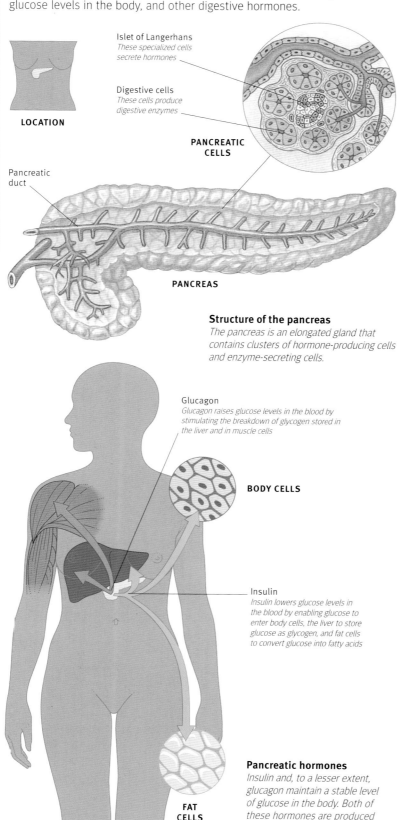

LOCATION

Islet of Langerhans
These specialized cells secrete hormones

Digestive cells
These cells produce digestive enzymes

PANCREATIC CELLS

Pancreatic duct

PANCREAS

Structure of the pancreas
The pancreas is an elongated gland that contains clusters of hormone-producing cells and enzyme-secreting cells.

Glucagon
Glucagon raises glucose levels in the blood by stimulating the breakdown of glycogen stored in the liver and in muscle cells

BODY CELLS

Insulin
Insulin lowers glucose levels in the blood by enabling glucose to enter body cells, the liver to store glucose as glycogen, and fat cells to convert glucose into fatty acids

FAT CELLS

Pancreatic hormones
Insulin and, to a lesser extent, glucagon maintain a stable level of glucose in the body. Both of these hormones are produced by cells in the pancreas.

 PROCESS

Metabolism

Thousands of chemical reactions and conversions take place continuously in body cells to keep the body alive and healthy and to generate energy. Metabolism is the collective term for all these chemical processes. The raw materials for metabolic processes are obtained from nutrients in food, which are broken down into simple molecules during digestion. These molecules are either recycled and built up into new complex molecules that can be used to repair or make new cells (anabolism) or are further broken down to release energy (catabolism).

Anabolism and catabolism

In anabolic processes, body cells are built up and repaired, or complex substances are constructed out of simpler ones. In catabolic processes, complex molecules are broken down into simple molecules, such as glucose and amino acids, and these simple molecules are broken down to supply the cells with energy and materials for renewing cell structures.

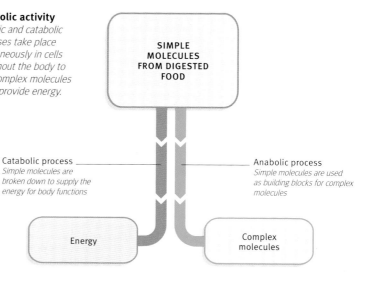

Metabolic activity
Anabolic and catabolic processes take place simultaneously in cells throughout the body to build complex molecules and to provide energy.

SIMPLE MOLECULES FROM DIGESTED FOOD

Catabolic process
Simple molecules are broken down to supply the energy for body functions

Anabolic process
Simple molecules are used as building blocks for complex molecules

Energy

Complex molecules

Basal metabolic rate

The amount of energy a person uses for essential functions, such as maintaining body heat, breathing, and heart rate, is called the basal metabolic rate (BMR). BMR decreases naturally with age, but it is raised in the short term by factors such as illness, pregnancy, breast-feeding, and menstruation. All forms of exercise increase the body's use of energy above the BMR.

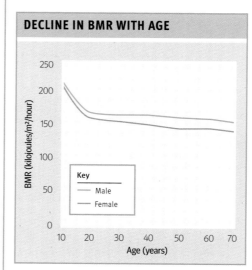

DECLINE IN BMR WITH AGE

BMR (kilojoules/m²/hour)

Key
— Male
— Female

Age (years)

Basal metabolic rate (BMR)
After about the age of 10, basal metabolic rate decreases with age and tends to be lower in females than in males. BMR is measured at rest and is often expressed as kilojoules used per square metre of body surface per hour (1 kilojoule equals about 4 kilocalories).

How the body uses food

Every living body cell depends on essential nutrients in food. Carbohydrates, proteins, and fats are converted into glucose, amino acids, and fatty acids respectively during digestion. These molecules enter the lymphatic system and the bloodstream and are converted into a usable form (metabolized) in the liver and in all body cells. Glucose is used to produce energy, as are fatty acids when glucose is in short supply. Amino acids are used to build the complex proteins needed to make and repair cells.

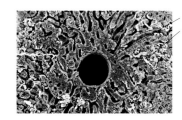

Liver tissue
The liver has a rich network of blood vessels. This magnified view of liver tissue shows a blood vessel surrounded by large liver cells (hepatocytes).

Mitochondrion
Each body cell contains many mitochondria. This magnified image of a mitochondrion, the cell "powerhouse", shows the folds (cristae) where energy-producing reactions take place.

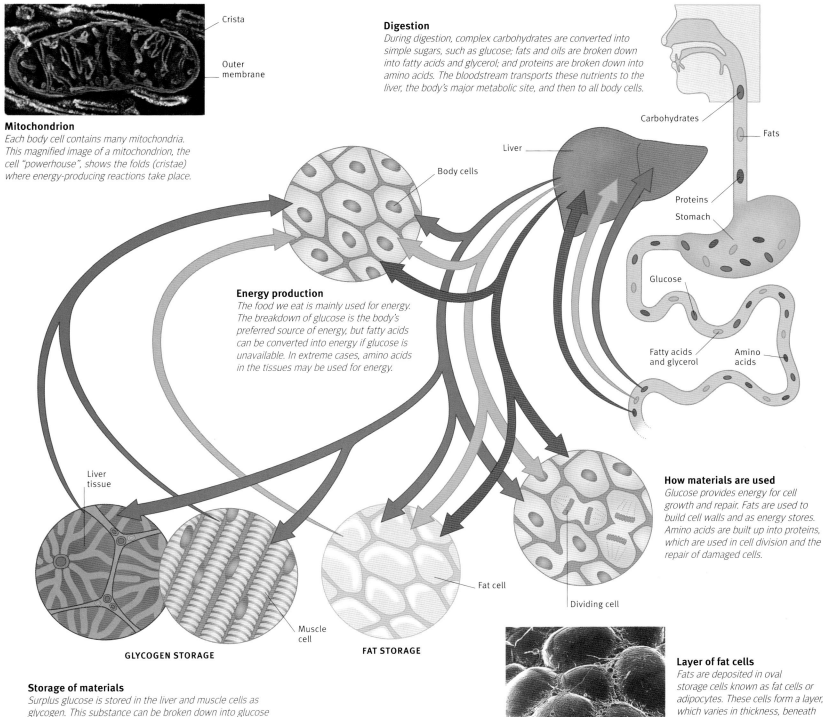

Digestion
During digestion, complex carbohydrates are converted into simple sugars, such as glucose; fats and oils are broken down into fatty acids and glycerol; and proteins are broken down into amino acids. The bloodstream transports these nutrients to the liver, the body's major metabolic site, and then to all body cells.

Energy production
The food we eat is mainly used for energy. The breakdown of glucose is the body's preferred source of energy, but fatty acids can be converted into energy if glucose is unavailable. In extreme cases, amino acids in the tissues may be used for energy.

How materials are used
Glucose provides energy for cell growth and repair. Fats are used to build cell walls and as energy stores. Amino acids are built up into proteins, which are used in cell division and the repair of damaged cells.

Storage of materials
Surplus glucose is stored in the liver and muscle cells as glycogen. This substance can be broken down into glucose and used for instant energy. Excess fats are stored as fatty acids in fat cells. Excess amino acids cannot be stored, but they can be converted into fatty acids for storage in fat cells. If glycogen stores are full, excess glucose is also converted into fatty acids for storage.

Layer of fat cells
Fats are deposited in oval storage cells known as fat cells or adipocytes. These cells form a layer, which varies in thickness, beneath the skin to insulate the body. A thin layer of adipose tissue surrounds the heart, kidneys, and other delicate internal organs. Fat cells also occur within organs, such as the pancreas.

Pituitary gland disorders

The pituitary gland is a small gland at the base of the brain that produces a large number of the hormones controlling growth, sexual development, and water balance. The gland also produces hormones that control many other hormone-secreting glands, such as the thyroid gland. Most pituitary disorders are caused by tumours that alter the output of particular pituitary hormones.

This section opens with a discussion of various tumours of the pituitary gland. Some types cause underproduction of particular hormones, and others cause overproduction. The abnormal hormone levels can have adverse effects elsewhere in the body; these effects are discussed in the articles that follow.

Particular pituitary hormones affect other hormone-secreting glands in the body; a pituitary disorder may thus lead to a disorder in another gland (see **Thyroid and parathyroid gland disorders**, pp.432–435, and **Adrenal gland disorders**, pp.435–436). Sex hormone disorders that may be caused by a problem with the pituitary gland are discussed elsewhere (see **Male hormonal disorders**, pp.465–466, and **Menstrual, menopausal, and hormonal problems**, pp.471–475), as are growth abnormalities in children that result from pituitary disorders (see **Growth disorders**, p.563).

KEY ANATOMY

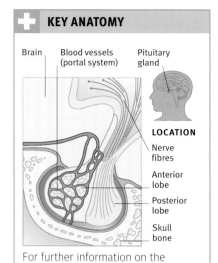

Brain | Blood vessels (portal system) | Pituitary gland

LOCATION

Nerve fibres

Anterior lobe

Posterior lobe

Skull bone

For further information on the structure and function of the pituitary gland, see pp.424–429.

Pituitary tumours

Abnormal growths in the pituitary gland, which may cause hormonal disturbances

 Age, gender, genetics, and lifestyle as risk factors depend on the type

The pituitary gland, located at the base of the brain, secretes hormones that either have a direct effect on the body or affect other hormone-secreting glands. For this reason, an abnormality in the pituitary gland may affect several body systems. Some pituitary tumours produce excessive amounts of hormones; others (called non-functioning tumours) do not produce hormones themselves but can disrupt the production of hormones from adjacent cells.

Tumours of the pituitary gland are rare. Usually, tumours occur in the front part of the gland and are noncancerous. The cause of most pituitary tumours is not known, although rarely they may be associated with the inherited disorder multiple endocrine neoplasia (p.434).

What are the types?

Nearly half of all hormone-secreting pituitary tumours make excess prolactin. Increased prolactin levels may lead to infertility in women and to erectile dysfunction in men (see **Prolactinoma**, right). Some pituitary tumours secrete growth hormone,

causing enlargement of some parts of the body (see **Acromegaly**, right). Others secrete hormones that overstimulate the adrenal glands, causing changes in body chemistry and physical appearance (see **Cushing's syndrome**, p.435).

As it grows, any pituitary tumour may press against the optic nerves, which lie above the gland. Such compression may cause headaches and loss of part of the field of vision (see **Visual field defects**, p.368). Growing pituitary tumours may also damage surrounding cells, thereby reducing secretion of one or more pituitary hormones (see

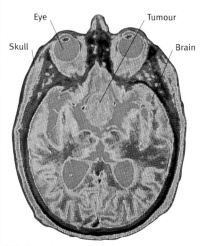

Eye | Tumour

Skull | Brain

Pituitary tumour
This MRI scan of the head reveals a large pituitary tumour, which may affect vision and produce headaches.

Hypopituitarism, opposite page). Reduced secretion of thyroid-stimulating hormone (TSH) may cause hypothyroidism (p.432). A tumour that presses on the posterior part of the pituitary gland may reduce secretion of vasopressin, which controls water balance (see **Diabetes insipidus**, opposite page).

What might be done?

You may have several blood tests to look for abnormal levels of pituitary hormones. You may also have MRI (p.133) or CT scanning (p.132) to look for a tumour and a visual field test (p.369) to check for blind areas. In some instances, a pituitary tumour is discovered during tests for another disorder. In this case, the tumour may be monitored without treatment unless symptoms develop.

Some tumours are treated with drugs (see **Pituitary drugs**, p.603). Others must be removed surgically. This is usually done by passing an endoscope (viewing tube) up through the nose to the pituitary gland. If it is not possible to remove the whole tumour, radiotherapy (p.158) may be given to prevent further growth of abnormal tissue. These treatments can result in hypopituitarism (underactivity of the pituitary), which may need hormone replacement for life.

Prolactinoma

A pituitary tumour causing excess secretion of prolactin, a hormone that influences fertility and breast milk production

 More common in females

 Age, genetics, and lifestyle are not significant factors

A prolactinoma is a noncancerous type of pituitary tumour. The tumour causes an excess of the hormone prolactin, which is essential for breast development and milk production in women. Although women's prolactin levels normally increase during pregnancy, an excessive level of the hormone can have adverse effects in both men and women. Prolactinomas occur more frequently in women. The cause is unknown.

What are the symptoms?

A prolactinoma usually develops over a period of several years, and the symptoms appear gradually. Symptoms that affect only women include:
■ Irregular or absent menstrual periods (see **Amenorrhoea**, p.471).
■ Infertility.
Some symptoms of prolactinoma affect only men, and these include:
■ Erectile dysfunction.
■ Breast enlargement.
There are some symptoms that affect both sexes, and these include:
■ Leakage of fluid from the nipples.
■ Reduced interest in sex.
An untreated tumour may grow large enough to put pressure on surrounding

areas of the brain. The pressure may cause headaches, loss of the normal field of vision (see **Visual field defects**, p.368), or hypopituitarism (opposite page).

What might be done?

If your doctor suspects that you have a prolactinoma, he or she will initially want to know if you could be pregnant or taking drugs, such as certain antipsychotics (p.592), that raise levels of prolactin and are not related to the presence of a prolactinoma. You will probably have a blood test to measure hormone levels. If the prolactin level is high, you may have imaging tests such as CT scanning (p.132) or MRI (p.133) to look for a pituitary tumour. If a tumour is found, drugs may be given to reduce production of prolactin (see **Pituitary drugs**, p.603). If treatment with drugs is unsuccessful, surgery to remove the tumour may be recommended.

What is the prognosis?

Drug treatment is successful in more than 3 in 4 cases. In the others, surgery is usually effective. Less commonly, the tumour may recur and treatment may need to be repeated.

If a woman becomes pregnant after treatment for a prolactinoma, she will be monitored carefully because the tumour may recur as a result of the hormonal changes. Drugs to lower prolactin levels may be discontinued during pregnancy.

Acromegaly

Excessive growth of parts of the body due to overproduction of growth hormone by the pituitary gland

 May occur at any age

 Occasionally runs in families

 Gender and lifestyle are not significant factors

Acromegaly is a rare condition that results from overproduction of growth hormone by the pituitary gland. Overproduction of growth hormone causes certain bones, particularly those in the face, hands, and feet, to enlarge. Soft tissues, such as the tongue, also become enlarged. Acromegaly may occur at any age. If excess growth hormone is produced during childhood, the condition causes exaggerated bone growth resulting in excessive height, and is called gigantism (see **Growth disorders**, p.563).

Acromegaly is usually caused by a pituitary tumour (left). In rare cases, acromegaly occurs as part of multiple endocrine neoplasia (p.434), an inherited disorder in which tumours develop in several of the endocrine glands around the body.

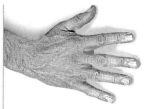

NORMAL

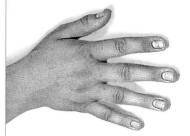

ACROMEGALY

Enlarged hand in acromegaly
Acromegaly can lead to enlarged hands, as shown in this comparison between the hand of an affected man and that of an unaffected man of similar build.

What are the symptoms?

If acromegaly develops in adulthood, the resulting physical changes occur almost imperceptibly over a period of years. Sometimes, the condition is detected by comparing old photographs with more recent ones. The following symptoms may become noticeable:

- Changes in the shape of the face, such as enlargement of the jaw.
- Enlargement of the hands or feet, resulting in a larger glove or shoe size.
- Deepening of the voice.
- Enlargement of the tongue.
- Tingling in the hands and feet.
- Excessive sweating.
- Increased growth of coarse body hair.

A growing pituitary tumour may press on the brain, causing headaches and loss of the normal field of vision (*see* **Visual field defects**, p.368) in addition to the symptoms of acromegaly. If not treated, acromegaly may cause serious disorders, such as diabetes mellitus (p.437) and enlargement of the heart (*see* **Dilated cardiomyopathy**, p.257), which may lead to chronic heart failure (p.247).

What might be done?

Your doctor may arrange for you to have several blood tests. If these tests reveal high growth hormone levels, you may also undergo imaging procedures, such as MRI (p.133) or CT scanning (p.132), to look for a pituitary tumour.

Small pituitary tumours may be removed completely by surgery. If a tumour is large or cannot be removed entirely, radiotherapy (p.158) may be necessary to destroy the remaining tumour cells, or drugs may be given to reduce the production of growth hormone (*see* **Pituitary drugs**, p.603).

Treatment is usually effective and prevents life-threatening complications from developing. Soft tissues will gradually decrease in size. However, changes in the size of bones cannot be reversed.

Hypopituitarism

Insufficient production of some or all of the pituitary hormones

 Age, gender, genetics, and lifestyle are not significant factors

Hypopituitarism is a rare condition in which the pituitary gland secretes inadequate amounts of one or more of its hormones. In some cases, the disorder is progressive, ultimately causing underproduction of all pituitary hormones.

Hypopituitarism is usually caused by a pituitary tumour that damages normal tissue in the gland as it grows. The disorder may also be due to other factors that damage the pituitary gland or the hypothalamus, the part of the brain directly above the pituitary gland. Such factors include surgery or radiotherapy (p.158) to treat a pituitary tumour or other head or neck tumour, head injury (p.322), or heavy blood loss that deprives the gland of oxygen.

What are the symptoms?

The symptoms may appear suddenly but more commonly develop gradually and can go unrecognized for months or years. They may include:

- Loss of interest in sex.
- Lack of menstrual periods in women.
- Loss of facial hair and shrinking of the testes in men.
- Loss of underarm and pubic hair.
- Dizziness, nausea, and vomiting.
- Paleness of the skin.
- Tiredness, constipation, weight gain, and intolerance to cold.

Left untreated, hypopituitarism can lead to coma and be fatal. This is because the body is unable to increase the output of hormones needed to respond to physical stresses such as injury or infection.

What might be done?

If your doctor suspects that you have hypopituitarism, he or she will probably arrange for blood tests to check your hormone levels. You may also need to undergo tests in hospital to determine hormone production in response to various chemical stimulants, and you may have MRI (p.133) or CT scanning (p.132) to look for a pituitary tumour.

If a tumour is detected, you may have surgery to remove it, followed by radiotherapy to prevent a recurrence. Hypopituitarism can be treated with lifelong hormone-replacement drugs. These drugs do not usually replace pituitary hormones; they replace hormones, such as thyroid hormones and corticosteroids, that are produced by other glands stimulated by the pituitary.

You may need additional doses of corticosteroid drugs (p.600) if you are injured or become ill. It is important for you to carry identification that provides information about the drugs you need in case a medical emergency arises.

Diabetes insipidus

Inadequate production of, or resistance to the effects of, the pituitary hormone involved in controlling water balance

 Age, gender, genetics, and lifestyle as risk factors depend on the type

Diabetes insipidus is a rare condition in which the kidneys produce large volumes of dilute urine. The condition is not related to diabetes mellitus (p.437), although both conditions cause thirst and excessive passing of urine.

In diabetes insipidus, the body lacks or cannot fully respond to the hormone vasopressin. This hormone is produced by the hypothalamus, the part of the brain directly above the pituitary gland. However, vasopressin is stored in and secreted by the pituitary gland, which is why it is usually considered a pituitary hormone. The role of vasopressin is to maintain the water balance of the body by controlling the amount of water excreted in the urine.

What are the types?

Diabetes insipidus occurs in two main forms: the more common form, called cranial diabetes insipidus, and a form known as nephrogenic diabetes insipidus.

Cranial diabetes insipidus is due to the reduced secretion of vasopressin. Possible causes of this condition include a pituitary tumour (opposite page), a tumour near the hypothalamus, surgery, radiotherapy (p.158), or head injuries (p.322). In some cases, the cause is not known.

In nephrogenic diabetes insipidus, there are normal levels of vasopressin but the kidneys fail to respond to it. In some cases, the condition is present from birth and is permanent. In these cases, it is more common in males because it is due to an inherited recessive gene carried on the X chromosome (*see* **Gene disorders**, p.151). The condition may also be due to chronic kidney disease (p.451) or to kidney damage resulting from the use of medications such as certain antibiotics (p.572) or lithium, a mood-stabilizing drug (p.593). In such cases, the condition may be reversible.

What are the symptoms?

Symptoms of both forms of diabetes insipidus usually develop over days or weeks, but they may appear suddenly if the pituitary gland has been damaged. Symptoms may include:

- Passing excessive amounts of urine.
- Insatiable thirst.
- Disturbed sleep due to the need to pass urine frequently.

If water lost from the body is not replaced, dehydration will occur. Severe dehydration may need immediate hospital treatment with intravenous fluids.

What might be done?

If your doctor suspects that you have diabetes insipidus, he or she may measure your urine volume over a 24-hour period. Also, urine output is measured after you have been deprived of fluids for several hours. If you have diabetes insipidus, you will continue to produce a large volume of urine. Your response to synthetic vasopressin is then measured. If vasopressin lowers your urine output, you probably have cranial diabetes insipidus; if output remains high, you probably have the nephrogenic form. If a tumour is suspected as the cause of the cranial form, you may also undergo imaging tests, such as MRI (p.133).

Cranial diabetes insipidus is most commonly treated with synthetic vasopressin (*see* **Pituitary drugs**, p.603). If there is an underlying cause, such as a pituitary tumour, this will be treated.

Nephrogenic diabetes insipidus that is inherited is usually treated with a low-sodium diet and thiazide diuretics (p.583), which paradoxically reduce urine volume. Treatment must be continued for life. Nephrogenic diabetes due to kidney damage may clear up as the kidneys recover; otherwise, drug treatment is needed. If you have diabetes insipidus, carry identification to alert others to the fact in an emergency.

Thyroid and parathyroid gland disorders

The thyroid and parathyroid glands are situated in the neck, where they produce and secrete hormones into the bloodstream. There are two types of thyroid hormone, both of which help to control the rate of metabolism (the chemical reactions constantly occurring in the body). The four small parathyroid glands produce a hormone that controls calcium levels in the blood.

Thyroid disorders are common, but their onset is often gradual and they may not be detected or diagnosed for months or even years. Low levels of thyroid hormones at birth can prevent normal development of the brain and, for this reason, a blood test for thyroid hormone levels is one of the first tests to be performed on a newborn baby (*see* Blood spot screening tests, p.561). Over- and underactivity of the thyroid gland are the most common thyroid disorders and are discussed first. Swellings and growths are covered next, followed by disorders in which there is over- or underproduction of hormones by the parathyroid gland.

The last article describes multiple endocrine neoplasia, a group of rare inherited disorders in which tumours develop in several endocrine glands, including the thyroid and parathyroid.

KEY ANATOMY

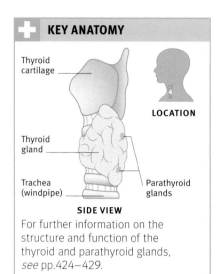

Thyroid cartilage

LOCATION

Thyroid gland

Trachea (windpipe)

Parathyroid glands

SIDE VIEW

For further information on the structure and function of the thyroid and parathyroid glands, *see* pp.424–429.

Hyperthyroidism

Overproduction of thyroid hormones, causing many body functions to speed up

 Most common between the ages of 20 and 50

 More common in females

 Sometimes runs in families

 Lifestyle is not a significant factor

When the thyroid gland produces an excess of hormones, many of the body's functions are stimulated by these hormones and speed up. This condition is known as hyperthyroidism and is one of the most common hormonal disorders. Hyperthyroidism is 7–10 times more common in women and often develops between the ages of 20 and 50.

About 3 in 4 cases of the condition are due to Graves' disease, an autoimmune disorder in which the immune system produces antibodies that attack the thyroid gland, resulting in overproduction of thyroid hormones. Graves' disease tends to run in families and is thought to have a genetic basis. In rare cases, hyperthyroidism may be associated with other autoimmune disorders, in particular the skin disorder vitiligo (p.198) and pernicious anaemia, a disorder

of the blood (*see* Megaloblastic anaemia, p.272). In some cases, thyroid nodules (p.433) that secrete hormones may be the cause of hyperthyroidism. Inflammation of the thyroid gland (*see* Thyroiditis, opposite page) may temporarily produce symptoms of hyperthyroidism.

What are the symptoms?
In most cases, symptoms of hyperthyroidism develop gradually over several weeks and may include:
- Weight loss despite increased appetite and food consumption.
- Rapid heartbeat, which is sometimes also irregular.
- Tremor (persistent trembling) affecting the hands.
- Warm, moist skin as a result of excessive sweating.
- Intolerance to heat.
- Anxiety and insomnia.
- Frequent bowel movements.
- Swelling in the neck caused by an enlarged thyroid (*see* Goitre, opposite page).
- Muscle weakness.
- In women, irregular menstruation.

People with hyperthyroidism caused by Graves' disease may also have bulging eyes (*see* Exophthalmos, p.363).

How is it diagnosed?
If your doctor suspects that you have hyperthyroidism, he or she may arrange for a blood test to check for abnormally high levels of thyroid hormones and for

antibodies that can attack the thyroid gland. Your doctor will also feel around your neck for lumps caused by enlargement of the gland. If swelling is detected, radionuclide scanning (p.135) or ultrasound scanning (p.135) may be used to investigate the cause.

What is the treatment?
Symptoms of hyperthyroidism can initially be relieved by beta-blocker drugs (p.581), which reduce tremor and anxiety but do not affect thyroid hormone levels. There are three main treatments aimed at reducing the production of thyroid hormones. The most common is antithyroid drugs (*see* Drugs for hyperthyroidism, p.602), which work by suppressing production of thyroid hormones. These drugs need to be taken daily for 12–18 months, after which the thyroid gland often functions normally. Radioactive iodine may be the most effective treatment for hormone-secreting thyroid nodules and may also be used for Graves' disease. Treatment usually involves taking a single oral dose of radioactive iodine. The radioactive iodine is absorbed by the body and accumulates in the thyroid gland, destroying part of it. Surgical removal of the thyroid is an alternative treatment. In most cases, the entire gland is removed to eliminate the possibility of a recurrence of hyperthyroidism.

What is the prognosis?
Many people recover fully following treatment. However, unless the thyroid has been completely removed, hyperthyroidism may recur. If the treatment involves surgery and the entire thyroid has been removed, thyroid hormone supplements will be needed for the rest of your life. If the treatment is with radioactive iodine, the remaining part of the thyroid may not be able to produce sufficient hormones (*see* Hypothyroidism, below) and therefore thyroid hormone levels need to be monitored regularly after treatment so that hormone supplements can be given if needed.

Hypothyroidism

Underproduction of thyroid hormones, causing many body functions to slow down

 May be present from birth but most common over the age of 40

 More common in females

 Sometimes runs in families

 Dietary iodine deficiency is a risk factor in developing countries

In hypothyroidism, the thyroid gland does not produce enough thyroid hormones. These hormones are important in metabolism (the chemical reactions constantly occurring in the body). A deficiency causes many of the body's functions to slow down. The condition may be present from birth down. The condition may be present from

birth, in which case treatment is begun immediately, but it is more common in people over the age of 40, particularly women.

What are the causes?
Hypothyroidism that is present from birth has no known cause. In adults, a common cause of hypothyroidism is thyroiditis (opposite page). The most common type of thyroiditis that leads to hypothyroidism is the autoimmune disorder Hashimoto's thyroiditis, which tends to run in families. In Hashimoto's thyroiditis, the body produces antibodies that attack the thyroid gland, damaging it permanently. Other forms of thyroiditis may lead to temporary or permanent hypothyroidism. Treatment for an overactive thyroid with radioactive iodine or surgery (*see* Hyperthyroidism, below left) can lead to permanent hypothyroidism.

Rarely, hypothyroidism is due to underproduction of thyroid-stimulating hormone (TSH) by the pituitary gland, often as the result of a pituitary tumour (p.430). TSH stimulates the thyroid gland to secrete its own hormones. Insufficient dietary iodine, essential for the production of thyroid hormones, can also cause hypothyroidism, but this is rare in developed countries.

What are the symptoms?
The symptoms of hypothyroidism vary in severity and usually develop slowly over months or years. They may include:
- Extreme tiredness.
- Weight gain.
- Constipation.
- Hoarseness of the voice.
- Intolerance to cold.
- Swelling of the face, puffy eyes, and dry, thickened skin.
- Generalized hair thinning.
- In women, heavy menstrual periods.

Some people with hypothyroidism develop a swelling in the neck due to an enlarged thyroid (*see* Goitre, opposite page).

What might be done?
Blood tests to measure the levels of thyroid hormones and antibodies that act against the thyroid gland are used to diagnose hypothyroidism. In the UK, all newborns are tested for hypothyroidism shortly after birth (*see* Blood spot screening tests, p.561).

Babies with an underactive thyroid are treated promptly with synthetic thyroid hormones, which need to be taken for life (*see* Drugs for hypothyroidism, p.602). Lifelong hormone treatment may also be needed if permanent hypothyroidism is diagnosed in adulthood, in which case symptoms should begin to improve about 3 weeks after starting treatment. Hormone treatment must be monitored regularly to ensure that the correct dose is maintained. If hypothyroidism is the result of a pituitary disorder, this will need to be investigated and treated.

Temporary hypothyroidism does not usually need to be treated. Supplements can be taken to correct iodine deficiency.

Goitre

A swelling in the neck due to enlargement of the thyroid gland

 Age, gender, genetics, and lifestyle as risk factors depend on the cause

If the thyroid gland becomes enlarged, it causes a swelling to appear in the neck. This swelling is known as a goitre. A goitre can range in size from a barely noticeable lump to a swelling the size of a grapefruit. In rare cases, a very large goitre may press against the oesophagus and trachea (windpipe) in the neck, which can cause difficulty in swallowing and breathing.

What are the causes?

The thyroid gland may enlarge without any disturbance of its function at certain times, particularly at puberty and during pregnancy. Disorders that may be associated with goitre include hyperthyroidism (opposite page), hypothyroidism (opposite page), thyroid nodules (right), and certain types of thyroiditis (right). Goitre is a known side effect of drugs such as lithium (*see* **Mood-stabilizing drugs**, p.593), which is used to treat bipolar affective disorder (p.344). Iodine deficiency may also be a cause of goitre, although this is extremely rare in developed countries. Rarely, goitre is due to thyroid cancer (p.434).

What might be done?

Your doctor will examine your neck to assess the size and shape of the thyroid gland. A blood sample may be taken to measure your thyroid hormone levels, and ultrasound (p.135) or radionuclide (p.135) scanning may be performed to look at the thyroid. Needle aspiration of the thyroid gland (right) may be performed for a more precise diagnosis.

Treatment with surgery, radioactive iodine, or antithyroid drugs (*see* **Drugs for hyperthyroidism**, p.602) is sometimes successful in shrinking a goitre in people with hyperthyroidism. Surgery may also be necessary if breathing or swallowing is obstructed or if thyroid cancer is suspected. A small goitre that has no effect on thyroid function may not need treatment and may decrease in size or disappear completely with time.

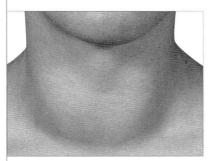

Goitre
This swelling in the neck, called a goitre, is due to enlargement of the thyroid gland. Most goitres are painless.

Thyroiditis

Inflammation of the thyroid gland, causing temporary or permanent damage

 More common in adults; rare in children

 Gender and genetics as risk factors depend on the type

 Lifestyle is not a significant factor

Inflammation of the thyroid gland is known as thyroiditis. This disorder can disrupt thyroid activity, causing underactivity (*see* **Hypothyroidism**, opposite page) or overactivity (*see* **Hyperthyroidism**, opposite page) of the thyroid gland. The under- or overproduction of thyroid hormones that results is usually temporary, but it can be permanent.

What are the types?

Thyroiditis may take a number of different forms, depending on its cause. The four most common types of thyroiditis are described below.

Hashimoto's thyroiditis The most common type of thyroid inflammation is Hashimoto's thyroiditis, an autoimmune disorder in which antibodies are produced that attack the thyroid gland. It often causes thyroid underactivity (*see* **Hypothyroidism**, opposite page) and sometimes swelling in the neck due to enlargement of the gland (*see* **Goitre**, left). Hashimoto's thyroiditis is eight times more common in women and sometimes runs in families. It may occur with other autoimmune disorders, such as the skin disorder vitiligo (p.198) or pernicious anaemia of the blood (*see* **Megaloblastic anaemia**, p.272).

Viral thyroiditis This form of thyroiditis can sometimes be mistaken for a throat infection because it causes pain on swallowing. There may also be pain in the jaws or ears, fever, and weight loss. Viral thyroiditis can cause overactivity followed by underactivity of the gland.

Postpartum thyroiditis About 1 in 10 women develops postpartum thyroiditis within a few months of giving birth. It is thought that it results from changes in a woman's immune system during pregnancy. Symptoms are uncommon but may include those of hyperthyroidism followed by those of hypothyroidism. Postpartum thyroiditis usually clears up after a few months but may recur after future pregnancies.

Drug-induced thyroiditis Certain medications may cause thyroiditis, producing either underactivity or overactivity of the gland, and sometimes also causing pain in the area around the gland. Drugs that may cause thyroiditis include amiodarone (used for heart arrhythmias), lithium (a mood-stabilizing drug), and interferon (a drug that alters the activity of the immune system).

What might be done?

Your doctor may arrange for a blood test to check your thyroid hormone levels and look for antibodies that attack the thyroid gland. Radionuclide scanning (p.135) may also be necessary to assess thyroid activity.

If you have Hashimoto's thyroiditis, you will usually need lifelong treatment with synthetic thyroid hormones (*see* **Drugs for hypothyroidism**, p.602). In severe cases of viral thyroiditis, corticosteroids (p.600) or aspirin may be used to relieve the inflammation. Postpartum thyroiditis is usually temporary. Drug-induced thyroiditis is usually short-lived and clears up when the medication is stopped.

Thyroid nodules

Growths that develop in the thyroid gland, which are usually noncancerous

 Most common between the ages of 40 and 60

 More common in females

 Genetics and lifestyle are not significant factors

Thyroid nodules are abnormal growths that develop in the thyroid gland. They are generally small and occur as single or multiple solid lumps or cysts. Some nodules produce excess thyroid hormones (*see* **Hyperthyroidism**, opposite page). All types of thyroid nodule are most common in people between the ages of 40 and 60 and are three times more common in women than in men.

What are the symptoms?

Nodules may cause no symptoms, but some people may develop the following:
- Lump or swelling in the neck.
- Difficulty in swallowing or breathing.
If nodules cause hyperthyroidism, additional symptoms may develop, such as rapid heartbeat and loss of weight.

What might be done?

Imaging of the thyroid gland with ultrasound scanning (p.135) or radionuclide scanning (p.135) may be necessary to diagnose a thyroid nodule. Needle aspiration of the thyroid gland (below) may be carried out to establish whether a nodule is a solid lump or a cyst or if it is cancerous. If the nodule is cancerous, further investigation and treatment are necessary (*see* **Thyroid cancer**, p.434).

▶ **TEST**

Needle aspiration of the thyroid gland

Also known as fine needle aspiration of the thyroid gland, this procedure is used to determine the cause of a lump and, if the lump is a cyst, to drain it. During the procedure, cells are removed from the abnormal area using a fine hollow needle attached to a syringe. Ultrasound guidance may be used to confirm the location of the lump. The sample is then examined in a laboratory for cancerous cells. This procedure is safe and almost painless and can be carried out in an outpatient clinic.

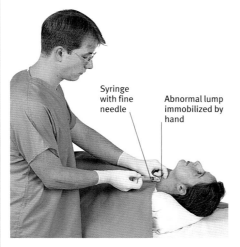

Syringe with fine needle

Abnormal lump immobilized by hand

Taking a sample
A pillow is placed under your neck to raise the thyroid area. The doctor withdraws cells from the abnormal area using a syringe with a fine needle.

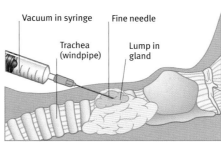

Vacuum in syringe

Fine needle

Trachea (windpipe)

Lump in gland

INSIDE THE NECK

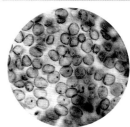

RESULTS

Cancerous thyroid cells
Abnormal thyroid cells obtained using needle aspiration are viewed through a microscope in the laboratory by a specialist. These cells, taken from an abnormal lump, are cancerous.

Noncancerous thyroid nodules that do not cause symptoms may not require treatment but should be monitored on a regular basis. Radioactive iodine will be used to treat a nodule that secretes excess thyroid hormones (see **Drugs for hyperthyroidism**, p.602).

Thyroid cancer

An uncommon, cancerous tumour occurring in the thyroid gland

 More common over the age of 40

 More common in females

 Previous exposure of the neck to radiation is a risk factor

 Genetics as risk factor depends on the type

Abnormal growths in the thyroid gland can sometimes be cancerous. Thyroid cancer is rare, accounting for only 1 in 100 of all cancers, but it is about twice as common in women as men. The condition is more common over the age of 40 but can occur at any age. Evidence suggests that previous exposure of the neck area to radiation increases the risk.

What are the types?
There are four main types of thyroid cancer: papillary, follicular, medullary, and anaplastic. About 7 in 10 thyroid cancers are papillary, and this type of thyroid cancer spreads most often to the lymph nodes. Follicular thyroid cancer is less common and may spread to the lungs or the bones. Medullary thyroid cancer is rare and is usually associated with multiple endocrine neoplasia (right), an inherited condition. Anaplastic thyroid cancer is also rare; it usually occurs in older people and tends to be more aggressive than other types of thyroid cancer.

What are the symptoms?
The symptoms depend on the type of thyroid cancer, but they often include:
- Painless, hard lump in the neck.
- Difficulty swallowing.
- Hoarseness.
The first symptom of papillary thyroid cancer may be a lump in the side of the neck due to enlarged lymph nodes.

What might be done?
If you develop a lump in your neck, your doctor will examine you and may arrange for a blood test to measure thyroid hormone levels. The thyroid gland may be imaged using ultrasound scanning (p.135) or radionuclide scanning (p.135). Needle aspiration of the thyroid gland (p.433) may be carried out to check for cancer.

Papillary, follicular, and medullary thyroid cancers are usually treated by surgical removal of the whole thyroid gland. With medullary cancer, it may also be necessary to remove nearby lymph nodes. Further treatment often involves an oral dose of radioactive iodine to destroy any cancer cells that may still be present. After treatment, you will need to take thyroid hormone drugs for the rest of your life (see **Drugs for hypothyroidism**, p.602). Treatment for anaplastic cancer involves radiation therapy and chemotherapy. Surgery is not usually beneficial because the cancer has often spread too extensively by the time it is diagnosed.

If papillary, follicular, or medullary cancers are diagnosed early, the survival rate is as high as 95 per cent after 5 years. Because it is so aggressive, anaplastic cancer has a poorer outlook, with less than 10 per cent of people surviving for 5 years or more after diagnosis.

Hyperparathyroidism

Overproduction of parathyroid hormone, which may lead to a high level of calcium in the blood

 More common over the age of 50

 More common in females

 In some cases, the condition is inherited

 Lifestyle is not a significant factor

Parathyroid hormone (PTH), which is produced by four pea-sized parathyroid glands embedded in the thyroid tissue, helps to regulate the body's calcium levels. Overproduction of PTH is called hyperparathyroidism and leads to high calcium levels in the blood. The condition rarely develops before the age of 50 and is much more common in women.

What are the causes?
The most common cause of hyperparathyroidism is a tumour in one or more of the four parathyroid glands. In some cases, development of parathyroid tumours is associated with the inherited disorder multiple endocrine neoplasia (right). Parathyroid tumours are rarely cancerous.

The parathyroid glands may become enlarged and overproduce PTH in an attempt to compensate for disorders that cause a low blood calcium level, such as chronic kidney disease (p.451) or severe vitamin D deficiency. In these cases, the condition is called secondary hyperparathyroidism.

What are the symptoms?
A slightly raised level of calcium in the blood due to hyperparathyroidism may not cause symptoms. However, people with a very high calcium level may develop the following symptoms:
- Abdominal pain.
- Nausea and vomiting.
- Constipation.
- Increased thirst and passing of urine.
- Depression.

An abnormally high level of calcium in the blood may also lead to dehydration, confusion, and unconsciousness, and it can even be life-threatening.

Serious complications of hyperparathyroidism include the formation of kidney stones (p.447), due to a build-up of calcium in the kidneys, and bone fractures (p.232), resulting from calcium gradually leaking out of the bone into the bloodstream.

What might be done?
If you develop symptoms of hyperparathyroidism, your doctor is likely to arrange for you to have blood tests to assess your kidney function and check for raised levels of calcium and PTH. If blood tests confirm hyperparathyroidism, you may have further tests, such as ultrasound, CT or other scans and possibly a biopsy of a gland (removal of a sample of gland tissue for analysis), to investigate the cause and check for complications.

If you have not experienced symptoms, hyperparathyroidism is usually detected by chance during a routine checkup or as a result of blood tests or other tests carried out to investigate another condition, such as the cause of kidney stones.

You may not require treatment if the level of calcium in your blood is only slightly raised; however, your blood calcium level and kidney function will need to be monitored annually. If your calcium levels are very high, you will be given fluids and drugs intravenously in hospital to lower blood calcium.

If a parathyroid tumour is accompanied by high blood calcium levels, the affected parathyroid gland will be removed surgically. You may need calcium supplements immediately after surgery, but body calcium levels usually return to normal after a few days. The underlying disorder causing secondary hyperparathyroidism will be treated if possible; alternatively, some of the parathyroid glands may be removed surgically.

Hypoparathyroidism

Underproduction of parathyroid hormone, which may lead to a low level of calcium in the blood

 More common in females

 Sometimes runs in families

 Age and lifestyle are not significant factors

Hypoparathyroidism occurs when the parathyroid glands, which are embedded in the thyroid tissue, produce too little parathyroid hormone (PTH). PTH regulates the amount of calcium in the body. A lack of PTH results in an abnormally low level of calcium in the blood and may lead to the development of disorders of the muscles and nerves, which need calcium to function properly. In rare cases, hypoparathyroidism is present from birth. It is twice as common in women as men and sometimes runs in families.

What are the causes?
Damage to the parathyroid glands during surgery on the thyroid gland is the most common cause of hypoparathyroidism. In this case, the disorder tends to develop suddenly. In rare cases, hypoparathyroidism is associated with autoimmune disorders, in which the body attacks its own tissues.

What are the symptoms?
If hypoparathyroidism develops after thyroid surgery, symptoms appear within a few hours. In other cases, symptoms develop gradually and are usually less severe. In either case, symptoms are due to low calcium levels and include:
- Tetany (muscular spasm) in the feet, the hands, and sometimes the throat.
- Tingling and numbness in the hands, the feet, and around the mouth.
- Seizures.
If the condition is left untreated, long-term complications, such as cataracts (p.357), may develop.

What might be done?
If your doctor suspects hypoparathyroidism from your symptoms, he or she will probably arrange for blood tests to measure the levels of PTH and calcium.

If the symptoms are severe, you may require emergency hospital treatment, including intravenous injections of calcium to relieve muscle spasms. Lifelong treatment with dietary supplements of calcium (see **Minerals**, p.599) and vitamin D (see **Vitamins**, p.598) may be necessary, as well as regular blood tests to monitor your blood calcium level.

Multiple endocrine neoplasia

A rare inherited disorder in which tumours develop in several of the endocrine glands

 Due to an abnormal gene inherited from one parent

 Age, gender, and lifestyle are not significant factors

In the rare disorder known as multiple endocrine neoplasia (MEN), tumours form in several of the endocrine glands around the body. The condition exists in many forms, each caused by a different abnormal gene. In each case, this abnormal gene is inherited in an autosomal dominant manner, which means that the condition can be inherited from just one parent (see **Gene disorders**, p.151). Each child of an affected person has a 1 in 2 chance of inheriting the abnormal MEN gene, and the condition can appear at any age.

Tumours may develop in several endocrine glands at the same time or at different times over a period of years. In the most common type of the disorder, known as MEN 1, tumours develop in the pancreas, parathyroid glands, and pituitary gland (*see* **Pituitary tumours**, p.430). Less commonly, a variant known as MEN 2 causes tumours to develop in the adrenal glands (*see* **Phaeochromocytoma**, p.436) and the thyroid gland. Thyroid tumours may be cancerous (*see* **Thyroid cancer**, opposite page), but tumours that develop in other endocrine glands are usually noncancerous. The affected glands may produce excess hormones.

What might be done?
If your doctor detects an abnormality in one gland, he or she may arrange for you to have blood tests to check the function of the other endocrine glands. If MEN is diagnosed, your family may be offered screening tests for the abnormal gene. Members with the abnormal gene can be monitored to detect tumours at an early stage.

Tumours are usually removed surgically. After treatment, you will probably be monitored periodically to check for endocrine abnormalities. If endocrine tumours are diagnosed early, they can usually be treated successfully.

Adrenal gland disorders

There are two adrenal glands, one situated above each kidney. Hormones produced by the adrenal glands are vital in controlling body chemistry. If adrenal hormone levels become imbalanced, the effects tend to be widespread throughout the body and are often serious, even life-threatening. However, these disorders are rare.

Adrenal gland disorders may involve either the over- or underproduction of adrenal hormones. This section first discusses disorders in which adrenal hormones are overproduced. The overproduction of adrenal hormones is most commonly due to the presence of an adrenal tumour. These tumours are usually noncancerous and can often be removed by means of surgery.

The final article discusses Addison's disease, a disorder in which the adrenal gland underproduces hormones. The lack of adrenal hormones is frequently caused by an autoimmune disorder that damages the gland. Addison's disease can be treated successfully with synthetic hormones.

Adrenal disorders are sometimes caused by changes in the levels of hormones that are produced by the pituitary gland (*see* **Pituitary gland disorders**, pp.430–431). There is also an extremely rare adrenal disorder that is caused by a genetic defect (*see* **Congenital adrenal hyperplasia**, p.561). Disorders that are due to the

abnormal production of sex hormones by the adrenal glands are described elsewhere in the book (*see* **Male hormonal disorders**, pp.465–466, and **Menstrual, menopausal, and hormonal problems**, pp.471–475).

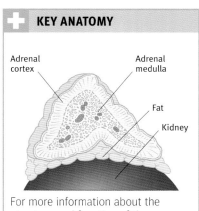

⊕ KEY ANATOMY

Adrenal cortex

Adrenal medulla

Fat

Kidney

For more information about the structure and function of the adrenal glands, *see* pp.424–429.

Adrenal tumours

Tumours in the adrenal glands, usually noncancerous, that may produce excess adrenal hormones

 Age, gender, genetics, and lifestyle as risk factors depend on the type

Tumours of the adrenal glands are rare, and in 9 out of 10 cases they are noncancerous. In almost all cases, tumours occur in only one adrenal gland, and their effects depend on which part of the gland is affected. Most adrenal tumours secrete excessive amounts of one or more of the adrenal hormones, which can upset metabolism (the chemical reactions constantly

occurring in the body) and water balance and may alter the body's response to physical stress such as injury.

What are the types?
Adrenal tumours can develop in either the cortex (outer layer) or the medulla (centre) of the adrenal gland.

Adrenal tumours in the cortex may secrete corticosteroids, aldosterone, or androgens (male sex hormones). Overproduction of corticosteroids leads to changes in physical appearance as well as in body chemistry (*see* **Cushing's syndrome**, right) and may cause serious complications. An excess of the hormone aldosterone, a condition known as hyperaldosteronism (p.436), disturbs the body's salt and water balance and is a rare

cause of high blood pressure (*see* **Hypertension**, p.242). A high level of androgens in women may lead to the development of male characteristics (*see* **Virilization**, p.474); in males, an excess often goes unnoticed.

Tumours that develop in the adrenal medulla are known as phaeochromocytomas (p.436). These tumours produce large amounts of either or both of the hormones epinephrine (adrenaline) and norepinephrine (noradrenaline), excessive levels of which cause sweating, high blood pressure, and palpitations.

What might be done?
Adrenal tumours are usually diagnosed by detecting abnormal levels of adrenal hormones in the blood. Imaging tests, such as MRI (p.133) and CT scanning (p.132), may also be carried out to look for abnormalities in the adrenal glands.

Most tumours can be treated by surgical removal. In the rare cases in which a tumour is found to be cancerous, chemotherapy (p.157) or radiotherapy (p.158) may also be necessary.

Cushing's syndrome

Changes in body chemistry and physical appearance caused by excessive amounts of corticosteroid hormones

 More common in females

 Age, genetics, and lifestyle are not significant factors

Corticosteroid hormones are involved in the regulation of metabolism (the chemical reactions that continually occur in the body) and play a part in the control of salt and water balance and blood pressure. In Cushing's syndrome, an excess of corticosteroids causes disruption of these control mechanisms. The distribution of fat around the body and the growth of body hair are affected, resulting in significant changes in physical appearance. Depression and other psychological problems may also develop. Cushing's syndrome is more common in women than in men.

What are the causes?
The most common cause of Cushing's syndrome is long-term treatment with oral corticosteroid drugs (p.600). These drugs mimic the effects of natural corticosteroids produced by the adrenal glands. Less commonly, Cushing's syndrome is due to the overproduction of corticosteroids by the adrenal glands. This may be caused by a hormone-secreting tumour in one of the adrenal glands (*see* **Adrenal tumours**, left) or by a tumour in the pituitary gland (*see* **Pituitary tumours**, p.430) that produces the hormone ACTH, which stimulates the adrenal glands.

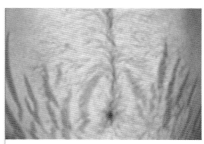

Stretch marks in Cushing's syndrome
Large, reddish-purple stretch marks on the trunk, especially the abdomen, are often seen in people with Cushing's syndrome.

Some cancers, such as primary lung cancer (p.307), produce hormones that mimic pituitary hormones and may cause Cushing's syndrome as a result.

What are the symptoms?
The symptoms of Cushing's syndrome appear gradually and become increasingly obvious over a period of weeks or months. Any of the following may occur:
■ Changes in the appearance of the face, which may become red and rounded.
■ Weight gain concentrated around the chest and abdomen.
■ Excessive growth of facial or body hair (more noticeable in women).
■ In women, irregular menstruation. Eventually, menstruation may stop.
■ Reddish-purple stretch marks on the abdomen, thighs, and arms.
■ Pads of fat between the shoulder blades at the base of the neck.
■ Difficulty climbing stairs, associated with muscle wasting and weakness of the legs. Arms may also be affected.
■ Tendency to bruise easily, especially on the limbs.
■ Acne (p.197).
■ Lack or loss of sexual drive; men may develop erectile dysfunction (p.494).
■ Depression and mood swings.
If the condition is left untreated, it may eventually lead to complications such as high blood pressure (*see* **Hypertension**, p.242), thinning of the bones (*see* **Osteoporosis**, p.217), diabetes mellitus (p.437), and chronic heart failure (p.247).

How is it diagnosed?
If you have been taking large doses of corticosteroid drugs, your doctor will probably be able to diagnose Cushing's syndrome from your symptoms. Otherwise, tests on blood or urine may be carried out to look for raised levels of natural corticosteroids. Abnormally high levels of corticosteroids may indicate that you have an adrenal tumour or that your adrenal glands are overstimulated.

Once the diagnosis is confirmed, the cause will be investigated. You may have tests in hospital to distinguish between raised hormone levels that may be due to a pituitary tumour and those possibly due to an adrenal tumour. MRI (p.133) or CT scanning (p.132) of the adrenal glands may be carried out.

What is the treatment?

The treatment of Cushing's syndrome depends on the underlying cause. If you are on a long-term course of corticosteroid drugs, your doctor will try to keep the dose to a minimum or, if possible, discontinue the treatment. However, you should not stop taking corticosteroid drugs without first consulting your doctor.

If the cause is a tumour in one of the adrenal glands, your doctor may initially prescribe drugs to lower corticosteroid levels. After that, it may be necessary to have the affected adrenal gland surgically removed.

If the adrenal glands have been over-stimulated by a pituitary tumour, the tumour may be surgically removed. In most cases the surgery is successful but radiotherapy (p.158) or drug treatment are sometimes necessary to destroy any remaining abnormal cells.

You may need to take small doses of corticosteroid drugs for several months after surgery until your adrenal gland or glands adapt and produce normal amounts of hormones. The symptoms of Cushing's syndrome should then improve gradually. In rare cases, if both adrenal glands are removed, you will need corticosteroid drugs for life.

Hyperaldosteronism

An excess of the hormone aldosterone that causes changes in body chemistry

 More common over the age of 30

 More common in females

 Genetics and lifestyle are not significant factors

Aldosterone is a hormone that is produced by the outer layers of the adrenal glands and acts on the kidneys to regulate the body's sodium balance and blood pressure. Overproduction of aldosterone by one or both adrenal glands is called hyperaldosteronism and leads to a high level of sodium in the body and loss of potassium in the urine. High sodium levels, in turn, cause high blood pressure (*see* **Hypertension**, p.242), although fewer than 2 in 100 people with high blood pressure have hyperaldosteronism.

Hyperaldosteronism is usually due to a noncancerous tumour in the adrenal cortex. It may also result from other conditions, such as chronic heart failure (p.247), cirrhosis (p.410), and nephrotic syndrome (p.447). Hyperaldosteronism due to an adrenal tumour is more common after the age of 30 and in women.

What are the symptoms?

Hyperaldosteronism causes high blood pressure but this rarely produces noticeable symptoms and may only be detected

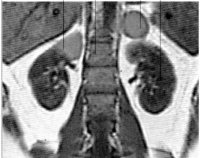

Aldosterone-producing tumour
This vertical CT scan through the upper abdomen shows an adrenal tumour. Such tumours may cause hyperaldosteronism.

during a routine health checkup. If symptoms do develop, they may include:
- Muscle weakness and cramps.
- Frequent passing of large amounts of urine, accompanied by thirst.
- Headaches and tiredness.

What might be done?

You may have arrange blood tests to measure sodium, potassium, and aldosterone levels, and CT scanning (p.132) or MRI scanning (p.133) to look for a tumour. If a tumour is found, the adrenal gland may be surgically removed. Treatment may include drugs to block aldosterone (such as spironolactone), and medication to control blood pressure (*see* **Antihypertensive drugs**, p.580).

Phaeochromocytoma

A tumour in the centre of the adrenal gland that produces an excess of certain adrenal hormones

 Most common between the ages of 30 and 60 but may occur at any age

 Sometimes runs in families

 Gender and lifestyle are not significant factors

A phaeochromocytoma is a tumour that develops in the medulla (centre) of one of the adrenal glands. Phaeochromocytomas produce excessive amounts of the hormones epinephrine (adrenaline) and norepinephrine (noradrenaline), which are normally produced by the adrenal glands to prepare the body for action or physical stress. Phaeochromocytomas are rare. Only 1 in 10 is cancerous. Such tumours may develop as part of multiple endocrine neoplasia (p.434), an inherited condition in which tumours occur in several hormone-secreting glands.

What are the symptoms?

Exercise, emotion, or even a change in body position can trigger the tumour to release hormones into the blood. When this happens, you may experience the following symptoms:

- Palpitations (awareness of an abnormally fast or irregular heartbeat).
- Pale, cold skin and profuse sweating.
- Nausea and vomiting.
- Feelings of intense anxiety.
- Headache.

Raised levels of epinephrine and norepinephrine also lead to a rise in blood pressure (*see* **Hypertension**, p.242).

What might be done?

If your doctor suspects a phaeochromocytoma, he or she may ask you to collect your urine over a 24-hour period so that tests can be performed on it. Chemicals in the urine provide information about levels of epinephrine and norepinephrine in the body. If the levels of these hormones are higher than normal, you will probably have MRI (p.133) or CT scanning (p.132) to look for a tumour.

Initially, drug treatment is used to lower your blood pressure. The tumour is then removed surgically. People who have had a noncancerous phaeochromocytoma removed usually make a full recovery. However, cancerous tumours are more likely to recur.

Addison's disease

Insufficient levels of corticosteroid hormones in the blood, causing changes in body chemistry

 Twice as common in females

 Sometimes runs in families

 Age and lifestyle are not significant factors

Corticosteroids are adrenal hormones involved in metabolism (the chemical reactions constantly occurring in the body). They also help to control blood pressure and sodium and water balance in the body. In the rare disorder Addison's disease, underproduction of corticosteroids leads to changes in body chemistry. The condition is twice as common in women and sometimes runs in families.

The usual cause of Addison's disease is damage to an adrenal gland by an autoimmune disorder (p.280), in which the body attacks its own tissues. Less common causes of the disorder include HIV infection and AIDS (p.169), tuberculosis (p.300), growth of cancer cells in the adrenal glands, lack of stimulation from the pituitary gland (*see* **Hypopituitarism**, p.431), and sudden, severe low blood pressure (*see* **Shock**, p.248).

Corticosteroid secretion is also suppressed if you take corticosteroid drugs (p.600) long term for another disorder. If you suddenly stop treatment, undergo surgery, or become ill, levels of natural corticosteroids will be too low.

What are the symptoms?

The symptoms of Addison's disease appear gradually but become increasingly obvious over a period of several weeks or months.

You may develop:
- Vague feeling of ill health.
- Tiredness and weakness.
- Gradual loss of appetite.
- Weight loss.
- Skin pigmentation similar to suntan, especially in the creases of the palms and on knuckles, elbows, and knees.

People with Addison's disease usually develop low blood pressure (*see* **Hypotension**, p.248). If you develop a serious illness or sustain an injury, corticosteroid levels may be too low for your body's needs, and this may result in a condition called an Addisonian crisis. In such a crisis, excessive loss of sodium and water results in dehydration, extreme weakness, abdominal pain, vomiting, and confusion. Without treatment, a crisis may lead to coma (p.323) and death.

How is it diagnosed?

The diagnosis will be obvious if you have suddenly stopped taking corticosteroid drugs. Otherwise, if your doctor suspects Addison's disease, you may have a blood test to measure sodium and potassium levels. Further tests may include blood tests to check levels of corticosteroids or to assess the response of the adrenal glands to an injection of a hormone that normally stimulates the glands.

What is the treatment?

Any underlying conditions will be treated if possible. In addition, people with Addison's disease usually need long-term treatment with oral corticosteroid drugs (p.600).

The dose of corticosteroid drugs will need to be increased in times of illness or stress. If you develop an infection while taking corticosteroid drugs long term, you should increase the dose as advised and consult your doctor. If you are vomiting or unable to take the drugs orally, you will need an injection of corticosteroids. Corticosteroid injections are also needed as emergency treatment in an Addisonian crisis along with intravenous fluids and glucose. If you are taking corticosteroid drugs long term for any reason, you should carry a card or wear a tag with this information.

Metabolic disorders

The chemical processes that take place in the body are known collectively as metabolism. These processes are largely controlled by hormones, and either overproduction or underproduction of a particular hormone can have wide-ranging effects on the body's internal chemistry. Metabolic disorders can also be caused by underlying conditions affecting major organs that regulate metabolism, such as the liver and the kidneys.

One important group of metabolic disorders is due to faulty or blocked chemical pathways, which cause the build-up of a chemical that is usually eliminated from the body. As the chemical accumulates, it may damage organs such as the brain and the liver. Many of these disorders, such as haemochromatosis, are due to genetic defects, some of which tend to run in families. If you have a close relative with one of these disorders, you may be at increased risk of developing the metabolic disorder yourself (see Gene disorders, p.151).

Most metabolic disorders can be diagnosed using blood or urine tests to measure levels of hormones or other specific chemicals. If the disorders are recognized early, they can sometimes be treated by a change in diet or the replacement of missing hormones or other chemicals. The sooner treatment is started, the better the prospects are for avoiding permanent damage.

The opening article in this section describes diabetes mellitus, the most common metabolic disorder. The next discusses hypoglycaemia, a condition sometimes associated with treatment for diabetes. The final articles cover disorders, including amyloidosis, in which abnormal levels of particular substances collect in the body.

Certain metabolic disorders are also disorders of particular endocrine (hormone-secreting) glands and are described elsewhere (see Pituitary gland disorders, pp.430–431; Thyroid and parathyroid gland disorders, pp.432–435; and Adrenal gland disorders, pp.435–436).

Diabetes mellitus

A disorder in which blood levels of glucose are raised due to low or absent production of the hormone insulin or resistance of body tissues to the hormone's effects

 Sometimes runs in families

 Age, gender, and lifestyle as risk factors depend on the type

Diabetes mellitus is one of the most common long-term diseases in the UK, affecting more than about 3.3 million people. In this disorder, either the pancreas produces insufficient amounts of the hormone insulin or body cells are resistant to the hormone's effects.

Normally, insulin is produced by the pancreas and enables the body's cells to absorb the sugar glucose (their main energy source) from the blood. In diabetes mellitus, glucose cannot be absorbed by the body's cells; as a result, glucose accumulates in the blood and passes into the urine, producing symptoms such as excessive urination and thirst.

Treatment is aimed at controlling glucose levels in the blood. Among people treated for diabetes mellitus, those with type 1 diabetes will require self-administered injections of insulin from the time the condition is diagnosed. Those with type 2 diabetes will require at least a carefully managed diet, and often oral drugs and sometimes insulin. These measures enable most affected people to lead normal lives. However, if blood glucose is not well controlled, complications can develop (see Are there complications?, right). Diabetes mellitus also weakens the immune system and thus increases susceptibility to infections, such as influenza (p.164).

Type 1 diabetes is usually permanent, although very rarely a transplant of the pancreas or of just insulin-producing pancreatic cells may be possible. In some cases, type 2 diabetes can be cured by weight loss in people who are severely overweight and whose diabetes is a result of the excessive weight.

What are the types?
The main types of diabetes mellitus are type 1 and type 2, although there are also several other types.

Type 1 diabetes Type 1 occurs when the pancreas is damaged by the body's immune system and is unable to produce any insulin. The disorder usually develops suddenly in childhood or adolescence but can occur at any age, including in the elderly. It must be treated with insulin injections. About 1 in 15 people with diabetes in the UK have this type of diabetes.

Type 2 diabetes Type 2 is by far the most common form of diabetes, affecting about 3 million people in the UK. In this condition, the pancreas initially continues to secrete insulin, but the cells of the body become resistant to its effects. Type 2 diabetes has traditionally affected people over the age of 40 but, with the increase in obesity at a younger age, it now affects even children. The condition develops slowly and is often detected by screening tests, although in some cases it remains undiagnosed for years. In the initial stages, weight loss, dietary measures, and exercise may control the condition. However, type 2 diabetes is usually progressive, and oral drugs and sometimes insulin injections may become necessary.

Other types Diabetes mellitus can sometimes develop during pregnancy (see Diabetes developing in pregnancy, p.509). This condition, called gestational diabetes, is more common in women who are overweight at the start of pregnancy. In many cases, it can be controlled by diet but sometimes it may require oral medication or insulin to maintain the health of the mother and baby. Gestational diabetes usually disappears after childbirth; however, women who have had it are at increased risk of developing gestational diabetes in subsequent pregnancies and type 2 diabetes in later life.

Maturity onset diabetes of the young (MODY) is a rare form of diabetes that is caused by an alteration (mutation) in a single gene. A child who inherits the mutation will typically develop diabetes before the age of 25, irrespective of other factors such as weight, lifestyle, or ethnicity. In some cases, the condition may not need specific treatment; in others, oral medication or insulin may be necessary.

What are the causes?
Type 1 diabetes is usually caused by an abnormal reaction in which the immune system destroys insulin-secreting cells (specifically, beta cells of the islets of Langerhans, often known simply as islet cells) in the pancreas. The cause of this reaction is unknown, but it may be triggered by a viral infection. In some cases, destruction of insulin-secreting tissues occurs following inflammation of the pancreas (see Acute pancreatitis, p.413).

Genetics may also play a role, but the pattern of inheritance is complicated. A child of a person with type 1 diabetes is at greater risk of developing the same type of diabetes, but most affected children do not have a parent with diabetes.

The causes of type 2 diabetes are less well understood, but genetics and obesity are important factors. About 1 in 3 affected people has a relative with the same type of diabetes. Type 2 diabetes is a major health problem in affluent societies and a growing problem in some developing countries. As food intake increases, more people become overweight and the prevalence of the condition rises.

In people who are predisposed to diabetes, the condition can be triggered by corticosteroid drugs (p.600) or by excessively high levels of natural corticosteroid hormones (see Cushing's syndrome, p.435), which act against insulin.

What are the symptoms?
Although some of the symptoms of both forms of diabetes mellitus are similar, type 1 diabetes tends to develop more quickly – usually over a few weeks – and become more severe. The symptoms of type 2 may not be obvious and may go unnoticed until a routine medical checkup. The main symptoms of both forms may include:

- Excessive passing of urine, including at night (nocturia).
- Thirst and a dry mouth.
- Tiredness and fatigue.
- Blurred vision.

Type 1 diabetes may also cause weight loss. In some people, the first sign of the disorder is ketoacidosis, a condition in which toxic chemicals called ketones build up in the blood. These chemicals are produced when the tissues of the body are unable to absorb glucose from the bloodstream, due to inadequate production of insulin, and have to use fats for energy. Ketoacidosis can also occur in people with type 1 diabetes who are taking insulin if they take insufficient insulin (for example, as a result of missing doses) or if they develop another illness (any illness increases the body's requirement for insulin) and the increased insulin requirement is not met. The symptoms of ketoacidosis may include:

- Nausea and vomiting, sometimes with abdominal pain.
- Deep, sighing breaths.
- Acetone smell to the breath (like nail-polish remover).
- Confusion.

The development of these symptoms is a medical emergency because they can lead to severe dehydration and coma (p.323) if they are not treated urgently. Emergency treatment for ketoacidosis includes intravenous infusion of fluids to correct dehydration and restore the chemical balance of the blood, and intravenous infusion of insulin to enable body cells to absorb glucose from the blood.

Are there complications?
Diabetes mellitus may give rise to short-term complications, which can usually be controlled, or long-term complications, which are more difficult to treat and can lead to premature death.

Short-term complications Poorly controlled or untreated type 1 diabetes may lead to ketoacidosis, the symptoms of which are described above.

A common complication of insulin treatment for either type of diabetes is hypoglycaemia (p.440), in which blood sugar falls to abnormally low levels. Hypoglycaemia is often caused by an imbalance between food intake and the dose of insulin, the result of exercise, or is associated with drinking alcohol. The disorder is more common in people with type 1 diabetes but may also affect people with type 2 diabetes who take sulphonylurea drugs or insulin (see Drugs for diabetes mellitus, p.601). Mild hypoglycaemia is

Living with diabetes

People with diabetes mellitus can lead normal lives, and they can continue to exercise and to eat most foods. However, it is very important to eat a healthy diet, maintain fitness, and, if necessary, lose weight. Following a healthy lifestyle helps to minimize the risk of developing complications over time, including heart disease, circulatory problems, and kidney failure.

A healthy diet

A healthy diet for people with diabetes is similar to that for those without diabetes. In general, you should eat a balanced diet with plenty of fruit and vegetables, and low levels of saturated fat and salt. You should also limit intake of rapidly absorbed carbohydrates. If you have type 1 diabetes, you will need to balance your carbohydrate intake with your insulin intake.

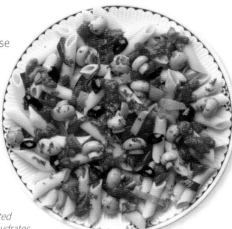

Eating healthily
A healthy diet should be low in saturated fats, salt, and rapidly absorbed carbohydrates.

Drinking and smoking

Alcohol in moderation is safe for most people, but in excess it may lower blood glucose levels. In addition, it is high in calories and may cause weight gain. Smoking is very harmful because it greatly increases the risk of long-term complications, such as heart disease and stroke. Various aids are available to help you stop smoking, including help from medical professionals, specialist advisers, and support groups as well as smoking cessation aids such as nicotine replacement therapy.

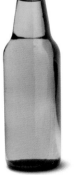
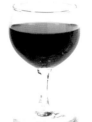
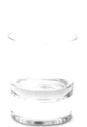

Alcohol
If you drink alcohol, there is no need to stop because you have diabetes but you should not drink more than the recommended limit. You should also be aware that alcohol makes hypoglycaemia more likely to occur.

Special care for your feet

Diabetes can increase the risk of skin infections and ulcers on the feet. You can reduce the risk by wearing shoes that fit comfortably, visiting a chiropodist regularly, not walking barefoot, and cutting your toenails straight across. You should inspect and clean your feet daily and consult your doctor promptly if you develop a sore on your foot.

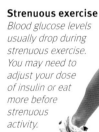

Foot care
Wash and dry your feet carefully. If the skin is dry, use a moisturizer every day.

Exercise and sports

Regular exercise makes you feel healthier, reduces the risk of heart disease, stroke, and high blood pressure, and can help if you need to lose weight. If you have type 1 diabetes, you may need to monitor your blood glucose before, during, and after exercise to check how the activity affects your requirements for both insulin and food.

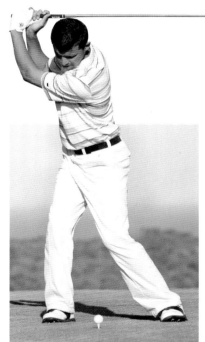

Strenuous exercise
Blood glucose levels usually drop during strenuous exercise. You may need to adjust your dose of insulin or eat more before strenuous activity.

Moderate exercise
Regular moderate exercise reduces the chance of developing coronary artery disease and may improve the control of your diabetes.

Your medical checkup

When you have just been diagnosed with diabetes you will be given a full medical examination, including measurements of your blood glucose, blood cholesterol, and blood pressure levels, height and weight measurement, an eye and foot examination, and blood and urine tests to check kidney, thyroid, and liver functions. Then every year you will have a medical review in which these checks are repeated to assess how well your blood glucose level is being controlled, and to look for any signs of complications.

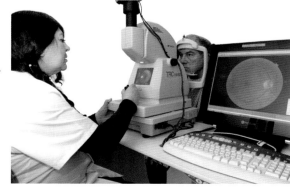

Retinal screening
Regular retinal screening with a special digital camera can detect any changes to the retina caused by diabetes at an early stage.

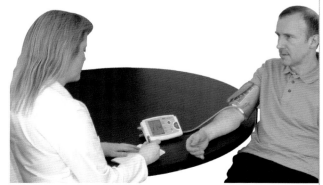

Blood pressure measurement
People with diabetes mellitus have an increased risk of high blood pressure, and regular monitoring is important.

Injecting insulin

If you need regular injections of insulin, you will be shown how to inject yourself. You can use a syringe and needle, but many people prefer insulin pens, which are easier to use and more discreet. Insulin can be injected into any fatty area, such as the upper arms, abdomen, or thighs. Insert the needle quickly and then inject the insulin slowly. You should try not to use exactly the same site each time for the injection.

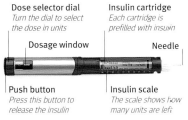

Dose selector dial
Turn the dial to select the dose in units

Insulin cartridge
Each cartridge is prefilled with insulin

Dosage window

Needle

Push button
Press this button to release the insulin

Insulin scale
The scale shows how many units are left

Insulin pen
This device for carrying and delivering insulin holds an insulin cartridge and has a dial that lets you set the required dose. Disposable needles attach to one end.

Learning to inject
From an early age, children who have diabetes can be taught how to inject themselves.

Injection site
For children, the thigh is often an easy site for injection

usually self-correcting as the liver automatically increases glucose production or it can be treated by eating or drinking something sugary. However, untreated severe hypoglycaemia can cause unconsciousness and seizures.

Long-term complications Certain longstanding problems pose the main health threat to people with diabetes and may eventually affect even people whose diabetes is well controlled. Close control of blood sugar and blood pressure reduces the risk of complications, and early recognition helps in their control. For these reasons, all affected people should see their doctor at least twice a year (*see* **Living with diabetes**, p.438). Type 2 diabetes is often not diagnosed until years after its onset. As a result, complications may be evident at the time of initial diagnosis.

People who have diabetes are at increased risk of cardiovascular disorders (*see* **Diabetic vascular disease**, p.260). Large blood vessels may be damaged by atherosclerosis (p.241), which is a major cause of coronary artery disease (p.243) and stroke (p.329). Raised amounts of cholesterol in the blood (*see* **Hypercholesterolaemia**, p.440), which accelerate the development of atherosclerosis, are more common in people who have diabetes. Diabetes is also associated with hypertension (p.242), another risk factor for cardiovascular disease.

Other long-term complications result from damage to the small blood vessels throughout the body. Damage to blood vessels in the light-sensitive retina at the back of the eye may cause diabetic retinopathy (p.361). Diabetes also increases the risk of developing cataracts (p.357). People with diabetes mellitus should have their eyes examined yearly as early treatment may prevent permanent loss of vision.

If diabetes affects blood vessels that supply nerves, it may cause nerve damage (*see* **Diabetic neuropathy**, p.336). There may be a gradual loss of sensation or a tingling feeling, starting at the hands and feet and sometimes gradually extending up the limbs. Symptoms may also include dizziness upon standing and erectile dysfunction (p.494) in men. Loss of feeling, combined with poor circulation, makes the feet more susceptible to ulcers and gangrene (p.262).

Damage to small blood vessels in the kidneys (*see* **Diabetic kidney disease**, p.450) may lead to chronic kidney disease (p.451) or end-stage kidney failure (p.452), which requires lifelong dialysis (p.451) or a kidney transplant (p.452).

How is it diagnosed?

Your doctor may first ask you to provide a urine sample, which will be tested for glucose. The diagnosis is confirmed by a blood test to check for a high glucose level. If you were unwell at the time, the blood test may need to be repeated. A blood test after fasting overnight or one performed 2 hours after a glucose drink may also be carried out. In addition, your blood may also be tested for glycosylated haemoglobin (HbA1c), an altered form of the pigment in red blood cells, which increases in concentration when the blood glucose level has been high for several weeks or months.

What is the treatment?

For anyone with diabetes mellitus, the aim is to maintain the level of glucose in the blood within the normal range without marked fluctuations. Treatment may involve dietary control, exercise, and pills or insulin injections to lower the blood glucose level. Treatment is usually lifelong, and with support, you will have to take some responsibility for the care of your diabetes.

Monitoring your blood glucose

You can monitor your blood glucose level using a digital meter. The method of use varies, depending on the type of meter, so you should follow the manufacturer's instructions. However, using most meters involves applying a drop of blood to a test strip impregnated with a chemical that reacts with glucose. Checking your blood glucose as often as recommended by your doctor or nurse allows you to monitor your treatment to confirm that it is effective and to alter it as necessary.

Typical blood glucose meter
There are many types of digital meter, with various features and methods of use. Most have a digital display screen that shows the blood glucose level, and a memory for storing readings. Some have a code button for calibrating the meter; some also have the ability to add notes and download readings.

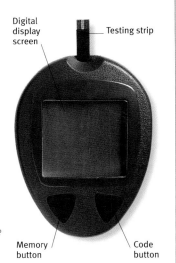

Digital display screen

Testing strip

Memory button

Code button

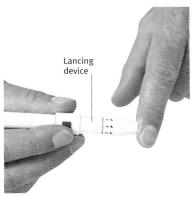

Lancing device

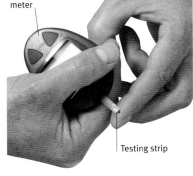

Blood glucose meter

Testing strip

1 *Before starting, test or calibrate your meter, if necessary. Wash and dry your hands, then obtain a drop of blood by using a spring-loaded lancing device against the side of your finger.*

2 *Apply the blood to the pad on the end of the testing strip. The meter analyses the blood and gives a rapid reading (typically within 5 seconds) of the blood glucose level.*

Type 1 diabetes This form is always treated with insulin injections; oral drugs alone are ineffective, and insulin cannot be absorbed from the intestines. Insulin is available in various forms, including short-acting, long-acting, and combinations of both (*see* **Drugs for diabetes mellitus**, p.601). Treatment regimens are individually tailored: your doctor or nurse will talk to you about your needs and arrange for you to learn how to inject yourself (*see* **Injecting insulin**, above). You will also have to control your diet and monitor your blood glucose (*see* **Monitoring your blood glucose**, above). If the diabetes is difficult to control, you may be offered an insulin pump, which dispenses insulin through a catheter (thin tube) inserted under the skin.

The only way to cure type 1 diabetes mellitus is by undergoing a pancreas transplant or a transplant of just the insulin-secreting islet cells, but such surgery is not routinely offered because the body may reject the transplanted tissue and also because lifelong treatment with immunosuppressant drugs (p.585) is needed afterwards. In some cases, people with diabetes who are receiving a kidney transplant are offered a pancreas transplant at the same time.

Type 2 diabetes Many people with this form of diabetes can control their blood glucose levels by taking exercise regularly and by following a healthy diet to maintain their ideal weight.

You should follow general guidelines for a healthy diet (*see* **Diet and health**, pp.16–20) and seek advice from a dietitian if necessary. You should try to keep fat intake low and obtain energy from complex carbohydrates (such as wholegrain bread and basmati or brown rice) to minimize fluctuations in the blood glucose level.

If you are taking insulin, you may be advised to check your blood glucose level regularly (*see* **Monitoring your blood glucose**, above). If the glucose level is higher or lower than recommended, you may need to alter your diet or adjust your insulin or drug dose with the help of your doctor. Blood glucose monitoring is particularly important if you develop another illness, such as influenza, because being ill can increase blood glucose levels even if you are not eating. You may also be advised to monitor your blood glucose in situations such as taking strenuous exercise and when your usual lifestyle has changed, for example, when on holiday. If you are taking insulin, you must check your glucose levels before driving and every 2 hours on long journeys.

When dietary measures are not sufficient to control your blood sugar, one or more drugs may be prescribed (*see* **Drugs for diabetes mellitus**, p.601). You are likely to begin with oral drugs, such as metformin, which is particularly useful for treating people with diabetes who are overweight, sulphonylureas, glitazones, gliptins, or drugs such as repaglinide, which stimulate the pancreas to release more insulin; in some cases, you may be prescribed injected medication, such as exenatide or liraglutide. Often, a combination of these drugs is prescribed. If these drugs are ineffective, you may need to have insulin injections.

It is important to keep your blood cholesterol and blood pressure at normal or even slightly lower than normal levels and you may therefore also be prescribed a statin (*see* **Lipid-lowering drugs**, p.603) and a drug to lower blood pressure (*see* **Antihypertensive Drugs**, p.580).

What is the prognosis?
Diabetes mellitus is not curable but a healthy lifestyle, good control of blood glucose levels, blood pressure, and blood cholesterol, together with support from diabetes care professionals have made the condition easier to control. As a result, people who have diabetes can often lead a relatively normal life. Children with diabetes quickly learn to manage their disease and can participate in sports and lead full social lives.

Hypoglycaemia

An abnormally low level of glucose in the blood, depriving body cells of glucose

 Age, gender, genetics, and lifestyle as risk factors depend on the cause

In hypoglycaemia, the body's cells are deprived of glucose, which is their main source of energy. As a result, symptoms such as sweating, nausea, and hunger develop. The condition is usually temporary, and occurs most often as a side effect of insulin treatment for diabetes (*see* **Diabetes mellitus**, p.437). Faintness or nausea that are sometimes attributed to hypoglycaemia are in fact usually due to other disorders, tiredness, or stress (p.31).

What are the causes?
In people with diabetes, hypoglycaemia is usually due to a dose of insulin that is excessive in relation to food intake and lowers blood glucose too much. The insulin dosage must be balanced with food intake, which raises blood glucose levels, and phys-

ical activity, which lowers blood glucose. If the balance is disturbed and the glucose level falls, hypoglycaemia may result.

Hypoglycaemia in people without diabetes is rare. It sometimes occurs as a rebound effect in which the blood glucose level temporarily falls after a sugar-rich meal – a condition known as reactive hypoglycaemia. Very rarely, non-diabetic hypoglycaemia may be due to a serious medical problem, such as severe liver disease, adrenal failure, or an insulin-secreting tumour of the pancreas. In babies, especially newborns, hypoglycaemia may occur because the liver does not yet have sufficient stores of glucose.

What are the symptoms?
When blood glucose levels become low, warning signs of hypoglycaemia may rapidly develop, including:
■ Sweating, nausea, hunger, and anxiety.
■ Rapid, forceful heartbeat.
If blood glucose continues to fall, further symptoms may develop, including:
■ Confusion.
■ Slurred speech and unsteady movements, similar to drunkenness.
■ Seizures (particularly in children).
Unconsciousness may result. If not treated promptly, the condition may cause permanent brain damage or death.

What is the treatment?
In many cases, mild hypoglycaemia corrects itself as the liver automatically increases glucose production to compensate, or it can be treated by eating or drinking something sugary. If you often experience reactive hypoglycaemia, you may be able to prevent episodes by limiting your sugar intake.

If you have diabetes mellitus and experience the symptoms of hypoglycaemia, take food or drink that contains sugar immediately. Always carry sweets or biscuits with you and wear an information tag to inform people that you have diabetes. If you develop hypoglycaemia and lose consciousness, you will need an immediate injection of glucagon, a hormone that raises blood glucose levels, or intravenous glucose.

Hypercholesterolaemia

Raised levels of cholesterol in the blood, which increase the risk of developing cardiovascular disease

 More common with increasing age

 More common in males

 Sometimes runs in families

 A diet high in saturated fats, obesity, and lack of exercise are risk factors

An estimated 2 in 3 adults in the UK have a high blood cholesterol level (above 5 mmol/L). Raised cholesterol levels are associated with increased risk of coronary

artery disease (p.243) and stroke (p.329) due to atherosclerosis (p.241).

Cholesterol is a substance known as a lipid. It is used in the manufacture of cell walls and in the production of bile acids (which aid the digestion of fat) and important steroid hormones. The liver produces most of the body's cholesterol, but some cholesterol is derived from food, such as eggs, meat, and shellfish. Diet (*see* **Diet and health**, p.16) and other lifestyle factors can affect the cholesterol level.

Cholesterol is carried in the blood in the form of lipid–protein particles known as lipoproteins. There are two main types: low-density lipoproteins (LDLs) and high-density lipoproteins (HDLs). LDLs carry larger amounts of cholesterol than HDLs and deposit it around the body. Raised levels of LDLs increase the risk of arterial disease. The excess LDLs form fatty deposits on the walls of arteries (atherosclerosis). As these deposits grow, they restrict blood flow and cause the formation of clots that block the vessels. HDLs pick up cholesterol molecules from the tissues and fatty deposits of atherosclerosis and return them to the liver to be broken down. A high level of HDLs thus protects against arterial disease.

What are the causes?
Cholesterol level is determined by a combination of genetic and lifestyle factors. A high level is associated with a diet that is high in fats, particularly saturated fats, being overweight, and lack of exercise. Although the condition often runs in families, some people have specific inherited hyperlipidaemias (right), which are associated with extremely high cholesterol levels.

A high cholesterol level does not usually cause symptoms until it leads to the development of another disorder, such as coronary artery disease.

How is it diagnosed?
Regular screening tests to measure the blood cholesterol level are recommended from early adult life for people with a family history of raised cholesterol levels, heart disease, or stroke. The tests may also be offered after the age of 40 as part of a general health checkup. Hypercholesterolaemia is frequently first diagnosed as a result of a routine screening test.

The optimal total cholesterol level for a healthy middle-aged person is less than 5 mmol/L. If the total cholesterol level exceeds 5 mmol/L, your doctor may carry out a further blood test to check your levels of LDL and HDL cholesterol.

What is the treatment?
Whether or not you require treatment depends on your risk of developing coronary artery disease. As well as your blood cholesterol level, it includes factors such as your body mass index, age, sex, whether or not you have high blood pressure (*see* **Hypertension**, p.242), medical history and any existing medical problems (diabetes, for example), ethnicity, and lifestyle factors such as whether or not you smoke. Even if

your cholesterol level falls within the normal range, you may be given treatment to lower cholesterol if you have heart disease or are at high risk of coronary heart disease.

If you are found to have a high cholesterol level, your doctor may initially advise you about changes in diet and exercise habits that should lower it. However, if these measures fail to lower the level sufficiently, your doctor may prescribe drugs, which you are likely to need to take for the rest of your life (*see* **Lipid-lowering drugs**, p.603).

Inherited hyperlipidaemias

Inherited conditions in which the blood contains abnormally high levels of cholesterol and/or triglycerides

 Present from birth but usually become apparent in early adulthood

 Due to an abnormal gene inherited from one or both parents

 A diet high in fats and lack of exercise aggravate the conditions

 Gender is not a significant factor

Many people have an elevated level of cholesterol in their blood (*see* **Hypercholesterolaemia**, left). In some of these people, levels of cholesterol and of lipids called triglycerides are high due to genetic disorders called hyperlipidaemias. The disorders create high levels of lipoproteins (lipid–protein particles), and may produce symptoms earlier in adulthood than other hypercholesterolaemias. High levels of lipids (especially cholesterol) increase the risk of complications of atherosclerosis (p.241), such as coronary artery disease (p.243).

There are several forms of inherited hyperlipidaemia. The most common form affects about 1 in 500 people of European descent, who inherit one copy of an abnormal gene and have a cholesterol level higher than normal. There is a one in a million risk that people will inherit the abnormal gene from both parents. If two copies are inherited, the cholesterol level is extremely high. Affected people have a very high probability of a heart attack (*see* **Myocardial infarction**, p.245) at a young age, even in childhood.

What are the symptoms?
Extremely high cholesterol levels associated with inherited hyperlipidaemias may cause the following symptoms, which develop gradually over years:
■ Yellow swellings of fat under the skin (xanthomas) on the back of the hands.
■ Swellings on the tendons around the ankle and wrist joints.
■ Yellow swellings on the skin of the eyelids (xanthelasmas).
■ White ring around the iris (the coloured part of the eye).

Raised triglyceride levels do not usually produce any symptoms but do increase the risk of acute pancreatitis (p.413).

People with these disorders can develop symptoms of coronary artery disease, such as chest pain (see **Angina**, p.244), in their 20s or 30s. In women, oestrogen usually gives some protection from these problems until after the menopause.

What might be done?

There is no cure for inherited hyperlipidaemias, but symptoms can be treated with a combination of exercise, a diet that is low in cholesterol and saturated fats, and lipid-lowering drugs (p.603). The outlook varies, but early lipid-lowering treatment can greatly reduce the risk of a heart attack. Relatives of an affected person should be offered screening for the disorder.

Haemochromatosis

A condition in which excessive amounts of iron accumulate in the body

 Age, gender, genetics, and lifestyle as risk factors depend on the cause

In haemochromatosis, the level of iron in the body is too high. The excess iron gradually accumulates in organs such as the heart and liver, eventually damaging the organs. Men are more likely to develop symptoms than women, because women regularly lose iron from their body when menstruating.

What are the causes?

Haemochromatosis may be caused by a genetic abnormality (primary, or inherited, haemochromatosis) or it may develop as a result of another condition or factor (secondary haemochromatosis).

Several gene abnormalities may cause primary haemochromatosis but a gene known as the HFE gene is responsible for more than 9 in 10 cases of the disorder. The effect of this gene is to increase the amount of iron the body absorbs from the diet. The HFE gene is inherited in an autosomal recessive manner, which means that a person must inherit two copies of the gene, one from each parent, to have the potential to develop symptoms (see **Gene disorders**, p.151). If a person has only one copy, he or she is a carrier but does not normally develop symptoms.

Secondary haemochromatosis may occur as a result of various underlying causes. These include having numerous blood transfusions, which may be given in the treatment of conditions such as thalassaemia (p.273) or sickle-cell disease (p.272); excessive dietary intake of iron (usually as a result of taking supplements or from drinking large amounts of beer that has been brewed in iron containers) or iron injections; chronic liver disease; and long-term kidney dialysis.

What are the symptoms?

The symptoms develop gradually and, at least initially, are often mild. Symptoms of primary haemochromatosis typically do not appear until after the age of about 40. Symptoms of secondary haemochromatosis may affect adults of any age. Initial symptoms may include:

- Weakness and lack of energy.
- Abdominal pain.
- In men, shrinking of the testes and erectile dysfunction.
- In women, infrequent or absent periods.
- Pain and stiffness in the joints, particularly in the hands.
- Bronzing of the skin.

As haemochromatosis progresses, damage to the organs can lead to conditions such as chronic heart failure (p.247), diabetes mellitus (p.437), and liver cirrhosis (p.410).

What might be done?

Haemochromatosis is diagnosed by testing blood for high levels of iron. MRI scanning (p.133) or ultrasound scanning (p.135) may be used to look for liver damage. A liver biopsy (p.410) may also be carried out to check for iron deposits in the liver. Relatives of an affected person should consult their doctor to see whether they should be screened for the condition.

Treatment is aimed at removing excess iron from the body. This is done by removing about 500 ml (1 pint) of blood each week until iron levels are normal. In a few cases where the underlying cause can be easily corrected, no further treatment may be necessary; for example, if the cause was simply too much dietary iron, restricting iron intake may be sufficient. However, usually it is necessary to continue to remove blood at regular intervals, although less frequently than once a week. People with haemochromatosis may also be treated with drugs that bind to iron in the body and enable it to be excreted.

It is also important to avoid alcohol, iron-rich foods, and iron supplements. Reducing your intake of vitamin C may also be helpful as this vitamin increases the amount of iron absorbed in the intestines.

What is the prognosis?

With early treatment, haemochromatosis is not thought to affect life expectancy. However, if organ damage has occurred, lifespan may be shortened, and in severe cases, an organ transplant may even be necessary.

Amyloidosis

A group of disorders in which abnormal proteins accumulate in internal organs

 More common in elderly people

 More common in males

 In some cases the condition is inherited

 Lifestyle is not a significant factor

The various rare conditions known as amyloidosis develop when deposits of abnormal proteins, called amyloid, collect in organs and interfere with their function. There are various forms of amyloidosis, each of which is caused by a different type of amyloid. The condition mainly affects elderly people and is more common in men than in women.

Amyloidosis may be due to an abnormal gene or have no apparent cause; in these cases it is called primary amyloidosis. More commonly, it occurs as a complication of another disorder and is therefore called secondary amyloidosis. Disorders associated with the condition include inflammatory disorders such as rheumatoid arthritis (p.222), long-term infections, and the bone marrow cancer multiple myeloma (p.277).

What are the symptoms?

Often, there are no symptoms in the early stages of amyloidosis. Over months or years, various symptoms develop, depending on which organs and tissues are affected. Diseased organs such as the kidneys, heart, liver, and nerves often become enlarged and cannot function properly. Resulting complications may include chronic kidney disease (p.451), chronic heart failure (p.247), chronic liver failure (p.411), or nerve damage (see **Peripheral neuropathies**, p.336). If amyloid deposits build up in the brain, Alzheimer's disease (p.331) may develop as a result.

What might be done?

Amyloidosis is diagnosed by examining a tissue sample from an affected organ under a microscope to detect deposits of amyloid. In some cases, a specialized scan to detect amyloid deposits in the body may also be carried out.

In cases of secondary amyloidosis, treating the underlying disorder may halt or even reverse the condition. However, amyloidosis that is associated with multiple myeloma tends to progress rapidly, and the outlook is poor. For primary amyloidosis, immunosuppressant drugs (p.585) or drugs that are more commonly used in the treatment of cancer (see **Anticancer drugs**, p.586) may be prescribed. If amyloidosis has already caused the failure of an organ, a transplant may be a treatment option, but the replacement organ could also be affected if the disease is not controlled.

Porphyria

A set of rare disorders in which chemicals called porphyrins accumulate in tissues

 Some types are inherited

 Excessive alcohol intake is a risk factor

 Age and gender are not significant factors

As the body makes haemoglobin, the red pigment in blood, it produces chemicals called porphyrins. Normally, porphyrins are turned into haemoglobin, but in porphyria this change is blocked and they build up in the body. There are several forms of porphyria. Most forms are due to abnormal genes. The most common is inherited in an autosomal dominant manner (see **Gene disorders**, p.151). Some forms are associated with sunlight exposure, liver disease, excessive alcohol use, or AIDS (see **HIV infection and AIDS**, p.169). In susceptible people, porphyria may be a side effect of some drugs.

What are the symptoms?

Each type of porphyria causes different symptoms. In some, the symptoms are persistent; in others, they are intermittent and triggered by sunlight, alcohol, or drugs. Symptoms may include:

- Dark, purplish urine.
- Rashes or blisters in areas that are exposed to sunlight.
- Abdominal pain.
- Pain or weakness in the arms or legs.

Severe intermittent porphyria can cause psychiatric problems such as delusions.

What might be done?

Porphyria is diagnosed by testing blood, faeces, or urine for porphyrins. Treatment varies according to the specific form of porphyria. It may include intravenous glucose or medication to prevent or alleviate attacks, venesection (removal of blood), splenectomy (removal of the spleen), or a stem cell transplant (p.276). Avoiding triggers may reduce the frequency of attacks.

Urinary system

The urinary system, also known as the urinary tract, acts as a filtering unit for the body's blood, excreting waste products and excess water as urine. The system consists of a pair of kidneys; the bladder; the ureters, which connect each kidney to the bladder; and the urethra, through which urine leaves the body. As the urinary system filters the blood, it regulates body water levels and maintains the balance of body fluids. The kidneys also produce hormones, one of which helps to control blood pressure. Every day the body's entire volume of blood passes through the kidneys over 300 times – a flow of about 1,700 litres (375 gallons).

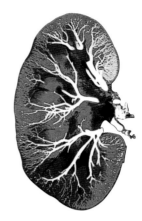

Rich blood supply
Numerous blood vessels supply the kidney with blood.

EVERY ACTION OF our daily lives, from eating and breathing to walking and running, is made possible by chemical reactions in our body cells. Wastes produced as a result of these reactions collect in the blood. In order for us to remain healthy, these wastes must be filtered out and excreted. This is the main function of the urinary system.

The kidneys are connected to the aorta, the body's main artery that runs directly from the heart. When the body is at rest, the kidneys receive about a quarter of the blood pumped by the heart. Filtered blood is returned to the heart through the inferior vena cava, the largest vein in the body.

red blood cells and proteins are much too large to pass through these pores and do not enter the filtered fluid. Smaller molecules pass into the renal tubule, where useful substances, such as glucose, are reabsorbed into the bloodstream. The fluid remaining in the tubule, called urine, is a mixture of wastes, such as urea, and other substances that are not required by the body, such as excess water and salts.

This constant filtration of blood not only removes harmful wastes from the body but also helps to regulate water levels. If, for example, you drink more water than is needed for the body's

requirements, the excess is excreted in urine. However, if you need to conserve water, the kidneys make the urine more concentrated and excrete as little water as possible. Furthermore, if your blood becomes too acidic or too alkaline, the kidneys change the urine's acidity level to restore the correct balance.

Hormone production

The kidneys produce a number of hormones, each with different roles. Their functions include stimulating the formation of blood cells and controlling blood pressure by helping to regulate the blood flow through arteries.

Blood filtration

Each kidney contains about 1 million nephrons, mini-filtering units that consist of a knot of capillaries called the glomerulus and a long, thin tube called the renal tubule. Pores in the glomerulus allow only some of the molecules in the blood to pass through, depending on their size and shape. For example,

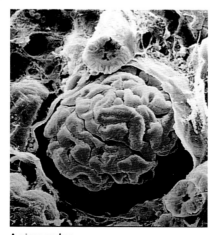

A glomerulus
This knot of capillaries is the glomerulus, which filters blood in the kidney.

✚ **STRUCTURE**

Sexual differences

The lower urinary tract is different in males and females. The urethra from the male bladder passes through the prostate gland, carrying either urine or semen to the opening at the tip of the penis. The female bladder sits under the uterus, and the urethra carries urine to the opening in front of the vagina. In both sexes, the passing of urine is partly controlled by muscles in the neck of the bladder.

Length of the urethra
The male urethra is usually about 20 cm (8 in) long. In females, the urethra is about 4 cm (1½ in) long.

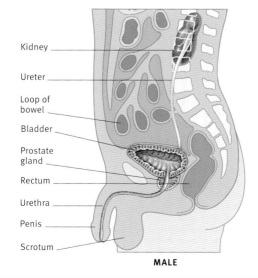

Kidney
Ureter
Loop of bowel
Bladder
Prostate gland
Rectum
Urethra
Penis
Scrotum

MALE

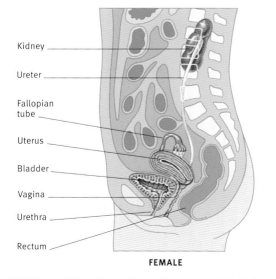

Kidney
Ureter
Fallopian tube
Uterus
Bladder
Vagina
Urethra
Rectum

FEMALE

✚ **STRUCTURE**

Urinary system

The urinary system consists of two kidneys, each linked by a ureter to the bladder, and a urethra, which connects the bladder to the outside of the body. The kidneys lie at the back of the abdomen, on either side of the spine. They are reddish-brown, bean-shaped organs, about 10–12.5 cm (4–5 in) long and 5–7.5 cm (2–3 in) wide. The ureters are thin, muscular tubes about 25–30 cm (10–12 in) long, and the bladder is a hollow, muscular organ located in the pelvis. The bladder's lower opening is surrounded by muscle that helps to control the release of urine through the urethra.

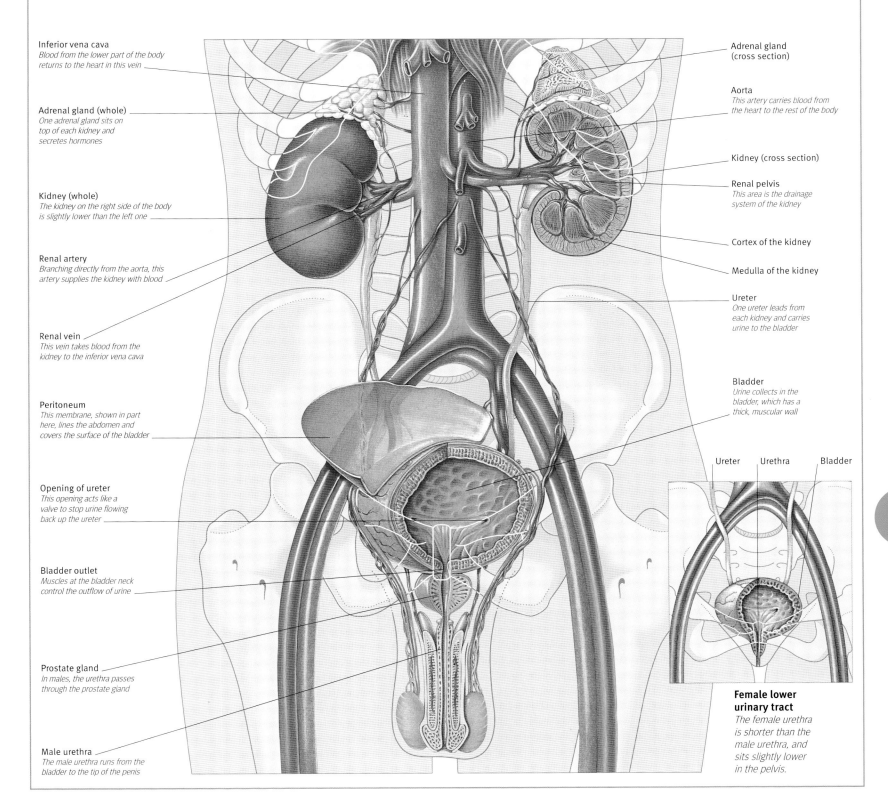

Inferior vena cava
Blood from the lower part of the body returns to the heart in this vein

Adrenal gland (whole)
One adrenal gland sits on top of each kidney and secretes hormones

Kidney (whole)
The kidney on the right side of the body is slightly lower than the left one

Renal artery
Branching directly from the aorta, this artery supplies the kidney with blood

Renal vein
This vein takes blood from the kidney to the inferior vena cava

Peritoneum
This membrane, shown in part here, lines the abdomen and covers the surface of the bladder

Opening of ureter
This opening acts like a valve to stop urine flowing back up the ureter

Bladder outlet
Muscles at the bladder neck control the outflow of urine

Prostate gland
In males, the urethra passes through the prostate gland

Male urethra
The male urethra runs from the bladder to the tip of the penis

Adrenal gland (cross section)

Aorta
This artery carries blood from the heart to the rest of the body

Kidney (cross section)

Renal pelvis
This area is the drainage system of the kidney

Cortex of the kidney

Medulla of the kidney

Ureter
One ureter leads from each kidney and carries urine to the bladder

Bladder
Urine collects in the bladder, which has a thick, muscular wall

Ureter   Urethra   Bladder

Female lower urinary tract
The female urethra is shorter than the male urethra, and sits slightly lower in the pelvis.

✚ **STRUCTURE**

The kidney

The kidney has three regions: the cortex, the medulla, and the renal pelvis. The outer layer, the cortex, contains filtering units called nephrons, each consisting of a glomerulus and a renal tubule. The middle layer, the medulla, consists of cone-shaped groups of urine-collecting ducts. The inner region, the renal pelvis, branches into cavities called major and minor calyces. Each minor calyx gathers urine from the medulla; the urine is then collected in major calyces and funnelled into the ureter.

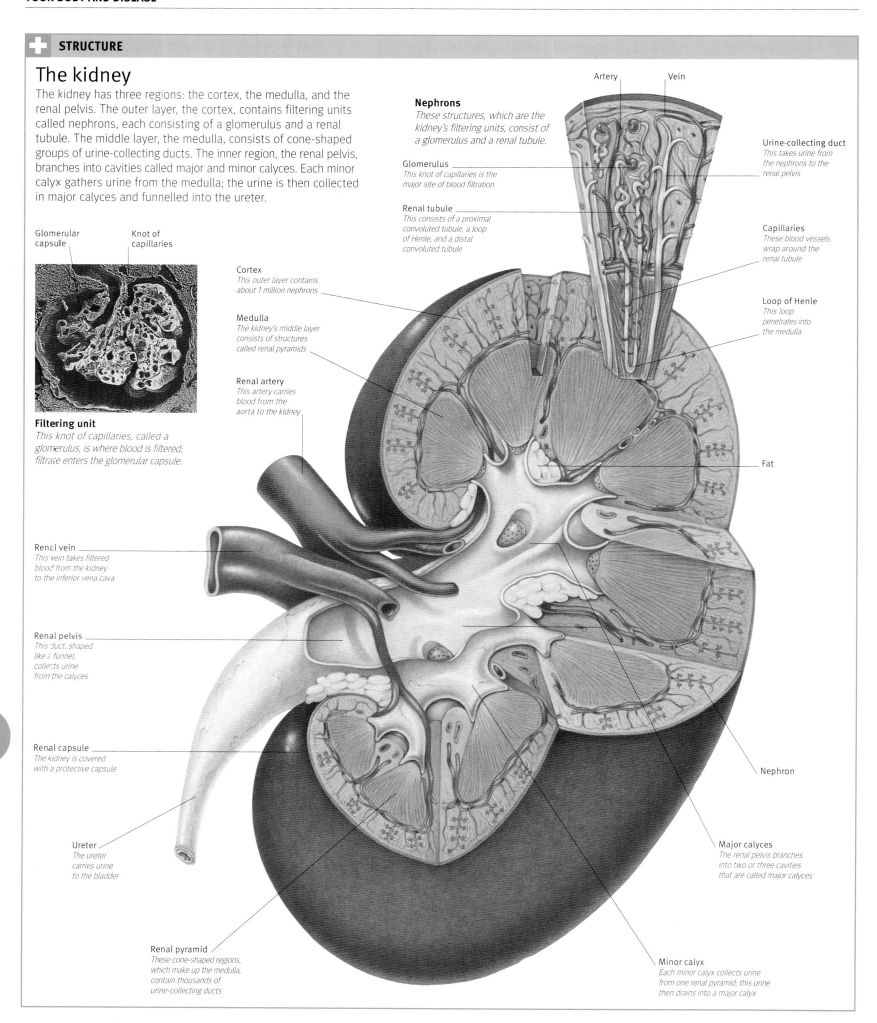

Glomerular capsule

Knot of capillaries

Filtering unit
This knot of capillaries, called a glomerulus, is where blood is filtered; filtrate enters the glomerular capsule.

Nephrons
These structures, which are the kidney's filtering units, consist of a glomerulus and a renal tubule.

Glomerulus
This knot of capillaries is the major site of blood filtration

Renal tubule
This consists of a proximal convoluted tubule, a loop of Henle, and a distal convoluted tubule

Artery   Vein

Urine-collecting duct
This takes urine from the nephrons to the renal pelvis

Capillaries
These blood vessels wrap around the renal tubule

Loop of Henle
This loop penetrates into the medulla

Cortex
This outer layer contains about 1 million nephrons

Medulla
The kidney's middle layer consists of structures called renal pyramids

Renal artery
This artery carries blood from the aorta to the kidney

Fat

Renal vein
This vein takes filtered blood from the kidney to the inferior vena cava

Renal pelvis
This duct, shaped like a funnel, collects urine from the calyces

Renal capsule
The kidney is covered with a protective capsule

Nephron

Ureter
The ureter carries urine to the bladder

Renal pyramid
These cone-shaped regions, which make up the medulla, contain thousands of urine-collecting ducts

Major calyces
The renal pelvis branches into two or three cavities that are called major calyces

Minor calyx
Each minor calyx collects urine from one renal pyramid; this urine then drains into a major calyx

FUNCTION

Urine formation and excretion

Urine is composed of unwanted substances that have been filtered from the blood by nephrons, the functional units of the kidneys. The urine formed in the kidneys passes through the ureters and is temporarily stored in the bladder. From here it is emptied, normally under voluntary control, through the urethra. A healthy adult excretes 0.5–2 litres (1–4 pints) of urine each day.

How a nephron makes urine

Blood entering the nephron is filtered through a cluster of capillaries called the glomerulus. The filtrate then enters the renal tubule, along which a complex process of secretion and reabsorption occurs. Useful substances such as glucose are reabsorbed; the acidity of the blood is regulated; and water levels are adjusted. The resulting fluid is called urine.

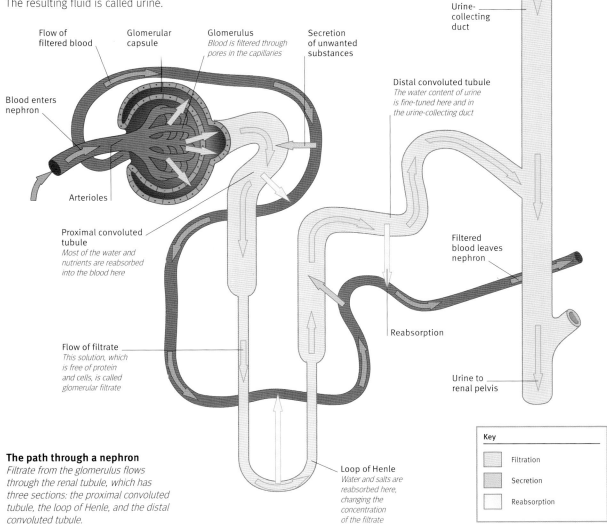

Flow of filtered blood

Glomerular capsule

Glomerulus
Blood is filtered through pores in the capillaries

Secretion of unwanted substances

Blood enters nephron

Arterioles

Proximal convoluted tubule
Most of the water and nutrients are reabsorbed into the blood here

Flow of filtrate
This solution, which is free of protein and cells, is called glomerular filtrate

Urine from other nephrons

Urine-collecting duct

Distal convoluted tubule
The water content of urine is fine-tuned here and in the urine-collecting duct

Filtered blood leaves nephron

Reabsorption

Urine to renal pelvis

The path through a nephron
Filtrate from the glomerulus flows through the renal tubule, which has three sections: the proximal convoluted tubule, the loop of Henle, and the distal convoluted tubule.

Loop of Henle
Water and salts are reabsorbed here, changing the concentration of the filtrate

Key	
	Filtration
	Secretion
	Reabsorption

What is urine made of?

Urine consists of a mixture of waste products and other substances. The mixture is balanced so that the body's internal environment remains constant. The water content of urine depends on whether there is too much or too little water in the body.

Sulphate   Creatinine

Phosphate

Uric acid

Potassium

Sodium

Chloride

Urea

Water

Mainly water
Urine is about 95 per cent water. The remainder includes wastes and other substances not needed by the body.

How urination is controlled

When the bladder is full, nerves in the bladder wall send signals to the spinal cord. Signals are then sent back to the bladder, making it contract and expel urine. In older children and adults, the timing of urination can be regulated because this process is controlled by the brain. Infants lack this control, and the bladder empties when full.

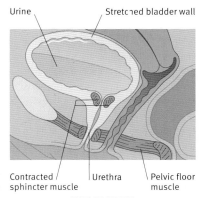

Urine

Stretched bladder wall

Contracted sphincter muscle

Urethra

Pelvic floor muscle

FULL BLADDER

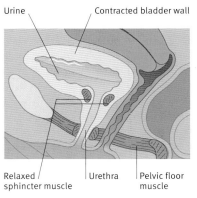

Urine

Contracted bladder wall

Relaxed sphincter muscle

Urethra

Pelvic floor muscle

EMPTYING BLADDER

Emptying the bladder
To empty the bladder, muscles in the bladder wall contract and the sphincter muscles relax, forcing urine out of the bladder and down the urethra.

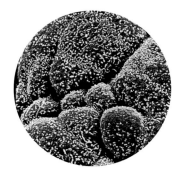

Inside the bladder
This highly magnified view shows the folds in the lining of the bladder wall. The folds in the wall stretch out as the bladder fills.

Kidney disorders

The kidneys keep the body's chemistry in balance by removing waste products and excess water. They also regulate blood pressure and stimulate red blood cell production. The body can stay healthy with one normal kidney, but many conditions affect both kidneys and it is therefore important that kidney disorders are treated promptly.

The first article in this section covers pyelonephritis, a common disorder in which kidney tissue becomes inflamed, usually due to a bacterial infection. Glomerulonephritis, which develops when inflammation damages the glomeruli (the kidneys' filtering units), is discussed in the second article. This condition nearly always results from the response of the kidneys to the activity of the immune system.

The next articles discuss stones and cysts in the kidneys. Kidney stones are often treated by a technique called lithotripsy in which shock waves are used to pulverize the stones. Cysts are usually harmless, but multiple cysts resulting from a genetic disorder may cause kidney failure. The final articles cover cancer of the kidneys and kidney failure. The latter disorder may occur suddenly, especially if it results from a reduction in the blood flow to the kidneys, but more often it develops gradually due to a chronic disease such as diabetes mellitus. Kidney infections in children and the rare kidney cancer called Wilms' tumour (p.565) are discussed in the section on infancy and childhood (pp.563–565).

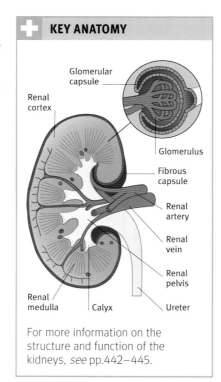

KEY ANATOMY

Glomerular capsule
Renal cortex
Glomerulus
Fibrous capsule
Renal artery
Renal vein
Renal pelvis
Renal medulla
Calyx
Ureter

For more information on the structure and function of the kidneys, *see* pp.442–445.

Pyelonephritis

Inflammation of one or both kidneys, usually due to bacterial infection

 Most common between the ages of 16 and 45

 Much more common in females

 In some cases, the cause is inherited from one parent

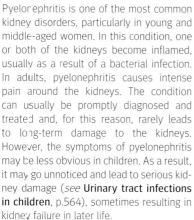 May be related to sexual activity in females

Pyelonephritis is one of the most common kidney disorders, particularly in young and middle-aged women. In this condition, one or both of the kidneys become inflamed, usually as a result of a bacterial infection. In adults, pyelonephritis causes intense pain around the kidneys. The condition can usually be promptly diagnosed and treated and, for this reason, rarely leads to long-term damage to the kidneys. However, the symptoms of pyelonephritis may be less obvious in children. As a result, it may go unnoticed and lead to serious kidney damage (*see* **Urinary tract infections in children**, p.564), sometimes resulting in kidney failure in later life.

What are the causes?
Pyelonephritis may be caused by bacteria entering the urinary tract through the urethra (the passage from the bladder to the outside of the body). Often the bacteria ascend to the kidneys through the ureters from an infection in the bladder (*see* **Cystitis**, p.453). Urinary infections, and therefore pyelonephritis, are much more common in females because the female urethra is shorter than that of the male, and its opening is nearer the anus. Bacteria from the anal area may enter the urethra during sex or if the area is wiped from back to front after a bowel movement. People with diabetes mellitus (p.437) are more likely to have urinary infections, partly because glucose in the urine may encourage bacterial growth.

In both sexes, pyelonephritis is more likely to develop if there is a physical obstruction anywhere in the urinary tract that prevents the normal flow of urine. In these circumstances, if bacteria have already contaminated the urine, they will not be flushed through the urinary tract as normal. Instead, they multiply in the stagnant urine. Obstruction to urine flow may result from pressure on the urinary tract. Common causes of blockage include the expanding uterus in pregnant women or an enlarged prostate gland (p.463) in men. Normal urine flow may also be obstructed by bladder tumours (p.456) or kidney stones

(opposite page). In addition, kidney stones may harbour bacteria and can therefore predispose to infection in the urinary tract. All of these conditions may lead to recurrent episodes of pyelonephritis.

Bacteria may also enter the bladder during bladder catheterization (p.455), a procedure in which a tube is passed up the urethra into the bladder to drain urine. In addition, bacteria may be carried in the bloodstream from elsewhere in the body to the kidneys.

What are the symptoms?
The symptoms of pyelonephritis may appear suddenly, often over a period of a few hours, and include:

- Intense pain that begins in the back just above the waist and then moves to the side and groin.
- Fever over 38°C (100°F), resulting in shivering and headache.
- Painful, frequent passing of urine.
- Cloudy, bloodstained urine.
- Foul-smelling urine.
- Nausea and vomiting.

If you develop these symptoms, consult your doctor immediately.

How is it diagnosed?
If your doctor suspects pyelonephritis, he or she will probably examine a sample of your urine to find out whether it contains bacteria. If there is evidence of infection, the urine sample will be sent for laboratory analysis to establish which type of bacterium has caused the infection. Men and children may need further tests to detect an underlying cause after a single episode of the disorder. Pyelonephritis is more common in women. For this reason, further tests are carried out for women only if they have recurrent episodes, or if the doctor suspects an underlying cause.

Further investigations may include a blood test to assess the function of the kidneys. Imaging procedures, such as ultrasound scanning (p.135) or CT urography (opposite page), may also be carried out to check for signs of kidney damage or of a disorder such as kidney stones.

What is the treatment?
Pyelonephritis is usually treated with a course of oral antibiotics (p.572), and symptoms often improve within 2 days of treatment. When the course of antibiotics is finished, further urine tests may be carried out to confirm that the infection has cleared up. However, if you are vomiting, in pain, or seriously ill, you may be admitted to hospital and given intravenous fluids and antibiotics.

If you experience repeated episodes of pyelonephritis, you may be advised to take low-dose antibiotics for a period of 6 months to 2 years to reduce the frequency of the attacks. If you have an underlying disorder, such as kidney stones, this may also need to be treated.

What is the prognosis?
In most cases, prompt treatment of pyelonephritis is effective, and the condition causes no permanent damage to the

kidneys. However, rarely, frequent episodes of pyelonephritis may lead to scarring of the kidneys and result in irreversible damage (*see* **End-stage kidney failure**, p.452).

Glomerulonephritis

Inflammation of the glomeruli, the tiny filtering units of the kidney

 Most common in children and young adults

 More common in males

 Genetics and lifestyle are not significant factors

Glomerulonephritis is an uncommon disorder in which many of the tiny filtering units of the kidneys, known as glomeruli, become inflamed. As a result, the kidneys are unable to carry out their usual function of removing waste products and excess water from the body efficiently. Blood cells and protein, which normally remain in the blood, leak through the glomeruli into the urine.

Glomerulonephritis can be a short-term (acute) or long-standing (chronic) disorder. An episode with a sudden onset is usually followed by complete recovery, but in severe cases damage to the glomeruli may be permanent. Chronic glomerulonephritis sometimes develops after an acute attack. Progressive kidney damage then occurs over several months or years as a result of continuing inflammation. Most people who develop glomerulonephritis have no previous history of kidney disease.

Although glomerulonephritis affects both kidneys, not all of the glomeruli may be affected to the same degree.

What are the causes?
Acute glomerulonephritis sometimes occurs as a complication of certain infectious diseases. The antibodies that are produced by the immune system to fight the infection attack the glomeruli in the kidneys, causing inflammation and damage. The most common cause of acute glomerulonephritis, especially in children, is a bacterial throat infection, such as a streptococcal infection. Occasionally, acute glomerulonephritis develops after a viral infection, such as infectious mononucleosis (p.166). In developing countries, the disorder may occur as a result of parasitic diseases, such as malaria (p.175).

Chronic glomerulonephritis is usually caused by a response of the immune system in which certain antibodies of the immunoglobulin A type are deposited in the kidney tissues. Chronic glomerulonephritis may also be associated with autoimmune disorders that affect many organs in the body, such as systemic lupus erythematosus (p.281).

▶ TEST

CT urography

CT urography is a procedure used to give a clear X-ray image of the urinary tract. It involves injection into the arm of a special dye (called a contrast medium) that shows up on X-rays. The dye is carried in the blood to the urinary system, where it is filtered through the kidneys and then passes into the ureters and bladder to be excreted in the urine. X-rays taken at intervals show outlines of the kidneys, ureters, and bladder. CT urography may be used to detect abnormalities, such as tumours and obstructions, and signs of kidney disease.

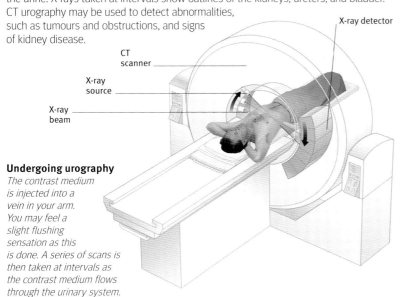

Undergoing urography
The contrast medium is injected into a vein in your arm. You may feel a slight flushing sensation as this is done. A series of scans is then taken at intervals as the contrast medium flows through the urinary system.

What are the symptoms?
In acute glomerulonephritis, symptoms develop rapidly over a few days. In contrast, the initial symptoms of chronic glomerulonephritis develop slowly and may only become apparent when the kidneys have already been severely damaged. The symptoms of both forms of the disorder may include:
- Frequent passing of urine.
- Frothy or cloudy urine.
- Blood in the urine.
- Puffiness of the face, with swelling around the eyes in the morning.
- Swollen feet and legs in the evening.
- Shortness of breath.
- Loss of appetite.

A serious complication of glomerulonephritis is high blood pressure (*see* **Hypertension**, p.242), which may result in further damage to the kidneys.

How is it diagnosed?
In the initial stages of chronic glomerulonephritis there may be no symptoms, and the condition may only be diagnosed during routine screening tests or investigations for another disorder. If you do develop symptoms of acute or chronic glomerulonephritis, the doctor may test a urine sample to detect blood and protein. Further urine tests and a blood test may be necessary to assess kidney function. In addition, your doctor may arrange for imaging tests to assess the size of your kidneys because the kidneys are likely to become larger in cases of acute glomerulonephritis and to shrink in chronic glomerulonephritis. The imaging

tests may include X-rays (p.131) or ultrasound scanning (p.135). A kidney biopsy (p.449) may also be needed to determine the cause of the kidney damage.

What is the treatment?
Treatment depends on the severity and, if known, the cause of the disorder. Some cases are so mild that they do not need treatment and are simply monitored. If the disorder follows a bacterial infection, antibiotics (p.572) and sometimes corticosteroids (p.600) may be prescribed. Glomerulonephritis due to an autoimmune disorder can usually be treated with immunosuppressants (p.585) and corticosteroids. If the condition is accompanied by high blood pressure, this will be treated with antihypertensive drugs (p.580) as good control of blood pressure is crucial to preserving kidney function.

What is the prognosis?
In most cases, the symptoms of acute glomerulonephritis disappear after 6–8 weeks. However, the outlook is variable. In some people, kidney function is reduced but does not deteriorate further. Others may develop chronic kidney disease (p.451), which can lead to end-stage kidney failure (p.452), an irreversible loss of kidney function that may be fatal if not recognized and treated promptly.

Nephrotic syndrome

A group of symptoms resulting from kidney damage that causes loss of protein into the urine and swelling of body tissues

 Most common in young children but can affect people of any age

 Gender, lifestyle, and genetics are not significant factors

The urine of a healthy person does not normally contain protein because the molecules are too large to pass across the glomeruli (the blood-filtering units in the kidneys). However, if the delicate glomeruli are damaged, large amounts of protein can leak into the urine from the blood. Eventually, this leakage results in low protein levels in the blood, an accumulation of fluid in body tissues, and widespread swelling.

What are the causes?
Nephrotic syndrome can be due to various kidney diseases, most commonly glomerulonephritis (opposite page) and diabetic kidney disease (p.450). It may also be a complication of infection elsewhere in the body, such as hepatitis B (*see* **Acute hepatitis**, p.408). Rarely, it can be due to amyloidosis (p.441), in which abnormal proteins collect in many organs throughout the body. Other possible causes include reactions to drugs and chemicals, as well as certain autoimmune disorders (in which the immune system attacks the body's own tissues), such as systemic lupus erythematosus (p.281).

What are the symptoms?
The symptoms of nephrotic syndrome appear gradually over days or weeks and worsen as more and more protein is lost. You may notice:
- Frothy urine.
- Decreased urine production.
- Puffiness of the face, with swelling around the eyes in the morning.
- Swollen feet and legs in the evening.
- Shortness of breath.
- Loss of appetite and weight loss.
- Swelling of the abdomen.

If you develop these symptoms, you should see a doctor immediately.

What might be done?
If your doctor suspects that you have nephrotic syndrome, he or she will first test your urine for the presence of protein. The doctor may also ask you to collect your urine over a 24-hour period so that daily protein loss can be measured. You will have a blood test to measure your protein level and to assess kidney function. In some cases, a kidney biopsy (p.449) is carried out to find the cause of the condition.

Your doctor may prescribe diuretics (p.583) to help to remove excess fluid from your body and may recommend a low-salt diet to prevent further fluid retention. If symptoms are severe, you may need treatment in hospital where you may be given

intravenous diuretics and possibly protein-rich intravenous fluids. You may also be given corticosteroids (p.600) and immunosuppressants (p.585) If possible, the underlying disorder will be treated.

What is the prognosis?
The outlook for someone with nephrotic syndrome depends on the extent of the kidney damage. Children usually respond well to corticosteroids and often make a full recovery, but adults may experience recurrent episodes. In the most severe cases, chronic kidney disease (p.451) and eventually end-stage kidney failure (p.452), an irreversible loss of kidney function, may develop.

Kidney stones

Crystal deposits of varying sizes that form in the kidney

 Most common between the ages of 30 and 50

 More common in males

In some cases, the cause is inherited

 Certain diets and living in a hot climate are risk factors

Normally, the waste products of the body's chemical processes pass out of the kidneys in the urine. Kidney stones occur when the urine is saturated with waste products that crystallize into stone-like structures, or when the chemicals that normally inhibit this crystallization process are not present. Kidney stones can take years to form.

If the stones are small, they may become dislodged from the kidney and move through the urinary tract, eventually passing out of the body in the urine. Larger stones stay in the kidney but may occasionally move into the ureter (the tube that takes urine from the kidney to the bladder). If a stone becomes lodged in the ureter, it can cause severe pain. A large stone in the kidney is not usually painful, but it increases the risk of urinary infection.

What are the causes?
The risk of stones forming in the kidneys is greatest when there is a high concentration of dissolved substances in the urine. Inadequate intake of fluid increases the risk of kidney stones. When there is too little water in the body, the kidneys conserve water by forming less urine, and as a result the urine they produce is highly concentrated. People who live in hot climates may be susceptible to kidney stones if they do not drink enough to replace the fluid lost through perspiration.

Different types of kidney stone can form, depending on the waste products that crystallize out of the urine. Most are made of calcium salts. These stones may be associated with a diet containing foods rich in calcium or a substance called oxalic acid. They may also develop if your body produces too much parathyroid hormone (see **Hyperparathyroidism**, p.434), a process causing high levels of calcium to build up in the bloodstream. A small percentage of stones contain uric acid and may occur in people who have gout (p.224).

Kidney stones may also result from a long-standing urinary tract infection. In such cases, the stones can grow into a staghorn shape and fill the central cavity of the kidney. Rarely, they are formed from cystine, a substance present in abnormally high levels in people who have the inherited disorder cystinuria. Kidney stones are also associated with some drugs, such as indinavir, which is used to treat HIV infection (see **Drugs for HIV infection and AIDS**, p.573).

What are the symptoms?
Very small kidney stones may pass unnoticed in the urine. Larger stones or small fragments of stones that pass into the ureter may cause painful spasms of the ureter wall. The symptoms usually appear suddenly and may include:
■ Excruciating pain that starts in the back, spreads to the abdomen and groin, and may be felt in the genitals.
■ Frequent, painful passing of urine.
■ Nausea and vomiting.
■ Blood in the urine.
If a kidney stone is passed in the urine, the pain will subside rapidly. However, if a stone lodges in a ureter, it may cause a build-up of urine, which will then result in swelling of the kidney (see **Hydronephrosis**, right).

How is it diagnosed?
If your doctor suspects that you have kidney stones, he or she will take a specimen of urine to look for blood, crystals, and evidence of an underlying infection. Stones that have been passed in the urine may be collected and analysed to determine their composition. An ordinary X-ray (p.131) may be used to look for calcium stones; other types of kidney stone can be detected by ultrasound scanning (p.135) or CT scanning (p.132). You may also have a blood test to assess kidney function, and to measure the levels of calcium, uric acid, and other substances in your blood. Collectively, these tests help the doctor to determine the presence and composition of kidney stones.

What is the treatment?
If the stones are small and remain in the kidney, you may simply be advised to take painkillers (p.589), and drink plenty of fluids to help flush the stones into the urine. For stones that need treatment, a common method is lithotripsy (below), in which shock waves are used to break them into small fragments that can be passed in the urine. Another is percutaneous lithotomy, in which an endoscope (viewing tube) is inserted into the kidney and instruments are passed through the tube to remove a stone. A very large stone may require treatment by both lithotripsy and endoscopic removal of the resulting stone fragments.

Rarely, a kidney contains a staghorn stone that has caused complete and irreversible loss of kidney function. This may necessitate removal of the entire kidney, which may be done by either conventional open surgery or keyhole surgery (laparoscopy).

If a stone moves into the ureter, it usually causes severe pain. You may need to go to hospital for strong painkillers. You may also

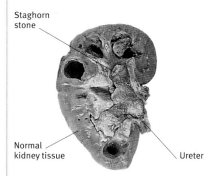

Staghorn
stone

Normal
kidney tissue

Ureter

Staghorn kidney stone
Named for its shape, this staghorn kidney stone has enlarged over many years to fill the entire centre of the kidney.

be given intravenous fluids to increase the volume of urine and help to flush out the stone. If a stone is lodged in the ureter, it may be pulverized or removed using instruments passed through a ureteroscope (a type of viewing tube that is passed into the ureter through the urethra and bladder).

The underlying cause needs to be treated to prevent the kidney stones from recurring. Your doctor will probably advise you to drink at least 2–3 litres (4–6 pints) of fluids every day and to avoid foods that may encourage the formation of stones (see **Preventing kidney stones**, below left).

What is the prognosis?
More than half the people treated for a kidney stone develop another within about 7 years. However, the self-help measures outlined below left may reduce the risk of recurrence. Kidney stones rarely cause permanent damage to the kidneys.

Hydronephrosis

Swelling of the kidney due to a blockage of the urinary tract

Most common in very young children and elderly people

Gender, genetics, and lifestyle are not significant factors

Hydronephrosis results from a blockage in the urinary tract that prevents urine from flowing normally through the system. As a result, the kidney becomes swollen with urine and pressure builds up within it, preventing normal function. The condition can affect one or both kidneys and may occur suddenly or gradually.

What are the causes?
The blockage that causes hydronephrosis may be due to an abnormality of the urinary tract that is present at birth or to narrowing of the ureter (the tube that takes urine from the kidney). This narrowing may develop as a result of pressure from outside the ureter, such as that caused by a tumour or by the enlargement of the uterus during pregnancy. Hydronephrosis may also occur if a ureter is blocked by a kidney stone (p.447) moving towards the bladder.

In addition, the disorder can be due to blockage of the urethra (the passage that leads from the bladder to outside the body). A blocked urethra is usually due to a urethral stricture (p.455) or an enlarged prostate gland (p.463).

What are the symptoms?
If hydronephrosis results from a sudden obstruction in the urinary tract, the following symptoms may develop:
■ Severe pain in the abdomen.
■ Acute lower back pain.
■ Nausea and vomiting.
However, hydronephrosis that develops gradually over a long period of time does not usually produce the symptoms listed above. In these cases, chronic kidney disease (p.451) may be the first sign that the condition exists.

People with hydronephrosis have an increased risk of urinary tract infection because bacteria are likely to multiply in urine that is not flowing freely.

How is it diagnosed?
If your doctor suspects that you have hydronephrosis, he or she may arrange for blood tests and urine tests to find out how well your kidneys are functioning. The

---

▶ **TREATMENT**

Lithotripsy

Lithotripsy is a procedure that is usually carried out in hospital. It uses high-energy shock waves to disintegrate stones in the kidneys, ureters, or bladder. The fragmented stones will then be passed in the urine, avoiding the need for surgery. Painkillers are given before the procedure since there may be some discomfort; children are usually given a general anaesthetic. For a few days after lithotripsy, you may have blood in your urine, and the treated area will feel bruised and tender. However, serious complications are uncommon.

Undergoing lithotripsy
The stone is located using X-rays. A machine called a lithotripter focuses high-energy ultrasonic shock waves on to the stone through a water- or gel-filled cushion placed under the back.

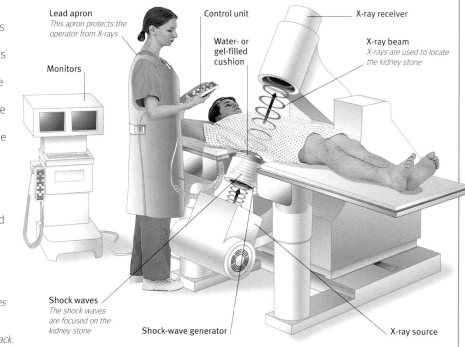

Lead apron
This apron protects the operator from X-rays

Monitors

Control unit

Water- or gel-filled cushion

X-ray receiver

X-ray beam
X-rays are used to locate the kidney stone

Shock waves
The shock waves are focused on the kidney stone

Shock-wave generator

X-ray source

doctor may also arrange for imaging tests, including ultrasound scanning (p.135) and CT urography (p.447). These tests will enable the blockage in your urinary tract to be located and the cause of the obstruction determined. In some instances, hydronephrosis is detected only when another disorder, such as an enlarged prostate gland, is being investigated.

What is the treatment?
Initially, the aim of treatment is to prevent permanent damage to the kidney by relieving the pressure that has built up inside it as soon as possible. If there is a blockage in the urethra, a tube will be inserted into the bladder to drain the urine (see **Bladder catheterization**, p.455). If the blockage is higher in the urinary tract, a tube may be inserted directly into the affected kidney to drain the urine. Once the pressure in the kidney has been relieved, the cause of the blockage can be treated.

Hydronephrosis associated with pregnancy is usually mild and does not require treatment. The condition improves spontaneously after the birth.

What is the prognosis?
If hydronephrosis is detected early, the affected kidney tissue normally recovers once the cause has been treated. However, hydronephrosis may lead to permanent kidney damage, and chronic kidney disease may develop if both kidneys are affected.

Kidney cyst

A fluid-filled swelling within the cortex, the outer part of the kidney

 More common over the age of 50

 Gender, genetics, and lifestyle are not significant factors

Kidney cysts form in the cortex (outer layer) of the kidney. They often occur singly, but three or four may develop. Kidney cysts are very common; up to half of all people over the age of 50 have at least one cyst, often without realizing it. The cause is not known.

Unlike the multiple cysts that occur in polycystic kidney disease (right), kidney cysts do not affect kidney function and are usually harmless. In most cases, they cause no symptoms. Rarely, a kidney cyst may become large enough to cause back pain, or it may bleed, causing blood to appear in the urine.

What might be done?
A kidney cyst is often detected by chance during ultrasound scanning (p.135), CT scanning (p.132), or CT urography (p.447) performed to investigate another condition. Rarely, a fluid sample may need to be taken from the cyst through a hollow needle to be examined for cancerous cells. This procedure is carried out under local anaesthesia using ultrasound to locate the cyst.

Kidney biopsy

A kidney biopsy is used to identify the nature and extent of kidney damage. The biopsy may be carried out as an outpatient procedure, or you may have to stay in hospital overnight. During the biopsy, a small piece of kidney tissue is removed. This tissue is then sent to a laboratory for microscopic examination. After the biopsy, you will be advised to rest for about 2 hours to minimize the risk of bleeding from the kidney.

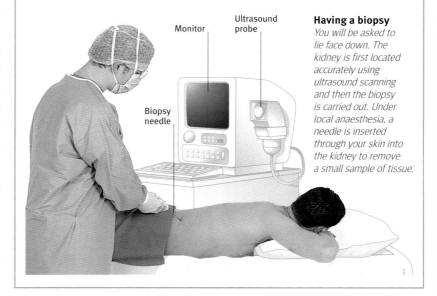

Monitor

Ultrasound probe

Biopsy needle

Having a biopsy
You will be asked to lie face down. The kidney is first located accurately using ultrasound scanning and then the biopsy is carried out. Under local anaesthesia, a needle is inserted through your skin into the kidney to remove a small sample of tissue.

A simple kidney cyst does not require treatment unless symptoms develop. However, if the cyst becomes painful, you may be sent to hospital to have fluid removed from it using a needle and syringe. Alternatively, the cyst can be removed surgically.

Polycystic kidney disease

An inherited disorder in which multiple fluid-filled cysts gradually replace the tissue in both kidneys

 Juvenile form usually evident at birth; adult form usually apparent by the age of 45

 Due to an abnormal gene inherited from one or both parents

 Gender and lifestyle are not significant factors

Polycystic kidney disease is an inherited condition in which the kidneys have a honeycomb appearance as a result of the presence of numerous fluid-filled cysts. The cysts gradually replace normal tissue so that the kidneys become larger and progressively less able to function until eventually they fail completely (see **End-stage kidney failure**, p.452). Polycystic kidney disease is not the same as simple kidney cysts (left), which are generally harmless.

Polycystic kidneys may affect adults or, rarely, infants. Adult polycystic kidney disease does not usually become apparent until about the age of 45, although

symptoms can appear as early as the age of 20. In children, the condition is known as juvenile polycystic kidney disease and is sometimes fatal.

What are the causes?
Polycystic kidney disease is caused by an abnormal gene. In the adult form, the gene is inherited in an autosomal dominant manner, and as a result the disease can be inherited from just one parent (see **Gene disorders**, p.151). Each child of such a parent has a 1 in 2 chance of developing the disorder in adulthood. The juvenile form is inherited in an autosomal recessive way; both parents must pass the faulty gene to the child for the disorder to develop. When both parents have one copy each of the faulty gene, each child has a 1 in 4 chance of developing the disorder.

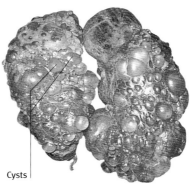

Cysts

Polycystic kidneys
Multiple fluid-filled cysts have replaced the normal tissue in both of these kidneys. As a result, the kidneys have become very large and irregularly shaped.

Can it be prevented?
The gene responsible for polycystic kidneys in adults has been identified, and genetic counselling (p.151) is available for people who have a family history of the disease. If both potential parents are aware that they carry the gene for the juvenile form, they will also need counselling before conceiving. It is possible to check the kidneys of a fetus for signs of the disorder using ultrasound scanning (see **Ultrasound scanning in pregnancy**, p.512). If an ultrasound scan reveals polycystic kidneys in the fetus, the parents can discuss the options available with the doctor.

What are the symptoms?
The symptoms of adult polycystic kidney disease may not appear for many years. The main symptoms are:
- Vague discomfort in the abdomen or aching in the lower back.
- Episodes of severe and sudden pain in the abdomen or lower back.
- Blood in the urine.

A baby with juvenile polycystic disease will have a very swollen abdomen due to enlargement of the kidneys.

In adults, as the disease progresses, high blood pressure (see **Hypertension**, p.242) may develop, which can lead to further kidney damage. Occasionally, one or more of the kidney cysts become infected, resulting in pain and fever. Sometimes, cysts develop in other organs, such as the pancreas and liver.

If you have abdominal pain and notice blood in your urine, you should consult your doctor as soon as possible.

What might be done?
Adult polycystic kidney disease is often first discovered during a routine physical examination. It may also be detected when family members are screened because a relative already has polycystic kidney disease. Blood and urine tests may be performed to assess kidney function, and ultrasound scanning (p.135) or CT scanning (p.132) may be carried out to confirm the diagnosis. Healthy children of people with polycystic kidney disease are usually advised to have an ultrasound scan at around the age of 20 to check for the development of the disorder.

If it has not been detected in the fetus, juvenile polycystic kidney disease may be obvious at birth because the baby will have a very swollen abdomen. The diagnosis can be confirmed by ultrasound scanning, which will show enlarged kidneys with cysts.

There is no effective way to prevent the cysts forming, but careful control of high blood pressure may slow the rate of the kidney damage. If the fluid in the cysts is infected, antibiotics (p.572) may be prescribed. If end-stage kidney failure occurs, dialysis (p.451) or a kidney transplant (p.452) will be needed.

What is the prognosis?
The progression of polycystic kidney disease in adults varies considerably. However, the outlook tends to be similar for affected

members of the same family. About 7 in 10 of the people who have polycystic kidney disease develop kidney failure by the age of 65.

In a child who has juvenile polycystic kidney disease, the kidneys will fail, and eventually the child will need dialysis or a kidney transplant. Some affected infants may die at only a few months of age due to kidney failure.

Kidney cancer

Cancerous tumours that either originate in the kidney or have spread from a cancer elsewhere in the body

> Age, gender, genetics, and lifestyle as risk factors depend on the cause

In most cases of kidney cancer, a tumour develops within the kidney tissue itself. Rarely, cancer may spread to the kidney from other organs in the body.

There are three main types of kidney cancer. The most common type, adenocarcinoma, develops from the cells that make up the main body of the kidneys. A second, rare form, known as transitional cell carcinoma, develops from the cells that line the urine-collecting system within the kidney, bladder, and ureters (the tubes that carry urine from the kidneys to the bladder). This form is more common in people who smoke, because tobacco contains carcinogens (cancer-inducing substances), and in people who have been exposed to other carcinogens, such as chemical dyes, even many years previously. A third type, called Wilms' tumour (p.565), is usually either present at birth or develops during the first 5 years of life.

What are the symptoms?
There are often no symptoms in the early stages of kidney cancer. If symptoms do develop, they may include:
- Painful, frequent passing of urine.
- Blood in the urine.
- Pain in the back or sides.
- Weight loss.

If you notice blood in your urine (indicated by a red, pink, or smoky colour), consult your doctor immediately.

What might be done?
If your doctor suspects kidney cancer, he or she may image the kidneys using ultrasound scanning (p.135) or CT scanning (p.132). The affected kidney will usually be removed by keyhole surgery (laparoscopy). (The other kidney can usually compensate.) If the cancer has spread, you may need systemic treatment. This is usually with targeted therapy, which involves giving drugs that disrupt the growth and spread of tumours. In a few cases, immunotherapy with drugs that stimulate the immune system to attack cancer cells may be helpful.

About 7 in 10 people who have a kidney tumour removed survive for more than 5 years, even if the tumour was large. If

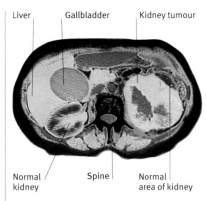

Liver   Gallbladder   Kidney tumour

Normal kidney   Spine   Normal area of kidney

Kidney cancer
This CT scan through the abdomen shows a large kidney tumour that has grown to replace most of the normal kidney tissue.

the cancer has spread to other organs before it is diagnosed, the length of survival decreases. However, systemic treatments may slow the spread of cancer considerably.

Diabetic kidney disease

Damage to the filtering units of the kidneys that occurs in people who have diabetes mellitus

 Usually occurs in adults who have had diabetes mellitus for many years

 Diabetes mellitus sometimes runs in families

 Poor control of diabetes mellitus is a risk factor

 Gender is not a significant factor

Long-term diabetes mellitus (p.437) may result in damage to various organs in the body. Kidney damage caused by diabetes mellitus is known as diabetic kidney disease. The disorder develops in about 4 in 10 of the people who have had diabetes for over 15 years.

Diabetes mellitus affects small blood vessels in the glomeruli (the filtering units of the kidney). Damage to these vessels causes protein to leak into the urine and reduces the kidneys' ability to remove wastes and excess water from the body. Symptoms do not usually appear until kidney damage is severe, and may include drowsiness, vomiting, and shortness of breath (*see* **Chronic kidney disease**, opposite page). Most people who have diabetes mellitus also have high blood pressure (*see* **Hypertension**, p.242), which may cause further damage to the kidneys.

What might be done?
People who have diabetes mellitus are monitored regularly by their doctor so that complications such as kidney damage can be detected at an early stage. The doctor will look for the first signs of diabetic kidney disease by arranging for urine tests to detect protein, and blood tests will

be performed to check how well the kidneys are functioning. Once the condition has been diagnosed, the primary aim of treatment is to slow the progression of the disease to kidney failure. Good control of blood glucose and blood pressure are crucial to slow the deterioration of kidney function. However, even if diabetes is under control, diabetic kidney disease may still progress. Drugs called ACE inhibitors (p.582) may be effective in slowing the progression of kidney disease due to diabetes mellitus. Nevertheless, the outcome may be end-stage kidney failure (p.452), in which there is a complete loss of function in both kidneys.

End-stage kidney failure due to diabetic kidney disease can often be treated with dialysis (opposite page) or a kidney transplant (p.452). It is sometimes possible to combine a kidney transplant with a transplant of the pancreas, treating both kidney failure and diabetes mellitus at the same time. However, the surgery involved is complex and is only carried out in certain specialist centres.

Kidney failure

Loss of the normal function of both kidneys due to a variety of causes

 Age, gender, genetics, and lifestyle as risk factors depend on the cause

In kidney failure, the kidneys do not function normally, and waste products and excess water build up in the body, disrupting the chemical balance of the blood. The condition may take one of three forms: acute kidney injury (below), chronic kidney disease (opposite page), or end-stage kidney failure (p.452).

Acute kidney injury is a sudden loss of kidney function that can be fatal if not treated rapidly. Chronic kidney disease is a gradual reduction in function of the kidneys over months or years. Some people have the condition for years without knowing it. End-stage kidney failure is a permanent and almost total loss of kidney function. Left untreated, the condition is fatal.

Treatment for kidney failure involves reversing or slowing the damage, restoring the chemical balance of the blood, and treating the underlying disorder. Methods of treatment for kidney failure may include drugs, dialysis (opposite page), or a kidney transplant (p.452).

Acute kidney injury

Sudden loss of the function of both kidneys, which is potentially life-threatening

 Age, gender, genetics, and lifestyle as risk factors depend on the cause

Acute kidney injury occurs when there is a sudden reduction of function in both kidneys. As a result, they can no longer

adequately filter waste products and excess water from the blood into the urine. The waste substances may build up to dangerous levels in the body, and the chemical balance of the blood is upset. The condition is life-threatening and requires immediate hospital treatment.

What are the causes?
The most common cause of acute kidney injury is a reduction in the blood supply to the kidneys. This reduction may be due to a fall in blood pressure associated with shock (*see* **Hypotension**, p.248), such as after severe bleeding, serious infection, or a heart attack (*see* **Myocardial infarction**, p.245). Acute kidney injury may also result from glomerulonephritis (p.446), toxic chemicals, drugs, or obstruction to the flow of urine (*see* **Hydronephrosis**, p.448).

What are the symptoms?
The symptoms of acute kidney injury may appear rapidly, sometimes over a period of hours, and include:
- Greatly reduced urine volume.
- Nausea and vomiting.
- Drowsiness and headache.
- Back pain.

If you develop these symptoms, you should call your doctor immediately. Without treatment, acute kidney injury may be fatal within a few days.

How is it diagnosed?
If your doctor suspects acute kidney injury, he or she will have you admitted to hospital for emergency treatment and tests to find the cause. In some cases, there may be an obvious cause, such as severe bleeding. In other cases, ultrasound scanning (p.135) or CT scanning (p.132) will be performed to look for a blockage of the urinary tract. A kidney biopsy (p.449) may also be performed to identify the cause.

What is the treatment?
If you have acute kidney injury, you will need immediate treatment for the disorder and any associated conditions. You will probably be treated in an intensive therapy unit (p.618). You may have to undergo dialysis (opposite page) for a short time so that the excess fluid and waste products can be removed from your bloodstream while the doctors investigate the cause of the kidney injury. If you have lost a large amount of blood, you may need to have a blood transfusion (p.272) to restore your normal blood volume. If an underlying disorder is diagnosed, treatment with drugs may be necessary. Finally, if there is a blockage anywhere in your urinary tract, you may need to undergo surgery to have the obstruction removed.

What is the prognosis?
If your kidneys have not already been damaged irreversibly, there is a good chance that you will make a complete

recovery, which may take up to 6 weeks. However, in some cases, the resulting damage is not completely reversible, and in this situation chronic kidney disease (below) may develop. If chronic kidney disease eventually progresses to end-stage kidney failure (p.452), in which there is a permanent and almost total loss of kidney function, you will need treatment that involves long-term dialysis or a kidney transplant (p.452).

Chronic kidney disease

Gradual and progressive loss of function in both kidneys

 Some causes are increasingly common with age

 Gender and genetics as risk factors depend on the cause

 Lifestyle is not a significant factor

In chronic kidney disease, progressive damage gradually reduces the ability of the kidneys to remove excess water and wastes from the blood. As a result, waste substances start to build up in the body. In many cases, kidney function is reduced by over 60 per cent before the build-up is detected; by this time, often after months or even years, the kidneys may be irreversibly damaged. Dialysis (right) or a kidney transplant (p.452) may therefore become necessary.

What are the causes?
Chronic kidney disease may result from disorders that progressively damage kidney tissue, such as polycystic kidney disease (p.449) or glomerulonephritis (p.446). The condition may also be the result of generalized disorders, such as diabetes mellitus (p.437) or high blood pressure (see Hypertension, p.242). People who have sickle-cell disease (p.272) are at risk of developing chronic kidney disease if abnormal blood cells block the small vessels that supply the kidneys. Chronic kidney disease can also follow prolonged blockage of the urinary tract, such as that caused by an enlarged prostate gland (p.463).

What are the symptoms?
The initial symptoms of chronic kidney disease appear gradually over weeks or months and are often vague, such as weakness and loss of appetite. As the condition progresses, other symptoms may then develop, including:
- Frequent passing of urine, particularly during the night.
- Pale, itchy, and easily bruised skin.
- Shortness of breath.
- Persistent hiccups.
- Nausea and vomiting.
- Muscular twitching.
- Pins and needles.
- Cramps in the legs.

▶ **TREATMENT**

Dialysis
Dialysis removes from the blood waste products and excess water, which are retained in people with kidney failure. It can be a temporary treatment for acute kidney injury (opposite page) or a long-term measure used in end-stage kidney failure (p.452). There are two forms: peritoneal dialysis, in which the peritoneal membrane in the abdomen is used as a filter; and haemodialysis, in which a kidney machine filters the blood.

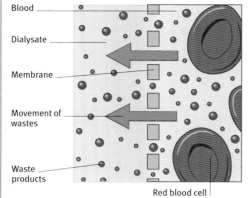

Blood
Dialysate
Membrane
Movement of wastes
Waste products
Red blood cell

How dialysis works
During dialysis, excess water and waste products from the blood pass across a membrane into a solution (the dialysate), which is then discarded.

Peritoneal dialysis
In peritoneal dialysis, the peritoneum, the membrane that surrounds the abdominal organs, is used instead of the kidneys to filter the blood. A procedure called an exchange is carried out four times a day at home. During an exchange, dialysis fluid that was infused into the abdomen 4–6 hours earlier is drained out of the peritoneum through a catheter in the abdominal wall. The fluid is replaced with fresh solution, then the equipment is disconnected and you can carry out normal activities. Between exchanges, wastes and excess water pass from the peritoneal blood vessels into the dialysis fluid.

Fresh dialysate
The bag of fresh dialysate is slowly emptied into the peritoneal cavity

Dialysate tubing

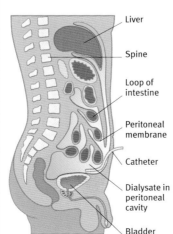

Undergoing peritoneal dialysis
In peritoneal dialysis, dialysis fluid is changed at regular intervals and is continually present in the abdomen. Once a fluid exchange has taken place, the bags and tubing are detached, and you can move freely.

Liver
Spine
Loop of intestine
Peritoneal membrane
Catheter
Dialysate in peritoneal cavity
Bladder

Bag of used dialysate
Used dialysate drains out of the body and collects in this bag before fresh fluid is allowed to flow in

Using the peritoneum as a filter
The abdominal organs are covered by the peritoneal membrane, which is rich in blood vessels. In peritoneal dialysis, waste products and water pass from the blood across the membrane and into dialysate fluid in the abdomen.

Haemodialysis
In haemodialysis, blood is pumped by a kidney machine through a filter attached to the side of the machine. Inside the filter, blood flows on one side of a membrane and dialysis fluid flows on the other. Waste products and water pass from the blood across the membrane and into the dialysate fluid, and the filtered blood returns to the body. Each treatment takes 3–4 hours and is usually repeated three times a week.

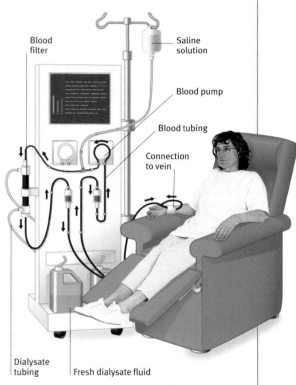

Blood filter
Saline solution
Blood pump
Blood tubing
Connection to vein
Dialysate tubing
Fresh dialysate fluid

Undergoing haemodialysis
During haemodialysis, you are attached to the kidney machine for several hours while waste products and water are removed from your blood. Haemodialysis is usually carried out in outpatient dialysis centres, but some people are able to treat themselves at home.

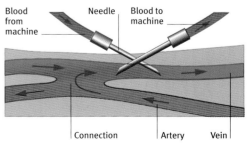

Blood from machine
Needle
Blood to machine
Connection
Artery
Vein

Access to the bloodstream
Dialysis requires fast blood flow. A vein and an artery near the skin surface are surgically joined so that the vein carries blood at high pressure. This vein can then be used for access to the circulatory system.

▶ **TREATMENT**

Kidney transplant

People with end-stage kidney failure may be treated with a kidney transplant, which can take over the function of both diseased kidneys. An organ may be donated by a living relative or spouse or by someone who has consented to the use of his or her organs after death. The new kidney is sited in the pelvis and the diseased kidneys are usually left in place. A successful kidney transplant avoids the need for dialysis and often allows a return to a normal lifestyle.

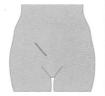

SITE OF INCISION

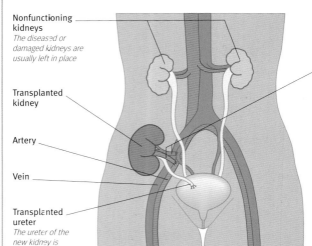

Nonfunctioning kidneys
The diseased or damaged kidneys are usually left in place

Transplanted kidney

Artery

Vein

Transplanted ureter
The ureter of the new kidney is connected directly to the bladder

Transplanted artery and vein
The artery and vein of the new kidney are attached to blood vessels in the pelvis

The operation
The new kidney is placed in the pelvis through an incision in the abdomen. The kidney is carefully positioned so that it can be connected easily to a nearby vein and artery and to the bladder.

The condition is associated with a number of complications, such as high blood pressure, which may be an effect as well as a cause of kidney failure; bone thinning (*see* **Osteoporosis**, p.217); hyperparathyroidism (p.434); and anaemia (p.271), in which the oxygen-carrying capacity of the blood is reduced.

How is it diagnosed?

If you have symptoms of chronic kidney disease, your doctor will probably arrange for tests of your blood and urine. You may also have ultrasound scanning (p.135), radionuclide scanning (p.302), or CT scanning (p.132) to assess the size of the kidneys; abnormally small kidneys are often a sign of chronic kidney disease. In addition, you may need to undergo a kidney biopsy (p.449), a procedure in which a small piece of kidney tissue is removed and examined under a microscope to determine the nature of kidney damage.

What is the treatment?

Treatment is directed at the underlying cause. Corticosteroids (p.600) may be used to treat some forms of glomerulonephritis. Drugs for high blood pressure (*see* **Antihypertensive drugs**, p.580) may also be given, whether the condition is the cause or result of chronic kidney disease. If there is an obstruction in the urinary tract, you will probably need surgery to relieve it. In addition, your doctor will monitor the progress of the disease and the effectiveness of your treatment with regular checkups.

What is the prognosis?

The outlook for chronic kidney disease depends on the cause and severity of the kidney damage. If your doctor is able to treat the cause and prevent further damage to your kidneys, you may not need dialysis. However, in many cases, treatment only slows the rate of deterioration. After several months or years, chronic kidney disease may develop into end-stage kidney failure (below), in which the damage is irreversible. At this stage, dialysis or a kidney transplant operation are the only treatment options.

End-stage kidney failure

Irreversible loss of the function of both kidneys, which is life-threatening

ⓘ Age, gender, genetics, and lifestyle as risk factors depend on the cause

End-stage kidney failure occurs when there is a permanent loss of over 90 per cent of kidney function. As a result, the kidneys are unable to filter waste products and excess water out of the blood for excretion as urine. End-stage kidney failure usually progresses from chronic kidney disease (p.451). If prompt action is not taken to replace the function of the failed kidneys with dialysis (p.451) or a kidney transplant (above), the condition is fatal.

What are the symptoms?

The main symptoms of end-stage kidney failure include:

- Swelling of the face, the limbs, and to abdomen.
- Severe lethargy.
- Weight loss.
- Headache and vomiting.
- Furred tongue.
- Very itchy skin.

Many people who have end-stage kidney failure also have breath that smells like ammonia, an odour similar to that of household bleach.

How is it diagnosed?

If your doctor suspects end-stage kidney failure, he or she will first arrange for urine tests and blood tests to detect abnormal levels of waste products. If the cause of kidney failure has not already been identified, you may also have to undergo imaging procedures such as ultrasound scanning (p.135), CT scanning (p.132), or radionuclide scanning (p.302) to detect abnormalities in your kidneys.

What is the treatment?

Kidney dialysis, the usual treatment for end-stage kidney failure, takes over the function of filtering harmful waste products and excess water from the blood. However, long-term dialysis may lead to complications such as gradual weakening of the bones (*see* **Osteoporosis**, p.217), hyperparathyroidism (p.434), and anaemia (p.271), in which the oxygen-carrying capacity of the blood is reduced. The anaemia may develop due to a lack of the hormone erythropoietin, which is made in the kidneys and stimulates red blood cell production; it may be treated by injections of erythropoietin.

A kidney transplant offers the best hope of returning to a normal lifestyle. The main drawback of a transplant is that you will need to take immunosuppressants (p.585) for the rest of your life to prevent your immune system from rejecting the donor organ. Occasionally, a second transplant is needed if the first kidney stops functioning. If you do not have a kidney transplant, you will need dialysis for the rest of your life.

Disorders of the bladder and urethra

Urinary disorders are very common. The symptoms may include an increased need to empty the bladder, urinary leakage, blood in the urine, and pain during and after urination. These symptoms can often disrupt daily routine. However, most disorders of the bladder and urethra (the passage from the bladder to the outside of the body) are curable or at least controllable by treatment.

The first article in this section deals with cystitis, a condition in which the bladder becomes inflamed. Cystitis is often due to infection by bacteria from the skin around the anus. Women are particularly susceptible to the disorder because the female urethra is short and close to the anus, allowing bacteria to enter easily. In men, bladder infections are often related to an obstruction due to an enlarged prostate gland.

The next three articles cover urinary incontinence. There are several types of incontinence, all of which are more common in women and in older people of both sexes. Structural disorders are covered in the next articles; they include stones that form in the bladder and strictures that narrow the urethra, making the passing of urine difficult. The last article in this section covers bladder tumours.

Sexually transmitted infections that affect the male urethra are discussed elsewhere (*see* **Sexually transmitted infections**, pp.491–493). Urinary tract problems that occur in children are covered in the section on infancy and childhood (pp.563–565).

➕ **KEY ANATOMY**

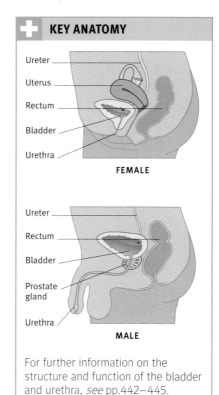

Ureter

Uterus

Rectum

Bladder

Urethra

FEMALE

Ureter

Rectum

Bladder

Prostate gland

Urethra

MALE

For further information on the structure and function of the bladder and urethra, *see* pp.442–445.

Cystitis

Inflammation of the bladder lining, causing painful, frequent passing of urine

 Rare in children; more common in teenage girls and women of all ages

 Much more common in females

 For some women, sexual intercourse may bring on an episode

 Genetics is not a significant factor

In cystitis, the lining of the bladder becomes inflamed, resulting in a frequent need to pass urine and pain when passing urine. In most cases, the condition is due to a bacterial infection.

Cystitis affects women much more commonly than men. About half of all women have at least one attack of bacterial cystitis in their lifetime, and some women have recurrent attacks. In men, cystitis is rare and is usually associated with a disorder of the urinary tract. In children, cystitis can be the result of an anatomical or structural problem and can damage the kidneys (*see* **Urinary tract infections in children**, p.564).

What are the types?

There are several types of cystitis. The most common form is bacterial cystitis, which is often caused by *Escherichia coli*, a bacterium that normally lives in the intestines. Cystitis usually occurs when bacteria from the anal or vaginal areas enter the bladder through the urethra (the tube from the bladder to the outside of the body), often during sex or when the anus is wiped after a bowel movement. Women are at much greater risk of infection than men because the female urethra is shorter than that of the male and the opening is nearer the anus. The risk of bacterial cystitis is increased if the bladder cannot be emptied fully. Incomplete emptying causes urine to be retained in the bladder, and bacteria can multiply in the trapped urine. Postmenopausal women are especially prone to bacterial cystitis because they have reduced levels of the hormone oestrogen, which leaves their urethral lining vulnerable. Women who use a diaphragm and spermicide for contraception are at increased risk because a diaphragm, which has to stay in place for several hours, can prevent complete bladder emptying, and spermicide may encourage the growth of bacteria in the vagina. People with diabetes mellitus (p.437) are also susceptible for several reasons: there may be glucose in their urine, which encourages the growth of bacteria; they may have reduced immunity to infection; or they may have nerve damage that prevents the bladder from emptying completely. Other disorders that prevent complete bladder emptying include an enlarged prostate gland (p.463) and urethral stricture (p.455), in which the urethra is narrowed.

Interstitial cystitis is a rare, chronic, non-bacterial inflammation of the lining and tissues of the bladder that may lead to ulceration. The cause is unknown, although some women find that certain foods or drinks trigger or worsen the symptoms. This type of cystitis may be responsible for chronic symptoms of pelvic pain and urinary frequency that do not improve with antibiotics, particularly in women.

In radiation cystitis, the lining of the bladder is damaged as a result of radiotherapy (p.158) to treat prostate cancer (p.464), bladder tumours (p.456), or cancer of the cervix (p.481).

What are the symptoms?

The main symptoms of all types of cystitis are the same and include:

- Burning pain when passing urine.
- Frequent and urgent need to urinate, with little urine passed each time.
- A feeling of incomplete emptying of the bladder.

If the cause of the cystitis is a bacterial infection, you may also notice:

- Pain in the lower abdominal region and sometimes in the lower back.
- Fever and chills.

A bladder infection can spread upwards to a kidney, causing severe pain in the back (*see* **Pyelonephritis**, p.446). In some severe cases of cystitis, complete or partial loss of control over bladder function can occur as a result of irritation of the muscle in the bladder wall (*see* **Urge incontinence**, p.454).

What might be done?

If you develop the symptoms of cystitis, arrange to see your doctor. You may be able to relieve symptoms by drinking ½ litre (about 1 pint) of fluid every hour for 4 hours. Taking an over-the-counter painkiller (p.589), such as paracetamol, may also help to relieve pain and discomfort. Self-help measures (*see* **Preventing bacterial cystitis**, below) may prevent a recurrence.

Your doctor will arrange for urine tests to detect any evidence of infection. While awaiting the results, he or she may prescribe antibiotics (p.572). Almost all attacks of bacterial cystitis are cured by a single course of antibiotics. Recurrent attacks in women or a single episode in men need further

SELF-HELP

Preventing bacterial cystitis

If you have had bacterial cystitis, the following measures can help you to avoid further attacks:

- Drink 2–3 litres (4–6 pints) of fluids each day. Drink even more in hot weather.
- Empty your bladder frequently and completely.
- Be careful about hygiene. After a bowel movement, wipe yourself from front to back to prevent bacteria around the anus from entering the urethra.
- Wash your genital area before sexual intercourse. Make sure your partner washes, too.
- Pass urine shortly after having sexual intercourse.
- Use unperfumed toiletries and avoid vaginal deodorants.
- Do not use a diaphragm or spermicide for contraception.

▶ **TEST**

Urodynamic studies

Urodynamic studies are carried out to investigate problems with bladder control, including incontinence and restricted urine flow. In these studies, probes are inserted into the bladder and rectum or vagina to monitor pressure changes while the bladder is being filled through a catheter and emptied. In some cases, the bladder is filled with a contrast medium (a dye that shows up on X-rays), which enables the doctor to view the shape of the bladder on an X-ray monitor. You will be asked to cough as the bladder fills, which may cause leakage of urine if you have stress incontinence.

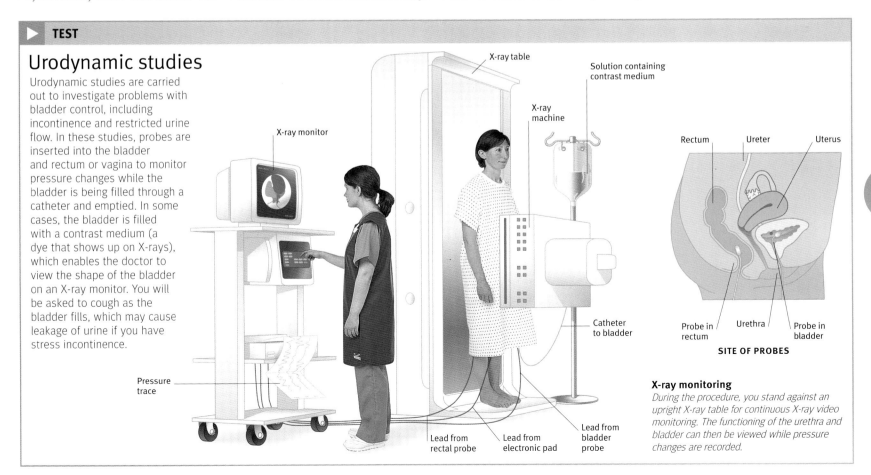

X-ray monitoring
During the procedure, you stand against an upright X-ray table for continuous X-ray video monitoring. The functioning of the urethra and bladder can then be viewed while pressure changes are recorded.

investigations, such as specialized imaging of the urinary tract (see **CT urography**, p.447), ultrasound scanning (p.135) of the urinary tract and sometimes cystoscopy (p.456). If there is no evidence of a disorder but the cystitis still recurs, your doctor may prescribe a long course of low-dose antibiotics. Women may be given a single high dose of antibiotics to be taken after intercourse or at the first sign of symptoms.

If urine tests show no infection but you have recurrent attacks of pain and frequent urination, your doctor may suspect interstitial cystitis. However, bacteria may be difficult to detect, and your doctor may prescribe antibiotics even though no infection has been found. He or she may suggest self-help measures, including avoiding foods or drinks that you find trigger symptoms. Some postmenopausal women find oestrogen-containing creams helpful.

Your doctor may arrange for cystoscopy to view inside the bladder, and a sample of bladder tissue may be taken. If these investigations reveal interstitial cystitis, your doctor may suggest one of several treatments, including a course of oral corticosteroids (p.600) or a procedure in which the bladder is stretched by filling it with water. This procedure, which is carried out under general anaesthesia, can relieve symptoms.

Urinary incontinence

Complete or partial loss of voluntary control over bladder function

 More common with increasing age

 More common in females

 Genetics and lifestyle as risk factors depend on the type

Normally, muscles in the bladder wall push the urine out of the bladder, while muscles in the neck of the bladder and urethra (the tube from the bladder to the outside of the body) control the opening and closing of the bladder outlet. Any disorder affecting these muscles or their nerve supply can result in a partial or complete loss of bladder control.

Urinary incontinence becomes more common with increasing age. The condition is more common in women than in men. It sometimes accompanies dementia (p.331) or stroke (p.329).

What are the types?

There are four main types of incontinence: stress, urge, overflow, and total. The symptoms and treatment are different for each type.

The most common type of incontinence is stress incontinence (right), in which small amounts of urine are expelled involuntarily.

People who have urge incontinence (right) feel an unexpected and urgent need to pass urine due to an involuntary contrac-

tion of the bladder, resulting in the uncontrollable and sudden passage of large amounts of urine.

In overflow incontinence, the bladder cannot empty because of a blockage at the bladder neck or in the urethra or because of a weak bladder muscle. The volume of urine then builds up in the bladder, causing an intermittent or continuous dribble. Urine outflow may be obstructed by a urethral stricture (opposite page), an abnormal narrowing of part of the urethra, or, in men, by an enlarged prostate gland (p.463), constricting the upper part of the urethra. Weakness of the bladder muscle may be due to an obstruction, diabetes mellitus (p.437), or pelvic surgery.

In total incontinence, there is no bladder control. The condition usually results from a nervous system disorder such as dementia or spinal injury (p.323). Surgery to treat pelvic cancers can also cause incontinence by damaging nerves that supply the bladder.

What might be done?

Urodynamic studies (p.453) can determine the type of incontinence. Pads to absorb urine can be worn to protect clothes. Pelvic floor exercises (opposite page) and physiotherapy (p.620) may help to improve bladder muscle tone. Incontinence due to incomplete bladder emptying can be relieved by intermittent self-catheterization to drain the urine or permanent bladder catheterization (opposite page) if the person is disabled.

Stress incontinence

Involuntary loss of urine during exertion, coughing, or sneezing

 More common with increasing age

 Almost exclusively affects females

 Genetics and lifestyle are not significant factors

Stress incontinence results from weakness of the urethra (the tube from the bladder to the outside of the body) and pelvic floor muscles. These muscles support the bladder and help to control the opening and closing of the bladder outlet when passing urine. Weakness of the muscles allows the bladder neck to drop. Involuntary loss of urine occurs when pressure in the abdomen is increased.

In mild stress incontinence, a small amount of urine leaks out of the bladder during strenuous activities, such as running. In severe cases, urine escapes during activities that cause increased pressure on the bladder, such as coughing or lifting. Stress incontinence is the most common type of incontinence and mostly affects women.

The disorder commonly occurs during and after pregnancy; after surgery in the pelvic area; during the menopause, when a

reduced level of the hormone oestrogen causes the pelvic muscles to lose elasticity; and with increasing age. Stress incontinence may also be linked to a prolapse of the uterus and vagina (p.479), rectal prolapse (p.422), or a prolapsed bladder. The condition is more likely to develop if you have a persistent cough. Rarely, men develop stress incontinence after prostate surgery.

How is it diagnosed?

Your doctor may diagnose stress incontinence after asking about your fluid intake, how often you pass urine, the amount of urine you pass, and when you leak urine. He or she will perform a pelvic examination to check your pelvic floor muscles and find out if you have a prolapsed uterus. The doctor may refer you to hospital for urodynamic studies (p.453) to assess your bladder function.

What is the treatment?

Your doctor will probably recommend pelvic floor exercises (opposite page) to strengthen the pelvic floor muscles, which are often effective in treating stress incontinence, whatever the cause. If the condition occurs after childbirth, muscle tone will gradually return but the exercises may speed recovery. In addition to pelvic floor exercises, you may be advised also to try other ways of exercising the pelvic muscles, such as electrical stimulation or vaginal cones. Electrical stimulation involves using a special electrical device to contract the pelvic floor muscles. A vaginal cone is a

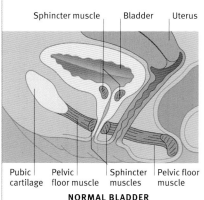

Sphincter muscle | Bladder | Uterus

Pubic cartilage | Pelvic floor muscle | Sphincter muscles | Pelvic floor muscle

NORMAL BLADDER

Dropped bladder neck | Uterus

Pubic cartilage | Sagging muscles

INCONTINENT BLADDER

Cause of stress incontinence
In stress incontinence, the muscles in the pelvic floor cannot support the bladder. The bladder neck drops, and the sphincter muscles become unable to keep it closed.

small plastic cone that you put inside the vagina for about 15 minutes twice a day. You need to use the pelvic floor muscles to keep the cone in. The cones come in different weights; you start with the lightest and, when you can hold it in comfortably, progress to a heavier weight, and so on. If you are overweight, your doctor may recommend a diet to help you lose weight (see **Controlling your weight**, p.19).

If these measures alone do not help, your doctor may prescribe a drug called duloxetine to be used in addition to pelvic floor exercises. If neither exercises nor drug treatment is effective, your doctor may suggest surgery to support your bladder or lift it back into the correct position, which is often successful in restoring normal or near-normal bladder control.

Urge incontinence

Repeated episodes of involuntary loss of urine preceded by a sudden, urgent need to empty the bladder

 More common with increasing age

 More common in females

 Genetics and lifestyle are not significant factors

A person with urge incontinence feels a sudden, urgent need to pass urine that is followed by involuntary loss of urine. This condition varies in severity. At its mildest, the person is usually able to reach a toilet before the bladder starts to empty. However, if the condition is severe, it can be impossible to stop the flow of urine voluntarily once the bladder has begun to empty.

What are the causes?

Urge incontinence is most commonly caused by overactivity of the muscle that forms the bladder wall. As a result, the muscle contracts involuntarily and empties the bladder. Overactivity of the bladder muscle can be due to infection or inflammation of the bladder lining (see **Cystitis**, p.453).

Urge incontinence can also be due to disorders such as bladder stones (p.456). Other causes are disorders that affect the nervous system, such as stroke (p.329), multiple sclerosis (p.334), or spinal injury (p.323). Some cases are thought to be linked to anxiety.

What might be done?

You will be asked to keep a record of how often you need to pass urine, the amount of urine passed each time, and how much fluid you drink. You may also need to provide a sample of your urine, which will be checked for evidence of infection. In addition, your doctor will carry out a physical examination to look for an underlying disorder and may refer you to hospital for further investigations.

Any underlying cause of urge incontinence should be treated first. If no underlying disorder is found, there are several self-help measures that you can try. For example, you can learn to control your bladder function by extending the intervals between the times when you pass urine. Pelvic floor exercises (below) strengthen the muscles that control the bladder outlet. If you smoke, you should try to stop since smoking is known to irritate the bladder. It is also advisable to avoid drinks containing caffeine and alcohol. In addition, you may be given an anticholinergic drug such as oxybutynin, which relaxes the muscle in the bladder wall and thereby increases bladder capacity and reduces the urge to urinate (*see* **Drugs acting on the bladder**, p.606).

Pelvic floor exercises

Exercises can be used to help to strengthen the pelvic floor muscles. These muscles support the bladder, uterus, and rectum. If performed regularly, pelvic floor exercises can help in both the treatment and prevention of incontinence.

You can perform pelvic floor exercises sitting, standing, or lying down. Do the exercises as often as you can, ideally for 5 minutes every hour throughout the day.

In order to identify the pelvic floor muscles, imagine that you are passing urine and have to stop suddenly midstream. The muscles that you feel tighten around your vagina, urethra, and rectum are the pelvic floor muscles. To strengthen these muscles, practise the following exercises:

- Contract the pelvic floor muscles and hold them for 10 seconds.
- Relax the muscles slowly.
- Repeat 5 to 10 times, as often as you can.

Urinary retention

Inability to empty the bladder completely or at all

 More common over the age of 50

 More common in males

 Genetics and lifestyle are not significant factors

Urinary retention may be either acute or chronic. In acute retention, the bladder cannot be emptied at all despite a desperate urge to do so, and a sudden and painful build-up of urine occurs. In chronic retention, some urine can be passed with difficulty, but the bladder cannot be emptied completely, and as a result a gradual and painless build-up of urine occurs. Both forms of urinary retention are more common in men.

What are the causes?

Anything that exerts pressure on the urethra (the tube from the bladder to the outside of the body) can restrict the flow of urine, causing acute or chronic urinary retention. The most common cause in men is an enlarged prostate gland (p.463). Sometimes, the flow of urine is restricted by a narrowed urethra (*see* **Urethral stricture**, right) or by a tightened foreskin of the penis (*see* **Phimosis**, p.461). In women, retention may occur during early pregnancy due to pressure by the enlarging uterus on the urethra, but it may disappear later as the uterus rises up into the abdomen. In both sexes, urinary retention may be caused by constipation because faeces in the rectum can press on the urethra. Rarely, the flow of urine from the bladder is restricted by conditions in which the neck of the bladder is obstructed, such as bladder stones (p.456) and bladder tumours (p.456).

Damage to the nerves supplying the bladder muscles can also cause urinary retention. Damage may occur in disorders such as multiple sclerosis (p.334) and diabetes mellitus (p.437), or it may be caused by spinal injury (p.323).

In some cases, chronic urinary retention can become acute because of a sudden increase in the amount of urine produced, which can be triggered by diuretic drugs (p.583), cold weather, or alcohol consumption. In other cases, acute urinary retention is a side effect of antidepressant drugs (p.592), drugs for Parkinson's disease (*see* **Parkinson's disease and parkinsonism**, p.333), or cold and flu remedies (p.588).

What are the symptoms?

Symptoms of acute urinary retention develop over a few hours and include:
- Abdominal pain.
- A distressing and painful urge to pass urine without being able to do so.

In contrast to acute retention, chronic retention is unlikely to cause any pain, although the condition can be uncomfortable. The symptoms tend to develop more slowly and include:
- A frequent urge to pass urine.
- Swelling of the abdomen.
- Difficulty starting to pass urine.
- A weak flow of urine that ends in a dribble. In some cases, there may be involuntarily dribbling of urine between visits to the toilet.

Urinary retention can cause kidney damage if urine cannot drain from the kidneys (*see* **Hydronephrosis**, p.448).

What might be done?

If you have acute urinary retention, you will probably need to have your bladder emptied in hospital (*see* **Bladder catheterization**, below). You will have a rectal or pelvic examination and may later have special tests (*see* **Urodynamic studies**, p.453, and **Cystoscopy**, p.456) to identify the underlying cause.

Chronic urinary retention may be suspected if a routine medical examination reveals that you have an enlarged bladder. Diagnostic tests are the same as those for acute retention. The cause of the retention is treated if possible, and, in most cases, bladder function returns to normal. If the condition results from nerve damage, permanent or intermittent catheterization to drain the urine may be necessary. You may be taught how to catheterize yourself.

Urinary retention that occurs during pregnancy usually disappears when the uterus enlarges and moves up and out of the pelvis into the abdominal area, relieving pressure on the urethra.

Urethral stricture

Abnormal narrowing of part of the urethra, the passage from the bladder to the outside of the body

 Can affect adults of any age but most common over the age of 50

 Almost exclusively affects males

 Unprotected sex with multiple partners is a risk factor

 Genetics is not a significant factor

In urethral stricture, scar tissue forms within the wall of the urethra, causing narrowing of the urethra and difficulty passing urine. In developed countries, scar tissue usually results from damage to the area during certain medical procedures, such as bladder catheterization (below, left), cystoscopy (p.456), or prostatectomy (p.464). Scarring from these procedures usually affects people over 50 years old. Worldwide, the most common causes of scarring are persistent urethral inflammation as a result of sexually transmitted infections, such as gonorrhoea (p.491) or nongonococcal urethritis (p.491), and accidental injury to the genital area, such as a fracture of the pelvis. Such conditions are usually more common in young adults.

What are the symptoms?

The symptoms of a stricture gradually get worse over time and may include:
- Difficulty passing urine.
- Poor flow of urine.
- Dribbling after passing urine.
- The sensation that the bladder has been only partly emptied.
- Frequent need to pass urine.

An untreated stricture may block the flow of urine from the bladder, causing urinary retention (left). Incomplete emptying of the bladder can result in cystitis (p.453). In a few cases, incomplete emptying may cause an abnormal build-up of pressure in the urinary tract that can damage the kidneys (*see* **Hydronephrosis**, p.448).

What might be done?

Your doctor will carry out a physical examination to find out if your bladder is enlarged. He or she may then arrange for specialized X-rays of the urinary tract to establish whether your bladder empties completely when you pass urine and to look for bladder abnormalities. A stricture may be suspected if X-rays reveal slow bladder emptying and an abnormally large volume of retained

---

▶ **TREATMENT**

Bladder catheterization

In this procedure, a catheter is inserted into the bladder through the urethra (urethral catheterization) or through an incision in the abdomen (suprapubic catheterization). The catheter allows urine to drain out of the body if passing urine is not possible, if a person is incontinent, or if urine flow needs to be measured for diagnostic reasons. The catheter is held in place by a small, water-filled balloon. Some people may be taught to insert a catheter themselves several times a day to drain urine.

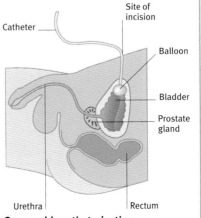

Urethral catheterization
The catheter is inserted along the urethra and into the bladder. Urine passes down the catheter into a drainage bag attached to a stand or worn around the thigh.

Suprapubic catheterization
This catheterization is used for drainage if the urethra is blocked. The catheter enters the bladder via an incision in the abdomen. Urine is collected in a bag.

urine. Further studies (*see* Urodynamic studies, p.453) may show whether or not a stricture exists, and cystoscopy and imaging may be used to locate it.

If a stricture is detected, treatment depends on its location and factors such as the age of the person. The simplest treatment is urethral dilation (widening). Under local anaesthesia, a slim, flexible instrument is passed into the urethra to stretch the narrowed area gently. The procedure may need to be repeated if the stricture recurs.

If the first attempt at dilation fails, or for more serious strictures, the scar tissue may be removed surgically during cystoscopy. If there is substantial scarring, the narrowed section may be removed and the urethra reconstructed by plastic surgery.

Bladder stones

Ball-like masses of variable size, made of chemical deposits, that gradually form within the bladder

 Can affect adults of any age but much more common over the age of 45

 More common in males

 Genetics and lifestyle are not significant factors

Stones can form in the bladder if waste products in the urine crystallize. About 8 in 10 stones consist of calcium, which comes from excess salts in the urine. Most are between 2 mm (1/16 in) and 2 cm (3/4 in) in diameter, but some grow much larger. Bladder stones are about three times more common in men than in women and are much more common in people over 45 years old.

The condition may develop if urine stagnates in the bladder as a result of incomplete emptying (*see* Urinary retention, p.455). It is also more likely to develop in people who have recurrent or persistent urinary tract infections (*see* Cystitis, p.453). Certain metabolic disorders, such as gout (p.224), can also give rise to increased levels of waste products in the urine and encourage the formation of bladder stones.

What are the symptoms?

A small bladder stone may not cause any symptoms. However, as a stone increases in size, it may start to irritate the bladder lining, causing some or all of the following symptoms:
■ Pain and difficulty passing urine.
■ Frequent and sometimes urgent need to pass urine.
■ Blood in the urine.

If you develop any of these symptoms, you should consult your doctor without delay. Left untreated, a stone may irritate the muscles in the bladder wall and cause urge incontinence (p.454). A stone that blocks the bladder outlet can cause urinary retention or cystitis, which may be intensely painful.

What might be done?

If bladder stones are suspected, you will be referred to hospital for tests such as an abdominal X-ray (p.131) or specialized X-rays of your urinary tract (*see* CT urography, p.447). You may also have samples of your blood and urine analysed to look for signs of infection and rule out an underlying metabolic disorder, such as gout. In addition, cystoscopy (right) may be carried out to examine the lining of your bladder.

Bladder stones can usually be broken into fragments and washed out during cystoscopy. Alternatively, a form of ultrasound (*see* Lithotripsy, p.448) is used to pulverize the stones, which are passed out in the urine soon after the procedure. If the stones are very large, surgery may be needed to remove them.

Bladder stones often recur. About 3 in 5 of the people successfully treated for bladder stones develop the condition again within 7 years.

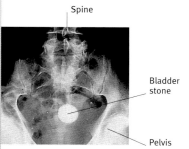

Spine

Bladder stone

Pelvis

Bladder stone
A large bladder stone can be seen in this X-ray. Stones, especially of this size, can make passing urine painful and difficult.

Bladder tumours

Cancerous growths that develop in the lining of the bladder

 Rare under the age of 50; more common with increasing age

 More common in males

 May be a significant factor

 Smoking and some occupations using chemicals are risk factors

Tumours in the bladder are all treated as cancerous. Most of these tumours begin as superficial, wart-like growths, called papillomas, which grow from the lining of the bladder and project into the bladder cavity. Bladder tumours are about three times more common in men than in women.

What are the causes?

More than half of all bladder tumours develop in people who smoke. About 1 in 6 tumours occurs in people who are employed in the rubber-manufacturing industry or work with industrial dyes or solvents. These people are susceptible to tumours since they handle carcinogens (cancer-causing substances), which are absorbed by the body and excreted in the urine. Carcinogens

▶ TEST AND TREATMENT

Cystoscopy

During cystoscopy, a thin, hollow viewing tube, known as a cystoscope, is inserted into the urethra and then into the bladder to look for tumours and other abnormalities affecting the urethra and bladder. The cystoscope may be rigid or flexible. Instruments to take tissue samples or destroy or remove tumours and stones can be inserted through the cystoscope. The procedure may be carried out under local or general anaesthesia.

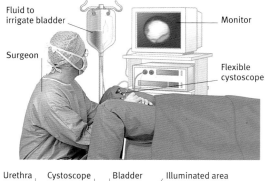

Fluid to irrigate bladder

Surgeon

Monitor

Flexible cystoscope

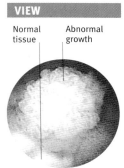

VIEW

Normal tissue

Abnormal growth

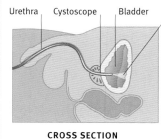

Urethra   Cystoscope   Bladder   Illuminated area

CROSS SECTION

During the procedure
An illuminated and magnified view of part of the bladder lining is transmitted from the cystoscope to a monitor.

Bladder lining
This magnified view through a cystoscope shows a growth in the lining of the bladder. Samples taken from such a growth will be analysed under a microscope to look for cancerous cells.

therefore come into contact with the bladder lining, where they can trigger the growth of abnormal tissue. The underlying cause of bladder tumours is unknown, but the possibility that they may be inherited is currently under investigation.

In tropical regions, a common cause of bladder tumours is the parasitic infestation schistosomiasis (p.179).

What are the symptoms?

Bladder tumours initially do not cause symptoms, but the following symptoms may develop over time:
■ Blood in the urine.
■ Dull ache in the lower abdomen.
■ Difficulty passing urine.

If urine flow is restricted, urine may stagnate, leading to infections in the urinary tract (*see* Cystitis, p.453). Large tumours may block the bladder outlet, causing urinary retention (p.455). Left untreated, the cancer may spread to nearby areas. Cancerous cells can also break away from the tumour and travel in the blood to other parts of the body.

What might be done?

Your doctor will have a urine sample tested in the laboratory for blood and cancerous cells. Ultrasound scanning (p.135), CT urography (p.447), CT scanning (p.132), or MRI (p.133) may be used to image the bladder and reveal abnormalities. Your doctor will also arrange for you to have cystoscopy (above), in which a viewing instrument is used to examine the bladder lining. If a tumour is found, surgical instruments are inserted through the cysto-

scope to take a tissue sample, remove the tumour, or destroy it by heat treatment. Tumours may also be treated by drugs that are delivered directly into the bladder through a catheter.

If a tumour is large or has spread deep into the tissues of the bladder, abdominal surgery may be necessary to remove the tumour along with part or all of the bladder. If the whole bladder must be removed, urine will be diverted through an opening on the skin in the abdominal area by way of a passage constructed from a piece of intestine. Radiotherapy (p.158) and chemotherapy (p.157) may be used for tumours that would be difficult to treat with cystoscopy or surgery or where a person is too ill or frail for surgery.

What is the prognosis?

Bladder tumours that have been diagnosed at an early stage can usually be treated successfully. However, lifelong monitoring will be necessary because further bladder tumours may develop. Regular checkups should ensure that, if more papillomas develop, they can be treated before they have the chance to become more serious.

If you smoke, giving up will greatly reduce your risk of developing a bladder tumour. Once you have had a tumour treated, giving up smoking will reduce the risk of recurrence. If you work with high-risk chemicals or have done so in the past, you should see your doctor for regular checkups because tumours can develop many years after exposure to carcinogenic chemicals.

Male reproductive system

Men reach their sexual peak between the ages of 16 and 18, shortly after puberty. Since they are able to produce sperm continuously from puberty onwards, men remain fertile for a longer period than women; some men can become fathers at the age of 70 or older. Sperm are produced in the testes, and, during sexual intercourse, the penis delivers them into the female reproductive system. The male reproductive system also manufactures sex hormones that are essential for sperm production and for sexual development during puberty.

THE MALE REPRODUCTIVE system begins to develop before a male baby is even born. The only visible parts of the male reproductive system are the penis and the scrotum, but inside the body there is a complicated network of ducts, glands, and other tissues that work together to make the production and transport of sperm possible.

Sperm production

Once puberty is reached, sperm are manufactured continuously in the two testes at a rate of about 125 million each day. Since sperm production is not efficient at body temperature, the testes are kept cool by being suspended outside the body in a sac of skin called the scrotum. Mature sperm leave each testis through an epididymis, a long

coiled tube that lies above and behind each testis. The sperm are stored in the epididymis and mature there before going to the vas deferens, the tube that connects an epididymis to an ejaculatory duct. During sexual activity, each vas deferens contracts and pushes sperm towards the urethra (the tube that connects the bladder to the outside of the body). The sperm are ejaculated during sexual activity or are reabsorbed into the body. Some dribble through the upper end of the vas deferens into the urethra and are later washed away in the urine.

The sperm are carried in a fluid consisting of secretions from various glands. Most of these secretions are produced by glands called seminal vesicles as the sperm leave the vas deferens. Fluid is also added by the prostate gland. In addition to acting as a vehicle for the sperm to help them to swim, the fluid provides nutrients that keep the sperm healthy. Together, these secretions and sperm form semen, containing about 50 million sperm per millilitre.

In order for reproduction to take place, sperm must enter the female reproductive system (*see* **Sex and reproduction**, pp.489–490). During arousal, the penis becomes enlarged and firm. Muscular contractions at the base of the penis then force sperm through the male urethra and into the vagina during male orgasm.

Male hormones

The principal male sex hormone, testosterone, is produced throughout life. Testosterone plays an important part in the development of the genitals and other male sexual characteristics. During puberty, there is a dramatic increase in the level of testosterone. This increase triggers the growth of the genitals and the development of secondary male sexual characteristics, such as body and facial hair, deepening of the voice, and muscle development.

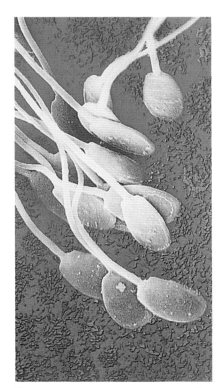

Sperm
Each sperm has a long tail that enables it to swim inside the female reproductive tract.

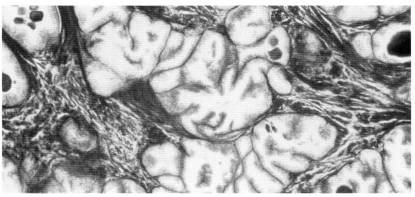

Prostate gland
The prostate gland secretes a milky fluid that helps the sperm to swim.

✚ **PROCESS**

Puberty

Puberty is the process of sexual development. In boys, puberty usually occurs between the ages of about 9 and 14 and lasts 3–4 years. Hormones secreted by the pituitary gland cause levels of the male sex hormone testosterone to rise, stimulating changes such as genital growth and the development of secondary sexual characteristics.

Physical development
During puberty, the penis, scrotum, and testes enlarge, and pubic hair grows. Hair also appears on the face and other parts of the body. Rapid growth occurs, the muscles develop, and the voice deepens.

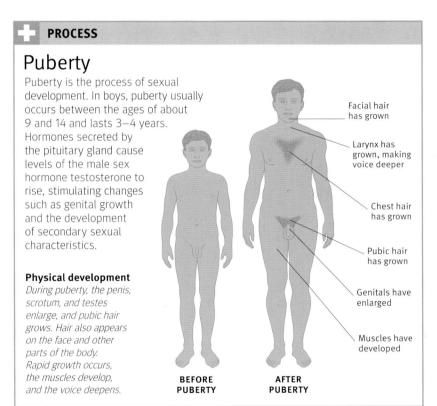

Facial hair has grown

Larynx has grown, making voice deeper

Chest hair has grown

Pubic hair has grown

Genitals have enlarged

Muscles have developed

BEFORE PUBERTY   **AFTER PUBERTY**

✚ **STRUCTURE**

Male reproductive system

The male genitals consist of the penis, scrotum, and the two testes, which are suspended in the scrotum. Above and behind each testis is an epididymis, a coiled tube that leads to another tube called the vas deferens. The upper end of each vas deferens is joined by a duct draining from a gland called the seminal vesicle. This duct and a vas deferens together form an ejaculatory duct. The two ejaculatory ducts then join the urethra where it is surrounded by the prostate gland, and the urethra passes through the penis to the outside.

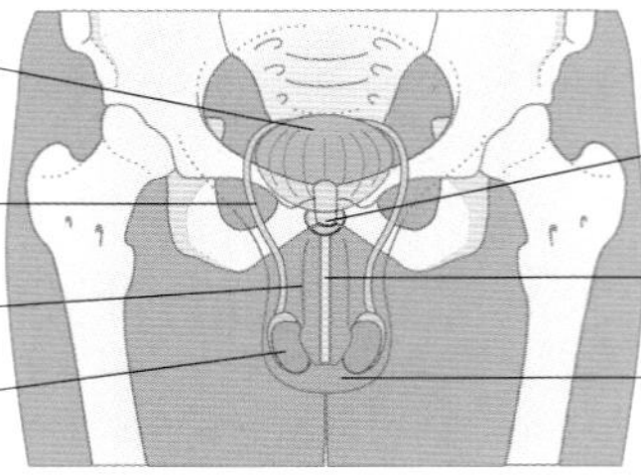

Bladder

Vas deferens

Penis

Testis

Prostate gland

Urethra

Scrotum

FRONT VIEW

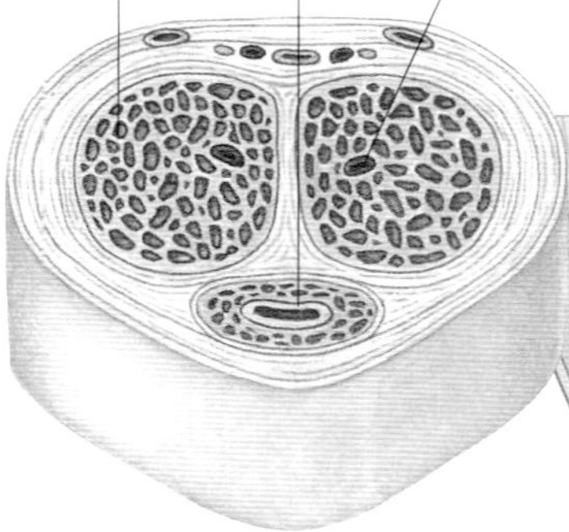

Spongy erectile tissue

Urethra

Artery

Vas deferens
This tube carries sperm to one of the ejaculatory ducts

Bladder

Ureter

Seminal vesicle
Each seminal vesicle adds fluid and nutrients to sperm

Ejaculatory duct
Each of these ducts joins one vas deferens to the urethra

Section through the penis
The penis contains three columns of spongy tissue and many blood vessels.

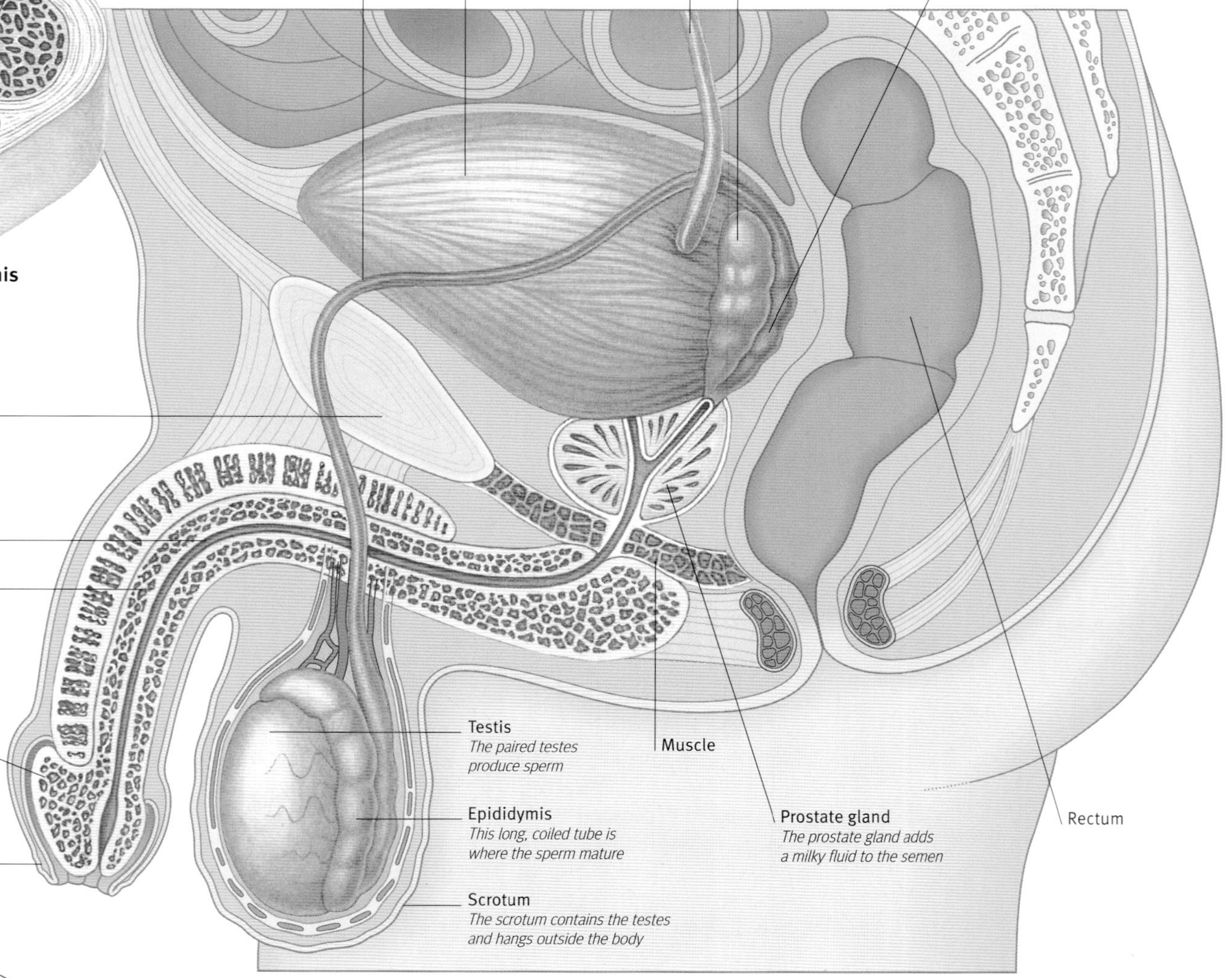

Pubic cartilage

Urethra
This tube carries urine and semen from the body

Spongy erectile tissue

Glans penis
This forms the bulbous end of the penis

Foreskin
The foreskin covers and protects the head of the penis

Testis
The paired testes produce sperm

Muscle

Epididymis
This long, coiled tube is where the sperm mature

Prostate gland
The prostate gland adds a milky fluid to the semen

Rectum

Scrotum
The scrotum contains the testes and hangs outside the body

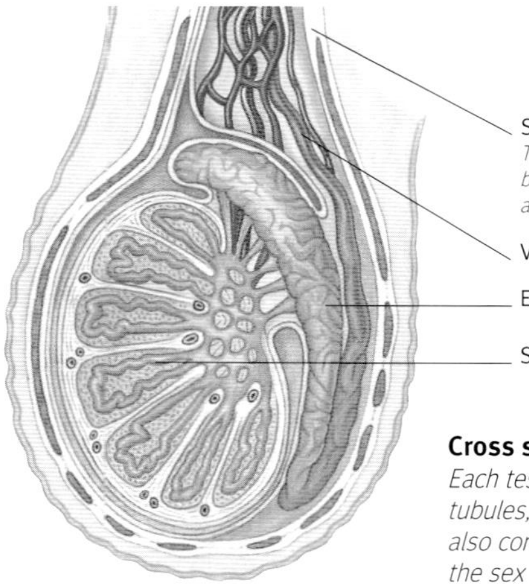

Spermatic cord
This cord contains muscle, blood vessels, nerves, and the vas deferens

Vas deferens

Epididymis

Seminiferous tubule

Cross section of the testis
Each testis is packed with seminiferous tubules, which make sperm. The testes also contain Leydig cells that manufacture the sex hormone testosterone.

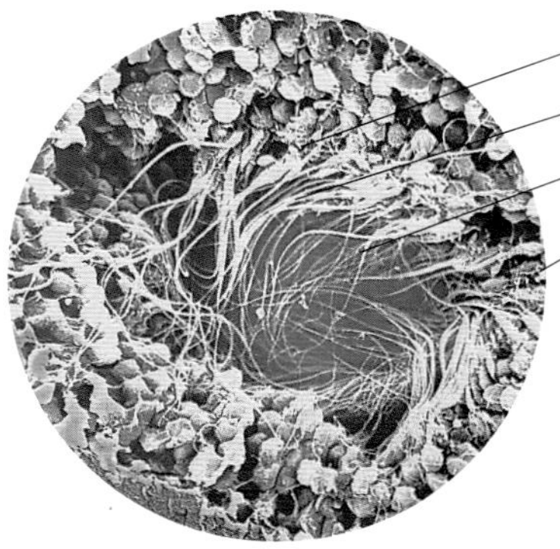

Developing sperm

Sperm tails

Centre of tubule

Tubule wall

Sperm production
This magnified image shows maturing sperm in a seminiferous tubule. The tails of developing sperm are near the centre.

Disorders of the testes, scrotum, and penis

Most of the male reproductive system – the penis, scrotum, and testes – is outside the abdomen. Consequently, symptoms of disorders in these structures are usually obvious at an early stage. Such symptoms should not be ignored out of embarrassment since most genital disorders can be cured by prompt treatment.

In this section, disorders that affect the epididymis (the coiled tube that carries sperm away from each testis) and the testes are described first. These disorders range from epididymal cysts, which are harmless collections of fluid, to cancer of the testis.

The next articles discuss disorders of the scrotum, the sac in which the testes are suspended. These disorders are usually not serious and include varicose veins in the scrotum, known as varicocele, and hydrocele, in which fluid collects around the testis.

Disorders caused by inflammation of the penis and foreskin are covered next, followed by two disorders of erectile function of the penis. The final article in this section discusses cancer of the penis, a very rare but distressing disorder that, if diagnosed early, responds well to treatment.

Skin conditions that may affect the penis and scrotum are discussed elsewhere (*see* **Skin, hair, and nails**, pp.189–210), as are male hormonal disorders (pp.465–466) including abnormal puberty, sexual problems (pp.494–496) such as erectile

dysfunction, infertility (pp.494–499), and sexually transmitted infections (pp.491–493). Conditions that develop in the male genitals during childhood are covered in disorders of the urinary and reproductive systems (*see* **Infancy and childhood**, pp.524–529).

KEY ANATOMY

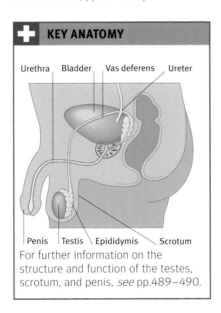

Urethra   Bladder   Vas deferens   Ureter

Penis   Testis   Epididymis   Scrotum

For further information on the structure and function of the testes, scrotum, and penis, *see* pp.489–490.

Epididymal cysts

Swellings in the epididymis, the coiled tube inside the scrotum that stores and transports sperm

 More common over the age of 40

 Genetics and lifestyle are not significant factors

Epididymal cysts, or spermatoceles, are harmless fluid-filled sacs that form in the epididymis, which stores and transports sperm away from the testis. Small epididymal cysts are common, particularly in men over the age of 40. The cysts develop slowly and are usually painless.

In many cases, there are multiple cysts, which can be felt as distinct, painless swellings like a tiny bunch of grapes on top of and behind the testis. The epididymal tubes in both testes may be affected by cysts at the same time.

If you detect a swelling on one or both sides of your scrotum, you should consult your doctor to rule out a serious condition,

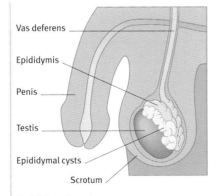

Vas deferens

Epididymis

Penis

Testis

Epididymal cysts

Scrotum

Epididymal cysts
Fluid-filled cysts that develop next to the testis in the epididymis are known as epididymal cysts and are usually painless.

such as cancer of the testis (p.460). He or she will probably be able to make a diagnosis from a physical examination, but further tests such as ultrasound scanning (p.135) may be necessary.

Epididymal cysts normally remain small and do not need treatment. Rarely, they become large and cause discomfort, in which case they can be removed.

Epididymo-orchitis

Inflammation of the epididymis, the coiled tube inside the scrotum that stores and transports sperm, and of the testis

 Rare before puberty

 Genetics and lifestyle are not significant factors

Infection of the testis and epididymis (the coiled tube that stores and transports sperm away from the testis) can lead to inflammation called epididymo-orchitis. This condition usually causes painful swelling of one testis and may be accompanied by fever.

What are the causes?
Epididymo-orchitis is usually caused by bacteria that have travelled from the urinary tract along the spermatic duct (vas deferens) to the epididymis. In men under 35 years of age, a common cause of the condition is a sexually transmitted infection (STI), such as nongonococcal urethritis (p.491). In older men, a urinary tract infection, prostatitis (p.463), or recently having had a catheter inserted to drain urine (*see* **Bladder catheterization**, p.455) are possible causes. In rare cases, an infection that is transmitted through the bloodstream, such as tuberculosis (p.300), leads to the development of epididymo-orchitis.

In boys and young men, the most common cause of epididymo-orchitis used to be inflammation as a result of mumps (p.167), but this has become less common since the introduction of routine immunization.

What are the symptoms?
The symptoms of epididymo-orchitis usually develop over a period of several hours and may include:

- Swelling, redness, and tenderness of the scrotum on the affected side.
- In severe cases, extreme pain in the scrotum, with fever and chills.

You may also have some symptoms of the underlying disorder, such as painful and frequent passage of urine in the case of a urinary tract infection.

The symptoms of epididymo-orchitis are similar to those of a more serious condition called torsion of the testis (right). For this reason, you should consult your doctor immediately if you have any of the symptoms listed above.

What might be done?
Your doctor will ask you to provide a urine sample to be tested for infection. If the doctor suspects an STI, he or she will take a swab from your urethra (the tube from the bladder to the outside of the body) to check for infection. If the diagnosis is unclear, you will need to go to hospital as

an emergency for tests to rule out torsion of the testis. In some cases, exploratory surgery is necessary.

Your doctor will probably prescribe antibiotics (p.572) unless the inflammation is caused by infection with the mumps virus, in which case antibiotics are ineffective. You may be advised to rest in bed and drink plenty of fluids. Taking painkillers (p.589) may help to ease the discomfort, and using an ice pack may reduce the swelling and pain in the scrotum. An athletic support can be worn to support the scrotum.

Pain is usually relieved in 1–2 days, but the swelling of the scrotum may take several weeks to subside.

Torsion of the testis

Twisting of the testis within the scrotum, causing severe pain

 Most common between the ages of 12 and 18 but can occur at any age

 Genetics and lifestyle are not significant factors

Each testis is suspended in the scrotum on a spermatic cord. The spermatic duct (vas deferens) and the blood vessels that supply the testis are contained in the spermatic cord. If the spermatic cord becomes twisted, the flow of blood to the testis is restricted, causing severe pain in the scrotum.

Torsion of the testis usually affects only one of the two testes. It sometimes occurs after strenuous activity but may develop for no apparent reason, even during sleep. Torsion of the testis most commonly occurs during adolescence, but it can develop at any age. The condition is potentially serious; torsion may result in permanent damage to the testis if not treated immediately.

What are the symptoms?
Symptoms of torsion of the testis usually appear suddenly. They may include:

- Sudden pain in the scrotum that tends to increase in severity.
- Pain in the groin and lower abdomen.
- Redness and extreme tenderness of the scrotum on the affected side.

The severity of the pain can cause nausea and vomiting. If you develop any of these symptoms, you should seek medical advice urgently.

What might be done?
Your doctor may arrange for ultrasound scanning (p.135) of the scrotum to exclude other disorders that cause similar symptoms, such as epididymo-orchitis (left). If you have torsion of the testis, an operation is carried out to untwist the spermatic cord. Both testes are then anchored in the scrotum with stitches to prevent a recurrence of the condition. If this operation is performed promptly, the testis is usually undamaged. However, if a testis is irreversibly damaged, it will be removed.

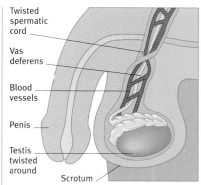

Torsion of the testis
In torsion of the testis, the spermatic cord, from which the testis hangs in the scrotum, becomes twisted, which restricts the flow of blood to and from the testis.

Occasionally, the spermatic cord will untwist spontaneously. If your symptoms disappear, you should still consult your doctor because they may recur.

What is the prognosis?
The testis is usually undamaged if the spermatic cord is untwisted within about 6 hours. Removal of one testis does not normally affect fertility because the remaining one is able to produce sufficient sperm. A testis can be replaced by an artificial implant for cosmetic reasons.

Cancer of the testis

A cancerous tumour that develops within a testis

 Most common between the ages of 20 and 40

 Sometimes runs in families

 Lifestyle is not a significant factor

Although cancer of the testis is a rare condition, it is one of the most common forms of cancer diagnosed in men between the ages of 20 and 40. It is also one of the most easily cured cancers if discovered at an early stage. However, cancer of the testis may spread to the lymph nodes and eventually to other parts of the body if left untreated, and it may ultimately be fatal. The condition usually affects only one testis.

Most testicular tumours develop in the sperm-producing cells of the testis. There are four types of tumour: seminoma, embryonal carcinoma, teratoma, and choriocarcinoma. Seminomas are the most common type of testicular tumour, and they are usually found in men between the ages of 35 and 45.

What are the causes?
The causes of cancer of the testis are not known, but certain factors increase the risk, such as having a family history of the condition or having had an undescended testis (p.564), a condition in which a testis fails to descend into the scrotum before birth.

What are the symptoms?
You may not notice the symptoms unless you examine your testes regularly (*see* **Examining your testes**, right). The symptoms may include:
- Hard, painless lump in the affected testis.
- Change in the usual size and texture of the testis.
- Dull ache in the scrotum.
- Rarely, a sudden, sharp pain in the affected testis.

In some cases, fluid may accumulate in the scrotum, causing a visible swelling in the scrotum (*see* **Hydrocele**, right). If you find any changes, consult your doctor immediately.

How is it diagnosed?
Your doctor will examine the affected testis and may arrange for you to have ultrasound scanning (p.135) of the testes. A special blood test may also be arranged to look for cancer. If a tumour is found, futher blood tests, CT scanning (p.132), and MRI (p.133) will be performed to determine whether the cancer has spread to other parts of the body.

What is the treatment?
If cancer of the testis is diagnosed, the affected testis will have to be surgically removed. If the cancer has not spread beyond the testis, no further treatment may be needed. However, even after the testis has been removed, blood tests to check tumour marker levels are usually carried out every 6 months to make sure that the cancer has not spread.

If the cancer has spread beyond the testes, you may be required to have further treatment, which may include surgery, radiotherapy (p.158), and chemotherapy (p.157). If the cancer has spread to the lymph nodes in the abdomen, surgery may be required to remove the nodes that are affected. Of the four types of testicular tumour, seminomas are the type most easily treated by surgery and radiotherapy.

What is the prognosis?
The outlook depends on the type of cancer and the stage at which it is diagnosed. Cancer of the testis has a very high cure rate.

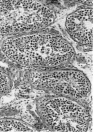 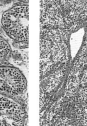

NORMAL   **ABNORMAL**
Cancer of the testis
These tissue samples from testes compare normal tissue structures in a healthy testis with the disordered tissue structures that are found in a cancerous testis.

▶ **SELF-HELP**

Examining your testes
Cancer of the testis is one of the most easily treated cancers if it is diagnosed at an early stage. For this reason, all men should examine their testes regularly to check for lumps or swellings. An early cancerous tumour can usually be felt as a hard lump embedded in the surface of the testis. This lump is not usually tender when pressed. Soft swellings in the testis may be harmless cysts, and painful swellings are often due to infection. You should also check for changes in the skin of the scrotum. If you detect any change in the normal appearance or texture of your testes or scrotum, consult your doctor immediately.

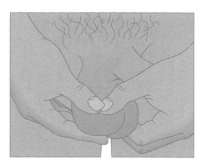

How to examine your testes
After a bath or shower, when the scrotum is relaxed, carefully feel across the entire surface of each testis by rolling each one slowly between fingers and thumb. Check for lumps or swellings and be thorough.

Most affected men are cured, even those in whom the cancer has spread outside the testes.

Surgical removal of a testis is not likely to affect sexual function or fertility if they were normal before surgery. However, both chemotherapy and radiotherapy reduce sperm production, and fertility may be temporarily or permanently affected by these treatments. For this reason, some men choose to have semen containing normal sperm frozen before treatment is started.

Varicocele

A collection of varicose veins in the scrotum

 Age, genetics, and lifestyle are not significant factors

A varicocele is a knot of dilated veins in the scrotum. The condition is caused by leaking valves in the testicular veins, which drain blood away from the testes, and it affects as many as 1 in 7 men. There is usually no identifiable reason for the leakage of these valves, but, in rare cases, a varicocele can result from pressure on a vein, usually in the pelvis, which prevents blood draining efficiently from the testis. This pressure may be due to a tumour in a kidney (*see* **Kidney cancer**, p.450). Varicoceles most commonly occur on the left-hand side of the scrotum.

If you develop a varicocele, you may notice some swelling of your scrotum and a dragging, aching discomfort. The affected side of your scrotum may hang lower than normal, and the swelling may feel like a bag of worms.

What might be done?
Your doctor will probably be able to make a diagnosis by examining your scrotum while you are standing up and again while you are lying on your back. If the swelling

is caused by a varicocele, it should disappear when you lie down because the veins will empty. Small, painless varicoceles do not need to be treated because they usually cause no other symptoms and often disappear. Wearing an athletic support or close-fitting underwear can relieve mild discomfort. If the varicocele is due to a kidney tumour, all or part of the kidney will be removed surgically.

A varicocele may reduce your fertility, but sexual performance should not be affected. If tests reveal that you have a low sperm count or if you have persistent discomfort, surgery may be needed to divide and tie off the swollen veins. Varicoceles sometimes recur.

Hydrocele

An abnormal accumulation of fluid between the double-layered membrane that surrounds the testis

 Most common in infants and the elderly

 Genetics and lifestyle are not significant factors

The double-layered membrane that surrounds each testis normally contains a small amount of fluid. If an excessive amount of fluid accumulates within this membrane, a swelling called a hydrocele will result. This condition is most common in infant boys and elderly men. In most cases, there is no apparent cause, but hydroceles have been linked to infection, inflammation, or injury to the testis. Rarely, a hydrocele that develops in adulthood is due to a tumour in the testis (*see* **Cancer of the testis**, left).

A hydrocele usually develops as a visible swelling in the scrotum. There may be a heavy, dragging sensation in the scrotum due to its increased size, but the swelling is not normally painful.

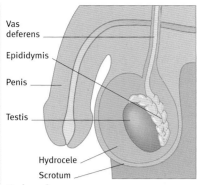

Hydrocele
If fluid accumulates in the double-layered membrane enclosing the testis, it forms a swelling in the scrotum called a hydrocele.

What might be done?

If you think you may have a hydrocele, you should consult your doctor. He or she will first try to identify a hydrocele by holding a torch against the affected area of your scrotum. If the swelling is due to excess fluid, light will shine through the swelling. Ultrasound scanning (p.135) of the scrotum may also be used to confirm the diagnosis and to exclude an underlying testicular disorder such as a tumour.

Hydroceles that develop in infants often subside by the age of 6 months without needing treatment. In all cases, if a hydrocele becomes uncomfortable or painful, it may be treated by a minor operation in which the sac containing the excess fluid is removed. Alternatively, the fluid may be drained using a hollow needle, and a sclerosant (a substance that

makes the layers of the membrane stick together) may be injected to prevent the hydrocele from recurring.

If the hydrocele is linked to an infection, an antibiotic (p.572) may be prescribed. If a tumour is found, you will be referred for further tests and treatment.

Phimosis

A foreskin that is tight or has a very small opening at the tip, preventing it from being retracted over the head of the penis

 More common in children but may occur at any age

 Genetics and lifestyle are not significant factors

In phimosis, the foreskin is too tight or the opening at its tip is too narrow, so that it cannot be retracted (pulled back) over the head of the penis (the glans). Phimosis may make it difficult to clean the head of the penis thoroughly and, as a result, infections may occur under the foreskin (*see* **Balanitis**, right). In some cases, the condition also interferes with the normal flow of urine.

What are the causes?

In most cases, phimosis is present at birth or becomes apparent during childhood, although it can occur at any age.

By the time a boy is 12 months old, it is usually possible to retract the foreskin. If it is not possible to pull a boy's foreskin back over the glans by the age of 5, he has

phimosis and probably needs treatment. The cause of the condition in babies and young children is unknown, but in older children and adults, it may result from scarring of the penile tissue due to recurrent episodes of balanitis.

What are the symptoms?

The only symptom of phimosis may be an inability to pull back the foreskin, but this may be accompanied by:
- Weak urinary stream.
- Gradual ballooning of the foreskin when passing urine.
- Painful erection.

If bacteria become trapped behind the foreskin, balanitis and recurrent urinary tract infections may occur.

A complication of phimosis called paraphimosis may occur. In this condition, it is not possible for a foreskin that has been retracted to be rolled forwards again. The condition needs immediate medical attention because it constricts the flow of blood to the head of the penis, causing the area to become swollen and extremely painful.

What might be done?

Boys under the age of 5 will probably not need treatment because the condition is likely to improve by itself. If the condition has resulted in a urinary tract infection or difficulty passing urine, or if it occurs in adolescent boys or men, the doctor will probably recommend that surgical removal of the foreskin (*see* **Circumcision**, p.462) is carried out.

Paraphimosis needs immediate treatment. The doctor may ease the foreskin forwards by applying an ice pack to the penis, then gently squeezing the head. Alternatively, the doctor may make a small incision in the foreskin to enable it to be pulled forwards. Circumcision is often required to prevent recurrence.

Balanitis

Inflammation of the head of the penis and foreskin

 More common in children

 Not being circumcised is a risk factor

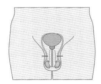 Genetics is not a significant factor

In balanitis, the head of the penis (the glans) and foreskin become itchy, sore, and inflamed. In addition, there may be a discharge, and a rash may develop.

The disorder can be caused by a bacterial infection, a fungal infection such as thrush (*see* **Candidiasis**, p.177), or an allergic reaction. It may also be due to a sexually transmitted infection (STI), such as the protozoal infection trichomoniasis (p.492). A tighter than normal foreskin (*see* **Phimosis**, left) may increase the risk of infection by preventing effective cleaning of the glans.

Men with diabetes mellitus (p.437) are more susceptible to the condition because their urine contains high levels of glucose, which can encourage the growth of microorganisms. This leads to infection and inflammation at the opening of the urethra (the tube leading from the bladder to the outside of the body). Excessive use of antibiotics (p.572) can increase the risk of a fungal infection by temporarily lowering the body's natural defences against this type of infection. Children are especially vulnerable to balanitis.

The condition may also occur as a result of sensitivity of the penis to certain chemicals, such as those found in some condoms, contraceptive creams, detergents, or washing powders.

What might be done?

If the head of your penis or your foreskin is inflamed, you should consult your doctor. He or she will examine the area and probably take a swab to look for evidence of infection. The doctor will also test your urine to check for glucose.

The treatment of balanitis depends on the cause. For example, if you have a bacterial infection, antibiotics may be prescribed, and, if the infection is due to a tight foreskin, circumcision (p.462) may be carried out to prevent balanitis from recurring. If the condition is the result of a sexually transmitted infection, your partner should be checked for evidence of infection and treated if necessary to prevent the condition from recurring (*see* **Preventing STIs**, p.491). If the cause seems to be sensitivity to a chemical, the irritant should be identified, if possible, so that you can avoid it.

The inflamed area should be kept clean, dry, and free of irritants. Most cases clear up once the cause is treated.

Priapism

Prolonged, painful erection of the penis, which may not be related to sexual desire

 More common in young adults

 Genetics and lifestyle are not significant factors

Priapism is a persistent erection of the penis occurring for 4 hours or longer, with or without any sexual arousal. The condition is usually painful, and it requires urgent treatment in hospital to avoid permanent damage to the erectile tissues of the penis.

Priapism develops if blood cannot drain away from the spongy tissues of the erect penis. Causes of the condition include damage to the nerves that control the supply of blood to the penis; disorders of the blood, including sickle-cell disease (p.272), leukaemia (p.276), and polycythaemia (p.278); and, in some instances, prolonged sexual intercourse. Priapism may also occur as a side effect of treatment with certain antipsychotic drugs (p.592). Drug treatments

---

▶ **TREATMENT**

Vasectomy

Vasectomy is a method of male sterilization. Counselling is given to make sure the man and his partner do not wish to have children in the future. The procedure has no effect on sex drive or ejaculation, but the semen no longer carries sperm, which are reabsorbed in each testis. Additional contraception is needed until 12–16 weeks later, when semen is tested to ensure sperm are no longer present. Although most vasectomies are successful, overall the operation has a failure rate of about 1 in 2,000.

SITES OF INCISIONS

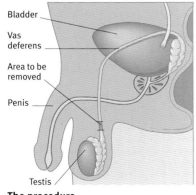

The procedure
A small section of each vas deferens (spermatic duct) is removed through small incisions on either side of the scrotum.

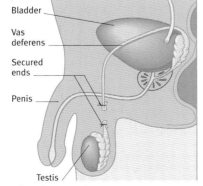

After the procedure
The open ends of the vas deferens have been turned back and secured with a stitch to prevent them from rejoining.

▶ **TREATMENT**

Circumcision

Circumcision is the surgical removal of the foreskin, the skin covering the head of the penis (the glans). This procedure is sometimes carried out in infancy for religious reasons. In the past, circumcision was often performed routinely in childhood in the belief that it would improve hygiene, but this practice is no longer recommended. In older boys and men, circumcision may be necessary if the foreskin becomes too tight to be pulled back fully (*see* **Phimosis**, p.461). When the operation is carried out in infancy, only local anaesthesia is required, but boys and men are usually given a general anaesthetic before undergoing surgery.

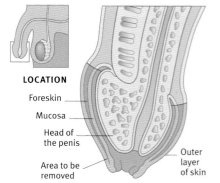

LOCATION

Foreskin
Mucosa
Head of the penis
Area to be removed
Outer layer of skin

The operation
The foreskin, which covers the head of the penis, consists of an inner layer of mucosa and an outer layer of skin. During the operation, both layers are removed.

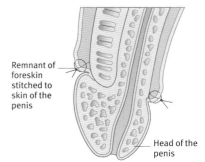

Remnant of foreskin stitched to skin of the penis

Head of the penis

After the operation
The remnant of the foreskin has been stitched to the skin just behind the head of the penis, leaving the head of the penis uncovered. These stitches either dissolve or fall out after a few days.

for erectile dysfunction (p.494), whether they are taken orally, such as the medication sildenafil, or injected into the penis, may rarely result in priapism.

What might be done?

If you develop a painful and very prolonged erection, particularly one that is not a result of sexual arousal, you must consult your doctor or go to your nearest accident and emergency department immediately. In most cases of priapism, blood can be drained from the erectile tissues of the penis by using a needle and syringe, which produces immediate relief of symptoms.

If priapism is a result of an underlying disorder, further treatment will depend on the cause. In all cases, there is a risk of permanent damage, and full erection of the penis may be adversely affected in the future.

Peyronie's disease

Scarring of the erectile tissue of the penis, causing it to bend at an angle when erect

 More common over the age of 40

 Sometimes runs in families

 Lifestyle is not a significant factor

In Peyronie's disease, the fibrous tissue of the penis becomes thickened, causing it to bend during erection. The penis may bend so much that sexual intercourse is difficult and painful. The disease occurs in 3–9 per cent of men, most commonly in those over 40.

In many cases, there is no apparent cause for the condition, but previous damage to the penis may be a risk factor. Peyronie's disease is also associated with Dupuytren's contracture (p.231), a condition in which fibrous tissue in the palm of the hand becomes thick and shortened.

Peyronie's disease sometimes runs in families, suggesting that a genetic factor is involved.

What are the symptoms?

The symptoms of Peyronie's disease develop gradually and may include:

- Curvature of the penis to one side during an erection.
- Pain in the penis on erection.
- Thickened area within the penis that can usually be felt as a firm nodule when the penis is flaccid.

Eventually, the thickened region may extend to the erectile tissue and the condition may lead to erectile dysfunction (p.494).

What is the treatment?

Peyronie's disease sometimes improves without any treatment. In mild cases, in which painless intercourse is still possible, treatment is often not necessary. However, in other cases, the condition becomes worse if left untreated.

If the condition is severe, the penis may be straightened surgically. If the disease has led to erectile dysfunction, a permanent implant may be surgically inserted into the penis to correct the deformity and restore erectile function.

Cancer of the penis

A rare, cancerous tumour that usually occurs on the head of the penis

 More common over the age of 40

 Smoking and not being circumcised are risk factors

 Genetics is not a significant factor

Cancer of the penis is a rare disorder that most commonly occurs in uncircumcised men, particularly those in whom the foreskin does not retract (*see* **Phimosis**, p.461). It is more common in men over the age of 40. Infection with the human papillomavirus, which causes genital warts (p.493), is thought to increase the risk of developing the cancer. Smoking is also a risk factor.

The tumour commonly develops on the head of the penis (the glans). It appears as a wart-like growth or flat, painless sore that may be hidden by the foreskin. Sometimes, the growth may bleed or produce an unpleasant-smelling discharge. The cancer usually grows slowly, but, if left untreated, it may spread to the lymph nodes in the groin and to other parts of the body.

A sore area on the penis should be examined by a doctor immediately.

What might be done?

Your doctor will carry out a physical examination and may take a swab to check for infections that can produce similar symptoms. He or she may also arrange for a biopsy, in which a sample of the growth is removed to be examined under the microscope for evidence of cancer.

If it is detected early, a tumour on the penis can often be treated successfully with surgery, radiotherapy (p.158), or a combination of both. Surgery involves either partial or complete amputation of the penis. In some cases, penile reconstruction may be possible following amputation. Radiotherapy may be recommended as the first choice treatment because it offers the chance of curing the cancer without loss of the penis.

The outlook depends on how far the cancer has advanced before treatment. About 9 in 10 men who have received treatment for penile tumours that have not spread survive for 5 years or more. If the cancer has spread only to lymph nodes in the groin, about 6 in 10 men survive for 5 years or more after treatment. If the cancer has spread beyond the groin, only about 2 in 10 men survive for 5 years or more after treatment.

Prostate disorders

The prostate gland is a firm, round organ about the size of a chestnut. It surrounds the upper part of the urethra (the tube through which urine is emptied from the bladder) and lies underneath the bladder and directly in front of the rectum. The secretions that are produced by the prostate gland are added to semen, the fluid that contains sperm.

Disorders affecting the prostate gland are very common, particularly in men over the age of 30. Prostatitis, in which the prostate gland is inflamed, is the first disorder discussed in this section. Enlargement of the prostate gland is covered next. Some degree of prostate enlargement occurs in most men over the age of 50 and is often viewed as a natural part of aging. The final article covers prostate cancer. In many cases, prostate cancer is not life-threatening, and in older men it may not require treatment because the tumour is often slow-growing and may not affect life expectancy. However, prostate cancer in younger men may spread to other parts of the body more quickly and can be life-threatening. There is therefore ongoing research aimed at developing tests to detect prostate cancer before symptoms start to appear. However, although tests may help to identify prostate cancer in its early stages, they cannot identify which cancers are more likely to spread and require early treatment.

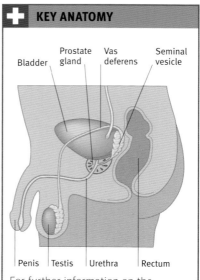

✚ **KEY ANATOMY**

Bladder
Prostate gland
Vas deferens
Seminal vesicle
Penis
Testis
Urethra
Rectum

For further information on the structure and function of the male reproductive system, *see* pp.457–458.

Prostatitis

Inflammation of the prostate gland, sometimes due to infection

 Most common between the ages of 30 and 50

 Unprotected sex with multiple partners is a risk factor

 Genetics is not a significant factor

Inflammation of the prostate gland, known as prostatitis, may be acute or chronic. Acute prostatitis is uncommon and tends to produce sudden, severe symptoms that clear up rapidly with treatment. By contrast, chronic prostatitis usually causes mild but persistent symptoms and can be difficult to treat. Both types are most common in sexually active men aged between 30 and 50.

What are the causes?

In many cases of acute or chronic prostatitis, an exact cause of the disorder cannot be determined. However, acute prostatitis tends to be the result of bacterial infection and chronic prostatitis is generally nonbacterial. Inflammation of the prostate gland may also develop in association with sexually transmitted infections (pp.491–493).

What are the symptoms?

The symptoms of acute prostatitis develop suddenly and are usually severe. They may include the following:

- Fever and chills.
- Pain around the base of the penis.
- Lower back pain.
- Pain during bowel movements.
- Frequent, urgent, and painful passing of urine.

Acute prostatitis sometimes causes urinary retention (p.455), painful swelling behind the testes, or the formation of an abscess in the prostate gland.

Chronic prostatitis may not produce symptoms. If symptoms do occur, they develop gradually and may include:

- Pain and tenderness at the base of the penis and in the testes, groin, pelvis, or back.
- Pain on ejaculation.
- Blood in the semen.
- Frequent, painful passing of urine.

If you suspect that you have either acute or chronic prostatitis, you should consult your doctor immediately.

How is it diagnosed?

Your doctor will perform a digital rectal examination, in which a finger is inserted into the rectum to feel the prostate. The doctor may also ask you to provide a urine sample and may obtain a sample of prostate gland secretions by massaging the prostate through the rectum and collecting secretions from the urethra. Both the urine sample and the prostate gland secretions will then be tested for the presence of

infectious organisms. Ultrasound scanning (p.135) may also be carried out to check for an abscess in the prostate gland.

What is the treatment?

If a bacterial infection is found, antibiotics (p.572) will be prescribed. It may take several months for the infection to clear up completely. In the meantime, your doctor may recommend painkillers (p.589) and may also give you drugs that soften the stools (*see* **Laxatives**, p.597) to make bowel movements more comfortable. If your symptoms are severe, your doctor may advise bed rest. Prostatitis that is not caused by a bacterial infection may be treated with painkillers to relieve the symptoms and with drugs that act to relax the muscle at the exit of the bladder (*see* **Drugs for prostate disorders**, p.605).

Although most affected men recover fully, both types of prostatitis can recur.

Enlarged prostate gland

Noncancerous enlargement of the prostate gland, causing difficulty in passing urine

 Rare before the age of 40; increasingly common after the age of 50

 Genetics and lifestyle are not significant factors

In most men over the age of 50, the prostate gland has become enlarged to some degree. Such prostate enlargement is known as benign prostatic hyperplasia. The condition is noncancerous and is not associated with prostate cancer (p.464). Minor prostate enlargement is considered a natural part of the aging process. The cause of the condition is unknown.

What are the symptoms?

As the prostate gland grows larger, it constricts and distorts the urethra (the tube from the bladder to the outside of the body). At first, this enlargement does not cause any symptoms. However, if the prostate gland continues to enlarge, it may cause difficulty in passing urine, resulting in the following symptoms:

- Frequent need to pass urine, during the day and night.
- Delay in starting to pass urine, especially at night or if the bladder is full.
- Weak, intermittent flow of urine.
- Dribbling at the end of urine flow.
- Feeling that the bladder has not completely emptied.

These symptoms may be worsened by cold weather; drinking large volumes of fluids (especially alcohol); taking drugs that increase urine production, such as diuretics (p.583); or taking drugs that may

---

▶ **TREATMENT**

Transurethral resection of the prostate (TURP)

There are several operations to treat an enlarged prostate gland. The most common procedure is a transurethral resection of the prostate (TURP), in which only the core of the gland is removed. The operation is performed under general or spinal anaesthesia and requires a hospital stay. Since the rest of the gland will continue to enlarge,

symptoms may recur and further surgery may be necessary later. About 8 in 10 men are infertile after this type of surgery because sperm pass into the bladder on ejaculation, but orgasm is normal. Transurethral prostatectomy can also result in erectile dysfunction.

1 *A specialized viewing instrument called a resectoscope is passed along the urethra (the tube leading from the bladder to the outside of the body) until it reaches the prostate. A heated wire (diathermy wire) is then introduced through the resectoscope and used to cut away prostate tissue, thus widening the urethra.*

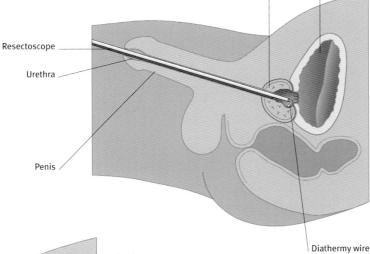

2 *After surgery, the diathermy wire and the resectoscope are withdrawn. A catheter is passed into the bladder to drain urine. An irrigation system is attached to the catheter to wash out urine and blood, with the aim of stopping clots from forming. The catheter is left in place for 2–3 days.*

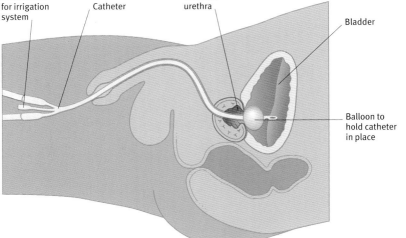

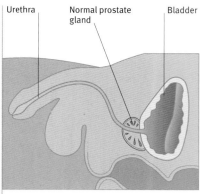

NORMAL PROSTATE

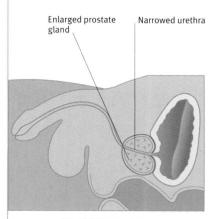

ENLARGED PROSTATE

Prostate enlargement

The prostate encircles the upper part of the urethra. An enlarged prostate may constrict the urethra, making it difficult to pass urine, and indent the base of the bladder, preventing it from emptying completely.

cause urinary retention, such as antispasmodics (*see* **Antispasmodics and motility stimulants**, p.598).

If the bladder does not empty completely, it may enlarge and make the abdomen swell visibly. Urine may collect in the bladder and stagnate. If the condition is left untreated, the urinary tract may become infected (*see* **Cystitis**, p.453) and there is an increased risk of bladder stones (p.456). Rarely, retained urine can produce a build-up of backward pressure from the bladder to the kidneys, leading to kidney damage (*see* **Hydronephrosis**, p.448), and kidney failure (p.450) may occur. Occasionally, an enlarged prostate gland may suddenly block the outflow of urine completely (*see* **Urinary retention**, p.455), causing rapidly increasing pain. This problem requires emergency treatment.

How is it diagnosed?

Your doctor will perform a digital rectal examination, in which a finger is inserted into the rectum to feel the prostate. The doctor may also arrange for blood tests to assess kidney function and rule out prostate cancer and urine tests to look for evidence of infection. Urine flow may also be assessed (*see* **Urodynamic studies**, p.453). Ultrasound scanning (p.135) may be carried out to measure the amount

of urine left in your bladder after passing urine and check that your kidneys are not abnormally enlarged.

What is the treatment?

The choice of treatment depends on factors such as age, general health, the degree of the prostate enlargement, and whether the obstruction of urine flow is having harmful effects on the bladder and kidneys. Treatment may affect sexual function, and you should discuss the available treatments with your doctor.

If your symptoms are mild, your doctor may simply advise you not to drink fluids in the evening so that urinary frequency is decreased at night, and to limit or stop consumption of alcohol and caffeine. If the symptoms persist, drugs, surgery, or catheterization may be necessary.

Alpha blockers are commonly used to treat prostate enlargement and can relieve the symptoms in some cases (*see* **Drugs for prostate disorders**, p.605). If your symptoms are more severe, your doctor may suggest prostate surgery to remove part of the gland through the urethra (*see* **Transurethral resection of the prostate (TURP)**, p.463). Only tissue that is obstructing urine flow is removed. If the prostate is considered to be too large for a TURP, the prostate may be removed through an abdominal incision. This procedure may result in infertility. It may also cause erectile dysfunction (p.494). Laser surgery is an alternative treatment that may sometimes be offered.

If surgery is not advisable due to old age or poor health, a catheter or urethral stent (a tube inside the urethra) may be left in permanently to drain the urine (*see* **Bladder catheterization**, p.455).

What is the prognosis?

The outlook varies greatly. Mild cases may be improved with drug treatment, but surgery is more effective for severe cases. About 1 in 7 men needs a second TURP after 8–10 years.

Prostate cancer

A cancerous tumour arising from the glandular tissue of the prostate gland

 Rare under the age of 40; increasingly common over the age of 65

 Sometimes runs in families; more common in certain ethnic groups

 Lifestyle is not a significant factor

Prostate cancer is the most commonly diagnosed male cancer in the UK, affecting about 1 in 8 men at some time in their lives. The disorder is more common in men of African or Afro-Caribbean descent. The number of cases of prostate cancer identified in the UK has been rising over the past few decades, not only in elderly men,

in whom it is most common, but also in men in their 40s and 50s. This increased identification has been largely due to increased public awareness and the availability of a test that measures the level of a protein called prostate-specific antigen (PSA) secreted by the prostate gland. Although prostate cancer is the cause of about 10,800 deaths each year in the UK, many tumours grow slowly, especially in elderly men, and may never cause symptoms. Treatment is more likely to be necessary in younger men.

What are the causes?

The exact cause of prostate cancer is not known, although the male sex hormone testosterone, produced by the testes, has been found to influence the growth and spread of the tumour. In some cases, the cancer is partly due to an inherited abnormal gene. In these cases, it is more likely to occur before the age of 60. There is also evidence that having had a vasectomy (p.461) increases the risk of prostate cancer, but only by a very small amount.

What are the symptoms?

Prostate cancer may not produce any symptoms, particularly in elderly men. If symptoms do occur, they are likely to develop when the tumour starts to constrict the urethra. The symptoms may then include:

- Weak urinary stream or inability to pass urine normally.
- Frequent urge to pass urine, especially during the night.
- Rarely, blood in the urine.

In some men, the initial symptoms of prostate cancer are due to the metastasis

---

▶ **TEST**

Prostate gland biopsy

A prostate gland biopsy is used to diagnose prostate cancer. In the most common type of biopsy, an ultrasound probe is inserted into the rectum in order to visualize the prostate. A hollow needle is passed through the probe and into the prostate several times, removing pieces of tissue for examination. After the biopsy, urine and semen may contain blood for several days.

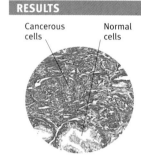

RESULTS

Prostate cancer

This prostate tissue sample shows normal and cancerous cells.

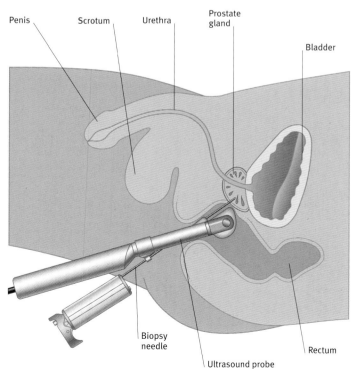

The procedure

A slight pricking sensation may be felt as each biopsy sample is taken. In most cases, a local anaesthetic may be given beforehand.

(spreading) of the cancer to other parts of the body, most commonly the bones, lymph nodes, and lungs. In these cases, the symptoms may include back pain, enlarged lymph nodes, shortness of breath, and significant weight loss

How is it diagnosed?

If you develop the symptoms of prostate cancer or if the disorder runs in your family, you should consult your doctor. The doctor will perform a digital rectal examination, in which a finger is inserted into the rectum to feel the prostate gland. He or she may also arrange for a blood test to measure your PSA level. A raised PSA level may indicate cancer but it is not a definitive indicator because other, noncancerous conditions may also raise the PSA level, such as benign prostatic hyperplasia (*see* **Enlarged prostate gland**, p.463). Conversely, the PSA level may be normal when cancer is present.

You may be referred to hospital to have a type of ultrasound scanning in which a probe is inserted into the rectum to visualize the prostate gland. This procedure enables the doctor to assess the size of the gland and to look for any abnormalities. During scanning, a prostate gland biopsy (opposite page) may also be carried out. In this procedure, some cells are removed from areas of the gland that appear abnormal and are examined under a microscope. If prostate cancer is confirmed, you may need imaging tests, such as MRI (p.133) and radionuclide scanning (p.135), to check whether the cancer has spread to other parts of the body.

What is the treatment?

The choice of treatment depends on age, general health, and whether the cancer has spread. If the cancer is confined to the prostate and your health is otherwise good, your doctor may recommend that the entire prostate gland be surgically removed, along with some of the surrounding tissues (*see* **Radical prostatectomy**, above right). Alternatively, radiotherapy (p.158) may be given. This involves either having a radioactive implant or radioactive seeds placed in the prostate or undergoing external radiotherapy. In elderly men in

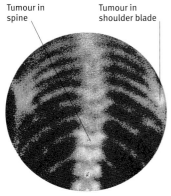

Metastatic cancer
This radionuclide bone scan of the chest shows "hot spots" in the spine and in the shoulder blade due to the spread of a cancer that originated in the prostate gland.

Tumour in spine | Tumour in shoulder blade

whom the cancer is confined to a small area of the prostate, no immediate treatment may be required, but the course of the disease will be monitored.

If the cancer has spread beyond the prostate, a cure may not be possible. However, progress of the disease can be slowed significantly with hormone ablation therapy. In this treatment, drugs that block the release or actions of testosterone are given to suppress the effects of the hormone on the cancer (*see* **Drugs for prostate disorders**, p.605). In some cases, part of both testes may be surgically removed to stop the production of testosterone. Rarely, treatments that block the actions or production of testosterone result in erectile dysfunction (p.494) and loss of interest in sex.

What is the prognosis?

A diagnosis of prostate cancer does not necessarily mean that the cancer will cause symptoms or be life-threatening. Sometimes the best policy, especially in elderly men, is to defer treatment and begin regular check-ups to monitor the disease. Men with certain types of small tumour do not need treatment and are likely to live for several years with no symptoms before dying from some other cause. For men who have had surgery for a tumour confined to the prostate, the outlook is good, with about 9 out of 10 men surviving for at least 5 years after diagnosis. However, surgery may result in erectile dysfunction and urinary incontinence.

Cancer that has spread beyond the prostate is unlikely to be cured completely, but hormone ablation therapy often controls the symptoms for years.

▶ **TREATMENT**

Radical prostatectomy

A radical prostatectomy may be done to treat prostate cancer if the cancer has not spread beyond the gland. The procedure is performed under general anaesthesia and usually requires a hospital stay of about 3–5 days. The operation removes the cancer in most men, but afterwards about 1 in 2 men will have erectile dysfunction, and some will have a degree of urinary incontinence.

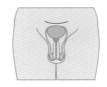

SITE OF INCISION

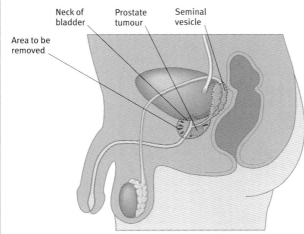

Neck of bladder | Prostate tumour | Seminal vesicle
Area to be removed

The procedure
The tumour is removed, together with the entire prostate gland, the seminal vesicles, and the neck of the bladder.

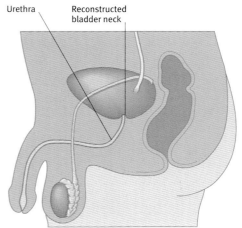

Urethra | Reconstructed bladder neck

After the procedure
The bladder neck has been reconstructed and rejoined to the urethra (the tube from the bladder to the outside of the body).

Male hormonal disorders

The most important male sex hormone is testosterone, which influences sperm production, fertility, and sex drive. Male sex hormones also promote the development of secondary sexual characteristics at puberty. Over- or underproduction of male sex hormones may be due to a variety of factors, including inherited disorders, long-term illnesses, tumours, or lifestyle factors.

Male sex hormones, or androgens, are produced mainly by the testes but also by the adrenal glands. The production of male sex hormones is controlled by hormones secreted by the pituitary gland. In turn, the pituitary gland is under the control of a part of the brain called the hypothalamus.

The changes that occur at puberty are controlled by the sex hormones. This section starts by discussing early or late onset of puberty in boys, which may be a symptom of under- or overproduction of male sex hormones. Hypogonadism, in which male sex hormones are underproduced, is covered next. In boys, this condition can suppress sexual development; in men, hypogonadism lowers sperm production and fertility. The final article discusses gynaecomastia, breast enlargement in males that temporarily affects nearly half of all boys during puberty.

Male hormonal disorders may lead to sexual problems (pp.494–496) and can sometimes be a cause of infertility (*see* **Male infertility**, p.499).

+ **KEY ANATOMY**

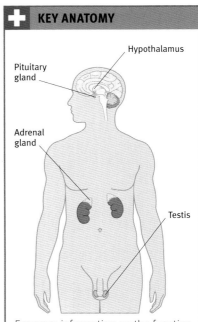

Pituitary gland | Hypothalamus
Adrenal gland | Testis

For more information on the function of male hormones, *see* pp.424–429 and pp.457–458.

Abnormal puberty in males

Very early or late onset of puberty, usually due to a hormonal imbalance

 Occurs before or after the normal age range for puberty

 Sometimes runs in families; rarely due to a chromosomal abnormality

 Excessive exercise and a poor diet may be risk factors in some cases

The natural process of sexual development and maturation that takes place over several years is known as puberty (p.457). In boys, puberty is normally characterized by enlargement of the genitals; development of hair on the face, in the armpits, and in the pubic region; a growth spurt, in which the body gets bigger and more muscular; and deepening of the voice. Puberty in boys usually begins between the ages of 9 and 14. Abnormal puberty starts either earlier than normal (precocious puberty) or later (delayed puberty).

Precocious puberty is rare and is usually an indication of an underlying hormonal disorder. Delayed puberty is more common and less likely to indicate a serious underlying condition.

What are the causes?

In boys, puberty is controlled by male sex hormones produced by the testes and adrenal glands. The production of these hormones is controlled by hormones from the pituitary gland and from the hypothalamus (the part of the brain that regulates the pituitary gland). Disorders in these organs may lead to abnormal early or late puberty.

Precocious puberty is caused by the overproduction of male sex hormones in a young boy. For example, congenital adrenal hyperplasia (p.561), in which the adrenal glands produce excessive amounts of male sex hormones, may lead to precocious puberty.

Boys in whom puberty is delayed are usually just late developers, a tendency that often runs in families. However, delayed puberty may also be caused by the underproduction of male sex hormones. Rarely, there is a more serious underlying cause, such as a brain tumour pressing on the hypothalamus or pituitary gland, or a chromosome disorder, such as Klinefelter's syndrome (p.534), in which the sex organs do not develop normally. Some long-term illnesses, such as Crohn's disease (p.417), kidney failure (p.450), cystic fibrosis (p.535), and diabetes mellitus (p.437), can also cause delayed puberty and growth. Certain lifestyle factors, such as excessive exercise and an inadequate diet, may delay the onset of puberty. Rarely, a pituitary tumour (p.430) may lead to either precocious or delayed puberty.

What might be done?

Early or late puberty should be investigated by a doctor, who will carry out a physical examination to see if puberty has started or how far it has progressed. A blood test may also be performed to measure hormone levels and to check for a chromosomal abnormality. X-rays (p.131) of the wrist and hand may be used to assess bone maturity, and ultrasound scanning (p.135) of the testes or adrenal glands may also be carried out to look for abnormalities. If a pituitary tumour is suspected, MRI (p.133) or CT scanning (p.132) may be performed.

If tests identify an underlying cause for abnormal puberty, it will be treated. For example, precocious puberty may be treated with drugs that block the production of male sex hormones or inhibit their action. These drugs may be given in the form of injections, implants under the skin, or nasal sprays. If delayed puberty runs in the family, treatment may not be needed. In many other cases, puberty is induced by giving injections of testosterone (*see* **Sex hormones and related drugs**, p.602). Some boys benefit from counselling for psychological problems caused by abnormal puberty.

Abnormal puberty is often treatable, but lifelong treatment may be needed. Future fertility depends on the cause.

Hypogonadism in males

Underactivity of the testes, resulting in low levels of the sex hormone testosterone and impaired production of sperm

 Sometimes caused by a chromosomal abnormality

 Alcohol abuse is a risk factor

 Age is not a significant factor

Reduced activity of the testes, known as hypogonadism, results in the underproduction of the male sex hormone testosterone and impaired sperm production. In boys who have not reached puberty, testicular growth and the development of secondary sexual characteristics (such as growth of facial, armpit, and pubic hair, muscle growth, and deepening of the voice) may be delayed or arrested. Hypogonadism is uncommon.

Abnormal development of the testes due to a chromosome disorder, such as Klinefelter's syndrome (p.534), may cause hypogonadism, as may failure of the pituitary gland to produce sufficient hormones, which may be the result of a pituitary tumour (p.430). There are also a number of disorders that may cause damage to the testes and lead to hypogonadism, such as torsion of the testis (p.459) and mumps (p.167). Excessive consumption of alcohol, chemotherapy (p.157), and radiotherapy (p.158) can also cause hypogonadism.

What are the symptoms?

If hypogonadism occurs after puberty, the only effect may be infertility (*see* **Male infertility**, p.499) due to the reduced production of sperm. However, some of the following symptoms may also be evident:

- Erectile dysfunction.
- Reduction in the size of the genitals.
- Lowered sex drive.
- Reduced growth of facial, underarm, and pubic hair.
- Reduced muscle strength.

When hypogonadism develops before adolescence, it may result in late onset of puberty (*see* **Abnormal puberty in males**, left).

What might be done?

The doctor will carry out a physical examination to determine whether the genitals and secondary sexual characteristics have developed normally. A blood test may be done to measure the levels of testosterone and other hormones and to look for a chromosomal abnormality.

Treatment is aimed at the underlying cause. For example, synthetic male hormones (*see* **Sex hormones and related drugs**, p.602) may be used to treat disorders of the testes. If underactivity of the pituitary gland is the cause, pituitary hormones may be given (*see* **Pituitary drugs**, p.603). A pituitary tumour may be removed surgically. In boys, hormone treatment stimulates puberty, including growth and sexual development; in men, it encourages growth of facial hair, muscle strength, potency, and sex drive. Side effects of treatment with hormones may include temporary breast development (*see* **Gynaecomastia**, below) and acne.

If the genitals are normal, treatment may improve sexual potency and fertility; if hypogonadism is due to a testicular disorder, fertility is rarely achieved.

Gynaecomastia

Noncancerous enlargement of one or both breasts in males

 Most common in newborn babies and adolescents

 Alcohol abuse and being overweight are risk factors in adults

 Genetics is not a significant factor

All males produce small amounts of the female sex hormone oestrogen. If too much oestrogen is produced, breast enlargement, called gynaecomastia, occurs. One or both breasts may be affected. The condition is common in newborn boys and affects 1 in 2 male adolescents. It is usually temporary in both of these age groups. Older men can also be affected.

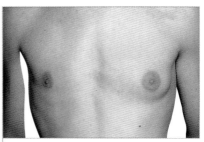

Gynaecomastia
An excess of the female sex hormone oestrogen in the blood may cause one or both male breasts to enlarge, as seen here.

What are the causes?

Gynaecomastia in the newborn occurs when the fetus has been exposed to the mother's oestrogen within the uterus. Increased levels of oestrogen, resulting in breast enlargement, are also common during puberty. In adults, alcohol abuse and being overweight are the most common causes of gynaecomastia.

Drugs that affect levels of female sex hormones, such as spironolactone (*see* **Diuretic drugs**, p.583) and corticosteroids (p.600), may lead to enlargement of the breasts. Some drugs for prostate cancer (*see* **Drugs for prostate disorders**, p.605) may have the same effect.

What are the symptoms?

The symptoms of gynaecomastia may include the following:

- Tender and swollen breast or breasts.
- Firm or rubbery button of tissue that can be felt underneath the nipple.
- Discharge from the nipple.

One breast may enlarge more than the other. The symptoms listed here should always be investigated so that breast cancer (p.486) can be excluded.

What might be done?

Newborn boys do not need treatment, and gynaecomastia usually disappears within a few weeks. In most adolescents, the condition disappears in less than 18 months without any treatment. In older men, the doctor will ask about lifestyle factors and carry out a physical examination. He or she may arrange for tests to measure hormone levels and to look for evidence of breast cancer. The treatment and outlook depend on the underlying cause, but, if gynaecomastia persists, the excess tissue may be removed surgically.

Female reproductive system

The central role of the female reproductive system is carried out by the ovaries, which produce sex cells, called ova or eggs, containing genetic material. When an egg fuses with a male sex cell, called a sperm, it has the potential to develop into a fetus. The ovaries also secrete sex hormones that control sexual development and the menstrual cycle. The breasts play a part in sexual arousal and produce milk after childbirth.

THE ONLY VISIBLE parts of the female reproductive system are the tissues that make up the vulva. The labia are folds of skin that protect the entrance to the vagina, which is lined with cells that produce a slightly acidic fluid to prevent infection. The vagina leads from the outside of the body to the uterus, the thick-walled organ in which a fetus develops. Two fallopian tubes lead from the uterus to the two ovaries, where eggs are stored.

Female fertility

Newborn girls have a supply of about 150,000 immature eggs, which are present in their ovaries before birth. The eggs are stored in the ovaries and do not begin to mature until a rise in the levels of female sex hormones at puberty triggers the start of monthly menstrual cycles.

Once a month, an egg matures for 14 days in its follicle and is released from the ovary into the fallopian tube in a process called ovulation. The egg survives for 24 hours after ovulation and can only be fertilized by a sperm during this time. It takes about 5–6 days for the egg, fertilized or not, to pass along the tube

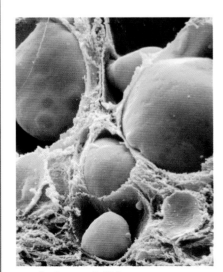

Developing egg follicles
A woman's eggs mature in fluid-filled follicles in the ovaries. This magnified image shows follicles at various stages of development.

to the uterus. If fertilized, the egg eventually implants in the lining of the uterus, which becomes thicker after ovulation, ready for an egg to implant. The egg then grows into an embryo. If not fertilized, the egg passes out of the vagina, along with the uterine lining. This blood loss is called menstruation.

The cycle of egg maturation, ovulation, and menstrual bleeding occurs at intervals of, on average, 28 days during a woman's reproductive life. At the menopause, which usually occurs between the ages of 45 and 55, eggs stop maturing and are no longer released by the ovaries. Menstruation stops, and the reproductive phase of a woman's life comes to an end.

Female hormones

The ovaries produce the hormones oestrogen and progesterone, but secretion of these is controlled by follicle-stimulating hormone and luteinizing hormone, which are produced in the pituitary gland, a tiny structure

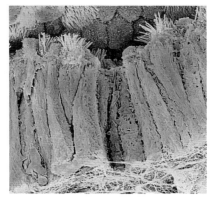

Inside the fallopian tube
Hair-like projections (cilia) in the fallopian tube propel the egg towards the uterus.

just below the brain. Sex hormones control sexual development at puberty, the menstrual cycle, and fertility. Oestrogen also stimulates the fat distribution that results in a woman's rounded shape. Changes in hormone levels during the menstrual cycle and at menopause may affect mood and behaviour.

✚ **PROCESS**

Puberty

Puberty is the period during which visible sexual characteristics develop and sexual organs mature. In girls, puberty usually starts between the ages of 8 and 14 and lasts for about 3–4 years. Girls tend to begin puberty about 1–2 years before boys, but there is considerable difference in its age of onset between individuals and on the rate of development.

Physical development
During puberty, the breasts start to develop, pubic hair grows, and there is a rapid increase in height. The hips also widen, hair grows in the armpits, and menstruation begins.

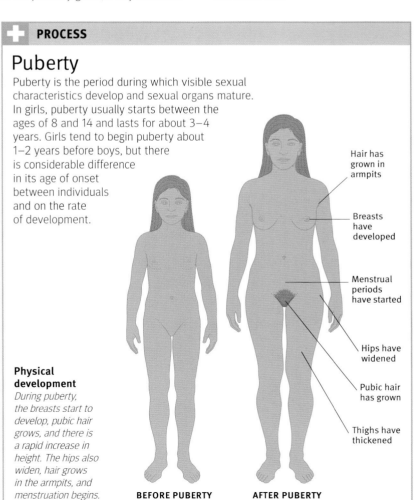

Hair has grown in armpits

Breasts have developed

Menstrual periods have started

Hips have widened

Pubic hair has grown

Thighs have thickened

BEFORE PUBERTY   **AFTER PUBERTY**

+ **STRUCTURE**

Female reproductive system

The internal organs of the female reproductive system are all located in the lower third of the abdomen. The ovaries store and release eggs, which pass along the fallopian tubes into the uterus. The vagina connects the uterus to the outside of the body. The visible external organs are collectively known as the vulva and consist of the sexually sensitive clitoris surrounded by folds of skin called the labia, which protect the entrances to the vagina and the urethra. Just inside the entrance to the vagina lie the two Bartholin's glands, which secrete a fluid that contributes to lubrication during sex.

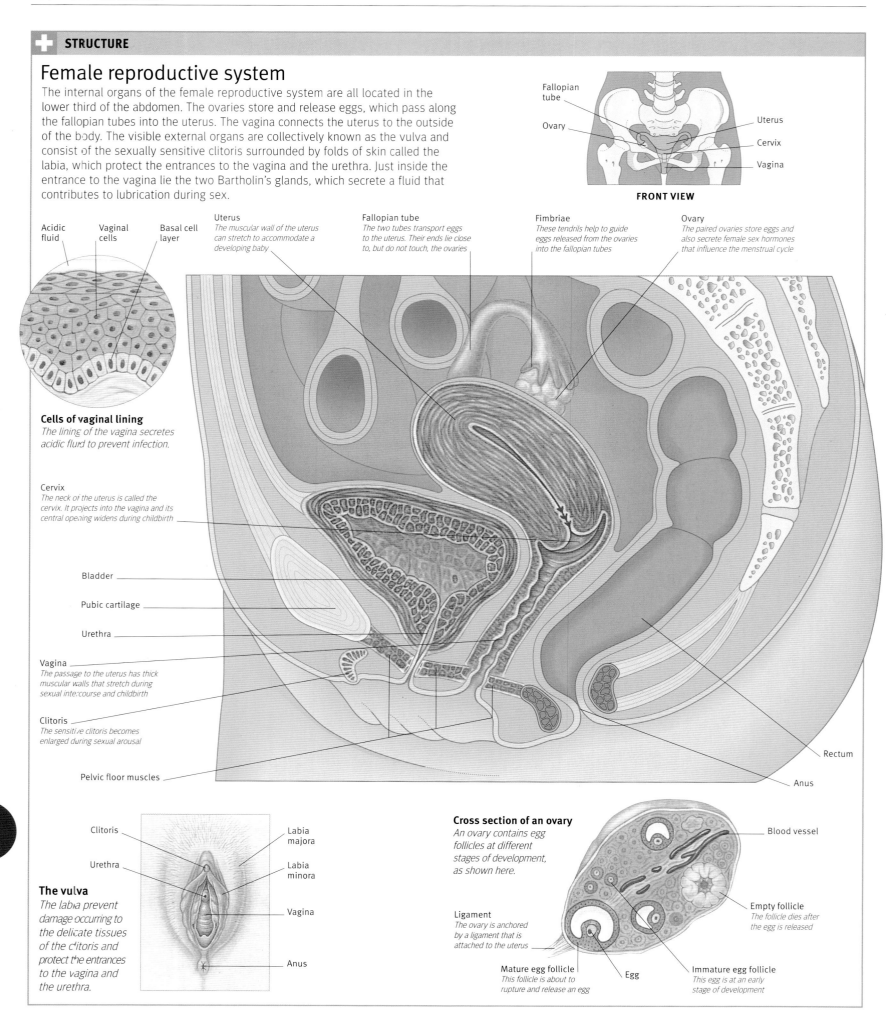

Fallopian tube

Ovary

Uterus

Cervix

Vagina

FRONT VIEW

Acidic fluid

Vaginal cells

Basal cell layer

Uterus
The muscular wall of the uterus can stretch to accommodate a developing baby

Fallopian tube
The two tubes transport eggs to the uterus. Their ends lie close to, but do not touch, the ovaries

Fimbriae
These tendrils help to guide eggs released from the ovaries into the fallopian tubes

Ovary
The paired ovaries store eggs and also secrete female sex hormones that influence the menstrual cycle

Cells of vaginal lining
The lining of the vagina secretes acidic fluid to prevent infection.

Cervix
The neck of the uterus is called the cervix. It projects into the vagina and its central opening widens during childbirth

Bladder

Pubic cartilage

Urethra

Vagina
The passage to the uterus has thick muscular walls that stretch during sexual intercourse and childbirth

Clitoris
The sensitive clitoris becomes enlarged during sexual arousal

Pelvic floor muscles

Rectum

Anus

Clitoris

Urethra

Labia majora

Labia minora

Vagina

Anus

The vulva
The labia prevent damage occurring to the delicate tissues of the clitoris and protect the entrances to the vagina and the urethra.

Cross section of an ovary
An ovary contains egg follicles at different stages of development, as shown here.

Blood vessel

Empty follicle
The follicle dies after the egg is released

Ligament
The ovary is anchored by a ligament that is attached to the uterus

Mature egg follicle
This follicle is about to rupture and release an egg

Egg

Immature egg follicle
This egg is at an early stage of development

Menstrual cycle

Each month between puberty and the menopause, a woman's body goes through the menstrual cycle in preparation for conception and pregnancy. A mature egg is released, and the lining of the uterus (the endometrium) becomes thicker, ready for a fertilized egg to implant. If the egg is not fertilized, it passes out of the body during menstruation. The menstrual cycle lasts 28 days on average but may not be the same length every month and varies from woman to woman. The cycle is regulated by a complex interaction between four sex hormones. Follicle-stimulating hormone (FSH) and luteinizing hormone (LH) are produced in the pituitary gland, and oestrogen and progesterone are secreted by the ovaries.

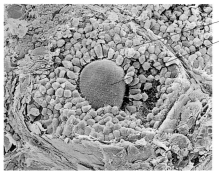

Nourishing cells in the follicle

Immature egg

Developing follicle
By absorbing nutrients from cells inside the follicle, an immature egg is able to develop and grow to maturity.

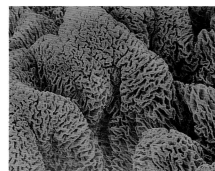

Fold of thickened endometrial tissue

Endometrium
After ovulation, the thickened endometrium tissue looks spongy and is ready to receive the fertilized egg.

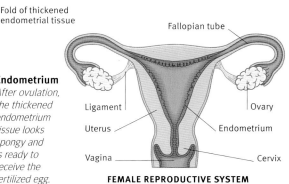

Fallopian tube

Ligament

Uterus

Vagina

Ovary

Endometrium

Cervix

FEMALE REPRODUCTIVE SYSTEM

CHANGES DURING THE MENSTRUAL CYCLE

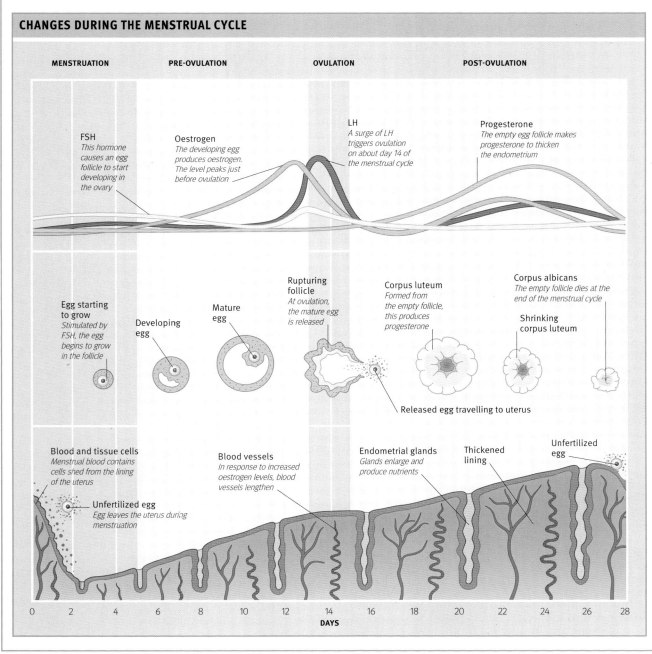

MENSTRUATION

PRE-OVULATION

OVULATION

POST-OVULATION

FSH
This hormone causes an egg follicle to start developing in the ovary

Oestrogen
The developing egg produces oestrogen. The level peaks just before ovulation

LH
A surge of LH triggers ovulation on about day 14 of the menstrual cycle

Progesterone
The empty egg follicle makes progesterone to thicken the endometrium

Hormones
Once a month, FSH causes an egg to mature and LH triggers its release. Just before ovulation, oestrogen levels peak. A rise in progesterone causes the lining of the uterus to thicken.

Egg starting to grow
Stimulated by FSH, the egg begins to grow in the follicle

Developing egg

Mature egg

Rupturing follicle
At ovulation, the mature egg is released

Corpus luteum
Formed from the empty follicle, this produces progesterone

Corpus albicans
The empty follicle dies at the end of the menstrual cycle

Shrinking corpus luteum

Released egg travelling to uterus

Inside the ovary
The cycle begins with an egg developing inside a follicle in the ovary. The mature egg is released into the fallopian tube, leaving the empty follicle, called the corpus luteum, in the ovary.

Blood and tissue cells
Menstrual blood contains cells shed from the lining of the uterus

Unfertilized egg
Egg leaves the uterus during menstruation

Blood vessels
In response to increased oestrogen levels, blood vessels lengthen

Endometrial glands
Glands enlarge and produce nutrients

Thickened lining

Unfertilized egg

Endometrium
Hormones cause the endometrium to double in thickness, to about 6 mm (¹/₄ in). If fertilization does not occur, some of the endometrial tissue is shed as menstrual blood, together with the unfertilized egg.

0   2   4   6   8   10   12   14   16   18   20   22   24   26   28
DAYS

✚ FUNCTION

Changes during the menopause

The menopause occurs between the ages of 45 and 55, when a woman's ovaries stop responding to follicle-stimulating hormone (FSH) and produce less of the female sex hormones oestrogen and progesterone. This drop in hormone levels brings an end to ovulation and menstruation. In the years just before and after the menopause, hormone changes produce physical symptoms such as hot flushes, vaginal dryness, and night sweats. The menopause is also associated with long-term physical changes, such as osteoporosis.

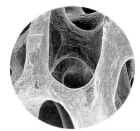
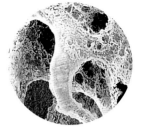

BEFORE THE MENOPAUSE　　　**AFTER THE MENOPAUSE**

Osteoporosis in bone tissue

Oestrogen is needed to give bones strength. After the menopause, when oestrogen levels are low, osteoporosis can develop. Bones lose density and may become thin and brittle, as shown in the microscopic image above.

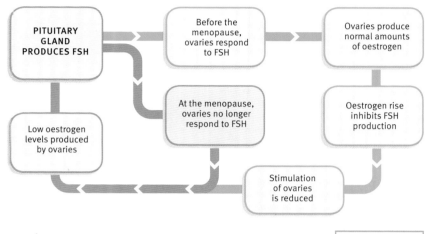

Hormone cycle

At the menopause, the ovaries no longer respond to FSH and produce little oestrogen. The pituitary gland reacts by increasing its production of FSH. The changes in the levels of the hormones cause symptoms such as hot flushes.

Key
☐ Before the menopause
☐ At the menopause

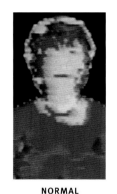

NORMAL　　　**HOT FLUSH**

Increased skin temperature

Hot flushes

These thermal images show increased skin temperature in a hot flush caused by the change in the levels of sex hormones.

✚ FUNCTION

Role of the breasts

Breasts have a role in sexual arousal, but their main function is to produce and deliver milk to a newborn baby. Hormonal changes in late pregnancy stimulate the production of milk in glands called lobules, which lead to ducts that converge and then open on to the surface of the nipple. The remaining breast tissue is mostly fat, with a small amount of connective tissue that helps to support the breasts. The variety in size and shape of breasts is determined by genetic factors, fat content, and muscle tone.

LOCATION

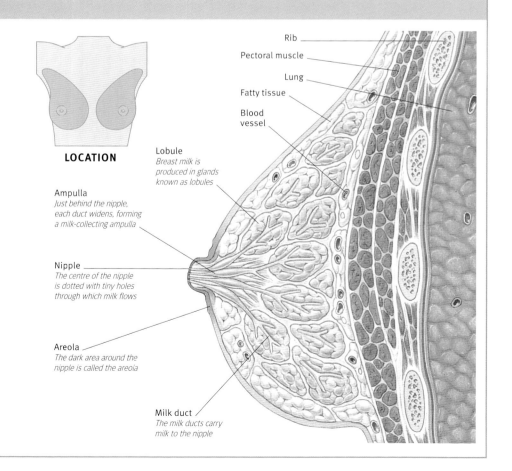

Rib

Pectoral muscle

Lung

Fatty tissue

Blood vessel

Lobule
Breast milk is produced in glands known as lobules

Ampulla
Just behind the nipple, each duct widens, forming a milk-collecting ampulla

Nipple
The centre of the nipple is dotted with tiny holes through which milk flows

Areola
The dark area around the nipple is called the areola

Milk duct
The milk ducts carry milk to the nipple

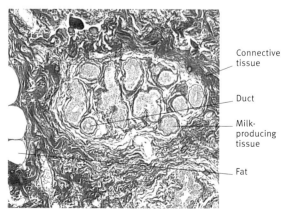

Connective tissue

Duct

Milk-producing tissue

Fat

Breast tissue

A milk-producing lobule of the breast and the drainage ducts leading from it are shown here. Each lobule is surrounded by fat and connective tissue.

Menstrual, menopausal, and hormonal problems

Menstruation usually starts at puberty and ceases at the menopause. These two stages in a woman's life are determined by the levels of female sex hormones in the body. The menstrual cycle itself is also governed by a combination of hormones, all of which are produced at varying levels throughout the cycle. Many conditions or disorders upset the balance of these hormones.

This section begins by discussing some common menstrual disorders. Several of these disorders are still not fully understood, but advances in diagnostic techniques have made investigation easier, and modern surgical methods have improved treatment. The articles that follow discuss health problems associated with the menopause and other disorders caused by an imbalance of the sex hormones. The widespread use of hormonal treatment has helped to relieve many of these disorders.

Related disorders that affect the female reproductive system are dealt with in other sections (*see* **Disorders of the female reproductive organs**, pp.475–483, and **Sex and reproduction**, pp.489–499), as are disorders involving hormones other than the sex hormones (*see* **Hormones and metabolism**, pp.424–441).

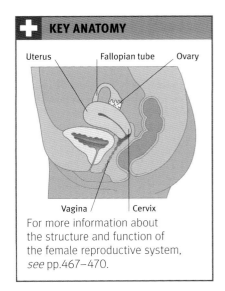

✚ KEY ANATOMY

Uterus · Fallopian tube · Ovary

Vagina · Cervix

For more information about the structure and function of the female reproductive system, *see* pp.467–470.

Irregular periods

A menstrual cycle that has wide variations in the length of time between periods

 Most common just after puberty and just before the menopause

 Stress, excessive exercise, and being underweight or overweight are all risk factors

 Genetics is not a significant factor

Periods start at puberty and continue until the menopause. The average menstrual cycle lasts 28 days, but periods may occur as often as every 24 days or as infrequently as every 35 days or more. After puberty, most women develop a regular menstrual cycle with a relatively consistent length of time between periods. In some women, however, periods remain irregular. Menstrual bleeding normally lasts between 2 and 7 days, with the average length of bleeding being 5 days.

What are the causes?

Variations in the length of the menstrual cycle are usually the result of a temporary hormonal imbalance. Fluctuations in hormone levels during puberty mean that periods are often irregular when they first start, and wide variations in a woman's normal pattern of bleeding are common in the first few months following childbirth and with the approach of the menopause.

Hormonal imbalances at other times may be caused by factors such as stress, depression, and severe or long-term illness. Excessive exercise and extreme loss of weight (*see* **Anorexia nervosa**, p.348) or a marked increase in weight are also common causes of hormonal disturbance that can cause menstruation to become irregular.

Occasionally, irregular menstruation may be a symptom of a disorder of the ovaries or of the uterus. For example, polycystic ovary syndrome (p.477), in which there is an imbalance of the sex hormones, or endometriosis (p.475), in which fragments of the tissue that normally lines the uterus are found attached to other organs in the pelvis, may disrupt periods.

In some cases, an unsuspected pregnancy produces irregular bleeding that could easily be mistaken for a period. A single, late, heavy period may be due to a miscarriage (p.511). If you have a late period that is accompanied by severe abdominal pain, you should seek medical attention urgently because it may be due to an ectopic pregnancy (p.511). In some cases, the cause of irregular menstruation is unknown.

What might be done?

Irregular periods due to the normal hormonal changes that follow puberty or childbirth usually become more regular with time. In women who are approaching the menopause, irregular periods will eventually cease altogether. In all these cases, treatment is not usually necessary. However, if the problem persists and interferes significantly with a woman's lifestyle, drugs, such as oral contraceptives, may sometimes be recommended to help regulate menstruation. Irregular menstruation that is due to extreme weight change, excessive exercise, stress, or depression should become more regular if these problems can be overcome.

If there is no obvious cause for your irregular periods and no apparent pattern to menstrual bleeding, your doctor may arrange for you to have tests to look for an underlying disorder. These may include a pregnancy test, blood tests to measure hormone levels, and ultrasound scanning (p.135) of the pelvic region to look at the ovaries and uterus. If an underlying disorder is discovered, treatment of that disorder should regulate periods in most cases.

Amenorrhoea

The absence of menstruation for at least 3 months in women who would otherwise be having periods

 Occurs between puberty and the menopause

 In some cases, due to a chromosomal abnormality

 Stress, excessive exercise, and being underweight are all risk factors

There are two types of amenorrhoea: primary and secondary. If a girl has not started to menstruate by the age of 16, she is said to have primary amenorrhoea. Once menstruation has become established during puberty, it is normal for periods to stop during pregnancy, for a few months following childbirth, while breast-feeding, temporarily after ceasing to take oral contraceptive pills, and permanently at the menopause. If menstruation stops at any other time for at least 3 months, the condition is known as secondary amenorrhoea.

What are the causes?

Amenorrhoea is often caused by a disturbance in the female sex hormones, which may be brought on by factors such as stress or depression. Excessive exercise and extreme or sudden weight loss (*see* **Anorexia nervosa**, p.348) may also lead to such hormonal disturbances and are common causes of amenorrhoea in athletes, gymnasts, and ballet dancers. Hormonal changes may lead to primary or secondary amenorrhoea, depending on when they occur.

Primary amenorrhoea is a characteristic feature of delayed puberty (*see* **Abnormal puberty in females**, p.474) and may be caused by a chromosomal abnormality. The failure of menstruation to start at puberty may also be due to a condition in which the hymen (the thin membrane over the vagina) has no opening, and menstrual blood cannot leave the body. In rare cases, the uterus is absent from birth, and therefore no menstruation can occur.

Secondary amenorrhoea may be due to a pituitary gland disorder, such as a pituitary tumour (*see* **Prolactinoma**, p.430). Some women have a premature menopause, in which periods cease before the age of 35. Other possible causes include disorders of the ovaries, such as polycystic ovary syndrome (p.477), and treatments such as radiotherapy (p.158) and chemotherapy (p.157), which can result in damage to the ovaries.

What might be done?

Treatment is not needed if amenorrhoea lasts for only a few months after stopping oral contraceptive pills or occurs during pregnancy or breast-feeding. Menstruation normally resumes within a few months of giving birth if you are not breast-feeding or within a month of stopping breast-feeding. After the menopause, amenorrhoea will be permanent.

Amenorrhoea that occurs at any other time should be investigated. Your doctor will examine you and may perform a pregnancy test. You may also need to have blood tests to measure hormone levels, ultrasound scanning (p.135) of the ovaries and uterus, and possibly CT scanning (p.132) of the pituitary gland.

Treatment of the underlying disorder induces menstruation in most cases. If the cause cannot be treated, hormonal treatment may be used to start menstruation. If periods are absent due to stress, weight loss, or excessive exercise, they should occur if the problem is overcome.

Menorrhagia

Menstrual bleeding that is heavier than normal

 More common over the age of 40

 Being overweight is a risk factor

 Genetics is not a significant factor

Some women have heavier periods than others. Menorrhagia is heavy bleeding that requires sanitary pads or tampons to be changed frequently and may include blood clots. Sometimes the bleeding may be so heavy that it cannot be controlled by pads or tampons and "flooding" occurs. Menorrhagia may be associated with a dragging pain in the lower abdomen. Menstruation may also be irregular (*see* **Irregular periods**, left). Severe menstrual bleeding may lead to iron-deficiency anaemia (p.271). About 1 in 20 women has menorrhagia regularly. It is more common in women approaching the menopause.

What are the causes?

Heavy or prolonged menstrual bleeding can be a symptom of disorders of the uterus, such as fibroids (p.477), uterine polyps (p.478), endometriosis (p.475), persistent pelvic infections, or, more rarely, cancer of the uterus (p.479). Menorrhagia is also a side effect of using an intrauterine contraceptive device (IUD). A single heavy period that is late may be a miscarriage (p.511). Menorrhagia may also be caused by a hormonal disorder, such as hypothyroidism (p.432). The condition is more common in overweight women.

Sometimes, the cause is not clear. If your periods have always been heavy, there is probably no need for concern. You should consult your doctor if the problem affects your lifestyle and to check there is no underlying disorder.

How is it diagnosed?

Your doctor will examine you and may arrange for blood tests to measure your hormone levels and to look for signs of anaemia. Further investigations, such as ultrasound scanning (p.135) to look for fibroids or polyps in the uterus, may be necessary. You may also have a hysteroscopy (p.478). A small sample of the endometrium (the lining of the uterus) may be taken for analysis (see Endometrial sampling, opposite page).

What is the treatment?

Treatment depends on the cause, your age, and the severity of the bleeding. Any underlying disorder will be treated. If no obvious cause is found, drugs may initially be given to reduce blood loss. You may want to consider changing your method of contraception if you use an IUD. If you are overweight, losing weight may help. In some cases, your doctor may recommend an IUS (intrauterine system, p.29), which reduces bleeding and provides contraception.

If initial treatments do not help or if menorrhagia is severe, you may require endometrial ablation, in which a laser or diathermy (heat treatment) is used to destroy the tissue lining the uterus, or an operation to remove the uterus (see Hysterectomy, p.479). These procedures are irreversible and are usually only offered to women who do not want to have children in the future. Endometrial ablation is a minor procedure, but it carries a small risk that problems will recur if any endometrial tissue remains. A hysterectomy is a major operation but ensures that menorrhagia will not recur.

Dysmenorrhoea

Lower abdominal pain and discomfort experienced just before or during menstruation

 Age, genetics, and lifestyle as risk factors depend on the type

Up to three-quarters of women have period pain, also known as dysmenorrhoea, at some time. In about a fifth of these women, the pain is severe and can seriously disrupt normal activities. Pain is usually experienced in the 24 hours before menstruation or over the first 1 or 2 days of the period.

What are the types?

There are two types of dysmenorrhoea: primary, which has no obvious cause; and secondary, which is the result of a disorder of the reproductive organs.

Primary dysmenorrhoea This form of dysmenorrhoea usually appears in the early teens and is associated with the hormones involved in the monthly release of eggs from the ovaries. Periods often become painful about 1–2 years after the start of menstruation, when ovulation begins. A rise in the level of hormone-like substances called prostaglandins in the body occurs some days after ovulation and makes the muscles of the uterus contract. This contraction interferes with the blood supply to the uterus and causes period pain. This type of menstrual pain tends to lessen after the age of 25, often disappearing by the age of 30, and it usually becomes less severe after childbirth, probably because the blood supply to the uterus increases.

Secondary dysmenorrhoea Painful periods in women who have not experienced menstrual pain before or have only had mild pain is called secondary dysmenorrhoea. This type of period pain usually affects women between the ages of 20 and 40. The cause is sometimes endometriosis (p.475), in which fragments of the tissue that normally lines the uterus are found attached to other organs in the pelvis, or a disorder of the uterus, such as fibroids (p.477). A persistent infection of the reproductive organs (see Pelvic inflammatory disease, p.475) and use of an intrauterine contraceptive device (IUD) may also cause painful periods.

What are the symptoms?

The symptoms of dysmenorrhoea begin either just before or at the start of menstruation and are worst when bleeding is heaviest. The pain may be described as either or both of the following:

- Cramping lower abdominal pain that comes in waves, radiating to the lower back and down the legs.
- Dragging pain in the pelvis.

This pain may be accompanied by any of the symptoms of premenstrual syndrome (right), such as headache.

What can I do?

Taking certain over-the-counter painkillers (p.589), such as ibuprofen, may help to alleviate the discomfort. Relaxing in a hot bath and applying a source of heat, such as a hot-water bottle, to your abdomen may also provide pain relief. However, consult your doctor if you are experiencing period pain for the first time or if the pain becomes severe.

What might the doctor do?

Your doctor will probably examine you, especially if you have secondary dysmenorrhoea. Various tests may be carried out, including a vaginal swab to look for infection, ultrasound scanning (p.135) of the lower abdomen, or examination of the uterus with an instrument called a hysteroscope (see Hysteroscopy, p.478).

Treatment depends on the type of dysmenorrhoea. If you have primary dysmenorrhoea, your doctor may prescribe a painkiller such as paracetamol and codeine or a nonsteroidal anti-inflammatory drug (p.578). In some cases, your doctor may prescribe oral contraceptive pills, which relieve period pain by preventing ovulation and can also decrease menstrual blood loss. Once ovulation has been suppressed, primary dysmenorrhoea should improve, but the pain may recur at any time if you stop treatment. Secondary dysmenorrhoea usually disappears if the underlying condition can be treated.

Premenstrual syndrome

Varying symptoms that may affect women in the days leading up to menstruation

 Usually develops in late adolescence; may occur in all menstruating females

 Stress and certain foods and drinks may aggravate symptoms

 Genetics is not a significant factor

As many as 1 in 3 women experiences symptoms of premenstrual syndrome (PMS) as her period approaches. In up to 1 in 20 women, these symptoms may be severe enough to disrupt activities.

The cause of PMS is uncertain, but it is thought that the symptoms are triggered by the changing levels of the female sex hormones in the body, particularly progesterone, before menstruation. Stress may make the symptoms worse, as may excessive consumption of chocolate, caffeine-containing drinks such as tea, coffee, and cola, and alcohol.

What are the symptoms?

The symptoms of PMS vary between women and may also differ from month to month. Symptoms may appear just a few hours before a period begins, but they can start up to 14 days beforehand. In most affected women, the symptoms disappear by the time menstruation has finished or a few days afterwards. The symptoms of PMS may include:

- Tenderness or generalized lumpiness of the breasts.
- A feeling of bloating caused by the retention of fluid.
- Mood changes, including feeling tense, irritability, depression, and anxiety.
- Tiredness.
- Difficulty concentrating and making everyday decisions.
- Headaches, including migraine.
- Backache and muscle stiffness.
- Disruption of normal sleep patterns.
- Unusual food cravings.

Less commonly, nausea, vomiting, cold sweats, dizziness, and hot flushes may also be experienced.

What might be done?

The diagnosis of PMS is usually easily made from the timing of your symptoms. Your doctor may ask you to keep a record of symptoms to confirm that they are related to menstruation.

There are several self-help measures you can take to try to prevent PMS (see **Preventing premenstrual syndrome**, above). If these are not effective or your symptoms are severe, you should seek medical advice. Certain nonsteroidal anti-inflammatory drugs (p.578), such as ibuprofen, can help to relieve headaches, backache, and muscle stiffness. Diuretic drugs (p.583) may help to relieve fluid retention, thereby relieving bloating and breast tenderness. Your doctor may also suggest hormone treatment, such as treatment with the combined oral contraceptive pill. If you have persistent psychological symptoms, such as depression, antidepressant drugs (p.592) may be helpful. No treatment is consistently successful, but the symptoms can usually be relieved.

Abnormal vaginal bleeding

Vaginal bleeding that is not related to menstruation

 Age and lifestyle as risk factors depend on the cause

 Genetics is not a significant factor

Normally, vaginal bleeding occurs only during a period. Bleeding that occurs outside menstruation is abnormal. In women under the age of 35, abnormal vaginal bleeding is often the result of starting oral contraceptives or of using an intrauterine contraceptive device (IUD). Abnormal bleeding caused by a disorder of the reproductive organs is more common in women over this age.

What are the causes?

Light bleeding between periods, known as spotting, is common in the first few menstrual cycles after starting oral contraceptives or changing to a different type of pill. Spotting is usually brought on by the body adjusting to changes in hormone levels, but this type of bleeding can also be associated with using an IUD.

Abnormal bleeding, especially within a few hours of sex, may indicate a disorder of the cervix, such as cervical ectopy (p.480), cervical polyps (see Uterine polyps, p.478) or, rarely, cancer of the cervix (p.481). In some cases, pelvic inflammatory disease (p.475) may cause bleeding after sex, although this condition can also cause abnormal vaginal bleeding that is not related to sex. In older women, sex may damage the vaginal wall, which becomes thinner and more fragile after the menopause, causing bleeding.

Abnormal vaginal bleeding that is not associated with sex or contraception may be caused by a disorder such as fibroids (p.477) or polyps in the uterus. Loss of blood from the uterus can also occur in early pregnancy and could indicate a miscarriage (p.511) or ectopic pregnancy (p.511). Various disorders of the reproductive organs may cause postmenopausal bleeding (right), such as cancer of the uterus (p.479).

If you notice abnormal bleeding, you should see your doctor immediately so that the cause can be investigated.

What might be done?

Your doctor may be able to make a diagnosis based on the timing of the bleeding and a physical examination. You may also need to have tests, such as a cervical screening test (p.480) to check for disorders of the cervix, ultrasound scanning (p.135) to look at the uterus, endoscopy to view the inside of the uterus (see Hysteroscopy, p.479), or endometrial sampling (below).

Treatment for abnormal vaginal bleeding depends on the cause. Spotting caused by oral contraceptives usually clears up spontaneously, or it may be necessary to change the dose or type of pill. Hormone treatments may be used to improve the elasticity of the vaginal walls in older women. Surgery may be required to treat cervical or uterine polyps or more serious underlying disorders. Cervical ectopy may be treated with cryotherapy (freezing), diathermy (cautery), or laser therapy. In most cases, the abnormal bleeding clears up once the cause has been treated.

Menopausal problems

Symptoms associated with the normal changes that take place in a woman's body as her period of fertility ends

 Most common between the ages of 45 and 55

 Sometimes runs in families

 Smoking may lower the age at which the menopause occurs

The menopause, the time at which a woman stops menstruating, is a normal consequence of the aging process. Around the menopause, about three-quarters of women experience symptoms, which tend to last for about 2 years. In the other quarter of women, symptoms persist for longer.

The onset of the menopause usually occurs between the ages of 45 and 55, although some women develop symptoms before or after this time (the time leading up to the menopause is known as the perimenopause). Smoking can lower the age at which the menopause takes place. A woman is generally considered to be menopausal if she has not had a period for at least 6 months and there is no other underlying cause. The tendency to have either an early or a late menopause can run in families.

What are the causes?

As women age, their ovaries gradually become less active and produce smaller amounts of the sex hormone oestrogen. The menopause occurs as a result of this reduction in oestrogen levels. As levels of oestrogen in the body decline, the pituitary gland begins to secrete more follicle-stimulating hormone (FSH) to try to stimulate the ovaries. Most of the symptoms associated with the menopause are a consequence of the reduced levels of oestrogen or increased levels of FSH. These tend to be more severe when the menopause takes place prematurely or abruptly. A sudden menopause can be brought about by surgical removal of the ovaries or anti-cancer treatments that can damage the ovaries, such as chemotherapy (p.157) and radiotherapy (p.158).

What are the symptoms?

Menopausal symptoms may begin up to 5 years before menstruation finally stops and usually last for a year or two. Many women find that one of the first signs of the menopause is irregularity in their menstrual cycle. Menstrual bleeding may also become heavier (see Menorrhagia, p.471). Other common menopausal symptoms include:

■ Hot flushes, in which the head, chest, and arms become red and feel hot, lasting from a couple of minutes to as long as an hour.
■ Heavy sweating, which is often especially troublesome at night.
■ Feelings of anxiety, panic, or depression, which may be made worse if the menopause coincides with a stressful life event such as the departure of adult children from the home.

The longer-term effects of a decline in oestrogen levels include:

■ Drying of the skin, which encourages the formation of wrinkles.
■ Vaginal dryness and discomfort during sexual intercourse as a result of thinning of the lining of the vagina.
■ Urinary infections that occur due to thinning of the lining of the urethra (the tube leading out of the bladder).

The decline in oestrogen levels following the menopause may also increase your risk of developing certain long-term conditions, such as coronary artery disease (p.243) and age-related thinning of the bones (see Osteoporosis, p.217).

What might be done?

Hormone replacement therapy (p.605), commonly known as HRT, may help to relieve many of the symptoms that occur at the menopause. However, HRT is usually only advised for short-term use around the menopause and is no longer normally recommended for long-term use nor for the treatment of osteoporosis because of the increased risk of disorders such as breast cancer (p.486) and thromboembolism (see Thrombosis and embolism, p.259).

Alternative treatments are available in the form of oestrogen creams, which help to control vaginal dryness and discomfort, and the drug clonidine, which can be used to relieve hot flushes. Some women find complementary therapies helpful.

The process of the menopause normally lasts between 1 and 5 years, after which symptoms usually disappear.

Postmenopausal bleeding

Bleeding from the uterus occurring at least 6 months after menstruation has stopped

 Occurs after the menopause

 Genetics and lifestyle are not significant factors

Menstrual bleeding should cease at the menopause. Postmenopausal bleeding is normal only with certain forms of hormone replacement therapy (p.605) that cause withdrawal bleeding, usually once a month. Other postmenopausal bleeding indicates an underlying disorder. In some cases, the causative disorder may be serious, such as a cancer of the reproductive tract, and so postmenopausal bleeding should always be investigated urgently by a doctor. Postmenopausal bleeding may range from light spotting to a heavier flow of blood and is usually painless.

What are the causes?

Postmenopausal bleeding can be a symptom of various disorders of the vulva, vagina, cervix, uterus, fallopian tubes, and ovaries. The most common

---

▶ **TEST**

Endometrial sampling

During endometrial sampling a small sample of tissue is removed from the endometrium (the lining of the uterus) to investigate symptoms such as heavy vaginal bleeding and to rule out cancer of the uterus. The sample is examined under a microscope for abnormalities. The procedure may be slightly uncomfortable but usually lasts for only a few minutes and does not require anaesthesia.

During the procedure

An instrument called a speculum is used to hold the vagina open while a thin, flexible tube is inserted into the uterus. A small sample of tissue is then drawn into the tube by vacuum suction.

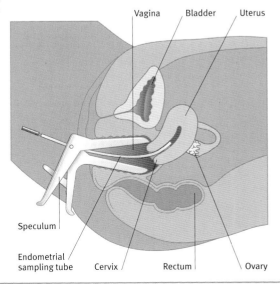

Vagina   Bladder   Uterus

Speculum

Endometrial sampling tube   Cervix   Rectum   Ovary

RESULTS

Endometrial tissue
This sample of tissue from the endometrium shows abnormal cells, indicating the presence of cancer of the uterus.

and least serious cause of such bleeding is atrophic vaginitis, in which the vagina becomes thinned due to low levels of oestrogen after the menopause (see **Vulvovaginitis**, p.482).

Postmenopausal bleeding could be caused by a disorder of the cervix, such as cervical ectopy (p.480) or cancer of the cervix (p.481). In these disorders, bleeding from the cervix may be more likely to occur after sexual intercourse. Postmenopausal bleeding may also be the result of a thickened endometrium (the lining of the uterus), precancerous or cancerous growths in the uterus (see **Cancer of the uterus**, p.479), or uterine polyps (p.478). Cancer of the vulva and vagina (p.483) may also lead to postmenopausal bleeding, although both of these disorders are very rare.

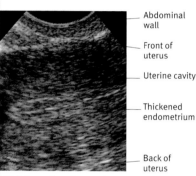

Abdominal wall
Front of uterus
Uterine cavity
Thickened endometrium
Back of uterus

Thickened endometrium
This ultrasound scan of the uterus shows that the endometrium (the lining of the uterus) is thickened. This may be a cause of postmenopausal bleeding.

What might be done?
Your doctor will examine the vagina and cervix to look for abnormalities. If abnormal areas are seen in the vagina, a small sample of tissue may be taken for examination under a microscope. Your doctor may also perform a cervical screening test (p.480) to check for abnormal cells in the cervix. In some cases, a sample of endometrial tissue may be taken for analysis (see **Endometrial sampling**, p.473).

Ultrasound scanning (p.135) may be carried out to image the uterus and to measure the thickness of the lining. The inside of your uterus may also be examined (see **Hysteroscopy**, p.478).

The treatment for postmenopausal bleeding varies depending on the underlying cause. Oestrogen creams that are applied to the vagina may be prescribed to relieve atrophic vaginitis. Surgery may be necessary to remove cancerous growths. Surgery may also be carried out to treat disorders of the cervix and uterus, such as a thickened endometrium. Postmenopausal bleeding should cease once the underlying disorder has been treated.

Hypogonadism in females

Underactivity, developmental failure, or absence of the ovaries, leading to low levels of female sex hormones

 Sometimes due to a chromosomal abnormality

 Age and lifestyle as risk factors depend on the cause

Female sex hormones control sexual development and the menstrual cycle. Underactivity of the ovaries, known as hypogonadism, leads to low levels of these hormones in the body. A decline in hormone levels occurs naturally during the menopause, but at other times it may indicate an underlying disorder. Hypogonadism may cause distressing symptoms but is often treatable.

What are the types?
There are two types of hypogonadism: primary and secondary. Either type can occur at any age. Primary hypogonadism is often caused by a disorder or failure of the ovaries, which may result from a chromosomal abnormality such as Turner's syndrome (p.534). It may also be caused by the surgical removal of the ovaries. In most cases, primary hypogonadism occurs as a natural consequence of the menopause.

Secondary hypogonadism is caused by an abnormality of the pituitary gland or of the hypothalamus (a part of the brain) that leads to underproduction of the hormones that stimulate the ovaries to function. This abnormality may be due to a disorder such as a pituitary tumour (p.430) or, rarely, to damage to the pituitary gland or the hypothalamus as a result of a head injury (p.322) or an infection such as viral encephalitis (p.326). Sometimes, it results from excessive exercise or sudden weight loss.

What are the symptoms?
Symptoms depend on the age at which hypogonadism develops and the amount of sex hormones produced. If the onset occurs before puberty, the condition causes abnormal puberty (right). If it is after puberty, symptoms may include:
- Reduced or absent menstruation (see **Amenorrhoea**, p.471).
- Reduced fertility.
- Hot flushes, excessive sweating, and anxiety, together with other symptoms associated with the menopause (see **Menopausal problems**, p.473).
- Rarely, the pubic hair may recede and the breasts may become smaller.

What might be done?
Your doctor may arrange for you to have blood tests to measure your hormone levels. You may also have CT scanning (p.132) of the brain to look for a pituitary abnormality or ultrasound scanning (p.135) of the ovaries.

The treatment depends on the cause. For example, a pituitary tumour may be removed by surgery. If the condition is due to weight loss, gaining weight may help. In some cases, hormone treatment may be prescribed to induce puberty. Women who go through premature menopause (before age 40) may be advised to have hormone replacement therapy (p.605) until age 50 to relieve symptoms and give protection from diseases associated with low levels of sex hormones, such as osteoporosis (p.217). For women under 50, the health risks of hormone replacement therapy are thought to be less than normal.

Abnormal puberty in females

Very early or late start of puberty, usually due to a hormonal imbalance

 Occurs before or after the normal age range for puberty

 In some cases, due to a chromosomal abnormality

 Excessive exercise and weight loss are risk factors

Puberty is the period during which sexual development occurs (see **Puberty**, p.457). In girls, it is characterized by a growth spurt, hair growth in the armpits and pubic region, development of the breasts and reproductive organs, and the onset of menstruation. Although there is some variation in the age of onset of puberty, girls tend to start this process between 8 and 14. Puberty may be considered abnormal if it starts either earlier than normal (precocious) or later (delayed). Puberty is early if a girl starts to develop breasts before the age of 8 or if menstruation starts before the age of 10. In extreme cases, puberty may begin at the age of 4. Puberty is delayed if menstruation has not started by the age of 14½ (see **Amenorrhoea**, p.471) or there are no signs of breast development by the age of 13.

Early puberty is rare and may be due to a hormone disorder. Delayed puberty is more common. Although there may be an underlying cause of delayed puberty, many girls who have not menstruated by the age of 14½ are simply late developers, a tendency that often runs in families.

Abnormal puberty can be disturbing for a girl and her family because physical and sexual development will not coincide with that of her peers. Medical advice should be sought as soon as abnormal puberty is suspected.

What are the causes?
Puberty in girls is controlled by female sex hormones produced by the ovaries. The production of these hormones is controlled by hormones from the pituitary gland and hypothalamus (both parts of the brain). Disorders of any of these organs may lead to an abnormally early or late puberty.

Early puberty may be due to a disorder that causes a premature rise in sex hormones. For example, an ovarian cyst (p.476) developing in childhood may produce sex hormones, causing early sexual development. A tumour of the hypothalamus or damage to the pituitary gland as the result of head injury (p.322) or an infection such as meningitis (p.325) may also cause early puberty. Rarely, early puberty may be caused by an adrenal gland tumour that produces sex hormones.

Delayed puberty may be caused by certain chromosome disorders, such as Turner's syndrome (p.534), or less commonly by a pituitary tumour (p.430). Excessive weight loss or exercise may create a temporary hormonal imbalance that can lead to delayed puberty.

In many cases of abnormal puberty, no underlying cause is found.

What might be done?
The doctor will carry out an examination to determine whether puberty has started or how far it has progressed. A blood sample may be taken to measure hormone levels or check for a chromosomal abnormality. The doctor may also arrange for MRI (p.133) or CT scanning (p.132) of the brain to look for a pituitary tumour, or ultrasound scanning (p.135) of the ovaries to check for cysts.

If there is an underlying condition, it will be treated. For example, an ovarian cyst may be surgically removed. Hormonal treatment may be prescribed to suspend precocious puberty or to promote sexual development if puberty is delayed. In some cases, delayed puberty is associated with infertility (see **Female infertility**, p.497), and further evaluation and treatment may be required in the future if a woman who has had a delayed puberty wants to have children.

Sometimes, puberty is simply late, and treatment is not necessary. Gaining weight and reducing strenuous activity may help if delayed puberty has been caused by weight loss or exercise.

Virilization

Development of male characteristics in a female due to a hormonal imbalance

 May be present at birth but usually develops later in life

 In some cases, the cause is inherited

 Lifestyle is not a significant factor

Normally, low levels of male sex hormones are present in females and are produced by the adrenal glands and the ovaries. However, if the production of these hormones increases significantly, various male characteristics begin to develop, a condition called virilization.

Virilization most commonly occurs in adulthood, causing symptoms such as deepening of the voice, excessive hair growth on the face and body known as hirsutism, and thinning of the hair on the temples and crown. These symptoms often cause psychological distress. Rarely, the condition is present at birth. If present at birth, virilization

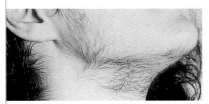

Excessive facial hair
This young woman has excessive facial hair (hirsutism), a common symptom of virilization, a condition caused by the excess production of male sex hormones.

is usually due to a genetic disorder that causes abnormal hormone levels (*see* Congenital adrenal hyperplasia, p.561).

What are the causes?
When virilization develops later in life, the possible causes include abnormalities of the ovaries, such as certain types of ovarian cysts (p.476), cancer of the ovary (p.477), and polycystic ovary syndrome (p.477). Hormone levels can also be increased by adrenal tumours (p.435) and the use of certain male hormone supplements by athletes.

What are the symptoms?
In the rare cases when virilization is present at birth, the most obvious feature is ambiguous-looking genitals. In other cases,

symptoms appear gradually as male sex hormone levels rise. They include:
- Excessive growth of hair on the face and body.
- Less regular or absent menstruation (*see* Amenorrhoea, p.471).
- Reduction in breast size or in rare cases failure of the breasts to develop.
- Enlargement of the clitoris.
- Irreversible enlargement of the larynx (Adam's apple), causing the voice to become deeper.
- Thinning of the hair around the temples and crown (*see* Male-pattern baldness, p.209).

The hormonal imbalance may lead to increased muscular development, producing a male body shape.

What might be done?
Your doctor will examine you and may arrange tests to determine the cause of your symptoms. These tests include blood tests to measure hormone levels, MRI (p.133) or CT scanning (p.132) to look for an adrenal tumour, and ultrasound scanning (p.135) to check the ovaries. Treatment of the cause, such as removal of a tumour, should reverse some of the changes. If no cause is found, combined oral contraceptives may be given to suppress hormone production by the ovaries and reduce male sex hormone levels. You may be given advice on how to manage excessive hair, perhaps by using electrolysis or waxing. Counselling (p.624) is often helpful.

Disorders of the female reproductive organs

The female reproductive organs are the ovaries, fallopian tubes, uterus, cervix, vagina, and vulva. Since the combined primary function of these organs is reproduction, disorders affecting them can result in infertility and should be treated as soon as possible, particularly if children are planned. Such disorders may be caused by infections, physical damage, or hormonal imbalances.

The first two articles in this section discuss pelvic inflammatory disease and endometriosis, disorders that may affect more than one female reproductive organ. The next articles discuss disorders of the ovaries, uterus, and cervix. Disorders affecting the vagina and vulva are covered last.

Disorders affecting the female reproductive organs are common, but many of them can be treated easily.

Disorders affecting menstruation, the menopause, or sexual development are covered in other sections (*see* Menstrual, menopausal, and hormonal problems, pp.471–475), as are sexual disorders of both sexes (*see* Sexually transmitted infections, pp.491–493, Infertility, pp.497–499, and Sexual problems, pp.494–496).

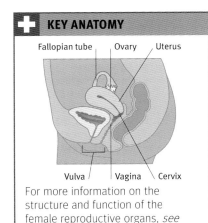

✚ KEY ANATOMY

Fallopian tube Ovary Uterus

Vulva Vagina Cervix

For more information on the structure and function of the female reproductive organs, *see* pp.467–470.

The infection spreads upwards from the vagina to the uterus and fallopian tubes. The ovaries may also be affected. An intrauterine contraceptive device (IUD) makes this spread of infection more likely if an infection is present at the time the IUD is inserted. If you think you may have an infection, tests will usually be performed so that you can be treated before PID develops. When PID is discovered during investigations for infertility, the original cause may remain unknown.

What are the symptoms?
PID may have no obvious symptoms, especially when caused by chlamydia. If there are symptoms, they may include:
- Pain in the pelvic region.
- Fever.
- An abnormal vaginal discharge.
- Heavy or prolonged periods (*see* Menorrhagia, p.471).
- Pain during sexual intercourse.
- Tiredness.

If PID develops suddenly, you may have severe pain, nausea, and vomiting, and urgent hospital attention is required.

If the condition is not treated, the fallopian tubes may be damaged. The infection may also spread to other organs in the pelvis and the abdomen.

What might be done?
If your doctor suspects that you have PID, he or she will carry out a pelvic examination. Swabs may be taken from both the cervix and the vagina to identify the organisms causing the infection. Ultrasound scanning (p.135) of the pelvis may also be performed. If you have severe symptoms, you will be admitted to hospital, and a laparoscopy (p.476) may be performed to view the abdominal and pelvic cavities.

Your doctor will probably prescribe antibiotics (p.572), which may be given intravenously in some cases. You may also be given painkillers (p.589).

You should not have sexual intercourse until your recovery is complete. Your sexual partners should have tests to look for sexually transmitted infections and

should be treated if necessary to prevent a reinfection (*see* Preventing STIs, p.491). If you use an IUD, your doctor may advise you to change to a different method of contraception.

If PID is detected and treated early, you should make a complete recovery. If PID is not treated, damage to the fallopian tubes can increase the risk of having an ectopic pregnancy (p.511) or may lead to infertility.

Endometriosis

A condition in which endometrial tissue, which normally lines the uterus, is attached to other organs in the abdomen

 Most common between the ages of 30 and 45

 Sometimes runs in families

 Not having had children is a risk factor

The lining of the uterus, known as the endometrium, is normally shed once a month during menstruation and then regrows. In endometriosis, some pieces of the lining are attached to organs in the pelvic cavity, such as the ovaries, fallopian tubes, vagina, cervix, bladder, or the lower intestine. These pieces of endometrial tissue react to the hormones of the menstrual cycle and bleed during menstruation. The blood cannot leave the body through the vagina and so, over time, it accumulates and forms blood-filled cysts. These cysts may be very small or may grow as large as a grapefruit and may cause pain.

Endometriosis is a common condition in the UK, affecting as many as 1 in 5 women of childbearing age. Women who do not have children until they are in their 30s and those who remain childless are more likely to develop the condition. In severe cases, endometriosis can often cause problems with fertility (*see* Female infertility, p.497).

Pelvic inflammatory disease

Inflammation of the female reproductive organs, most often due to a sexually transmitted infection

 Most common between the ages of 15 and 24; rare before puberty

Lifestyle as a risk factor depends on the cause

 Genetics is not a significant factor

Pelvic inflammatory disease (PID) is a common cause of pain in the pelvic region in women. In this condition, some of the

female reproductive organs become inflamed, usually as a result of an infection. Young and sexually active women are most likely to be affected. PID may have no obvious symptoms, and some women are unaware that they have had the condition until, years later, they are investigated for infertility (*see* Female infertility, p.497).

PID is usually caused by a sexually transmitted infection (STI), such as gonorrhoea (p.491) or chlamydial infection (p.492). PID may also be caused by an infection developing after a termination of pregnancy (p.510) or after childbirth. In rare cases, PID can occur as a result of tuberculosis (p.300) developing in the pelvis or from the spread of a severe infection from the large intestine.

▶ **TEST AND TREATMENT**

Laparoscopy

During laparoscopy, a rigid viewing instrument called a laparoscope is used to view the inside of the pelvis and the abdomen through small abdominal incisions. Laparoscopy may be used to look for disorders of the female reproductive organs, such as endometriosis, and to investigate other abdominal disorders, such as appendicitis. Some types of surgery, such as female sterilization (right), and surgery for endometriosis, ectopic pregnancy, and to remove ovarian cysts, may also be carried out laparoscopically. Laparoscopy is always performed under general anaesthesia. Recovery is usually faster than after conventional surgery.

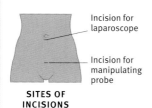

SITES OF INCISIONS

Incision for laparoscope

Incision for manipulating probe

The procedure

The laparoscope and a tool to manipulate the internal organs are inserted through incisions. Gas is pumped through the laparoscope so that the organs separate and can be seen clearly. In women, a second tool may be inserted through the vagina.

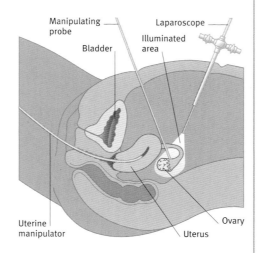

Manipulating probe

Laparoscope

Bladder

Illuminated area

Uterine manipulator

Ovary

Uterus

VIEW

Uterus

Probe

Area of endometriosis

Ovary

Endometriosis

This view through a laparoscope shows areas of endometriosis on the lining of the pelvic cavity next to the uterus. The tip of a manipulating probe and one of the ovaries can also be seen.

The exact cause of endometriosis is not known, but there are many theories. One theory is that fragments of endometrium shed during menstruation do not leave the body in the usual way through the vagina. Instead, they travel along the fallopian tubes, from where they may pass into the pelvic cavity and become attached to the surfaces of nearby organs.

What are the symptoms?

Endometriosis may not produce symptoms. If symptoms do develop, their severity varies from woman to woman. Symptoms may also vary depending on which organs are affected by the condition. They may include:

■ Pain in the lower abdomen, which often becomes more severe just before and during menstrual periods (*see* **Dysmenorrhoea**, p.472).
■ Heavier menstrual bleeding.
■ Pain during sexual intercourse.

If the endometrium grows on the lower intestine, you may develop diarrhoea or constipation, pain during bowel movements, and, in rare cases, bleeding from the rectum or blood in the faeces during menstruation.

What might be done?

In women who do not have symptoms, endometriosis may only be suspected following investigations for infertility. To help make a diagnosis, your doctor may carry out a pelvic examination. The diagnosis may be confirmed by ultrasound scanning (p.135). If ultrasound is inconclusive, laparoscopy (above) may also be carried out.

There are many different treatments for endometriosis, and the one chosen depends on your age, which organs are affected, the severity of symptoms, and whether you wish to have children in the future. You may be offered hormonal or surgical treatment. In mild cases, treatment may not be necessary.

If your symptoms are troublesome, your doctor may prescribe one of several different hormonal treatments that stop menstruation for several months. These drugs may include the synthetic hormone gonadorelin (*see* **Sex hormones and related drugs**, p.602), which suppresses production of oestrogen and has the effect of stopping menstruation. Alternatively, you may be given the combined oral contraceptive pill or progesterone-only medication for approximately 6 months, during which time the endometriosis should improve. If the condition does recur, it may be milder than before.

▶ **TREATMENT**

Female sterilization

Female sterilization involves blocking the fallopian tubes so that sperm cannot travel through them to fertilize eggs. It may be performed through two small incisions in the abdomen (laparoscopic sterilization) or through a single incision in the pubic area (minilaparotomy). The tubes may be blocked by using clips or rings, or by cutting and tying the tubes. Less commonly, a small metal implant (called a microinsert) may be placed into each tube using a hysteroscope (p.478) inserted through the cervix, a procedure that does not require incisions. The microinserts cause the fallopian tubes to form scar tissue, which eventually blocks the tubes. Female sterilization procedures are difficult to reverse so should be considered permanent. Overall, they are more than 99 per cent effective.

SITES OF INCISIONS

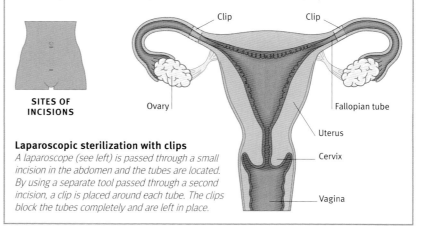

Clip

Clip

Ovary

Fallopian tube

Uterus

Cervix

Vagina

Laparoscopic sterilization with clips

A laparoscope (see left) is passed through a small incision in the abdomen and the tubes are located. By using a separate tool passed through a second incision, a clip is placed around each tube. The clips block the tubes completely and are left in place.

Small fragments of endometrial tissue that do not respond to a period of hormonal treatment may be destroyed during a laparoscopy. However, endometriosis sometimes recurs after this treatment, and further operations may be necessary.

If you have severe endometriosis and do not plan to have children, your doctor may suggest that you have a hysterectomy (p.479) to remove the uterus. Both ovaries will also be removed, together with other areas affected by endometriosis. If the ovaries are removed before you have reached the menopause naturally, you will develop menopausal symptoms. To alleviate these symptoms, your doctor may recommend hormone replacement therapy (p.605).

What is the prognosis?

Although treatment is usually successful, endometriosis may recur until the menopause occurs and menstrual cycles end. Endometriosis is unlikely to recur if the ovaries are removed.

Ovarian cysts

Fluid-filled swellings that grow on or in one or both ovaries

 Most common between the ages of 30 and 45

 Genetics and lifestyle are not significant factors

Ovarian cysts are fluid-filled sacs that grow on or in the ovaries. Most ovarian cysts are noncancerous and not harmful, but a cyst may sometimes become cancerous (*see* **Cancer of the ovary**, opposite page). Cancerous cysts are more likely to develop in women over the age of 40.

What are the types?

There are many types of ovarian cyst. The most common is a follicular cyst, in which one of the egg follicles grows and fills with fluid. This type of cyst may grow to 5 cm (2 in) in diameter and usually occurs singly. Multiple small cysts that develop in the ovaries are thought to be caused by a hormonal disorder known as polycystic ovary syndrome (opposite page).

Less commonly, cysts may form in the corpus luteum, the yellow tissue that develops from a follicle after the release of an egg. These cysts can fill with blood and can grow to 6 cm ($2\frac{1}{2}$ in).

A dermoid cyst is a cyst that contains cells that are normally found elsewhere in the body, such as skin and hair cells. A cystadenoma is a cyst that grows from one type of cell in the ovary. In rare cases, a single cystadenoma can fill the entire abdominal cavity.

What are the symptoms?

Often, ovarian cysts do not cause symptoms, but when there are symptoms, they may include:

■ Discomfort in the abdomen.
■ Pain during sexual intercourse.
■ A change in your usual menstrual pattern.

Large cysts can put pressure on the bladder, leading to urinary retention (p.455) or a frequent need to pass urine.

Are there complications?

If an ovarian cyst ruptures or becomes twisted, severe abdominal pain, nausea, and fever may develop. Cysts may grow so large that the abdomen is distended. In rare cases, a cyst producing the sex hormone oestrogen may develop before puberty, which leads to early sexual development (see **Abnormal puberty in females**, p.474). Some ovarian cysts produce male sex hormones, which can cause the development of male characteristics, such as growth of facial hair (see **Virilization**, p.474).

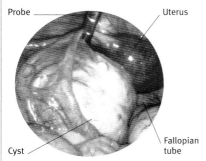

Probe — Uterus
Cyst — Fallopian tube

Ovarian cyst
This view through a laparoscope shows a large ovarian cyst next to the uterus. Most ovarian cysts are noncancerous.

What might be done?

Sometimes, ovarian cysts are only discovered when a pelvic examination is carried out during a routine checkup. If you have symptoms of a cyst, your doctor will perform a pelvic examination. You may also be sent for ultrasound scanning (p.135) or for a laparoscopy (opposite page) to confirm the diagnosis and determine the size and position of the cyst. You may also have blood tests to give an indication of whether a cyst might be cancerous.

Ovarian cysts may disappear without treatment, although the size of a cyst may be monitored with regular ultrasound scans. Large or persistent cysts may be drained or removed. If there is a chance that the cyst is cancerous, it will be removed, leaving the ovary and fallopian tube if possible. Ovarian cysts may recur if the ovary is not removed.

Polycystic ovary syndrome

Multiple, small, fluid-filled cysts in the ovaries associated with a sex hormone imbalance

 Affects females of childbearing age

 Sometimes runs in families

 Lifestyle is not a significant factor

Many women have multiple fluid-filled cysts in their ovaries but most of these women do not have polycystic ovary syndrome (PCOS), which is the presence of multiple ovarian cysts associated with an imbalance of the sex hormones and certain other characteristics, such as acne, exces-

sive body hair (see **Virilization**, p.474), and menstrual irregularities. The sex hormone imbalance, which may include higher than normal levels of the male sex hormone testosterone, may prevent ovulation (egg release), thus reducing fertility (see **Female infertility**, p.497).

The underlying cause of PCOS is not fully understood but the increased resistance of body tissues to the hormone insulin that is a feature of the syndrome is thought to play an important part. To compensate for the increased insulin resistance, the pancreas produces excessive insulin, which, in turn, may lead to overproduction of testosterone, high levels of which disrupt normal functioning of the ovaries. PCOS sometimes runs in families.

What are the symptoms?

The symptoms vary in severity, depending on the degree of hormone imbalance. PCOS may go unnoticed until a woman is tested for infertility. Symptoms include:
■ Infrequent or absent periods (see **Amenorrhoea**, p.471).
■ Obesity.
■ Excessive hair growth on the face, around the nipples, and/or on the lower abdomen.
■ Thinning of the hair on the head.
■ Long-lasting acne.
Women with PCOS have an increased risk of developing diabetes mellitus (p.437), high blood pressure (see **Hypertension**, p.242), coronary heart disease (p.243), and cancer of the uterus (p.479).

What might be done?

If your doctor suspects that you have PCOS, he or she will take blood samples to measure your levels of sex hormones. You will also have ultrasound scanning (p.135) to look for ovarian cysts.

Treatment depends on the severity of your symptoms and whether you want to conceive. Infertility can be treated with drugs, such as clomifene (see **Drugs for infertility**, p.604). If drugs are unsuccessful in treating infertility, the cysts may be treated with diathermy (a type of heat treatment) carried out during laparoscopy (p.476). If necessary, assisted conception (p.498) may then be considered. If you do not want to have children, abnormal periods can be treated with a combined oral contraceptive pill.

To treat insulin resistance, if necessary, and reduce your risk of developing diabetes, you may be prescribed an antidiabetic drug (see **Drugs for diabetes mellitus**, p.601), such as metformin. Such drugs may also restore ovulation and regulate menstrual periods. If you are overweight, losing weight may help to relieve symptoms. Excessive hair growth may respond to an anti-androgen drug such as cyproterone. Cosmetic hair-removal treatments, which may be combined with eflornithine cream (which slows growth of facial hair) may also help.

Cancer of the ovary

A cancerous tumour that can develop in one or both ovaries

 Most common between the ages of 50 and 70; rare under the age of 40

 Sometimes runs in families

 Not having had children is a risk factor

Cancer of the ovary is the fifth most common type of cancer in women and causes about 4,300 deaths each year in the UK, more than any other cancer of the female reproductive tract. This high death rate is usually explained by the fact that symptoms do not develop until late in the progress of the disease, which delays the diagnosis and treatment.

The cause of cancer of the ovary is not known, but the tumour sometimes develops from an ovarian cyst (opposite page). There seem to be hormonal and genetic risk factors for developing the disease. Women who have never had children or have had a late menopause are more likely to develop cancer of the ovary. Women with a close relative who developed ovarian cancer before the age of 50 are also at greater risk.

What are the symptoms?

Ovarian cancer rarely produces symptoms in the early stages, although there may be symptoms similar to those of an ovarian cyst, such as irregular periods. In most cases, symptoms occur only if the cancer has spread to other organs and may include:
■ Pain in the lower abdomen.
■ Swelling in the abdomen caused by excess fluid.
■ Frequent need to pass urine.
■ Rarely, abnormal vaginal bleeding.
There may also be general symptoms of cancer, such as loss of weight, nausea, and vomiting. Left untreated, the cancer may spread to other organs in the body, such as the liver or lungs.

How is it diagnosed?

If a close relative has had cancer of the ovary, you should consult your doctor about testing for this type of cancer. Testing may detect cancerous changes before symptoms develop and allows treatment to be given in the early stages of the disease. You may be offered ultrasound scanning (p.135) through the vagina or abdomen to look for a tumour or blood tests to look for a specific protein produced by this cancer.

If you have symptoms and your doctor suspects cancer of the ovary, he or she will examine your abdomen for the presence of swellings or lumps. You will also have an ultrasound scan of your ovaries and possibly also a laparoscopy (opposite page). Other tests that may be carried out include MRI (p.133) and/or CT scanning (p.132) of the lungs or liver to see if the disease has spread. Unfortunately, there is no effective screening test for the general population.

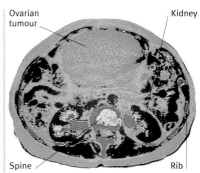

Ovarian tumour — Kidney
Spine — Rib

Cancer of the ovary
Most of the abdominal cavity seen in this colour-enhanced CT scan is filled by a large cancerous ovarian tumour.

What is the treatment?

If cancer of the ovary is diagnosed in a woman who wishes to have children, if possible, only the affected ovary and fallopian tube are removed, although the surgery that will be recommended will depend on the precise type of cancer and the stage of the disease. If the cancer has spread to other parts of the reproductive tract or the woman does not wish to have children, a total hysterectomy may be performed, in which the uterus and both the fallopian tubes and ovaries are removed. Surgery is followed by chemotherapy (p.157) to kill any remaining cancer cells. Radiotherapy (p.158) is not usually used to treat ovarian cancer, although it may occasionally be recommended in specific cases. After treatment, blood tests and physical examinations are carried out regularly to check for recurrence.

What is the prognosis?

The outlook depends on how advanced the cancer is at the time of diagnosis. A complete recovery is possible only if the condition is diagnosed and treated while in the early stages. However, the disease has spread in up to 3 in 4 women by the time of diagnosis. In these women, chemotherapy can prevent further spread of the cancer, sometimes for years, but it can rarely eliminate the cancer completely.

Fibroids

Common, noncancerous tumours that grow slowly within the muscular wall of the uterus

 Most common between the ages of about 30 and 50

 More common in women of Afro-Caribbean origin

 Lifestyle is not a significant factor

Fibroids are nonmalignant growths in the uterus that consist of muscular and fibrous tissue. Fibroids develop in about 1 in 3 women at some time during their life, most often between the ages of about 30 and 50. They are more common in women of Afro-Caribbean origin. Fibroids occur singly or in groups and may be as small as a pea or as big as a grapefruit. Small fibroids may not cause problems, but larger ones may affect menstruation or fertility (*see* **Female infertility**, p.497).

What is the cause?
The cause of fibroids is unknown, but they are thought to be related to an abnormal response by the uterus to the female sex hormone oestrogen. Fibroids do not occur before puberty (when the ovaries first begin to increase oestrogen production) and usually stop growing or shrink after the menopause. They also enlarge when there are increased levels of oestrogen, such as during pregnancy, although they do not seem to be affected by the combined contraceptive pill. In women who are taking hormone replacement therapy (p.605), fibroids do not shrink and may even continue to grow.

What are the symptoms?
Most small fibroids do not cause symptoms, but the common symptoms of larger fibroids include:
- Prolonged menstrual bleeding.
- Abdominal pain during periods (*see* **Dysmenorrhoea**, p.472).
- Heavy bleeding during periods (*see* **Menorrhagia**, p.471).

Heavy blood loss may lead to anaemia (p.271) Large fibroids may distort the uterus, which can sometimes result in infertility and possibly recurrent miscarriages (p.511) During pregnancy, a large fibroid may cause the fetus to lie in an abnormal position (*see* **Abnormal presentation**, p.517). Fibroids may also press on the bladder, causing a need to pass urine often, or on the rectum, causing back pain. Rarely, a fibroid may become twisted, resulting in sudden pain in the lower abdomen.

How are they diagnosed?
The doctor will perform an abdominal and internal pelvic examination to look for the presence of fibroids in your uterus. You may also have ultrasound scanning (p.135) of the uterus or a hysteroscopy (below), in which a viewing instrument is inserted into the uterus through the cervix. A sample of the fibroid may be removed during the hysteroscopy to check that the growth is not cancerous. Sometimes, fibroids show up on X-rays (p.131) that are taken for other reasons.

What is the treatment?
Small, symptomless fibroids often do not need treatment but should be checked regularly by your doctor to make sure that they have not grown. Fibroids that are causing symptoms may be treated with medication to relieve the symptoms, such as an IUS (p.30), tranexamic acid (*see* **Drugs that promote blood clotting**, p.583), nonsteroidal anti-inflammatory drugs (p.578), an oral contraceptive pill, or progestogen (a synthetic form of the hormone progesterone). If these are ineffective, medication to shrink the fibroids may be recommended. This is usually with drugs such as goserelin (*see* **Drugs for infertility**, p.604), which may sometimes be combined with hormone replacement therapy. Alternatively, ulipristal (more commonly used for emergency contraception, p.30) may be prescribed.

If medication has proved ineffective, removal of the fibroids may be advised. This may involve either conventional surgery or may be performed during a hysteroscopy (below) or by laparoscopy (p.476). Before the surgery, you may be given hormones that suppress oestrogen production to make the fibroids shrink. Alternative techniques that may sometimes be used include uterine artery embolization (cutting off the blood supply to the fibroids) and endometrial ablation (removal of the lining of the uterus). If you have persistent, large fibroids and do not want children, you may consider having a hysterectomy (opposite page). Removal of fibroids usually results in regained fertility, but the fibroids may recur.

Uterine polyps

Noncancerous growths that develop in the uterus or the cervix

 Most common between the ages of 30 and 50

 Not having had children is a risk factor

 Genetics is not a significant factor

Uterine polyps are painless growths that are attached to the cervix or to the inside of the uterus. The polyps may occur singly or in groups and vary in length up to about 3 cm (1 in). They are usually harmless, but may become cancerous in rare cases. Uterine polyps are common, especially in premenopausal women over the age of 30.

The reason why uterine polyps form is unknown, but they may develop on the cervix if it is already affected by cervical ectopy (p.480), in which the cells on the surface of the cervix are more delicate than usual. Polyps also sometimes form on the cervix following infection of the area. Women who have not had children are more likely to develop uterine polyps.

Symptoms of uterine polyps include a watery, bloodstained discharge from the vagina and bleeding after sexual intercourse, between periods, or after the menopause. Such bleeding may also be a sign of a more serious disorder, such as cancer of the cervix (p.481).

What might be done?
Your doctor will usually be able to see polyps that are on the cervix by looking at the cervix while holding your vagina open with an instrument called a speculum. If polyps in the uterus are suspected, further investigations will be arranged, such as ultrasound scanning (p.135) or hysteroscopy (below),

Treatment of polyps is usually quick and easy. Polyps on the cervix may be removed surgically during examination through the speculum, and uterine polyps can be removed during a hysteroscopy. Mild pain and slight vaginal bleeding are likely for a few days after surgery. Samples of tissue from the polyps are examined under a microscope to make sure that there are no cancerous cells. Uterine polyps may recur after treatment, and then further surgery is usually required.

Retroverted uterus

A usually harmless condition in which the uterus is tilted backwards

 Having had children is a risk factor

 Age and genetics are not significant factors

The uterus is normally inclined upwards and forwards. However, in about 1 in 10 women the uterus is tilted backwards, lying close to the rectum. This condition is known as a retroverted uterus and is a harmless variation of the normal position. There is often no cause for a retroverted uterus, although the condition may occur after childbirth or because an ovarian cyst (p.476) pushes the uterus backwards. A retroverted uterus could also be the result of pelvic inflammatory disease (p.475) or endometriosis (p.475) in which the uterus becomes adhered to the back part of the pelvis.

A retroverted uterus usually causes no symptoms and you may be unaware that you have the condition. It does not affect fertility, pregnancy, or childbirth.

What might be done?
Your doctor may be able to feel that the uterus is retroverted while carrying out a pelvic examination. If an underlying disorder is thought to be causing the condition, laparoscopy (p.476) may be performed to view the pelvis and abdominal cavity. If there is an underlying cause, such as a cyst, this may be treated, allowing the uterus to return to its normal position.

▶ **TEST AND TREATMENT**

Hysteroscopy

A hysteroscope is an instrument used to see inside the uterus. Hysteroscopy is used to diagnose disorders such as uterine fibroids and can be performed under general or local anaesthesia in an outpatient clinic. Minor surgery, such as the removal of fibroids, may also be carried out through the hysteroscope. The procedure usually lasts 15 minutes or less.

The procedure
After the hysteroscope is inserted into the vagina, the uterus is filled with gas or fluid passed through the hysteroscope. This allows it to be seen easily. Light provides a clear view.

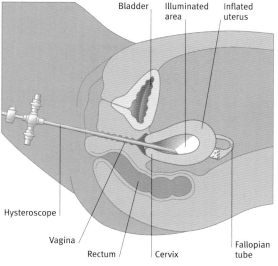

Bladder — Illuminated area — Inflated uterus — Hysteroscope — Vagina — Rectum — Cervix — Fallopian tube

VIEW

Polyp — Lining of uterus

Uterine polyp
This view of the uterus through a hysteroscope shows a polyp attached to the uterine lining.

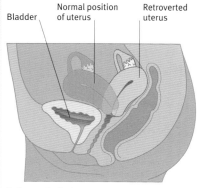

Bladder — Normal position of uterus — Retroverted uterus

Retroverted uterus
The uterus usually tilts forwards, resting close to and just above the bladder. A retroverted uterus tilts backwards so that it lies close to the rectum.

Prolapse of the uterus and vagina

Downward displacement of the uterus and/or wall of the vagina

 More common after the menopause

 Being overweight and having had children are risk factors

 Genetics is not a significant factor

The uterus and vagina are held in place by ligaments and muscles in the pelvis. If these supporting structures become weakened or stretched, often as a result of childbirth, the uterus and/or vaginal walls may be displaced downwards. This condition, called a prolapse, usually occurs after the menopause, when low levels of the hormone oestrogen lead to weakening of the ligaments. The risk of prolapse of the uterus and/or vagina is increased by conditions that put extra pressure on the muscles and ligaments in the pelvis, such as obesity, a persistent cough, or straining during bowel movements.

What are the types?
In uterine prolapse, the uterus moves down into the vagina. The amount of movement ranges from slight displacement into the vagina to projection of the uterus outside the vulva.

There are two main types of vaginal prolapse: cystocele and rectocele. In a cystocele, the bladder presses inwards against the weak front vaginal wall. In a rectocele, the rectum bulges against the weakened back vaginal wall. Both types of vaginal prolapse may occur together with or without uterine prolapse.

What are the symptoms?
The symptoms of any type of uterine or vaginal prolapse may include:
- A feeling of fullness in the vagina.
- A lump protruding into or even out of the vagina.
- A dragging sensation or mild pain in the lower back.
- Difficulty passing urine or stools.
- Passing urine more frequently.

A cystocele can cause leakage of urine when laughing or coughing (*see* **Stress incontinence**, p.454). It also increases the risk of an infection in the bladder (*see* **Cystitis**, p.453) because the bladder may not empty properly.

What might be done?
Your doctor may be able to see that you have a prolapse by looking at the position of the uterus and the walls of the vagina while using a speculum to hold the vagina open. He or she may ask you to cough or strain so that the prolapse can be assessed. A sample of urine may also be taken to check for infection.

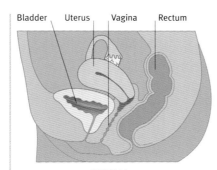

Bladder   Uterus   Vagina   Rectum

NORMAL

Cystocele   Rectocele   Prolapsed uterus

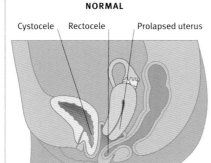

PROLAPSE

Prolapse of the uterus and vagina
In this prolapse, the uterus is displaced, the bladder bulges into the front vaginal wall (cystocele), and the rectum bulges into the back vaginal wall (rectocele).

Pelvic floor exercises (p.455), which strengthen the supporting muscles, can help prevent the condition from developing and should be continued indefinitely. Weight control, avoiding constipation (to avoid straining during bowel movements), and not smoking (to minimize coughing) will also reduce the likelihood of a prolapse. Some women may be offered treatment in which a plastic ring pessary is inserted into the vagina to help keep the uterus in place; the ring needs to be replaced every 6 months. Surgical techniques may also be used to treat a prolapse. The aim of surgery is to restore the uterus and/or the vagina to their normal positions. However, if a uterine prolapse is severe and surgical repositioning is not possible, you may be offered a hysterectomy (above, right) to completely remove the uterus.

Cancer of the uterus

A cancerous tumour that grows in the lining of the uterus

 Most common between the ages of 55 and 65

 Being overweight and not having had children are risk factors

 Genetics is not a significant factor

Cancer of the uterus is one of the most common cancers of the female reproductive organs in the UK, with 8,475 new cases diagnosed in 2011. Most uterine cancers develop in the endometrium (the lining of the uterus). More rarely, cancer occurs in the muscular wall of the uterus.

▶ **TREATMENT**

Hysterectomy

A hysterectomy is an operation in which the uterus is removed. There are two main types: in a total hysterectomy the uterus and cervix are removed; in a subtotal hysterectomy only the uterus is removed. Occasionally, the ovaries and fallopian tubes may also be removed. In all types, the operation is carried out under general anaesthesia. The operation may be performed through an incision in the abdomen (abdominal hysterectomy) or through the vagina (vaginal hysterectomy). Less commonly, a hysterectomy may be performed by "keyhole surgery" using a laparoscope (a viewing tube); this normally involves several small incisions in the abdomen through which the surgeon performs the operation. After a hysterectomy, you may have vaginal bleeding and some pain. You will need to stay in hospital for several days, and recovery may take 6–8 weeks, depending on your health.

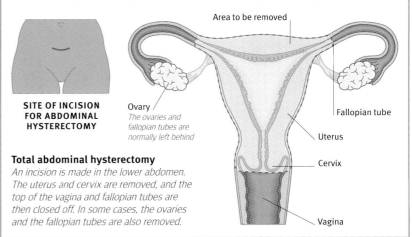

SITE OF INCISION FOR ABDOMINAL HYSTERECTOMY

Area to be removed

Ovary
The ovaries and fallopian tubes are normally left behind

Fallopian tube

Uterus

Cervix

Vagina

Total abdominal hysterectomy
An incision is made in the lower abdomen. The uterus and cervix are removed, and the top of the vagina and fallopian tubes are then closed off. In some cases, the ovaries and the fallopian tubes are also removed.

What are the causes?
The causes of cancer of the uterus are unclear. The disorder is more common in women aged 55–65 and in those who have or have previously had abnormally high levels of the female sex hormone oestrogen. Raised oestrogen levels may be caused by being overweight and by certain disorders, such as polycystic ovary syndrome (p.477). The disorder is also more likely in women who have had a late menopause (after the age of 52) or who have not had children.

What are the symptoms?
The symptoms of cancer of the uterus vary depending on whether it develops before or after the menopause. These symptoms may include:
- In premenopausal women, heavier than normal periods (*see* **Menorrhagia**, p.471) or bleeding between periods or after sexual intercourse.
- In postmenopausal women, vaginal bleeding that may vary from spotting to heavier bleeding.

Left untreated, cancer of the uterus may spread to the fallopian tubes and the ovaries and to other organs, including the lungs and sometimes the liver.

How is it diagnosed?
If your doctor suspects cancer from your symptoms, he or she will perform a pelvic examination. During the examination, a small sample of tissue may be taken from the endometrium to check for the presence of cancerous cells (*see* **Endometrial sampling**, p.473). Your doctor will also arrange for ultrasound scanning (p.135) to assess the thickness of the lining of the uterus. A thicker than normal lining may indicate cancer of the uterus.

If these tests are not conclusive, a hysteroscopy (opposite page) may be needed to remove a larger amount of tissue from the uterus. Samples of the endometrial tissue are then microscopically examined for cancerous cells. During the hysteroscopy, your doctor is also able to directly view the endometrium to check for any obvious abnormalities.

If cancer of the uterus is diagnosed, tests will be carried out to see if the cancer has spread. For example, you may have a chest X-ray (p.300) or MRI (p.133) of the pelvis and abdomen. You may also have blood tests to assess the function of the liver.

What is the treatment?
The treatment for cancer of the uterus depends on the stage at which the cancer is diagnosed and whether or not it has spread elsewhere in the body.

In most women, the tumour can be treated by a hysterectomy (above), in which the uterus, ovaries, and fallopian tubes are removed. In addition, samples from nearby pelvic lymph nodes are usually taken and examined under a microscope to see if the disease has spread and to check whether further treatment s required. Surgery is often followed by radiotherapy (p.158) to destroy any cancer cells that remain.

If cance-ous cells are found in the lymph nodes, you will be treated with chemotherapy (p.157) and the female hormone progesterone (see **Sex hormones and related drugs**, p.602), which slows down the growth of cancer cells. After treatment, you will have regular follow-ups to check for signs of cancerous changes in the pelvis.

The outlook for cancer of the uterus depends on whether the tumour is treated at an early stage before the condition has spread to other parts of the body. About 4 in 5 women who are treated when the cancer is at an early stage survive for 5 years or longer.

Choriocarcinoma

A cancerous tumour that develops from the placenta after a pregnancy

 Affects females of childbearing age

 Genetics and lifestyle are not significant factors

A choriocarcinoma is a rare cancerous tumour that occurs in 1 in every 50,000 pregnancies. The tumour develops from the placental tissue and usually arises from a noncancerous placental tumour called a hydatidiform mole (see **Molar pregnancy**, p.510). A choriocarcinoma may also occur after an ectopic pregnancy (p.511) or rarely after childbirth or termination of pregnancy (p.510) if some placenta cells remain. Occasionally, the tumour may not develop until months or even years after pregnancy. The main symptom is persistent vaginal bleeding. If left untreated, the tumour grows quickly, and the disease spreads first to the walls of the uterus and then to other organs such as the liver.

What might be done?

Choriocarcinoma is usually diagnosed by blood or urine tests to measure levels of the hormone human chorionic gonadotropin (HCG). HCG is normally produced by the placenta in pregnancy, but extremely high levels of the hormone are associated with a choriocarcinoma. Women who have had a molar pregnancy, and are therefore at particular risk of the disease, are given regular tests to measure the levels of HCG. Women who have had persistent bleeding after childbirth, a termination, or an ectopic pregnancy may also have their HCG levels checked. If HCG levels are found to be high, ultrasound scanning (p.135) will be carried out to look for a tumour. If choriocarcinoma is confirmed, further tests, such as CT scanning (p.132) of the abdomen and blood tests to assess liver function, may be arranged to check whether the disease has spread.

Choriocarcinoma is usually treated with chemotherapy (p.157), whether or not the disease has spread to other organs.

Rarely, a hysterectomy (p.479) may be necessary. Most women recover completely following treatment.

Cervical ectopy

Extension of cells that normally line the inside of the cervical canal or uterus on to the surface of the cervix

 More common after puberty

 Long-term use of oral contraceptives is a risk factor

 Genetics is not a significant factor

In cervical ectopy (formerly called cervical erosion), the layer of delicate cells that line the cervical canal or uterus extend on to the outer surface of the cervix, which is usually covered with stronger tissue. Because the cervix is covered with delicate tissue, it is more easily damaged than normal and has a tendency to bleed.

In many cases, there is no obvious reason for cervical ectopy, but the disorder may occur in association with long-term use of oral contraceptives or after the cervix has been stretched during childbirth. In most cases, cervical ectopy does not result in any obvious symptoms. However, a few women may notice increased vaginal discharge and bleeding between menstrual periods. A non-irritating discharge and bleeding may also occur after sexual intercourse.

What might be done?

Cervical ectopy is often detected during a routine cervical screening test (below). Treatment is usually not necessary, but if troublesome symptoms develop, the abnor-

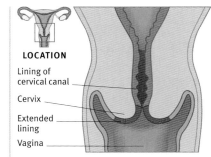

LOCATION
Lining of cervical canal
Cervix
Extended lining
Vagina

Cervical ectopy
In cervical ectopy, the delicate cells that line the inside of the cervical canal or uterus extend on to the surface of the cervix.

mal cells can be destroyed using a freezing technique called cryotherapy. The cells can also be treated with an electrical current, a technique known as diathermy, or by laser treatment (p.613). Following treatment, you may have a discharge for 2–3 weeks, and you will be advised to avoid sexual intercourse during this period. The disorder does not usually recur after treatment.

Cervical intraepithelial neoplasia (CIN)

Changes in the surface cells of the cervix that may become cancerous

 Most common between the ages of 25 and 35

 Unprotected sex at an early age, unprotected sex with multiple partners, and smoking are risk factors

 Genetics is not a significant factor

In some women, the cells of the cervix gradually change from normal to cancerous. The condition between these two extremes, when the cells are abnormal

and have the potential to become cancerous, is known as cervical intraepithelial neoplasia, or CIN (also sometimes called cervical dysplasia). There are three grades of CIN, depending on the severity of the changes in the abnormal cells: mild (CIN1), moderate (CIN2), and severe (CIN3). Mild CIN usually returns to a normal state by itself but moderate or severe CIN may progress to cancer of the cervix (opposite page) if not treated.

Many countries, including the UK, have screening programmes that check for CIN using the cervical screening test (below left). Regular testing to detect abnormal cells on the cervix helps to ensure that CIN is diagnosed and treated before abnormal cells become cancerous.

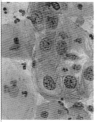 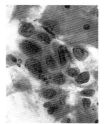
MILD CIN   SEVERE CIN

Cervical intraepithelial neoplasia (CIN)
These highly magnified images of cells taken from the cervix illustrate the degree of cell distortion that is present in mild and severe CIN.

What are the causes?

Not all of the causes of CIN have been identified, but the main cause is thought to be infection with certain strains of human papillomavirus (HPV). Risk factors for the development of CIN include smoking, and having unprotected sex at an early age and unprotected sex with many partners because these activities are associated with an increased risk of HPV infection.

How is it diagnosed?

CIN does not produce symptoms. Normally, the condition is only diagnosed after a cervical screening test, during which a sample of cells is taken from the cervix and sent for microscopic examination. If you are found to have abnormal cells, your doctor may arrange for you to have a colposcopy (opposite page), in which the cervix is viewed through a magnifying instrument to examine abnormal-looking areas. A small sample of tissue may be removed from the cervix for examination under the microscope.

What is the treatment?

If you are diagnosed with CIN, the treatment depends on the degree of abnormality of the cells. Mild CIN may not require treatment because the abnormal cells revert to normal in most cases. However, the disorder will be regularly monitored with cervical screening tests. If CIN persists or worsens, treatment to destroy or remove the abnormal cells will be needed (see **Treating CIN**, opposite page).

▶ **TEST**

Cervical screening test

Previously known as a cervical smear, a cervical screening test is a usually painless procedure used to detect abnormal cells on the cervix. The vagina is held open with a speculum, and cells are collected from the cervix using a brush. The cells are then sent for examination under a microscope. Women are advised to have regular screening, the interval between tests depending on the woman's age. More frequent tests may be advised if abnormal cells are detected. Early treatment of some cervical abnormalities helps to prevent cervical cancer (see **Treating CIN**, opposite page).

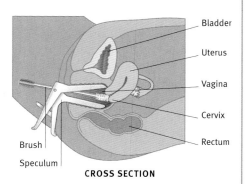
Brush
Speculum
Bladder
Uterus
Vagina
Cervix
Rectum
CROSS SECTION

RESULTS

Normal cervical cells
This highly magnified image shows cervical cells of regular shape and size. This pattern of cells indicates a normal test result.

▶ **TEST AND TREATMENT**

Colposcopy

A colposcope is a binocular viewing instrument used to magnify the cervix for examination. Colposcopy is often performed after an abnormal cervical screening test (p.480) to look for signs of CIN. During the procedure, which is painless and lasts for about 15–30 minutes, your doctor may paint solutions on to the cervix to highlight abnormal areas. A sample of cervical tissue may also be taken, or abnormal areas of the cervix may be treated (*see* **Treating CIN**, right).

During the procedure
You will need to put your legs in supports. The doctor uses an instrument called a speculum to open the vagina and allow the cervix to be seen with the colposcope.

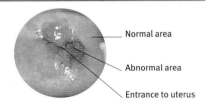

Colposcope　Leg support

Monitor
The view through the colposcope may be shown on a screen

VIEW

View of the cervix
Normal and abnormal areas of tissue can be seen on this cervix. The abnormal area close to the centre of the cervix proved to be due to moderate CIN (CIN2).

Normal area

Abnormal area

Entrance to uterus

The main methods of treatment are LLETZ (large loop excision of the transformation zone) and cone biopsy. After treatment, your condition will be monitored for the next few years to ensure that no further abnormalities develop.

Vaccination that protects against some of the strains of HPV is offered to all girls aged 12–13 as part of the routine immunization programme. However, vaccination does not protect against all strains of HPV and so regular cervical screening tests are still important to detect CIN at an early stage.

Cancer of the cervix

A cancerous growth occurring in the lower end of the cervix

 Most common between the ages of 25 and 65

 Unprotected sex at an early age, unprotected sex with multiple partners, and smoking are risk factors

 Genetics is not a significant factor

Cervical cancer is the 12th most common cancer in women in the UK, with about 3,100 new cases being diagnosed in 2011. It is one of the few cancers that can be largely prevented by regular screening before symptoms appear. The HPV (human papillomavirus) vaccine also helps to protect against the disease.

Cancer of the cervix usually develops slowly. In the precancerous stage, cervical cells gradually change from being mildly to extremely abnormal, a condition that is known as cervical intraepithelial neoplasia (opposite page). These changes in the cervical cells can be detected with the cervical screening test (opposite page), allowing treatment to be carried out before cancer develops.

What are the causes?
In almost all cases, the cause of cervical cancer is thought to be infection with certain strains of the human papillomavirus (HPV) as more than 99 per cent of cases of the cancer occur in women who have previously been infected with HPV. This virus is transmitted through unprotected sexual intercourse, and the risk of cervical cancer is increased if you have unprotected sex from an early age or with many partners. Smoking is also a risk factor for cervical cancer. Women who have reduced immunity or who are taking immunosuppressants (p.585) are at increased risk of developing cancer of the cervix.

▶ **TREATMENT**

Treating CIN

Mild CIN may not require treatment but more severe CIN or persistent mild CIN may need treatment to destroy or remove the area of abnormal tissue (the transformation zone). The main methods are LLETZ (large loop excision of the transformation zone) and cone biopsy. All treatments are carried out through the vagina, and it is usual to have slight bleeding or a discharge for a few days afterwards.

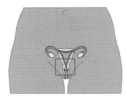

LOCATION

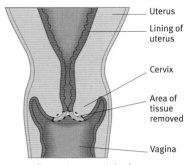

Uterus

Lining of uterus

Cervix

Area of tissue removed

Vagina

LLETZ (large loop excision)
This is used mainly when the abnormal tissue is localized around the opening of the cervix. It uses a heated wire loop to remove the abnormal tissue, and is usually done under local anaesthesia.

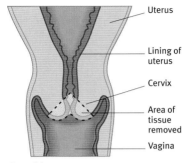

Uterus

Lining of uterus

Cervix

Area of tissue removed

Vagina

Cone biopsy
This method is used when the abnormal tissue extends in towards the uterus. In the procedure, done under either local or general anaesthesia, a larger cone-shaped area of the cervix is removed.

What are the symptoms?
Cancer of the cervix does not always cause symptoms. However, in some women, there may be abnormal vaginal bleeding, especially after sexual intercourse. As the cancer progresses, further symptoms may include:
■ A watery, bloodstained, and offensive-smelling vaginal discharge.
■ Pelvic pain.
Left untreated, cancer of the cervix may spread to the uterus and then to the lymph glands in the pelvis. Eventually, cancer may spread to other parts of the body, such as the liver and lungs.

How is it diagnosed?
If your doctor suspects that you have cancer of the cervix from your symptoms, he or she may perform a cervical screening test and should arrange for you to have a colposcopy (above left), in which the cervix is viewed through a magnifying instrument and checked for abnormal areas. A sample of tissue will probably be taken from the cervix during the procedure and later examined under a microscope for evidence of cancerous cells.

If cancer of the cervix is diagnosed, you may have further tests to see if the condition has spread to other parts of the body. These tests may include a chest X-ray (p.300) or MRI (p.133) of the chest to look at the lungs and blood tests and CT scanning (p.132) of the abdomen to assess liver function.

What is the treatment?
The treatment for cancer of the cervix depends on the stage of the disease and your individual circumstances.

If the cancer is at a very early stage, is confined to the cervix, and you would like to have children at a later date, it may sometimes be possible to remove only the cervix and upper part of the vagina; the uterus is then reattached to the remaining part of the vagina. However, in most cases a hysterectomy (p.479) is recommended. If the cancer is large, the tissues around the cervix, the top of the vagina, and the lymph nodes around the uterus, will also probably be removed. In women who are premenopausal, the ovaries are left if possible because they produce sex hormones and removing them causes premature menopause. If the cancer has spread to other organs in the body, radiotherapy (p.158) and/or chemotherapy (p.157), may be needed.

Hip joint　Bladder　Cancerous tumour

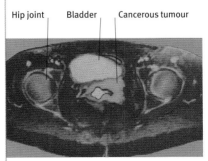

Cancer of the cervix
This colour-enhanced MRI through the pelvis shows a large cancerous tumour of the cervix lying just behind the bladder.

What is the prognosis?
If cervical cancer is diagnosed and treated at the earliest stage, about 95 per cent of women survive for at least 5 years

after diagnosis. Overall, of all women with cervical cancer, about 67 per cent survive for 5 years or more after diagnosis. In 2012, 919 women in the UK died from the disease.

Can it be prevented?

Routine cervical screening tests can help to ensure the early diagnosis and treatment of abnormal cervical cells and have greatly reduced the incidence of cervical cancer. In addition to having regular cervical screening, it is advisable to try to reduce the risk of developing cervical cancer by not smoking and by using barrier methods of contraception (p.28).

A vaccine is available to protect against the two strains of HPV that cause most cases of cervical cancer. The vaccine is offered to girls aged 12–13 as part of the routine immunization programme. However, this vaccine does not protect against all strains of the virus associated with cervical cancer and it is therefore important for girls who have been vaccinated to have regular cervical screening tests later in life.

Vulvovaginitis

Inflammation of the vulva and vagina, causing itching and soreness

 Age and lifestyle as risk factors depend on the cause

 Genetics is not a significant factor

Vulvovaginitis is a very common disorder affecting most women at some time during their life. In this condition, the vulva and the vagina become inflamed, itchy, and sore. There may also be pain during sexual intercourse and a discharge from the vagina. The condition can also affect children.

What are the causes?

Most cases of vulvovaginitis are caused by an infection, either with the fungus *Candida albicans*, which causes vaginal thrush (right), or with the protozoan *Trichomonas vaginalis*, which is the cause of the sexually transmitted infection trichomoniasis (p.492). Women with diabetes mellitus (p.437) have an increased risk of fungal vulvovaginitis. Overgrowth of the harmless bacteria that normally live in the vagina (*see* **Bacterial vaginosis**, right) may also lead to vulvovaginitis.

In some cases, the condition may be caused by irritation from perfumed bath products, detergents, deodorants, or contraceptive creams. Following the menopause, the disorder may develop as the vaginal tissues become thinner, drier, and more susceptible to irritation. These changes in the tissues of the vagina occur when levels of oestrogen fall.

In rare cases, vulvovaginitis may be the result of cancerous changes in the cells that line the surface of the vulva or the vagina (*see* **Cancer of the vulva and vagina**, opposite page).

In children, the cause of the disorder is often unclear. In some cases, a foreign body in the vagina or sexual abuse may be the cause.

What might be done?

Your doctor will take a swab from the inflamed area to look for an infection and to identify the causative organism. If you have repeated episodes of fungal vulvovaginitis, your urine may also be tested for glucose to exclude diabetes mellitus. If cancerous changes are suspected, a tissue sample will be taken and examined for abnormal cells.

Treatment of vulvovaginitis depends on the cause of the inflammation. If you have bacterial vaginosis, you will be prescribed antibiotics (p.572); if necessary, your sexual partner should also be treated to avoid reinfecting you. Hormone replacement therapy (p.605) or topical creams that contain oestrogen can relieve vulvovaginitis that is caused by low levels of oestrogen following the menopause. If vulvovaginitis is caused by a particular bath product, detergent, deodorant, or contraceptive cream, you should change to another product.

Your doctor will advise you to avoid sexual intercourse until your symptoms have cleared up. Most affected people recover completely after treatment, but the condition may recur.

Vaginal thrush

Inflammation of the vagina caused by infection with the candida fungus

 Most common in females of childbearing age

 Stress may trigger the condition

 Genetics is not a significant factor

Vaginal thrush affects many women at some point in their adult lives, most commonly at some time during the childbearing years, and can recur regularly. The condition develops when a fungus called *Candida albicans*, which can occur naturally in the vagina, grows more rapidly than usual. Vaginal thrush is not serious, but it may cause unpleasant itching of the vulva and vagina and a discharge. Candida infections may occur in other areas, such as the mouth (*see* **Oral thrush**, p.559) and around the anus.

What are the causes?

The candida fungus is found in the vagina of about half of all women and does not usually cause disease. The growth of the

SELF-HELP

Preventing vaginal thrush

If you often have vaginal thrush, the following self-help measures may help to prevent further episodes of infection:

- Wash the vaginal area with water only. Try to avoid using bath additives, perfumed soaps, or vaginal deodorants or douches, and do not wash inside the vagina.
- Avoid spermicidal creams, lubricants, and latex condoms if you find they irritate the vagina.
- Avoid scented sanitary towels or tampons, change tampons frequently, and use sanitary towels instead of tampons as often as possible.
- Keep your external genital area clean, dry, and cool. Wear cotton underwear and loose-fitting clothes if possible.
- If thrush seems to be triggered by stress, try to avoid stressful situations whenever possible.

fungus is suppressed by both the immune system and harmless bacteria that normally live in the vagina. If these bacteria are destroyed by antibiotics or spermicides, the fungus can multiply, which may lead to symptoms. Harmless bacteria in the vagina may also be destroyed as a result of changes in levels of female sex hormones. Such changes may occur during pregnancy or before periods or may be due to drugs that affect female sex hormone levels, such as the oral contraceptive pill. Vaginal thrush may also develop after having sexual intercourse with a partner who has a candida infection.

Women who have diabetes mellitus (p.437) are more susceptible to vaginal thrush. Sometimes, stress can trigger an episode of the condition.

What are the symptoms?

The symptoms usually develop gradually over several days and may include:

- Intense irritation and itching of the vagina and vulva (*see* **Vulvovaginitis**, left).
- Thick, white vaginal discharge that is cheesy in appearance.

Left untreated, vulvovaginitis may lead to redness and eventually cracking of the delicate skin of the vulva.

What can I do?

If you are confident that your symptoms are due to vaginal thrush because you have had the condition before, you can treat yourself with over-the-counter drugs. Antifungal drugs (p.574) are readily available and include vaginal pessaries and creams or pills. It is advisable not to have sexual intercourse for the next few days until your symptoms have cleared up. Your sexual partner should also be treated in order to avoid reinfection.

If you get vaginal thrush regularly, some simple measures can be taken to avoid the condition (*see* **Preventing**

vaginal thrush, left). If you are not sure about the cause of your symptoms or if treatment with over-the-counter preparations does not help, you should consult your doctor.

What might the doctor do?

Your doctor may diagnose thrush from the vaginal discharge. He or she will perform a pelvic examination and may take a swab from your vagina for examination. If vaginal thrush is diagnosed, your doctor may advise you on self-help measures or prescribe a stronger antifungal drug. Although treatment for vaginal thrush is usually successful, the condition tends to recur.

Bacterial vaginosis

Bacterial infection of the vagina that sometimes causes an abnormal discharge

 Can affect sexually active females of any age

 Unprotected sex with multiple partners is a risk factor

 Genetics is not a significant factor

Bacterial vaginosis is caused by excessive growth of some of the bacteria that normally live in the vagina, particularly *Gardnerella vaginalis* and *Mycoplasma hominis*. As a result, the natural balance of these organisms in the vagina is altered. The reason for this is unknown, but the condition is more common in sexually active women and often, but not always, occurs in association with sexually transmitted infections. Vaginal infections can also be caused by an excessive growth of the candida fungus (*see* **Vaginal thrush**, left) and the protozoan *Trichomonas vaginalis* (*see* **Trichomoniasis**, p.492).

Bacterial vaginosis often causes no symptoms. However, some women may have a greyish-white vaginal discharge with a fishy or musty odour and vaginal or vulval itching. The disorder may lead to pelvic inflammatory disease (p.475), in which some of the reproductive organs become inflamed.

What might be done?

Your doctor may be able to diagnose bacterial vaginosis from your symptoms. Swabs of any discharge may be taken and tested to confirm the diagnosis. Vaginosis is usually treated with antibiotics (p.572), either orally or as a gel or cream applied inside the vagina. Sexual partners should also be checked for infection and treated if necessary. Vaginosis usually clears up completely within a few days of starting treatment, but the condition does tend to recur.

Bartholinitis

Infection of one or both Bartholin's glands, located in the vulva, and/or of their ducts

 More common after puberty

 Poor hygiene and unprotected sex with multiple partners are risk factors

 Genetics is not a significant factor

Bartholin's glands are two pea-sized glands with ducts that open into the vulva. The glands produce a fluid that lubricates the genital area during sexual intercourse. In bartholinitis, one or both of the glands and/or their ducts become infected. In some cases, the disorder is caused by bacteria from faeces entering the glands as a result of poor hygiene. A sexually transmitted infection may also cause the condition. The condition causes swelling in the surrounding tissues and a painful abscess may develop. One or both ducts may also become blocked, causing a painless swelling called a Bartholin's cyst.

Your doctor will prescribe antibiotics (p.572) to treat bartholinitis, and the disorder should clear up within a few days. Painkillers (p.589) may help to relieve discomfort. An abscess may be drained under local anaesthesia. Bartholin's cysts are not usually removed unless they are very large or cause discomfort. Bartholinitis may recur.

Cancer of the vulva and vagina

Cancerous growths occurring on the vulva or in the vagina

 More common over the age of 60

 Unprotected sex at an early age, unprotected sex with multiple partners, and smoking are risk factors

 Genetics is not a significant factor

Cancers of the vulva and vagina are rare and usually affect women over the age of 60. They account for about 1 in 20 cancers of the female reproductive organs. Although these cancers do not usually occur together, they may both be associated with certain types of the human papillomavirus (HPV), which is sexually transmitted. Smoking may also be a risk factor. If not treated, these cancers may spread to the pelvic lymph nodes and to other parts of the body.

Cancer of the vulva may cause vulval itching, but often the first symptom is a hard lump or ulcer on the vulva. If the ulcer is not treated, it may produce an offensive, bloody discharge. Cancer of the vagina often causes no symptoms until the tumour is at an advanced stage, although bleeding and pain may occur after sexual intercourse. If you develop any of these symptoms, you should consult your doctor at once.

What might be done?

Your doctor may make a diagnosis of cancer of the vulva or vagina from your symptoms. A sample of tissue may also be removed from the affected area and examined to look for cancerous cells.

Cancer of the vulva is usually treated surgically by removing the affected area. The nearby lymph nodes are also usually removed and examined to see if the disease has spread and if further treatment is necessary. Radiotherapy (p.158) and/or chemotherapy (p.157) may also sometimes be used.

Cancer of the vagina is usually treated with radiotherapy. However, it may also be necessary to remove part of the vagina and the nearby lymph nodes. Chemotherapy may also sometimes be used to help control symptoms.

The outlook for both these cancers depends on whether they have spread. Overall, about 60 per cent of women with either type of cancer survive for at least 5 years after diagnosis.

Breast disorders

The breasts consist of fatty tissue that gives them their size and shape, lobules that secrete milk after childbirth, and milk ducts that carry the milk to the nipple during breast-feeding. The nipples are sensitive to touch and play a role in sexual arousal. Most disorders of the breasts are not serious, although breast cancer is becoming increasingly common.

Throughout life, the breasts change size and shape in response to varying levels of female sex hormones. The breasts usually enlarge during puberty, before periods, and during pregnancy and breast-feeding. This enlargement can be associated with breast pain and with generalized lumpiness.

This section opens with an overview of the causes of breast lumps, both normal and abnormal. Many women associate a breast lump with breast cancer, but in fact most lumps are noncancerous. Two of the common causes of noncancerous lumps in the breasts, fibroadenomas and breast cysts, are discussed next in this section.

The following articles cover breast pain, abnormalities in breast size, and problems that affect the nipples. The final article deals with breast cancer. Since early diagnosis of this disease significantly improves the chances of long-term survival, this section includes information about screening for breast cancer and how to examine your breasts so that abnormalities are detected as soon as possible.

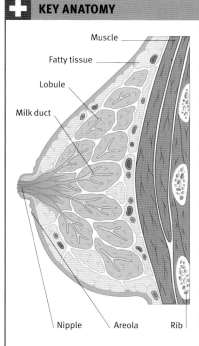

KEY ANATOMY

- Muscle
- Fatty tissue
- Lobule
- Milk duct
- Nipple
- Areola
- Rib

For more information about the structure and function of the breast, *see* pp.467–470.

Breast lumps

Any masses or swellings that can be felt in the breast tissue

 Age, genetics, and lifestyle as risk factors depend on the cause

Breast lumps are a common problem. Many women notice generalized breast lumpiness, especially when the breasts enlarge during puberty and pregnancy and before menstruation. This generalized lumpiness is a variation in normal breast development and does not increase the risk of breast cancer. A single, discrete breast lump may cause concern, but in fact only about 1 in 10 breast lumps is due to cancer.

What are the causes?

Generalized lumpiness, often associated with breast tenderness, is thought to be related to the hormonal changes that occur during the menstrual cycle. The lumpiness usually becomes worse just before a period; the worsening may be due to oversensitivity of the breast tissue to female sex hormones at this time.

A discrete lump is often a fibroadenoma (p.484). This noncancerous lump is caused by overgrowth of one or more breast lobules (the structures that produce milk). Breast cysts (p.484) are fluid-filled sacs in the breast tissue. There may be one or more cysts, and both breasts may be affected. Sometimes, a breast lump is caused by an infection that has developed into an abscess. A breast abscess may develop if mastitis (p.523) is not treated, and may be associated with inflammation and localized pain. A lump may also be a symptom of breast cancer (p.486).

What might be done?

You should become familiar with the appearance and feel of your breasts so that you can recognize any changes (*see* **Breast awareness**, p.484). Consult your doctor promptly if you notice a new lump, a change in an existing lump, or any other change described in the box.

Your doctor will probably give you a physical examination and refer you to a breast clinic. At the clinic you will usually undergo a triple assessment: examination by a doctor; breast imaging by ultrasound scanning (p.135) and/or mammography (p.487); and fine-needle aspiration (p.484) and/or a core biopsy of the lump. In a fine-needle aspiration, a sample of cells is taken and examined microscopically for cancerous cells. In a core biopsy a sample of tissue is taken and examined for cancerous cells.

Generalized breast lumpiness tends to decrease after the menopause but may continue if you take hormone replacement therapy (p.605). Most noncancerous lumps do not need treatment, although breast cysts usually need to be drained. Modern screening techniques and treatment mean that breast cancer can often be diagnosed early and treated successfully. If a breast tumour is found, further treatment will be planned.

Fibroadenoma

A firm, round, noncancerous growth in the breast tissue

 Most common between the ages of 15 and 30

 Genetics and lifestyle are not significant factors

A fibroadenoma is an overgrowth of a breast lobule (the part of the breast that produces milk) and the surrounding connective tissue. Although the cause of this condition is not fully understood, the development of a fibroadenoma is thought to be linked to the sensitivity of breast tissue to female sex hormones. Fibroadenomas tend to grow more quickly during pregnancy, probably because of the increased levels of female sex hormones during this period. Fibroadenomas are most common in women aged between 15 and 30.

Fibroadenomas are usually painless. These lumps can develop in any part of the breast and can be up to about 6 cm (2½ in) in size. There may be more than one lump and sometimes both breasts are affected. In some women, multiple fibroadenomas develop together with a generalized thickening of the breast tissue.

It is important to become familiar with your breasts so that you can recognize any abnormal changes (*see* **Breast awareness**, right). Fibroadenomas are harmless but you should consult your doctor promptly if you detect any new lump so that the possibility of breast cancer (p.486) can be investigated.

What might be done?

Your doctor will probably give you a physical examination and refer you to a breast clinic. At the clinic you will usually undergo triple assessment: examination by a doctor; breast imaging by ultrasound scanning (p.135) and/or mammography (p.486); and fine-needle aspiration (right) and/or a core biopsy of the lump.

In a fine-needle aspiration, a sample of cells is taken from the lump and examined microscopically for the presence of cancerous cells. In a core biopsy, a sample of tissue is taken from the lump and examined for cancerous cells.

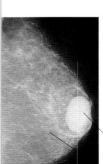

Fibroadenoma
A fibroadenoma can be seen as a large pale area in the breast tissue in this mammogram (breast X-ray).

Fibroadenoma

Normal breast tissue

Small fibroadenomas do not usually need treatment. About 1 in 3 fibroadenomas become smaller or disappear completely within 2 years. If you are worried about the fibroadenoma, or if it grows larger, surgical removal may be recommended. After removal, the lump will be examined under a microscope for the presence of cancerous cells. In most cases, fibroadenomas do not recur after treatment.

Breast cyst

A firm, round, fluid-filled swelling within the breast tissue

 Most common between the ages of 30 and 50

 Genetics and lifestyle are not significant factors

A breast cyst is a firm, round lump in the breast tissue that forms when a lobule (the part of the breast that produces milk) fills with fluid. The development of cysts is influenced by levels of female sex hormones. Breast cysts most often affect women aged 30–50, particularly those approaching the menopause.

A cyst may be felt just under the skin or may occur deeper within the breast tissue. Cysts are usually not painful, although some can be and the pain can come on suddenly.

Breast cysts may occur singly, but in about half of all cases there is more than one cyst, and both breasts may be affected. Some women also have generalized lumpiness of the breast tissue.

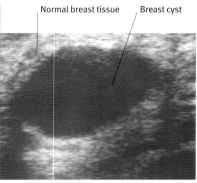

Normal breast tissue   Breast cyst

Breast cyst
This ultrasound scan of a breast shows a fluid-filled breast cyst, visible as a dark area within the breast tissue.

You should always consult your doctor if you detect a lump so that the possibility of breast cancer (p.486) can be investigated. In rare cases, cancerous cells may be found in the wall of a cyst.

What might be done?

If your doctor suspects a cyst, he or she may refer you to a breast clinic, where you may have a physical examination and breast imaging by ultrasound scanning (p.135) or mammography (p.486).

The usual treatment is to drain the cysts of fluid (*see* **Fine-needle aspiration of a breast lump**, below), which may then be examined for cancerous cells. Cysts usually disappear after aspiration but may recur, requiring further drainage. If cysts recur frequently, they may be removed surgically, but this is not usually necessary.

▶ **TEST AND TREATMENT**

Fine-needle aspiration of a breast lump

Aspiration of a breast lump is used as a diagnostic procedure to detect breast cancer and as a treatment for fluid-filled breast cysts. If aspiration confirms that a breast lump is solid tissue, a sample of cells is withdrawn and examined under a microscope for evidence of cancer. If the lump is a cyst, the fluid will be drained and the lump should disappear. If it does not disappear, a cell sample will be taken and examined, as for a solid lump. Aspiration may be uncomfortable but usually takes only a few seconds.

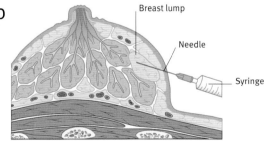

Breast lump

Needle

Syringe

CROSS SECTION

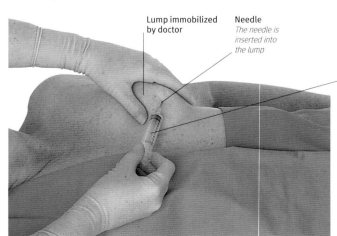

Lump immobilized by doctor

Needle
The needle is inserted into the lump

Syringe
The syringe is used to withdraw cells and/or fluid from the lump

During the procedure
The doctor immobilizes the breast lump with one hand and inserts a needle attached to a syringe into the lump. Cells or fluid are then withdrawn through the needle for analysis.

RESULTS

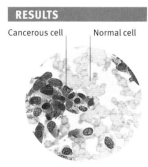

Cancerous cell   Normal cell

Cells withdrawn from a breast lump
In this sample of cells, both normal and cancerous cells are visible. The cancerous cells have large nuclei.

Breast pain

Pain or discomfort usually affecting one or both breasts

 Most common between the ages of 15 and 50

 Genetics and lifestyle as risk factors depend on the cause

Breast pain is an extremely common problem. In most women, the pain is cyclical, varying in severity in response to the hormonal changes of the menstrual cycle. This cyclical pain is usually most severe before periods and tends to affect both breasts.

Cyclical breast pain affects as many as 1 in 2 women and is commonly a long-term problem. Women who experience cyclical breast pain frequently also have generalized breast lumpiness, which tends to become worse before a period. The pain may be aggravated by stress, caffeine in certain drinks, and smoking.

In some women, breast pain is not related to menstruation. Possible causes of noncyclical breast pain include muscle strain or a breast cyst (opposite page). It may also be due to inflammation of, or an abscess in, the breast tissue caused by an infection (*see* **Mastitis**, p.523) or engorgement of the breasts with milk after childbirth (*see* **Breast engorgement**, p.522). Sometimes, the cause of breast pain is not known. Only very rarely is it due to breast cancer. If you have large breasts, you are more likely to suffer from both cyclical and noncyclical breast pain.

What might the doctor do?

Your doctor will ask you about your breast pain to see if there is a pattern. He or she will examine your breasts to look for an underlying cause, such as a breast cyst, or any tender areas in the surrounding muscles. If it is apparent from the consultation and examination that you do not have an underlying disorder, your doctor may ask you to keep a record of when you experience breast pain to help to confirm that the pain is cyclical. If your doctor suspects that an underlying disorder may be causing the pain, he or she will probably refer you to a breast clinic for mammography (p.486) and/or ultrasound scanning (p.135) to look for any abnormalities in the breast tissue.

Mild cyclical pain does not normally require treatment. However, in about 1 in 10 women, the pain is so severe that it can interfere with everyday life. In such cases, your doctor may prescribe danazol, a drug that reduces the effects of female sex hormones acting on the breast (*see* **Sex hormones and related drugs**, p.602). Although this drug is effective in relieving pain, it can have side effects such as acne and weight gain. Cyclical breast pain tends to diminish following the menopause. If you are taking hormone replacement therapy (p.605), the pain may continue after the menopause, but it often improves after a few months.

If your breast pain is noncyclical, the cause will be treated if necessary. Cysts are usually drained (*see* Fine-needle aspiration of a breast lump, opposite page), and antibiotics (p.572) can be used to treat infection. Nonsteroidal anti-inflammatory drugs (p.578) may help to relieve muscle pain.

What can I do?

Breast pain may be eased by wearing a bra that supports your breasts properly. If your breasts are heavy and the pain is severe, you may need to wear a bra at night. Pain may be relieved by cutting down on caffeine, stopping smoking, practising relaxation exercises (p.32) to help to control stress, and losing weight to reduce the size of the breasts.

Various complementary remedies have been advocated for the treatment of cyclical breast pain, but there is no conclusive evidence that they are effective.

Abnormality of breast size

Abnormally large, small, or asymmetrical breasts

 Develops during puberty

 Genetics and lifestyle are not significant factors

There is considerable variation in breast size among women. A slight asymmetry in the size of the breasts in an individual woman is also common. However, having abnormally large, small, or asymmetrical breasts can lead to emotional distress and, in the case of very large breasts, may cause pain (*see* **Breast pain**, left) and discomfort.

Breasts that grow abnormally large often develop rapidly during puberty and are thought to be the result of oversensitivity of the breast tissue to the female sex hormone oestrogen. Large breasts may lead to pain in the back, shoulders, and neck, and in some cases a skin infection may develop in the fold under the breast. Women who have abnormally large breasts may experience discomfort when running or playing sports. They may also have difficulty in finding clothes that fit.

In some women, the breasts develop to only a very small size. A woman who has very small breasts may find her appearance unfeminine. However, having small breasts does not cause any physical problems and does not affect a woman's ability to breast-feed.

Occasionally, there is a marked difference in size between the two breasts because one breast develops more than the other at puberty. This asymmetry may cause embarrassment and anxiety.

What might be done?

Women with large breasts can benefit from a well-fitting, supportive bra. You may also find that wearing a bra at night

▶ TREATMENT

Breast reduction

Breast reduction operations relieve the discomfort of very large, heavy breasts. The procedure takes place under general anaesthesia and involves a short hospital stay. During the operation, some skin and breast tissue are removed, and the breast is reshaped. The nipple and areola (the dark area around the nipple) may be moved up and made smaller. After surgery, your breasts will be smaller and firmer. The scarring is usually minimal and is mostly hidden under the breast. However, sensation in the nipple will be reduced, and breast-feeding will not be possible.

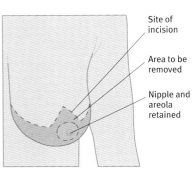

Site of incision

Area to be removed

Nipple and areola retained

1 *A substantial area of skin and tissue is removed from the lower part of the breast. The nipple and areola are retained, along with the blood vessels and some of the nerves that supply the area.*

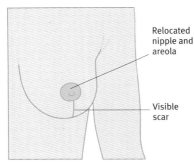

Relocated nipple and areola

Visible scar

2 *The nipple and areola are repositioned higher up, and the V-shaped part of the incision is sewn together below it. The remaining skin edges are rejoined under the breast and are not visible.*

makes you feel more comfortable. If this does not relieve your discomfort or distress, you may wish to consider the possibility of a surgical operation to permanently reduce the size of your breasts (*see* **Breast reduction**, above).

Women who have small breasts may find that a padded bra improves their body shape under clothes. However, the only permanent way to enlarge small breasts is by surgically inserting an implant behind the breast tissue. Breast implants consist of a flexible silicone shell filled either with silicone gel or with saline (a sterile salt water solution).

Some women who experience distress as a result of having abnormally large, small, or asymmetrical breasts may find counselling (p.624) of benefit.

Abnormal nipples

Change in the appearance of a nipple or the area around it (areola)

 Age, genetics, and lifestyle as risk factors depend on the cause

There are two main types of nipple abnormality: retraction into the breast (nipple inversion) and disorders affecting the skin on or around the nipple. Although these abnormalities are most often caused by minor problems that are easily treatable, any changes in the condition of the nipples should receive medical attention because, in rare cases, they may indicate breast cancer (p.486).

What are the causes?

Inversion of the nipples may occur during puberty if the breasts do not develop properly. This type of inversion is usually harmless, although it may later make breast-feeding difficult. Nipple inversion may also occur as a result of inflammation of the milk ducts behind the nipple. This condition most often affects nonpregnant women who smoke. Changes in the structure of the breasts as they age may cause the nipple to be drawn into the breast in older women. Less commonly, nipple inversion that develops in adulthood may be due to breast cancer.

Many women develop fine cracks and tender areas on their nipples during the first few weeks of breast-feeding (*see* **Cracked nipples**, p.523). These cracks are most often the result of the baby not taking the whole nipple into his or her mouth properly when feeding. Leaving the nipples wet after a feed can also cause them to become sore and cracked. Cracked nipples often cause stabbing or burning pain as the baby starts or stops feeding and may become infected, causing inflammation of the breast tissue (*see* **Mastitis**, p.523).

Dry, flaky patches of skin that occur on or around both nipples may be due to eczema (p.193). Eczema is usually itchy and tends to occur in several sites on the body. However, occasionally, skin changes on the nipples that resemble eczema are in fact caused by Paget's disease of the breast, a rare form of cancer that originates in the milk ducts. Unlike eczema, Paget's disease rarely develops on both nipples and does not heal. This type of breast cancer often causes soreness and bleeding from the nipple. It may also cause a breast lump, although if diagnosed early enough, a breast lump is unlikely to have developed when the diagnosis is made.

What might be done?

Your doctor will examine your breasts, and if nipple inversion has occurred in adulthood but is not related to breast-feeding, may refer you to a breast clinic, where you may have ultrasound scanning (p.135) or mammography (opposite page) to look for breast abnormalities. If a breast lump is found, cells or fluid may be taken from it (*see* **Fine-needle aspiration of a breast lump**, p.484) and examined for cancer cells. A skin sample may also be tested for cancer cells.

Occasionally, it is possible to correct nipple inversion that has been present since puberty by gently drawing the nipples out between your thumb and forefinger every day for several weeks. Suction devices, such as nipple shells, which are temporarily worn in your bra, can also help to draw out the nipple. There is also a simple surgical procedure to correct inverted nipples but it is not always successful and may also damage the milk ducts so that breast-feeding becomes impossible.

If your nipples have become cracked, washing and drying them carefully and applying a moisturizer may help. Make sure that you wash the moisturizer off before breast-feeding. You should also avoid plastic-lined breast pads, which may become damp and encourage infection. Infection is usually treated with antibiotics (p.572), and eczema can be improved by hydrocortisone cream (*see* **Topical corticosteroids**, p.577).

If cancer of the breast is discovered, you will be referred for additional tests and treatment (*see* **Breast cancer**, right).

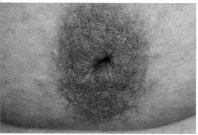

Inverted nipple
This nipple has become drawn into the breast (inverted), which may be due to shortening of the milk ducts with age.

Nipple discharge

Discharge of fluid from one or both nipples

Age, genetics, and lifestyle as risk factors depend on the cause

It is normal for women to release milk from their nipples during late pregnancy and while breast-feeding. At any other time, a nipple discharge may be due to hormonal changes in the menstrual cycle or a symptom of a minor disorder. However, because the condition may be a sign of a more serious disorder,

such as breast cancer (right), you should see your doctor if you notice an unusual discharge, if the discharge is bloodstained, or if you are at all concerned.

What are the causes?

The main causes of nipple discharge are hormonal changes, enlargement of the mammary ducts, infection within the breast, or, more rarely, a breast tumour. Fluid discharged from the nipples can vary considerably in colour and consistency, and its appearance is not always a good indication of the cause.

Hormonal changes Changes in the levels of female sex hormones may produce a discharge, usually from both nipples, just before a period. This type of discharge is usually clear and watery.

A watery, milky discharge in women who are not pregnant or breast-feeding is known as galactorrhoea. This may be a result of overproduction of prolactin, a hormone produced by the pituitary gland. The condition may be due to a noncancerous tumour of the pituitary gland, called a prolactinoma (p.430), or may be an effect of a hormonal disorder such as hyperthyroidism (p.432). Some drugs, including some antipsychotics (p.592), can cause galactorrhoea as a side effect.

Mammary duct enlargement In this condition, known medically as mammary duct ectasia, one or more milk ducts under the areola become enlarged and may produce a discharge, which may sometimes be bloodstained. The cause is not known, but the condition is more common in older women, particularly those who smoke.

Breast infection In breast-feeding women, blocked milk ducts may become infected and produce a discharge of pus from the nipples (*see* **Mastitis**, p.523). In nonbreast-feeding women, smoking may be associated with inflammation of the milk ducts, producing a pus-containing nipple discharge. This is most common in women under 40. Mastitis may also occur for no obvious reason.

Breast tumours A bloodstained discharge from the nipple may be a symptom of cancer, although, more commonly, this type of discharge is the result of a noncancerous tumour (called a papilloma) forming within a duct.

What might be done?

Your doctor will carry out a physical examination of your breasts. He or she may take a sample of the discharge to be examined for evidence of infection or cancerous cells. X-rays of the breast (*see* **Mammography**, opposite page) and ultrasound scanning (p.135) may be performed. A blood sample may also be taken to measure hormone levels.

In most cases, a discharge that is caused by mammary duct enlargement does not need treatment. In rare cases your doctor may recommend surgery to remove the affected duct or ducts, which usually stops the discharge. A discharge due to normal hormonal changes is usually harmless and does not require treatment. Galactorrhoea

can often be treated successfully using drugs, such as cabergoline (*see* **Pituitary drugs**, p.603), which reduce the production of prolactin by the pituitary gland. If galactorrhoea is due to a tumour in the pituitary gland, surgery and radiotherapy (p.158) may be required. A discharge of pus usually clears up after treatment with antibiotics (p.572). A bloodstained discharge caused by a noncancerous tumour (papilloma) of a milk duct is normally treated by surgical removal of the duct.

If initial tests reveal that your nipple discharge has been caused by a cancerous growth in the breast, you will be referred for further tests and treatment.

Breast cancer

A cancerous growth that originates in the breast

 Risk increases with age

 In some cases, due to an abnormal gene

 Obesity, smoking, and delaying or avoiding pregnancy are risk factors

Breast cancer is the most common cancer in the UK, with about 49,900 women being diagnosed with the disease in 2011. It can also occur in men, although it is rare, with about 350 cases being diagnosed in the UK in 2011.

The risk of breast cancer is negligible under the age of 30 and then increases with age, doubling every 10 years; 8 out of 10 cases are diagnosed in women over the age of 50. Overall, about 1 in 8 women will develop the disease during their lifetime. The number of cases diagnosed each year in the UK has been increasing since the mid-1970s. However, there has been a drop in the number of deaths from breast cancer in recent years, and now about 8 in 10 women who receive treatment for the disease survive for at least 10 years after diagnosis. The improved survival rate is due to better treatment and the increased use of mammography (opposite page) to screen for breast cancer, which means that tumours can be detected early, when they usually respond well to treatment. Early treatment also reduces the likelihood of the cancer spreading to other parts of the body. Screening reduces the number of breast cancer deaths in women over the age of 50, and in the UK all women aged 50–70 are offered a mammogram every 3 years.

What are the causes?

The underlying cause of most breast cancers is unclear. However, some risk factors have been identified, many of which suggest that the female hormone oestrogen is an important factor in the development of the disease. Many cancerous breast tumours are oestrogen-sensitive, and oestrogen encourages them to grow once they have formed. Women who have their first

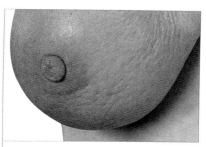

Appearance of the skin in breast cancer
A cancerous growth in this breast has caused the skin to become swollen with fluid, giving an "orange peel" appearance.

period before the age of 11 or who have a late menopause seem to be at increased risk of developing breast cancer, probably because their breasts are exposed to oestrogen for longer. Similarly, the number of menstrual cycles before a first pregnancy has some influence on the risk of breast cancer; for example, a woman who never has children is about twice as likely to develop breast cancer as a woman who has her first child before the age of 20. Breast-feeding has an additional protective effect.

Obesity increases the risk of breast cancer because excess body fat causes an increase in oestrogen levels. Artificial oestrogen in some medications may also influence susceptibility to breast cancer. Combined oral contraceptive pills slightly increase the risk of developing breast cancer. Hormone replacement therapy (p.605) in postmenopausal women is associated with a significant increase in risk, especially if it is continued for more than 10 years.

In a small minority of cases, breast cancer is linked to an inherited abnormal gene, and several of these genes have now been identified (notably the BRCA1, BRCA2, TP53, and PTEN genes). The risk of developing breast cancer increases the more close relatives have had breast or ovarian cancer before age 40 and also the younger the affected relatives were when they were diagnosed with either of the cancers. (If close relatives have had breast or ovarian cancer after age 40, the risk is only slightly increased.) However, in the majority of cases there is no family history of the disease. Noncancerous breast lumps do not increase the risk of developing breast cancer.

What are the symptoms?

It is very unusual for breast cancer to produce symptoms in its early stages. When symptoms do occur, they usually affect only one breast and may include:

- A lump in the breast, which is usually painless and may be situated deep in the breast or just under the skin.
- A lump or swelling in the armpit.
- A change in breast shape or size.
- Dimpling of the skin in the area of the lump, or swelling of the skin with an "orange peel" appearance.
- A rash around the nipple.

- A change in the appearance of the nipple, such as becoming inverted.
- An unusual nipple discharge, which may contain blood.

In Paget's disease of the breast, a rare form of breast cancer that originates in the milk ducts, the only symptom may be a patch of dry, flaky skin on the nipple, although there is also soreness and bleeding from the nipple (*see* **Abnormal nipples**, p.485).

Although these symptoms may result from noncancerous conditions, you should consult your doctor if you notice a change in your breasts. If breast cancer is not treated early, it can spread to the lymph nodes in the armpit and then to other organs, such as the lungs, liver, or bones.

How is it diagnosed?

You should become familiar with your breasts so that you can recognize any abnormal changes (*see* **Breast awareness**, p.484). Screening using mammography enables tumours to be detected before symptoms have appeared. Although this procedure is reliable, it may not detect every case and it is therefore important that you remain breast-aware even after a normal mammogram. Mammography may also produce a false-positive result; that is, it may indicate cancer when cancer is not, in fact, present. For this reason, if mammography does produce a positive result, further tests are done to check.

If you visit your doctor because you have noticed a lump or other abnormality of your breast, he or she will carry out a breast examination and check for signs of spread to the lymph nodes in the armpit. If your doctor finds a lump or other sign that might indicate breast cancer, he or she will refer you to a breast clinic. At the clinic you will usually undergo triple assessment: a physical examination by a specialist; breast imaging by ultrasound scanning (p.135) and/or mammography (below); and a fine-needle aspiration (p.484) and/or core biopsy. In a fine-needle aspiration, a sample of cells is taken from the lump; in a core biopsy, a sample of tissue is taken. The cells or tissue are then examined microscopically for the presence of cancer.

If the diagnosis of cancer is confirmed, further tests may be performed to find out whether the cancer is sensitive to oestrogen and if it has spread. A chest and abdominal CT scan (p.132) will be arranged to look for evidence of spread to the lungs, liver, and/or other organs, and a bone scan (*see* **Radionuclide scanning**, p.135) may be carried out to see if the bones have been affected. An MRI scan (p.133) of the breasts may also be performed to accurately assess the extent of the cancer in the breast, especially in young women whose breasts are too dense for adequate mammographic assessment.

What is the treatment?

The extent of the cancerous growth within the breast, whether it has spread to other parts of the body, and whether it is oestrogen-sensitive are the main considerations when deciding on the most appropriate course of treatment. Once a full assessment has been made, your doctor will discuss your treatment options with you. Treatment of breast cancer may include surgery, radiotherapy, chemotherapy, hormone therapy, immunotherapy, or, most frequently, a combination of these. Counselling may help you to come to terms with cancer, and some complementary therapies can be used to promote a sense of well-being. While you are undergoing treatment, you will be allocated a key person (often a breast-care nurse) who will be your main contact with the medical team looking after you.

Surgery Surgery is normally the first stage of breast cancer treatment. There are many possible types of operation used to treat breast cancer (*see* **Surgery for breast cancer**, p.488).

If the tumour is small, a lumpectomy (also known as a wide local excision) may be carried out, in which the tumour and about 1 cm (½ in) of surrounding tissue are removed. This is almost always followed by radiotherapy. In some cases, it may be necessary to have a second operation if sufficient tissue was not removed on the first occasion.

In some cases, all of the tissue from the affected breast is surgically removed in a procedure known as a mastectomy. Some women choose to have a mastectomy because they think that this is the only way to make sure all of the tumour has been removed but medical studies have shown that this operation is not necessary for treating most single, small breast tumours.

For some breast cancers, a type of chemotherapy called neo-adjuvant chemotherapy may be given before surgery. The main benefit of this treatment is to shrink the tumour so that it becomes small enough for breast-conserving surgery rather than requiring a mastectomy. However, not all tumours are suitable for this type of chemotherapy.

During surgery, a number of lymph nodes from the armpit on the same side as the affected breast will be removed and examined to look for signs of cancer, a procedure known as a sentinal node biopsy. If the lymph nodes are found to be free of cancerous cells, the cancer is unlikely to have spread from the tumour site and it will not be necessary to remove further lymph nodes. If the nodes do show signs of cancer, this indicates that the cancer has spread and the remaining lymph nodes will need to be removed, a procedure called axillary node clearance.

Surgery will affect the appearance of your breast. If one breast looks smaller after surgery, you may want to have the other breast reduced to the same size (*see* **Breast reduction**, p.485). After a mastectomy, many women have a breast reconstruction. The breast may be reconstructed using a silicone implant, tissue from another part of the body (such as the abdomen or back), or a combination of both. Breast reconstruction can either be performed at the same time as the mastectomy or at a later date.

Radiotherapy Treatment with radiotherapy (p.158) is given to almost all women after lumpectomy, regardless of the size of the tumour. It may also be used after a mastectomy if the removed tumour was growing close to the underlying muscle or the skin, or if the cancer is a fast-growing type or has spread to more than 1 or 2 lymph nodes. Treatment usually begins 1 or 2 months after surgery and is given 5 days a week for a period of 3 or 4 weeks. The aim is to destroy any cancer cells that may remain after surgery.

Drug treatments Tumours that are oestrogen-sensitive usually respond to drugs that block the action of oestrogen (endocrine therapy), whereas cytotoxic chemotherapy (p.137) can be effective for many other types of tumour. Treatment with synthetic forms of substances made naturally in the body called monoclonal antibodies (known as immunotherapy or biological therapy) can be useful in the treatment of breast cancer in which the cancer cells are of a particular type. Often a combination of drug therapies is used.

Endocrine therapy inhibits the effects of oestrogen, with the result that oestrogen-sensitive tumours shrink or do not

---

▶ **TEST**

Mammography

A mammogram is an X-ray of the breast and is used to screen for signs of breast cancer and to investigate lumps. Mammograms can show benign or precancerous tumours as well as malignant ones but may not detect every case of breast cancer. For this reason, it is important to examine your breasts regularly. You should have routine mammograms from the age of 50 because the risk of developing breast cancer increases with age. The procedure is often uncomfortable but lasts only a few minutes. Two X-rays are usually taken of each breast.

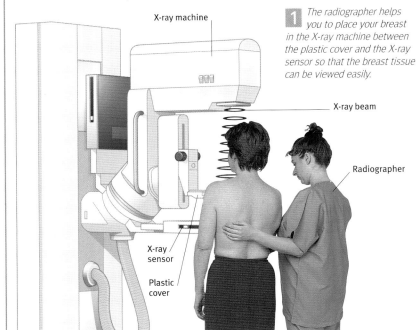

X-ray machine

X-ray beam

Radiographer

X-ray sensor

Plastic cover

1 *The radiographer helps you to place your breast in the X-ray machine between the plastic cover and the X-ray sensor so that the breast tissue can be viewed easily.*

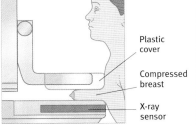

Plastic cover

Compressed breast

X-ray sensor

2 *The breast is firmly compressed between the plastic cover and the X-ray sensor. X-rays pass through the breast and on to the sensor.*

RESULTS

Cancerous growth

Normal breast tissue

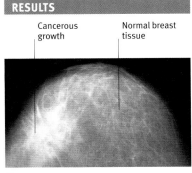

Mammogram
In this X-ray image, a tumour is visible within the breast. The tumour is denser than normal breast tissue and appears opaque on the X-ray.

grow as quickly. Tamoxifen (*see* **Sex hormones and related drugs**, p.602) is an oestrogen-inhibitor that is used mainly to treat breast cancer in premenopausal women, although it may also be used in some postmenopausal women; it is also effective in preventing breast cancer in women at increased risk. It is usually taken for 5 years. Drugs known as aromatase inhibitors also inhibit oestrogen production but are effective only in postmenopausal women.

Cytotoxic chemotherapy involves using combinations of drugs that destroy rapidly dividing cancerous cells. Treatment is usually given at intervals of 3–4 weeks over a period of 4–6 months. In most cases, cytotoxic chemotherapy is used in addition to surgery. These drugs can also kill normal cells, and commonly cause side effects such as hair loss and mouth ulcers.

Biological therapy is a form of chemotherapy that uses synthetic monoclonal antibodies (such as Herceptin) to boost the body's immune response to cancer cells. It is given for at least a year and generally has fewer side effects than other chemotherapy drugs. However, it is only effective against specific types of cancer cells, and it is not suitable for women who have certain heart or circulatory problems.

Complementary therapies Women with breast cancer may choose to complement conventional treatments with other therapies, such as relaxation exercises (p.32), meditation, homeopathy, or acupuncture. These therapies should not be regarded as alternatives to conventional treatment. If you are considering using complementary therapies, you should consult your doctor. Counselling (p.624), in which people are encouraged to express their feelings, may also be helpful in coping with cancer.

What is the prognosis?
If breast cancer is diagnosed before it has spread to other organs, treatment is very likely to be successful. Combinations of treatments usually give the best results, and the success rate of treatment has improved dramatically in recent years. Following treatment, you will have follow-up examinations at the hospital and annual mammograms to check for a recurrence of the disease. About 1 in 4 women treated for breast cancer has a recurrence within 5 years, usually those who had advanced cancer when they were first diagnosed. Cancer may recur close to the site of the original tumour or in a different area, and any recurrence requires further treatment.

Overall, about 8 in 10 women who receive treatment for breast cancer survive for more than 10 years after diagnosis, and more than 6 in 10 women survive for 20 years or more.

▶ **TREATMENT**

Surgery for breast cancer
The aim of surgery is to remove all cancerous tissue. The procedure varies depending on the size and position of the tumour. Two operations are described here: lumpectomy (also known as wide local excision), commonly used to treat small tumours; and mastectomy, sometimes used to treat larger or multiple tumours. The surgeon will also remove some lymph nodes from the armpit. These are checked to *see* whether the cancer has spread.

Lumpectomy
In a lumpectomy, the small area of breast tissue containing the tumour is removed, along with a small number of lymph nodes from the armpit. This procedure takes place under general anaesthesia. After the operation, the shape of the breast remains essentially unchanged.

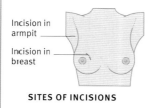

Incision in armpit

Incision in breast

SITES OF INCISIONS

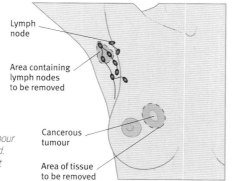

Lymph node

Area containing lymph nodes to be removed

Cancerous tumour

Area of tissue to be removed

During the procedure
An incision is made in the breast. The tumour and some surrounding tissue are removed. Some of the lymph nodes from the armpit are removed through a separate incision.

Mastectomy
In a mastectomy, the whole breast is removed. This operation is used to treat large or multiple cancerous breast tumours. The procedure takes place under general anaesthesia, and you will need to stay in hospital for several days. You may choose to have plastic surgery to reconstruct your breast at the same time as you have the mastectomy or at a later time.

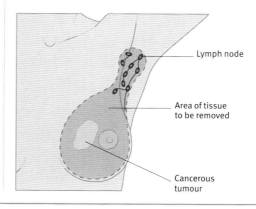

Lymph node

Area of tissue to be removed

Cancerous tumour

SITE OF INCISION

During the procedure
A single incision is made, through which are removed the tumour, all of the breast tissue, and, if necessary, all of the lymph nodes in the armpit. A scar is left on the chest.

Sex and reproduction

In biological terms, the urge to reproduce is one of the strongest basic drives. Producing a new generation to ensure the continuation of the species fulfils one of the primary functions of the human body. However, in humans, sexual intercourse is not only the means by which males and females reproduce but also an outlet for emotional expression. A sexual relationship can therefore play an important role in creating and maintaining the bond between partners.

ALL LIVING ORGANISMS maintain their populations by reproduction. Most simple organisms, such as bacteria, reproduce asexually, usually by cell division, resulting in offspring that are genetically identical.

In humans, reproduction is sexual, involving the fusion of two cells: a sperm and an egg. Eggs are produced by the ovaries in women, and sperm are produced by the testes in men. These cells are normally brought into contact through sexual intercourse. If a sperm succeeds in fertilizing an egg, DNA (genetic material) from each parent combines to create a unique individual.

Sexual reproduction results in an infinite variety of offspring. The only exceptions are identical twins, which develop when a fertilized egg divides equally to produce two individuals with the same genetic make-up.

Human sexuality

In many animals, the urge to reproduce is largely instinctive, but, in humans, many social and psychological factors also significantly influence sexuality and reproduction. Changing social attitudes towards sexual behaviour in the last few decades have enabled both men and women to express their sexual needs more freely to each other.

Sex drive varies widely between individuals of both sexes and ranges from a complete lack of sexual interest to very powerful urges. The ease with which sexual arousal can be achieved also varies between individuals.

Human beings are probably unique among animals in seeking to engage in sexual intercourse as a pleasurable experience separate from the act of reproduction. Most people have a preference for a sexual partner of the opposite sex (heterosexual). Others have a preference for members of the same sex (homosexual), and some individuals experience attraction to members of either sex (bisexual).

Fertility

Reproduction depends on an egg being fertilized and embedding in the uterus of the woman. Sexual behaviour and fertility affect the likelihood that these events will occur. If a fertile man and a woman at the fertile stage of her menstrual cycle have sex without contraception, a sperm has about a 1 in 5 chance of fertilizing an egg.

With medical advances, the process of reproduction can increasingly be controlled. Couples can choose to prevent conception by using a form of contraception. On the other hand, if a couple is unable to conceive naturally, conception can be assisted in a number of different ways.

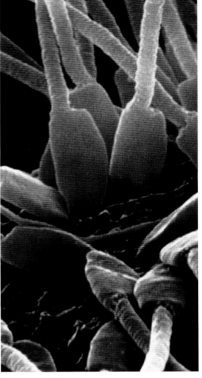

Sperm meet egg
Many sperm attempt to penetrate the surface of an egg to fertilize it.

➕ **FUNCTION**

Sexual response

Sexual thoughts, the sight of a partner's body, and foreplay all contribute to sexual arousal. Excitement makes breathing quicken, heart rate increase, and blood pressure rise. In a male, the penis becomes firm and erect. In a female, the labia and clitoris swell, the vagina lengthens and becomes lubricated, and the breasts enlarge. The time taken for sexual arousal varies between men and women.

Phases of sexual arousal
In men, sexual excitement rises rapidly to reach a plateau; in women, arousal is more gradual. In both sexes, arousal peaks at orgasm, which may not occur simultaneously, and wanes in the resolution phase.

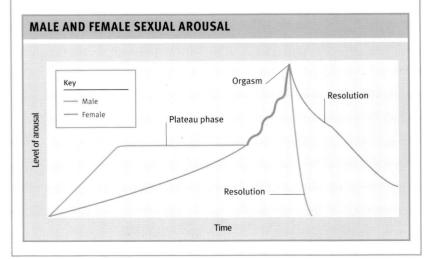

MALE AND FEMALE SEXUAL AROUSAL

Key
— Male
— Female

Orgasm
Resolution
Plateau phase
Resolution

Level of arousal

Time

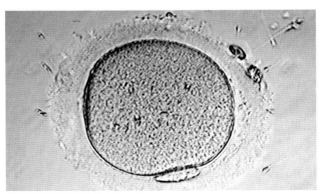

Unfertilized egg
This highly magnified image shows a human egg surrounded by several, much smaller sperm, just before fertilization.

✚ **FUNCTION**

Sexual intercourse

When a couple is sexually aroused
(*see* **Sexual response**, p.489),
the man's penis becomes erect and the
woman's vagina is lubricated. During sexual
intercourse, also called coitus, the penis
is inserted into the vagina and the man
begins thrusting pelvic movements.
At orgasm, which the partners may
experience simultaneously or at different
times, intense, pleasurable sensations
spread throughout the body. The woman's
vaginal walls contract rhythmically and
the man ejaculates, releasing sperm.

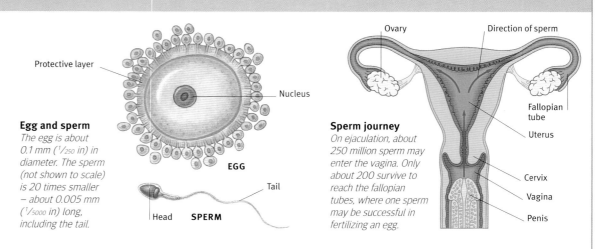

Egg and sperm
*The egg is about
0.1 mm ($^1/_{250}$ in) in
diameter. The sperm
(not shown to scale)
is 20 times smaller
– about 0.005 mm
($^1/_{5000}$ in) long,
including the tail.*

Sperm journey
*On ejaculation, about
250 million sperm may
enter the vagina. Only
about 200 survive to
reach the fallopian
tubes, where one sperm
may be successful in
fertilizing an egg.*

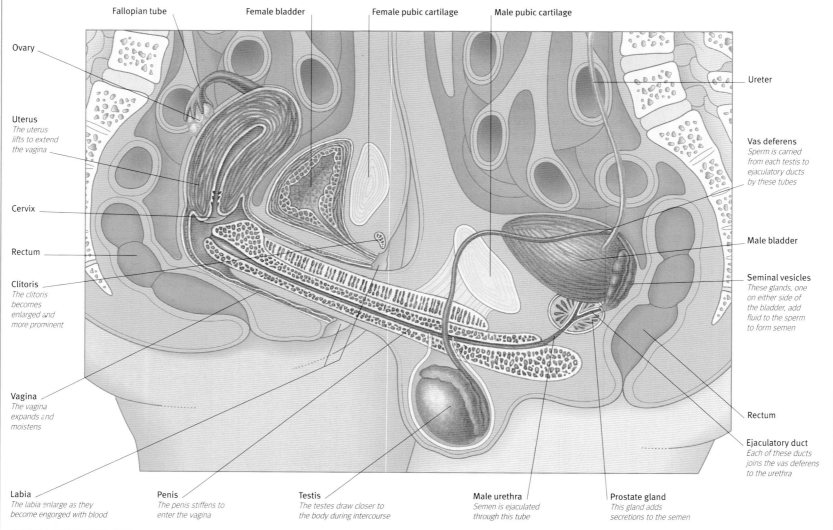

Ovary

Uterus
*The uterus
lifts to extend
the vagina*

Cervix

Rectum

Clitoris
*The clitoris
becomes
enlarged and
more prominent*

Vagina
*The vagina
expands and
moistens*

Labia
*The labia enlarge as they
become engorged with blood*

Penis
*The penis stiffens to
enter the vagina*

Testis
*The testes draw closer to
the body during intercourse*

Male urethra
*Semen is ejaculated
through this tube*

Prostate gland
*This gland adds
secretions to the semen*

Fallopian tube

Female bladder

Female pubic cartilage

Male pubic cartilage

Ureter

Vas deferens
*Sperm is carried
from each testis to
ejaculatory ducts
by these tubes*

Male bladder

Seminal vesicles
*These glands, one
on either side of
the bladder, add
fluid to the sperm
to form semen*

Rectum

Ejaculatory duct
*Each of these ducts
joins the vas deferens
to the urethra*

✚ **FUNCTION**

Fertilization

Fertilization, which can only occur when the woman is ovulating
(*see* **Menstrual cycle**, p.469) takes place in one of the fallopian
tubes. Many sperm reach the egg and try to penetrate its outer
covering. If a sperm succeeds, its head enters the egg and its tail is
then shed. A membrane then rapidly forms around the egg, creating
a barrier to prevent other sperm from entering. Fertilization occurs
when the head of the sperm fuses with the nucleus of the egg.

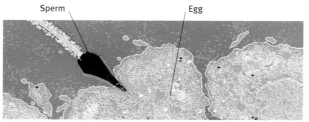

Sperm penetrating egg
*The head of the sperm
pushes through the egg's
outer coating in order to
reach the nucleus.*

Sexually transmitted infections

Sexually transmitted infections (STIs) are infections that are passed primarily from person to person during sexual activity. Many people delay seeking medical help for STIs because of embarrassment, but early diagnosis often prevents complications. Most STIs can be treated successfully with drugs.

The diseases covered in this section are grouped according to the type of organism that causes them. The first few articles discuss bacterial infections such as gonorrhoea. The protozoal infection trichomoniasis is then described, and the following articles deal with viral infections, such as genital warts. The final article looks at parasitic infestation with pubic lice.

Early treatment of STIs is essential because some, such as chlamydial infection, may cause infertility. Sexually active people who change their partners should have tests because some STIs may not cause symptoms, and many people are unaware that they have an STI. Syphilis, a progressive and once fatal disease, can now usually be

fully cured if it is treated in its early stages. STIs such as genital herpes and genital warts can often recur. Some types of genital wart virus increase the risk of cancer of the cervix. Pregnant women with an STI must carefully follow their recommended treatment because STIs can pass to the baby during pregnancy or in the birth canal during childbirth.

HIV infection and AIDS (p.169) and certain forms of hepatitis (pp.408–409) are viral infections that can also be transmitted by sexual contact.

The risk of contracting STIs can be reduced by using the safe sex practices, covered here and in detail elsewhere (see **Sex and health**, pp.27–30).

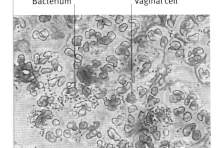
Bacterium   Vaginal cell

Cells infected by gonorrhoea bacteria
The vaginal cells in this image have been infected by Neisseria gonorrhoeae, *the bacterium that causes gonorrhoea.*

What might be done?

If you suspect that you or your partner has gonorrhoea, go to a clinic specializing in STIs or to your doctor. To confirm the diagnosis, a swab will be taken from areas that are likely to be infected and tested for the bacteria. You will also have tests for other STIs, such as chlamydial infection. Gonorrhoea is treated with antibiotics (p.572) and usually clears up in 3–4 days. If bacteria have spread throughout the body, treatment with intravenous antibiotics in hospital is necessary. All sexual partners should be tested and offered treatment.

Can it be prevented?

You can take steps to reduce your risk of contracting gonorrhoea (see **Preventing STIs**, right). If you are infected, avoid sex until you and your partner have finished treatment and your doctor says that you are free of infection.

SELF-HELP

Preventing STIs

There are several safe sex measures that you can follow to reduce the risk of acquiring an STI:

- Avoid sex with multiple partners.
- In a new sexual relationship, you or your partner should use a condom.
- If you use lubricants, use water-based types; oil-based lubricants damage the rubber in condoms.
- Avoid sexual activity that may split a condom or sex that causes breaks in the skin or the tissues of the vagina or anus.

If you suspect that you or your partner has an STI, you should both consult an STI clinic or a doctor. Complete your course of treatment and avoid sexual contact until your doctor confirms that you are free of infection (see **Sex and health**, pp.27–30).

the protozoan *Trichomonas vaginalis*, which also causes trichomoniasis (p.492); and the fungus *Candida albicans*, which can cause candidiasis (p.177). The viruses that cause genital warts (p.493) and genital herpes (p.493) can also result in NGU. Often, no cause is found.

What are the symptoms?

About 1–6 weeks after you have become infected with NGU, the following group of symptoms may develop:

- Pain on passing urine, especially the first time in the morning.
- Discharge from the penis.
- Redness and soreness at the opening of the urethra.

If you have any of these symptoms, you should go to a clinic specializing in STIs or consult your doctor.

Are there complications?

Various complications may result from NGU, including inflammation of the prostate gland (see **Prostatitis**, p.463), symptoms of which include pain at the base of the penis and frequent, painful urination. Occasionally, the testes and the epididymides (the tubes carrying sperm from the testes) become inflamed (see **Epididymo-orchitis**, p.459). The infection may trigger an immune response that causes inflammation of the joints (see **Reactive arthritis**, p.224).

What might be done?

Your doctor will take a swab from your urethra, together with a urine sample, to check for the presence of an infectious organism that could cause NGU. Tests for other STIs will probably be carried out at the same time.

Depending on the organism found, your doctor may then prescribe antibiotics (p.572), antifungal drugs (p.574), or antiviral drugs (p.573). With treatment, NGU usually clears up in about a week; however, it sometimes returns, and treatment may need to be repeated. You can also be

---

Gonorrhoea

A bacterial infection that causes genital inflammation and discharge

 Can affect sexually active people of any age

 More common in males

 Unprotected sex with multiple partners is a risk factor

 Genetics is not a significant factor

The bacterium *Neisseria gonorrhoeae* (gonococcus), which causes gonorrhoea, can be transmitted by various forms of sexual contact, including vaginal, oral, and anal sex. The infection is usually confined to the site where the bacteria enter the body, such as the vagina or the mouth, but can spread through the bloodstream to other parts of the body. A baby who is exposed to the infection in the birth canal during delivery may develop neonatal ophthalmia, a severe eye infection that can cause blindness.

Gonorrhoea is one of the most common sexually transmitted infections in the UK, with more than 32,000 new cases in 2013. It is more common in young adults, although it can affect sexually active people of any age, and males are more commonly affected than females.

What are the symptoms?

Gonorrhoea often causes no symptoms. If symptoms occur, they usually appear 1–14 days after sex with an infected person. In men, they may include:
- Discharge of pus from the penis.
- Pain on passing urine.

Without treatment, the symptoms may start to disappear after about 2 weeks, but the person remains infectious.

About 1 in 2 infected women has symptoms, which may include:
- Yellowish-green discharge of pus from the vagina.
- Pain on passing urine.
- Lower abdominal pain.
- Irregular vaginal bleeding.

In both sexes, if gonorrhoea occurs as a result of anal intercourse, the anus and the rectum may become inflamed (see **Proctitis**, p.422), but usually there are no symptoms. If the infection has been transmitted during oral sex, the first symptom may be a sore throat.

Are there complications?

Gonorrhoea in men can lead to inflammation of the testes and epididymides (the tubes that carry sperm from the testes), a condition called epididymo-orchitis (p.459). Gonorrhoea may also result in inflammation of the prostate gland (see **Prostatitis**, p.463) or of the bladder (see **Cystitis**, p.453). Rarely, the disorder results in urethral stricture (p.455), scarring and blockage of the urethra (the tube from the bladder) that causes difficulty in passing urine.

In women, the infection may spread from the vagina to the fallopian tubes and cause pelvic inflammatory disease (p.475). Left untreated, the disorder increases the risk of ectopic pregnancy (p.511) and can also make women infertile (see **Female infertility**, p.497).

Occasionally, gonorrhoea spreads in the bloodstream, causing fever, rash, and, rarely, infection of the joints (see **Septic arthritis**, p.225).

Nongonococcal urethritis

Inflammation of the urethra in men that may be caused by several different organisms

 Can affect sexually active males of any age

 Affects men. Women can carry the infection

 Unprotected sex with multiple partners is a risk factor

 Genetics is not a significant factor

Inflammation of the male urethra (the tube leading from the bladder to the tip of the penis) that is not due to the bacterium causing gonorrhoea (left) is known as nongonococcal urethritis (NGU). Worldwide, NGU is one of the most common sexually transmitted infections (STIs) in men.

What are the causes?

About half of all cases of NGU are due to a bacterium, *Chlamydia trachomatis*, which can also infect the female reproductive organs (see **Chlamydial pelvic infection**, p.492). NGU can also be due to the bacterium, *Ureaplasma urealyticum*;

reinfected if your sexual partner has the disease. Sexual partners must be tested and treated even if they have no symptoms because in women the infection causes pelvic inflammation, which can lead to infertility (*see* **Female infertility**, p.497).

Can it be prevented?
The risk of contracting NGU can be reduced by following safe sex measures (*see* **Preventing STIs**, p.491). To avoid spreading the infection, it is important that you do not have sexual contact until you and your partner have finished your treatment and your doctor confirms that you are no longer infected.

Chlamydial pelvic infection

An infection of the genital tract in women that is usually symptomless

 Can affect sexually active women of any age

 Affects women. Men can carry the infection

 Unprotected sex with multiple partners is a risk factor

 Genetics is not a significant factor

The bacterium *Chlamydia trachomatis* is the most common sexually transmitted infection (STI) in the UK, with about 236,000 new cases in 2013. In women, the most common site of infection is the cervix, and the bacterium can cause serious inflammation of the reproductive organs. In men, chlamydial infection is the most common cause of nongonococcal urethritis (p.491). A baby exposed to chlamydial infection during delivery may develop conjunctivitis (p.355), an inflammation of the membrane covering the white of the eye and the inside of the eyelids, and lung infections such as pneumonia (p.299).

What are the symptoms?
Most women are symptom-free, but if symptoms do occur, they may include:
■ Abnormal vaginal discharge.
■ Bleeding between periods or after sex.
■ Frequent urge to pass urine.
■ Pain in the lower abdomen.
■ Pain on deep penetration during sex.
Left untreated, chlamydial infection can spread from the cervix to the fallopian tubes (*see* **Pelvic inflammatory disease**, p.475), and is a common cause of infertility in women. The infection sometimes triggers a form of arthritis (*see* **Reactive arthritis**, p.224).

What might be done?
Chlamydial infection may not be suspected until symptoms develop or a partner is tested for an STI. It may also be suspected during investigations for infertility, which can be a complication of untreated infection. For this reason, screening is important for

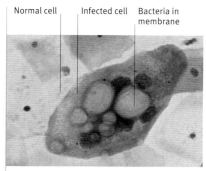

Normal cell · Infected cell · Bacteria in membrane

Cervical cell infected by chlamydia
The magnified view of a cervical specimen shows an infected cell in which chlamydia bacteria are enclosed within a membrane.

sexually active women at high risk, including those who have been treated previously for an STI or who have multiple partners.

If you think that you or your partner has a chlamydial infection, you should go to a clinic that specializes in STIs or consult your doctor. In women, diagnosis is confirmed by a urine test or by taking a swab from the cervix or vagina. Treatment is with antibiotics (p.572). Even if symptom-free, partners should also be tested and, if necessary, treated.

Can it be prevented?
You can reduce your risk of infection by following safe sex measures (*see* **Preventing STIs**, p.491). If you and/or your partner is infected, you should abstain from sexual contact until treatment has been completed.

Syphilis

A bacterial infection initially affecting the genitals that, left untreated, can damage other parts of the body years later

 Can affect sexually active people of any age

 Unprotected sex with multiple partners is a risk factor

 Gender and genetics are not significant factors

Syphilis is caused by the bacterium *Treponema pallidum*. This organism enters the body through the mucous membranes of the genital area or the skin. Left untreated, the disease may be fatal.

Syphilis was once a widespread disease throughout the world but became less common with the introduction of penicillin in the 1940s. Today, it rarely reaches its most advanced stage. A rise in incidence in homosexual men in the 1960s and 1970s was reversed by safe sex practices to combat HIV in the 1980s. The incidence fell very low, but has since risen again, from about 140 new cases in the UK in 1995 to about 3,500 new cases in 2013.

A pregnant woman with syphilis can pass the disease to the fetus, causing it to develop congenital syphilis (*see*

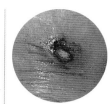

Chancre on penis
In primary stage syphilis, a hard, painless sore, called a chancre, appears. It usually develops on the genitals.

Congenital infections, p.530). However, screening during pregnancy has now made congenital syphilis very rare.

What are the symptoms?
The symptoms of syphilis develop in three stages. The primary and secondary stages are infectious for up to 2 years. The tertiary stage is not infectious.

Primary stage Within 1–12 weeks of infection, the following may develop:
■ Hard, painless, and highly infectious sore known as a chancre. The chancre usually appears on the penis or vulva but may occur in the mouth or rectum as a result of oral or anal sex.
■ Painless enlargement of the lymph nodes in the groin or neck.
The chancre may go unnoticed and disappears after 1–6 weeks.

Secondary stage About 6–24 weeks after the appearance of the chancre, the following symptoms may develop:
■ Nonitchy, infectious rash over the whole body, including the palms of the hands and soles of the feet.
■ Thickened, grey or pink, moist, wartlike patches in the skin folds of the genitals and anus.
■ In rare cases, patchy hair loss.
■ Fever and tiredness.
■ Headaches and muscle pain.
After about 4–12 weeks, these symptoms disappear, and the disease then enters a symptomless stage of indefinite length.

Tertiary stage Some people remain without further symptoms for the rest of their lives. However, if treatment is not given, tertiary syphilis may develop 10–20 years after the initial infection. The symptoms vary and may include changes in personality; mental illness; meningitis (p.325); tabes dorsalis (destruction of the spinal cord), which causes weakness and difficulty in walking; and aortic aneurysm (p.259).

What might be done?
If you think you or your partner has syphilis go to a clinic specializing in STIs or consult your doctor. In the primary stage, you may have a swab of the chancre taken for microscopic examination. Diagnosis of both primary and secondary syphilis may be confirmed by a blood test. At the same time you will probably be tested for other STIs. If tertiary syphilis is suspected, a lumbar puncture (p.326) may be carried out to look for antibodies to the bacterium in the cerebrospinal fluid.

Syphilis is treated with injections of antibiotics (p.572). In the primary or secondary stages, treatment usually results in complete recovery. Damage due to tertiary syphilis may be permanent.

Can it be prevented?
The risk of contracting syphilis is reduced by taking safe sex measures (*see* **Preventing STIs**, p.491). If you have the disease, or your partner has it, avoid sexual contact until you have both finished your treatment and your doctor confirms that you are free of infection.

Trichomoniasis

A genital tract infection that may cause inflammation and a discharge in women or, less commonly, in men

 Can affect sexually active people of any age

 Unprotected sex with multiple partners is a risk factor

 Gender and genetics are not significant factors

Trichomoniasis is an infection caused by the protozoan *Trichomonas vaginalis*. In women, this infection may cause vulvovaginitis (p.482), inflammation in and around the vagina, which may lead to a profuse vaginal discharge and to cystitis (p.453). In men, the infection may cause mild inflammation of the urethra (the tube from the bladder to the outside of the body) and occasionally results in nongonococcal urethritis (p.491). In most cases, trichomoniasis is a sexually transmitted infection, but an infected pregnant woman may pass the infection to her baby, which may cause the baby to be born prematurely or to have a low birth weight.

What are the symptoms?
Some women have no symptoms, and the infection may only be detected on a routine cervical screening test (p.480). If symptoms do occur, they may include:
■ Profuse, yellow, frothy, and offensive-smelling discharge from the vagina.
■ Painful inflammation of the vagina.
■ Itching and soreness of the vulva (the skin around the vagina).
■ Burning sensation on passing urine.
■ Discomfort during intercourse.
Men usually have no symptoms but, if present, they may include:
■ Discomfort on passing urine.
■ Discharge from the penis.
If you or your partner develop any of these symptoms, go to a clinic specializing in STIs or consult your doctor.

What might be done?
Swabs will be taken from infected areas and tested for the presence of the protozoan. You will probably be tested for other STIs at the same time. If you have trichomoniasis, you will be prescribed antibiotics (p.572). Sexual partners should also be tested and treated, even if they have no symptoms. Babies who are born infected do not normally need treatment as the infection usually clears up by itself.

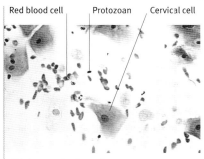

Trichomoniasis protozoan
This magnified image of cells from the cervix shows the presence of Trichomonas vaginalis, *the protozoan responsible for causing trichomoniasis.*

Can it be prevented?
You can reduce your risk of contracting trichomoniasis by practising safe sex (*see* Preventing STIs, p.491). If you or your partner have been infected, you should avoid spreading the infection further by abstaining from sexual contact until you have both finished your course of drug treatment and your doctor has confirmed that the infection has cleared up completely.

Genital herpes

A viral infection that causes painful blisters on and around the genitals that can recur

 Can affect sexually active people of any age

 Unprotected sex with multiple partners is a risk factor

 Gender and genetics are not significant factors

Genital herpes is caused by the herpes simplex virus, of which there are two forms, known as type 1 (HSV-1) and type 2 (HSV-2). Genital herpes is usually due to type 2; type 1 mainly causes blisters around the mouth (*see* Cold sore, p.205). However, HSV-1 can be transmitted from the mouth to the genitals during oral sex, producing genital herpes. In England, there were about 32,200 new cases of genital herpes in 2013.

The disease can recur, especially in the first few years after the initial attack. In women, it tends to recur 5–12 days before a period and to clear up in a few days. Subsequent attacks are milder, but still infectious. A pregnant woman with genital herpes should inform her midwife of the fact because, very rarely, the infection causes serious illness in a baby exposed to it during birth (*see* Congenital infections, p.530)

What are the symptoms?
The first attack of genital herpes is usually the most severe and occurs within about 5 days of contact with an infected person. The symptoms may include:
- Painful, fluid-filled blisters on the genitals. Blisters may occur on the thighs and buttocks and, rarely, in the mouth or rectum due to oral or anal sex.

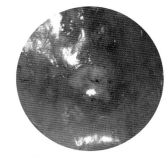

Genital herpes
The fluid-filled blisters shown in this close-up of a penis are caused by the genital herpes virus.

- Tingling, burning, soreness, and redness of the affected area.
- Enlarged and painful lymph nodes in the groin.
- Pain on passing urine.
- Headache, fever, and muscle aches.
- In women, vaginal discharge.

After 10–21 days the symptoms usually disappear. There may be further milder attacks, often affecting the same areas.

What might be done?
If you suspect genital herpes in yourself or your partner go to a clinic specializing in STIs or consult your doctor. A diagnosis will probably be made from your symptoms and a physical examination. Swabs of the blisters may be taken to test for the virus. You may also have tests for other STIs. Partners need to attend for a checkup even if they have no obvious symptoms.

Your doctor may prescribe aciclovir or another antiviral drug (p.573) during an attack. If aciclovir is taken early, it usually reduces the severity of symptoms but it does not rid the body of the virus.

What is the prognosis?
About 2 in 10 infected people have only one attack. However, the virus remains in the body, and some people have recurrent attacks a few times a year for several years. Symptoms are usually less severe in subsequent attacks and the time between attacks increases.

Can it be prevented?
The risk of contracting genital herpes can be reduced by practising safe sex (*see* Preventing STIs, p.491). However, a condom may not always provide total protection since areas of skin around the genitals may have blisters or be less obviously infected. The virus can be passed on even if no blisters are present. If you have an attack, avoid sex until the symptoms have gone.

If you have repeated attacks, your doctor may prescribe preventive treatment with an antiviral drug to reduce the risk of a recurrence. Treatment is rarely needed for more than a year.

A pregnant woman who has a genital herpes attack close to delivery may need a caesarean section to prevent the infection passing to the baby.

Genital warts

Fleshy, painless growths on and around the genitals caused by a virus

 Can affect sexually active people of any age

 Unprotected sex with multiple partners is a risk factor

 Gender and genetics are not significant factors

Genital warts are skin growths caused by the human papillomavirus (HPV). There are many different types of HPV, each of which affects particular parts of the body. Certain forms of the virus affect the genital area and are spread by sexual contact. Some of these HPV forms cause genital warts. Certain other types of HPV affecting the genitals have been associated with cancer of the cervix (p.481).

Genital warts is one of the most prevalent sexually transmitted infections (STIs), with about 73,400 new cases in England in 2103. The disorder is reported more often by men than by women, probably because warts are more visible on the penis. An infected person can transmit the virus to sexual partners even if he or she has no symptoms of infection.

The warts appear from a few weeks to as long as 20 months after infection. They are usually soft with a rough surface and are painless. A few may have a hard surface. Genital warts become larger rapidly, and in some instances the growths cluster together in one area.

In men, warts may occur on the shaft of the penis, on the foreskin, on the glans (head of the penis), and around the anus. In women, warts may appear on the vulva (the external part of the female genitals) or may develop inside the vagina, on the cervix, and around the anus. The warts may also occur in the rectum due to infection through anal intercourse. If a pregnant woman has genital warts, she should make sure that her midwife is aware of the fact because there is a risk of passing the infection to the baby during delivery.

What might be done?
If you or your partner has genital warts, or if you have been exposed to infection, you should go to a clinic that specializes in STIs or consult your doctor. Diagnosis is based on a physical examination. Tests may also be performed to check for other STIs.

There are several ways of treating genital warts. You may be prescribed a cream containing imiquimod or podophyllotoxin, which is for use on external genital areas and applied directly to the warts. The treatment is repeated until the warts have gone. Other techniques include cryotherapy, in which the warts are destroyed by freezing; electrocautery, which burns them off; laser treatment; and surgical removal. Genital warts may recur, but in most cases the body's immune system controls them eventually.

Can it be prevented?
You can reduce your risk of contracting genital warts by practising safe sex measures (*see* Preventing STIs, p.491). People are often advised to avoid sexual contact at times when the warts are visible. However, genital warts can be acquired from someone who is a carrier of the virus but has no symptoms. To prevent a short-term recurrence of warts, condoms should be used for 12 weeks after treatment has finished. However, condoms may not give total protection since they may not cover all of the affected areas.

Vaccination against certain strains of HPV is offered to all girls aged 12–13 as part of the routine childhood immunization programme (p.13). This helps to protect against strains of HPV responsible for most cases of genital warts and also against HPV strains linked to many cases of cervical cancer. However, the vaccine does not protect against all types of HPV and it is therefore important still to have cervical screening tests (p.480).

Pubic lice

Infestation of pubic hair by a type of small wingless parasite causing irritation

 Can affect sexually active people of any age

 Sex with multiple partners is a risk factor

 Gender and genetics are not significant factors

Pubic lice, often called "crabs", are usually spread by sexual contact. The lice usually live in the pubic hair but may also sometimes occur in other hairy areas of the body, although rarely on the scalp. The adult lice are about 2 mm ($1/12$ in) long, feed on blood, and lay eggs called nits.

The most common symptom is itching in the affected area (most commonly the pubic area and around the anus), especially at night, although some people have no symptoms. Normal washing does not remove nits.

If you think that you or your partner has pubic lice, you should consult your doctor or go to a clinic specializing in sexually transmitted infections (STIs).

What might be done?
Your doctor will probably prescribe a preparation containing permethrin or malathion (*see* Preparations for skin infections and infestations, p.577). The preparation usually needs to be applied over the whole body, including the scalp, taking care to avoid getting any in the eyes. A second application is usually needed 3–7 days after the first to destroy any freshly hatched lice. To prevent the spread of lice, everybody who has close bodily contact with the affected person should also be treated. The clothing and bed linen used by an infested person should be machine-washed in hot water.

Sexual problems

Most men and women experience a sexual problem at some time in their lives. Some problems, such as decreased sex drive and pain during intercourse, may be experienced by either partner, while others, such as erectile dysfunction and vaginismus, are specific to men or women. Sexual problems have many causes, including physical and psychological disorders and certain drug treatments.

The most common sexual problem that affects both sexes is decreased sex drive. This is often a natural response to changing hormone levels, although there are many other causes. Other common problems include failure of orgasm in women, and, in men, erectile dysfunction and premature ejaculation, which affect most men at some time. A sexual problem may begin with an underlying physical cause, but anxiety about sexual performance can often develop and compound the original problem. Sometimes, a sexual problem experienced by one partner may be caused by the response or behaviour of the other partner. For these reasons, doctors and sex therapists often

prefer to involve both partners in discussions and therapy sessions to promote mutual understanding and appreciation. This is particularly important when the recommended treatment involves exercises to be practised at home by both partners.

A variety of treatments is currently available, and there are many doctors and therapists who specialize in treating sexual problems. Sources of specialized help include urologists, gynaecologists, sex therapists, and counsellors. For some problems, assistance from a psychiatrist or psychologist may be helpful. Treatments for sexual problems have a high success rate.

Decreased sex drive

A temporary or long-term reduction of interest in sex

 More common with increasing age

 In rare cases, due to an extra chromosome

 Physical and mental stress and the use of certain drugs may be risk factors

 Gender is not a significant factor

Someone whose sex drive has decreased loses interest in sex, does not fantasize about sex, and feels little or no pleasure during sexual activity. It is common for a person to experience a temporary loss of sex drive, or libido, at some point in his or her life. However, a long-term decrease in a person's sex drive may become a problem if it causes d stress either to the individual concerned or to his or her sexual partner.

Sex drive is partly controlled by sex hormones, which decrease gradually as you grow older. As a result, sex drive also declines naturally with age. However, men and women have different patterns of sexual desire. Sex drive is most intense in young men in their teens and 20s, whereas women tend to reach their sexual peak later in life, often not until their 30s. Different people have different levels of sex drive and activity. For this reason, a decrease in your sex drive should be judged only in comparison with your own normal sex drive and activity, not in comparison with the claims of other people.

What are the causes?
Many women experience a temporary decline in sex drive after childbirth or gynaecological surgery, and sometimes during pregnancy. Menopausal women may also be affected both because of fluctuations in the levels of their sex hormones and because of their emotional responses to the menopause. Many women experience regular fluctuations in sexual desire that reflect the normal changes in hormone levels that occur during the menstrual cycle.

A number of psychological problems may trigger a loss of interest in sex in either men or women. Such problems may include anxiety disorders (p.341), depression (p.343), stress (p.31), and general problems with the relationship.

A reduction in sex drive may be a side effect of certain drugs, including some contraceptive pills; some types of antidepressant drug (p.592); and certain antihypertensive drugs (p.580), such as beta-blockers (p.581). Heavy drinking may also decrease sex drive.

Other possible causes include illness and tiredness as well as a few rare genetic disorders, such as Klinefelter's syndrome (p.534), which affects only males and results in low levels of sex hormones.

What can I do?
You may be able to identify the reason for your loss of sex drive. If you suspect that stress or heavy drinking may be the cause, try changing your lifestyle. If you think that the cause is an underlying problem in your relationship, it may help to discuss the issue with your partner (*see* **Communicating your sexual needs**, opposite page). If you cannot improve the situation, consult your doctor.

What might the doctor do?
Your doctor will discuss your lifestyle and relationship with you to determine which factors are contributing to the problem. If your doctor suspects that your decreased sex drive is the result of a physical condition, he or she may examine you and arrange for tests to look for a disorder. For example, blood tests may be used to check for abnormally low hormone levels in men. If your decreased sex drive is a side effect of a particular drug, your doctor may give you a different medication. The doctor may also suggest changes in your lifestyle, such as reducing stress or cutting down on alcohol intake. If the cause seems to be psychological, your doctor may recommend that you and your partner have sex therapy (p.496)..

Most people who consult a doctor about a decrease in their sex dtive can be treated successfully.

Failure of orgasm

Inability to reach the peak of sexual excitement

 Can affect sexually active people of any age

 Common in females; rare in males

 Stress, alcohol, and the use of certain drugs are risk factors

 Genetics is not a significant factor

Failure to reach orgasm, called anorgasmia, is the most frequently reported sexual problem in women and affects up to half of all women at some time in their lives. However, It is less common in men, being reported by fewer than 1 in 10 men.

What are the causes?
Psychological factors that can inhibit orgasm include anxiety about sexual performance, fear of pregnancy, a previous unpleasant sexual experience, physical or mental abuse during childhood, and sexual inhibitions as a result of a strict upbringing regarding sex.

Poor sexual technique on the part of one or both partners may lead to failure of orgasm. Most often, insufficient time is allowed for the woman to become fully aroused. Poor sexual technique is common between new partners who know little about each other's sexual responses. The problem may also be due to inexperience or by a lack of communication between partners.

Some long-term disorders that result in damage to nerves, including diabetes mellitus (p.437), may lead to failure of orgasm. Certain drugs, such as particular antidepressants (p.592) and some antihypertensive drugs (p.580), including beta-blockers (p.581), can cause a decreased sex drive (left) that may result in anorgasmia. Heavy drinking may also cause failure of orgasm.

What might be done?
If you or your partner repeatedly fail to reach orgasm, it is important to discuss the matter together (*see* **Communicating your sexual needs**, opposite page). Your doctor should be consulted if the situation does not improve. If the problem is psychological or due to poor sexual technique, you will probably be referred to a sex therapist (*see* **Sex therapy**, p.496). If the problem is caused by drug treatment, the doctor may change your medication. However, if you have nerve damage, the problem is usually permanent and cannot be treated.

Sex therapy is effective in most cases, but, if you or your partner have deep-rooted problems such as difficulties due to abuse in childhood, some form of psychological therapy (pp.622–624) may be needed. Failure of orgasm can be treated successfully in many people

Erectile dysfunction

Inability to achieve or sustain an erection

 More common with increasing age

 Smoking, alcohol, stress, and the use of certain drugs are risk factors

 Genetics is not a significant factor

Most men experience temporary difficulty in achieving or maintaining an erection at some time in their lives. Such occasional erectile dysfunction is normal. Persistent, long-term difficulty in achieving an erection may indicate a physical cause and should prompt you to seek medical advice. Erectile dysfunction over a long period often results in distress for both the individual and his partner. Despite this, only a minority of men with the condition seek medical advice.

What are the causes?
Erectile dysfunction can be due to a physical or a psychological disorder and in many cases may be a combination of the two. Anxiety disorders (p.341) and depression (p.343) can lead to erectile dysfunction, and may themselves be a reflection of stress in a man's life, a relationship difficulty, or fear of sexual failure. The condition may also be a side effect of drugs, including certain antidepressants (p.592) and antihypertensives (p.580). The risk of erectile dysfunction can be increased by factors such as tiredness, heavy drinking, and smoking.

The condition is more common in middle-aged and elderly men and often has a physical cause. The most common cause is a vascular disease, such as atherosclerosis (p.241), that reduces the blood supply to the penis. Occasionally, the blood supply may be reduced as a result of pelvic injury. Erectile dysfunction can also result if the nerves supplying the penis are damaged due to surgery, such as operations on the prostate gland (*see* **Transurethral resection of the prostate**, p.463, and **Radical prostatectomy**, p.465), or to conditions such as multiple sclerosis (p.334) or diabetes mellitus (p.437). Rarely, it is due to low levels of the sex hormone testosterone.

What might be done?

If you have persistent problems with erectile dysfunction, you should consult your doctor. He or she will ask if you have full morning erections. If you do, it is more likely that your erectile dysfunction has a psychological cause. Your doctor will also ask about your lifestyle and about any medication that you use to see if there are factors contributing to your problem that can be altered.

The doctor may give you a physical examination and may take a blood sample to check for diabetes mellitus and to measure your testosterone level. You may also be referred to a specialist for Doppler ultrasound scanning (p.259) to assess the blood flow to your penis.

If the blood vessels to the penis are damaged by pelvic injury, surgery may restore normal blood flow and allow you to achieve an erection. Your doctor may change your medication if drug treatment is a likely cause. If you have diabetes, your doctor should make sure that it is well controlled to prevent further nerve damage.

If your doctor suspects that an aspect of your lifestyle is causing your condition, he or she may suggest changes, such as reducing stress or your alcohol intake.

If the erectile dysfunction appears to have a psychological basis or if you have difficulties in your relationship, your doctor may suggest that you and your partner consult a sex therapist or a counsellor (*see* **Sex therapy**, p.496).

In cases where the underlying cause cannot be treated, a range of drug treatments and physical aids is available.

Communicating your sexual needs

Many people feel that the sexual side of their relationship could be better. The key to improving your sex life is communication with your partner and mutual understanding. Bear the following points in mind when you discuss your problems with your partner:

- Think carefully about your words and timing to avoid sounding hostile or critical.
- Talk about the positive aspects of your sex life.
- Suggest things that you would like to do or would like to spend more time on; watch your partner's reaction carefully.
- Keep your comments open and your suggestions positive.
- Listen to what your partner says.
- Create an action plan together, and include the points that you would both like to work on.

Drug treatments The oral medications sildenafil, tadalafil, vardenafil, and avanafil have proved effective in treating erectile dysfunction in many men. A medical assessment is needed before taking these drugs as they may cause serious side effects in some men and may also interact with other medications.

The drug alprostadil may also help you to achieve an erection. This drug can be inserted into the urethra (the tube through which urine and semen leave the body). Alternatively, the drug is injected directly into the penis. However, alprostadil can sometimes have serious side effects. For the small number of men with low testosterone levels, testosterone injections may be effective.

Physical treatments There are many physical aids that can help you to achieve and maintain an erection. The vacuum constriction device consists of a cylinder that is fitted over the penis. A hand-held pump is used to create a vacuum in the cylinder, causing the penis to fill with blood and become erect. The cylinder is then removed and the erection is maintained by a special rubber band fitted on the base of the penis.

An alternative is a penile prosthesis, which is surgically implanted into the penis. One type consists of paired rods that enable the position of the penis to be adjusted manually. However, once the rods are implanted, the size of the penis cannot be altered. Another device is the inflatable penile implant, which consists of paired cylinders and a small pump. The pump can be triggered to inflate the cylinders, which then hold the penis erect. When not in use, this implant enables the erection to subside.

The outlook for the condition is good. In many men, the cause can be treated, but if this is not treatable, drugs and physical aids are usually effective.

Premature ejaculation

Release of seminal fluid from the penis that occurs before or immediately after penetration and with minimal stimulation

 Most common in young, sexually inexperienced males

 Early sexual encounters in rushed conditions may be a risk factor

 Genetics is not a significant factor

Premature ejaculation is a very common sexual problem, particularly for young men. Ejaculation is considered to be premature when semen is released from the penis before or very shortly after penetration and with minimal sexual stimulation. Most sex therapists agree that the experience of premature ejaculation is part of the normal sexual learning curve; inexperienced men, particularly if they are young, often ejaculate prematurely. The problem may also occur in experienced men when they have intercourse after a long period of abstinence from sex.

Squeeze technique

The squeeze technique can be used to prevent premature ejaculation. Just before ejaculation, the shaft of the penis is firmly squeezed between the thumb and forefinger. The squeezing causes the erection to be partially lost, thus preventing ejaculation. Repeated regularly, the exercise can dramatically improve control of ejaculation.

Applying pressure

The thumb and forefinger are used to apply pressure just behind the head of the penis, on the upper and lower sides. This pressure prevents ejaculation.

Recurrent premature ejaculation can be a frustrating problem. Repeated episodes may make a man anxious about his performance and possibly result in erectile dysfunction (opposite page). If premature ejaculation occurs repeatedly, medical advice should be sought.

What are the causes?

The causes of premature ejaculation are usually psychological. Problems may include anxiety about performance or result from early sexual experiences in which there was a fear of being discovered. Some men cannot recognize the physical sensations that they experience immediately before they ejaculate and therefore cannot control the timing of their orgasm. Premature ejaculation is more common during the early stages of a sexual relationship, when the partners may lack confidence and may be nervous about their performance.

Rarely, premature ejaculation may be caused by a physical disorder such as inflammation of the prostate gland (*see* **Prostatitis**, p.463) or may result from damage to the spinal cord.

What might be done?

If you experience recurrent problems with premature ejaculation, you should discuss the matter with your doctor. You will have an examination to look for a physical cause, and any underlying disorder will be treated.

If premature ejaculation does not have a physical cause, treatment of the disorder is aimed at teaching you how to recognize and control sexual arousal. Your doctor will probably recommend that you see a sex therapist, who can teach you exercises for managing arousal (*see* **Sex therapy**, p.496).

Exercises may include the start/stop technique, in which the man's penis is stimulated by his partner. When the man feels that he is close to ejaculation, he asks his partner to stop stimulating him. After a few minutes, stimulation is resumed by his partner and then stopped again. When the stop/start exercise is repeated many times over a period of weeks, it can help men to achieve better control. The squeeze technique (above) can be used together with the start/stop technique or the two techniques can be used separately.

Some antidepressant drugs (p.592), such as sertraline, have the side effect of delaying ejaculation. They may be prescribed as a short-term measure to treat premature ejaculation because delaying ejaculation can boost confidence and assist in solving the problem.

The outlook is excellent: most men who seek help vastly improve their control over the timing of ejaculation.

Painful intercourse in men

Pain experienced in the genital area during sexual intercourse

 Can affect sexually active males of any age

 Unprotected sex is a risk factor

 Genetics is not a significant factor

Painful sexual intercourse, known as dyspareunia, is rare in men. The cause is usually physical, but in some cases it may be psychological. Pain in the penis during intercourse may be accompanied by a burning sensation during and after ejaculation.

What are the causes?

The most common cause of painful intercourse in men is an infection of the genitals, the prostate gland, or the urethra (the tube through which urine and semen pass out of the body). These infections, which include genital herpes (p.493) and nongonococcal urethritis (p.491), are often transmitted through unprotected sex. Friction on the penis during sexual intercourse can aggravate the pain of an infection. Other possible causes of pain during intercourse include inflammation of the head of the penis (*see* **Balanitis**, p.461) and persistent inflammation of the prostate gland (*see* **Prostatitis**, p.463), which may result in pain on ejaculation. Dyspareunia may also be due to

Peyronie's disease (p.462), a condition in which the shape of the penis is abnormal when erect. A tight foreskin is another possible cause (see **Phimosis**, p.461).

In some instances, discomfort during penetration results from skin irritation caused by an allergic reaction to a particular brand of condom or spermicide. Less commonly, sharp pain during penetration can be caused by threads of an intrauterine contraceptive device that protrude from the woman's cervix (see **Using contraceptives**, p.28). Rarely, there may be a psychological reason, such as sexual abuse in childhood.

What might be done?

If you think that the pain is due to an allergy to condoms or spermicide, try changing to another brand. If the pain persists, consult your doctor. The doctor will examine you and may take a swab from the tip of the penis to test for infection. If you have an infection, the doctor may prescribe antibiotics (p.572) for both you and your partner so that you do not reinfect each other, or may refer you to a clinic that specializes in sexually transmitted infections.

Any disorder that interferes with the erection of the penis may require surgery if it is causing pain. If your partner has an intrauterine contraceptive device that causes you discomfort, her doctor may trim its threads so that they do not protrude as far through the cervix.

If no physical cause is found, your doctor may refer you to a sex therapist, who will help you to work through any psychological problems together with your partner (see **Sex therapy**, right). Painful sexual intercourse in men can usually be treated successfully.

Painful intercourse in women

Pain experienced in the genital area or the lower abdomen during sexual intercourse

 Can affect sexually active females of any age

 Unprotected sex is a risk factor

 Genetics is not a significant factor

Many women experience painful sexual intercourse, known as dyspareunia, at some point in their lives. The pain may be superficial, in the vulva or vagina, or deep in the pelvis. It may have either a psychological or a physical cause.

What are the causes?

For many women, superficial pain during sexual intercourse may be caused by psychological factors, such as anxiety disorders (p.341), guilt, or fear of sexual penetration. These factors can also result in vaginismus (right).

There are many physical causes of superficial pain during intercourse. A fairly common cause is vaginal dryness. This may result from insufficient arousal before penetration. It may also be a side effect of certain drugs, such as some antidepressants (p.592), or be due to hormonal changes after childbirth or the menopause (see **Menopausal problems**, p.473). Many women find intercourse painful after giving birth, especially if they had a vaginal tear or if a tear has healed poorly. Pain during a woman's first sexual experience is common, particularly if the hymen is intact. Occasionally, a remnant of the hymen subsequently causes difficulty and pain with sexual penetration.

Superficial pain during intercourse may also be caused by infections of the urinary tract or the genitals, including cystitis (p.453), trichomoniasis (p.492), and vaginal thrush (p.482); certain skin conditions affecting the vulva, such as lichen sclerosus, which may cause narrowing of the opening into the vagina; or excessive sensitivity of the nerve endings in the vulva. In rare cases, an abnormally shaped vagina may make sexual intercourse painful.

Pain that is felt deep within the pelvis during intercourse may be due to a disorder of the pelvic cavity or of the pelvic organs, such as pelvic inflammatory disease (p.475), fibroids (p.477), or endometriosis (p.475). In some cases, deep pain may occur after vaginal surgery or a hysterectomy (p.479) as a result of scar tissue formation, or after radiotherapy for cancer of the uterus (p.479) due to narrowing of the vagina. Another possible cause of pain may be an intrauterine contraceptive device that is incorrectly positioned in the uterus (see **Using contraceptives**, p.28).

Despite common belief, a large penis does not make sex painful, although certain sexual positions can cause pain in the vagina and vulva or deep in the pelvis.

What can I do?

If you think your pain is due to vaginal dryness caused by lack of arousal, you may need to talk to your partner about spending more time on foreplay (see **Communicating your sexual needs**, p.495). Alternatively, you may find it helpful to use a lubricant, particularly after childbirth and during and after the menopause. If certain sexual positions cause discomfort, try other ones.

What might the doctor do?

If you consult your doctor, he or she may take swabs from your vagina and cervix to test for infection and may arrange for ultrasound scanning (p.135) of the pelvis to look for abnormalities. If pain is due to an underlying disorder, the disorder will be treated if possible. If the pain is due to vaginal dryness caused by a drug, your doctor may prescribe an alternative. If no physical cause is found, your doctor may refer you for sex therapy (right) with your partner. In most cases, the pain ceases following treatment.

Vaginismus

Spasm of the muscles around the entrance to the vagina, making sexual intercourse painful or impossible

 Can affect sexually active females of any age

 Genetics and lifestyle are not significant factors

In vaginismus, the pelvic floor muscles go into painful involuntary spasm and reduce the size of the vaginal opening. As a result, sexual intercourse may be very painful and vaginal penetration can often be impossible. The condition varies in severity for different women. Some women are affected by vaginismus to such an extent that they cannot insert even a finger or a tampon into the vagina and may need an anaesthetic for a vaginal examination. Other women may be able to tolerate a vaginal examination by a doctor or nurse but cannot tolerate sexual intercourse.

What are the causes?

Vaginismus is usually psychological in origin and often occurs in women who fear that penetration may be painful. This fear may result from a previous traumatic sexual experience, such as a rape or sexual abuse in childhood. Another cause of vaginismus may be the fear of pregnancy. Anxiety or guilt concerning sex may also be a contributing factor to this condition.

Certain physical disorders can also lead to vaginismus. Inflammation of the vagina (see **Vulvovaginitis**, p.482) may make intercourse painful and lead to vaginismus. Some women develop the condition because they expect that sex will be painful after childbirth or that they will experience sexual difficulties during or after the menopause (see **Menopausal problems**, p.473).

What might be done?

Your doctor will examine you gently to look for any physical problem that could make penetration painful or difficult. If there is an underlying physical cause, he or she will treat it. If the problem is psychological, you may need some form of psychological therapy (pp.622–624) or, alternatively, you may be referred to a sex therapist (see **Sex therapy**, below). The sex therapist will explain that the vaginal wall is elastic and may teach you relaxation exercises. He or she may then show you how a small dilator can be inserted into the vagina. By practising this technique and gradually using larger dilators, you should lose your fear that penetration will be painful. Treatment for vaginismus is successful in about 9 out of 10 women.

▶ **TREATMENT**

Sex therapy

Sex therapy is often helpful when a sexual problem has a psychological basis rather than a physical cause. The type of therapy used depends on your problem but often involves discussions with a sex therapist. To overcome particular problems, the therapist may set exercises for you to practise at home, either by yourself or with your partner.

Discussion sessions

Discussing sexual problems with a trained sex therapist or counsellor can often help a couple to analyse and understand their relationship and sexual needs more clearly. It is important that both partners attend the therapy sessions. Each visit lasts about 1 hour, and several sessions may be necessary.

Counselling
Talking with a counsellor can help you to understand your relationship and deal with sexual problems.

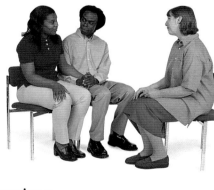

Exercises

A sex therapist may assign you exercises to practise at home to improve the way in which you and your partner communicate. Exercises may include techniques such as sensate focus. This technique involves experiencing your partner simply through touch and is helpful for problems stemming from anxiety about performance.

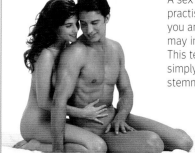

Sensate focus technique
This technique involves discovering pleasure in your own body and that of your partner by means of touch rather than sexual intercourse.

Infertility

Infertility affects 1 in 10 couples who want children. Fertility declines in both sexes after the ages of 25–30, and because more and more couples are delaying starting a family until their 30s, infertility is becoming more common in the developed world. If conception has not occurred after a year of unprotected, regular sex, one or both partners may have a fertility problem.

For every 10 couples who try to have a child, 8 conceive within a year and 9 conceive within 2 years. The remainder may have fertility problems. Some problems may be temporary or can be treated medically, but certain problems can prevent a couple from ever having children. Infertility can also affect people who have children already.

It is important that both partners visit the doctor together if they are worried about an inability to conceive. In about half of all couples who have difficulty conceiving, the problem lies with the female partner, and in about a third of couples it lies with the male partner. However, in some couples, no cause can be found.

In this section, the first article covers the advice that a doctor might give to a couple who are having difficulties in conceiving. The following two articles describe specific infertility problems in women and in men. Each article describes the tests that a doctor may carry out to identify fertility disorders and discusses how specific problems may be treated. Other conditions that can lead to infertility are covered elsewhere in the book. Such conditions include polycystic ovary syndrome (p.477) and endometriosis (p.475) in women, and varicocele (p.460) and hypogonadism in men (p.466).

In many couples, the cause of infertility can be identified and treated. If a specific cause cannot be found or is untreatable, assisted conception may be advised. This section discusses some of the techniques that may be used, including developments in embryo testing.

Problems conceiving

When pregnancy does not result after a couple have had regular, unprotected sex for more than a year

 Age, gender, genetics, and lifestyle as risk factors depend on the cause

The average time taken by a couple who are trying to conceive is 6 months, and 8 in 10 couples will be successful within a year. It is very common for a couple to feel anxious if pregnancy does not occur in the first few months, but most young couples are advised to continue trying for a year before seeking medical help. Older couples may decide to ask for medical help earlier because fertility in both sexes declines with age. Women over the age of 35 may find it particularly difficult to conceive.

What might be done?
If you are having problems conceiving, you and your partner should consult a doctor together. The doctor will ask about your sex life and whether you are having any specific difficulties with sexual intercourse (*see* **Sexual problems**, pp.494–496). He or she will also check whether you have been having sexual intercourse around the middle of the woman's menstrual cycle, when conception is most likely to take place.

Your doctor will take a medical history from both of you because previous illnesses or operations may be relevant. You will be asked how often you drink alcohol and how much, whether you smoke, and if you use any prescribed or recreational drugs. You may also be given a physical examination that includes your genitals.

If you are both relatively young and there is no obvious problem, your doctor may give you advice about measures that you can take to improve your likelihood of conceiving (*see* **Maximizing your chance of conception**, below) and suggest that you keep trying. If you have not had preconcep-

SELF-HELP

Maximizing your chance of conception
The overall health of both partners has an important effect on fertility. You may find that following the self-help measures below improves your chance of conception:

- Make sure your weight is in or near the normal range (*see* **Are you a healthy weight?**, p.19).
- Eat a healthy diet.
- Do not smoke.
- Cut down on alcohol, which is known to reduce the sperm count and can damage the fetus if pregnancy occurs.
- Have sex every day at the woman's most fertile time, in the middle of the menstrual cycle.
- Try not to worry, because stress can lower fertility. Learn relaxation exercises (p.32) to lower stress levels.
- Men should avoid taking hot baths or using saunas, and should wear loose-fitting underwear.

tion counselling for advice on a healthy pregnancy, the doctor may discuss your health, diet, and lifestyle with you.

If your doctor suspects there may be a problem responsible for preventing conception, you may be referred to a specialist for a series of tests (*see* **Female infertility**, below, and **Male infertility**, p.499).

What is the prognosis?
For most couples, it is only a matter of time before they conceive, and 9 in 10 couples are successful within 2 years.

If a problem is detected, the treatment and outlook will depend on the cause. Assisted conception (p.498) or artificial insemination (right) may be suitable for some couples if no cause is discovered or if the problem cannot be treated successfully.

Female infertility

Inability of a woman to conceive with a partner of normal fertility

 Increases with age; most common over the age of 35

 In rare cases, may be due to a chromosomal abnormality

 Stress, excessive exercise, and low or excess body weight are risk factors

About half of all couples who experience difficulties conceiving do so as a result of female infertility. Fertility in women decreases with age and is generally lower after the age of 35, making conception more difficult.

For conception to occur, all of the following steps must take place: ovulation (the production and release of a mature egg by an ovary), fertilization of the egg by a sperm, transport of the fertilized egg along the fallopian tube to the uterus, and implantation of the fertilized egg in the lining of the uterus. If any stage does not occur or is interrupted, conception cannot take place.

What are the causes?
There are a number of fertility problems in females that may affect one or more of the processes required for conception. The problems can develop at different stages of conception.

Problems with ovulation A common cause of female infertility is failure of the ovaries to release a mature egg during each monthly cycle. Ovulation is controlled by a complex interaction of hormones, including those produced by the hypothalamus (an area of the brain), the pituitary gland, and the ovaries. A common and usually treatable cause of female infertility is polycystic ovary syndrome (p.477), which may cause a hormonal imbalance that prevents ovulation from taking place. Very rarely, disorders of the thyroid gland, such as hypothyroidism (p.432), may also lead to a hormonal imbalance that can affect the frequency of ovulation. Pituitary

▶ **TREATMENT**

Artificial insemination

Also known as intrauterine insemination, artificial insemination is a procedure to introduce sperm into a woman's uterus. Sperm from the woman's partner or from a donor is washed and filtered to remove dead sperm. The fastest-moving sperm are then selected to produce a sample of the best sperm. This sample is drawn into a syringe and injected through a fine, flexible tube into the uterus. The procedure is painless and takes only minutes, and the woman can go home after half an hour of rest.

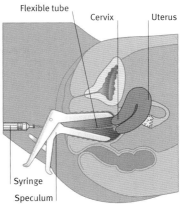
Flexible tube | Cervix | Uterus | Syringe | Speculum

Artificial insemination
The vagina is held open by a speculum so that sperm can be injected through the cervix and into the uterus.

gland disorders, such as prolactinoma (p.430), a noncancerous tumour, may cause a similar imbalance. Ovulation does not always occur in some women for reasons that are unclear. In some cases, women who have been using oral contraceptives for a number of years may take time to re-establish a normal hormonal cycle after discontinuing them. Excessive exercise, stress, and obesity or low body weight may be other factors that affect hormone levels and cause temporary infertility.

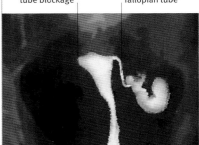
Site of fallopian tube blockage | Distorted fallopian tube

Damaged fallopian tubes
In this X-ray, a contrast dye has been used to show the female reproductive organs. One fallopian tube is blocked and is not visible; the other is narrowed and distorted.

Premature menopause also results in a failure to ovulate. It can occur for no apparent reason or may be the result of pelvic surgery, chemotherapy (p.157), or radiotherapy (p.158). In rare cases, the ovaries do not develop normally due to a chromosomal abnormality, such as Turner's syndrome (p.534).

Problems with egg transport and fertilization The passage of the egg from the ovary to the uterus may be impeded by damage to one of the fallopian tubes. This damage may be due to pelvic infection (*see* **Pelvic inflammatory disease**, p.475), which may in turn result from a sexually transmitted infection such as chlamydial infection (p.492). Such disorders may exist with no symptoms and may be detected only if you have difficulty conceiving.

Endometriosis (p.475), a condition that can lead to the formation of scar tissue and cysts within the pelvis, may prevent the passage of an egg.

Problems with implantation If the lining of the uterus has been damaged by an infection, such as gonorrhoea (p.491), the implantation of a fertilized egg may not be possible. Hormonal problems may also result in the uterine lining not being adequately prepared for successful implantation. Noncancerous tumours that distort the uterus (*see* **Fibroids**, p.477) and, rarely, structural abnormalities present from birth may make it difficult for a fertilized egg to embed itself in the uterine lining.

What might be done?

Your doctor will ask you about your general state of health, your lifestyle, your medical and menstrual history, and your sex life before recommending particular tests and treatments.

Most causes of female infertility can now be identified through testing. You can find out if and when you ovulate by using an ovulation prediction kit, available over the counter, or by recording your body temperature daily (*see* **Using contraceptives**, p.28). If your doctor suspects that you are not ovulating regularly, you may have to undergo repeated blood tests during your menstrual cycle to assess the level of the hormone progesterone, which normally rises after ovulation.

If tests show that you are not ovulating, you may need further blood tests to check the levels of certain hormones, including prolactin, and drugs may be prescribed to stimulate ovulation (*see* **Drugs for infertility**, p.604). However, if you are ovulating, the next step is for your doctor to find to find out whether your partner is producing sufficient normal sperm. This can be done by microscopic examination of samples of semen (*see* **Semen analysis**, opposite page).

If you are ovulating normally and your partner's sperm are healthy, your doctor will check to see if there is a problem preventing the egg and sperm from meeting. He or she may arrange for further investigations to look for a blockage in the fallopian tubes

or an abnormality of the uterus. One such test is laparoscopy (p.476), in which an endoscope containing a camera is inserted through a small incision in the abdomen. Another test that may be used to look for abnormalities in the fallopian tubes or uterus is hysterosalpingography, in which a dye is injected through the cervix and X-rays are taken as the dye enters the reproductive organs.

The treatment depends on the problem. For example, a blockage of the fallopian tubes may sometimes be corrected by microsurgery (p.613), and endometriosis may be treated with drugs (*see* **Sex hormones and related drugs**, p.602) or, in some cases, by laparoscopy (p.476).

▶ **TREATMENT**

Assisted conception

Infertility treatments that involve mixing eggs and sperm outside the body include in vitro fertilization, gamete intrafallopian transfer (GIFT), and intra-cytoplasmic sperm injection (ICSI, *see* **Male infertility**, opposite page). IVF may also be used when couples are affected by certain genetic disorders because the embryo can be tested for abnormalities before implantation, a procedure known as preimplantation genetic diagnosis (PIGD).

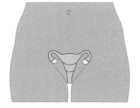

LOCATION

In vitro fertilization

IVF may be performed if the cause of infertility cannot be determined or treated or if there is a blockage in a fallopian tube. It may be done using a couple's own eggs and sperm or with donated sperm and/or eggs.

1 *Drugs are given to stimulate several eggs to mature in the ovaries. Under ultrasound guidance, the eggs are collected with a needle inserted through the vaginal wall.*

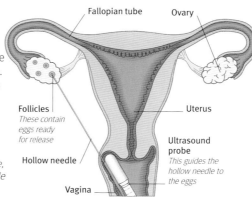

Fallopian tube — Ovary

Follicles
These contain eggs ready for release

Hollow needle

Ultrasound probe
This guides the hollow needle to the eggs

Uterus

Vagina

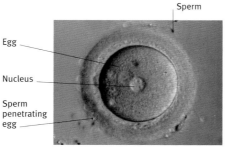

Sperm

Egg

Nucleus

Sperm penetrating egg

2 *A sperm sample is combined with the collected eggs and the mixture is incubated at body temperature (37°C/98.6°F) to allow fertilization to take place. The fertilized eggs (now called embryos) are then checked and the best are selected for transfer. In some cases, they may also be checked for genetic abnormalities (known as preimplantation genetic diagnosis)*

3 *The selected embryos are introduced into the woman's uterus. Up to three eggs are injected through a thin tube that is fixed to a syringe and passed through the cervix. This procedure takes around 20 minutes. If one or more fertilized eggs implant, conception occurs.*

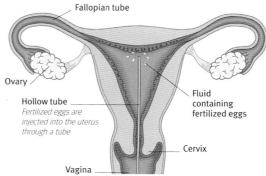

Fallopian tube

Ovary

Hollow tube
Fertilized eggs are injected into the uterus through a tube

Fluid containing fertilized eggs

Cervix

Vagina

GIFT

Gamete intrafallopian transfer (GIFT) may sometimes be used to help couples who have fertility problems. In GIFT, eggs are collected as in IVF, mixed with sperm, then returned to the fallopian tube rather than the uterus.

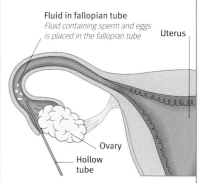

Fluid in fallopian tube
Fluid containing sperm and eggs is placed in the fallopian tube

Uterus

Ovary

Hollow tube

GIFT replacement method
In GIFT, eggs are mixed with sperm outside the body. The egg–sperm mixture is then returned to the fallopian tube for fertilization to occur.

Preimplantation genetic diagnosis

A procedure that may be carried out on embryos at an early stage of development to determine whether they are affected by a genetic disorder. It may be performed during assisted conception, before transfer of embryos to the woman's uterus, to help ensure that only unaffected embryos are transferred. The process involves taking a single cell from each embryo once it has grown to a cluster of about eight cells. The DNA (genetic material) in the removed cell is then analysed to identify healthy embryos suitable for transfer to the woman.

What is the prognosis?

Treatments for female infertility have greatly increased the chance of pregnancy. Success rates vary, depending on the cause of the infertility and the type of treatment carried out. Microsurgery to correct a tubal blockage can be successful but this procedure increases the risk of ectopic pregnancy (p.511), a pregnancy that develops outside the uterus, usually in a fallopian tube.

Success rates for assisted conception methods (above) vary according to the method used and also the age of the woman. For example, for IVF or intracytoplasmic sperm injection (*see* **Male infertility**, opposite page), the chance of a

woman conceiving in one cycle ranges from about 32 per cent for women under 35 to about 5 per cent or less from women aged 43 or older. Assisted conception techniques also carry various risks, including ectopic pregnancy, multiple pregnancy (p.512), premature birth (p.515), and a condition called ovarian hyperstimulation syndrome, in which the drugs used to stimulate egg production cause the ovaries to become swollen and fluid to accumulate in the abdomen and chest.

Male infertility

Inability of a man to produce or deliver sufficient numbers of healthy sperm to achieve fertilization

 In rare cases, may be due to a chromosomal abnormality

 Smoking and drinking alcohol are risk factors

 Age is not a significant factor

In about 1 in 3 couples who have difficulty conceiving, the problem results from male infertility. In men, fertility depends partly on the production of enough normal sperm to make it likely that one of them will fertilize an egg and partly on the ability to deliver the sperm into the vagina during sexual intercourse. If either of these processes is faulty, infertility may result.

What are the causes?

Unlike the causes of female infertility, which are more easily identifiable, the cause of infertility can be difficult to determine in some men. A cause is discovered in only 1 in 3 men investigated.

Problems with sperm production A low sperm count or the production of abnormal sperm may have various causes. One is a rise in the temperature of the testes. Normally, the testes are about 2°C (4°F) cooler than the rest of the body. Any factors that raise their temperature may reduce the sperm count.

Sperm production can be adversely affected by certain long-term illnesses, such as chronic kidney disease (p.451) and by the infectious disease mumps (p.167). Conditions affecting the scrotum, such as a varicocele (p.460), in which there are varicose veins in the scrotum, may also reduce fertility. In addition, fertility problems may occur if the testes are damaged by medical procedures including surgery, chemotherapy (p.157), or radiotherapy (p.158) for disorders such as cancer of the testis (p.460).

Low sperm production may also be due to a hormonal deficiency. Insufficient production of the sex hormone testosterone by the testes (*see* **Hypogonadism in males**, p.466) can cause a low sperm count. Since the pituitary gland controls testosterone secretion, pituitary disorders, such as a tumour (*see* **Prolactinoma**, p.430), may also lead to reduced sperm production. Rarely, low testosterone levels are due to a chromosomal abnormality such as Klinefelter's syndrome (p.534). The most common cause of a low sperm count is idiopathic oligospermia, in which there is a reduced sperm count for no identifiable reason.

Problems with sperm delivery A number of factors may prevent sperm from reaching the vagina. The most easily identifiable factor is erectile dysfunction (p.494), which is the inability to achieve or maintain an erection. Other factors include damage to the epididymides and vas deferens (tubes that transport sperm). This type of damage is often due to a sexually transmitted infection such as gonorrhoea (p.491). It may also be caused by retrograde ejaculation, in which semen flows back into the bladder when the valves at the outlet of the bladder neck do not close properly. Retrograde ejaculation can also occur following surgery of the prostate gland (*see* **Transurethral resection of the prostate**, p.463, and **Radical prostatectomy**, p.465).

What might be done?

Your doctor will ask about your health, medical history, and sex life. He or she will

▶ TEST

Semen analysis

Microscopic examination of several samples of a man's semen is carried out to investigate male infertility. If there are too few sperm or if many are deformed or unable to swim properly, fertility will be reduced. An abnormally small volume of semen may also indicate a fertility problem.

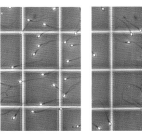

NORMAL SPERM COUNT   **LOW SPERM COUNT**

The sperm count

A sperm count is usually considered normal if there are over 20 million sperm per millilitre of semen with over 50 per cent able to swim effectively and over 30 per cent of normal shape.

give you a physical examination, including an examination of your genitals. You will also need to provide samples of your semen (*see* **Semen analysis**, above). If your sperm count is low or if many of your sperm are abnormal, you may have further investigations such as blood tests to check your hormone levels.

The underlying cause will be treated, if possible. For example, low testosterone levels can be treated with injections of hormones (*see* **Sex hormones and related**

drugs, p.602). Various treatments are available for erectile dysfunction. Damage to the epididymides or vas deferens can be treated by microsurgery (p.613). If the underlying cause of the infertility cannot be treated, there are various measures that can be taken to increase the chance of conception. For example, artificial insemination (p.497) may be used in cases of erectile dysfunction that do not respond to treatment. Artificial insemination may also be used for retrograde ejaculation; alternatively, sperm may be taken from the urine. If you produce only a few healthy sperm, single sperm may be taken from the semen or directly from the epididymis or testis. A process called intracytoplasmic sperm injection (ICSI) may then be used to fertilize an egg. In ICSI, an individual sperm is injected directly into an egg, which is obtained in the same way as in IVF. The fertilized egg is then placed in the woman's uterus. In some cases, donor sperm may be considered.

What is the prognosis?

If the infertility is treatable, the chance of regaining fertility is high. However, the chance of achieving a successful conception also depends on other factors, notably the age of the woman: in general, a woman's ability to conceive diminishes with age. Artificial insemination (using donor sperm) gives about a 16 per cent chance of conceiving in one menstrual cycle for women aged under 35, and an 11 per cent chance for women aged 35–39; however, for women aged 43–44, there is only about a 1 per cent chance of successful conception in a single cycle. Each attempt at IVF (opposite page) or ICSI is successful in about 32 per cent of cases for women under 35, falling to about 21 per cent for women aged 38–39 and 5 per cent for women aged 43–44.

Pregnancy and childbirth

From the moment of conception, when an egg is fertilized, to the moment of birth, complex changes take place within a pregnant woman's body. Genetic material from the father and the mother fuses together, eventually forming a new, genetically distinct individual. During this time, the mother provides a nourishing and protective environment in which the fetus can develop. When the baby is born, he or she is able to survive outside the mother's body and begin a separate existence.

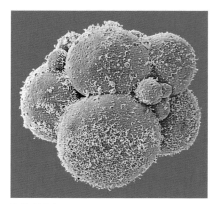

Cell division
In the days after fertilization, the egg has divided to form a cluster of cells called a morula.

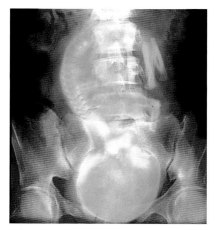

A fully grown fetus
This X-ray shows the skeleton of a fetus at full term. Its head is low in the mother's pelvis.

ABOUT A WEEK after fertilization, the egg embeds itself securely in the lining of the uterus, at which stage it is known as an embryo. Only 8 weeks later, the embryo is recognizable as a human being and has developed all its vital organs, including the heart and brain. From this stage onwards, it is called a fetus. Over the next 32 weeks, the fetus continues to grow and develop, and by the time the baby is born at about week 40, it weighs just over 3 kg (7 lb) on average.

The pregnant woman

Changes in the mother's hormone levels control the physical changes necessary for a healthy pregnancy and for birth.

First, menstruation ceases, and later the ligaments and joints in the mother's pelvis begin to soften and become more flexible in preparation for the birth of the baby. In addition, the mother's breasts enlarge as their milk-producing glands increase in number, ready for breast-feeding the newborn baby.

Each new pregnancy runs a slightly different course. Many prospective mothers feel well throughout their pregnancies. Others experience uncomfortable symptoms such as nausea, vomiting, heartburn, indigestion, and tiredness. These are a result of the biological changes, such as pressure of the fetus on surrounding organs and hormone changes, occurring in the body as the fetus grows. Such symptoms develop at particular stages during the pregnancy.

The baby's birth

After about 37 weeks, the fetus is fully formed and is able to survive independently outside its mother's body. Around the 40th week, the first of the three stages of labour begins. After the baby is born, the mother begins to produce breast milk in preparation for breast-feeding, and her body gradually returns to its state before pregnancy.

✚ PROCESS

From egg to embryo

Pregnancy begins when an egg is fertilized by a sperm. This takes place in the outer third of one of the fallopian tubes, when a single sperm fuses with an egg following sexual intercourse. After fertilization, the egg starts its journey towards the uterus, propelled by the muscular action of the fallopian tube. As the egg travels, its cells gradually divide to form a cluster of cells called a morula.

After about 4 days, the morula arrives in the uterus and then by day 7 begins to embed securely in the uterine lining. From this moment onwards, the pregnancy is properly established, and the morula is known as an embryo.

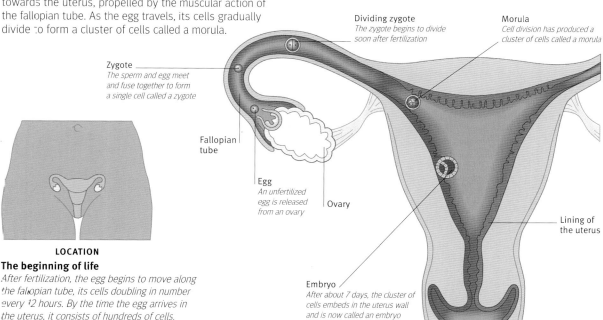

Dividing zygote
The zygote begins to divide soon after fertilization

Morula
Cell division has produced a cluster of cells called a morula

Zygote
The sperm and egg meet and fuse together to form a single cell called a zygote

Fallopian tube

Egg
An unfertilized egg is released from an ovary

Ovary

Lining of the uterus

Embryo
After about 7 days, the cluster of cells embeds in the uterus wall and is now called an embryo

LOCATION

The beginning of life
After fertilization, the egg begins to move along the fallopian tube, its cells doubling in number every 12 hours. By the time the egg arrives in the uterus, it consists of hundreds of cells.

✚ STRUCTURE AND FUNCTION

Pregnancy

Inside the uterus, the fetus is surrounded by a protective, fluid-filled bag known as the amniotic sac. Nourishment is provided through the placenta, an organ attached to the wall of the uterus and connected to the fetus by the umbilical cord. As the fetus grows, the uterus increases in size and weight and gradually expands into the mother's abdomen. Many of the mother's organs, such as the bladder and the intestines, are pushed out of their normal positions by the enlarging uterus. By the end of pregnancy, the fetus is usually tightly curled up with its head pointing downwards towards the mother's pelvis.

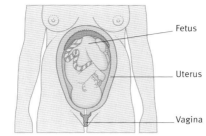

Fetus

Uterus

Vagina

LOCATION

Placenta
Oxygen and nutrients are carried from the mother to the fetus via the placenta and umbilical cord

Umbilical cord
The cord allows nutrients and waste products in the blood to travel between the fetus and the placenta

Fetus at 40 weeks
The fully grown fetus is tightly curled up and usually in a head-down position

Umbilical cord   Fetal foot

Uterus
The thick, muscular wall of the uterus stretches greatly as the fetus grows during pregnancy

Amniotic sac
This fluid-filled sac cushions the fetus against injury

Amniotic fluid
At 40 weeks, about 800 ml (1½ pints) of fluid has accumulated in the sac

Cervix
The cervix is closed until childbirth, when it widens to let the baby through

Mucus plug
A plug of thick mucus sits in the cervix entrance and protects against infection

Rectum

Bladder
As the fetus grows larger in size, the bladder becomes compressed

Vagina
The walls of the vagina soften and relax in preparation for the baby's birth

Nourishing the fetus
The umbilical cord provides a link to the placenta and the mother's nourishing blood supply.

✚ PROCESS

Multiple pregnancy

Most multiple pregnancies produce twins; birth of three or more babies is rare. The majority of twins are nonidentical and develop when two eggs are released from an ovary and are fertilized by two separate sperm. These twins may or may not be the same sex. Less commonly, fertilization of a single egg takes place as normal, but the fertilized cell divides to form two identical, same-sex embryos.

Twins in the uterus
Nonidentical twins develop in their own amniotic sacs and have their own separate placentas. Identical twins may share an amniotic sac or a placenta, or both. Twins can lie in any position in the uterus.

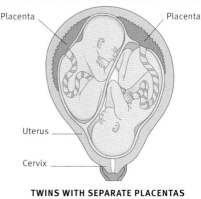

Placenta   Placenta

Uterus

Cervix

TWINS WITH SEPARATE PLACENTAS

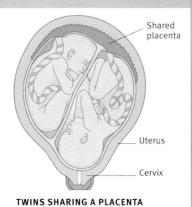

Shared placenta

Uterus

Cervix

TWINS SHARING A PLACENTA

✚ PROCESS

Stages of pregnancy

Pregnancy lasts about 40 weeks and is divided into three stages, or trimesters, each about 3 months in duration. Each trimester brings about significant changes in the mother's body and progressive development and growth of the baby. During the first 8 weeks of pregnancy, the developing baby is called an embryo. After 8 weeks, it is called a fetus.

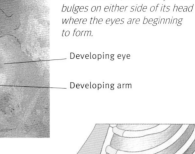

Embryo at 4 weeks
At 1 month old, the embryo has bulges on either side of its head where the eyes are beginning to form.

Developing eye

Developing arm

Placental blood vessel

First trimester (weeks 1–12)

There are few visible changes in the mother's body during this trimester but major adaptations are occurring and her heart rate increases by up to 15 beats per minute to increase the blood circulation. Most of the growing fetus's major organs, such as the heart and the brain, become fully developed during the first 3 months.

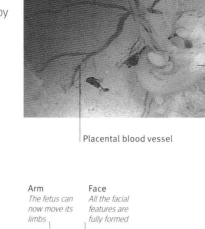

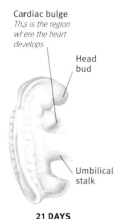

Cardiac bulge
This is the region where the heart develops

Head bud

Umbilical stalk

21 DAYS
3 mm (⅛ in) long

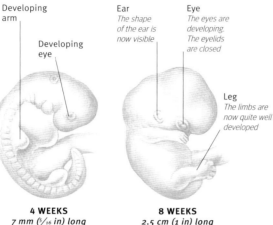

Developing arm

Developing eye

4 WEEKS
7 mm (⁵⁄₁₆ in) long

Ear
The shape of the ear is now visible

Eye
The eyes are developing. The eyelids are closed

Leg
The limbs are now quite well developed

8 WEEKS
2.5 cm (1 in) long

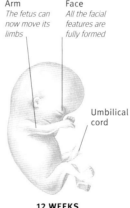

Arm
The fetus can now move its limbs

Face
All the facial features are fully formed

Umbilical cord

12 WEEKS
6 cm (2½ in) long

Nipple

Lobule (milk-producing gland)

Stomach

Slightly thickened waistline

Intestine

Uterus

Fetus

Bladder

From embryo to fetus
The first trimester is crucial in the baby's development; 8 weeks after fertilization, the embryo has developed most of its organs and is now called a fetus. During the third month, it more than doubles in length.

The mother at 12 weeks
At 12 weeks, the mother's waistline is only slightly thickened. The breasts are tender and the areola, the area around the nipple, becomes darker in colour.

Second trimester (weeks 13–28)

The mother may experience backache as she copes with the growing weight of the fetus. Her appetite tends to increase. Fetal movements are first perceived at 18–20 weeks as fluttering sensations in the mother's abdomen.

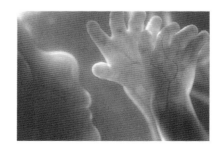

Fetus at 20 weeks
At this stage, the hands are well developed and the fetus is able to flex its fingers. The fetus now has recognizable features and the profile of the face shows the forehead, nose, lips, and chin.

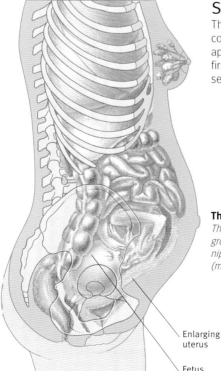

The mother at 24 weeks
The mother's abdomen swells as the fetus grows. There may be discharge from the nipples, caused by enlarging lobules (milk-producing glands) in the breasts.

Enlarging uterus

Fetus

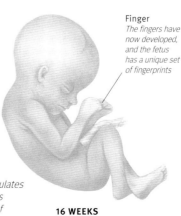

Finger
The fingers have now developed, and the fetus has a unique set of fingerprints

Hand
The hands are fully developed, and the fetus can suck its thumb

The fetus
The fetus grows in size and accumulates a layer of fat, and its internal organs become more complex. Its sense of hearing is now developed.

16 WEEKS
18 cm (7 in) long

28 WEEKS
30.5 cm (12 in) long

Umbilical cord

Third trimester (weeks 29–40)

During the third trimester, the mother gains weight as the fetus undergoes a growth spurt. The top of the uterus is high in the abdomen, almost to the level of the breastbone. This can cause slight shortness of breath due to compression of the mother's lungs.

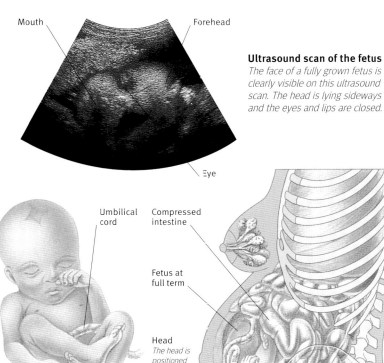

Mouth

Forehead

Ultrasound scan of the fetus
The face of a fully grown fetus is clearly visible on this ultrasound scan. The head is lying sideways and the eyes and lips are closed.

Eye

Umbilical cord

Compressed intestine

Fetus at full term

Head
The head is positioned just over the pelvis

The fetus at 37 weeks
The fetus is now fully formed, weighs about 3 kg (7 lb), and is about 50 cm (20 in) in length.

Mucus plug
A plug of mucus protects the fetus from infection

The mother at 37 weeks
The growing uterus presses on the intestines. The stomach may also be compressed, causing heartburn.

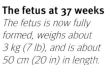

PROCESS

Engagement

A few weeks before labour begins, the head of the fetus moves down to sit snugly in the pelvis. The head is then said to be engaged. In women who have given birth before, this process may not occur until labour begins.

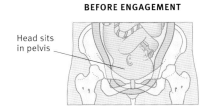

Head   Uterus   Pelvis

BEFORE ENGAGEMENT

Head sits in pelvis

AFTER ENGAGEMENT

Fetus at 40 weeks
In preparation for the birth, the fetus drops lower in the mother's abdomen so that its head sits low in her pelvic cavity.

PROCESS

Nourishing the fetus

The fetus is dependent on the mother for nourishment and oxygen. These substances are transferred from the mother's blood to the fetus's blood inside the placenta, an organ attached to the uterus and connected to the fetus by the umbilical cord. About 600 ml (1.1 pints) of maternal blood passes through the placenta every single minute, carrying a continuous supply of nutrients.

Umbilical cord

Placenta

Fetus

LOCATION

Maternal artery
This artery circulates blood, which contains oxygen and nutrients for the fetus, around the chorionic villi

Chorionic villus
Tiny projections, called villi, form from a thin membrane called the chorion and contain the fetal blood vessels

Flow of oxygen and nutrients

Wall of uterus

Maternal vein
This vein carries waste products away from the fetus

Lining of uterus (endometrium)

Flow of wastes

Pool of mother's blood

Umbilical vein
Blood, oxygen, and nutrients pass to the fetus from this vein

Umbilical artery
This artery carries waste products away from the fetus

Amniotic fluid

Umbilical cord

Blood vessels of the placenta
Inside the placenta, various substances are exchanged between the mother's blood and that of the fetus through a thin membrane called the chorion. Oxygen, nutrients, and antibodies pass from the mother's blood to the fetus's blood, and waste products pass in the opposite direction.

Fetal blood vessel
The blood vessels of the fetus are surrounded by the mother's blood

Lining of the uterus
The placenta is firmly attached to the uterine lining

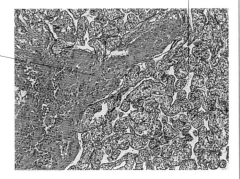

Placental tissue
This magnified image of a section of placenta shows tissue from both the mother and the fetus. In the placenta, their blood circulations do not mix but are in very close proximity.

Childbirth

The process of childbirth, known as labour, begins at about the 40th week of pregnancy. There are three distinct stages of labour: first, the contractions in the uterus and the widening of the cervix; second, the birth of the baby; and finally, the delivery of the placenta. The length of each stage varies between women and may depend on the number of previous pregnancies.

The first signs of labour

Labour begins when regular contractions start. The passing of the mucus plug from the cervix may occur several days before contractions start. The amniotic sac that surrounds the baby ruptures either shortly before or at any time during the first stage of labour. The first stage of labour lasts on average 6–12 hours.

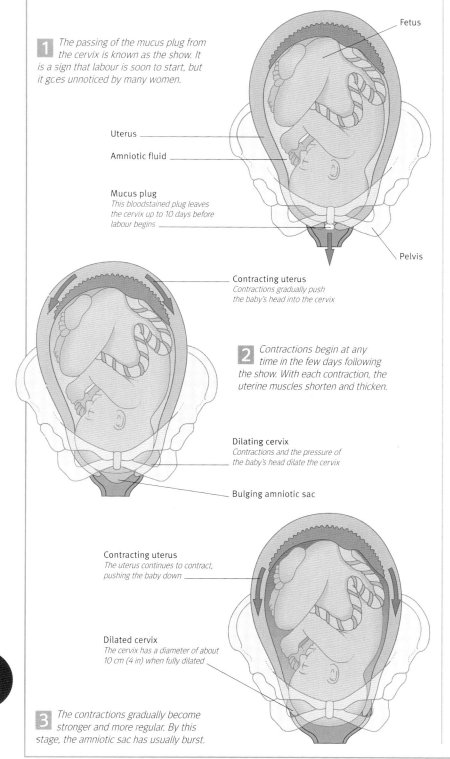

1 *The passing of the mucus plug from the cervix is known as the show. It is a sign that labour is soon to start, but it goes unnoticed by many women.*

Fetus

Uterus

Amniotic fluid

Mucus plug
This bloodstained plug leaves the cervix up to 10 days before labour begins

Pelvis

Contracting uterus
Contractions gradually push the baby's head into the cervix

2 *Contractions begin at any time in the few days following the show. With each contraction, the uterine muscles shorten and thicken.*

Dilating cervix
Contractions and the pressure of the baby's head dilate the cervix

Bulging amniotic sac

Contracting uterus
The uterus continues to contract, pushing the baby down

Dilated cervix
The cervix has a diameter of about 10 cm (4 in) when fully dilated

3 *The contractions gradually become stronger and more regular. By this stage, the amniotic sac has usually burst.*

Delivery of the baby

During the second stage of labour, the baby travels from the uterus down the vagina and is born. This stage is much quicker than the first stage and usually lasts 1–2 hours. The cervix is fully dilated, and the uterine contractions are very strong and usually painful. The baby's head presses down on the pelvic floor, which causes the mother to have an overwhelming urge to push down. Once the baby's head is visible at the vaginal opening, the birth is imminent.

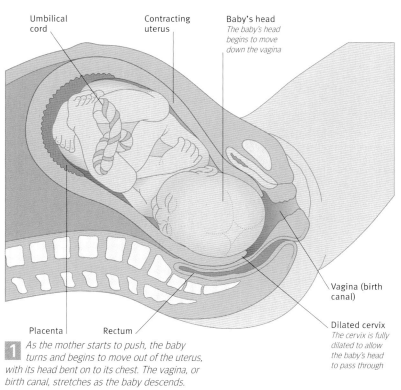

Umbilical cord

Contracting uterus

Baby's head
The baby's head begins to move down the vagina

Vagina (birth canal)

Dilated cervix
The cervix is fully dilated to allow the baby's head to pass through

Placenta

Rectum

1 *As the mother starts to push, the baby turns and begins to move out of the uterus, with its head bent on to its chest. The vagina, or birth canal, stretches as the baby descends.*

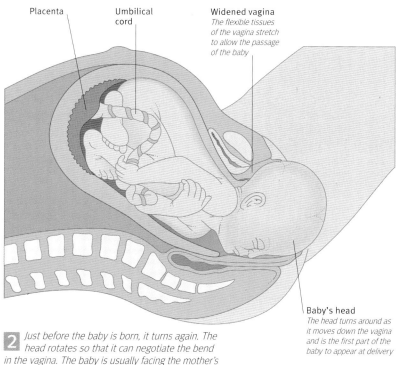

Placenta

Umbilical cord

Widened vagina
The flexible tissues of the vagina stretch to allow the passage of the baby

Baby's head
The head turns around as it moves down the vagina and is the first part of the baby to appear at delivery

2 *Just before the baby is born, it turns again. The head rotates so that it can negotiate the bend in the vagina. The baby is usually facing the mother's anus as it leaves the vagina.*

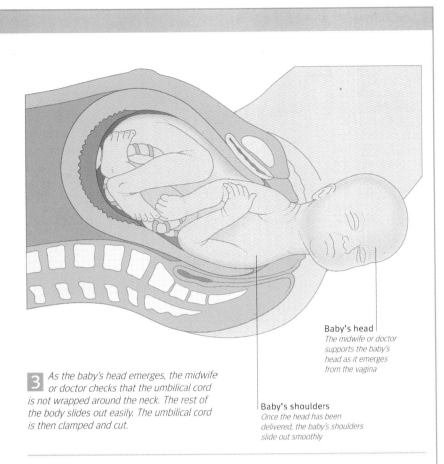

3 *As the baby's head emerges, the midwife or doctor checks that the umbilical cord is not wrapped around the neck. The rest of the body slides out easily. The umbilical cord is then clamped and cut.*

Baby's head
The midwife or doctor supports the baby's head as it emerges from the vagina

Baby's shoulders
Once the head has been delivered, the baby's shoulders slide out smoothly

Delivery of the placenta

During the third stage of labour, the placenta is expelled from the uterus. The placenta peels away from the lining of the uterus and is gently pushed through the vagina and out of the body. Often, the mother is injected with a drug that helps the muscles of the uterus to contract and so stop any bleeding from the site where the placenta was attached.

Uterus
The uterus resumes mild contractions shortly after the baby is born

Placenta
The placenta separates from the uterus 5–15 minutes after delivery

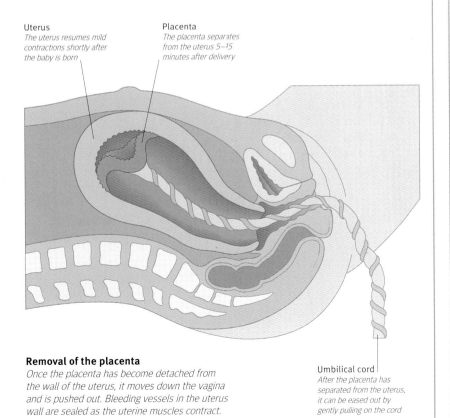

Removal of the placenta
Once the placenta has become detached from the wall of the uterus, it moves down the vagina and is pushed out. Bleeding vessels in the uterus wall are sealed as the uterine muscles contract.

Umbilical cord
After the placenta has separated from the uterus, it can be eased out by gently pulling on the cord

After the birth

After birth, the mother's breasts produce colostrum, a fluid rich in nutrients and antibodies, before milk production begins. The mother's uterus, cervix, vagina, and abdomen, which enlarged during pregnancy, begin to return to their normal sizes.

Preparing for lactation

During pregnancy, the lobules (milk-producing glands), which are dormant in nonpregnant women, gradually become able to produce milk in preparation for nourishing the newborn baby. At the same time, they increase in number so that enough milk is produced.

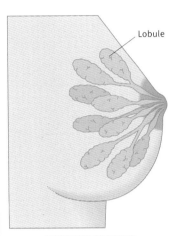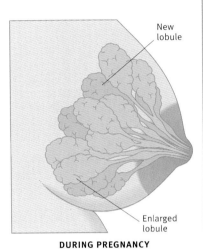

Lobule · New lobule · Enlarged lobule

BEFORE PREGNANCY · **DURING PREGNANCY**

Changes in the breasts
The number of lobules (milk-producing glands) in the breasts increases during pregnancy. After 3 months, they are able to produce colostrum, and after the baby is born, they can produce around 1 litre (1¾ pints) of milk each day.

The uterus returns to normal

The uterus begins to shrink immediately after birth and continues to decrease in size for the next 6–8 weeks, helped by hormones circulating in the mother's body. There may be some mild pains as the uterus shrinks, but these usually disappear soon after delivery.

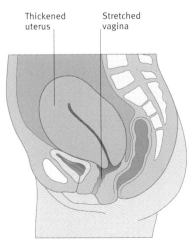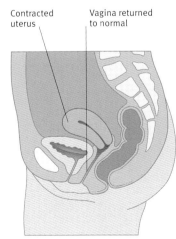

Thickened uterus · Stretched vagina · Contracted uterus · Vagina returned to normal

One week after childbirth
By 1 week after the birth, the uterus is already about half the size it was immediately after delivery of the baby.

Six weeks after childbirth
After 6 weeks, the uterus has contracted, although not quite to its original size, and returned to its usual position.

Problems in pregnancy

Pregnancy normally lasts about 40 weeks from conception to delivery of the baby. During this time, a single fertilized cell develops into a fully grown fetus that is able to survive outside the uterus. For the fetus to develop, it must be protected in the uterus and nourished by the mother. Although this process usually progresses smoothly, sometimes problems may develop.

Problems during pregnancy may affect the mother, the fetus, or both. Many of the most common disorders are mild and short-lived, but others may be severe or even life-threatening to the mother or the fetus.

The first article in this section deals with common complaints that occur at some time during most pregnancies. These complaints are usually minor and can often be relieved by simple self-help measures. High-risk pregnancies and pre-existing conditions that should be taken into consideration when planning a pregnancy are discussed next. The remaining articles in this section cover various problems that may occur at different stages of pregnancy.

In developed countries, pregnancy is no longer a major health risk for most women. In some cases, problems in pregnancy can be averted by good antenatal care and a healthy lifestyle before and during pregnancy. Pregnant women can stay healthy by eating a nutritious diet and exercising regularly (see **Exercise and relaxation in pregnancy**, p.508).

KEY ANATOMY

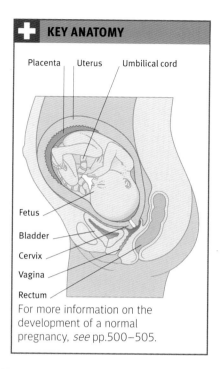

Placenta   Uterus   Umbilical cord

Fetus
Bladder
Cervix
Vagina
Rectum

For more information on the development of a normal pregnancy, see pp.500–505.

Common complaints of normal pregnancy

Minor problems commonly experienced during pregnancy

 Age, genetics, and lifestyle are not significant factors

Most of the common complaints that occur during pregnancy are not serious and are a result of the normal changes in the body that take place as the pregnancy progresses. Some problems are caused by changes in the levels of sex hormones in the mother, others by the weight and pressure of the developing fetus on the organs around the uterus. Although many pregnant women experience some or all of these complaints, others have only a few problems, and some feel even healthier than usual.

What are the symptoms?

Some symptoms that occur in pregnancy are due to the hormonal changes taking place in the body. They often develop early and may include:

- Breast tenderness.
- Nausea, often with vomiting (known as morning sickness).
- Tiredness.
- Constipation (p.398).

- Heartburn (see **Gastro-oesophageal reflux disease**, p.403).
- Skin changes, such as increased pigmentation and dryness.

The weight and pressure of the growing fetus and its surrounding fluid may also cause symptoms. These usually develop later in pregnancy and may include:

- An increased urge to pass urine.
- Increased constipation, which sometimes leads to haemorrhoids (p.422).
- Swollen ankles.
- Varicose veins (p.263).
- Stretch marks (p.203).
- Backache.
- Sciatica (p.338).
- Shortness of breath.
- Difficulty sleeping due to discomfort.

You may also feel very tired, feel faint on occasion, and have headaches.

It is normal to have several different symptoms during pregnancy and often to have more than one problem at a time. If you are worried about a specific symptom, you should obtain medical advice. You should also speak to your doctor or midwife if you are having problems with severe vomiting and cannot keep any food or fluids down (see **Hyperemesis**, p.510). If you find it painful to pass urine or your urine appears cloudy, you should consult your doctor or midwife to make sure that you do not have a urinary tract infection, such as cystitis (p.453).

TESTS

Routine antenatal care

Antenatal care is essential to make sure that a pregnancy is progressing well. The table below lists tests that may be offered to a woman during pregnancy. However, the precise tests offered will depend on the individual woman's situation. Antenatal genetic tests (p.509) may also be carried out to look for a gene or chromosome disorder in the fetus.

Routine tests
Antenatal care usually starts at about 10 weeks into the pregnancy. Follow-up visits to check progress of the pregnancy then occur at regular intervals until delivery.

When done	Type of test	Reason for test
First visits (before 12 weeks)	Medical history and examination	To look for pre-existing risk factors, such as long-term illnesses
	Urine tests	To check the urine for glucose, which may indicate diabetes developing in pregnancy (p.509), and for protein, which may indicate pre-existing kidney disease
	Blood tests	To determine the woman's blood type, and to check for anaemia (p.271); antibodies to rubella (p.168); hepatitis B virus (see **Acute hepatitis**, p.408); Down's syndrome (p.533); sickle-cell disease (p.272); thalassaemia (p.273); and, after discussion, HIV infection (p.169). Genetic counselling may be offered to couples with a family history of inherited disease or from ethnic groups at high risk
	Weight and blood pressure	To provide initial measurements against which later ones can be compared
Between 12 and 20 weeks	Ultrasound scans	At 12 weeks: to check dates and look for multiple pregnancy; also, together with blood test results, to assess the risk of fetal abnormalities. At 20 weeks: to check for anatomical fetal abnormalities and to check the position of the placenta (see **Ultrasound scanning in pregnancy**, p.512). Additional scans may also be recommended
Follow-up visits at regular intervals from 12 weeks to delivery	Weight (not routine in women of normal weight) and abdominal examination	To assess the growth of the fetus and determine which way it is lying in the uterus
	Urine tests	To detect diabetes mellitus, pre-eclampsia (p.513), and urine infection
	Blood pressure	To detect developing pre-eclampsia
	Blood tests (at some visits only)	To look for anaemia and, in combination with ultrasound scanning, to assess the risk of fetal abnormalities. A test to screen for diabetes mellitus in the mother may also be necessary
	Fetal heartbeat check	To assess whether the fetus's heart is beating normally

What can I do?

There is little that you can do to relieve some of the symptoms associated with pregnancy, such as breast tenderness. However, some other complaints may be eased by self-help measures (see **Coping with pregnancy**, opposite page). For example, eating frequent snacks rather than a few larger meals may help to reduce nausea and heartburn. If heartburn is severe, you may be prescribed antacid drugs (p.596).

You should check with your doctor or midwife before you take any over-the-counter drugs or complementary remedies because there are several common medications that can harm a developing baby and should not be taken at any time during pregnancy.

High-risk pregnancy

A pregnancy with a higher than average risk for the mother or the fetus

 Most common under the age of 15 or over the age of 35

 Smoking and alcohol or drug abuse during pregnancy are risk factors

 Genetics as a risk factor depends on the cause

For most women, pregnancy progresses well except for minor problems, such as tiredness and swollen ankles (see **Common complaints of normal pregnancy**, p.506).

▶ **SELF-HELP**

Coping with pregnancy

It is normal to experience a variety of complaints during pregnancy. These are usually caused by hormonal changes within the body and by the increasing weight of the fetus. Although such complaints may cause discomfort, they are usually not serious. Many symptoms can be relieved by self-help measures, but you should consult your pharmacist, doctor, or midwife before using any over-the-counter drugs or complementary remedies and see your doctor if symptoms are severe.

Digestive complaints

A healthy diet is important throughout pregnancy. It not only provides the fetus with the correct nutrients for growth but also helps to prevent you having digestive problems associated with pregnancy, such as nausea, heartburn, and constipation. Avoid spicy foods because they can cause heartburn, and always have something plain available to eat in case you feel hungry.

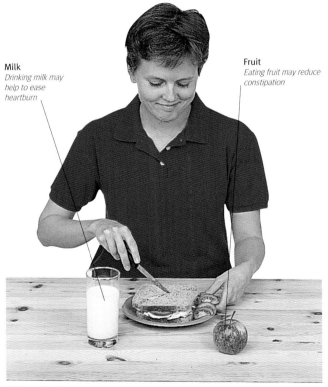

Milk
Drinking milk may help to ease heartburn

Fruit
Eating fruit may reduce constipation

Eating during pregnancy
Small, frequent meals may help to reduce nausea, and milky drinks may ease heartburn. Plenty of fruit, vegetables, and other fibre-rich foods in your diet should help to reduce constipation.

Circulatory complaints

Increased pressure on the blood vessels in the pelvis may lead to varicose veins, swollen ankles, and feeling faint in late pregnancy. To relieve symptoms, avoid standing still for long periods of time and sit or lie down whenever you feel faint. Support tights may help to relieve varicose veins.

Support for back

Pillow under legs

Feet raised above hip level

Sitting comfortably
Try to rest and put your feet up whenever possible. Support your back and always try to elevate your feet above the level of your hips.

Backache and sciatica

Backache is an increasingly common problem as pregnancy progresses, and poor posture may place pressure on the sciatic nerve, causing a shooting pain from the buttock down one leg (sciatica). Both of these problems may be eased by adopting good posture when standing, using a chair with good back support, sleeping on a firm mattress, and wearing flat shoes.

Shoulders held back

Straight spine

Buttocks tucked in

Abdomen tucked in

Knees relaxed

Shoulders hunched

Curved spine

Buttocks protruding

Abdomen protruding

Knees locked

CORRECT   **INCORRECT**

Standing correctly
Stand with your feet apart and your weight equally balanced on each foot. Hold your back straight and your shoulders back. Tuck in your buttocks and abdomen and relax your knees.

Tiredness and difficulty sleeping

You will probably feel tired from early pregnancy onwards. As your pregnancy progresses and your abdomen enlarges, you may also find it more difficult to get into a comfortable position in which to sleep. Before going to bed, try to relax, have a warm bath and a milky drink, and watch television, listen to the radio, or read until you feel sleepy.

Sleeping comfortably
Try to sleep on your side, with a pillow between your legs. You may feel more comfortable if you place another pillow under your abdomen.

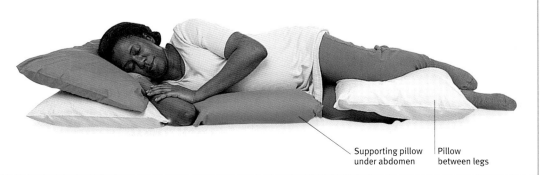

Supporting pillow under abdomen

Pillow between legs

However, pregnancy is not without risks. Although the risk of death for both mother and fetus is low, it increases in certain situations. Some women are at higher risk of developing problems in pregnancy, and one of the functions of routine antenatal care (p.506) is to identify these women so that they can be monitored and receive additional treatment if needed.

What are the risk factors?
There are many different risk factors that may lead to a high-risk pregnancy. Women under the age of 15 or over the age of 35 are more likely to have problems, as are women who have a small build or who are overweight. Other risk factors in pregnancy include certain lifestyle factors, such as smoking; a history of problems in previous pregnancies; and pre-existing illnesses.

Age Women under the age of 15 who become pregnant are at increased risk of going into labour before the end of the pregnancy (see **Premature labour**, p.515). They are also at risk of certain complications during pregnancy, such as pre-eclampsia and eclampsia (p.513) in which blood pressure is high.

Women over the age of 35 are more likely to have pre-existing disorders, such as noncancerous tumours in the uterus (see **Fibroids**, p.477) or diabetes mellitus (p.437). They are also at greater risk of developing pre-eclampsia or diabetes while pregnant (see **Diabetes developing in pregnancy**, p.509), which may place the pregnancy at risk. There is also an increased likelihood of the fetus having a chromosomal abnormality, such as Down's syndrome (p.533).

Physical factors Women who have a small build and a small pelvis are at greater risk of a delayed first stage of labour (p.517), particularly if they are carrying a large baby who cannot easily fit through the pelvis.

Women who weigh less than 47.5 kg (105 lb) before pregnancy are more likely to have small babies. Conversely, women who are overweight are at increased risk of developing diabetes mellitus during pregnancy, which increases their risk of having a large baby. Overweight women are also at greater risk of high blood pressure (see **Hypertension**, p.242).

Lifestyle factors Having a poor diet, smoking, and abusing alcohol or drugs during pregnancy all increase the risk of problems occurring, including miscarriage (p.511), premature labour, and intra-uterine growth retardation (p.514).

Problems in previous pregnancies Any problems in a previous pregnancy, such as a premature labour or stillbirth (p.520), increase the risk for the current pregnancy. A woman who had a small baby in a previous pregnancy will be more likely to have another baby who is underweight.

Pre-existing illnesses Any disorder that is already present (see **Pre-existing diseases in pregnancy**, right), such as diabetes mellitus, epilepsy (p.324), or high blood pressure, may lead to problems for

mother and fetus. Changes to the mother's medication and additional monitoring of mother and fetus may be necessary both before and during the pregnancy.

What might be done?
At your first antenatal visit, your doctor or midwife will ask you questions to determine whether or not you are at increased risk. If you are, you will need additional monitoring and possibly specialized treatment.

If you have a high-risk pregnancy, you will probably need more frequent antenatal visits. You may be offered additional tests if you are at increased risk of having a baby with a gene or chromosome disorder (see **Antenatal genetic tests**, opposite page). Blood tests may be needed to monitor any pre-existing diseases, and additional ultrasound scans may be needed to monitor the growth of the fetus (see **Ultrasound scanning in pregnancy**, p.512). You may be supervised by several doctors and specialists.

What is the prognosis?
With monitoring and modern delivery techniques, most problems can be treated successfully. Although complications are more likely to occur in a high-risk pregnancy, modern treatments have improved the outlook.

Pre-existing diseases in pregnancy

Long-term pre-existing diseases that could affect the progress of pregnancy or the health of the fetus

 More common over the age of 35

 Genetics and lifestyle as risk factors depend on the specific condition

If a woman who becomes pregnant has a long-term medical condition, she will need specialist care throughout pregnancy and labour. Pre-existing disorders that could adversely affect pregnancy or the health of the fetus are more common in women over the age of 35. For example, such women are more likely to have pre-existing disorders, such as noncancerous tumours in the uterus (see **Fibroids**, p.477) or diabetes mellitus (p.437), which may affect the progress of the pregnancy and the development of the fetus.

Long-term pre-existing disorders and their treatment may affect the progress of the pregnancy. For example, women who have diabetes mellitus (p.437) are more prone to problems such as high blood pressure (see **Hypertension**, p.242) or premature labour (p.515), particularly if the condition is not well controlled. Changes in hormone levels during pregnancy can have adverse effects on diabetes mellitus, which often worsens. However, in some women who have mild asthma (p.295), symptoms improve during pregnancy.

▶ HEALTH ACTION

Exercise and relaxation in pregnancy
Antenatal and other gentle exercises help to keep you fit, prepare you for the physical demands of labour, and speed recovery after the birth. Relaxation exercises relieve stress of the mind and the body and conserve energy to allow you to cope more effectively with labour.

Exercise
You can maintain your previous level of exercise during pregnancy, but you may need to modify some exercises because you are more vulnerable to injury. Drink lots of water and try not to push your heart rate over 140 beats per minute.

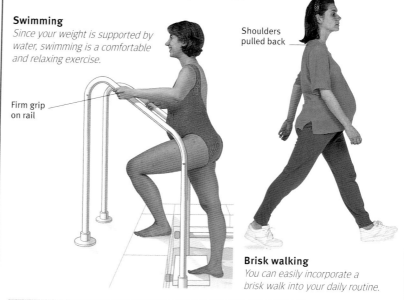

Swimming
Since your weight is supported by water, swimming is a comfortable and relaxing exercise.

Shoulders pulled back

Firm grip on rail

Brisk walking
You can easily incorporate a brisk walk into your daily routine.

Antenatal exercises
Exercises can help to relieve some of the discomforts of pregnancy, such as backache, and in most cases are very beneficial for both mother and baby. For example, pelvic tilt exercises are an excellent way to improve posture. Antenatal exercise classes can teach you how to exercise safely.

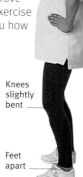

Straight back

Pelvic tilt exercises
Tighten your buttocks and tuck your pelvis under, then relax the buttocks and rock the pelvis back; repeat several times. Do this a number of times a day.

Knees slightly bent

Feet apart

Relaxation
Certain breathing and relaxation techniques, such as massage, can help you to cope better with labour. Antenatal or yoga classes may teach you how to contract and relax muscle groups all over your body (see **Relaxation exercises**, p.32).

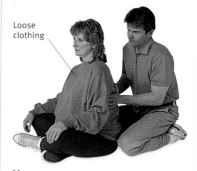

Loose clothing

Massage
Massage can help you to relax and can lessen pain in the early stages of labour.

The fetus may also be affected by pre-existing diseases in the mother. Some maternal disorders, such as chronic high blood pressure and kidney failure (p.450), may affect the function of the placenta and lead to malnourishment of the fetus, affecting its development and growth. For example, a mother who has high blood pressure is at an

increased risk of having a smaller than average baby (see **Intra-uterine growth retardation**, p.514). A baby who is born to a mother with diabetes mellitus may have low blood sugar levels immediately after birth.

If you have a long-term pre-existing condition, and are planning to start a family, you should consult your doctor before

▶ **TEST**

Antenatal genetic tests

You may be offered blood tests and/or ultrasound scanning to determine whether you are at increased risk of having a baby with a genetic or chromosomal disorder. Ultrasound can detect thickening of the tissues at the back of the neck of the fetus (nuchal translucency) and absence of the nasal bone, which indicate a risk of a chromosomal disorder such as Down's syndrome (p.533). If tests suggest a disorder, you may be offered chorionic villus sampling or amniocentesis.

Chorionic villus sampling

Chorionic villus sampling is usually carried out between the 11th and 14th weeks of pregnancy. Tissue from the edge of the placenta (chorionic villi) is taken and then analysed to look for a chromosomal or genetic abnormality. The risk of miscarriage is increased slightly by having this test.

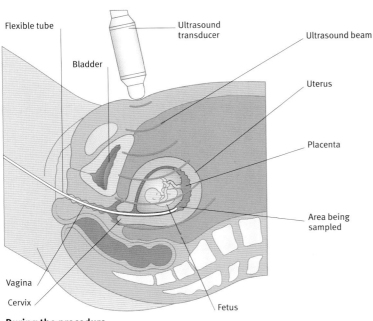

Flexible tube · Ultrasound transducer · Ultrasound beam · Bladder · Uterus · Placenta · Area being sampled · Vagina · Cervix · Fetus

During the procedure
A small sample of the placenta is taken either by inserting a needle through the abdominal wall or, as shown here, using a flexible tube that is passed through the cervix. Ultrasound is used to guide the tube, and the sample is removed using gentle suction.

Non-invasive prenatal diagnosis

This is based on a blood test carried out on a sample of the mother's blood. The test is usually performed at about the 10th week of pregnancy and is carried out on a blood sample taken from the mother's arm. Genetic material from the unborn baby occurs naturally in the mother's blood, and this can be analysed to check for the baby's sex, as well as certain genetic and chromosomal disorders, such as achondroplasia (p.540), Duchenne muscular dystrophy (p.536), and Down's syndrome (p.533). The test does not carry any risk for the pregnancy.

Amniocentesis

Amniocentesis is usually carried out between the 15th and 20th weeks of pregnancy. A small sample of the amniotic fluid surrounding the fetus is removed and analysed for genetic abnormalities. The procedure is associated with a small risk of miscarriage (about 1 in 200 women).

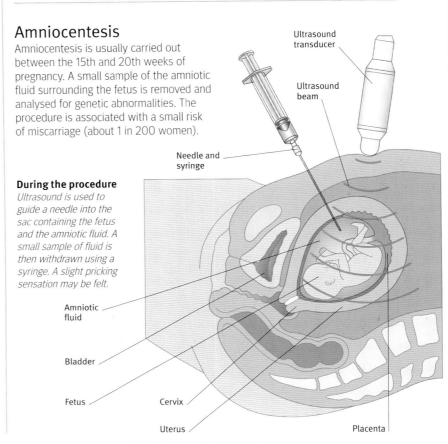

Ultrasound transducer · Ultrasound beam · Needle and syringe

During the procedure
Ultrasound is used to guide a needle into the sac containing the fetus and the amniotic fluid. A small sample of fluid is then withdrawn using a syringe. A slight pricking sensation may be felt.

Amniotic fluid · Bladder · Fetus · Cervix · Uterus · Placenta

---

becoming pregnant. Your condition, and that of your fetus, will need careful monitoring throughout the term of your pregnancy. Your doctor will work with your obstetrician to make sure that you remain as healthy as possible and that the progress of your pregnancy is successful.

What might be done?
If you have a long-term disorder, your doctor will review your condition carefully before you become pregnant to make sure that it is as well controlled as possible.

Your usual treatment may need to be altered while you are pregnant because some drugs can affect the fetus. For example, if you normally take tablets to control your diabetes mellitus, you may have to change to insulin injections (*see* **Drugs for diabetes mellitus**, p.601). The dose of some treatments may need to be altered, and additional measures may be required to control the pre-existing disorder. For example, women who have epilepsy (p.324), and who are taking

anticonvulsant drugs (p.590) to prevent any seizures, will usually be prescribed a higher than normal dose of folic acid in order to reduce the risk of their medication causing neural tube defects (p.547), abnormalities of the brain and spinal cord which may occur during pregnancy, in the fetus.

You may have antenatal checkups at more frequent intervals than usual, and your doctor may refer you to an obstetrician specializing in your condition. You may be required to have additional tests, including extra ultrasound scans (*see* **Ultrasound scanning in pregnancy**, p.512). Additional monitoring may be necessary during labour, and after the delivery your baby may be given a series of tests to ensure that he or she is healthy.

What is the prognosis?
With regular monitoring and carefully adjusted treatment, both before and during a pregnancy, as well as during the birth, pre-existing conditions can be controlled, and they usually carry little risk for either the

mother or the fetus. Any changes in the mother's condition that may have developed as a result of the pregnancy will normally be reversed soon after the baby has been born.

> ## Diabetes developing in pregnancy
>
> *Inability of the tissues to absorb glucose from the bloodstream during pregnancy due to a lack of the hormone insulin*
>
> More common over the age of 30
>
> A family history of diabetes mellitus is a risk factor
>
> Being overweight is a risk factor

During the course of pregnancy, up to 1 in 50 women temporarily develops diabetes mellitus (p.437). The condition

is called gestational diabetes. Normally, the hormone insulin, which is produced by the pancreas, enables body cells to absorb glucose from the bloodstream. During pregnancy, additional hormones, which have an anti-insulin effect, are produced by the placenta. If the body does not produce enough insulin to counter this effect, the result is high levels of glucose in the blood and gestational diabetes.

Diabetes developing in pregnancy is more common in women over the age of 30, women who are overweight, and those who have a family history of diabetes mellitus. Gestational diabetes can usually be controlled by a special diet.

In most cases, gestational diabetes disappears after the birth of the baby, but about 1 in 3 women who has had gestational diabetes develops permanent type 2 diabetes mellitus, often within 5 years of pregnancy.

What are the symptoms?

Most women with gestational diabetes do not develop symptoms. Others may develop the same symptoms that occur in non-gestational diabetes, including:

- Tiredness.
- Dry mouth and increased thirst.
- Frequent urination, and passing large amounts of urine.

If gestational diabetes is not controlled, the fetus may gain an excessive amount of weight and have difficulty passing through the mother's pelvis. Labour may then be particularly difficult (*see* **Problems during delivery**, p.518). Babies born to mothers with gestational diabetes are also at risk of having low blood sugar levels at birth. Women whose diabetes cannot be controlled have a greater risk of a stillbirth (p.520).

How is it diagnosed?

Diabetes mellitus is usually detected when urine and/or blood tests reveal the presence of glucose. Your urine will be tested for glucose at each antenatal visit. If glucose is found in your urine, your doctor may arrange for a glucose tolerance test, in which you are given a sugar solution to drink and a sample of your blood is tested. If your blood shows higher than expected glucose levels, the diagnosis of gestational diabetes is confirmed. Your doctor may also suggest that you have the glucose tolerance test if you have had an unexplained stillbirth in the past; if you have given birth to a larger than average baby; or if diabetes mellitus runs in your family because this may increase your risk of developing gestational diabetes.

What is the treatment?

If you have gestational diabetes, your doctor will recommend that you follow a modified diet that contains less sugar than normal. Some women also need metformin (*see* **Drugs for diabetes mellitus**, p.601) or insulin injections. You may be advised to test your blood sugar levels at home (*see* **Monitoring your blood glucose**, p.439). More frequent antenatal visits than usual may be necessary, and you may also need to have extra ultrasound scans (*see* **Ultrasound scanning in pregnancy**, p.512).

For most women with gestational diabetes, pregnancy progresses safely. Labour is often induced (*see* **Induction of labour**, p.515) at about 38 weeks and vaginal delivery is possible. However, if diabetes becomes difficult to control, early induction of labour may be necessary. If the fetus is very large, the doctor may carry out a caesarean section (p.518).

After delivery, your blood sugar levels and those of your baby will be monitored. If the baby's blood sugar level is low, he or she may need to be admitted to a special care baby unit (p.619) for treatment. Since you may be at risk of developing permanent diabetes mellitus after pregnancy, you will be given a glucose tolerance test at your 6-week postnatal checkup.

▶ TREATMENT

Termination of pregnancy

A termination of pregnancy may be carried out if the pregnancy threatens the woman's physical or emotional health or if tests show a severe fetal disorder. All types of termination cause some abdominal pain for a few hours and a brown discharge for several days. Sexual intercourse should be avoided for 2 weeks afterwards.

Methods of termination
There are several different methods of termination, depending on the stage of the pregnancy. The main methods and their usual timing are outlined in the table below.

Method	When done	Procedure used
Early medical abortion	Up to the 9th week of pregnancy	This method involves taking two drugs to cause an early miscarriage. First, oral mifepristone is given then, about 48 hours later, a prostaglandin drug is also given, usually as a vaginal pessary. These drugs induce the uterus to contract and expel the embryo and placenta, usually within a few hours.
Medical abortion	Between the 9th and 20th weeks of pregnancy	This method, which is similar to an early medical abortion, involves giving an initial dose of oral mifepristone then, about 48 hours later, also giving a prostaglandin drug, usually as vaginal pessary. However, several doses of prostaglandin may be needed to make the uterus contract and expel the embryo and placenta.
Suction termination	Between the 7th and the 12th weeks of pregnancy. Sometimes used before the 7th week and up to the 15th week	This procedure involves dilating the cervix and removing the contents of the uterus with a suction device. It may be carried out under either local or general anaesthesia. Before the procedure, the cervix may be softened by administering medication (for example, a prostaglandin pessary inserted into the vagina).
Surgical dilatation and evacuation	Between the 15th and end of the 23rd weeks of pregnancy	This procedure involves dilating the cervix and removing the contents of the uterus with forceps; any remaining uterine contents are then removed with a suction device. The procedure is carried out under general anaesthesia.

What is the prognosis?

Usually, glucose levels return to normal soon after the birth, and you should be able to resume your normal diet. If you were having insulin injections, they can be stopped. However, you are likely to develop diabetes in future pregnancies and may be at risk of developing diabetes in later life.

Hyperemesis

Severe vomiting associated with early pregnancy

 More common in younger women

 May sometimes run in families

 Stress may aggravate the condition

Hyperemesis is vomiting that occurs in early pregnancy and is so extreme that no food or fluids can be kept down. The condition is more severe than common morning sickness (*see* **Common complaints of normal pregnancy**, p.506). In morning sickness, nausea and vomiting also occur in early pregnancy, as a result of hormonal changes in the body, but are usually not serious.

When morning sickness occurs in pregnancy, the mother continues to gain weight steadily as the pregnancy progresses. In contrast, a mother who has hyperemesis will lose weight. The excessive vomiting eventually leads to dehydration, which, in turn, decreases urine volume and causes an imbalance of chemicals in the blood. If hyperemesis is allowed to continue without treatment, dehydration may become life-threatening for both the mother and the fetus.

Hyperemesis is generally more common in younger mothers, and in some cases it seems to run in families. However, the underlying cause is usually not known, although it is thought that very high amounts of human chorionic gonadotropin (HCG), a hormone that is produced by the placenta in pregnancy, may contribute to excessive nausea and vomiting in the mother. High levels of HCG occur if more than one fetus is present (*see* **Multiple pregnancy and its problems**, p.512). Less commonly, very high amounts of HCG are produced if a tumour develops from part of the placenta (*see* **Molar pregnancy**, p.510). Occasionally, a urinary tract infection may cause vomiting in pregnancy. Psychological factors, such as emotional stress, may aggravate hyperemesis in some women.

What might be done?

If you are unable to keep any food or fluids down, you will need to be admitted to hospital for treatment. You may need to have blood tests so that the doctors can assess the degree of dehydration that has occurred as a result of severe vomiting, and a urine test in order to check for a urinary tract infection. You may also undergo ultrasound scanning (*see* **Ultrasound scanning in pregnancy**, p.512) to investigate the possibility of a multiple or molar pregnancy.

Usually, dehydration is treated in hospital with intravenous fluids. You may also be given drugs that help to stop the vomiting (*see* **Antiemetic drugs**, p.595). If the urine tests have confirmed the presence of a urinary tract infection, antibiotics will probably be given to treat it.

Once the vomiting has been treated, and you can begin to keep down food and fluids, you should be able to start eating small quantities of plain food and gradually build up to a normal diet. However, the vomiting often recurs, and further stays in hospital may be necessary so that adequate measures may be taken to prevent dehydration. Hyperemesis usually subsides after the 14th week of pregnancy, although the condition is likely to recur in subsequent pregnancies.

Molar pregnancy

A rare condition in which there is abnormal overgrowth of all or part of the placenta

 More common over the age of 35

 More common in Asian women

 Lifestyle is not a significant factor

In about 1 in 700 pregnancies, part of the placenta develops into a hydatidiform mole, a tumour (abnormal growth) that resembles a small bunch of grapes. Although a hydatidiform mole is noncancerous, in a few cases it develops into a cancerous tumour (*see* **Choriocarcinoma**, p.480). A hormone called human chorionic gonadotropin (HCG), which is normally produced by the placenta in pregnancy, is present in very high levels in molar pregnancy. In most molar pregnancies, the tumour prevents a fetus from developing, but occasionally an abnormal fetus develops. Placental cells left after a miscarriage or pregnancy can develop into a hydatidiform mole.

In about 1 in 10 molar pregnancies, a hydatidiform mole invades the wall of the uterus. In about 3 in 100 cases, a hydatidiform mole becomes cancerous, and the cancer may spread. Molar pregnancy occurs more often in women over the age of 35 and is more common in Asian women. The cause is unknown. In many cases, molar pregnancy is detected during a routine ultrasound scan in early pregnancy (*see* **Ultrasound scanning in pregnancy**, p.512).

What are the symptoms?

A hydatidiform mole exaggerates some of the symptoms of a normal, healthy pregnancy, such as tiredness, and it may also produce the following:

- Bleeding from the vagina and passing material that looks like grapes.
- Extreme nausea and vomiting (*see* **Hyperemesis**, p.510).

A hydatidiform mole grows faster than a normal fetus, making the uterus larger than normal for the stage of pregnancy. If the pregnancy progresses, additional problems, including pre-eclampsia (p.513) and anaemia (p.271), may develop.

What might be done?

If you are experiencing severe nausea and vomiting or if your uterus appears much larger than normal for the stage of your pregnancy, your doctor may suspect a molar pregnancy. He or she will arrange for an ultrasound scan to look for signs of a molar pregnancy, and your blood will be tested to measure levels of HCG. If a hydatidiform mole is diagnosed, the abnormal tissue will be removed from the uterus under general anaesthesia.

What is the prognosis?

Most women recover fully and need no further treatment once the molar pregnancy has been removed. However, a choriocarcinoma sometimes develops and further treatment, such as chemotherapy (p.157), is required.

It is important that women who have had a molar pregnancy should have regular urine tests for at least 2 years to measure HCG levels and ensure that any cancerous changes are detected early. It is advisable not to conceive for at least 1 year after treatment for a hydatidiform mole because the risk of choriocarcinoma is greatest during this time and a pregnancy will interfere with HCG monitoring. In up to 3 in 100 subsequent pregnancies, a hydatidiform mole recurs.

Ectopic pregnancy

A pregnancy that develops outside the uterus, usually in a fallopian tube

 Age, genetics, and lifestyle are not significant factors

About 2 in 100 pregnancies is ectopic. In an ectopic pregnancy, a fertilized egg becomes implanted in tissues outside the uterus instead of in the uterine lining. The egg then begins to develop into an embryo. In most ectopic pregnancies, the fertilized egg lodges inside one of the two fallopian tubes. Rarely, the egg implants in the cervix, in one of the ovaries, or in the abdominal cavity. The embryo is not able to grow normally in an ectopic pregnancy and only rarely survives.

If the placenta develops inside a fallopian tube and the embryo grows, the fallopian tube will eventually rupture, caus-ing life-threatening bleeding into the mother's abdominal cavity. Ectopic pregnancies need to be treated as soon as possible after detection because of the risk to the mother.

What are the causes?

Ectopic pregnancy may occur as a result of previous damage to the fallopian tubes, which may obstruct the passage of a fertilized egg along a tube to the uterus. The egg then implants in the wall of the tube instead of in the uterus. This damage is most commonly due to previous pelvic inflammatory disease (p.475) but may also have occurred as a result of surgery on the fallopian tubes, such as reversal of sterilization (*see* **Female sterilization**, p.476).

What are the symptoms?

An ectopic pregnancy usually produces symptoms in the first 6–7 weeks, sometimes even before the woman realizes she is pregnant. However, most women who have an ectopic pregnancy will have missed a menstrual period by the time symptoms appear. The symptoms may include:

- Pain that is low down on one side of the abdomen.
- Irregular vaginal bleeding that may be confused with menstruation.

If the ectopic pregnancy is not detected and a fallopian tube ruptures, further symptoms may develop that include:

- Sudden, severe pain that gradually spreads throughout the abdomen.
- Shoulder pain (referred pain due to irritation of the diaphragm).

Sudden internal bleeding follows the rupture of the fallopian tube and may cause shock (p.248). If you are in shock, you may sweat profusely and feel faint. It is important to see your doctor at once if you have abdominal pain or vaginal bleeding and might be pregnant. If you experience severe pain or shock, call an ambulance immediately.

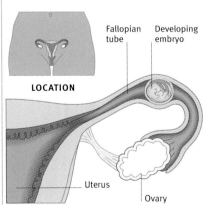

LOCATION

Fallopian tube / Developing embryo / Uterus / Ovary

Ectopic pregnancy
In most ectopic pregnancies, the fertilized egg implants in a fallopian tube and starts to develop there, rather than in the uterus.

What might be done?

If you are not sure whether or not you are pregnant, a pregnancy test will be performed. If the test is positive, your doctor may arrange for you to have an ultrasound scan to find out the position of the embryo.

You may also have a blood test to measure blood levels of human chorionic gonadotropin (HCG), a hormone that is produced in lower amounts than normal in ectopic pregnancies. To confirm the diagnosis, an examination of the inside of the abdominal cavity may be performed under general anaesthesia (*see* **Laparoscopy**, p.476).

If an ectopic pregnancy is confirmed, the embryo and surrounding tissue are usually removed. This may be done by laparoscopy or by conventional surgery. A damaged fallopian tube will be repaired if possible, but, if it is badly damaged, the tube may be removed to prevent another ectopic pregnancy from occurring at the same site. If an ectopic pregnancy is diagnosed early, it may be treated with the drug methotrexate rather than by surgery.

What is the prognosis?

Although approximately 1 in 10 women will have a further ectopic pregnancy, most affected women can have normal pregnancies even if one fallopian tube has been removed. If both tubes have been damaged, in-vitro fertilization (*see* **Assisted conception**, p.498) may help a woman to become pregnant.

In subsequent pregnancies, an ultrasound scan (*see* **Ultrasound scanning in pregnancy**, p.512) may be carried out at an early stage to check that the fetus is developing in the uterus.

Vaginal bleeding in pregnancy

Bleeding from the vagina at any time during pregnancy

 Age, genetics, and lifestyle are not significant factors

If you experience vaginal bleeding in pregnancy, you should seek immediate advice from your doctor. If you develop heavy bleeding, particularly late in pregnancy, you should call an ambulance. Severe bleeding may be life-threatening for both you and your baby, so it is vital that you receive emergency care.

What are the causes?

The causes of vaginal bleeding in pregnancy vary, depending on the stage of the pregnancy.

Bleeding before 14 weeks Bleeding in early pregnancy can be caused by a miscarriage (right) and may be accompanied by cramping, period-like pain. Light to heavy bleeding and severe pain before about 7 weeks may be due to a pregnancy outside the uterus (*see* **Ectopic pregnancy**, left).

Rarely, light, painless vaginal bleeding called spotting persists during the first 14 weeks of pregnancy. In most of these cases, the pregnancy continues.

Bleeding at 14–24 weeks After week 14 of pregnancy, bleeding may be due to a late miscarriage, the causes of which can include a weak cervix (*see* **Cervical incompetence**, p.513). Bleeding due to miscarriage at this stage may be painful.

Bleeding after 24 weeks After the 24th week of pregnancy, painful, light to heavy vaginal bleeding may be caused by placental abruption (p.516), in which the placenta becomes partially separated from the wall of the uterus. Painless vaginal bleeding after 24 weeks may be due to placenta praevia (p.516), in which the placenta covers some or all of the opening of the cervix.

What might be done?

A manual examination is rarely carried out, particularly if you are in late pregnancy, because the examination could damage the placenta if it is lying low in the uterus. Using a speculum to hold the vagina open, your doctor will examine your cervix to look for a local cause of the bleeding. You will also have an ultrasound scan (*see* **Ultrasound scanning in pregnancy**, p.512) and fetal heartbeat monitoring may be carried out (*see* **Fetal monitoring**, p.519).

Treatment depends on the cause and extent of the bleeding and the stage of your pregnancy. If you have light to moderate bleeding in early pregnancy, your doctor may suggest that you rest in bed. Most of these pregnancies continue normally. However, surgery may be necessary in some cases of miscarriage or if the cause of the bleeding is found to be an ectopic pregnancy. If you have heavy vaginal bleeding later in your pregnancy, your baby may have to be delivered by an emergency caesarean section (p.518). If you have lost a large amount of blood, you may need to have a blood transfusion (p.272).

Miscarriage

The spontaneous end of a pregnancy before week 24, also known as a spontaneous abortion

 Most common under the age of 16 and over the age of 35

 In some cases, due to a genetic or chromosomal abnormality in the fetus

 Smoking and alcohol or drug abuse during pregnancy are risk factors

More than 1 in 4 of all pregnancies end in miscarriage, the loss of a fetus before the 24th week of pregnancy. Most miscarriages occur in the first 14 weeks of pregnancy, and some occur so early that the woman may not be aware that she is pregnant. Generally, women who miscarry have abnormal vaginal bleeding and abdominal cramps.

What are the causes?

About 3 in 5 miscarriages in the first 14 weeks of pregnancy are caused by a genetic disorder or an abnormality in the fetus. Early miscarriage is more common in multiple pregnancies (*see* **Multiple pregnancy and its problems**, p.512).

Later miscarriages (between weeks 14 and 24) may be due to a weak cervix (see Cervical incompetence, p.513) or to a severe infection in the mother. An abnormally shaped uterus or noncancerous tumours in the wall of the uterus (see Fibroids, p.477) may also cause a late miscarriage. Smoking and alcohol or drug abuse in pregnancy are also risk factors. Women who have diabetes mellitus (p.437) are at increased risk of a late miscarriage.

Any of the above factors may cause recurrent miscarriages. Generally, miscarriage is more common in women under the age of 16 or over 35. It is a commonly held belief that stress or minor injuries may lead to miscarriage, but there is no evidence to support this.

What are the types?
A miscarriage can be classified into one of several different types: threatened, inevitable, and missed miscarriage.

In a threatened miscarriage, the fetus is alive and the cervix remains closed. There is some vaginal bleeding, which is usually painless, but the pregnancy often continues for its full term of about 40 weeks. However, sometimes a threatened miscarriage develops into an inevitable miscarriage.

In an inevitable miscarriage, the fetus is usually dead and the cervix is open. An inevitable miscarriage is frequently painful because the uterus contracts to expel the fetus. Pain varies from mild, menstrual period-type pains to severe pain, and there may be heavy vaginal bleeding with clots. An inevitable miscarriage may be either complete (all the contents of the uterus are expelled) or incomplete (some contents remain in the uterus after the miscarriage).

In a missed miscarriage, the fetus is dead, but there is usually no bleeding or pain. The uterus does not contract, and the cervix is closed with the fetus still inside. Although pregnancy symptoms, such as nausea, come to an end, a missed miscarriage is often not detected until a routine ultrasound scan is carried out (see Ultrasound scanning in pregnancy, right).

You should consult your doctor if you have vaginal bleeding or pain in pregnancy. If bleeding or pain is severe, call an ambulance immediately.

How is it diagnosed?
Your doctor will examine your cervix using a speculum. If your cervix is closed, an ultrasound scan will be performed and, if the fetus is alive, the pregnancy often continues. However, if the cervix is open, miscarriage is usually inevitable. An ultrasound scan will be carried out to check that all the contents of the uterus have been expelled.

How might the doctor treat it?
If you have a threatened miscarriage, your doctor will probably suggest that you

rest for a few days until the bleeding has stopped and any identifiable cause, such as an infection, is treated. In the event of an inevitable miscarriage, your treatment will depend on whether the miscarriage is complete or incomplete. Normally, no further medical treatment is needed for a complete miscarriage, although you may be given painkillers (p.589) if necessary. If a miscarriage was incomplete, you may need to be admitted to hospital so that any tissue left behind in the uterus can be removed. This procedure is also used for an early missed miscarriage. The doctor may also prescribe antibiotics (p.572) to prevent an infection developing. If a missed miscarriage occurs in later pregnancy, you may require induction of labour (p.515).

What can I do?
The loss of a baby is always distressing, and you should take time to grieve and talk about your feelings. You may want to discuss your concerns about future pregnancies with your doctor. If you want to become pregnant again, it is best to wait several months to give yourself time to recover from your loss.

What is the prognosis?
Most women who have a miscarriage do not have problems with subsequent pregnancies. Some women have recurrent miscarriages, but with specialist investigation and treatment they may eventually have a successful pregnancy.

Multiple pregnancy and its problems

The presence of more than one fetus in the uterus and the problems that may arise

 Multiple pregnancy more common over the age of 30

 Multiple pregnancy sometimes runs in families

 Lifestyle is not a significant factor

Multiple pregnancy occurs when more than one fetus develops in the uterus. Although most multiple pregnancies progress smoothly, the risk of problems is increased for both mother and fetuses.

Nonidentical fetuses may develop if two or more eggs are fertilized at the same time, whereas two or more identical fetuses may develop if an egg splits after fertilization. Fetuses may share a placenta or each fetus may have its own.

In the UK, twins occur naturally in about 15 in 1,000 births and triplets occur in about 1 in 4,400 births.

Natural pregnancies of more than three fetuses are extremely rare, but there has been a dramatic increase in multiple pregnancies as a result of fertility treatment.

You are more likely to have nonidentical twins if you are over the age of 30 or if there are multiple births in your family history on your mother's side. However, these factors do not increase your chance of having identical twins.

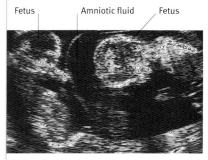

Fetus   Amniotic fluid   Fetus

Twins in the uterus
Two fetuses, each in its own sac of fluid, can be seen lying at right angles to each other in this colour-enhanced ultrasound scan.

What are the causes of multiple pregnancy?
Multiple pregnancies may occur naturally, but 2 in 3 pregnancies with three or more fetuses result from infertility treatments

---

▶ **TEST**

Ultrasound scanning in pregnancy

Ultrasound scanning uses sound waves to produce an image of the internal organs. The procedure is routinely used during pregnancy to assess the health of the fetus, determine the fetus's age, and measure fetal growth. Scanning may also be used to investigate problems, such as vaginal bleeding, and diagnose fetal abnormalities. For example, the procedure may identify neural tube defects and can sometimes detect heart problems. A scan takes about 20–30 minutes and is painless and safe. Doppler ultrasound scanning may be used to measure blood flow to the fetus.

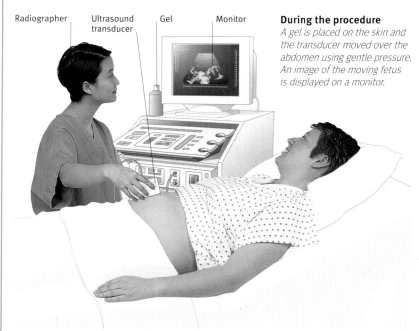

Radiographer   Ultrasound transducer   Gel   Monitor

During the procedure
A gel is placed on the skin and the transducer moved over the abdomen using gentle pressure. An image of the moving fetus is displayed on a monitor.

RESULTS

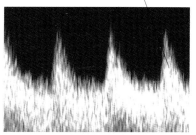

Hand   Face

ULTRASOUND SCAN

Pulse of blood through artery

DOPPLER ULTRASOUND SCAN

Fetal scans
The top image shows a healthy 24-week-old fetus inside the uterus. The bottom image shows normal pulses of fetal blood through the artery in the umbilical cord.

(see **Assisted conception**, p.498). This is because drugs for infertility (p.604) stimulate the ovaries to release more than one egg each month, and more than one fertilized egg is inserted into the uterus during in-vitro fertilization.

What are the problems?

The common problems associated with normal pregnancy (see **Common complaints of normal pregnancy**, p.506) are sometimes more severe in a multiple pregnancy. This is partly due to the increased size of the uterus and partly because the placenta or placentas produce a higher level of hormones.

Women who are carrying more than one fetus are more likely to have certain problems, such as high blood pressure during pregnancy (see **Pre-eclampsia and eclampsia**, p.513). Such women are also more likely to develop excessive vomiting during early pregnancy (see **Hyperemesis**, p.510), have greater than normal amounts of fluid surrounding the fetus (see **Polyhydramnios**, p.514), and have a low-lying placenta or placentas (see **Placenta praevia**, p.516). Iron-deficiency anaemia (p.271) is also more likely because the mother must supply iron to more than one fetus.

A multiple pregnancy is more likely to result in a miscarriage (p.511) or in premature labour (p.515). The fetuses in a multiple pregnancy are often smaller than single babies, and there is a greater risk of one baby not being in the normal position for labour (see **Abnormal presentation**, p.517). Since there may be more than one placenta, bleeding after the delivery may be heavy (see **Postpartum haemorrhage**, p.521).

What might be done?

Your doctor or midwife may suspect a multiple pregnancy if your abdomen is larger than would be expected for the stage of the pregnancy. The diagnosis is usually confirmed by ultrasound scanning (see **Ultrasound scanning in pregnancy**, opposite page). You may be monitored with ultrasound scans every month, possibly with Doppler ultrasound scanning every 2 weeks to check that each fetus is receiving adequate blood. Some hospitals have multiple pregnancy clinics.

Additional treatment may be needed if problems develop. For example, you may be prescribed iron supplements to treat anaemia. You should rest often, especially after the 28th week, to help to reduce the risk of a premature labour. Multiple fetuses are usually delivered in hospital because of the risks of a difficult or premature labour. Twins may be delivered vaginally if the first baby is in the head-down position. A caesarean section (p.518) is usually necessary for the delivery of three or more babies.

Since the babies are often premature and small, they may need to be looked after in a special care baby unit (p.619).

Cervical incompetence

Weakness of the cervix, which may result in a late miscarriage

 Age, genetics, and lifestyle are not significant factors

The cervix normally stays closed until labour begins. However, if the cervix has become weak, a condition known as cervical incompetence, the weight of the growing fetus and its surrounding amniotic fluid may cause the cervix to open early, resulting in a miscarriage (p.511). Cervical incompetence is the cause of about 1 in 4 miscarriages that occur after the 14th week of pregnancy.

The cervix may be weakened by previous surgery, such as a cone biopsy (see **Treating cervical intraepithelial neoplasia**, p.481), or by any procedure that involves artificial opening of the cervix. For example, a woman who has had more than three pregnancy terminations (p.510) at an early stage is more likely to develop cervical incompetence.

Often there are no symptoms of cervical incompetence before miscarriage occurs. At this stage, the mother may feel pressure in the lower abdomen or a "lump" in the vagina.

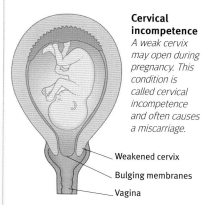

Cervical incompetence
A weak cervix may open during pregnancy. This condition is called cervical incompetence and often causes a miscarriage.

— Weakened cervix
— Bulging membranes
— Vagina

What might be done?

If you have had a previous miscarriage after the 14th week of pregnancy, your doctor may arrange for you to have ultrasound scanning (p.135) to check for cervical incompetence. The scan is performed through the vagina to measure the length of the cervix and may be carried out at an early stage in your next pregnancy. If you are at high risk of cervical incompetence, possibly as a result of previous surgery on the cervix, for example, you may also be investigated for cervical incompetence before or early in pregnancy.

If the cervix is weak, a stitch can be inserted in it to hold it closed. The procedure is carried out under general or epidural anaesthesia between weeks 12 and 16 of pregnancy. The stitch is usually removed at 37 weeks, before the beginning of labour. If labour starts while the stitch is still in place, it will be removed immediately to prevent the cervix from becoming torn. If the stitch fails to prevent a miscarriage, another pregnancy may be successful if a stitch is inserted higher in the cervix, sometimes during an abdominal operation.

Cervical incompetence is likely to recur in subsequent pregnancies, so the cervix may need to be stitched each time to prevent miscarriage.

Pre-eclampsia and eclampsia

High blood pressure, fluid retention, and protein in the urine in pregnancy, which may lead to seizures and coma

 Most common under the age of 19 or over the age of 35

 Sometimes runs in families

 Being overweight is a risk factor

Pre-eclampsia, also called pre-eclamptic toxaemia, develops in about 1–2 out of 20 pregnancies, most often in the second half of pregnancy. The condition is a combination of high blood pressure with excessive fluid retention and/or protein in the urine. Mild pre-eclampsia is common in the last weeks of pregnancy and is usually easy to treat. Severe pre-eclampsia may threaten the life of the mother and/or the fetus. If it is left untreated, severe pre-eclampsia may lead to a potentially fatal disorder known as eclampsia that causes seizures and may bring on a coma (p.323).

The cause of pre-eclampsia is not yet understood, but it may be due in part to the mother developing an immune reaction to the fetus. The condition is most likely to develop in a first pregnancy, a subsequent pregnancy with a new father, or a multiple pregnancy. Pre-eclampsia can run in families and is most common in women under the age of 19 or over 35. There is also an increased risk of pre-eclampsia in overweight women and in women who have chronic kidney disease, diabetes mellitus (p.437), or pre-existing high blood pressure (see **Hypertension**, p.242).

What are the symptoms?

Initially, pre-eclampsia may produce no symptoms. As the condition progresses, the symptoms tend to develop gradually, but occasionally the onset is rapid. Symptoms may include:

■ Swollen feet, ankles, and hands and excessive weight gain due to retention of fluid
■ Headaches.
■ Visual disturbances, such as blurred vision and seeing flashing lights.
■ Vomiting.
■ Upper abdominal pain.

You should consult your doctor or midwife immediately if you develop any of the above symptoms during pregnancy. Without immediate hospital supervision, the condition may worsen rapidly.

How is it diagnosed?

Your doctor or midwife will examine you for evidence of pre-eclampsia at every antenatal checkup. He or she will examine you for signs of fluid retention, take your blood pressure, and test your urine for protein. If pre-eclampsia is suspected, various blood tests may be arranged, including tests to check your kidney function and blood clotting.

What is the treatment?

Treatment for pre-eclampsia depends on the stage of your pregnancy and the severity of your symptoms. If you have mild to moderate pre-eclampsia and are less than 36 weeks pregnant, you will probably be advised to rest at home. Your blood pressure will be taken frequently to check that it is not raised. In some women, monitoring in hospital and bed rest may be needed. You may also be prescribed medication to lower your blood pressure.

If pre-eclampsia becomes severe and the fetus is mature enough to survive an early delivery, induction of labour (p.515) or a caesarean section (p.518) may be recommended. Before an early delivery, you may have injections of corticosteroids to help the lungs of the fetus to mature. In rare cases, severe pre-eclampsia that develops before the 24th week requires a termination of pregnancy (p.510) to save the mother.

Regardless of the severity, if you have pre-eclampsia later than 36 weeks into your pregnancy, your doctor is likely to recommend that labour be induced at once or that a caesarean section be performed to deliver the baby.

If eclampsia develops, you may be given antihypertensive drugs (p.580) to lower your blood pressure and intravenous anticonvulsant drugs (p.590) to stop seizures. Delivery by emergency caesarean section is then performed.

What is the prognosis?

If pre-eclampsia is treated before it becomes severe, the outlook is usually good. If eclampsia develops, the lives of the mother and fetus are at risk. High blood pressure usually returns to normal within about a week of delivery, but there is an increased risk of the mother developing high blood pressure in later life. About 1 in 10 affected women has pre-eclampsia in a future pregnancy.

Polyhydramnios

An excessive amount of amniotic fluid surrounding the fetus in the uterus

 Genetics as a risk factor depends on the cause

 Age and lifestyle are not significant factors

Normally, the amount of amniotic fluid surrounding the fetus does not exceed 1.5 litres (3 pints). In polyhydramnios, more than 2 litres (4 pints) of amniotic fluid build up, causing abdominal discomfort or pain in the mother.

Excess fluid makes it easier for the fetus to move in the uterus. For this reason, the fetus may not lie in the normal head-down position at the end of pregnancy (*see* **Abnormal presentation**, p.517). Excess fluid also increases the likelihood of premature labour (opposite page) or premature rupture of membranes (opposite page).

What are the types?
There are two types of polyhydramnios: chronic, in which the amniotic fluid accumulates slowly over several weeks; and acute, in which the amniotic fluid accumulates over a few days.

Chronic polyhydramnios is the more common form. It develops from about week 32 of pregnancy and causes gradually worsening abdominal discomfort. Breathing difficulties and indigestion may also occur. In many women, no cause is found for chronic polyhydramnios. However, it occurs more often in mothers who have pre-existing diabetes mellitus (p.437), in women carrying more than one fetus (*see* **Multiple pregnancy and its problems**, p.512), and in pregnancies where there is Rhesus incompatibility (right) between the mother and fetus.

The acute form of polyhydramnios develops from 22 weeks and is typically associated with an identical twin pregnancy. It is also more likely if the fetus has a developmental defect in which there is a blockage in the fetus's small intestine. The symptoms are similar to but more severe than those of chronic polyhydramnios. Frequently, there is severe abdominal pain, nausea, and vomiting.

What might be done?
Your doctor may suspect that you have polyhydramnios if your abdomen is larger than would be expected for the stage of your pregnancy. You will probably undergo ultrasound scanning (*see* **Ultrasound scanning in pregnancy**, p.512) to confirm the diagnosis and to look for fetal abnormalities. You may also need a blood test to check whether you have diabetes mellitus.

If troublesome symptoms occur late in pregnancy, induction of labour (opposite page) may be recommended.

If you have acute polyhydramnios, your doctor may recommend induction of labour if the fetus or fetuses are mature enough. If the fetus is immature, you may be given corticosteroid injections to help the lungs of the fetus mature so that it can be delivered early. Abdominal pain may be relieved temporarily by removing some of the amniotic fluid from the uterus using a needle inserted into the abdomen. If required, the procedure can be repeated.

If you have diabetes mellitus, polyhydramnios may recur in subsequent pregnancies. However, careful control of your diabetes should reduce this risk. If you have polyhydramnios due to other causes, you are not at increased risk in future pregnancies.

Rhesus incompatibility

A mismatch between the Rh blood group of a pregnant woman and that of her fetus

 Due to incompatibility of genetically determined blood groups

 Age and lifestyle are not significant factors

One of the systems for classifying blood is the Rhesus (Rh) group. This system classifies blood according to the presence or absence of certain proteins on the surface of red blood cells. About 17 in 20 people in the UK have Rh proteins on the surface of their red blood cells and are Rh positive. The remaining 3 in 20 people do not have these proteins and are therefore Rh negative.

Rh incompatibility occurs when a mother is Rh negative and her fetus is Rh positive. The situation rarely causes problems in a first pregnancy. However, the mother may develop antibodies if stray blood cells from the baby enter her circulation. These antibodies may attack red blood cells in an Rh-positive fetus in a future pregnancy. The destruction of fetal blood cells may result in severe anaemia (p.271) in the fetus and in anaemia and yellowing of the skin and whites of the eyes (*see* **Neonatal jaundice**, p.531) in the newborn baby.

Women who are Rh negative and have no antibodies are now routinely given preventive treatment at 28 weeks of pregnancy and soon after the delivery, and fewer than 1 in 100 women develop problems in future pregnancies.

What is the cause?
Blood groups are inherited from both parents. A baby who is Rh positive can be born to an Rh-negative mother only if the baby's father is Rh positive. The circulatory systems of the mother and the fetus are separate, and red blood cells do not usually cross from one to the other. However, there are circumstances in which stray red blood cells from the fetus can enter the mother's circulation. The fetus's blood cells may leak into the mother's system during delivery, miscarriage (p.511), or termination of pregnancy (p.510).

There is also a risk of blood mixing when an amniocentesis test is carried out (*see* **Antenatal genetic tests**, p.509) or after a placental abruption (p.516), in which part or all of the placenta detaches from the uterus before delivery. The mother's immune system reacts by producing antibodies to destroy the fetal red blood cells in her circulation. In future pregnancies in which the fetus is Rh positive, these antibodies cross the placenta and destroy fetal red blood cells. Untreated, these effects become increasingly severe in each subsequent Rh-incompatible pregnancy.

What are the effects?
The mother remains well and is usually unaware that there is a problem. The effects on the fetus depend on the level of antibodies present and when in the pregnancy they are produced.

The fetus may develop swelling and progressive anaemia, in which destruction of the red blood cells leads to low levels of oxygen-carrying pigment in the blood. Rarely, a severely anaemic fetus develops acute heart failure (p.247) and may die in the uterus (*see* **Stillbirth**, p.520). After an Rh-incompatible pregnancy, a baby may be born with severe anaemia. Jaundice in the newborn baby occurs due to build-up of bilirubin, a pigment produced from the destruction of fetal red blood cells. Rarely, severe jaundice may cause brain damage.

What might be done?
If Rh antibodies develop, treatment depends on the amount of antibodies and their effect on the fetus. A sample of the fluid in the uterus is tested for evidence of high bilirubin in the fetus. A sample of fetal blood may also be taken from the umbilical cord and tested for haemolysis (destroyed red blood cells). Additional ultrasound scanning (*see* **Ultrasound scanning in pregnancy**, p.512) may be used to check whether the fetus is swollen. If antibody levels are low, the pregnancy may continue until labour is induced at 38 weeks (*see* **Induction of labour**, opposite page); if levels are high, labour may be induced earlier. A fetus that is too immature for delivery may have a transfusion of Rh-negative blood into the umbilical cord or abdominal cavity. After birth, the baby may need more transfusions and treatment for jaundice.

Can problems be prevented?
All women are tested at their first antenatal visit to determine their Rh blood group. If you are Rh negative, you will have a blood test at about 28 weeks to see if you have developed antibodies. You will also be given an injection of antibodies against Rh-positive blood at about week 28 and soon after the birth to destroy any fetal red blood cells in your blood. This prevents you from developing antibodies that might react against future Rh-positive fetuses. You may also have this injection after a miscarriage or other procedure that causes fetal and maternal blood to mix. With this treatment, you are very unlikely to develop antibodies that will cause problems in the future.

Intra-uterine growth retardation

Failure of the fetus to grow properly in the uterus so that it is smaller than expected

 Most common under the age of 17 or over the age of 34

 Smoking, alcohol or drug abuse, and an inadequate diet during pregnancy are risk factors

 Genetics as a risk factor depends on the cause

Also sometimes known as intra-uterine growth restriction or IUGR, intra-uterine growth retardation affects about 1 in 20 babies and occurs when a fetus fails to put on sufficient weight during pregnancy. On average, a baby weighs just over 3 kg (7 lb) at full term. A baby who has intra-uterine growth retardation may weigh less than 2.5 kg (5½ lb) at full term and is usually thinner than average rather than shorter in length. Underweight, thin babies are more commonly born to mothers who are under the age of 17 or over the age of 34.

What are the causes?
Poor fetal growth is usually caused by lack of nourishment, which may be due to a disorder in the mother or a factor in her lifestyle. The condition may also be caused by a problem with the placenta or a fetal abnormality.

Maternal disorders that may affect the functioning of the placenta and lead to malnourishment of the fetus include pre-eclampsia (*see* **Pre-eclampsia and eclampsia**, p.513), in which high blood pressure and other symptoms develop during pregnancy, chronic high blood pressure (*see* **Hypertension**, p.242), or pre-existing kidney failure (p.450). Poor fetal growth can also be caused by a serious infection in the mother, such as rubella (p.168). In addition, several factors in the mother's lifestyle are thought to be linked to intra-uterine growth retardation. Smoking, abusing alcohol or drugs, and eating an inadequate diet may all affect levels of nutrients passing across the placenta to nourish the fetus.

In addition, there are problems with the placenta itself that may lead to fetal malnourishment. For example, part of the placenta may separate from the wall of the uterus (*see* **Placental abruption**, p.516). Rarely, an inherited or a chromosomal abnormality in the fetus, such as Down's syndrome (p.533), leads to intra-uterine growth retardation.

What might be done?
You will probably have no symptoms, but your doctor may be concerned if measurements of your abdomen during pregnancy show that your uterus is not increasing in size at the normal rate. You will have regular ultrasound scans to monitor the rate of growth of the fetus and may be given special ultrasound scans (called Doppler scans)

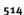

that measure blood flow through the umbilical cord to the fetus (*see* **Ultrasound scanning in pregnancy**, p.512).

If intra-uterine growth retardation is diagnosed, you may need to be admitted to hospital for observation. You will be treated for any underlying condition, if possible. For example, you may be given drugs to treat high blood pressure. If your diet is inadequate, you may be offered dietary advice. The fetus's heartbeat will probably be monitored twice daily. If the fetus continues to grow slowly, it may be delivered early, either by induction of labour (right) or by caesarean section (p.518).

What is the prognosis?

After they are born, small babies may initially need to be monitored and cared for in a special care baby unit (p.619) because they tend to be more susceptible to problems such as infections, low blood glucose, and low body temperature (hypothermia). Most small babies gain weight rapidly and reach a normal size. Having a small baby slightly increases the risk of your next baby also being small.

Premature rupture of membranes

Rupture of the membrane sac surrounding the fetus that is not closely followed by labour or that occurs before labour is due

 Age, genetics, and lifestyle are not significant factors

The fetus is protected in the uterus inside a filled bag called the amniotic sac. The membranes that form this sac normally rupture during or just before the start of labour, but in about 1 in 14 women they rupture early. It is not known exactly what causes membranes to break early, although in some pregnancies, premature rupture of membranes may be due to an infection that spreads upwards to the uterus from the vagina.

Rupture of the membranes causes the amniotic fluid to leak from the vagina. The amount of fluid lost varies from a trickle to a heavy gush. If your membranes rupture at night, you may wake in a wet bed, which can easily be mistaken for urine. If you think that your membranes may have broken, you should contact your doctor or midwife.

What are the complications?

If labour does not commence within a few hours of the membranes rupturing, there is a risk of infection or of the fetus becoming distressed. There is also a possibility of a cord prolapse, in which the umbilical cord drops down into the vagina. If this occurs, the supply of oxygen to the fetus may be reduced, causing distress (*see* **Fetal distress**, p.513). If the lungs have not yet reached maturity, premature rupture of the membranes may lead to premature labour (right). In this event, the risk to the fetus of an early delivery must be balanced against the risk of an infection developing if labour is stopped.

What might be done?

You may need to be admitted to hospital and monitored for evidence of an infection. Your doctor will feel your abdomen and examine you internally using a speculum to hold the vagina open. He or she will also take your temperature because a fever may indicate an infection. Your doctor may also take a vaginal swab and arrange for blood tests to look for signs of an infection. You will be treated with antibiotics (p.572), either to treat an infection or, if you do not have an infection, as a preventive measure. The heart rate of the fetus may be monitored (*see* **Fetal monitoring**, p.519) to look for indications of fetal distress. If you are at least 37 weeks into your pregnancy, labour usually begins within 24 hours of rupture of the membranes. Labour will usually be induced (*see* **Induction of labour**, above) if it fails to start.

If you are 36 weeks pregnant or the fetus is mature enough for delivery, labour may be induced; otherwise, you may be kept in hospital and monitored for any signs of infection. You may be given injections of corticosteroids to help the fetus's lungs mature.

After birth, the baby may need to be monitored in a special care baby unit (p.619), but most babies are healthy and have no ill effects from early delivery.

▶ TREATMENT

Induction of labour

If a pregnancy continues beyond 42 weeks or if the health of the mother or fetus is at risk, labour may need to be artificially induced. Various methods may be used. If the cervix is closed, usually a pessary is inserted into the vagina to encourage the cervix to open. If labour seems to have started, the membranes surrounding the fetus may be ruptured. If the membranes have ruptured but labour is slow, the hormone oxytocin may be given by intravenous drip to accelerate labour.

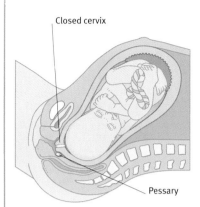

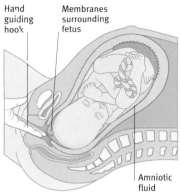

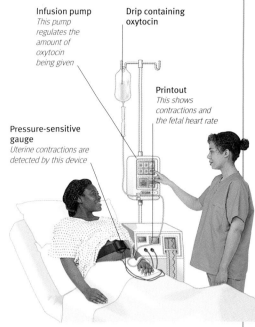

Infusion pump
This pump regulates the amount of oxytocin being given

Drip containing oxytocin

Printout
This shows contractions and the fetal heart rate

Pressure-sensitive gauge
Uterine contractions are detected by this device

Insertion of a pessary
If the cervix is closed, a prostaglandin pessary is placed at the top of the vagina to soften the cervix, which then thins and begins to open.

Rupture of membranes
If the cervix is already open, a small hook may be used to rupture the membranes that contain the fetus and its surrounding amniotic fluid.

Stimulating uterine contractions
If the cervix is open and the membranes have ruptured, oxytocin may be given intravenously to encourage the uterus to contract. The contractions and the fetal heart rate will be monitored.

Premature labour

The onset of labour before the 37th week of pregnancy

 Most common under the age of 17 or over the age of 35

 Smoking and alcohol or drug abuse during pregnancy are risk factors

 Genetics is not a significant factor

The normal duration of pregnancy is about 40 weeks. Labour that starts before 37 weeks is considered premature. Premature labour involves few extra risks for the mother, but premature babies often have problems because of their small size and immaturity (*see* **Problems of the premature baby**, p.530).

If premature labour is diagnosed early, there is a chance that it can be stopped and that the pregnancy will continue. If labour cannot be stopped completely, it may be delayed for a day or two so that corticosteroids (p.600) can be given to help the fetus to mature. Premature labour occurs in approximately 1 in every 10 births and is more common in very young mothers and those who are over the age of 35.

What are the causes?

Often, the cause of premature labour is not known, but triggering factors can sometimes be identified.

A multiple pregnancy often results in premature labour, possibly because the uterus is stretched (*see* **Multiple pregnancy and its problems**, p.512). An excessive amount of fluid around the fetus (*see* **Polyhydramnios**, opposite page) has the same effect.

Factors that increase the risk of premature labour include smoking and alcohol or drug abuse during pregnancy, heavy work, stress, a previous premature labour, and long-term disorders such as diabetes mellitus (p.437).

What are the symptoms?

The symptoms of premature labour may be mistaken initially for the backache and painless contractions that commonly occur in late pregnancy. They include:

■ Intermittent pain in the lower back.
■ Tightenings felt in the abdomen that become regular painful contractions.
■ A discharge of blood and mucus from the vagina.

If you think you are going into premature labour, you should contact your doctor or midwife immediately. The earlier premature labour is diagnosed, the greater the chances of stopping it. You may be admitted to hospital and transferred to a centre with a special care baby unit (p.619) in case it is impossible to stop labour and you deliver your baby early.

What might be done?

You will be examined to make sure that you are in labour and to assess how far it has advanced. The uterine contractions and the heartbeat of the fetus will be monitored regularly (*see* **Fetal monitoring**, p.519). Tests may also be carried out to try to find the cause of the premature labour.

If the fetus is not mature enough to be delivered safely, your doctor may try to stop labour by giving you an intravenous infusion of drugs (*see* **Drugs for labour**, p.605) that sometimes stop the muscles of the uterus from contracting. Your doctor may also prescribe antibiotics to reduce any risk of infection in the fetus.

If your labour cannot be stopped, the doctor may try to postpone it for a couple of days so that you can be given two injections of corticosteroid drugs, which help the lungs of the fetus to mature. This procedure reduces the risk of breathing problems in the baby after delivery. The fetus will be monitored for signs of fetal distress (p.519). In many cases, a carefully monitored vaginal delivery is possible, but, if there are risk factors such as a multiple pregnancy, it may be necessary to carry out a caesarean section (p.518).

What is the prognosis?
In many cases, labour can be stopped and the pregnancy then progresses to about 40 weeks. Otherwise, postponing labour for a day or two allows time for corticosteroid drug treatment to improve the fetus's chance of survival. Babies born before 37 weeks may need to be cared for and monitored in a special care baby unit until they are more mature. Premature labour often recurs in subsequent pregnancies.

Placenta praevia

A condition in which the placenta covers or partially covers the opening of the cervix into the uterus

 More common over the age of 35

 Genetics and lifestyle are not significant factors

In some pregnancies, the placenta is implanted lower down in the uterus and closer to the cervix than is normal. Although a placenta that is lying low will usually move upwards gradually as the uterus expands, the placenta may remain in this position and cover some or all of the opening of the cervix. This condition, known as placenta praevia, occurs in about 1 in 200 pregnancies and is more common in women over the age of 35. Placenta praevia causes up to 1 in 5 cases of vaginal bleeding that occurs after week 24 of pregnancy.

The severity of this condition is related to how much of the opening of the cervix is covered by the placenta. In marginal placenta praevia, the placenta lies low in the uterus and just reaches the edge of the cervix. When complete placenta praevia occurs, the whole of the cervix is covered. Symptoms caused by the condition vary, and mild cases may cause no adverse effects. In other cases, intermit-

tent light to heavy vaginal bleeding occurs from week 24 of pregnancy onwards. Complete placenta praevia may cause severe bleeding that can be life-threatening to the mother and/or fetus. Women who have placenta praevia are at increased risk of developing postpartum haemorrhage (p.521) because the lower part of the uterus may not be able to contract sufficiently to constrict the blood vessels of the uterus and stop bleeding after birth.

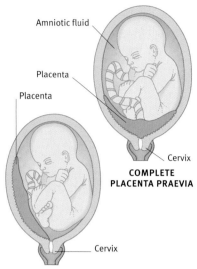

Placenta
Placenta
Amniotic fluid

Cervix

COMPLETE PLACENTA PRAEVIA

Cervix

MARGINAL PLACENTA PRAEVIA

Placenta praevia
In marginal placenta praevia, the placenta implants low in the uterus but only just reaches the opening of the cervix. In complete placenta praevia, the placenta covers the entire opening of the cervix.

What are the causes?
There is an increased risk of placenta praevia in women who have had several pregnancies or if the uterus has been scarred by previous surgery, such as a caesarean section (p.518). The placenta may also develop low in the uterus if there are noncancerous tumours present (*see* **Fibroids**, p.477). The risk of placenta praevia is increased in a multiple pregnancy because there may be more than one placenta or because the placenta may be larger than in a normal pregnancy (*see* **Multiple pregnancy and its problems**, p.512).

What might be done?
Usually, placenta praevia is detected after week 20 by routine ultrasound scanning (*see* **Ultrasound scanning in pregnancy**, p.512). If the placenta is lying low, you will be given follow-up scans to monitor its position. The problem may disappear because, in many cases, the placenta moves upwards and away from the cervix by week 34.

If the placenta remains low and you develop vaginal bleeding, you may be admitted to hospital. If you have light bleeding, you may need only bed rest, but if bleeding is heavy, you may need to

have an emergency caesarean section and possibly a blood transfusion (p.272) to replace the blood you have lost.

Even if there are no problems, when placenta praevia is complete your baby will be delivered by caesarean section at 38 weeks. With marginal placenta praevia, it may be possible to have a vaginal delivery or you may be advised to have a caesarean section, depending on the details of your individual case.

What is the prognosis?
With careful monitoring, most women with placenta praevia have a successful pregnancy. The condition is unlikely to recur in future pregnancies.

Placental abruption

Separation of the placenta from the wall of the uterus before the baby is delivered

 Smoking and alcohol or drug abuse during pregnancy are risk factors

 Age and genetics are not significant factors

The placenta normally separates from the wall of the uterus after the baby has been born. In placental abruption, part or all of the placenta separates from the uterus before the baby has been delivered. The condition occurs in about 1 in 120 pregnancies and is potentially life-threatening, especially for the fetus. Placental abruption is the most common cause of vaginal bleeding in pregnancy after the 28th week.

There are two basic types of placental abruption: revealed and concealed. A revealed placental abruption causes mild to severe vaginal bleeding. In a concealed placental abruption, there is no visible bleeding from the vagina because blood collects between the placenta and the wall of the uterus.

What are the causes?
The exact cause of placental abruption is not known. However, the condition appears to be more common in women who have long-term high blood pressure (*see* **Hypertension**, p.242). The risk is also increased if a woman smokes during pregnancy, drinks large amounts of alcohol, and/or abuses drugs. The disorder occurs more often after several previous pregnancies or in women who have had a placental abruption in a previous pregnancy. Abdominal injury sometimes leads to placental abruption.

What are the symptoms?
Symptoms usually occur suddenly and depend on how much of the placenta has separated from the wall of the uterus. If only a small part of the placenta has pulled away, bleeding may be minor, a large separation can cause severe

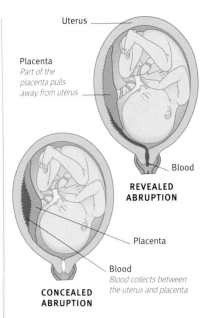

Uterus

Placenta
Part of the placenta pulls away from uterus

Blood

REVEALED ABRUPTION

Placenta

Blood

CONCEALED ABRUPTION

Blood collects between the uterus and placenta

Placental abruption
In a placental abruption, part of the placenta separates from the uterine wall before birth. A revealed abruption causes vaginal bleeding; in a concealed abruption, blood collects behind the placenta.

orrhage. In increasing order of severity, symptoms may include:
- Slight to heavy vaginal bleeding.
- Abdominal cramps or backache.
- Severe, constant abdominal pain.
- Reduced fetal movements.

If you develop vaginal bleeding a' stage of pregnancy, you should your doctor or midwife immediate bleeding is heavy, it is advisable ambulance without delay be may need emergency care.

What might be done?
Your doctor will examine using a speculum, which that holds the vagin also have ultrasou **Ultrasound scanni** p.512), and the fe checked. If the s may stay in hos' for monitoring **Fetal monitor'**

If bleeding labour may **labour**, p abruption section the fe sion/

T' de t'

Problems in labour

Labour is the process of birth, from the first strong contractions of the uterus to the delivery of the baby and placenta. Labour may last up to 24 hours for a first pregnancy but tends to be shorter in subsequent pregnancies. In most cases, the stages of labour progress smoothly. When problems do occur, they are rarely serious if they are identified and treated promptly.

Improvements in monitoring and more effective pain relief have made labour a safer and much less traumatic experience than it once was. In the past, little relief was available to help mothers cope with the extreme pain of a difficult labour, and complications often threatened the life of the mother or baby, or sometimes both.

The first article in this section looks at abnormal presentation, a condition in which the fetus is not lying in the normal position in the uterus, the easiest position for delivery. Problems that may complicate labour and delivery, usually because the fetus is unable to pass through the mother's pelvis, are covered next.

Two relatively rare conditions are discussed in the final part of this section. Fetal distress arises when the fetus is deprived of sufficient oxygen for its needs. This condition may occur at any stage of pregnancy, but is more common during labour. The final article discusses stillbirth, a rare and distressing situation that occurs when a fetus dies in the womb later than 24 weeks into a pregnancy or, even more rarely, when a baby dies during labour.

KEY ANATOMY

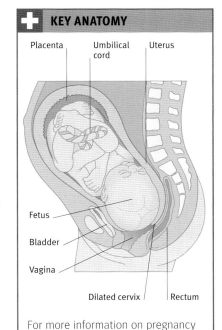

Placenta | Umbilical cord | Uterus

Fetus

Bladder

Vagina

Dilated cervix | Rectum

For more information on pregnancy and the stages of childbirth, *see* pp.500–505.

Abnormal presentation

Any deviation from the normal position of the fetus for delivery

 Age, genetics, and lifestyle are not significant factors

In most normal pregnancies, the fetus settles into the mother's pelvic cavity from week 36 onwards, ready for labour and birth. In labour, about 8 in 10 fetuses are head downwards, facing the mother's back, with the chin resting on the chest. In this presentation, the fetus is in the optimum position for birth, and a normal vaginal delivery is usually possible. All other fetal positions are considered to be abnormal and may cause problems during labour.

When a fetus is lying in an abnormal position in the uterus, a vaginal delivery may be possible, but the labour may be prolonged (*see* **Problems during delivery**, p.518). If the fetus becomes stuck, it may need an assisted delivery (p.520) or caesarean section (p.518).

Most abnormal presentations can be diagnosed before labour begins, and arrangements to deliver the fetus safely can be discussed in advance.

What are the causes?

Abnormal presentation may occur if the fetus is able to move more freely within the uterus than usual, either because the fetus is small and does not fit closely into the pelvis (*see* **Premature labour**, p.515) or because there is excess amniotic fluid surrounding the fetus (*see* **Polyhydramnios**, p.514). There is also an increased risk of an abnormal presentation when there is more than one fetus in the uterus (*see* **Multiple pregnancy and its problems**, p.512).

Occasionally, the fetus cannot settle into the pelvic cavity because of an obstruction, such as the placenta lying low in the uterus (*see* **Placenta praevia**, opposite page) or a noncancerous growth in the uterine wall (*see* **Fibroids**, p.477). An unusually shaped uterus may also contribute to an abnormal presentation.

What are the types?

The most common abnormal presentations are the breech position and the occipitoposterior position. Rarer types include face, compound, brow, and shoulder presentations, named according to the parts of the fetus that are over the dilated cervix at delivery.

Breech In a breech birth, the fetus presents buttocks first. Many fetuses lie in a breech position before week 32 of pregnancy but

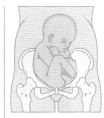

BREECH

most turn by 36 weeks. The 3 in 100 that do not turn are in one of three types of breech presentation. A complete breech is one in which the fetus is curled up. In a frank breech, the legs are extended and the feet are close to the face. In a footling breech, one or both feet are positioned over the cervix. Often one twin fetus is a breech.

Occipitoposterior At the beginning of labour, about 1 in 5 fetuses lies in

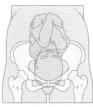

OCCIPITOPOSTERIOR

an occipitoposterior position, which is head-down but facing the mother's abdomen instead of her back. Most fetuses will turn at some stage during labour, but 2 in 100 do not and are still in this presentation when they are delivered.

Rare presentations In a face presentation, the neck of the fetus is bent backwards so that the face is positioned over the cervix. This type of presentation occurs in 1 in every 400 births. In a compound presentation, which occurs in 1 in every 700 births, an arm or leg lies over the cervix in addition to the head or buttocks. In a brow presentation, the fetus's head is bent slightly backwards with the brow over the cervix; this occurs in about 1 in every 1,000 births. A shoulder or oblique presentation, in which the fetus lies across the uterus with its shoulder over the cervix, occurs in 1 in every 2,500 births.

Are there complications?

If the fetus lies in an abnormal position just before delivery, there may be complications that place both the fetus and mother at risk. A fetus in the normal head-down position blocks the cervix and prevents the umbilical cord from passing out of the uterus before the fetus. Some abnormal presentations leave space for the cord to drop through the cervix when the membranes surrounding the fetus rupture. When this occurs, the cord may be compressed by the fetus, or, rarely, its blood vessels may go into spasm because of the drop in temperature outside the uterus. As a result, the fetus may be deprived of oxygen (*see* **Fetal distress**, p.519). This may cause brain damage or fetal death.

A breech delivery may cause problems if the legs and body of the fetus are able to pass through the cervix when it is not completely dilated, but the head becomes stuck. If, in a footling breech, one foot drops through the cervix, this may prompt the mother to try to push too early. An abnormal presentation may also increase the risk of the cervix or vagina being torn during delivery.

How is it diagnosed?

Normally, the position of the fetus in the uterus is assessed at each antenatal visit. Your doctor will usually be able to tell if your baby is lying in an abnormal position at the end of your pregnancy. If your doctor suspects an abnormal presentation, you will be given ultrasound scanning to confirm the position (*see* **Ultrasound scanning in pregnancy**, p.512).

What is the treatment?

Abnormal presentation is usually diagnosed towards the end of a pregnancy, and, if necessary, a caesarean section is arranged. A vaginal birth may be possible for some abnormal presentations. Sometimes, a mother with a fetus in a breech presentation is offered a procedure to turn the fetus around after week 37 of pregnancy. The doctor attempts to manipulate the fetus into the correct position by pushing gently on the wall of the abdomen. This technique is performed using ultrasound guidance. It does not require an anaesthetic and is successful in about 50 per cent of cases.

If the abnormal presentation was due to a structural problem, such as an unusually shaped uterus, there is an increased risk of recurrence in a subsequent pregnancy. However, if the presentation was caused by a condition associated with that particular pregnancy, such as placenta praevia, the risk of recurrence is not increased.

Delayed first stage of labour

Prolonged or complicated labour in the predelivery stage

 Age, genetics, and lifestyle are not significant factors

The first stage of labour begins with the onset of regular, strong contractions of the uterus and ends when the cervix is fully dilated. In this period, the cervix widens until it is 10 cm (4 in) in diameter to allow the fetus to pass into the vagina. The average length of the first stage of labour is 6–12 hours, but it can take much longer in a first pregnancy. Labour is delayed when the first stage is prolonged and the cervix is not dilating normally. A prolonged labour occurs in about 3 in 10 first births and about 1 in 8 subsequent births.

When it has been recognized that the first stage of labour is not progressing, the problem can usually be treated successfully with modern techniques and monitoring. The mother may become exhausted during a long first stage of labour and this can cause problems during delivery (p.518). Left untreated, a delay in the first stage may threaten the life of the mother and/or the fetus.

What are the causes?

A delay in the first stage of labour may be due to uterine contractions that are too weak to fully dilate the cervix. In first pregnancies, weak uterine contractions are especially common, and the cervix often takes longer to dilate than normal. Drugs given to relieve pain in labour, such as epidural anaesthesia (*see* **Epidural anaesthesia in labour**, right), may also weaken contractions.

Sometimes, the cervix fails to dilate because it is scarred from surgery. In some labours, the fetus is in an unusual position and cannot put enough pressure on the cervix to assist dilation (*see* **Abnormal presentation**, p.517).

What can I do?
If your labour is taking an abnormally long time, try to keep changing position and walking around because gentle movement encourages the uterus to contract more effectively, and gravity increases the pressure from the fetus on the cervix. If you cannot get out of bed, try to sit upright. A prolonged labour can be exhausting and may cause dehydration. It is therefore important that you keep your fluid intake up.

What might the doctor do?
At regular intervals during your labour, a midwife will measure your blood pressure and check whether your cervix is dilating. Your contractions and the heart rate of the fetus will be monitored (*see* **Fetal monitoring**, opposite page). If the fetal heart rate is abnormal, a blood sample may be taken from the fetus's scalp to check for signs of distress. An intravenous drip may be used to maintain your fluid levels. If your uterine contractions cannot dilate the cervix effectively, your doctor may be able to speed up labour by using a number of different methods (*see* **Induction of labour**, p.515). If labour is still delayed, you may need to have a caesarean section (right).

What is the prognosis?
With careful monitoring and management, a delayed first stage of labour is unlikely to cause problems.

The chance of having a delayed first stage of labour in future pregnancies depends on the cause. Weak or ineffective uterine contractions are less likely to occur in subsequent pregnancies, and dilation of the cervix is usually quicker. However, if the cervix has been scarred by surgery or damaged by a difficult delivery, a caesarean section may be necessary in future births.

Problems during delivery

Any problem that prolongs the second stage of labour or prevents normal delivery

 Age, genetics, and lifestyle are not significant factors

The second stage of labour begins as soon as the mother's cervix has fully dilated to 10 cm (4 in) and ends when the baby

---

▷ **TREATMENT**

Epidural anaesthesia in labour

Epidural anaesthesia is a method of pain relief in labour. The anaesthetic is given through a catheter inserted between two of the vertebrae (bones in the spine) in the lower back. The tip of the catheter is put into the epidural space formed by membranes surrounding the spinal cord. The other end is taped to the shoulder, so that further doses can be given. The anaesthetic numbs nerves from below the waist, including those from the uterus. Intravenous fluids are given, and the baby's heart rate is monitored.

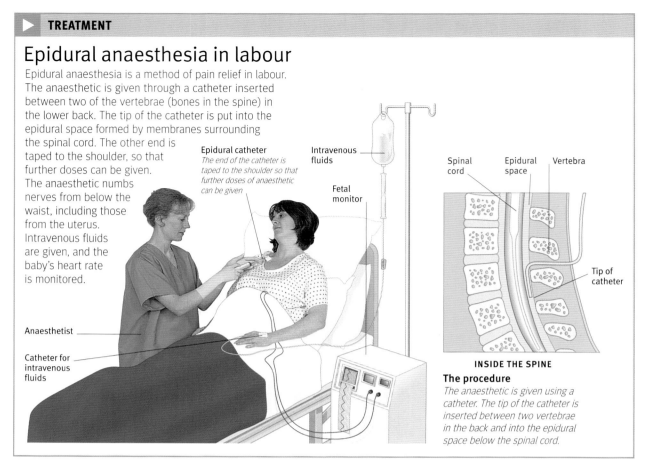

Epidural catheter
The end of the catheter is taped to the shoulder so that further doses of anaesthetic can be given

Intravenous fluids

Fetal monitor

Anaesthetist

Catheter for intravenous fluids

Spinal cord · Epidural space · Vertebra

Tip of catheter

INSIDE THE SPINE

The procedure
The anaesthetic is given using a catheter. The tip of the catheter is inserted between two vertebrae in the back and into the epidural space below the spinal cord.

▷ **TREATMENT**

Caesarean section

In a caesarean section, the baby is delivered through an incision in the mother's abdomen. The operation is carried out when circumstances make it safer than a vaginal birth for the mother and baby. It may be planned (elective) or may be performed as an emergency procedure, for example, if there are signs of fetal distress (*see* opposite page). A caesarean section is usually carried out using an epidural anaesthetic injected into the mother's lower back, which numbs her body below the waist (*see* **Epidural anaesthesia in labour**, above). An incision is made in the lower abdomen and the baby and placenta are delivered within minutes.

During the procedure
A caesarean section may be performed under epidural anaesthesia so that you can remain awake. Your partner can be with you during the operation, and you can hold the baby immediately afterwards.

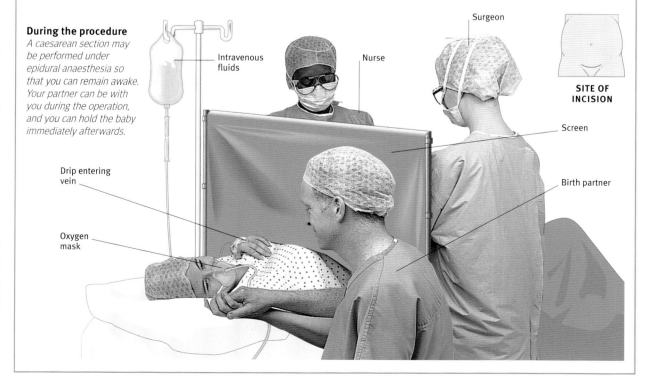

Intravenous fluids

Drip entering vein

Oxygen mask

Surgeon

Nurse

SITE OF INCISION

Screen

Birth partner

▶ **TREATMENT**

Fetal monitoring

In low-risk pregnancies, the fetus is monitored intermittently in labour with a hand-held device that measures the fetal heart rate. In high-risk pregnancies, electronic fetal monitoring, also known as cardiotocography, is used to detect fetal distress. During labour, changes in the fetal heart rate in response to uterine contractions are recorded. An abnormal heart rate may be a sign of fetal distress. A more accurate reading may be taken using a probe attached to the fetus's head. A blood sample may be taken from the fetus's scalp to check the level of oxygen. As well as being used in labour, monitoring may also be used during pregnancy to detect problems.

External fetal monitoring
Two devices are strapped to your abdomen: an ultrasound transducer to detect the fetus's heartbeat and a movement sensor to measure your contractions.

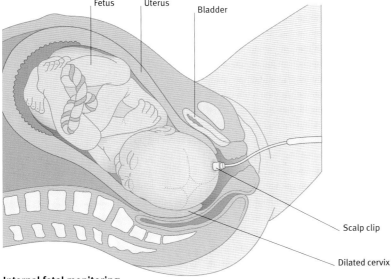

Movement sensor

Ultrasound transducer

Cardiotocograph
This machine gives a printout of readings

Fetus Uterus Bladder

Scalp clip

Dilated cervix

Internal fetal monitoring
A clip is attached directly to the skin of the fetus's head, and the heart rate is monitored continually. This device produces a more accurate reading than an ultrasound transducer, but it can only be attached when the cervix has started to dilate.

RESULTS

Cardiotocograph during labour
Readings from the two devices around the mother's abdomen are converted into tracings on a cardiotocograph. The heart rate of a healthy fetus usually speeds up at the start of a contraction, as the peaks show, then rapidly returns to a normal level.

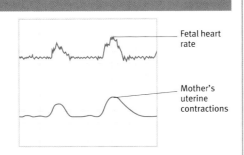

Fetal heart rate

Mother's uterine contractions

---

is born. About 4 in 10 mothers have problems during the delivery, and the risk is higher for a first pregnancy. With careful management, it may be possible to carry out a normal vaginal delivery, but if the second stage of labour is long, and the fetus's oxygen supply becomes insufficient, there is an increased risk of fetal distress (right). The doctor may then carry out an assisted delivery (p.520), using vacuum suction or forceps, or a caesarean section (opposite page).

What are the causes?
Any of the problems that cause a delayed first stage of labour (p.517) can prevent a normal delivery. However, even if the first stage has progressed smoothly, a problem may arise at the second stage.

Weak or ineffective uterine contractions may slow down the delivery. Pain relief, such as epidural anaesthesia during labour (opposite page), may also affect the strength of contractions. If the mother is exhausted as a result of a long first stage of labour or because of poor general health, contractions may be weak and delivery may be difficult.

There may be a delay in the baby's passage through the cervix and vagina if the baby is not in the normal position (*see* **Abnormal presentation**, p.517). Normal delivery may also be difficult if the baby cannot pass easily through the pelvis, either because the baby is large or because the mother has a narrow or irregularly shaped pelvis.

Once the baby has reached the vaginal opening, there may be problems in delivery if the surrounding tissues cannot stretch enough to let the head out.

How is it diagnosed?
When your cervix has dilated fully and the second stage of labour begins, your midwife will monitor the baby's passage through the cervix and into the vagina and will check the heartbeat (*see* **Fetal monitoring**, left) for signs of distress. The strength and frequency of uterine contractions are monitored. This information is then used to help determine whether a vaginal delivery is possible.

What is the treatment?
If your uterine contractions are too weak, the doctor may give an intravenous drip of oxytocin, a hormone that stimulates strong contractions (*see* **Induction of labour**, p.515). When a baby is slow to pass through the cervix and vagina, the doctor may perform an assisted delivery using forceps or vacuum suction. Just before an assisted delivery, an incision, called an episiotomy (right), is usually made in the tissue between the vagina and the anus. This cut eases the baby's passage and prevents the tissues around the vaginal opening from tearing. An episiotomy is also used to help delivery when a mother's vaginal opening is too small for the baby's head to pass through.

A caesarean section will be necessary if the baby cannot pass easily through your pelvis or if an assisted delivery would put either of you at risk.

What is the prognosis?
You may feel disappointed if you need an assisted delivery, a caesarean section, or an episiotomy, but these methods are only used to ensure that your baby is delivered safely. Your ability to have normal vaginal deliveries in the future is not usually affected by any of these procedures. Many women who have a difficult first birth have no problems with subsequent births. However, if there is a physical reason why normal childbirth is difficult for you, such as an abnormally shaped pelvis or one that is too narrow, a caesarean birth will usually be required for future pregnancies.

Fetal distress

Physical stress experienced by a fetus due to a lack of oxygen

 Age, genetics, and lifestyle are not significant factors

Fetal distress develops when there is an insufficient supply of oxygen reaching the fetus. Although this condition usually

---

▶ **TREATMENT**

Episiotomy

An episiotomy is an incision made in the perineum (the area of tissue between the vagina and anus) to enlarge the birth opening and prevent a ragged tear. The cut may be used before an assisted delivery or if the perineum fails to stretch sufficiently for the baby's head.

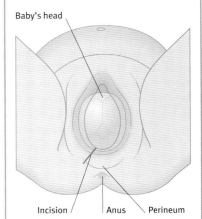

Baby's head

Incision Anus Perineum

Having an episiotomy
A local anaesthetic is injected into the perineum and a small cut is made during a contraction. The cut is usually made at an angle to avoid the anus, enabling the baby's head to pass through the vaginal opening more easily.

▶ **TREATMENT**

Assisted delivery

When a vaginal delivery does not progress smoothly, a baby may need an assisted delivery. This sometimes occurs if the mother is too exhausted to push the baby out or the baby becomes stuck or distressed. In these circumstances, the doctor may use vacuum suction or forceps to assist the delivery. An episiotomy (p.519) to enlarge the birth opening is usually carried out just before an assisted delivery.

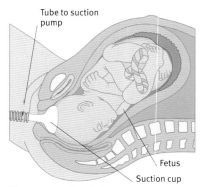

Vacuum suction delivery
A suction cup is placed on the baby's scalp, and the baby is pulled out while the mother pushes. The suction cup leaves a temporary swelling on the baby's head.

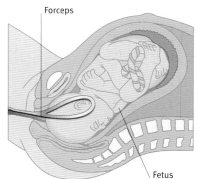

Forceps delivery
Metal forceps are inserted into the vagina and placed on each side of the baby's head. The doctor pulls with the forceps as the mother pushes the baby out.

occurs during labour, it can develop at any time. Fetal distress occurs in approximately 1 in 20 pregnancies, but the fetus is usually delivered before lasting harm occurs. However, left untreated, fetal distress may cause fetal brain damage or even death.

What are the causes?

A common cause of fetal distress in pregnancy is a problem with the placenta, the organ that supplies oxygen and nutrients via the umbilical cord to the fetus. The function of the placenta may be affected if the mother develops pre-eclampsia (see **Pre-eclampsia and eclampsia**, p.513). The oxygen supply to the fetus may also be reduced if part or all of the placenta separates from the uterus during pregnancy (see **Placental abruption**, p.516).

Frequently, the cause of fetal distress during labour is unknown. There may be a placental abruption during labour, or the umbilical cord may become tangled, preventing oxygen from reaching the fetus. Another, less common, cause of fetal distress is cord prolapse. This condition may develop if the fetus is not securely fitted into the mother's pelvis because it is not lying in the normal head-down position facing the mother's back (see **Abnormal presentation**, p.517). An abnormal position may create space for the umbilical cord to drop through the cervix into the vagina. Once it is outside the uterus, the blood vessels in the cord may become compressed or, rarely, may go into spasm. Both of these situations can reduce the oxygen supply to the fetus.

The risk of fetal distress is increased if the fetus is weak or smaller than average (see **Intra-uterine growth retardation**, p.514) or if your labour starts before the 37th week of pregnancy (see **Premature labour**, p.515).

How is it diagnosed?

If your doctor is concerned that there is a risk of fetal distress during your pregnancy, he or she may decide to refer you for an additional ultrasound scan (see **Ultrasound scanning in pregnancy**, p.512). This scan enables your doctor to observe fetal movements and also to look at the blood flow in the vessels carrying blood from the placenta to the fetus. Reduced fetal movements may indicate oxygen deficiency. Your doctor may also recommend fetal monitoring (p.519). This monitors the fetus's heart rate, which may be abnormal if the fetus is not getting enough oxygen.

During labour, the fetal heartbeat may be monitored continuously, and a sample of blood may be taken from the fetus's scalp to assess blood oxygen levels. The amniotic fluid from the uterus may be examined regularly for signs of staining from fetal faeces (meconium), which are sometimes released from the fetus when it is under stress.

What is the treatment?

Treatment for fetal distress depends on the cause, the severity of the distress, whether it occurs before or in labour, and how far labour has progressed.

If there are signs of even mild fetal distress during late pregnancy or early labour, your doctor will probably recommend a caesarean section (p.518). If labour is advanced and the fetus is experiencing only mild levels of distress, an assisted delivery (left) may be a possible option. However, if fetal distress is severe, or there is a cord prolapse, your doctor will probably advise an emergency caesarean section.

What is the prognosis?

If fetal distress is diagnosed and treated promptly, there is a good chance that your baby will be delivered safely and with no permanent harm. However, in some situations – for example, when a baby is premature (see **Problems of the premature baby**, p.530) – your baby will need careful monitoring after birth (see **Special care baby unit**, p.619).

Stillbirth

The delivery of a dead fetus after week 24 of pregnancy

 More common over the age of 35

 Smoking and alcohol or drug abuse during pregnancy are risk factors

 Genetics as a risk factor depends on the cause

The death of a fetus in the uterus or during birth is a very distressing event. Bereaved parents may experience confused feelings of anger, shock, guilt, and inadequacy, in addition to overwhelming grief. Stillbirths are rare, with fewer than 5 in 1,000 babies being stillborn in the UK each year. Stillbirth is slightly more common in mothers over the age of 35.

What are the causes?

Often, the precise cause of fetal death is unknown. The death may be caused by a decrease in the fetus's oxygen supply (see **Fetal distress**, p.519) due to a problem with the umbilical cord or the placenta. For example, the umbilical cord may be tangled or knotted, or the placenta may separate from the uterus before the baby is born (see **Placental abruption**, p.516). If the mother has very high blood pressure or poorly controlled diabetes mellitus (p.437), the risk of stillbirth is increased.

Stillbirth may also occur if the fetus has a severe genetic disorder or, rarely, if the blood groups of the mother and fetus are not compatible (see **Rhesus incompatibility**, p.514). Certain infectious diseases that pass from the mother to the fetus, such as listeriosis (p.172), may harm the fetus and, if they are severe, may be fatal. Women who smoke or abuse drugs or alcohol are at greater risk of a stillbirth.

What might be done?

The first sign that a fetus may have died in the uterus is the absence of movement. If, after week 20 of pregnancy, you are aware that fetal movements have decreased or ceased altogether, you should call your doctor or midwife without delay. The doctor will listen for the fetal heartbeat and then confirm his or her findings with an ultrasound scan (see **Ultrasound scanning in pregnancy**, p.512). In most cases, the results of the scan confirm that the fetus is well and the pregnancy is progressing normally. Rarely, if the fetus has died and labour has not started, induction of labour (p.515) will probably be necessary.

If there is no immediate risk to your health, such as an infection or internal bleeding, you may be given time to come to terms with the loss of the baby before it is delivered. A caesarean section is not usually used to deliver the baby because of the risks associated with any operation and the small risk of the scar reopening during a subsequent vaginal delivery. In the very rare event of a baby dying during labour, delivery will continue.

Parents are encouraged to see and hold their stillborn baby after the birth as part of the grieving process. After the delivery, the mother and baby undergo tests to determine the cause of death. Before leaving hospital, the mother may be given drugs to inhibit her milk production and provide pain relief.

Your doctor may recommend professional counselling to help you to recover from your loss (see **Loss and bereavement**, p.32). You should not be afraid to seek support from family and friends. You may also find it helpful to join a self-help group and meet people who have been through a similar experience. Some people may find comfort in a funeral ceremony. About 6 weeks after the birth, your doctor will review the results of tests and the postmortem (if one was carried out) with you and discuss the cause of the death, if it is known.

What is the prognosis?

After a stillbirth, you may feel strongly that you want to begin another pregnancy straight away. However, it may be better to wait until you are emotionally ready for a new baby and are fully recovered from your pregnancy. If you do decide on another pregnancy, your doctor will ensure that you are given extra care because you will be considered to be at high risk (see **High-risk pregnancy**, p.506). The risk of having a further stillbirth depends on the original cause, if one can be found, but most subsequent pregnancies are successful. As with all grief, the pain of losing a baby lessens with time.

Problems after childbirth

Childbirth is an exhilarating experience for many women, but it can also be difficult and painful. In addition to recovering from physical trauma, the body has to adapt to the abrupt changes in hormone levels after the birth. This hormonal fluctuation, which causes physiological changes, particularly in the breasts in preparation for breast-feeding, often leads to emotional swings.

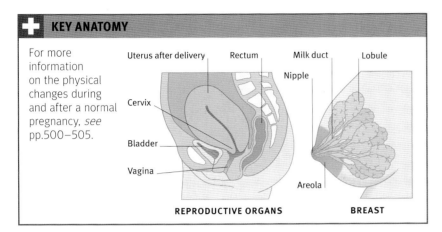

KEY ANATOMY

For more information on the physical changes during and after a normal pregnancy, see pp.500–505.

Uterus after delivery · Rectum · Milk duct · Lobule · Nipple · Cervix · Bladder · Vagina · Areola

REPRODUCTIVE ORGANS · **BREAST**

Once the baby and the placenta have been delivered, the uterus starts to revert to its size before pregnancy. This process takes about 6 weeks. However, it may take several months for muscle tone to be regained in the abdomen, and any excess weight gained during pregnancy will have to be lost through a careful diet and exercise. The breasts remain enlarged while breast-feeding and only return to their normal size once the baby has been weaned.

The first article covers excessive bleeding occurring immediately after the delivery of the baby or in the first few weeks following childbirth.

Depression, which is covered next, is very common after the birth of a baby. Feelings range from mild baby blues to severe depression that requires hospital treatment. The final articles in this section cover breast disorders that can occur after childbirth, often in association with breast-feeding.

Postpartum haemorrhage

Excessive loss of blood immediately after delivery of a baby or in the first few weeks following childbirth

 More common over the age of 35

 Genetics and lifestyle are not significant factors

Almost all women have some degree of blood loss in the days after childbirth, and most women have some light vaginal bleeding for up to 4 weeks afterwards. Postpartum haemorrhage is defined as the loss of more than 500 ml (1 pint) of blood after childbirth.

After delivery of the baby, the placenta normally separates from the wall of the uterus and is then expelled from the body through the vagina. The site where the placenta was attached continues to bleed until strong contractions of the uterus constrict the blood vessels in the wall of the uterus and gradually stop the flow of blood. The majority of postpartum haemorrhages,

especially if severe, are the result of bleeding from the uterus. However, bleeding may also come from the cervix or the vagina.

Postpartum haemorrhage occurs in about 1 in 50 births, usually immediately after delivery (early postpartum haemorrhage). Only a few women have a late postpartum haemorrhage, in which excessive bleeding occurs more than 24 hours after delivery. Severe postpartum haemorrhage may be life-threatening, but is uncommon.

What are the causes?
In most cases, early postpartum haemorrhage occurs because the uterus is unable to contract sufficiently to constrict the blood vessels in its wall. This may be due to exhaustion of the muscles of the uterus after a prolonged labour, overstretching of the uterus as a result of a multiple pregnancy (see **Multiple pregnancy and its problems**, p.512), excess amniotic fluid (see **Polyhydramnios**, p.514), or a large baby.

Contraction of the uterus may also be impaired by noncancerous growths in the uterus (see **Fibroids**, p.477) or if some or all of the placenta remains in the uterus after birth. Occasionally, a general anaesthetic given for a caesarean section (p.518) can impair contractions. Early postpartum

haemorrhage may also occur if the placenta has implanted in the lower uterus (see **Placenta praevia**, p.516).

Less commonly, a tear in the cervix or vagina during childbirth may cause early postpartum haemorrhage. Such tears are more likely to occur if the baby is born rapidly, is not born head first (see **Abnormal presentation**, p.517), or is delivered with forceps or suction (see **Assisted delivery**, opposite page).

Late postpartum haemorrhage is usually caused by fragments of the placenta left in the uterus or by an infection.

What are the symptoms?
The main symptom of early postpartum haemorrhage is excessive loss of bright red blood through the vagina after birth.

A late postpartum haemorrhage may occur between 24 hours and 6 weeks after the birth. Symptoms may include:
- Sudden, heavy vaginal bleeding that is bright red in colour.
- Lower abdominal pain.
- Fever.

Sudden, severe loss of blood may lead to shock (p.248). Early postpartum haemorrhage almost always occurs while you are hospitalized. If you are not in hospital and develop severe bleeding through the vagina after giving birth, you should seek medical advice immediately.

How is it diagnosed?
If you are not already in hospital, you will probably be admitted immediately. Your pulse and blood pressure will be monitored to look for any evidence of shock. If an early postpartum haemorrhage has occurred, your doctor will feel your lower abdomen to see if the uterus is contracted. The placenta will be checked to ensure that it is complete. If the uterus appears to be contracted but bleeding continues, your cervix and vagina will be examined. This may be carried out under general anaesthesia or epidural anaesthesia.

If you are having a late postpartum haemorrhage, your doctor may arrange for an ultrasound scan, using a probe inserted into the vagina, to check for remaining pieces of placenta in the uterus. A vaginal swab may be taken to check for evidence of infection.

What is the treatment?
If an early postpartum haemorrhage is due to poor contraction of the uterus, you may be given an injection to help the uterus to contract. Your doctor may also massage your abdomen. If these measures do not work, further drugs may be given to help the uterus to contract. If the bleeding continues, surgery may be required. In rare cases, a hysterectomy (p.479) may be necessary. Bleeding caused by a retained placenta is treated by manually removing the remaining placenta through the vagina. If the blood loss is due to tears in the cervix or vagina, these will be stitched.

If a late postpartum haemorrhage is the result of an infection, antibiotics (p.572) will be prescribed. If the bleeding continues, surgery may be needed to examine the

uterus and remove any remaining fragments of placenta. Blood lost due to a postpartum haemorrhage may have to be replaced by a blood transfusion (p.272).

Depression after childbirth

Depressive feelings or psychological disturbances in the first few weeks or months after childbirth

 Sometimes runs in families

 Lack of emotional support and additional stressful life events are risk factors

 Age is not a significant factor

It is very common for a new mother to feel low or miserable during the first few days or weeks after childbirth. A new baby leads to major changes in lifestyle, and adjustments will need to be made. This mild mood change is commonly known as the "baby blues" and affects up to 8 in 10 women following the birth of a child.

More severe postpartum depression is a relatively common disorder in the first few weeks or months after childbirth and affects about 1 in 10 women. About 1 in 1,000 women develops a serious psychiatric condition known as postpartum psychosis that requires immediate treatment in hospital.

What are the causes?
Baby blues are thought to be caused by the sudden fall in hormone levels (particularly of oestrogen and progesterone) that occurs after a baby is born. These hormonal changes may also cause postpartum depression and possibly also postpartum psychosis.

Women who have suffered from depression (p.343) before are at increased risk of becoming depressed after childbirth. Postpartum depression may run in families. Other factors, such as feelings of isolation and inadequacy and concerns about the new responsibilities of motherhood, can cause stress and contribute to depression. Lack of sleep due to caring for the baby, exhaustion from a long labour, or painful wounds, such as tears in the vagina or scars from a caesarean section, may aggravate the problem. Mothers who have had a difficult labour are more likely to experience postpartum depression. Extra stresses or problems with a partner can make feelings of depression worse. Some women experience anxiety after childbirth, and they may have panic attacks with palpitations and shortness of breath (see **Anxiety disorders**, p.341). If recurrent panic attacks are untreated, they may lead to postpartum depression.

Although the precise cause of postpartum psychosis is not understood, a previous history of episodes of depression that alternate with episodes of mania (see **Bipolar affective disorder**, p.344) significantly increases the risk. Women who have close relatives with a medical history of bipolar affective disorder or severe depression are at greater risk of postpartum psychosis.

What are the symptoms?
The symptoms of baby blues start 3–10 days after giving birth. They are often worse by about day 5 and include:
- Dramatic mood swings.
- Weeping.
- Tiredness and irritability.
- Lack of concentration.

Postpartum depression may begin any time in the first 6 months after childbirth. The condition is similar to baby blues but much more severe, and, unlike baby blues, it can interfere with the mother's ability to carry out day-to-day activities. The symptoms include:
- Constantly feeling exhausted.
- Having little interest or no interest at all in the new baby.
- Sense of anticlimax.
- Feeling inadequate and overwhelmed by new responsibilities.
- Difficulty sleeping.
- Loss of appetite.
- Feelings of guilt.

The symptoms of postpartum psychosis usually develop rapidly about 2–3 weeks after childbirth. They often include:
- Insomnia and overactivity.

- Extreme mood swings from depression to mania.
- False beliefs of being disliked and persecuted by people.
- Hallucinations.
- Confusion.

Sometimes, threats of suicide or of harming the baby may be made by women who develop symptoms of postpartum psychosis.

What can I do?
You should try to get as much support as possible from medical staff, friends, and family after childbirth. Make sure you are not left alone until you feel happy caring for your baby, and rest as much as possible. You may also wish to find out about local self-help groups or mother-and-baby groups.

Baby blues do not usually require medical treatment and, with emotional support and time, almost always disappear. If you develop severe depression and find it hard to carry out day-to-day activities and look after your baby, you should consult your doctor.

What might the doctor do?
If postpartum depression is interfering with your life and simple reassurance and support are not helping to relieve your symptoms, your doctor may prescribe antidepressant drugs (p.592) and advise counselling (p.624).

If you have very severe postpartum depression or postpartum psychosis, you will need to be admitted to hospital. The hospital will make sure that your baby can stay with you. To treat severe depression, you may be given a higher dose of antidepressant drugs or a different type of antidepressant drug. Antipsychotic drugs (p.592) are usually prescribed for postpartum psychosis, and psychotherapy, in which you are encouraged to talk freely about your feelings, may be recommended to help you to overcome your problem. You will also be offered practical help looking after your baby.

You may not be able to breast-feed while you are taking antidepressant or antipsychotic drugs because of the risk of the drugs passing into your breast milk and harming your baby.

What is the prognosis?
The mildest form of depression, baby blues, usually improves within a few weeks, especially if the mother is given reassurance and support. Postpartum depression is likely to start responding to antidepressant drugs within 2–4 weeks, but full recovery may take up to a year. Antipsychotic drugs are usually helpful for postpartum psychosis within 2–3 months.

However, the drugs may need to be taken for a period of several months and long-term follow-up and support will be given.

Any form of depression may recur after subsequent pregnancies. Women who have an increased risk of developing either postpartum depression or psychosis will be offered extra support during and after future pregnancies. They will also be monitored for signs of depression and may be given hormone patches after birth to counter the sudden fall in their hormone levels.

Breast engorgement

Swollen, painful breasts caused by congestion with milk after childbirth

 Age, genetics, and lifestyle are not significant factors

All mothers normally produce breast milk after childbirth and develop some degree of breast engorgement before feeding is established and milk production adapts to match the needs of their baby. During engorgement, the breasts become full of milk and may swell to up to twice their normal size. They also become hard, red, and painful.

▶ **HEALTH OPTIONS**

Feeding your infant

Doctors advise that breast-feeding should be continued for at least 6 months and ideally for a year. Breast milk is better for your baby than milk formula. This is because breast milk contains the ideal balance of nutrients for a baby and also provides valuable antibodies (proteins made by the immune system), which protect against infections. Another good reason for breast-feeding your baby is that in the first few days after childbirth, the breasts produce a fluid called colostrum, which is especially rich in vitamins, minerals, and antibodies to protect the baby from infection. Bottle-feeding is a

satisfactory alternative feeding method, as long as the formula is prepared according to the instructions. The formula is a milk preparation usually based on modified cows' milk and contains valuable nutrients, similar to those found in breast milk. However, it lacks protective antibodies. Weaning is advised from about 6 months of age, when you can gradually introduce solid foods into your baby's diet. However, you should avoid giving your baby certain foods (see below) while he or she is weaning, and your baby should also continue to receive breast milk or formula throughout the first year of life.

Breast- or bottle-feeding
If possible, all mothers should breast-feed for the first month. Every extra month brings more benefits, but bottle-feeding may be a solution if you are taking drugs that pass into the breast milk and might pose a danger to your baby or if there are other considerations. Breast-fed babies are less susceptible to infections, asthma, allergies, and sudden infant death syndrome, and are less likely to become obese when they get older.

Weaning
During weaning, gradually introduce solid foods, first as purées and later in mashed or minced form. To reduce the risk of allergies and digestive upsets, do not give wheat-based foods, raw eggs, raw cows' milk, citrus foods, fatty foods, or strong spices before the age of 6 months, and avoid nut products and honey before a year. You should also avoid giving your baby sweet foods and should not add salt to your baby's food.

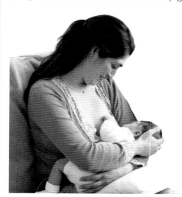

Natural protection from breast milk
Breast milk contains natural antibodies that protect against infections and also reduce the risk of allergies developing.

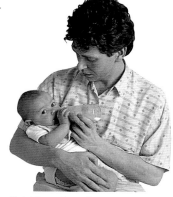

Nutritious formula
Most milk formulas are approximately as nutritious and digestible as breast milk but lack the protective antibodies that breast milk provides.

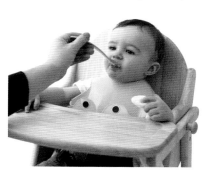

Diet at 6 months
Start by giving your baby a diet of baby rice or purées of vegetables or fruit during or after a milk feed. Slowly increase the amount of solid food, including puréed meat, fish, poultry, and pulses.

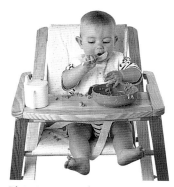

Diet at 7–9 months
You can now give mashed or minced food before the milk. At 9 months, peeled apple and bread encourage self-feeding and provide chewing practice.

▶ **SELF-HELP**

Avoiding cracked nipples

Cracked nipples are usually caused by the baby not taking the nipple into his or her mouth properly. To avoid cracked nipples, make sure that your baby is positioned on your nipple correctly each time you breast-feed. Dry your nipples thoroughly after each feed and avoid plastic-lined breast pads, which may become damp and encourage soreness and infection. Emollient creams can prevent the skin from drying out but should be washed off before breast-feeding.

Correct position of baby

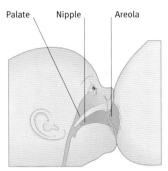

Palate   Nipple   Areola

SUCKING POSITION

Positioning your baby on the nipple
When breast-feeding, the entire nipple and most of the areola (the darker area around the nipple) should be taken into the baby's mouth to prevent the skin around the nipple becoming cracked.

Breast engorgement may occur if a woman stops breast-feeding or if her baby needs special care in an incubator and she is unable to breast-feed. In these situations, milk accumulates inside the breasts until milk production ceases. In women who are breast-feeding, breast engorgement may develop because the baby is weak and unable to feed properly, so that the initial milk supply exceeds demand. In all cases, the accumulation of excess milk may lead to the development of infection in one or both breasts, causing a painful inflammation (*see* **Mastitis**, right).

What can I do?

After childbirth, you should wear a firm, supportive bra, whether or not you are going to breast-feed your baby. Local heat treatment may ease discomfort in the breasts, as may taking painkillers (p.589) such as paracetamol. Do not try to express milk if you are not going to breast-feed because this may stimulate further milk production. Your breasts should gradually become less painful after a few days of not breast-feeding. Rarely, you may be prescribed a drug to stop milk production.

If you decide to breast-feed, try to encourage your baby to feed as soon as possible. You can remove some of the excess milk by gently expressing it using your hands or a breast pump. Once your baby is feeding regularly, the production of milk should adapt to match the demands of your baby, and your breasts will become less engorged.

When you stop breast-feeding, cut out feeds one at a time over several days or weeks in order to help prevent your breasts from becoming engorged.

Cracked nipples

Fine cracks in the nipple caused by breast-feeding

ⓘ Age, genetics, and lifestyle are not significant factors

During the first few weeks of breast-feeding, fine cracks and raw areas may develop in the skin on and surrounding the nipple. These cause a stabbing or burning pain, usually as the baby starts or stops feeding. Cracked nipples are most often caused by the baby failing to take the whole nipple into his or her mouth properly when feeding, which itself is usually due to poor positioning of your baby at the breast. Leaving your nipples wet after each feed may also cause them to become tender and cracked. Occasionally, cracked nipples can become infected and inflamed (*see* **Mastitis**, right).

Your doctor or breast-feeding counsellor will advise you on the correct technique for positioning and feeding your baby properly. You can also take preventive measures to help stop cracks forming (*see* **Avoiding cracked nipples**, above) and to avoid infection.

Cracked nipples will heal over time after you have learned how to position your baby correctly at the breast. However, if your nipples are very painful or if discomfort develops only after several weeks of successful breast-feeding, you should consult your doctor. If your doctor suspects that the sore area has become infected, he or she will probably prescribe a course of antibiotics (p.572) for you. Your doctor will also possibly prescribe

---

treatment for your baby if his or her mouth has become infected. This treatment should clear up the infection in a few days.

Mastitis

Painful inflammation of breast tissue in part of one or both breasts

ⓘ Age, genetics, and lifestyle are not significant factors

Inflammation of one or both breasts is called mastitis. The condition usually occurs in the first 6 weeks of breast-feeding. However, mastitis may also develop after this time if breast-feeding is stopped suddenly and the breasts become over-filled with milk (*see* **Breast engorgement**, opposite page). Mastitis in women who are not breast-feeding may be related to smoking, which can cause inflammation of the milk ducts, resulting in discharge of fluid from one or both nipples (*see* **Nipple discharge**, p.486).

Mastitis is caused by infection of a blocked milk duct or an area of the breast that is inadequately drained of milk. The infection is commonly caused by the bacterium *Staphylococcus aureus*, which enters the breast through broken skin, most often on the nipple (*see* **Cracked nipples**, left). Mastitis affects up to 1 in 10 women who breast-feed. Women breast-feeding for the first time are particularly likely to develop the condition because they may not have learned how to position their baby correctly on the breast to make sure that the entire nipple is taken into the baby's mouth, which will prevent the skin around the nipple from becoming cracked (*see* **Avoiding cracked nipples**, left).

What are the symptoms?

Mastitis usually affects only one area of a breast. Symptoms of the condition develop gradually over a period of several days and may include:

■ Tender, red area that spreads away from the nipple.
■ Swelling and pain in the affected part of the breast.

A severe, flu-like illness with fever and chills may also develop together with the breast inflammation.

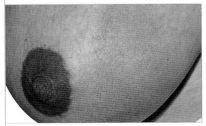

Mastitis
The red triangular area of inflammation radiating away from the nipple indicates mastitis, a condition that may develop in women who are breast-feeding.

If it is left untreated, inflammation of the breast gradually becomes worse and a pus-filled cavity, called a breast abscess, may develop, causing a firm lump that is painful to the touch. However, such breast abscesses are now relatively uncommon because antibiotics (p.572) are usually prescribed at the first sign of an infection to destroy the bacteria before a breast abscess has had a chance to develop.

What can I do?

You should keep breast-feeding if you develop mastitis because stopping may cause the breasts to become engorged with milk and encourage an abscess to develop. However, you should check your breast-feeding technique with your breast-feeding counsellor. The infection will not harm your baby because the bacteria in your milk will be destroyed by the baby's stomach acid. The regular flow of milk will help to keep your breast well drained and thereby prevent the condition from becoming worse. Any milk that still remains in the affected breast following breast-feeding should be expressed if possible.

A heat pad or a well-wrapped hot water bottle placed on the affected area of the breast may help to encourage the flow of milk and relieve the pain. Mild painkillers (p.589), such as paracetamol, may be useful to ease the discomfort. You should try to rest as much as possible and also try to drink plenty of nonalcoholic fluids.

If an abscess develops, you should not breast-feed with the affected breast. Instead, you should empty the breast of milk by gently expressing it with your hands or using a breast pump, a suction device that is designed to extract and collect milk from the breasts.

What might the doctor do?

A diagnosis of mastitis is usually obvious from the symptoms, especially if you are currently breast-feeding your baby or if you have recently stopped breast-feeding. Your doctor will examine your breasts and may arrange for a sample of your milk to be sent to a laboratory in order to identify the bacteria that are causing the infection. He or she may also arrange for you to have ultrasound scanning (p.135) to examine any lumps that may be present in the breast. Your doctor will probably prescribe a course of oral antibiotics to treat the infection.

Mastitis usually clears up within 2 or 3 days of beginning a treatment regimen with antibiotics but you should finish the entire course, even if your symptoms start to improve, in order to eradicate the infection. However, if a breast abscess has already developed, the pus that has collected may have to be drained from the breast, either under local or general anaesthesia. Once all the pus has been removed, a recurrence of the abscess is unlikely.

Infancy and childhood

From the moment of birth, babies grow and develop physically, mentally, and socially. In the first year, a baby grows faster than at any other time in later life. Within the first few years, children learn basic skills and go on to acquire a wide range of physical and intellectual accomplishments.

CHILDREN PASS THROUGH predictable patterns of growth and development, but each child progresses at a different rate. Physical growth and intellectual development are partly determined by genetic factors, but these processes are also affected by general health and stimulation from the environment.

Growth and development

Babies are born with various primitive reflexes: they communicate by crying and instinctively suck when offered a nipple. At first, babies grow fast, tripling in weight and growing in length by about 25 cm (10 in) in the first year. After about the age of 2, children begin a long, slower period of growth, which allows time for complex skills to be acquired.

A child's intellectual skills and physical coordination depend on the healthy development of the muscular and nervous

systems. The earliest accomplishments are basic skills such as walking, talking, and feeding themselves. As independence grows, children recognize themselves as individuals, interact more actively with their surroundings, and develop close relationships. By the age of 12, they have usually acquired sophisticated language and numeracy skills and wide-ranging physical abilities.

Between the ages of about 8 and 14, children undergo the dramatic changes of puberty, with maturation of the reproductive organs and the development of secondary sexual characteristics such as breasts and body hair. These physical changes occur some time before emotional maturation, and adolescence is therefore a time of adjustment to adulthood. At the age of 18, young people are considered adults in most societies, although they continue to develop psychologically for many years.

✚ STRUCTURE AND FUNCTION

The heart before and after birth

In the fetus, only a little blood passes through the lungs because the task of adding oxygen to the blood and filtering out waste gases is done by the mother's placenta. Before birth, most blood bypasses the lungs by flowing through two openings in the heart. With a baby's first breath the lungs expand, triggering

changes so that all blood flows through the lungs to be oxygenated.

Changes in the heart's circulation
An opening in the fetal heart, the foramen ovale, diverts blood from the right atrium (chamber) to the left, and a duct, the ductus arteriosus, diverts blood into the aorta. The openings close soon after birth.

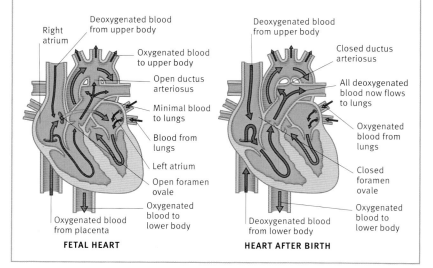

FETAL HEART

HEART AFTER BIRTH

✚ **STRUCTURE AND FUNCTION**

The newborn baby

A full-term newborn baby weighs on average 3.5 kg (7 lb 11 oz), measures 51 cm (20 in) in length, and is well prepared for survival. Many aspects of a newborn's appearance, such as the shape of the skull, are a result of the transition from the uterus to the outside world and are different from those of a fetus or older child. Such differences are normal and usually disappear relatively quickly. Other structures, such as the long bones, are not yet fully formed. The baby also has primitive reflexes, such as a grasp reflex, which are important to survival but disappear with increasing age.

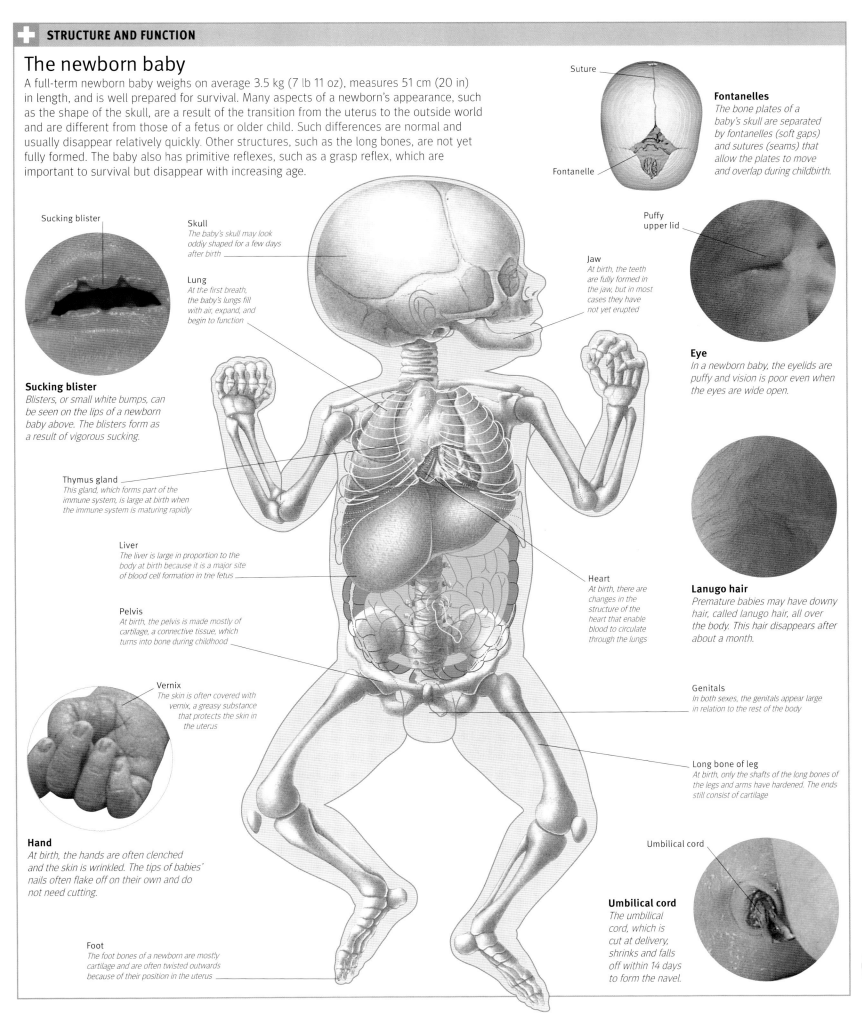

Sucking blister

Skull
The baby's skull may look oddly shaped for a few days after birth

Lung
At the first breath, the baby's lungs fill with air, expand, and begin to function

Sucking blister
Blisters, or small white bumps, can be seen on the lips of a newborn baby above. The blisters form as a result of vigorous sucking.

Thymus gland
This gland, which forms part of the immune system, is large at birth when the immune system is maturing rapidly

Liver
The liver is large in proportion to the body at birth because it is a major site of blood cell formation in the fetus

Pelvis
At birth, the pelvis is made mostly of cartilage, a connective tissue, which turns into bone during childhood

Vernix
The skin is often covered with vernix, a greasy substance that protects the skin in the uterus

Hand
At birth, the hands are often clenched and the skin is wrinkled. The tips of babies' nails often flake off on their own and do not need cutting.

Foot
The foot bones of a newborn are mostly cartilage and are often twisted outwards because of their position in the uterus

Suture

Fontanelle

Fontanelles
The bone plates of a baby's skull are separated by fontanelles (soft gaps) and sutures (seams) that allow the plates to move and overlap during childbirth.

Puffy upper lid

Jaw
At birth, the teeth are fully formed in the jaw, but in most cases they have not yet erupted

Eye
In a newborn baby, the eyelids are puffy and vision is poor even when the eyes are wide open.

Lanugo hair
Premature babies may have downy hair, called lanugo hair, all over the body. This hair disappears after about a month.

Heart
At birth, there are changes in the structure of the heart that enable blood to circulate through the lungs

Genitals
In both sexes, the genitals appear large in relation to the rest of the body

Long bone of leg
At birth, only the shafts of the long bones of the legs and arms have hardened. The ends still consist of cartilage

Umbilical cord

Umbilical cord
The umbilical cord, which is cut at delivery, shrinks and falls off within 14 days to form the navel.

The developing body

A child's body grows and changes continuously from birth to adulthood through processes that are largely controlled by hormones. The most dramatic changes take place during infancy, when rapid growth occurs, and during puberty, when the body is approaching sexual maturity. At certain times, some parts of the body develop faster than others, which is why body proportions change throughout childhood. A child's brain is almost fully grown by the age of 6, while the rest of the body remains relatively undeveloped.

Changing body proportions

At birth, a baby's head is as wide as the shoulders and appears large in relation to the rest of the body. The head continues to grow quickly, and by the age of 2, the brain is four-fifths of its adult size. As the child gets older, the rate of growth of the head decreases compared with the rest of the body. Eventually, usually by the age of 18, the proportion of the head with the rest of the body stays the same and growth stops.

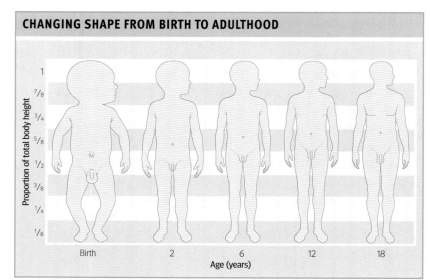

CHANGING SHAPE FROM BIRTH TO ADULTHOOD

Proportion of total body height

1, 7/8, 3/4, 5/8, 1/2, 3/8, 1/4, 1/8

Birth   2   6   12   18

Age (years)

How proportions change
A newborn baby's head makes up about a quarter of total body length, and the legs three-eighths. By 18 years, proportions have changed; the head is an eighth of total body length and the legs a half.

How bones develop

Hard-bone formation (ossification) commences before birth at sites in the bone shafts known as primary ossification centres. In a newborn baby, only the shafts (diaphyses) are ossified. The ends of these bones (epiphyses) consist of tissue called cartilage, which is gradually replaced by bone that develops from secondary ossification centres. Between the shaft and the ends is a zone called the growth plate, which produces more cartilage to elongate the bones.

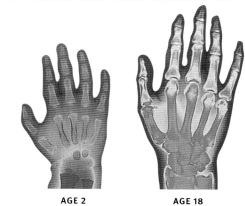

Hand growth
At the age of 2, ossified hand bone shafts look opaque on an X-ray. The growing cartilage looks transparent. By 18 years, all bone is ossified.

AGE 2   **AGE 18**

Articular cartilage
This smooth tissue protects the end of a long bone

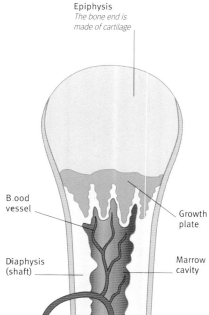

Epiphysis
The bone end is made of cartilage

Blood vessel

Growth plate

Diaphysis (shaft)

Marrow cavity

Long bone of a newborn baby
The shaft (diaphysis) is mostly bone, while the ends (epiphyses) are made of cartilage that gradually hardens.

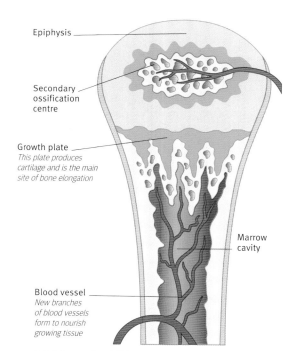

Epiphysis

Secondary ossification centre

Growth plate
This plate produces cartilage and is the main site of bone elongation

Marrow cavity

Blood vessel
New branches of blood vessels form to nourish growing tissue

Long bone of a child
The epiphyses contain secondary ossification centres from which bone forms. A growth plate near the ends produces new cartilage.

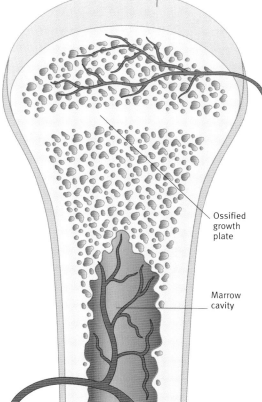

Ossified growth plate

Marrow cavity

Long bone of an adult
By the age of 18, the shafts, growth plates, and epiphyses have all ossified and fused into continuous bone.

How the skull and brain develop

At birth, a newborn's brain has its full complement of billions of neurons (nerve cells) that transmit and receive messages along axons (nerve fibres). At first, these neural networks are partially developed. In the first 6 years, the networks expand, and the brain grows rapidly to allow new skills to be learned. The skull expands to accommodate this growth. Between the ages of 6 and 18, neural pathways develop at a slower rate.

How the brain and skull grow
During infancy, the part of the skull around the brain (cranium) grows rapidly at the seams (sutures) and soft gaps (fontanelles) between the bone plates. By the age of 6, the brain is almost full size.

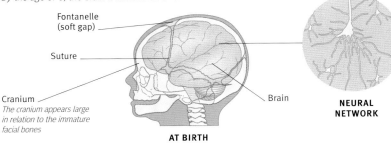

Fontanelle (soft gap)

Suture

Cranium
The cranium appears large in relation to the immature facial bones

Brain

NEURAL NETWORK

AT BIRTH

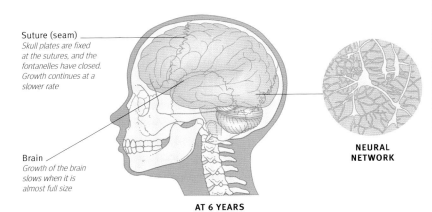

Suture (seam)
Skull plates are fixed at the sutures, and the fontanelles have closed. Growth continues at a slower rate

Brain
Growth of the brain slows when it is almost full size

NEURAL NETWORK

AT 6 YEARS

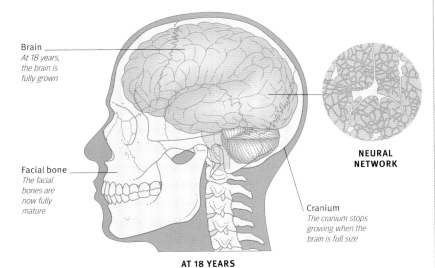

Brain
At 18 years, the brain is fully grown

Facial bone
The facial bones are now fully mature

Cranium
The cranium stops growing when the brain is full size

NEURAL NETWORK

AT 18 YEARS

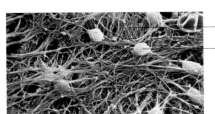

Axon (nerve fibre)

Neuron cell body

Neural network
This highly magnified view of adult brain tissue shows neurons within a complex network of neural pathways.

How nerves develop

Early in life, most nerve fibres (axons) become wrapped in insulating sheaths made of a fatty substance known as myelin. This insulation speeds up nerve transmission by as much as 100 times and is essential for the body to grow and function normally.

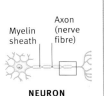

Myelin sheath

Axon (nerve fibre)

NEURON

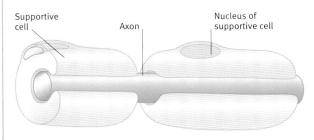

Supportive cell

Axon

Nucleus of supportive cell

1 *Supportive cells, composed mainly of fatty material known as myelin, wind around an axon to form a protective and insulating sheath.*

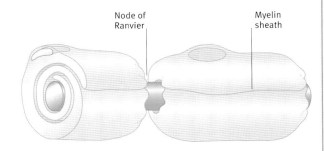

Node of Ranvier

Myelin sheath

2 *The axon is now wrapped in sections of myelin sheath separated by gaps (nodes of Ranvier). Nerve signals jump from one gap to the next.*

Factors affecting growth

A child's potential maximum growth is determined by genes, but achieving the maximum depends on a number of other factors, such as nutrition and general health. Girls and boys have similar patterns of yearly growth in childhood (below). A growth spurt at puberty is triggered by sex hormones, which also speed up the fusion of growth plates in the bone. Growth is complete by about the age of 18.

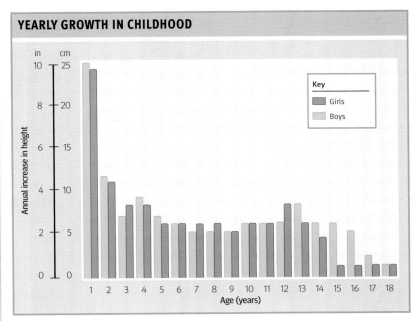

YEARLY GROWTH IN CHILDHOOD

in / cm

Annual increase in height

Key
Girls
Boys

Age (years)

Why boys grow taller than girls
In boys, the growth spurt occurs later in puberty than in girls, giving them longer to grow in childhood before their full growth is complete.

✚ **DATA**

Gaining skills during the first five years

During their first 5 years, children learn the basic skills necessary for their future development. The four main areas are physical skills, manual dexterity, language, and social skills. Although children progress at different rates, developmental milestones occur in a predictable order. This is partly because the ability to learn particular skills depends upon the maturity of the child's nervous system. In addition, for some complex skills, children need to develop a lesser skill first; for example, babies must learn to stand before they can walk.

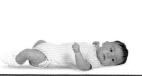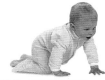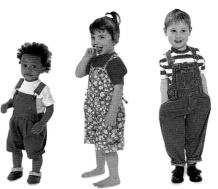

DEVELOPMENTAL MILESTONES

Age (years)

| 0 | 1 | 2 | 3 | 4 | 5 |

Physical skills
Babies first master control of their body posture and head, then go on to develop physical skills, including standing, crawling, and walking.

- Can lift head to 45°
- Can roll over
- Can bear weight on legs
- Can crawl
- Can stand by hoisting up own weight
- Can sit unsupported
- Can walk without help
- Can stand without help
- Can walk holding on to furniture
- Can throw a ball
- Can kick a ball
- Can walk up stairs without help
- Can catch a bounced ball
- Can balance on one foot for a second
- Can pedal a tricycle
- Can hop on one leg

Manual dexterity and vision
Children have to coordinate their movement and vision to perform manipulative tasks, such as picking up objects or drawing.

- Holds hands together
- Reaches out for a rattle
- Plays with feet
- Passes rattle from hand to hand
- Can pick up a small object
- Can grasp object between finger and thumb
- Likes to scribble
- Can build a tower of four bricks
- Can draw a straight line
- Can copy a circle
- Can draw rudimentary likeness of a person
- Can copy a square

Hearing and language
Early on, babies turn towards voices and respond to sounds by cooing. At about 1 year, children speak their first word.

- Startled by loud sounds
- Squeals
- Makes cooing noises
- Turns towards voice
- Says "dada" and "mama" to anyone
- Says "dada" and "mama" to parents
- Can point to parts of the body
- Starts to learn single words
- Can put two words together
- Can talk in full sentences
- Knows first and last names
- Can name a colour
- Can define seven words

Social behaviour and play
Self-care begins with basic skills, such as dressing and toilet training. Social skills range from smiling to making the first new friends.

- Smiles spontaneously
- Looks at own hands
- Plays peekaboo
- Eats with fingers
- Can drink from a cup
- Mimics housework
- Can eat with a spoon and fork
- Can undress without help
- Stays dry in the day
- Separates easily from parent
- Can dress without help
- Stays dry at night
- Can eat with a knife and fork

Age (months)

| 0 | 2 | 4 | 6 | 8 | 10 | 12 | 14 | 16 | 18 | 20 | 22 | 24 | 30 | 36 | 42 | 48 | 54 | 60 |

| 0 | 1 | 2 | 3 | 4 | 5 |

Age (years)

+ FUNCTION

Puberty

Puberty is a period of rapid growth and physical change, during which adolescents become sexually mature. The age at which puberty begins and the rate of growth are influenced by genetics, general health, and weight. Puberty begins when the pituitary gland, located at the base of the brain, secretes hormones that stimulate the production of sex hormones. Within about 2 years of the start of puberty, sexual reproduction is possible, but it takes longer for adolescents to become mature enough emotionally for adult relationships.

Changes in girls during puberty

In girls, puberty begins between the ages of 8 and 14, when luteinizing hormone (LH) and follicle-stimulating hormone (FSH) stimulate the ovaries to secrete the sex hormones oestrogen and progesterone. These hormones prompt physical changes and, later, stimulate ovulation and menstruation.

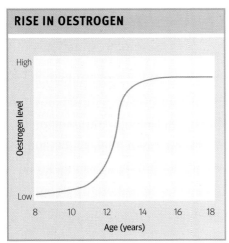

RISE IN OESTROGEN

Oestrogen and puberty
The oestrogen level rises sharply during puberty then levels out until the menopause, when it declines.

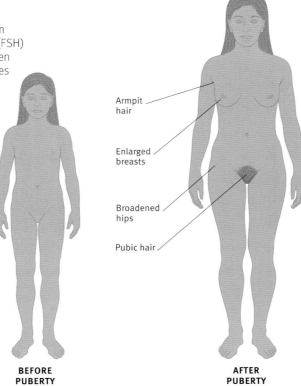

BEFORE PUBERTY

AFTER PUBERTY

- Armpit hair
- Enlarged breasts
- Broadened hips
- Pubic hair

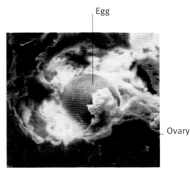

Milk duct — Milk-producing cells

Magnified breast tissue
At puberty, the breasts start to enlarge as they develop the milk glands and ducts that supply milk after a baby is born.

Egg

Ovary

Ovulation
Late in puberty, ovulation begins; every month an egg is released from the ovary (as shown here) and travels to the uterus.

Changes in boys during puberty

In boys, puberty usually begins between the ages of about 9 and 14, when the pituitary gland starts to secrete the hormones LH and FSH. These hormones stimulate the testes to secrete the male sex hormone testosterone, which prompts physical changes and, later, sperm production and increased sex drive.

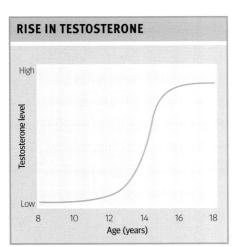

RISE IN TESTOSTERONE

Testosterone and puberty
The testosterone level rises sharply during puberty, levels out, then begins to decline gradually frcm about the age of 30.

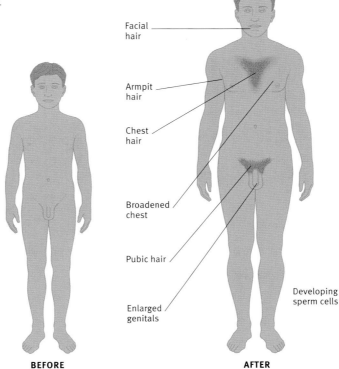

BEFORE PUBERTY

AFTER PUBERTY

- Facial hair
- Armpit hair
- Chest hair
- Broadened chest
- Pubic hair
- Enlarged genitals
- Developing sperm cells

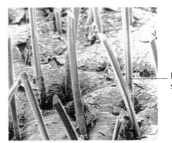

Hair shaft

Facial hair
Hair on the face is part of the typical male pattern of hair growth triggered by increasing levels of testosterone.

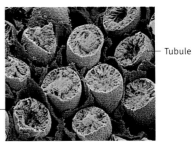

Tubule

Cross section of testis tissue
In each testis, there are about 1,000 tubules. During puberty, these tubules begin to produce sperm cells.

Problems in babies

Many problems in babies are associated with their immaturity and adjustment to a new environment. Premature babies are at particular risk of life-threatening conditions, but medical advances have greatly increased the number of babies that survive.

The first article in this section covers problems experienced by premature babies, those born more than 3 weeks before their expected birth date, who may have special problems as a result of their immaturity. The next article discusses congenital infections, which are transmitted from the mother to the fetus either during pregnancy or at birth as the baby passes through the birth canal. Although these infections are rare, they may have serious effects. Neonatal jaundice, which is discussed next, occurs in many newborn babies. In most cases, the jaundice is normal, but rarely there is a serious cause, such as the underdevelopment of the bile ducts in the baby's liver. Problems experienced with sleeping, feeding, crying, colic, and teething are also covered. These minor problems can be stressful for parents but rarely require medical treatment. The section ends with an article on sudden infant death syndrome (SIDS), also known as cot death, and advice on how to reduce the risk of it occurring. The cause of SIDS is not known, but its incidence has decreased since parents were advised to position babies on their backs to sleep. Other conditions that affect babies from birth are discussed in chromosome and gene disorders (pp.533–537) and endocrine and metabolic disorders (pp.561–563).

Problems of the premature baby

Problems experienced by babies born more than 3 weeks earlier than their expected birth date

 Present from birth

 Gender, genetics, and lifestyle are not significant factors

Pregnancy usually lasts about 40 weeks. Babies born before 37 weeks of pregnancy (*see* **Premature labour**, p.515) are called premature, and these babies may have problems because of their small size and immaturity. The severity of these problems will depend on how far the pregnancy has progressed and the baby's weight at birth. With specialist care, babies born as early as 23 weeks now have a chance of survival.

What are the problems?

All premature babies lose heat easily because they are smaller than full-term babies and have thin skin and little fat. In addition, respiratory problems may occur because the lungs are immature and may not produce enough surfactant, a chemical that is required for the lungs to function properly. This problem is known as respiratory distress syndrome. Temporary cessation of breathing is a common problem due to immaturity of the brain. Premature babies are also particularly vulnerable to injury and infection. The trauma of birth, lack of oxygen, and infection can all affect the developing brain. In very premature babies (born before 28 weeks), tiny blood vessels in the brain may rupture and bleed. There are usually no lasting problems, but specific learning disabilities (p.553) and problems with movement and posture (*see* **Cerebral palsy**, p.548) may occur.

About 8 in 10 premature babies are affected by neonatal jaundice (opposite page), due to immaturity of the liver. In this condition, there is yellowing of the skin and the whites of the eyes.

What might be done?

The doctor will assess your baby's condition at birth and start treatment if necessary. A baby who is only a few weeks premature may not need specialist care. However, you will be advised to feed your baby frequently and to make sure that he or she is kept warm.

Other premature babies may be looked after in a special care baby unit and are placed in an incubator so that their environment can be carefully controlled. They may also be given fluids and fed intravenously or through a tube that is passed through the nose and into the stomach. A premature baby may need to spend several weeks or months in the unit, and parents will be encouraged to take part in the baby's care. Tests may also be performed, such as ultrasound scanning (p.135) of the brain and chest X-rays (p.300), to look for abnormalities that may require treatment.

If your baby has respiratory distress syndrome, mechanical ventilation may be necessary, and surfactant will probably be

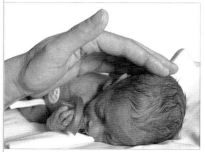

A premature baby
This baby was born prematurely and is smaller than normal. Premature babies need specialist care and monitoring.

given directly into the airways to help the lungs to function. A ventilated baby may be given sedatives to make him or her more comfortable. However, the high levels of oxygen that are sometimes needed to treat respiratory problems in premature babies may be associated with damage to the retina (the light-sensitive layer at the back of the eye), resulting in visual impairment.

A baby who has jaundice may have treatment with a specific wavelength of fluorescent light (*see* **Phototherapy**, opposite page). Antibiotics (p.572) may also be given to treat or prevent infection.

When your baby leaves hospital, the doctor will continue to give you advice and support. Your baby may be given a vision test to look for retinal damage (*see* **Vision tests in children**, p.555) and also a hearing test (*see* **Hearing tests in children**, p.557) to check for any hearing loss. The growth and development of your baby will also be carefully monitored.

What is the prognosis?

The success of treatment depends on how early the baby was born and the weight at birth. About 4 in 10 babies born at 23–24 weeks survive, but they may have long-term problems, such as visual impairment, lung disorders, or cerebral palsy. Most babies born after 30 weeks develop normally with no long-term health problems. Premature babies are more susceptible to sudden infant death syndrome (p.532).

Congenital infections

Infections contracted before or at birth from the mother

 Present from birth

 Lifestyle as a risk factor depends on the cause

 Gender and genetics are not significant factors

Most infections contracted by a mother during pregnancy do not affect the fetus, but some cross the placenta and cause harm. These infections are often minor illnesses for the pregnant mother, and she may not even be aware of them. Serious infections such as HIV (*see* **HIV infection and AIDS**, p.169) may also be passed on to the fetus.

The effect on the baby depends on the stage of pregnancy at which the infection occurs. In early pregnancy, the development of organs may be disrupted, and a miscarriage (p.511) could occur. Infections in later pregnancy may result in premature labour (p.515) and a baby who is seriously ill at birth. Infections may also be transmitted as the baby passes through the birth canal.

What are the causes?

In the first 3 months of pregnancy, the viral disease rubella (p.168) can lead to fetal heart abnormalities (*see* **Congenital heart disease**, p.542) and impaired hearing and

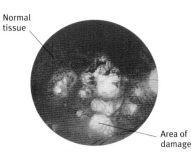

Normal tissue

Area of damage

Toxoplasmosis
The pale patches in this view of the retina at the back of a baby's eye indicate the congenital infection toxoplasmosis.

vision. Cytomegalovirus (CMV) infection (p.167) and toxoplasmosis (p.176), which is caused by a protozoal parasite found in cats' faeces or undercooked meat, may cause miscarriage or malformations of the fetus in early pregnancy. CMV is the leading cause of congenital deafness (p.556) and toxoplasmosis can damage the retina (the light-sensitive cells at the back of the eye). Later in pregnancy, these infections may lead to premature labour, stillbirth (p.520), and serious illness in the newborn baby. Listeriosis (p.172), a bacterial infection that can be contracted from eating soft cheese and pâté, may cause miscarriage, stillbirth, or serious infection in the newborn baby.

Long-term viral infections that can be passed from mother to fetus include HIV infection and hepatitis B and C (*see* **Acute hepatitis**, p.408). The bacterial infection syphilis (p.492) may also be passed on. These infections do not always produce symptoms at birth but can cause serious illness later in life.

Some infections can be transmitted from mother to baby during labour. Some of these infections, such as herpes simplex virus (*see* **Genital herpes**, p.493) and streptococcal bacteria, can be life-threatening in a newborn baby. The risk of contracting an infection is increased if the mother's waters break prematurely (*see* **Premature rupture of membranes**, p.515).

What might be done?

If a baby is seriously ill at birth and a congenital infection is suspected, blood and urine samples are taken to identify the infection. Babies are usually nursed in a special care baby unit and treated intravenously with appropriate drugs. Ultrasound scanning (p.135) may be used to image the baby's brain and echocardiography (p.255) may be arranged if there is a heart problem. In the UK, newborn babies at high risk of hepatitis B infection are routinely immunized against it. If the mother is known to be infected with hepatitis B, the newborn baby is given antibodies against the virus in addition to immunization.

Can they be prevented?

Women can minimize the risk of contracting many of these infections during pregnancy. For example, they can ensure they are immunized against rubella before starting a pregnancy. To avoid toxoplasmosis infection, pregnant women should avoid eating under-cooked meat, wash their hands after handling raw meat or food contaminated with soil, and avoid contact with cat faeces (in cat litter, for example). Pregnant women should also avoid eating foods linked with listeriosis.

Pregnant women with HIV infection are monitored, and they may be prescribed antiviral drugs to keep them healthy and to reduce the risk of transmitting the virus to the fetus. In some cases, a caesarean section (p.518) may be recommended for pregnant women with HIV or active herpes infection at the time of the birth.

Mild congenital infections may have no lasting effect on the baby, but severe infections can be life-threatening. Congenital abnormalities may also result in long-term health and learning problems.

Neonatal jaundice

Yellow discoloration of the skin and the whites of the eyes in a newborn baby

 Present from or shortly after birth

 Genetics as a risk factor depends on the cause

 Gender and lifestyle are not significant factors

More than half of all newborn babies develop slight yellowing of the skin in the first week of life, giving them a tanned appearance. This condition is known as neonatal jaundice. In most cases, neonatal jaundice is normal, lasts only a few days, and does not indicate a serious underlying illness.

Neonatal jaundice is caused by high levels of a yellowish-green pigment in the blood known as bilirubin, which is a breakdown product of red blood cells. The liver, which removes bilirubin from the blood, may not function properly in a newborn baby for several days. As a result, the level of bilirubin rises as fetal blood cells are broken down. Breast-feeding may make neonatal jaundice worse, but it can be continued without harming the baby.

Neonatal jaundice may be more severe if it is caused by an underlying condition, for example if the mother and baby have incompatible blood groups because of Rhesus (Rh) incompatibility (p.514). Incompatibility of ABO blood groups is also a common cause of jaundice, as is G6PD deficiency (an inherited enzyme deficiency). Rare conditions that may produce jaundice include congenital infections (opposite page) and biliary atresia, in which a baby is born with underdeveloped bile ducts (the tubes that drain bile from the liver).

What are the symptoms?
In most full-term babies with neonatal jaundice, the skin and the whites of the eyes appear yellow, but there are no other symptoms. However, if bilirubin levels rise, symptoms may include:
- Lethargy.
- Reluctance to feed.

Severe, abnormal jaundice may lead to impaired hearing or brain damage. If the bile ducts are underdeveloped due to biliary atresia, there is a risk of fatal liver damage unless the condition is treated.

What might be done?
Your baby will probably have a blood test to measure the level of bilirubin and exclude underlying disorders. If biliary atresia is suspected, imaging tests such as ultrasound scanning (p.135) and MRI (p.133) of the liver may be performed. A liver biopsy, in which a small sample of liver tissue is removed for examination, usually confirms the diagnosis.

Most babies with mild jaundice do not require treatment. However, if the level of bilirubin in the blood is high, phototherapy

(below, left) may be necessary, whatever the cause of the jaundice. In phototherapy, bilirubin is converted into a harmless substance that can be excreted. Treatment of Rh incompatibility may involve exchange transfusion, in which a large proportion of the baby's blood is replaced. Biliary atresia is corrected by surgery in the first weeks of the baby's life to prevent liver damage.

Neonatal jaundice does not usually have long-term effects and tends to disappear during the first week of life, or slightly later if the baby is breast-fed. Babies who have had severe jaundice will have a hearing test (*see* **Hearing tests in children**, p.557) and will be monitored for the first few months of life.

Sleeping problems in babies

Night-time wakefulness in babies, especially during the first months of life

 More common under the age of 12 months

 An unsettled environment is a risk factor

 Gender and genetics are not significant factors

Most newborn babies take time to establish a sleeping pattern that fits in with their parents' sleep and a normal 24-hour day. A baby's sleeping pattern will depend on how frequently he or she needs to feed. Premature babies tend to feed more often than full-term babies and therefore sleep for shorter periods. In older infants, problems may be caused by temperament, an unsettled or stressful environment, or a minor illness such as a common cold (p.164). Some sleeping problems are inevitable with a baby, but they can be stressful for parents.

What can I do?
Although your baby will have an irregular sleeping pattern at first, there are some self-help measures that may be useful. During the day, give your baby plenty of stimulation and try to nap when your baby is asleep. If you are breast-feeding, lactation is established, and your baby is gaining weight at the expected rate, from 6 weeks onwards you can express milk so that you can share night feeding with your partner. When your baby is about 10 weeks old, you can begin to establish a bedtime routine. Give your baby's last feed in a quiet, darkened room. Check that your baby is comfortable, not hungry, and wearing a clean nappy. Put your baby to bed before he or she has fallen asleep so that your baby gets used to going to sleep without being held. Do not play with him or her during night-time feeds. If you think your baby's wakefulness may be due to an illness, consult your doctor.

In most babies, night-time wakefulness will improve with time. However, a few may develop sleeping problems later in childhood (*see* **Sleeping problems in children**, p.551).

Feeding problems in babies

Feeding difficulties experienced during the first years of life

 More common in early infancy

 Gender, genetics, and lifestyle as risk factors depend on the cause

Problems with feeding are common in young babies until a routine is established, but if a baby is gaining weight there is usually no need to worry. However, when a baby who normally feeds well becomes reluctant to feed or vomits, there may be an underlying illness.

What are the causes?
Breast-feeding may not come naturally to mother or baby and takes time to be learned. Problems with bottle-feeding are less common but may be due to the brand of milk or teat size used. A minor illness may cause temporary difficulties. Most babies regurgitate after each feed, but in some babies regurgitation is persistent (*see* **Gastro-oesophageal reflux disease in infants**, p.559). A few babies vomit forcefully after feeds, which may indicate that the outlet of the stomach is narrowed or blocked (*see* **Pyloric stenosis in infants**, p.559).

What might be done?
If you bottle-feed, you should avoid frequently changing the brands of milk or the teats because such changes may make the problem worse. Wind your baby after a feed and, if he or she tends to vomit, try propping him or her up after feeds. If you are worried, weigh your baby to make sure that he or she is gaining weight. You should seek medical advice if you are still concerned or have problems with breast-feeding.

Your doctor will be able to exclude problems that require treatment, such as gastro-oesophageal reflux disease or pyloric stenosis, and will give you advice on breast-feeding. Your child may need to have regular weight and measurement checks to assess his or her growth. With time, most feeding problems disappear.

Excessive crying

Prolonged, inconsolable crying in babies that may indicate an underlying illness

 More common in early infancy

 Gender, genetics, and lifestyle are not significant factors

Babies let adults know they are hungry or uncomfortable by crying. Prolonged, inconsolable crying, especially at night, is very stressful and tiring for parents. Newborn babies are more likely to cry excessively

---

▶ **TREATMENT**

Phototherapy

In phototherapy, blue fluorescent lights are used in the treatment of neonatal jaundice (above), a disorder in which the skin and whites of the eyes become yellow due to high levels of the pigment bilirubin in the blood. In order to maximize exposure, your baby will be undressed and placed under the lights in an incubator to keep him or her warm. You will be allowed to take your baby out of the incubator for feeding, but otherwise he or she will continue phototherapy until blood tests show that bilirubin levels are normal. In most cases, treatment is needed for a couple of days.

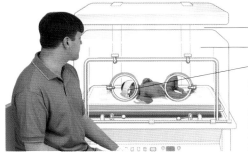

Blue fluorescent light

Incubator

Eye shield

During the procedure
The baby is undressed and sleeps in the incubator under the fluorescent lights. An eye shield is used to protect the baby's eyes.

because they have yet to establish a routine. Regular episodes of crying are called colic (below). Babies also cry more when they are teething (right). However, if the crying is persistent or sounds different from normal, you should consult your doctor because it may indicate that your baby has an underlying infection or disorder.

If your baby is crying but is otherwise well and has been feeding, make sure that you have excluded causes such as wind or a dirty nappy. Holding a crying baby will often soothe him or her, and offering a dummy may help. Many parents find it stressful if their baby cries for hours on end and may feel unable to cope. If you are afraid that you may harm your baby in an attempt to keep him or her quiet, you should put the baby in his or her cot and call someone for support. These feelings are a normal reaction and do not mean that you are a bad parent. Most babies grow out of excessive crying by the age of 6 months.

Colic

Regular episodes of inconsolable crying, usually at the same time every day

 Most common between the ages of 3 weeks and 3 months

 Gender, genetics, and lifestyle are not significant factors

From the age of about 3 weeks, many babies start to cry vigorously at approximately the same time each day, usually in the evening. This crying may sound different from crying at other times, and the baby may also draw up his or her legs. During these episodes, the baby may not respond to any form of comfort, such as feeding or holding, for more than a few minutes. The baby may continue crying for up to 3 hours. Episodes of crying that do not have this regular pattern are not called colic (*see* **Excessive crying**, p.531).

Although the baby may appear to be in pain, colic is not due to an illness, and the crying does not cause permanent harm. However, parents may find the condition distressing. The cause of colic is unknown, but the crying may be made worse by tiredness or an unsettled environment.

What might be done?

You should try to arrange your day so that you can comfort your baby when he or she is crying. If you have difficulty coping and require advice and support, consult your doctor or health visitor. You should consult your doctor if your baby develops additional symptoms, such as fever, which may indicate an underlying infection. The doctor will examine your baby in order to exclude other causes of the crying. Occasionally, the doctor may suggest that you try giving your baby an over-the-counter remedy to relieve the colic. However, this type of treatment is only helpful in some cases. Colic disappears suddenly, on its own, usually when a baby reaches about 3 months of age.

Teething

Discomfort during early childhood caused by the eruption of the primary teeth

 Most common between the ages of 6 months and 3 years

 Gender, genetics, and lifestyle are not significant factors

An infant's first tooth usually appears at about the age of 6 months. Although the primary teeth have usually all erupted by about the age of 3 years, teething is an almost continuous process until the mid-teens, when the primary teeth are completely replaced by secondary teeth.

The eruption of a tooth can be uncomfortable and will probably make your baby irritable and restless. He or she may also be less willing to feed and may sleep poorly at night. Other symptoms include flushed cheeks, dribbling, and red, swollen gums around the site of the new tooth. You may also be able to feel the emerging tooth if you stroke the gum with your finger. Symptoms such as high fever, vomiting, or diarrhoea are not due to teething and you should take your baby to see the doctor if these symptoms appear.

What can I do?

Babies who are teething often like chewing on a cold, hard object such as a teething ring. Over-the-counter local anaesthetic teething gels can be soothing if applied to the affected gums. Babies over 3 months can be given liquid paracetamol to relieve pain (*see* **Painkillers**, p.589).

You should avoid using sweet drinks to comfort your baby. Begin to clean his or her teeth with a soft baby toothbrush and fluoride toothpaste as soon as the first tooth appears. Regular brushing will help to prevent decay and establish a routine of good oral hygiene (*see* **Caring for your teeth and gums**, p.384).

Sudden infant death syndrome

The sudden and unexpected death of a baby for which no cause can be found

 Most common between the ages of 1 and 6 months

 Slightly more common in boys

 Parental smoking and drug abuse are risk factors

 Genetics is not a significant factor

Sudden infant death syndrome (SIDS), also known as cot death, is devastating for parents of an affected baby. SIDS occurs when healthy babies are put to bed and later found dead for no identifiable reason.

▶ **SELF-HELP**

Positioning your baby for sleep

It is important to position your baby for sleep in a way that minimizes the risk of SIDS. You should make sure that your baby sleeps on his or her back near the foot of the cot so that he or she cannot wriggle under the bedcovers. The cot should have a firm mattress but no pillow and no cot bumper. The number of bedcovers should be appropriate for the room temperature.

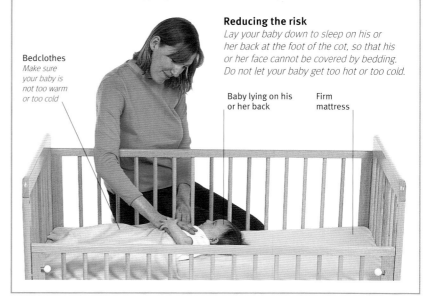

Bedclothes
Make sure your baby is not too warm or too cold

Reducing the risk
Lay your baby down to sleep on his or her back at the foot of the cot, so that his or her face cannot be covered by bedding. Do not let your baby get too hot or too cold.

Baby lying on his or her back

Firm mattress

What are the causes?

The cause of SIDS is unknown. However, several risk factors have been recognized, such as parental smoking and drug abuse. Evidence suggests that putting babies to sleep on their fronts and bottle-feeding increase the risk. Babies who are overwrapped, particularly during an illness, can become overheated and may be at increased risk. Parents sometimes report minor symptoms of infection in the hours or days beforehand, but whether these symptoms are significant is not known. The risk of SIDS is slightly higher for siblings of an infant who has died of SIDS and is slightly more common in babies born before 37 weeks (*see* **Problems of the premature baby**, p.530).

What might be done?

If possible, parents should begin resuscitation immediately after calling for an ambulance. On arrival at hospital, the doctors will attempt to resuscitate the baby, but they are rarely successful. Very occasionally, an infant will be revived, and tests will then be done to try to discover the cause. The baby will receive follow-up care and monitoring to prevent a recurrence.

The sudden death of a baby is an extremely distressing and shocking event. Bereaved parents will need support from doctors, family, and friends, and they may be offered professional counselling (*see* **Loss and bereavement**, p.32). A postmortem examination of the baby is always carried out to exclude any other causes of death and to reassure

the family that the death could not have been prevented. During this period, everyone concerned may experience intense emotions, including guilt, and relationships can be disrupted. These feelings are quite normal. Many bereaved parents find it helpful to contact a support group. If the parents decide to have another child, the doctor will provide advice and support and can arrange for special monitoring.

Can it be prevented?

Many parents feel that SIDS is a threat over which they have no control, but there are ways to reduce the risk. All babies should be placed on their backs to sleep, and pillows should not be used until a baby is over 1 year old (*see* **Positioning your baby for sleep**, above). You should prevent your baby from becoming too cold or overheated. Make sure the baby's room is at the right temperature (about 16–18°C/61–64°F); do not swaddle or overdress your baby; keep your baby's head uncovered; and avoid using duvets, quilts, and cot bumpers. You should not sleep with your baby on an armchair or sofa, and neither should you share a bed with your baby, especially if you are very tired or have been drinking or using drugs. Other measures include not exposing your baby to cigarette smoke, and putting your baby's cot in your bedroom for the first 6 months. Breast-feeding your baby also reduces the risk of SIDS. Alarms that alert parents if their baby stops breathing are available but there is no firm evidence that these devices reduce the risk of SIDS.

Chromosome and gene disorders

The 46 chromosomes (22 pairs plus two sex chromosomes) in human body cells contain about 20,000 to 25,000 pairs of genes, and several thousand disorders are directly the result of a defect in a gene or a chromosomal abnormality. Such genetic defects or chromosomal abnormalities vary enormously in their effects, from unnoticeably minor to severe physical and/or mental problems.

This section covers a few examples of chromosome and gene disorders that affect many body systems and become apparent during childhood. Some of these conditions are caused by an extra or absent chromosome or an abnormality in a chromosome. For example, Down's syndrome is due to an extra chromosome, and Turner's syndrome is due to an absent chromosome. Other conditions in this section are caused by defective genes. These include cystic fibrosis, muscular dystrophy, and neurofibromatosis.

Genetic disorders that mainly affect one part of the body are covered in the relevant sections of the book. The principles of chromosome and gene disorders, including how and why they occur and patterns of inheritance, are discussed elsewhere (*see* **Genetic disorders**, pp.150–151).

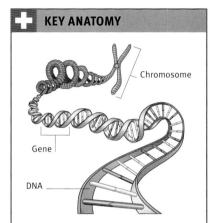

✚ KEY ANATOMY

Chromosome

Gene

DNA

For information on the structure and function of chromosomes and genes, *see* pp.144–149.

Down's syndrome

A chromosome disorder affecting mental development and physical appearance

 Present at birth

 Most commonly due to an extra chromosome

 Gender and lifestyle are not significant factors

Down's syndrome, also called trisomy 21, is the most common chromosomal abnormality. Approximately 1 in 600 babies born each year in the UK is affected. The condition usually occurs because a baby has three copies of chromosome 21 instead of the normal two copies, giving a total of 47 chromosomes instead of the usual 46. In most cases, the extra chromosome is inherited from the mother due to an abnormality in the egg; less commonly, it is inherited from the father due to a sperm abnormality. Rarely, Down's syndrome is due to a chromosomal abnormality called a translocation, in which an extra piece of chromosome 21 attaches itself to another chromosome. In this situation, there are the normal number of chromosomes (46) in each cell but one of the chromosomes has extra genetic material. Although every person with Down's syndrome is affected in a slightly different way, they typically share certain physical characteristics and also have generalized learning disabilities (p.553).

The risk of a baby having Down's syndrome becomes greater with increasing age of the mother. In women who conceive at the age of 20, there is a risk of 1 in 1,500 that the baby will have the condition. For women aged 40, the risk of Down's syndrome rises to 1 in 100. A woman who has already had an affected child has a slightly increased risk of having other children with the condition.

What are the symptoms?

Many of the physical characteristics of Down's syndrome are present at birth and may include:

- Floppy limbs.
- Round face with full cheeks.
- Eyes that slant up at the outer corners with folds of skin covering the inner corners of the eyes.
- Protruding tongue.
- Flattening of the back of the head.
- Excess skin on the back of the neck.
- Short, broad hands that have a single transverse crease on the palm.

Children with Down's syndrome have abnormalities that vary in severity. They are slow in learning to walk and talk, have learning disabilities ranging from mild to severe, and are typically short in stature. However, these children are usually cheerful and affectionate.

Are there complications?

More than 1 in 3 children with Down's syndrome have an abnormality of the heart (*see* **Congenital heart disease**, p.542), usually a hole in the wall (septum) that divides the main chambers of the left and right sides of the heart. Sometimes, abnormalities can occur in the digestive tract, causing the tract to become narrowed or blocked. Affected children are also more likely to have ear infections and an accumulation of fluid in the ear, which may lead to impaired hearing (*see* **Chronic secretory otitis media**, p.557). Eye problems, such as cataracts (p.357) are also common. The neck joints may become unstable, which can prevent children with Down's syndrome from taking part in sports. Affected children also have an increased risk of developing cancer of the white blood cells (*see* **Acute leukaemia**, p.276) and a higher than average risk of having an underactive thyroid gland (*see* **Hypothyroidism**, p.432). In later life, people with Down's syndrome are at increased risk of developing Alzheimer's disease (p.331), a progressive disorder of the brain that results in a gradual decline in mental abilities.

How is it diagnosed?

An increased risk of Down's syndrome can be determined by tests early in pregnancy (*see* **Antenatal genetic tests**, p.509). These tests include blood tests and ultrasound scanning. Ultrasound can detect thickening at the back of the neck of the fetus (called nuchal translucency), which indicates an increased risk of Down's syndrome. A definitive diagnosis can only be made by examining the chromosomes from fetal cells obtained at amniocentesis or CVS.

Sometimes, Down's syndrome may not be diagnosed until after the baby is born. The condition is usually recognized by the distinctive appearance of the face. The diagnosis is confirmed by taking a sample of the baby's blood and performing a blood test to look for an extra copy of chromosome 21. Further tests, such as ultrasound scanning of the heart (*see* **Echocardiography**, p.255) or a contrast X-ray (p.132) of the intestines, called a barium enema, may then be carried out to look for complications.

What is the treatment?

In the past, many children with Down's syndrome were given institutional care and lacked the necessary stimulation and support to maximize their mental development. Today, improved facilities mean that it is possible to make the most of their mental capabilities and to treat any physical problems as they arise. In the majority of cases, children are able to remain in their home environment.

Children who have Down's syndrome and their families usually receive medical care and long-term support from a team of professionals. Specialized care may include physiotherapy (p.620) and speech therapy (p.621). Special educational programmes may be adopted to help affected children to develop intellectually as much as possible. In some cases, surgery is necessary to correct abnormalities of the heart or intestine. Parents of affected children may find it helpful to contact a support group.

What is the prognosis?

Most children with Down's syndrome lead happy and fulfilling lives. Although intellectual ability varies widely, affected children are now able to achieve much more because of the improvement in teaching methods and availability of special educational programmes. Some children learn to read and write, and some young adults are able to pursue further education. As adults, some also gain employment. However, most people with Down's syndrome are unable to live completely independently and need long-term supervision, provided either by their parents or in a special residential home.

Although many people who have Down's syndrome now survive into late middle age or beyond, the syndrome carries an increased risk of dying in childhood, often as a result of congenital heart disease. In addition, the average life expectancy of a person with Down's syndrome is about 50–60 years, but there is a significant chance of developing Alzheimer's disease in later life: about a third of people with Down's syndrome develop Alzheimer's in their 50s, and it affects more than half of those who live to 60 or older.

Fragile X syndrome

A defect in a specific gene on the X chromosome, causing learning difficulties

 Present at birth

 Much more common in boys

 Due to an abnormal gene on the X chromosome

 Lifestyle is not a significant factor

Fragile X syndrome is caused by an abnormality of a specific gene on the X chromosome, one of the two sex chromosomes. This abnormality results in learning difficulties, and the condition is associated with a characteristic physical appearance. In the UK, about 1 in 4,000 boys is affected; the condition is far less common in girls since many women who carry the gene for the condition remain unaffected.

Girls with fragile X syndrome tend to have milder symptoms than affected boys because they have a second copy of the X chromosome that is normal and compensates for the abnormal gene on the other chromosome. However, any woman who carries this gene can pass it on to her sons, who would develop more severe symptoms of the disorder.

What are the symptoms?

The initial symptoms are learning disabilities, which vary from mild to severe and become more obvious as the child grows older (*see* **Generalized learning disabilities**, p.553). Affected children tend to be taller than normal. Other characteristic physical features of fragile X syndrome often do not appear until puberty and include:

- Large head and a long, thin face with a prominent jaw and large ears.
- In boys, large testes.

Affected children are also susceptible to seizures and behaviour problems (see **Autism spectrum disorders**, p.552).

What might be done?

If your child's doctor suspects fragile X syndrome, he or she will arrange for a blood test to look for the gene abnormality on the X chromosome. Although the condition cannot be treated, affected children may benefit from speech therapy (p.621), specialized teaching, and help from a psychologist for behaviour problems. Some affected children need to take anticonvulsant drugs (p.590) to prevent seizures. Parents of an affected child may wish to join a support group.

Genetic counselling (p.151) is offered to couples who already have a child with fragile X syndrome to assess the risk of having another child with this condition. Antenatal testing can be performed in subsequent pregnancies (see **Antenatal genetic tests**, p.509).

The life expectancy for affected children is normal, but boys usually require lifelong care, either from their parents or in a residential home.

Klinefelter's syndrome

A chromosomal abnormality in boys, causing tall stature and small genitals

 Present at birth

 Affects only boys

 Due to an extra chromosome

 Lifestyle is not a significant factor

Klinefelter's syndrome affects only boys. In the UK, about 1 in every 600 boys has the condition, but it is thought that many cases are never detected. Affected boys have two copies of the X chromosome instead of the usual one. This may lead to insufficient levels of the male sex hormone testosterone and cause infertility and characteristic physical features.

What are the symptoms?

A boy with Klinefelter's syndrome often appears normal at birth. However, as he reaches puberty, the physical characteristics of the condition become more obvious and include:

- Tall stature.
- Long legs.
- Small penis and testes.

In some cases, breast enlargement also develops (see **Gynaecomastia**, p.466). Almost all men with Klinefelter's syndrome are infertile because they are unable to pro-

duce sperm. A small number of those who have the condition have generalized learning disabilities (p.553).

What might be done?

Klinefelter's syndrome is often suspected from an affected boy's physical characteristics. The diagnosis is confirmed by a blood test to look for the extra X chromosome. If the condition is diagnosed in childhood, treatment with a testosterone supplement may encourage the development of male characteristics and prevent gynaecomastia. However, if gynaecomastia does occur and causes psychological distress, an operation may be done to reduce breast size. Most boys with Klinefelter's syndrome lead a normal life, although they will not be able to father children. Genetic counselling (p.151) is offered to parents of an affected child who plan to have more children.

Turner's syndrome

A chromosome disorder in which a girl has only one X chromosome

 Present at birth

 Affects only girls

 Due to an absent chromosome

 Lifestyle is not a significant factor

Normally, girls have two copies of the X sex chromosome. In Turner's syndrome, only one X chromosome is present, giving a total of 45 chromosomes instead of the normal complement of 46. Girls without a second X chromosome have ovaries that do not function normally. As a result, certain hormones that are needed for normal growth and sexual development, such as oestrogen and progesterone, are not produced, leading to infertility. Turner's syndrome affects about 1 in 2,500 girls in the UK.

What are the symptoms?

Some symptoms of Turner's syndrome may be present at birth and include:

- Puffy hands and feet.
- Broad chest.
- Short, broad neck.
- Low-set ears.

However, in some girls, there may be no symptoms except short stature. In some cases, Turner's syndrome is recognized only when a girl fails to reach puberty at the normal age (see **Abnormal puberty in females**, p.474). If the condition is recognized and treated before adolescence, a girl is more likely to attain a greater height and will develop normal female sexual characteristics, such as breasts, and have menstrual periods.

Are there complications?

About 3 in 10 girls with Turner's syndrome also has an abnormal narrowing of the

aorta, the main artery of the body (see **Congenital heart disease**, p.542). About 1 in 3 girls with Turner's syndrome has a mild kidney abnormality. Hearing impairment is common and is usually sensorineural (see **Hearing loss**, p.376). Vision problems, including squints, are also common (see **Strabismus**, p.555). In later life, other possible complications include infertility (see **Female infertility**, p.497) and osteoporosis (p.217), in which the bones progressively become thin and brittle.

Girls with Turner's syndrome are of normal intelligence, but some may have minor learning disabilities, especially with respect to mathematics and activities requiring hand–eye coordination. Psychological problems may also arise when a girl becomes aware of her sexual immaturity and short stature.

How is it diagnosed?

Turner's syndrome may be diagnosed in the fetus during routine ultrasound scanning in pregnancy (p.512). Antenatal genetic tests (p.509) can confirm the diagnosis. Most fetuses with severe Turner's syndrome die before birth. If the fetus survives and the condition is suspected in infancy or childhood due to short stature, a blood test will be carried out to analyse the chromosomes. Mild Turner's syndrome may not be suspected until adolescence, when puberty and menstruation do not occur.

What might be done?

There is no cure for Turner's syndrome, and treatment for the disorder is aimed at relieving some of the symptoms. Growth hormone and oestrogen may be given to encourage growth, allow normal puberty, and prevent the early onset of osteoporosis. Growth hormone is usually given only until the child reaches the usual age of puberty. Oestrogen is then given from this age and is continued for life.

Other treatments focus on associated complications. The ears will be checked regularly for fluid build-up. Narrowing of the aorta can be corrected surgically if necessary. Women who have Turner's syndrome are extremely unlikely to conceive naturally.

Genetic counselling (p.151) is usually offered to the parents of a daughter with Turner's syndrome, although the risk of having another affected child is low. Affected individuals and their parents may find it useful to contact a support group.

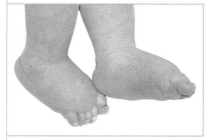

Turner's syndrome
Newborn baby girls with the chromosome disorder Turner's syndrome are sometimes born with temporary puffiness of the feet.

What is the prognosis?

Although affected girls do not grow to the average height for their age, most should be able to have a normal childhood and eventually to become healthy and independent women. Even serious complications that are associated with Turner's syndrome, such as a narrowed aorta, can now be treated successfully.

Marfan's syndrome

An inherited condition in which a protein is deficient, resulting in tall stature and defects of the eyes, heart, and arteries

 Present at birth

 Due to an abnormal gene often inherited from one parent

 Gender and lifestyle are not significant factors

In Marfan's syndrome, a protein that is a component of the connective tissue between the structures and organs of the body is deficient. The condition most often affects the bones, eyes, heart, and main arteries of the body. Marfan's syndrome is due to an abnormal gene that is inherited in an autosomal dominant manner (see **Gene disorders**, p.151). However, not everyone with this condition is affected to the same extent. In the UK, about 1 in 5,000 people has Marfan's syndrome.

What are the symptoms?

The symptoms of Marfan's syndrome usually appear at about the age of 10 but may be seen earlier. They may include:

- Very tall stature.
- Long, thin limbs, fingers, and toes.
- Weak joints and ligaments.
- Inward curving of the chest.
- Curvature of the spine.
- Impaired vision.

The risk of complications depends on which tissues are affected and the severity of abnormalities. Most people with Marfan's syndrome are shortsighted (see **Myopia**, p.365), and some have other eye defects, such as an incorrectly placed lens. Marfan's syndrome can lead to heart valve disorders (p.253). The aorta, the main artery of the body, may also become weakened and may swell and rupture (see **Aortic aneurysm**, p.259), a condition that is life-threatening.

What might be done?

Marfan's syndrome is usually diagnosed when the visible features of the condition begin to appear. There is no cure, but an affected child is monitored carefully, and complications are treated as they arise. Many affected children need glasses and should have an eye test once a year. Some people with the condition are given beta-blockers (p.581) to help to prevent weakening of the aorta. In rare cases, affected girls under the age of 10 are given hormone treatment to promote the early

▶ TEST

Sweat testing

A sweat test is used to diagnose cystic fibrosis by measuring the levels of salt in sweat. The procedure is painless and is performed in hospital on an outpatient basis. The production of sweat is stimulated for about 3 minutes using two electrodes. The electrodes are then replaced with a pad, which collects the sweat for the next 30 minutes.

Technician

Electrical source

Electrodes

During the test
A small electrical current passes to gel-filled electrodes on the arm to stimulate sweat production.

---

onset of puberty and to reduce their growth, preventing excessive height in adulthood. Defects in the heart valves or aorta can be corrected by surgery. Affected individuals may wish to join a support group for advice.

What is the prognosis?

In the past, people with the condition were restricted in their activities and often died before the age of 50. Today, many affected people can lead active lives, although some may be advised to avoid certain sports, such as contact sports, and overall life expectancy may be shortened.

Cystic fibrosis

An inherited condition that causes body secretions to be thick and abnormal

 Present at birth

 Due to an abnormal gene inherited from both parents

 Gender and lifestyle are not significant factors

Cystic fibrosis is the most common severe inherited disease among white people of European and North American origin. In the UK, about 1 in 2,500 babies is born with the disorder. Cystic fibrosis is much less common in people of African or Asian descent. The disorder affects all the fluid-and mucus-secreting glands in the body, leading to production of abnormally thick secretions, especially in the lungs and pancreas. As a result, children with cystic fibrosis experience recurrent chest infections and may have difficulty absorbing nutrients from food.

In the past, severe chest infections were a major cause of death in children with cystic fibrosis. Today, with better understanding of the disease and recent advances in treatment, most affected children survive into adulthood.

What are the causes?

Cystic fibrosis is caused by an abnormal gene, which is carried by about 1 in 25 people and inherited in an autosomal recessive manner (*see* **Gene disorders**, p.151). The abnormal gene occurs on chromosome number 7. Over 1,500 different mutations (abnormalities) in the gene have now been identified. Of these, the most common is called delta F508, and this is the cause of more than 7 in 10 cases of cystic fibrosis.

What are the symptoms?

A newborn baby with cystic fibrosis may have a swollen abdomen and may not pass meconium (thick, sticky faeces passed by newborn infants) for the first few days following birth. Other symptoms of cystic fibrosis usually develop later in infancy and may include:

- Failure to put on weight or grow at the normal rate.
- Pale, greasy faeces that float and have a particularly offensive smell.
- Recurrent chest infections.

In many cases of cystic fibrosis, a constant cough develops, producing large amounts of sticky mucus.

Are there complications?

As cystic fibrosis progresses, the lung disorder bronchiectasis (p.303) may occur, in which the main airways are abnormally widened. Abscesses may also form in the lungs. Further complications may include liver damage (*see* **Cirrhosis**, p.410) and persistent inflammation of the sinuses (*see* **Sinusitis**, p.290). About 1 in 20 children who have cystic fibrosis develop diabetes mellitus (p.437). In all affected children, abnormally high levels of salt are excreted in the sweat, which may lead to dehydration in hot weather.

Children with cystic fibrosis sometimes develop psychological problems as a result of the many difficulties that are associated with lifelong illness. Affected children may

---

be unable to participate in normal childhood and school activities due to continual bad health and may therefore feel isolated.

In later life, almost all males with cystic fibrosis are infertile as a result of a birth defect in which the two vasa deferentia (the tubes through which sperm are propelled) are absent. About 1 in 5 affected females are infertile because the mucus secretions produced by the reproductive organs are abnormally thick.

How is it diagnosed?

All newborn babies are routinely screened for cystic fibrosis as part of the blood spot screening tests (p.561). An early diagnosis improves the long-term outlook by helping to prevent damage to the lungs in infancy. If the doctor suspects that a child has the condition later in infancy, a sweat test (left) may be carried out to look for abnormally high levels of salt in the baby's sweat. A sample of blood may also be tested to look for the abnormal gene. If the test result is found to be positive, siblings of the affected child can also be tested.

What is the treatment?

Treatment for cystic fibrosis is aimed at slowing the progression of lung disease and maintaining adequate nutrition.

Chest physiotherapy (p.620) is usually performed twice a day to remove secretions from the lungs. Parents and older affected children are often taught how to carry out this procedure at home. If an affected child develops a chest infection, he or she will require immediate treatment with antibiotics (p.572). In addition, long-term use of antibiotics may be necessary to prevent other chest infections from

---

developing. Older children sometimes require regular courses of intravenous antibiotics to eliminate bacteria that become established in the lung secretions. In this case, a permanent catheter may be inserted under general anaesthesia just below the chest wall so that antibiotics can be administered more easily (*see* **Antibiotic delivery system**, below). Some children with cystic fibrosis can be helped by inhaled drugs that reduce the stickiness of the secretions in the lungs. If the lungs are very severely damaged, it may be possible to carry out a heart–lung transplant.

A high-calorie diet helps to ensure that a child with cystic fibrosis grows normally. Most children also need to take pancreatic enzymes and vitamin supplements with every meal.

An affected child and his or her family will be offered psychological support, particularly during adolescence, when long-term illness is especially difficult to cope with. Family members may also find it helpful to join a support group.

Can it be prevented?

Genetic testing means that carriers can be identified and the condition can be detected antenatally. This form of testing may be offered to adults with a family history of cystic fibrosis and to partners of people who have the disease. If these test results are positive, the couple will be offered genetic counselling (p.151). A couple who are at risk may opt to use assisted conception (p.498), which enables the embryo to be tested for the abnormal gene before the embryo is implanted. Pregnant women may be offered antenatal genetic tests (p.509).

▶ TREATMENT

Antibiotic delivery system

This system enables the easy and regular delivery of intravenous antibiotics and is particularly useful for children with cystic fibrosis (left). Under general anaesthesia, the internal part of the system is placed on the chest wall just under the skin so that it does not interfere with the child's normal activities. A catheter carries the injected antibiotics from the injection site to a vein in the chest just above the heart. The external part of the system is removable.

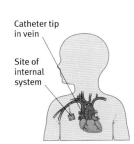

Catheter tip in vein

Site of internal system

POSITION OF SYSTEM

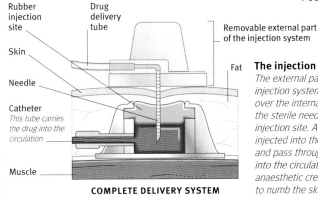

Rubber injection site

Drug delivery tube

Removable external part of the injection system

Skin

Needle

Catheter
This tube carries the drug into the circulation

Fat

Muscle

COMPLETE DELIVERY SYSTEM

The injection procedure
The external part of the injection system is positioned over the internal part so that the sterile needle pierces the injection site. Antibiotics are injected into the delivery tube and pass through the catheter into the circulation. Local anaesthetic cream is often used to numb the skin beforehand.

In the future, cystic fibrosis may be treated with gene therapy, in which a normal gene is introduced into relevant tissues to prevent cystic fibrosis from developing.

What is the prognosis?

The average life expectancy of a person with cystic fibrosis has increased over the past 35 years. Due to advances in the specialized treatment of cystic fibrosis, most people with the disorder now survive into their third decade.

Muscular dystrophy

A group of genetic conditions in which muscles become weak and wasted

 Present at birth

 The most common types almost always affect only boys

 Due to an abnormal gene

 Lifestyle is not a significant factor

The two main types of muscular dystrophy almost exclusively affect boys. The most common type is Duchenne muscular dystrophy, which affects about 1 in 3,500 boys in the UK and causes serious disability from early childhood. A second, rarer type is Becker muscular dystrophy, which affects about 1 in 10,000 boys. The onset of Becker muscular dystrophy is slower, and the symptoms tend to start later in childhood. Other rare forms of muscular dystrophy can affect both girls and boys.

What are the causes?

Both Duchenne and Becker muscular dystrophies are caused by an abnormal gene carried on the X chromosome (*see* **Gene disorders**, p.151). Girls may carry the defective gene, but they do not usually have the disorder because they have two X chromosomes, and the normal X chromosome usually compensates for the defect in the gene on the other. However, in a small number of female carriers the heart may be affected and so female carriers may be advised to have their heart checked.

Normally, this gene is responsible for the production of a protein called dystrophin, which is necessary for healthy muscles. In Duchenne and Becker muscular dystrophies, the gene is abnormal, resulting in a deficiency of the protein and damage to muscle. In Duchenne muscular dystrophy, almost no dystrophin is produced. However, in Becker muscular dystrophy some dystrophin is present, accounting for the difference in severity between the two conditions.

What are the symptoms?

The symptoms of Duchenne muscular dystrophy usually appear around the time a child would begin to walk. Late walking is common; often an affected child does not begin to walk until about 18 months and then will fall more frequently than other children. The more obvious symptoms of the disorder may not appear until the child is between 3 and 5 years old and may include:

- Waddling gait.
- Difficulty climbing stairs.
- Difficulty getting up from the floor. Characteristically, a child will use his hands to "walk up" the thighs.
- Large calf muscles and wasted muscles at the tops of the legs and arms.
- Mild learning disabilities.

The symptoms are progressive, and a child may be unable to walk by the age of 12. The symptoms of Becker muscular dystrophy are similar but usually do not appear until later in childhood or adolescence. This condition progresses more slowly; some of those affected are still able to walk until their 30s or later.

Are there complications?

In Duchenne muscular dystrophy, the heart muscle may become thickened and weakened. The limbs may also become deformed, and abnormal curvature of the spine may develop (*see* **Scoliosis**, p.219). In the later stages, a child may have difficulty breathing, and there is an increased risk of chest infections that can be life-threatening.

How is it diagnosed?

If a pregnant woman is known to be a carrier, she may be offered antenatal testing to determine whether the fetus is affected (*see* **Antenatal genetic tests**, p.509).

In most cases, muscular dystrophy is suspected only when symptoms appear. A blood test to look for the abnormal gene may be used to confirm the diagnosis. If the result is positive, a further blood test may be performed to look for evidence of muscle damage. Electromyography (*see* **Nerve and muscle electrical tests**, p. 337), which records electrical activity in muscles, may be performed. A muscle biopsy may be carried out, in which a small piece of muscle is removed for examination. Tests will also be done to find out if the heart is affected, including a recording of the heart's electrical activity (*see* **ECG**, p.243) and ultrasound scanning (*see* **Echocardiography**, p.255).

What is the treatment?

The treatment for muscular dystrophy is directed at keeping an affected child mobile and active for as long as possible. A team of professionals, including a physiotherapist, a doctor, and a social worker, can provide support for the whole family. Physiotherapy (p.620) is important to keep the limbs supple, and supportive splints may be used. Some children require mobility aids. If a child develops scoliosis, surgery may be necessary to straighten the spine.

Children with muscular dystrophy and their families usually need a great deal of psychological support. Genetic counselling (p.151) is offered to parents of an affected child who wish to have another baby and to sisters of boys affected by the disorder.

Duchenne muscular dystrophy may be fatal before the age of 20. Becker muscular dystrophy has a better outlook; people usually live into their 40s or later.

Congenital immunodeficiency

Defects of the immune system present from birth, leading to recurrent infection and failure of normal growth

 Present at birth

 Due to an abnormal gene

 Gender as a risk factor depends on the type

 Lifestyle is not a significant factor

In immunodeficiency, the immune system is defective and therefore unable to combat infections effectively. As a result, infections are more frequent and severe and may be life-threatening. A child's growth may also be affected. In children, immunodeficiency is usually caused by an underlying illness (*see* **Acquired immunodeficiency**, p.280). In rare cases, the condition is inherited and is present at birth, in which case it is called congenital immunodeficiency.

What are the types?

Congenital immunodeficiencies are due to an abnormal gene. This gene is either linked to the X chromosome or inherited in an autosomal recessive manner (*see* **Gene disorders**, p.151). The type of immunodeficiency depends on which part of the immune system is affected.

The most common type of immunodeficiency is agammaglobulinaemia, a disorder that affects only boys. In this condition, severe bacterial infections, especially of the chest, frequently occur because antibody production is greatly reduced. Other, less serious, types of immunodeficiency may be caused by failure of the immune system to produce some specific types of antibody.

Chronic granulomatous disease is another type of congenital immunodeficiency. In this disease, the phagocytes, the white blood cells that are responsible for engulfing and killing bacteria and fungi, are unable to function properly. As a consequence, a child who has this disorder may have frequent bacterial and fungal infections, especially of the skin, lungs, and bones.

Severe combined immunodeficiency (SCID) is a disorder in which a child is unable to fight most forms of infection because both the antibodies and the white blood cells are deficient.

What might be done?

It is possible to screen for congenital immunodeficiency during pregnancy if the fetus is thought to be at risk (*see* **Antenatal genetic tests**, p.509). More often, congenital immunodeficiency is suspected when a child has persistent unusual infections or fails to grow normally. The doctor may then arrange for blood tests to measure the levels of antibodies and white blood cells and assess the function of the child's immune system. Sometimes, it is possible to detect the abnormal gene by a blood test.

All infections in a child who has a congenital immunodeficiency should be treated as soon as possible. Antibiotics (p.572) will be given if appropriate. If antibodies are deficient, they can be replaced intravenously every few weeks. In some severe types of congenital immunodeficiency, such as SCID, a stem cell transplant (p.276) may be necessary, and this will be done if a suitable donor can be found. If the transplant is successful, the transplanted stem cells will start to produce normal white blood cells that can fight infection.

If treatment for congenital immunodeficiencies is started sufficiently early, many children affected with these disorders can lead a normal life and have an average life expectancy.

In the future, treatment of congenital immunodeficiency may include gene therapy. The aim of this new treatment is to correct the genetic defects that affect the function of the immune system.

Genetic tests may be offered to relatives of affected people. Genetic counselling (p.151) is offered to couples who are found to have the abnormal gene or who have an affected child and plan to have more children.

Neurofibromatosis

The development of noncancerous tumours along nerve fibres

 Present at birth

 Due to an abnormal gene often inherited from one parent

 Gender and lifestyle are not significant factors

Neurofibromatosis is the collective term for a group of genetic disorders that cause soft, noncancerous growths, known as neurofibromas, to grow along nerves.

There are two main types of neurofibromatosis. The more common of the two, known as neurofibromatosis 1, affects about 1 in every 2,500 babies born in the UK. The other type, neurofibromatosis 2, is extremely rare, and the symptoms do not usually appear until adulthood. Both types are caused by an abnormal gene that is inherited in an autosomal dominant manner (*see* **Gene disorders**, p.151). The abnormal gene for neurofibromatosis 1 is located on chromosome 17, and the gene for neurofibromatosis 2 is located on chromosome 22.

What are the symptoms?

The symptoms of neurofibromatosis 1 usually appear during early childhood.

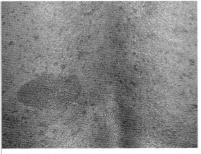

Café au lait spot in neurofibromatosis
This pale-brown, flat patch on the skin is known as a café au lait spot. The development of patches such as this is typical of neurofibromatosis 1.

The symptoms may include:
- Numerous pale-brown, flat patches with irregular edges, known as café au lait spots, that develop on the skin.
- Soft growths underneath the skin (neurofibromas), which can range in size from hardly noticeable to large and disfiguring.
- Freckles in the armpit and groin areas.

People with neurofibromatosis 2 tend to develop tumours in the inner ear, which can affect hearing and balance. They may also develop mild cataracts (which often do not significantly impair vision), and small, raised, coloured patches on the skin.

Are there complications?
Complications may occur when growing tumours press on the surrounding organs or nerves. For example, vision may be affected if a tumour develops on the optic nerve, which connects the eye to the brain. Tumours can also cause curvature of the spine (*see* **Scoliosis**, p.219). Other possible complications include high blood pressure (*see* **Hypertension**, p.242), epilepsy (p.324), and learning difficulties. In rare cases, the tumours become cancerous.

What might be done?
Neurofibromatosis 1 is normally diagnosed in childhood when the symptoms appear. Neurofibromatosis 2 is usually diagnosed in adulthood. The doctor will arrange for CT scanning (p.132) or MRI (p.133) of the brain to look for tumours, and hearing and vision may be tested.

There is no cure for either form of neurofibromatosis and neither can their progression be slowed. Many cases are mild, but long-term care may be needed for severely affected children. Tumours that are large, painful, or disfiguring can sometimes be surgically removed. Complications are usually treated as they arise. For example, a child with learning problems may need special education. Parents of an affected child who want to have more children may be offered genetic counselling (p.151).

In mild cases of neurofibromatosis, life expectancy is normal, but, if tumours are extensive and cancer develops as a complication, lifespan may be reduced.

Skin and hair disorders

Young skin is sensitive and particularly susceptible to irritation or allergies. Most skin disorders in children are minor, affect only a small area of skin, and disappear as the child grows older. Many skin and hair disorders that affect children can be treated successfully at home with over-the-counter preparations.

Skin and hair disorders that mainly or exclusively affect children include a number of rashes and viral infections. The section begins with disorders that may affect young babies: birthmarks, which are present at birth or develop soon afterwards, and two skin rashes, cradle cap and nappy rash. The next article discusses eczema, which is sometimes caused by an allergy and may persist for many years. Viral infections that cause a rash and affect only young children are also covered. The section concludes with an article on infestation with head lice. Children are especially vulnerable to this problem due to close contact with other children at school.

Skin and hair disorders that affect people of any age are covered either in the main section on skin, hair, and nails (pp.189–210) or, if the disorders are caused by viruses, in the section on viral infections (pp.164–170).

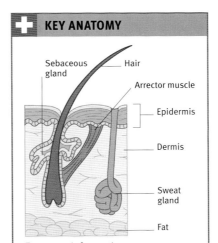

KEY ANATOMY
Sebaceous gland
Hair
Arrector muscle
Epidermis
Dermis
Sweat gland
Fat

For more information on the structure and function of the skin and hair, *see* pp.189–191.

Birthmarks

Coloured patches of skin that are present at birth or appear soon afterwards

 Present at or shortly after birth

 Genetics as a risk factor depends on the type

 Gender and lifestyle are not significant factors

Many babies have patches of coloured skin, known as birthmarks, that may be present at birth or appear during the first weeks of life. Although they can be unsightly and distressing to the parents, most birthmarks are not harmful, and they rarely cause discomfort.

What are the types?
There are two types of birthmark: haemangiomas, which form from the small blood vessels just under the surface of the skin; and pigmented naevi, which form from densely pigmented skin cells.

Haemangiomas This group of birthmarks includes stork marks, strawberry naevi, and port-wine stains.

Stork marks are very common birthmarks and can occur in up to half of babies at birth. A stork mark appears as a flat, pale pink patch, usually between the eyebrows or on the nape of the neck. This type of birthmark usually disappears by the age of 18 months.

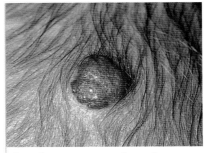

Strawberry naevus on the scalp
This red swelling, known as a strawberry naevus, is a common birthmark that usually disappears by the age of 5.

Strawberry naevi are common birthmarks, occurring in about 1 in every 50 babies. The naevus appears as a small, flat, red spot at birth. The spot enlarges rapidly and becomes raised during the first year of life but usually disappears completely by the time the child reaches about 5 years of age.

Port-wine stains occur in about 1 in 3,000 babies, and they are usually permanent. The birthmark is visible as an irregularly shaped red patch and may be distressing, particularly if the mark is on the baby's face. In rare cases, a port-wine stain on the face is associated with abnormal blood vessels in the brain that can cause epilepsy (p.324).

Pigmented naevi This group of birthmarks includes Mongolian blue spots and moles. Mongolian blue spots are irregular, bluish areas on the skin. They are commonly seen at birth over the backs and buttocks of darker-skinned babies and

may be mistaken for bruises. The spots usually disappear by the time the child is 10 years of age.

A mole is a permanent, raised, dark-brown patch on the skin. The presence of a mole at birth is very unusual. Rarely, such birthmarks may become cancerous in later life.

What might be done?
Most birthmarks fade as the baby grows. However, a strawberry naevus on the eyelid is usually treated soon after birth before it can enlarge and affect vision. Corticosteroids (p.600) may be given to shrink it, or it may be removed with laser treatment (p.613). Permanent birthmarks can also be treated with laser surgery, usually during infancy to minimize scarring. All moles should be checked for changes in size, shape, and colour. If moles cause concern, they can be removed by surgery. Treatment for permanent birthmarks usually provides good cosmetic results.

Cradle cap

A thick, scaly rash that appears on the scalp during the first months of life

Occurs between the ages of 1 month and 1 year

Gender, genetics, and lifestyle are not significant factors

Babies with cradle cap have reddened skin and thick, yellowish scales on the scalp. Scaly areas may also appear on the baby's forehead and eyebrows and behind the ears. The cause of the condition is unknown. Although cradle cap can be unsightly, it is harmless. Rarely, the rash may become inflamed or infected by bacteria (*see* **Impetigo**, p.204) or fungi (*see* **Candidiasis**, p.177).

What might be done?
Cradle cap eventually disappears on its own without any treatment. However, washing your baby's hair and scalp regularly will help to prevent scale build-up. You can also massage baby oil into your baby's scalp at night and then brush out the softened scales in the morning.

You should consult your doctor if these measures are not effective or the rash becomes inflamed or infected. If there is no

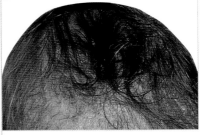

Cradle cap
The reddened skin and thick patches of yellowish scales on top of this baby's head are typical of cradle cap.

inflammation or infection, a lotion may be prescribed to dissolve the scales, but such products can cause skin irritation and should be used with care. An infected rash may be treated with topical antibiotics or antifungal drugs (see **Preparations for skin infections and infestations**, p.577) and an inflamed rash with topical corticosteroids (p.577). The condition should start to improve within a few weeks of treatment but may take longer to disappear.

Nappy rash

A red rash in the area covered by a nappy, caused by irritation or infection

 May affect babies from birth until they stop wearing nappies

 Poor hygiene and infrequent nappy changes increase the risk

 Gender and genetics are not significant factors

Nearly all babies are affected by nappy rash at some time. The rash causes inflammation and soreness in the area of skin covered by a nappy, and the discomfort can make a baby irritable.

What are the causes?
Nappy rash is most commonly caused by urine or faeces irritating the skin. It usually occurs only where the skin and soiled nappy have been in direct contact and does not spread to creases in the baby's skin. The rash is made worse if the baby's nappy is not changed frequently or the nappy area is not cleaned thoroughly. Perfumed skin products and some washing powders used to clean fabric nappies can cause a similar rash.

A fungal infection of the skin such as candidiasis (p.177) or, less commonly, a bacterial infection such as impetigo (p.204) can also cause nappy rash. A rash caused by infection will affect the whole nappy area, including the creases in the baby's skin.

SELF-HELP

Managing nappy rash
Nappy rash can usually be managed successfully using the measures described below, which also help to prevent recurrence.

- Change your baby's nappies often to prevent skin irritation.
- When changing nappies, clean the nappy area gently with water and allow it to dry thoroughly.
- Use a barrier cream, such as zinc and castor oil cream.
- Avoid perfumed skin products.
- Leave your baby without a nappy as much as possible.
- Wash fabric nappies with a nonbiological washing powder and rinse them thoroughly.
- Use absorbent nappy liners with fabric nappies.

Sometimes, a scaly rash similar to cradle cap (p.537) develops in the baby's nappy area (see **Seborrhoeic dermatitis**, p.194).

What might be done?
Your baby's nappy rash will usually clear up within a few days without any medical treatment if you follow simple self-help measures (see **Managing nappy rash**, below left).

You should take your baby to the doctor if these self-help measures do not produce an improvement or if you think the nappy rash may be infected. Your baby's doctor will examine the rash and may prescribe topical corticosteroids (p.577) to reduce the inflammation. Oral or topical antibiotics (p.572) may be prescribed to treat a bacterial infection, and topical antifungal drugs may be given to treat candidiasis (see **Preparations for skin infections and infestations**, p.577).

An infected nappy rash should improve with treatment and clear up completely within a week. Nappy rash may recur if preventive self-help measures are not followed regularly throughout the time your child is wearing nappies.

Eczema in children

Itching and inflammation of the skin, sometimes accompanied by scaling

 Can occur at any age but most commonly develops under 18 months

 Sometimes runs in families

 Exposure to irritants aggravates the condition

 Gender is not a significant factor

Eczema affects up to 1 in 5 children under school age in the UK. The condition may last for many years but usually disappears in late childhood. A child with eczema has dry, red, inflamed, itchy skin that may make him or her irritable.

What are the causes?
The cause of eczema in children is not fully understood, but it is thought to be at least partly due to the skin being abnormally "leaky" and unable to retain moisture. Allergens or irritants in the environment may be trigger factors. Common allergens (substances that provoke an allergic reaction) include cows' milk (see **Cows' milk protein allergy**, p.560), soya, wheat, and eggs (see **Food allergy**, p.284). Affected children are also susceptible to allergic conditions such as hay fever (see **Allergic rhinitis**, p.283) and asthma (see **Asthma in children**, p.544). Close relatives sometimes have similar allergic disorders, suggesting that a genetic factor is involved.

What are the symptoms?
The symptoms of eczema vary in severity and usually affect particular areas of the body. The symptoms may include:
- Red, scaly rash.
- Intense itching.
- Gradual thickening of the skin.

In babies, the rash of eczema tends to occur on the face and neck and then on the knees and elbows as the children begin to crawl. In older children, the rash usually appears on the insides of the elbows and wrists and on the backs of the knees. The intense itching causes children to scratch the rash, which may break the skin and lead to bacterial infection. If an infection does occur, the inflammation becomes more severe, and weeping may occur.

A rare but serious complication of eczema is eczema herpeticum, which occurs if a child with eczema is also infected with a type of herpes simplex virus (see **Herpes simplex infections**, p.166). Eczema herpeticum produces a widespread rash with blisters and fever.

How is it diagnosed?
Your child's doctor will probably diagnose eczema from the inflamed, itchy rash. In some cases, he or she may arrange for a blood test and a skin prick test (p.284) to try to identify a specific food or substance to which your child is allergic. The doctor may also take swabs of the eczema rash to check for signs of bacterial infection.

What is the treatment?
Parents play a major part in treating children with eczema, mostly by preventing the affected skin from becoming dry (see **Managing eczema in children**, above). Your child's doctor will advise you on day-to-day care and how to moisturize your child's skin with unperfumed emollients (see **Emollients and barrier preparations**, p.575). He or she may prescribe a topical corticosteroid (p.577) to reduce inflammation and oral antibiotics (p.572) or antibiotic creams (see **Preparations for skin infections and infestations**, p.577) if the rash is infected. Your child may also be prescribed an oral antihistamine (p.585) to take at night, which helps to reduce itching and also acts as a sedative.

Reddened skin   Scaly rash

Eczema in children
A red, scaly eczema rash is seen here on the inside of a child's elbow. The inflamed skin is often very itchy and uncomfortable.

SELF-HELP

Managing eczema in children
Parents play an important role in managing eczema in their children, and the following measures may help to control symptoms and to keep your child comfortable.

- Avoid perfumed skin products.
- Wash your child with emollient cream instead of soap.
- Bathe your child at least once a day using moisturizing bath oil.
- After washing, moisturize your child's skin with a chilled emollient cream.
- Use prescribed corticosteroid ointments regularly on the affected areas of skin.
- If your child scratches, make sure his or her fingernails are cut short and he or she wears cotton mittens at night.

In very rare cases, a child with severe eczema may be admitted to hospital. Treatment usually consists of applying a corticosteroid cream to the inflamed rash and wrapping the affected areas in bandages soaked in emollient cream.

If your child develops eczema herpeticum, he or she will be admitted to hospital and treated with intravenous antiviral drugs (p.573).

If the cause of eczema is found to be related to something your child eats, elimination of that food from the diet should improve the eczema. However, you should only give your child a special diet under medical supervision. In babies, breast-feeding can help to protect against future food allergies.

Since eczema is a long-term disorder with no reliable cure, you may wish to try alternative treatments. Before trying any such treatments, discuss them with your doctor, who may advise you on reliable sources and caution you against purchasing treatments that may have serious side effects.

What is the prognosis?
Eczema may last throughout childhood. Although there is no reliable cure, the symptoms of the condition can usually be controlled. Eczema usually disappears by adolescence without leaving scars, but in a few cases the rash continues to flare up (see **Atopic eczema**, p.193). Some affected children develop another allergic disorder later in life.

Roseola infantum

A viral infection that causes a high fever followed by a rash of tiny pink spots

 Most common between the ages of 6 months and 2 years

 Gender, genetics, and lifestyle are not significant factors

Roseola infantum is a common illness in early childhood that affects about 3 in 10 children in the UK. The infection is caused by strains of the herpes virus that are spread by close contact with other children. One attack of the infection gives lifelong immunity.

What are the symptoms?

The symptoms of roseola infantum develop in two stages. The first and main symptom is a high fever, which appears 5–15 days after infection and develops rapidly over a few hours. Some children also have:

- Mild diarrhoea.
- Dry cough.
- Swollen lymph nodes in the neck.

In some children, the high fever causes febrile convulsions (p.550). After about 4 days, the fever subsides and a rash of tiny pink spots develops on the face and trunk. This rash usually disappears within a few days.

What might be done?

Roseola infantum does not require specific treatment, and your child will feel better as soon as his or her temperature drops and the spots appear. However, you should contact the doctor at once if the self-help measures for bringing down a fever (p.165) are not effective, if a baby under 6 months old is feverish, if your child has a febrile convulsion, or if he or she seems ill even after the fever has been lowered.

Hand, foot, and mouth disease

A common viral infection that causes small blisters in the mouth and blisters on the hands and feet

 More common in children under the age of 10

 Gender, genetics, and lifestyle are not significant factors

Hand, foot, and mouth disease is a common childhood infection that occurs in epidemics during the summer and early autumn. The infection is caused by the coxsackie virus and lasts a few days.

What are the symptoms?

The symptoms develop 3–5 days after infection and may include:

- Blisters inside the mouth that may develop into painful ulcers.

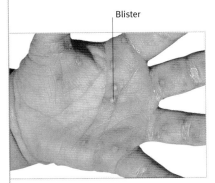

Hand, foot, and mouth disease
The small blisters on this child's hand are characteristic of the viral infection hand, foot, and mouth disease.

- Blisters on the hands and feet that typically develop 1–2 days after those in the mouth and disappear spontaneously after 3–4 days.
- Fever.

Children often seem well but may not want to eat if mouth ulcers develop.

What might be done?

There is no specific treatment for hand, foot, and mouth disease, but self-help measures should relieve the symptoms. You should make sure that your child drinks plenty of fluid, such as chilled milk. However, fruit juices should be avoided because they are acidic and can aggravate mouth ulcers. Liquid paracetamol (*see* **Painkillers**, p.589) will help in bringing down a fever (p.165) and reduce discomfort. If your child is reluctant to drink, watch for signs of dehydration, such as abnormal drowsiness, and consult your child's doctor immediately if you become concerned.

You should also consult a doctor if your child has severe symptoms of hand, foot, and mouth infection. Your child's doctor may prescribe a medicated mouthwash to soothe the ulcers and prevent bacterial infection. Blisters clear up in a few days, but ulcers can persist for up to 1 week.

Head lice

Infestation of tiny, wingless insects on the scalp that may cause intense itching

 Most common between the ages of 4 and 11

 More common in girls

 Genetics and lifestyle are not significant factors

Infestation with head lice is common among young schoolchildren, particularly girls, between the ages of 4 and 11 years. These tiny, almost transparent insects are transmitted by close contact and by sharing personal items such as combs and hats. Head lice are not a result of poor hygiene.

The insects live by sucking blood from the scalp and may be seen as they fall off a child's head when the hair is washed or combed. The eggs, known as nits, are visible as tiny white specks attached to the base of the hairs. An infestation of head lice usually causes intense itching, but there may be no other obvious symptoms.

What can I do?

If you think that your child has head lice, check for eggs at the bases of hairs and comb the hair over a piece of white paper to see if adult lice fall out. If head lice are present, you should check the rest of the family for infestation and alert your child's school.

You can normally treat head lice at home using over-the-counter lotions or shampoos containing an insecticide (*see* **Preparations**

▶ **SELF-HELP**

Treating head lice

Infestations of head lice can be treated with an over-the-counter lotion or shampoo, and the lice can then be removed with a nit comb. Hair conditioner may make it easier for you to comb out the dead lice and eggs, especially if your child's hair is long, thick, or curly. All combs and towels should be washed in very hot water after use to prevent reinfestation.

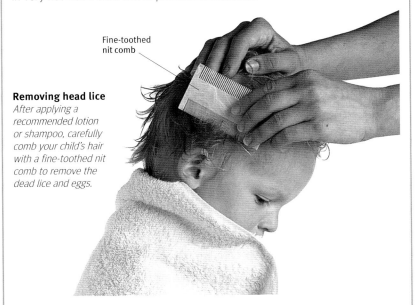

Fine-toothed nit comb

Removing head lice
After applying a recommended lotion or shampoo, carefully comb your child's hair with a fine-toothed nit comb to remove the dead lice and eggs.

for skin infections and infestations, p.577). You should use the type that is currently recommended because lice develop resistance to insecticides. If your child is under the age of 2 or has allergies, eczema, or asthma, discuss treatment with the doctor. To avoid reinfestation, wash bedlinen and combs in very hot water and discourage your child from sharing combs and hats.

Musculoskeletal disorders

In addition to everyday injuries and fractures, most bone, muscle, and joint problems in children fall into two broad categories: problems that are present at birth and those associated with the changes that occur during the growth spurt of puberty. Early treatment of most of these conditions improves the likelihood of recovery and reduces the risk of complications.

This section begins with articles on three conditions that may be present at birth: developmental dysplasia of the hip, clubfoot, and achondroplasia, which is caused by an abnormal gene. These are followed by musculoskeletal conditions that may develop later in childhood and around puberty. These conditions include two that affect the femur (thighbone), Perthes' disease and slipped femoral epiphysis, as well as Osgood–Schlatter disease, which causes inflammation of the tibia (shinbone). Minor foot and leg problems, such as flat feet and bow legs, which are often part of normal development, are also covered. The final article discusses the joint disorder juvenile chronic arthritis. Musculoskeletal disorders that affect adults in addition to children are included in the main section on the musculoskeletal system (pp.211–234).

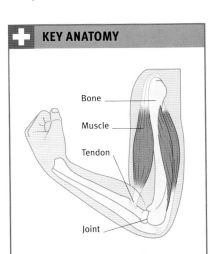

✚ **KEY ANATOMY**

Bone

Muscle

Tendon

Joint

For more information on the structure and function of the musculoskeletal system, *see* pp.211–216.

Developmental dysplasia of the hip

Problems affecting the hip joint, ranging from mild looseness to dislocation

 Present at birth

 More common in girls

 Sometimes runs in families

 Rarely persists in babies who are carried astride the mother's back

Developmental dysplasia of the hip (DDH) is a term that covers a range of problems with the hip joint in the newborn. In mild cases, the hip joint moves excessively when manipulated. In moderate cases, the head of the femur (thighbone) slips out of the hip socket when manipulated but can be eased back in. In severe cases, the dislocation is permanent, and the head of the femur lies outside the hip socket.

Mild cases may be the result of loose ligaments, but in severe cases, the dislocation is related to abnormal development of the hip socket. DDH occurs more often in the left hip and rarely affects both hips About 1 in 500 babies is affected. Carrying a baby astride the mother's back may correct mild DDH. DDH is more common in girls and in babies who are born in the breech position. It may also be associated with clubfoot (right).

The cause of DDH is not fully understood. In about 1 in 5 babies affected, there is a family history of hip dysplasia, suggesting a genetic factor. It may also be due to the effect of maternal hormones that relax the mother's own ligaments in preparation for labour.

What are the symptoms?

Mild forms of DDH may have no symptoms. In severe cases, the symptoms may include:
- Asymmetrical creases in the skin on the backs of the baby's legs.
- Inability to turn the affected leg out fully at the hip.

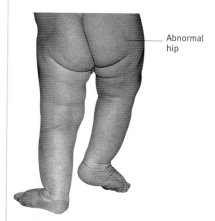
Abnormal hip

Developmental hip dysplasia
This infant has a dislocated right hip. The right leg appears shorter than the left and cannot be fully straightened.

- Shorter appearance of the affected leg.
- Limping when older.

If DDH is not corrected early, it may lead to permanent deformity and to the early onset of the joint disorder osteoarthritis (p.221).

What might be done?

The doctor will check your baby's hips for stability and range of movement shortly after birth and then regularly at routine checkups until your child is walking normally. If your doctor suspects DDH, he or she may arrange ultrasound scanning (p.135) to confirm the diagnosis.

The less severe forms of DDH often correct themselves during the first 3 weeks of life. However, if the problem persists, prompt treatment is essential because the head of the femur must be positioned correctly if the socket is to develop normally. In a very young baby, the hip joint may be positioned in a harness for 8–12 weeks to hold the head of the femur in the hip. In an older baby, the hip may need holding in a cast for up to 6 months to correct the problem. If treatment is unsuccessful, surgery may be necessary to correct the hip dysplasia.

If DDH is diagnosed early and treated immediately, most babies develop normal hip joints and there is no permanent damage.

Clubfoot

A condition, in which a baby is born with one or both feet twisted out of shape or position; also called talipes equinovarus

 Present at birth

 Sometimes runs in families

 Gender as a risk factor depends on the type

 Lifestyle is not a significant factor

Babies are often born with their feet in awkward positions (*see* **Minor leg and foot problems**, opposite page). In severe cases, the defect is known as clubfoot. There are two types of clubfoot: positional clubfoot, in which the twisted foot is flexible and can be manipulated into a normal position, and structural clubfoot, in which the deformity is rigid.

In positional clubfoot, the foot is a normal size but appears twisted, possibly due to compression in the uterus. Most cases are mild and correct themselves. Structural clubfoot occurs in about 1 in 1,000 babies and is more serious. In this disorder, the foot turns downwards and inwards and is usually abnormally small in size. In about half of these babies, both feet are affected. Structural clubfoot may be related to low levels of fluid in the uterus during pregnancy or may be caused by an underlying condition such as spina bifida (*see* **Neural tube**

defects, p.547), and is sometimes associated with developmental dysplasia of the hip (left). Structural clubfoot is twice as common in boys and can run in families.

What might be done?

Clubfoot is usually diagnosed during a routine examination after birth. Positional clubfoot may not need treatment, but physiotherapy (p.620) may help to straighten the foot, and a cast may be used to move the foot into position. A normal position can usually be achieved within 3 months. Structural clubfoot requires physiotherapy and a cast for a long period. In more than half of cases, this treatment is successful. If not, surgery may be needed at the age of 6–9 months. Surgery is usually successful, enabling most children to walk normally.

Achondroplasia

Defective bone growth due to an abnormal gene, causing short stature

 Present at birth

 Due to an abnormal gene

 Gender and lifestyle are not significant factors

Achondroplasia causes abnormal body proportions and short stature. The disorder affects the bones of the limbs and base of the skull and prevents normal growth. As a result, although the child's trunk and head grow at a near normal rate, the arms and legs are disproportionately short and the forehead often protrudes. However, the child's intelligence is not usually affected. In the UK, about 2,000 people are affected.

Achondroplasia is caused by an abnormal gene inherited in an autosomal dominant manner (*see* **Gene disorders**, p.151). Usually, the gene abnormality occurs spontaneously, and there is no family history of the condition. When there is a family history of the disorder, people with achondroplasia have a 1 in 2 chance of passing the disorder on to a child. They may wish to have genetic counselling (p.151) if they are planning a pregnancy.

What are the symptoms?

Symptoms such as short, bowed legs and a prominent forehead are usually apparent at birth. Other symptoms develop as the baby grows and include:
- Short stature.
- Short, broad hands and feet.
- Forward curve to the lower spine (*see* **Kyphosis and lordosis**, p.218).
- Waddling gait.

Psychological difficulties may develop when a child starts to realize that other children are different. Rarely, a baby also has hydrocephalus (p.548), in which there is excess fluid around the brain.

What might be done?

Achondroplasia is sometimes diagnosed during routine ultrasound scanning in pregnancy (p.512) at about 18–20 weeks, but more often the condition is diagnosed at birth. The doctor may arrange for X-rays (p.131) to be taken to confirm the diagnosis, and CT scanning (p.132) or MRI scanning (p.133) may be carried out to look at the baby's head.

There is no cure for achondroplasia, and treatment is rarely needed. The legs can be lengthened slightly by surgery, but many children prefer their natural height. A baby with hydrocephalus may need an operation to drain excess fluid from the brain (*see* **Shunt for hydrocephalus**, p.547). Affected children usually have a normal life expectancy, but may have spinal problems as adults.

Perthes' disease

Gradual breaking down and re-forming of the head of the femur (thighbone)

 Most common between the ages of 4 and 8

 Five times more common in boys

Genetics and lifestyle are not significant factors

Perthes' disease is a rare condition in which the head of the femur (thighbone) softens and breaks down, and is gradually replaced by new bone over 18 months to 2 years. The disease causes pain in the hip and sometimes in the knee. An affected child may walk with a limp and have restricted movement of the hip. Perthes' disease occurs mainly in boys between the ages of 4 and 8 and is more severe in older children. The disease affects 1 in 10,000 children. Of these, 1 in 10 has the disease in both hips.

The cause of Perthes' disease is not known. The condition requires treatment, and you should consult your doctor if your child develops a limp or has a painful hip or knee.

What might be done?

The doctor will examine your child and will probably arrange for X-rays (p.131) of the hip. MRI scanning (p.133) and radionuclide scanning (p.135) of the hip may also be performed.

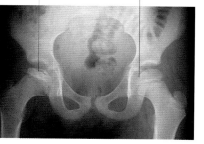
Damaged femur   Normal femur

Perthes' disease
The head of one femur (thighbone) is flattened compared to the other, as a result of Perthes' disease.

Initial treatment is bed rest until the pain subsides. In younger children, bed rest may be sufficient, but sometimes traction is used to place the femur under tension and hold it in the correct position. In more severe cases, casts or braces may be used to protect the hip joint and hold the head of the femur securely in the hip socket while the bone reforms. Occasionally, surgery is required. Your child's progress will be monitored by X-rays every few months while the head of the femur recovers. He or she will probably have physiotherapy (p.620) to encourage mobility of the joint during healing.

About 3 in 10 of those affected develop the joint condition osteoarthritis (p.221) later in life. In general, a complete recovery is more likely in a child under the age of 8 years.

Slipped femoral epiphysis

Displacement of the head of the femur (thighbone) at the hip joint

 Most common in girls aged 11–13 and boys aged 14–16

 More common in boys

 Sometimes runs in families

 Being overweight increases the risk

In children, the epiphysis (the area at the end of a long bone) is separated from the main shaft of the bone by a soft, flexible layer of cartilage where new bone is formed. In the condition known as slipped femoral epiphysis, the epiphysis at the head of the femur (thighbone) becomes displaced. This displacement can happen suddenly as a result of an injury that damages the soft cartilage, or gradually for reasons that are unknown. In 20–40 per cent of cases, both hips are affected but usually at different times. Slipped femoral epiphysis occurs in children growing rapidly at puberty. The disorder affects 30–60 in 100,000 children in the UK each year, and overweight children are particularly at risk. Slipped femoral epiphysis can run in families, suggesting a genetic factor.

What are the symptoms?

Symptoms may appear suddenly but usually develop over several weeks and may include the following:

- Pain in the hip, knee, or thigh.
- Limping with an out-turned foot.
- Restricted hip movement.
- Reluctance and eventually inability to bear weight on the affected leg.

If your child has any of these symptoms, you should contact your doctor within 24 hours.

What might be done?

If your doctor suspects that the child has slipped femoral epiphysis, he or she will arrange for X-rays (p.131) of the affected hip. If there is displacement, your child will need surgery to fix the epiphysis in place

and, possibly, to strengthen the other hip joint to prevent displacement occurring in both hips. If treated promptly, most children recover completely and the condition is unlikely to recur. Rarely, osteoarthritis (p.221) develops later in life.

Osgood–Schlatter disease

Inflammation of the front of the tibia (shinbone) below the knee

 Most common between the ages of 10 and 14

 Much more common in boys

 Strenuous activity aggravates the symptoms

 Genetics is not a significant factor

In Osgood–Schlatter disease, fragments of cartilage become loose at the front of the tibia (shinbone) just below the knee at the point where a large tendon is attached. The condition is caused by repetitive strong pulls on the tendon that attaches the muscle at the front of the thigh to the tibia. The symptoms include tenderness, swelling, and pain in the affected area and appear slowly over several weeks or months. Physical exercise tends to make the symptoms worse. Osgood–Schlatter disease is most common in boys aged 10–14 who take regular strenuous exercise. The disease usually occurs in only one leg, but in about 1 in 5 cases both legs are affected.

If your doctor suspects that your child has Osgood–Schlatter disease, he or she may arrange for X-rays (p.131) of the affected area to confirm the diagnosis. In most cases, no treatment is required apart from rest and painkillers (p.589) to ease the discomfort. In rare cases, if the condition persists, the affected knee may be immobilized in a cast for 6–8 weeks. Treatment is usually successful, and the disorder rarely recurs. Severely affected children may be advised to avoid strenuous exercise until they are over the age of 14 and the musculoskeletal system has matured.

Minor leg and foot problems

Variations in the position and shape of the feet and legs during childhood

 Sometimes run in families

 Age and lifestyle as risk factors depend on the type

 Gender is not a significant factor

When a young child stands and walks, the position of the legs or feet may look odd or awkward. Different minor foot problems are common at different ages. However,

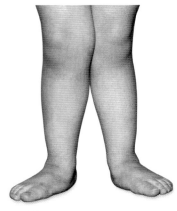

Knock-knees
This child's legs curve inwards, a position known as knock-knees. The condition is common in young children and rarely needs treatment.

these problems rarely interfere with walking or require treatment. Specific minor problems with the legs and feet can run in families, suggesting that a genetic factor may be involved.

What are the types?

Minor leg and foot problems include in-toeing and out-toeing, bow legs and knock-knees, and flat feet.

In-toeing and out-toeing The condition known as in-toeing, in which the feet point inwards, is common, particularly in infancy and early childhood. Out-toeing, in which the feet point away from each other, is less common but may occur from 6 months.

Bow legs and knock-knees If both tibias (shinbones) curve outwards, a child's knees cannot touch when he or she stands with the feet together. This condition, known as bow legs, is common in children up to 3 years. Severe bowing is uncommon but may be caused by a deficiency of vitamin D (*see* **Osteomalacia and rickets**, p.217). In knock-knees, the child's legs curve in at the knees, so that the feet are wide apart even when the knees are touching. Knock-knees is common in children between the ages of 3 and 7 years.

Flat feet Most children have flat feet until the arch develops between 2 and 3 years of age. Children also have a pad of fat beneath the foot that accentuates the flat-footed appearance. However, some children have persistent flat feet.

What might be done?

Your child's legs and feet will be examined regularly during routine medical checkups. However, you should consult your doctor if you are worried by the appearance of your child's legs or feet or if your child has difficulty in walking, has a limp, or complains of pain.

Most children with minor leg and foot problems do not need treatment because walking is rarely affected and the problems disappear as a child grows up. Out-toeing disappears first, usually within a year of a child starting to walk. Bow legs

usually disappears by the age of 2–3 years; in-toeing by the age of 7–8; and knock-knees by the age of about 6. Persistent flat feet do not often need treatment unless they cause pain.

Your doctor may recommend physiotherapy (p.620) if your child experiences difficulty in walking or the shape of his or her legs is abnormal. Rarely, if your child's legs or feet are seriously affected, he or she may need to have orthopaedic surgery to correct the problem.

Juvenile chronic arthritis

Persistent inflammation of one or more joints that occurs only in childhood

 Sometimes runs in families

 Age and gender as risk factors depend on the type

 Lifestyle is not a significant factor

Children may be affected by the same types of arthritis (p.220) as adults, but juvenile chronic arthritis (JCA) is found only in children. In the UK, about 1 child in 1,000 is affected. The condition is the result of an abnormal response of the body's immune system, leading to inflammation, swelling, and pain in the lining of an affected joint. Although the cause is not known, juvenile chronic arthritis sometimes runs in families, which suggests a genetic factor may be involved. In mild cases, the child is still able to carry out normal activities. In severe cases, there may be joint deformities and reduced mobility.

What are the types?

Juvenile chronic arthritis is divided into three types according to the number of joints affected by the disease and the specific symptoms involved.

Polyarticular arthritis This type affects more girls than boys and can occur at any age. Symptoms include inflammation, stiffness, and pain in five or more joints. The joints commonly affected include those in the wrists, fingers, knees, and ankles.

Pauciarticular arthritis This is the commonest type of JCA and most frequently affects girls under school age. Symptoms include inflammation, stiffness, and pain in four or fewer joints, and there is a risk of developing the eye disorder uveitis (p.357). The joints in the knees, ankles, and wrists are commonly involved.

Systemic arthritis Also known as Still's disease, this type of JCA affects boys and girls equally. The disorder occurs at any age during childhood but mostly commonly around the age of 3–6 years. Any number of joints may be affected

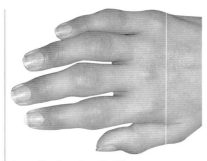

Juvenile chronic arthritis
The joints of this young child's hand are swollen due to the inflammatory disorder polyarticular arthritis.

by pain, swelling, and stiffness. The other symptoms include fever, swollen glands, and a rash. Some children recover completely, but others develop polyarticular JCA.

What might be done?

If the doctor suspects that your child has a type of juvenile chronic arthritis, he or she may arrange for X-rays (p.131) of the affected joints and blood tests to look for particular antibodies associated with the condition.

The goal of treatment is to reduce inflammation, minimize damage to the joints, and relieve pain. If your child is mildly affected, he or she may only need to take nonsteroidal anti-inflammatory drugs (p.578) to reduce inflammation and relieve pain. In more severe cases, your child may be prescribed locally acting corticosteroids (p.578), which are injected into the affected joints, or oral corticosteroids (p.600). Sometimes, the inflammation can be reduced by using antirheumatic drugs (p.579), such as methotrexate and sulfasalazine.

Other treatments for JCA include physiotherapy (p.620), to help to maintain joint mobility, and occupational therapy (p.621). Splints may be used for support and to help to prevent deformity. Special devices are also available and may help with daily activities such as dressing. If damage to the joints is severe and has caused deformity, joint replacement (p.223) may be necessary.

Juvenile chronic arthritis can clear up within a few years, but severely affected children may be left with deformed joints, and some may have arthritis that persists into adult life.

Disorders of the cardiovascular and respiratory systems

Disorders of the heart and lungs are relatively common in children. The heart is affected by birth defects more than any other organ, and all children have recurrent bacterial and viral infections of the throat and lungs. Usually these infections are mild and play a role in developing a healthy immune system.

The first articles in this section cover disorders of the cardiovascular system, such as congenital heart disease. Many heart abnormalities correct themselves without medical intervention as a child grows. Many of the more serious heart defects can now be treated successfully because of recent advances in surgical techniques. A rarer disorder that can affect the heart in children is Kawasaki disease, which damages the heart and blood vessels. In Henoch–Schönlein purpura, which is due to an abnormal response by the immune system, small blood vessels are damaged. In some cases, Henoch–Schönlein purpura can eventually cause kidney failure.

The final articles address respiratory disorders, of which asthma is the most common, affecting about 1 in 11 of all children in the UK. Respiratory tract infections, such as bronchiolitis and croup, are common in young children. The inflammatory disorder epiglottitis can be dangerous but is now rare in developed countries because of routine immunization of infants against *Haemophilus influenzae* type B, the bacterium responsible for causing the condition.

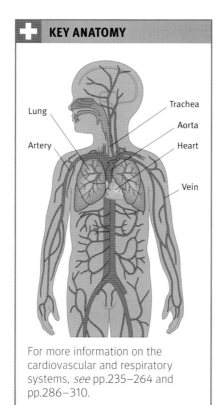

Lung · Artery · Trachea · Aorta · Heart · Vein

For more information on the cardiovascular and respiratory systems, *see* pp.235–264 and pp.286–310.

Congenital heart disease

One or more defects of the heart that are present at birth

 Present at birth

 Use of certain drugs and alcohol during pregnancy are risk factors

 Gender and genetics as risk factors depend on the type

The heart is a complex organ that can develop abnormally in a fetus, leading to defects that affect a baby from birth (congenital heart defects). Congenital heart disease affects about 4–9 in 1,000 babies and is one of the most common birth defects. Many of these abnormalities disappear naturally as the baby grows, but more serious defects require complex corrective surgery.

Congenital heart disease may cause shortness of breath in affected children, which may inhibit their feeding, growth, and activity.

What are the causes?

In most cases, the cause of congenital heart disease is unknown. However, it can sometimes run in families, suggesting that a genetic factor may be involved. Heart defects at birth may also be associated with genetic disorders, such as Down's syndrome (p.533). Exposure of the fetus to excessive alcohol or drugs such as the anticonvulsant phenytoin increases the risk of congenital heart disease. In early pregnancy, certain infections, such as rubella (p.168), in the mother can lead to fetal heart defects (*see* **Congenital infections**, p.530). More than 1 in 10 babies with congenital heart disease are also found to have a defect elsewhere in the body, commonly in the digestive tract.

What are the types?

Most types of congenital heart disease affect only one part of the heart or one of the major blood vessels, such as the aorta, connected to the heart. Less commonly, several parts of the heart or more than one blood vessel are affected. These multiple heart defects are more serious and can be life-threatening.

Septal defects The most common type of congenital heart abnormality is a septal defect, also known as a hole in the heart. In this defect, there is a hole in the septum (the inner wall that divides the heart) either between the two lower chambers (ventri-

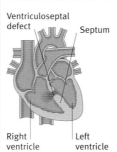

Ventriculoseptal defect · Septum · Right ventricle · Left ventricle

culoseptal defect, pictured left) or alternatively between the two upper chambers (atrioseptal defect). In both cases, some oxygen-rich blood passes from the left side to the

right side of the heart and is sent back to the lungs instead of going around the body. About 1 in 3 cases of congenital heart disease is due to a ventriculoseptal defect, which is often small and may close naturally. About 1 in 4 cases of congenital heart disease is caused by an atrioseptal defect, which usually produces few symptoms but is likely to require surgical treatment. Both septal defects are common in children with Down's syndrome.

Patent ductus arteriosus The ductus arteriosus is a small blood vessel that connects the pulmonary artery to the aorta in the fetus so that blood bypasses the lungs. If this vessel fails to close up soon after birth, normal circulation is prevented. This disorder is often found in premature babies.

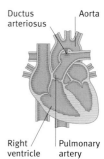

Ductus arteriosus · Aorta · Right ventricle · Pulmonary artery

Coarctation of the aorta In this congenital heart disorder there is a narrowing of an area in the aorta, which restricts the flow of blood to the lower part of the body. As a result, the heart muscle works harder to compensate, and the pressure of blood in the upper part of the body is raised. The disorder requires surgical treatment. Children with coarctation of the aorta may additionally have an abnormality of one or more of the four heart valves.

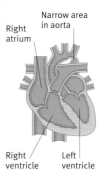

Narrow area in aorta · Right atrium · Right ventricle · Left ventricle

Valve defects Any of the four heart valves may develop abnormally. The most common valve disorder is pulmonary stenosis. In this condition, the pulmonary valve, which opens to allow blood to flow from the right ventricle into the pulmonary artery, is narrowed so that blood flow is restricted. Defects of the aortic valve, which opens to allow blood to flow from the left ventricle into the aorta, are less common.

Multiple defects Sometimes, several heart defects occur together. In addition to placing extra strain on the heart, the defects usually prevent blood from passing through the lungs normally so that blood oxygen levels become very low. Tissues throughout the body may then become oxygen-starved. The most common multiple defect is Fallot's tetralogy, in which four heart abnormalities occur together. These consist of a ventriculoseptal defect, obstruction to blood flow from the right ventricle (known as right ventricular outflow obstruction), a displaced aorta, and a thickened right ventricle. Another type of multiple defect is hypoplastic left heart syndrome, in which the chambers and valves on the left side of the heart are underdeveloped. This was once a fatal condition but can now sometimes be treated. A rarer multiple defect involves reversal of the positions of the aorta and the pulmonary artery.

What are the symptoms?
Minor congenital heart defects may not cause symptoms. When symptoms do occur, they vary depending on the severity and type of the heart defect. The symptoms of all types of congenital heart disease may include:
- Shortness of breath, leading to difficulty in feeding and sweating.
- Slow weight gain and growth.

Symptoms of severe heart defects may develop suddenly in the first weeks of life. If there are low levels of oxygen in the blood, the tongue and lips may appear bluish in colour. Children with heart defects may be susceptible to chest infections and are at increased risk of infection of the lining of the heart (see **Infective endocarditis**, p.256), especially after surgery or dental treatment. Over a period of several years, congenital heart defects may lead to irreversible damage to the lungs (see **Pulmonary hypertension**, p.309).

How is it diagnosed?
In some cases, congenital heart disease is diagnosed during routine ultrasound scanning in pregnancy (p.512). Otherwise, defects may be found after birth when symptoms develop or during a routine examination. The doctor may hear a sound (heart murmur) caused by turbulent blood flow while listening to your child's heart. Although many heart murmurs are normal, the doctor is likely to arrange for an ECG (p.243), which monitors the electrical activity of the heart. Your child may also have the imaging technique echocardiography (p.255), which is used to assess the structure and function of the heart.

What is the treatment?
Many heart defects correct themselves or need no treatment. Only about 1 in 3 children requires surgery. Affected children are usually monitored throughout childhood and, if necessary, surgery is performed when the child is older and the operation easier. Rarely, an emergency operation is necessary to save a young baby's life. A heart transplant (p.257) is now a possibility for children who have multiple heart defects. Chest infections need to be treated promptly, and, if the child has dental treatment or surgery, antibiotics (p.572) may be necessary to prevent infection of the lining of the heart. Some children will need drugs, such as diuretics (p.583), to control the symptoms of a heart defect.

What is the prognosis?
The outlook depends on the type of heart defect and its severity. Septal defects either close naturally or are corrected surgically. As a result of surgical advances over the last 20 years, even very severe defects can often be corrected, and many severely affected children are leading normal, active lives.

Kawasaki disease

A prolonged fever during which the heart and blood vessels may be damaged

 More common under the age of 5

 Slightly more common in boys

 More common in people of Asian descent

 Lifestyle is not a significant factor

First observed in Japan in the 1960s, Kawasaki disease is a rare condition in which a prolonged fever is associated with damage to the heart and blood vessels. In the UK, fewer than 1 in every 25,000 children under the age of 5 are affected each year. The disorder is now being diagnosed more often in Western countries, and it occurs more frequently in people of Asian descent. Heart damage occurs in about 1 in 5 of all cases of Kawasaki disease. Early diagnosis is very important because the condition can become life-threatening.

The cause of Kawasaki disease is not known, although it is suspected that a viral or bacterial infection may be involved. However, despite a great deal of research, there is as yet no conclusive evidence to confirm this theory.

What are the symptoms?
The symptoms develop over about 2 weeks and may include:
- Prolonged, constant high fever that lasts more than 5 days.
- Sore or itchy eyes and redness of the white of the eye (see **Conjunctivitis**, p.355).
- Cracked, painful, and swollen lips.
- Reddening of the mouth and throat.
- A blotchy red rash.
- Swollen glands, especially in the neck.
- Reddening of the palms of the hands and soles of the feet, usually followed by peeling skin on the tips of the fingers and toes.

Kawasaki disease may lead to serious complications. For example, balloon-like swellings, called aneurysms, can develop in the walls of the coronary arteries, which supply the heart muscle. Inflammation of the heart muscle (see **Myocarditis**, p.256)

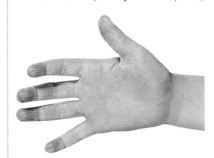

Kawasaki disease
One of the symptoms of the rare disorder Kawasaki disease is reddening of the hands with peeling skin on the tips of the fingers.

may also occur. Kawasaki disease can also damage blood vessels throughout the body.

What might be done?
Diagnosis of Kawasaki disease can be difficult because the symptoms are very similar to those of minor viral infections, such as the common cold. You should consult a doctor if your child develops a fever that cannot be lowered by taking paracetamol and other simple self-help measures (see **Bringing down a fever**, p.165). If Kawasaki disease is suspected, your child will be admitted to hospital immediately because treatment is most effective if started within 10 days of the onset of the disease. Your child will probably have blood tests to look for evidence of Kawasaki disease. The imaging technique echocardiography (p.255) may also be carried out to look for damage to the heart muscle and coronary blood vessels.

If Kawasaki disease is confirmed, the child will probably be given intravenous immunoglobulin. This substance is a blood product containing antibodies that fight infection. Immunoglobulin also reduces the risk of aneurysms and inflammation of the heart muscle in Kawasaki disease for reasons that are not fully understood. High doses of aspirin are usually prescribed until the fever subsides. Lower doses are then continued over a period of several weeks.

What is the prognosis?
Most children who have Kawasaki disease recover completely within 3 weeks but need regular follow-up visits, and possibly echocardiography, over the next few months. Aneurysms and myocarditis, if present, usually disappear over a period of several months. Kawasaki disease is fatal in about 1 in 100 affected children. In children who survive, there is a small risk of developing coronary artery disease (p.243) later in life.

Henoch–Schönlein purpura

Inflammation of small blood vessels, the kidneys, and joints, caused by an abnormal immune response

 Most common between the ages of 2 and 8

 Twice as common in boys

 Genetics and lifestyle are not significant factors

In Henoch–Schönlein purpura, small blood vessels are damaged by an abnormal reaction of the immune system, possibly triggered by an infection. Antibodies, which are a component of the immune system and normally fight infection, are deposited in the small blood vessels throughout the body, causing them to become inflamed. The inflammation results in blood leaking out of the vessels into the skin, causing distinctive

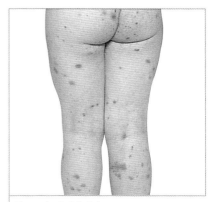

Henoch–Schönlein purpura
The raised purple lesions that have developed over the back of this child's legs and buttocks are one of the symptoms typical of Henoch–Schönlein purpura.

lesions, mainly on the buttocks and the backs of the legs. Bleeding may also occur from the lining of the intestines. The inflammation may also affect the joints and the kidneys.

Henoch–Schönlein purpura is most common in children between the ages of 2 and 8. The disorder occurs more frequently in the winter months and is more common in boys.

What are the symptoms?
The symptoms usually develop over several days and may include:
- Numerous raised, purple lesions that typically appear on the buttocks and legs and sometimes also on the arms and feet.
- Periodic attacks of abdominal pain, often with vomiting.
- Sometimes, blood in the faeces.
- Painful, swollen joints, most often the knees and ankles.

In many children with the condition, the kidneys become inflamed, leading to loss of blood and protein in the urine (see **Glomerulonephritis**, p.446). The blood is usually present in amounts too small to be seen with the naked eye. If the kidneys are badly affected, they may be damaged permanently, which may result in a rise in blood pressure. If the intestines become inflamed, a condition known as intussusception (p.560) may develop, in which part of the intestine "telescopes" in on itself, causing intestinal obstruction.

How is it diagnosed?
The diagnosis of Henoch–Schönlein purpura is based on the symptoms. Your doctor will probably arrange for a urine test to look for blood or protein, indicating that the kidneys are inflamed. Blood tests will be carried out to assess the function of your child's kidneys and to rule out other possible causes of the symptoms. In some cases, a small sample of tissue may be removed from the kidney (see **Kidney biopsy**, p.449) or skin (see **Skin biopsy**, p.199) for examination.

What is the treatment?
There is no specific treatment for Henoch–Schönlein purpura. Your doctor will probably advise that your child rests in bed and may

prescribe painkillers (p.589), such as para-cetamol. If the abdominal pain is very severe, he or she may also prescribe corti-costeroids (p.600). Joint pain usually disappears without permanent damage, and the rash should go away without treatment. Symptoms normally take 2–6 weeks to dis-appear completely. Kidney function is monitored by checking your child's blood pressure and by performing blood tests. Urine tests are carried out for months or even years, until no traces of blood or protein remain in the urine. If the kidneys are severely damaged, the doctor may prescribe immunosuppressants (p.585). Children with kidney damage require long-term follow-up.

What is the prognosis?
Most children with Henoch–Schönlein pur-pura make a full recovery with no long-term effects. The symptoms may recur over about a year but are rare thereafter. In rare cases, there is long-term kidney damage that may lead to kidney failure (p.450).

Asthma in children

Attacks of breathlessness, coughing, and/or wheezing in children due to reversible narrowing of the airways

 Most common under the age of 6; becomes less common with age

 More common in boys

 Exposure to furry animals, air pollution, viral respiratory infections, and parental smoking are risk factors

 Sometimes runs in families

In children with asthma, the airways in the lungs tend to narrow temporarily. Narrowing occurs when the linings of the airways become swollen and inflamed and produce excess mucus, which may block the smaller airways.

Asthma affects about 1 in 11 children in the UK and is the most common long-term respiratory disease in children. The reason for the high prevalence of asthma in chil-dren is not known, but allergies and other environmental factors may be involved.

Asthma attacks in children are a common cause of absence from school and admis-sion to hospital. However, between attacks, children can be perfectly well. Severe attacks of asthma are distressing for both children and their parents and can be life-threatening.

What are the causes?
Asthma is more likely to develop in children with a family history of the condition, sug-gesting that a genetic factor may be involved. Other respiratory disorders, espe-cially those associated with premature birth (*see* **Problems of the premature baby**, p.530), may also increase the risk of devel-oping asthma. Regular exposure to cigarette

▶ TREATMENT

Giving inhaled drugs to children
The drugs that are used to treat asthma are often inhaled. Devices that administer these drugs are tailored to suit the age of the child (*see* **Taking inhaled asthma drugs**, p.297). Because small children cannot coordinate their breathing to inhale the drugs, they require special inhalers that incorporate a face mask and a spacer. The spacer retains the drug while the face mask allows the child to inhale the drug while breathing normally.

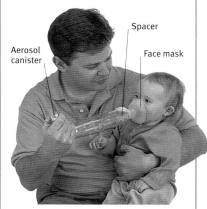

Aerosol canister · Spacer · Face mask

Giving drugs to a young child
A dose of the drug is dispensed from the canister into a spacer, such as the one shown, and the mask is placed over the child's nose and mouth.

smoke in the home and pollution from car exhaust and factory fumes may also be risk factors for asthma.

In children under the age of 5, attacks of asthma are usually triggered by a viral infec-tion, such as the common cold (p.164). In older children, asthma attacks are often caused by an allergic reaction to substances such as pollens, moulds, house dust mites, and the fur or dander from animals. Exercise, especially outside in cold, dry conditions, may also trigger an asthma attack. In rare cases, certain foods, such as milk, nuts, and eggs, can provoke asthma. In some affected children, emotional stress may make the attacks more severe.

What are the symptoms?
Symptoms vary in severity from day to day and week to week and with the age of the child. They appear rapidly and may per-sist for a few hours or longer. Symptoms may include:
■ Wheezing.
■ Shortness of breath.
■ Tightness in the chest.
■ Dry cough that may be worse at night and disturb sleep.
Very young children with asthma often have a dry cough at night and no other symptoms. Older children often feel tired

due to disturbed sleep and may have dif-ficulty participating in strenuous sports due to shortness of breath. Children with asthma are also predisposed to the aller-gic disorders eczema (*see* **Eczema in children**, p.538) and hay fever (*see* **Allergic rhinitis**, p.283).

A severe asthma attack may cause very rapid breathing, difficulty speaking, and indrawing of the chest wall. If the level of oxygen in the blood is low, a child may develop a bluish tinge to the lips and tongue, a condition known as cyanosis. You should call an ambulance immediately if your child has such an attack, because he or she needs emergency treatment.

Left untreated, severe asthma may impair a child's growth (*see* **Growth disorders**, p.563) and development. Because children who have asthma often have difficulty sleep-ing, many become chronically tired, which can lead to poor performance at school.

How is it diagnosed?
Diagnosis of the condition is based on a description of your child's symptoms. The doctor will listen to your child's chest with a stethoscope. An older child may be asked to breathe out through a peak flow meter, a special device that measures the child's capacity to exhale (*see* **Monitoring your asthma**, p.296). To confirm the diagnosis, the doctor may prescribe a trial of a quick-relief drug that opens up the airways in the lungs (*see* **Bronchodilator drugs**, p.588). If your child's symptoms are caused by asthma, they should improve significantly after administration of the drug.

Once the diagnosis has been confirmed, your child may have a skin test to look for specific allergies that may be the trigger fac-tors for his or her asthma attacks (*see* **Skin prick test**, p.284).

What is the treatment?
The aim of treatment for asthma is to ena-ble your child to live as active a life as possible with a minimum of drug treatment. The doctor may give you a detailed plan for managing your child's asthma with advice on when to change treatments and what to do if your child has a sudden attack. It is important that children who have asthma understand their condition and are confi-dent about dealing with their symptoms. Some children will need to take regular peak flow readings at home to monitor their asthma over a period of time. Since the nor-mal peak flow values are determined according to a child's height, growth should also be measured regularly.

Environmental measures There are many ways in which you can modify your child's environment to minimize contact with fac-tors that may trigger an attack (*see* **Reducing the risk of asthma attacks in children**, right).

Drug treatment The drugs that are used to treat children with asthma fall into two groups: reliever drugs and preventer drugs, which are usually corticosteroids (*see* **Corticosteroids for respiratory disease**,

p.588) although leukotriene antagonists (*see* **Antiallergy drugs**, p.585) may also be used. The reliever drugs act rapidly to open up the airways and relieve wheezing. They usually work within 10 minutes, but their effect lasts for only a few hours. Children who have mild asthma attacks once or twice a week may be prescribed a reliever drug for use when symptoms occur.

Children who have frequent asthma attacks also need to take regular doses of preventer drugs. These drugs take effect slowly over several days and should be taken regularly, even if there are no symp-toms of asthma. Preventer drugs reduce inflammation of the airways and prevent the symptoms from occurring. Respiratory corticosteroids are commonly prescribed as preventer drugs, but other drugs, such as sodium cromoglicate, may be given to dampen the allergic response and help to keep the airways open. Leukotriene antagonists may be used in addition to inhaled corticosteroids to treat moder-ately severe asthma.

Drugs to treat asthma are usually administered with an inhaler. A spacer device attached to an inhaler may be nec-essary for young children who find an inhaler difficult to use effectively (*see* **Giving inhaled drugs to children**, left). A nebulizer, a device that delivers a drug in aerosol form through a face mask, may be used during a severe asthma attack. It is crucial to learn the correct technique for using inhalers and nebulizers. The doctor or a nurse will show you and your child how to use the devices properly. After a severe asthma attack, oral corticosteroids may be prescribed for your child in addition to the inhaled drugs.

Managing an asthma attack You or your child should always carry a reliever inhaler in case it is needed to treat an asthma attack. An inhaler should also be kept at

SELF-HELP

Reducing the risk of asthma attacks in children

Asthma attacks are often triggered by contact with allergy-producing substances, such as cat hair. By adopting simple measures, you can reduce the likelihood of your child having an attack.

■ Do not allow people to smoke in the house.
■ Do not keep furry animals or birds as pets.
■ Dust furniture using a damp cloth and vacuum carpets regularly, if possible when your child is out of the house.
■ Do not use fluffy, dust-collecting blankets and make sure pillows and duvets contain artificial fibres and not feathers.
■ Enclose mattresses completely in plastic covers.
■ If pollen is a problem, keep windows closed, especially while grass is releasing pollen, and use an air purifier.
■ Avoid products that have strong odours, such as air fresheners, mothballs, and perfume.

your child's school and you should ensure that his or her teachers understand its use. If your child's symptoms are not eased by a single dose of a reliever drug, a repeat dose should be taken. If that fails to improve the symptoms, call for an ambulance immediately or take your child to the nearest accident and emergency department. It is important to remain calm and reassure your child. Once in hospital, your child will probably be given oxygen and high doses of reliever drugs through a spacer or with a nebulizer to relieve the symptoms. He or she may need to stay in hospital to recover completely from a severe attack of asthma and may also require a course of oral corticosteroids.

What is the prognosis?

Children with asthma are usually able to lead active lives through careful use of drugs and avoidance of trigger factors, such as animal fur. About half of all children with asthma grow out of the condition by the time they are teenagers. Asthma that persists past the age of 14 is likely to continue into adulthood (*see* **Asthma**, p.295).

Despite the ease with which asthma can be controlled, severe attacks of asthma can cause death. In most cases, fatalities are caused by a delay in getting an affected child to hospital and a lack of understanding about potentially life-threatening symptoms.

Bronchiolitis

Inflammation of the small airways in the lungs caused by a viral infection

 Most common under the age of 12 months

 Parental smoking and living in overcrowded conditions are risk factors; babies who are not breast-fed are also at increased risk

 Gender and genetics are not significant factors

Bronchiolitis is a common and usually mild condition that mainly occurs in babies under the age of 12 months. The small airways in the lungs, called bronchioles, become inflamed due to a viral infection and restrict the flow of air in and out of the lungs. In about 9 in 10 cases, the infection is caused by the respiratory syncytial virus, which can be transmitted from person to person in the airborne droplets from coughs and sneezes. By the age of 5, almost all children in the UK have been infected with this virus. Most of those affected only develop the symptoms of a common cold (p.164), but occasionally the infection leads to more severe breathing difficulties. During winter, bronchiolitis tends to occur in epidemics. The risk of a child having bronchiolitis is increased if his or her family lives in overcrowded conditions, in which a viral infection can spread more quickly, or if the child's parents

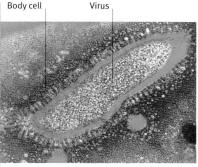

Respiratory syncytial virus
This virus is the most common cause of bronchiolitis, in which small airways in the lungs are inflamed. In some cases, the infection causes severe breathing difficulties.

smoke. Babies who have never been breast-fed are also more likely to develop the condition.

What are the symptoms?

Initially, an affected child may have symptoms resembling a common cold, such as a runny nose, fever, and sneezing. However, the following symptoms may develop after 2–3 days:

- Cough.
- Rapid breathing.
- Wheezing.
- Feeding difficulties.

If your child is under 1 year old and has these symptoms, you should contact the doctor. Occasionally, babies may experience severe breathing difficulties, especially if they are very young or have an underlying condition such as congenital heart disease (p.542). These babies may develop a blue tinge on the tongue, lips, and skin, a condition called cyanosis. In very small babies who have bronchiolitis, intervals of more than 10 seconds may occur between breaths. You should call an ambulance immediately if your baby is having difficulty breathing, if his or her tongue, lips, or skin become blue-coloured, or if he or she becomes drowsy at unexpected times because of the extra effort that is needed to breathe.

How is it diagnosed?

The doctor will probably suspect bronchiolitis from the symptoms and by listening to your child's chest with a stethoscope. A chest X-ray (p.300) may be arranged and the doctor may take samples of your child's nasal secretions to look for evidence of infection with the respiratory syncytial virus.

What is the treatment?

If the bronchiolitis is mild, you will probably be able to treat your child at home. The doctor may prescribe inhaled bronchodilators (p.588) to widen the airways and ease breathing. You may be advised to give your child liquid paracetamol (*see* **Painkillers**, p.589) to bring down a fever. You can help to ease your child's breathing by increasing humidity in the bedroom.

This can be done by placing a wet towel or a dish of water in the room close to a source of heat, such as a radiator. You should give your child small, frequent drinks and feeds so that he or she receives an adequate quantity of fluids to avoid dehydration, which can be serious.

Children with severe symptoms need to be treated in hospital, where they may be given an inhaled bronchodilator drug, sometimes via a nebulizer (a device that delivers a drug in aerosol form through a face mask). Intravenous fluids may be administered if the child is unable to feed. Oxygen is given if blood oxygen levels are low. Premature babies and those with problems such as heart disease may be given antiviral drugs (p.573) to treat the infection and may need temporary mechanical ventilation to help them to breathe.

What is the prognosis?

Mild bronchiolitis usually improves within 5 days and clears up completely in about 10 days. Severe bronchiolitis may require several weeks of hospital treatment but usually causes no permanent damage. However, many children who have had bronchiolitis tend to suffer from wheezing when they have a cold.

Croup

Inflammation and narrowing of the main airway (trachea) due to a viral infection

 Most common between the ages of 6 months and 3 years

 Slightly more common in boys

 Genetics and lifestyle are not significant factors

Croup is a common disorder that usually affects children between the ages of 6 months and 3 years. During an attack of croup, the airway that leads from the back of the throat to the lungs becomes inflamed because of a viral infection, restricting the flow of air and causing noisy breathing. Although symptoms are usually mild, croup may occasionally cause severe breathing difficulties that require treatment in hospital. Boys appear to be more susceptible to the condition, but the reason for this is not known. Croup occurs more frequently in the autumn and winter months.

What are the symptoms?

Croup usually begins with the symptoms of a common cold, such as a runny nose. About 1–2 days later, the following symptoms may develop:

- Barking cough.
- Harsh, noisy breathing, particularly when inhaling.
- Hoarseness.

In severe cases, breathing may become rapid and difficult. This may cause a lack of oxygen and lead to the development of a bluish colour to the tongue and lips, a condition called cyanosis. If cyanosis develops, you should call an ambulance immediately.

What might be done?

The doctor will probably diagnose croup from the symptoms. He or she will assess the severity of your child's condition and may suggest self-help measures to ease your child's breathing. For example, sitting with your child in a steamy bathroom can relieve minor breathing difficulties. You can increase the humidity in your child's room by placing a dish of water near a source of heat, such as a radiator. Taking your child outside in the cool night air for a few minutes may also help to ease your child's breathing. The doctor may prescribe an inhaled or oral corticosteroid drug (*see* **Corticosteroids for respiratory disease**, p.588) to reduce inflammation in the airways. If the symptoms are very severe, your child will need to be admitted to hospital. In rare cases, mechanical ventilation may also be necessary.

What is the prognosis?

Most children with croup recover completely within a few days. However, the condition may recur until your child reaches about the age of 5. At this age, the airways are wider and therefore less likely to become severely narrowed by inflammation after an infection.

Epiglottitis

Inflammation of the epiglottis, a flap of cartilage that closes over the main airway to the lungs when food is swallowed

 Most common between the ages of 1 and 6

 Gender, genetics, and lifestyle are not significant factors

In this rare condition, the epiglottis, a flap of tissue behind the tongue that prevents food from entering the airways of the lungs during swallowing, becomes inflamed due to infection. Inflammation causes the epiglottis to swell so that the main airway is partially blocked. The swelling can be so severe that the child is unable to breathe. This situation is life-threatening and needs urgent hospital treatment.

Epiglottitis is caused by infection with the bacterium *Haemophilus influenzae* type B (Hib). Children between 1 and 6 years old are most commonly affected. Epiglottitis is now rare in the UK due to routine immunization (p.13) of babies.

What are the symptoms?
In most cases, the symptoms of epiglottitis develop suddenly over a period of 1–2 hours and may include:
- High fever.
- Severe sore throat.
- Difficulty swallowing.
- Saliva dribbling from the mouth.
- Restlessness and anxiety.
- Rapid, laboured breathing.
- Harsh noise on inhaling.

If there is severe obstruction of the airway, your child may become short of oxygen, possibly causing his or her lips, tongue, and skin to become blue-tinged. If your child develops difficulty swallowing or breathing, you should call for an ambulance immediately.

What might be done?
Initially, your most important tasks are to get immediate medical help then to reassure your child and try to keep him or her calm. You should not attempt to examine your child's throat because this may increase distress, resulting in further blockage of the airway. Your child will probably be more comfortable sitting upright with his or her chin jutting out to maintain an unobstructed flow of air into the lungs.

The doctor will probably make a diagnosis from your child's symptoms. Humidified oxygen will need to be given through a mask held near to his or her face. In hospital, your child will probably be taken to the operating theatre and given an inhaled anaesthetic so that a tube can be inserted into the main airway to keep it open. To maintain breathing, your child may need mechanical ventilation. To treat the Hib infection, your child will be given intravenous antibiotics (p.572).

What is the prognosis?
Most children recover in about a week. The tube that keeps the airway open is usually removed after about 2–3 days. There are usually no long-term problems, and the condition does not recur.

Enlarged adenoids

Enlargement of the adenoids, tissue at the back of the nasal cavity that forms part of the body's defence system

 Most common under the age of 7

 Gender, genetics, and lifestyle are not significant factors

The adenoids, which are located at the back of the nasal cavity, consist of lymphatic tissue that forms part of the body's defences against infection. In some children, particularly those under the age of 7, the adenoids become enlarged, which may lead to difficulties with breathing and speech. This enlargement is sometimes a result of recurrent respiratory infections or can be caused by allergies. In other cases, the cause is unknown. Infected adenoids are sometimes associated with infection of the tonsils (*see* **Tonsillitis**, below).

What are the symptoms?
In most children with enlarged adenoids, symptoms are mild and appear gradually. The symptoms may include:
- Breathing through the mouth and snoring during sleep.
- Persistently blocked or runny nose.
- Nasal-sounding voice.

Difficulty in breathing may cause your child to wake frequently during the night, leading to tiredness and inability to concentrate. Enlarged adenoids may cause partial blockage of one or both of the eustachian tubes connecting the throat to the middle ear, which may cause recurrent middle-ear infections (*see* **Acute otitis media in children**, p.557) or a build-up of fluid in the middle ear that results in impaired hearing (*see* **Chronic secretory otitis media**, p.557). In an older child, enlarged adenoids may cause chronic sinusitis (p.290).

What might be done?
The doctor will probably examine your child's throat. If the symptoms are mild, no treatment for enlarged adenoids is required because adenoids shrink naturally with age, and usually disappear before puberty. However, if your child has constantly disrupted sleep, recurrent middle-ear infections, or chronic secretory otitis media, the doctor may advise surgical removal of the adenoids. The tonsils are sometimes removed at the same time (*see* **Tonsillectomy and adenoidectomy**, right). A build-up of fluid in the middle ear may be relieved by inserting a tiny drainage tube called a grommet (p.558) into the eardrum.

The symptoms tend to diminish as a child gets older, and have usually gone by the time adolescence is reached.

Tonsillitis

Inflammation of the tonsils, two areas of tissue at the back of the throat that form part of the body's defence system

 Most common under the age of 10

 Gender, genetics, and lifestyle are not significant factors

The tonsils are two areas of lymphatic tissue at the back of the throat that form an important part of the body's defences against infection. A condition known as tonsillitis develops if the tonsils become inflamed and painful. This usually occurs as a result of infection. Infections may be caused either by viruses, such as those that cause the common cold (p.164), or bacteria, such as streptococci.

▶ TREATMENT

Tonsillectomy and adenoidectomy

Surgical removal of the tonsils is performed on children who have frequent episodes of tonsillitis. Enlarged adenoids may also be removed at the same time if they are causing breathing difficulties and recurrent ear problems.

The operation is performed in hospital under general anaesthesia. A child should be able to return home the day after the operation, and he or she should make a full recovery in about 2 weeks.

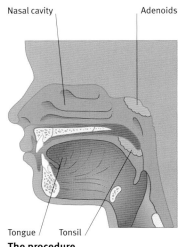

Nasal cavity — Adenoids
Tongue — Tonsil

The procedure
Surgical removal of the tonsils and adenoids is performed through the mouth under general anaesthesia.

In children under the age of 10, tonsillitis is common because the tonsils are exposed to many infections for the first time. Children who have tonsillitis may also have enlarged adenoids (left). Tonsils become smaller with age and therefore tonsillitis occurs far less frequently in adults (*see* **Pharyngitis and tonsillitis**, p.293).

What are the symptoms?
The symptoms of tonsillitis usually develop over a period of about 24–36 hours. The symptoms of the condition may include:
- Sore throat and discomfort when swallowing.
- Enlarged and tender lymph nodes in the neck.
- Fever.
- Headache.
- Abdominal pain.

Babies and children who are too young to talk are unable to tell their parents they have a sore throat, but they may refuse to eat or drink because of the discomfort when swallowing. They may also be lethargic and irritable.

Sometimes, a painful abscess called quinsy (also known as peritonsillar abscess) forms next to a tonsil, causing difficulty in

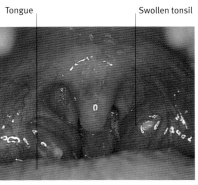

Tongue — Swollen tonsil

Tonsillitis
These tonsils have become swollen and inflamed as a result of an infection, a condition known as tonsillitis.

opening the mouth and swallowing. In young children, the rapid rise in temperature at the start of tonsillitis may cause a convulsion (*see* **Febrile convulsions**, p.550).

What can I do?
You may be able to make your child more comfortable by practising simple self-help measures at home. To bring down a fever, you can give your child liquid paracetamol or ibuprofen at the recommended dose, and you should encourage your child to drink small amounts of fluid at regular intervals, particularly if he or she has been vomiting (*see* **Bringing down a fever**, p.165). This will help to prevent dehydration, which can be serious. Cold, nonacidic drinks such as milk can help to relieve a sore throat, but older children may prefer ice cream or ice lollies. Older children may also find that sucking throat lozenges or gargling with warm salt water helps to relieve a sore throat.

You should consult the doctor if self-help measures do not bring down body temperature, if your child is taking very little fluid, or if symptoms do not improve in 24 hours.

What might the doctor do?
The doctor will examine your child's throat and may take a swab to test for bacterial infection. He or she may also look inside your child's ears to check for an ear infection (*see* **Otoscopy**, p.374). If the doctor suspects a bacterial throat infection, a course of antibiotics (p.572) will be prescribed.

Most children recover fully from tonsillitis within a few days. However, if your child is not drinking adequate amounts of fluid, he or she may become dehydrated and need to be admitted to hospital for treatment with intravenous fluids and antibiotics. If quinsy has developed, the abscess may need to be surgically drained.

What is the prognosis?
Some children have frequent episodes of tonsillitis, but by the age of 10 these bouts are usually rare. If a child misses school regularly because of tonsillitis, the doctor may recommend surgical removal of the tonsils (*see* **Tonsillectomy and adenoidectomy**, above, left).

Disorders of the nervous system

The nervous system consists of the brain, the spinal cord, and the network of nerves that extends throughout the body. Serious disorders of this system are uncommon in children, although disabling conditions may be present from birth due to defects that occur during pregnancy. The nervous system is sometimes affected by minor disorders and, rarely, by infections and cancers.

Damage to the nervous system, either before birth or in early childhood, can result in varying degrees of physical disability. The first articles in this section describe defects that occur during the development of the spinal cord and brain, causing disorders such as spina bifida and cerebral palsy.

Children are commonly affected by minor disorders of the nervous system, such as headache and migraine, which are described next. Migraine may be more difficult to recognize in young children than in adults because the main symptom is often abdominal pain or vomiting rather than headache. Further articles discuss serious disorders of great concern to parents, including meningitis, which is a dangerous infection of the coverings of the brain and spinal cord, and Reye's syndrome, an inflammation of the brain and liver. The final articles describe tumours of the brain and of the spinal cord, both of which are rare in children.

Epilepsy (p.324), which usually develops in childhood, is discussed in general nervous system disorders.

KEY ANATOMY

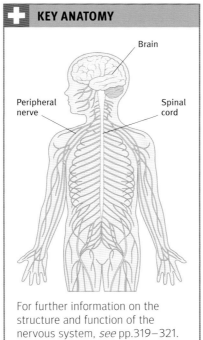

For further information on the structure and function of the nervous system, see pp.319–321.

Neural tube defects

Developmental abnormalities of the brain and spinal cord and their protective coverings

 Present from birth

 Sometimes run in families

 Taking certain drugs during pregnancy is a risk factor

 Gender is not a significant factor

Neural tube defects occur during pregnancy as a result of abnormalities in the embryo's development. The neural tube, which develops along the back of the embryo by about the third week of pregnancy, later becomes the brain and spinal cord and their coverings. If this tube fails to close completely, defects in any of these body parts can result.

Most commonly, the spinal cord and vertebrae are affected, causing a disorder known as spina bifida. The effects of spina bifida vary from dimpling or a tuft of hair at the base of the spine and a minor abnormality of the vertebrae to complete exposure of part of the spinal cord, known as a myelomeningocele. Rarely, the brain and skull are affected. Since the discovery in 1992 that folic acid taken during early pregnancy provides protection against neural tube defects, spina bifida is becoming less common.

The cause of neural tube defects is not fully understood, but they tend to run in families, which suggests genetic factors. Certain types of anticonvulsant drug (p.590), such as sodium valproate, are associated with neural tube defects if they are taken during pregnancy.

What are the symptoms?

The symptoms of a neural tube defect depend upon its severity. Often, there are no obvious symptoms, and spina bifida may be diagnosed only if minor conditions, such as backache, occur in adult life. The symptoms of a severe defect will become apparent at varying stages in childhood; they mainly affect the lower body and include:

■ Paralysis or weakness of the legs.
■ Absence of sensation in the legs.
■ Abnormalities in the functioning of the bladder and bowels.

About 8 in 10 children who have severe spina bifida also have a build-up of fluid within the brain (see **Hydrocephalus**, p.548). Occasionally, learning difficulties may develop. In some cases, neural tube defects lead to meningitis, a serious infection of the membranes covering the brain and spinal cord (see **Meningitis in children**, p.549).

How is it diagnosed?

Most neural tube defects are detected during routine antenatal blood tests and ultrasound scanning (see **Ultrasound scanning in pregnancy**, p.512). If a neural tube defect is detected, the implications will be explained to the parents and they may be asked whether they wish to continue with the pregnancy.

After birth, a baby with a neural tube defect will probably have CT scanning (p.132) or MRI (p.133) of the spine to assess the severity of the defect.

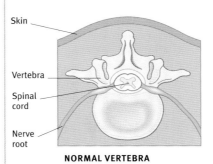

NORMAL VERTEBRA

Skin
Vertebra
Spinal cord
Nerve root

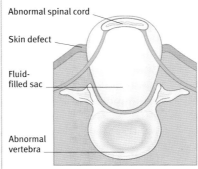

MYELOMENINGOCELE

Abnormal spinal cord
Skin defect
Fluid-filled sac
Abnormal vertebra

Neural tube defect
A myelomeningocele, a severe neural tube defect, occurs when the vertebrae are not fully formed. The spinal cord, contained in fluid-filled membranes, bulges outwards through a defect in the skin.

▶ TREATMENT

Shunt for hydrocephalus

A shunt is a drainage tube inserted into the brain to treat hydrocephalus, a disorder in which cerebrospinal fluid builds up in the brain cavities. The shunt diverts the excess fluid to another part of the body where it can be absorbed into the bloodstream. The fluid is released through a valve when pressure increases and drains into either the abdominal cavity or, rarely, a chamber in the heart.

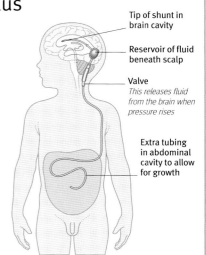

Tip of shunt in brain cavity

Reservoir of fluid beneath scalp

Valve
This releases fluid from the brain when pressure rises

Extra tubing in abdominal cavity to allow for growth

Inserting the shunt
The tip of the shunt is inserted through the skull into the fluid-filled cavity in the brain. The drainage tube is then passed under the skin and ends in the abdomen.

What is the treatment?

If the defect is minor, no treatment is necessary. However, if a baby has a serious defect, he or she is likely to require surgery shortly after birth. If hydrocephalus is present, a drainage tube will probably be inserted to release excess fluid and also to prevent further fluid build-up in the cavities of the brain (see **Shunt for hydrocephalus**, above).

Even with surgery, children who are born with severe defects will be permanently disabled and will need lifelong care. Practical and emotional support will be provided for the whole family. An affected child will often need regular physiotherapy (p.620) to keep as mobile as possible, and some children may need a wheelchair. Training in the regular use of a urinary catheter may be necessary for children who cannot pass urine normally (see **Bladder catheterization**, p.455). Some children may need special teaching. Many families find support through joining a self-help group.

Can it be prevented?

You can reduce the risk of your baby having a neural tube defect by taking the recommended dose of folic acid supplements before conception and during the first 12 weeks of pregnancy. Your doctor may recommend that you take a higher dose if you already have an affected child. If a close blood relative has a neural tube defect, a couple who are planning a pregnancy may wish to seek genetic counselling (p.151) because their children may be at increased risk of the disorder.

What is the prognosis?

Children with only minor defects have a normal life expectancy. If symptoms affecting posture develop, there may be an increased risk of developing osteoarthritis (p.221). Children with extensive damage to the brain and/or the spinal cord may have a reduced life expectancy.

Hydrocephalus

An abnormal build-up of fluid within the skull, also known as water on the brain

 Age and genetics as risk factors depend on the cause

 Gender and lifestyle are not significant factors

Hydrocephalus is an uncommon condition that occurs mainly in premature babies or with other disorders present from birth, such as spina bifida (*see* **Neural tube defects**, p.547).

Cerebrospinal fluid (CSF) is produced in the cavities of the brain and flows around the brain and spinal cord, protecting them from injury. Hydrocephalus develops if CSF builds up in the cavities of the brain, causing them to enlarge. This build-up occurs when the system that drains the CSF away from the brain is damaged or blocked or if excess CSF is produced. In such cases, the resulting increase in pressure in the skull may lead to brain damage.

Hydrocephalus may be caused by a brain defect that is present from birth. The disorder also sometimes develops as a result of meningitis, a serious infection of the membranes covering the brain and spinal cord (*see* **Meningitis in children**, opposite page), or a brain tumour (*see* **Brain and spinal cord tumours in children**, p.550).

What are the symptoms?

The symptoms vary according to the age of the child, but the following may occur in all affected children:

■ Vomiting.
■ Drowsiness.
■ Reluctance to settle down.

In young babies, the skull bones are not yet fused and are able to separate to some extent to accommodate excess fluid. For this reason, the first signs of hydrocephalus in babies may be an enlarged head that grows too fast and widening of the fontanelles (the soft areas on the top of a baby's skull). In older children with hydrocephalus, the head does not enlarge because the skull bones have fused, and headache due to pressure may be an early symptom.

Left untreated, hydrocephalus may lead to seizures and to cerebral palsy (right), in which movement and posture are affected. The disorder may also affect vision and hearing and can result in poor intellectual development.

How is it diagnosed?

Hydrocephalus can sometimes be diagnosed during pregnancy with routine ultrasound scanning (*see* **Ultrasound scanning in pregnancy**, p.512).

If the condition is suspected after birth, the doctor will arrange for ultrasound scanning (p.135) or CT scanning (p.132) of the child's head to look for obstructions or other abnormalities.

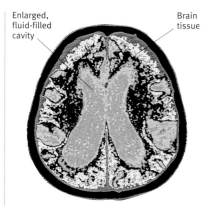

Enlarged, fluid-filled cavity / Brain tissue

Hydrocephalus
In this CT scan, the small cavities in the centre of the brain have been enlarged by an abnormal build-up of fluid, a condition known as hydrocephalus.

What is the treatment?

A child who has hydrocephalus usually needs surgery. During the operation, a narrow flexible tube, called a shunt, is inserted into a cavity in the brain to drain away the excess fluid (*see* **Shunt for hydrocephalus**, p.547). The tube is normally left in place permanently.

In addition, the child may be prescribed drugs that will slow down the production of CSF in the brain. Underlying causes of obstruction, such as a brain tumour, will be treated.

Some children with hydrocephalus are able to lead normal lives if they are given treatment before significant brain damage occurs. However, if the condition is severe or is left untreated, resulting in physical disabilities or difficulties with learning, affected children and their families will need long-term practical and psychological support.

Parents who have a child with hydrocephalus may wish to consider genetic counselling (p.151) because there is an increased risk of the condition occurring in subsequent children.

Cerebral palsy

Abnormalities of movement and posture caused by damage to the immature brain

 Age as a risk factor depends on the cause

 Gender, genetics, and lifestyle are not significant factors

Cerebral palsy is not a specific disease but a general term used to describe a group of disorders affecting movement and posture. These disorders all result from damage to the developing brain either before or during birth or during a child's early years. Children with cerebral palsy lack normal control of limbs and posture, but their intellect is often unaffected. Although the damage to the brain does not progress, the disabilities it causes change as a child grows. Many children have symptoms that are hardly noticeable, but other children may be severely disabled. Cerebral palsy affects about 1 in 400 children born in the UK.

What are the causes?

In many cases of cerebral palsy, there is no obvious cause. However, the fetus can be damaged by an infection, such as rubella or cytomegalovirus, transmitted from the mother during pregnancy (*see* **Congenital infections**, p.530). Cerebral palsy may also result if a baby is deprived of oxygen during a difficult birth (*see* **Problems during delivery**, p.518). The disorder can develop in premature babies, whose immature brains are often prone to abnormal bleeding (*see* **Problems of the premature baby**, p.530). During early childhood, cerebral palsy can develop after meningitis, an infection of the membranes around the brain (*see* **Meningitis in children**, opposite page), or after a head injury (p.322).

What are the symptoms?

If brain damage has occurred during pregnancy or birth, a newborn baby may be limp and unable to feed properly. Even if the symptoms are vague, such as a reluctance to settle down, parents may suspect that there is a problem from an early age. More commonly, symptoms do not appear until after 6 months of age and may include:

■ Weakness or stiffness affecting one or more limbs.
■ Reluctance to use a limb.
■ Abnormal, uncontrolled movements.
■ Delay in achieving normal milestones in motor development (*see* **Developmental delay**, p.553).
■ Difficulty in swallowing.
■ Speech problems.
■ Chronic constipation (*see* **Constipation in children**, p.560).

Many children have vision disorders, such as squint (*see* **Strabismus**, p.555), and impaired hearing (*see* **Congenital deafness**, p.556). About 1 in 2 children has a learning disability (*see* **Generalized learning disabilities**, p.553).

Are there complications?

If a child with cerebral palsy has stiff limbs, he or she may experience difficulty in walking and have an abnormal posture. The disorder can also increase the risk of

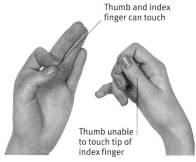

Thumb and index finger can touch

Thumb unable to touch tip of index finger

NORMAL   **ABNORMAL**

Poor coordination in cerebral palsy
A person with cerebral palsy often cannot coordinate movement in some parts of the body. The right hand shown here has poor coordination but the left hand is normal.

dislocated joints, particularly the hips. Sometimes, children with cerebral palsy develop epilepsy (p.324). Behavioural problems may develop if a child becomes frustrated because of his or her physical disabilities and inability to communicate clearly. Children with severe cerebral palsy are particularly susceptible to chest infections because they cannot cough effectively.

What might be done?

The diagnosis of cerebral palsy is often difficult to make in a very young child. As a child becomes older, the symptoms become more obvious. Once the condition is suspected, tests such as CT scanning (p.132) or MRI (p.133) may be carried out to identify brain damage.

Once the diagnosis is confirmed, the whole family has to adjust to the lifestyle changes that are often associated with caring for a child with cerebral palsy. Many affected children have only mild disabilities, requiring some physiotherapy (p.620), but children who have more severe disabilities usually need long-term therapy and specialist support. Emphasis is placed on assessing individual needs and helping a child to achieve his or her maximum potential. Physiotherapy to encourage normal posture plays a major part in the care of an affected child. Parents can encourage a child to play in a way that exercises the muscles and develops coordination.

If a child has only a minor physical disability, he or she may be able to attend a normal school. Children who have more severe disabilities or whose intellectual ability is affected may benefit from special schooling.

Complications and problems associated with cerebral palsy will be treated as necessary. For example, if your child has impaired hearing, he or she may require a hearing aid. Caring for a disabled child at home is stressful, and occasional residential care or residential schools can provide respite.

What is the prognosis?

Children with mild physical disabilities can usually lead active, full, and long lives and often live independently as adults. Severely disabled children, especially those with swallowing difficulties who are more prone to serious chest infections, have a lower life expectancy.

Headache in children

Pain of variable severity affecting the head, sometimes due to an underlying disorder

 More common in school-age children

 Gender, genetics, and lifestyle as risk factors depend on the cause

Headaches are a common symptom in childhood. They normally cause no more than temporary discomfort, but, if severe or recurrent, they may indicate an underlying condition that requires prompt medical treatment.

Young children, particularly those under the age of 5, are often unable to identify the precise location of pain. They may therefore complain of a headache when the problem is toothache, earache, or even a pain located elsewhere in the body, such as in the abdomen.

What are the causes?
There are many causes of headaches in children, most of which are not serious. In older children especially, the reasons for most headaches are often similar to those in adults (*see* **Headache**, p.320). However, parents may be understandably worried that their child is suffering from a serious illness such as meningitis, an inflammation of the membranes covering the brain (*see* **Meningitis in children**, right), or a brain tumour (*see* **Brain and spinal cord tumours in children**, p.550). These two disorders account for only a tiny percentage of childhood headaches, but it is important that parents are aware of the main symptoms so that they know when they should seek medical advice (*see* **Symptom chart 7: Headache**, p.50).

Short-lived headaches in children are usually caused by a viral infection, such as a common cold (p.164). These infections normally clear up within a few days without needing treatment. Many school-age children suffer from recurrent tension headaches (p.320). In the majority of cases, tension headaches last no longer than 24 hours and may be related to emotional stress either at school or at home. Problems with vision, such as shortsightedness (*see* **Myopia**, p.365), can sometimes result in persistent headaches. By the age of 15, about 1 in 10 children has experienced one or more migraine attacks (*see* **Migraine in children**, right).

What can I do?
If a severe headache occurs with vomiting or drowsiness, contact your doctor without delay. A child who has lost consciousness after a head injury, however briefly, should be taken to hospital immediately. If the headache is mild, encourage your child to rest and relieve his or her discomfort with paracetamol or ibuprofen (*see* **Painkillers**, p.589).

If you suspect that your child has headaches because of tension, you may be able to help him or her by identifying the particular anxiety. Recurrent headaches that have no obvious cause should be investigated by the doctor.

What might the doctor do?
If the doctor cannot find a cause for concern following a physical examination of your child, further tests are not usually necessary. If the doctor suspects meningitis, he or she will have the child admitted to hospital immediately for treatment. Rarely, your child may need CT scanning (p.132) or MRI (p.133) of the brain to investigate an injury or rule out the presence of a tumour.

If your child is normally well but has regular, persistent headaches, an eye test may be needed to exclude vision problems, and the doctor may refer him or her to an optician.

Migraine in children

Recurring symptoms that may include headache and abdominal pain

 Can occur as early as 2 years of age

 More common in girls

 Sometimes runs in families

 May be triggered by certain foods, fumes, and perfume

Migraine is a significant cause of headache in children, particularly girls, and by the age of 15 about 1 in 10 children has experienced an attack. The condition is known to occur in children as young as 2 years of age. However, childhood migraine often differs from that experienced by adults, and the disorder can sometimes be difficult to recognize. In younger children, the symptoms frequently include recurrent episodes of abdominal pain or vomiting, and the one-sided headaches and nausea that are typical of the condition in adults (*see* **Migraine**, p.320) may not occur.

What are the causes?
Why some children develop migraine is not fully understood, but the condition sometimes runs in families, suggesting that genetic factors may be involved. Migraine is thought to be associated with changes in the blood flow through the blood vessels inside the skull. There may also be temporary alterations in the levels of chemicals in the brain, which are probably responsible for triggering some of the symptoms elsewhere in the body.

Certain substances are known to trigger attacks of migraine. These include some types of food, commonly chocolate, cheese, citrus fruits, and alcohol, and inhaled substances such as perfume, petrol fumes, and tobacco smoke.

What are the symptoms?
In children under 8 years, the symptoms of migraine may not include headache. Symptoms develop gradually over a few hours, and a child may experience:
■ Pain in the centre of the abdomen.
■ Pale skin.
■ Tiredness.
■ Vomiting.
Often, these symptoms persist for several days. If children continue to have attacks of migraine as they grow older, they are likely to have symptoms more similar to those experienced by adults. These symptoms develop over a few hours and may include:

■ Visual disturbances, such as seeing flashing lights.
■ Headache, typically on one side.
■ Nausea and vomiting.
■ Dislike of bright lights.
Rarely, a child may experience temporary weakness in one arm or leg.

What might be done?
The doctor may be able to diagnose migraine from your child's symptoms. Occasionally, he or she may arrange for tests, such as CT scanning (p.132) or MRI (p.133) of the head, or, in young children, ultrasound scanning of the abdomen, to exclude other disorders.

Resting quietly in bed in a darkened room may make your child feel better. Taking painkillers (p.589) will also help to relieve a headache or abdominal pain. If the symptoms are severe, the doctor will probably prescribe specialized drugs (*see* **Antimigraine drugs**, p.590). Drugs such as beta-blockers (p.581) may also be prescribed as a long-term treatment to help to prevent continuing attacks of migraine. Your child's diet may also be reviewed by a dietitian to identify foods that may trigger migraine attacks.

With treatment, the symptoms of childhood migraine can usually be controlled. Often, the condition disappears completely as a child becomes older, although in some cases migraine attacks continue throughout adulthood.

Meningitis in children

Inflammation of the membranes that cover the brain and spinal cord, usually caused by a bacterial or viral infection

 Living in close communities is a risk factor

 Age as a risk factor depends on the cause

 Gender and genetics are not significant factors

Meningitis is a serious infection of the meninges (the membranes that cover the brain and spinal cord). Bacterial meningitis is a potentially fatal condition and causes between 150 and 200 deaths each year in the UK. Most cases of bacterial meningitis occur in infants under the age of 3 and in young people between the ages of about 15 and 25. Outbreaks of the infection can occur in communities where children are in close contact with one another, such as nurseries and schools.

Meningitis that is caused by a viral infection is a much less severe disorder and is rarely life-threatening.

What are the causes?
Bacterial meningitis in children is most often due to infection with *Neisseria meningitidis* (meningococcus), of which there are several types, or *Streptococcus pneumoniae*. Until recently, another major cause of meningitis

was the bacterium *Haemophilus influenzae* type b (Hib). In the UK, the introduction of routine immunization (p.13) for Hib and meningococcus type C has made these particular infections uncommon. A vaccine for meningococcus type B and a separate one for meningococcus types A, C, W, and Y are also available and were introduced as part of the routine immunization programme in 2015. Tuberculosis (p.300) can also cause bacterial meningitis but this form of the disease is uncommon in children.

Viral meningitis can be caused by a number of different viruses, including those responsible for chickenpox (p.165) and mumps (p.167).

What are the symptoms?
The symptoms of bacterial and viral meningitis are similar. However, bacterial meningitis tends to develop much more rapidly, and can cause serious illness within a few hours. Unlike adults, young children, especially those under 2 months of age, may not have obvious symptoms, and it is often difficult to distinguish the disease from other less serious infections. Symptoms likely to appear in young children include:
■ Fever.
■ Drowsiness or restlessness and high-pitched crying.
■ Vomiting and/or diarrhoea.
■ Reluctance to feed.
■ In meningococcal meningitis, a distinctive rash of flat, reddish-purple lesions varying in size from pinheads to large patches that do not fade when pressed (*see* **Checking a red rash**, p.57).
Older children may, in addition, have the characteristic symptoms of meningitis in adults, which are:
■ Severe headache and an extremely stiff neck, particularly when bending the head forwards.
■ Dislike of bright lights.
If bacterial meningitis is left untreated, seizures may occur, followed by loss of consciousness, coma (p.323), and possibly death. Rarely, pus may collect in the brain (*see* **Brain abscess**, p.327).

What might be done?
A child with meningitis needs urgent hospital treatment, often in an intensive therapy unit (p.618). When bacterial meningitis is suspected, one or more intravenous antibiotics (p.572) will be given before any tests are carried out. A lumbar puncture (p.326),

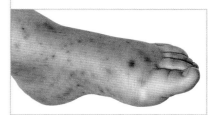

Rash of meningococcal meningitis
This distinctive rash, which can develop anywhere on the body and does not disappear when pressed, is a hallmark of meningococcal meningitis.

to remove a sample of fluid from around the spinal cord, will be performed to confirm the diagnosis. The antibiotics will be discontinued if the spinal fluid does not contain bacteria associated with meningitis. The child will be given fluids intravenously to prevent dehydration, and anticonvulsant drugs (p.590) may be prescribed if he or she has seizures.

Close contacts, such as family members and children in the same class as the child, may be given oral antibiotics as a precaution.

What is the prognosis?
Children with viral meningitis usually recover fully in about 2 weeks. Bacterial meningitis proves fatal in about 1 in 10 cases. About 1 in 10 children who recovers has long-term problems such as impaired hearing or epilepsy (p.324).

Febrile convulsions

Seizures caused by a high fever as a result of infection in a part of the body other than the brain

 Most common between the ages of 6 months and 5 years

 Slightly more common in boys

 Sometimes runs in families

 Lifestyle is not a significant factor

A febrile convulsion is the most common type of seizure in childhood and may affect as many as 1 in 20 children. The disorder occurs slightly more often in boys. Usually, a febrile convulsion occurs in the first 24 hours of a viral infection, such as a sore throat or common cold (p.164). Sometimes, a seizure may occur in association with a bacterial infection, such as an infection of the ears or upper respiratory tract. The convulsion develops in response to a rapid increase in body temperature that triggers an abnormal burst of electrical activity in the cells of the child's brain.

A febrile convulsion causes jerking body movements and is alarming for parents. However, the disorder is rarely serious, and it does not indicate a brain defect or epilepsy (p.324). Febrile convulsions sometimes run in families.

What are the symptoms?
The symptoms of a febrile convulsion may include:
- Loss of consciousness.
- Stiffening of the arms and legs and arching of the back.
- Abnormal movements of the limbs.
- Rolling upwards of the eyes.
- A slight pause in breathing, which may result in a bluish tinge to the skin.

A febrile convulsion usually lasts for less than about 5 minutes but may sometimes last longer. Your child will probably fall asleep afterwards. If your child has a seizure of any kind, you should contact the doctor immediately. If the convulsion lasts for longer than 5 minutes, call an ambulance at once.

What can I do?
You should not try to restrain a child who is having a febrile convulsion but protect him or her from injury by placing nearby objects out of reach and surrounding the child with pillows or rolled-up towels or blankets. After the convulsion is over, and when the child is fully conscious and awake enough to be able to swallow, he or she should be given a dose of liquid paracetamol (*see* **Painkillers**, p.589), which also helps to lower body temperature.

What might the doctor do?
The convulsion is likely to be over by the time the doctor sees your child. He or she will perform a physical examination to make sure that your child's temperature is coming down and to look for possible sources of the fever. The doctor may arrange for your child to be admitted to hospital, particularly if his or her body temperature remains high. A sample of cerebrospinal fluid may be extracted from around the spine (*see* **Lumbar puncture**, p.326) to check that the seizure was not caused by meningitis (*see* **Meningitis in children**, p.549). Other tests, such as urine tests or throat swabs, may also be performed to look for a bacterial infection.

If your child has prolonged or recurrent febrile convulsions, he or she may need to be given anticonvulsant drugs (p.590). The doctor will prescribe antibiotics (p.572) f a bacterial infection is present. Up to 1 in 3 children who have had a febrile convulsion will have another within a year. About 1 per cent of affected children will go on to develop epilepsy in later life.

Reye's syndrome

A rare illness in which there is sudden inflammation of the brain and liver

 Most common between the ages of 5 and 12

 Taking aspirin in childhood is a risk factor

 Gender and genetics are not significant factors

Reye's syndrome is an extremely rare condition, affecting fewer than 1 in 100,000 children each year in the UK. The disorder causes inflammation of the brain (*see* **Viral encephalitis**, p.326) and the liver (*see* **Acute hepatitis**, p.408) and can be fatal. It almost always occurs in children under the age of 12. The exact cause of Reye's syndrome is not known, but it is thought that in some cases the disorder may be associated with a viral infection, such as chickenpox (p.165). Aspirin is linked to Reye's syndrome and is no longer recommended for children under the age of 16.

The symptoms develop very rapidly over a few hours and may include vomiting, drowsiness, and seizures. As the disorder progresses, there may be loss of consciousness, coma (p.323), and eventually cessation of breathing.

What might be done?
If a child is very sick, he or she will be admitted to an intensive therapy unit (p.618). Tests to confirm the diagnosis include blood tests to assess liver function, a tracing of the electrical activity in the brain (*see* **EEG**, p.324), and CT scanning (p.132) or MRI (p.133) to look for brain swelling. A sample of the liver may be removed for microscopic examination (*see* **Liver biopsy**, p.410).

There is no specific cure for Reye's syndrome, but supportive treatment, such as mechanical ventilation, will be given until the condition improves. More than half of all children who have Reye's syndrome recover spontaneously. However, for those who lapse into a deep coma, the outlook is poor, and the condition may be fatal. In some cases, Reye's syndrome leads to long-term developmental problems, such as speech and learning difficulties.

Brain and spinal cord tumours in children

Abnormal growths in the brain or spinal cord that are usually cancerous

 Slightly more common in boys

 The underlying cause may be inherited

 Age and lifestyle are not significant factors

Tumours of the brain and spinal cord are rare in children but still account for almost 1 in 4 cases of all childhood cancers. The disorder is slightly more common in boys. Most of these tumours originate in the nerve cells of the brain or spine or in the cells surrounding the nerves. The tumours are usually cancerous but rarely spread elsewhere. The cause of such tumours is not fully understood, but the risk is increased if a child has the inherited disorders neurofibromatosis (p.536), in which tumours grow along the nerves, or tuberous sclerosis, in which growths form on the brain and become hardened over time.

What are the symptoms?
The symptoms of brain tumours usually develop gradually and at first may be vague, such as failure to gain weight in babies or unsatisfactory school performance in older children. Brain tumours are therefore often not diagnosed until they are quite large, when symptoms may include:
- Headache and vomiting, especially in the morning.
- Clumsiness and unsteadiness.
- Abnormal alignment of the eyes (*see* **Strabismus**, p.555).
- Change in personality.

Sometimes, excess fluid builds up in the brain cavities (*see* **Hydrocephalus**, p.548). If a tumour is in the spinal cord, the symptoms may include:
- Back pain.
- Inability to pass urine.
- Difficulty in walking.

Children with back pain should be seen by a doctor as soon as possible.

What might be done?
If the doctor is concerned that a child may have a brain or spinal cord tumour, he or she will arrange for imaging tests such as CT scanning (p.132) or MRI (p.133) to look for abnormalities. If a tumour is found, a small piece of tissue may be removed under general anaesthesia for microscopic examination.

Once the diagnosis has been confirmed, surgery is usually carried out to remove the tumour. Radiotherapy (p.158) may also be given, and in some cases, chemotherapy (p.157) may be used. If there is an accumulation of excess fluid around the brain, a shunt (a small drainage tube) may be inserted into the brain to divert the fluid into the abdomen (*see* **Shunt for hydrocephalus**, p.547).

If a child has a tumour, a team of professionals will be available to offer his or her whole family psychological support (*see* **Counselling**, p.624).

What is the prognosis?
Although brain and spinal tumours are serious and often diagnosed late, 1 in 2 children is alive 5 years after diagnosis. The outlook depends on the type of tumour. Some children who survive after treatment may have long-term physical disabilities or learning problems.

Neuroblastoma

A cancerous tumour that develops from nervous tissue, often in the adrenal gland

 More common under the age of 5

 Slightly more common in boys

 May be due to an abnormal gene

 Lifestyle is not a significant factor

Although rare, neuroblastomas are still the most common cancerous tumours in children under 1 year. The disorder is

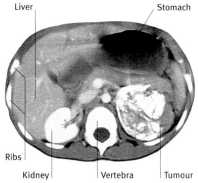

Neuroblastoma
This cross-sectional CT scan of a child's upper abdomen shows a neuroblastoma that has developed from the nervous tissue in one of the adrenal glands.

slightly more common in boys. Most of these tumours originate from nerve tissue that has not developed beyond the embryonic stage. Neuroblastomas may occur in the abdomen or, less commonly, in the chest or pelvic cavity and often spread elsewhere. About half of all neuroblastomas develop in the adrenal glands, above the kidneys. The cause of these tumours is not known, although a genetic factor is thought to be involved.

What are the symptoms?
The symptoms of neuroblastoma may be present from birth or develop gradually in childhood. They may include:
■ Lump in the abdomen.
■ Painless, bluish lumps on the skin.
■ Tiredness.
■ "Dancing" eye movements.
If a neuroblastoma spreads through the body, other symptoms may occur, such as bone pain or, if the lymph nodes are affected, swellings in the neck or armpits. Anaemia (p.271) may result if the cancer spreads to the bone marrow.

What might be done?
If the doctor suspects a neuroblastoma, he or she may arrange for a urine test to check for substances that indicate the presence of a tumour. The diagnosis is confirmed by a biopsy, in which a tissue sample is removed for examination. MRI (p.133) or radionuclide scanning (p.135) may be needed to find out if the cancer has spread elsewhere in the body. A bone marrow aspiration and biopsy (p.274) may also be performed to look for the spread of cancer to the bones. If possible, the tumour is removed surgically. Treatment with chemotherapy (p.157) and radiotherapy (p.158) may also be necessary.

If a tumour has not spread, about 9 in 10 children remain well 5 years after surgery. When a tumour has spread, the outlook is poor, with only about 2 in 10 children surviving more than a year after the diagnosis. In babies under 1 year of age, neuroblastomas may disappear without requiring treatment.

Developmental and psychological disorders

A child's development is a continuous process, marked by identifiable advances in skills and behaviour. The rate at which an individual develops is influenced by many factors, including the family environment and physical health. In some children, psychological disorders may cause developmental delays.

The first two articles in this section cover sleeping and eating problems, which can be very disruptive to the whole family but which can often be overcome with simple self-help measures. The following article covers childhood obesity, a problem that is becoming increasingly common in developed countries and one that could have long-term health consequences. Soiling (encopresis) is dealt with next, followed by an article that covers the more serious problems that may be caused by autism spectrum disorders, which result in failure to develop normal communication and social skills. Autism, which may be linked to brain abnormali-

ties, is a life long condition, but its effects can usually be reduced by appropriate education and therapy.

The next articles describe disorders that may delay children's achievement of certain developmental milestones. These range from generalized learning disabilities, which can affect all areas of development, to specific learning disabilities and speech difficulties in an otherwise normal child.

Attention deficit hyperactivity disorder and conduct disorder, covered in the last two articles, are behavioural disorders that tend to have underlying medical, psychiatric, or social causes. Affected children usually respond to skilled guidance and therapy.

Many children sleep through the night by the age of 12 months, but about 1 in 3 children has frequent wakeful nights until the age of 5 or even later. Sleeping problems rarely cause ill health but may disrupt family life and can affect school performance in older children.

Disrupted sleep in children is usually temporary and may occur only because of a lack of or change to daily routine. Sleeping problems may also be related to illnesses, such as ear infections or those causing a cough, or to anxiety, such as that caused by family quarrels.

What are the types?
Sleeping problems in children take various forms. In toddlers, one of the most common problems is an inability to settle down and go to sleep after being left alone at bedtime. Such restlessness is sometimes caused by anxiety about separation from a parent. Difficulty settling down can also be due to a noisy environment or fear of the dark. The problem may simply be due to bedtime being too early; children vary in the amount of sleep they need.

Most children wake briefly several times during the night without needing attention. However, sudden wakefulness is sometimes caused by nightmares, particularly in children about 5 years of age. Nightmares are commonly triggered by frightening or unusual experiences and, if they occur frequently, may be a sign that a child has a particular worry.

Night terrors are another type of sudden sleep disturbance, which may occur for no apparent reason. During an episode of night terror, a child experiences acute fear and may scream. Although the child seems to be awake, he or she is actually still asleep. If a child wakes from a night terror, he or she usually has little or no memory of the episode. Night terrors usually occur within about 2 hours of falling asleep and last only a few minutes. Just before a night terror, a child may appear restless.

Sleepwalking most often occurs in preschool and school-age children. A sleepwalking child will get out of bed and wander around aimlessly, usually finding his or her own way back to bed.

What might be done?
Simple measures are often effective in overcoming a sleeping problem. You should try to establish regular routines, with a bath and a story at the same time every night. There is no need to go to a child as soon as he or she cries; often, the crying will stop within a few minutes. If you think that poor sleeping or nightmares are related to an underlying anxiety, such as a frightening television programme or family stress, you should discuss the problem with your child.

If your child has night terrors, it may be possible to wake him or her in the restless period that precedes the terror. Once a

terror begins, there is little you can do except stay with the child until the fear recedes. In the case of sleepwalking, try not to wake the child but gently guide him or her back to bed.

You should consult the doctor if your child's sleep problem disrupts the family or if you think that nightmares or night terrors have a particular cause.

In most cases, providing a child with reassurance and introducing a routine will help to establish a normal sleeping pattern within a few weeks. Most children eventually learn to settle down at night and outgrow nightmares, night terrors, or sleepwalking. By the age of 8, few children have sleeping problems.

Eating problems in childhood are very common, affecting about 1 in 10 young children. Usually, the problem is part of growing up and disappears as the child matures. However, persistent problems may be linked to stresses in family life.

What are the types?
Some children appear to eat too little or are fussy about their food. Other children may overeat or have cravings for strange non-food substances.

Refusing food is often the way in which toddlers try to assert their independence, and the problem is serious only if normal growth or weight gain is affected. Food

SELF-HELP

Encouraging your child to eat
If your child is overly fussy about certain food or refuses to eat, the following hints may be helpful:
■ Keep the atmosphere relaxed at mealtimes. Do not put pressure on your child to eat everything on his or her plate.
■ Serve small portions. You can always give second helpings.
■ Avoid too many snacks and excessive fluids between meals.
■ Be imaginative when preparing food. Cut sandwiches into decorative shapes and create "pictures" on the plate with fruit and vegetables.
■ Do not persist in offering rejected foods. Keep them off the menu for a week or two.
■ Avoid distractions, such as toys or television, at mealtimes.

refusal in older children may be due to emotional distress and, in very severe cases, may be a sign of anorexia nervosa (p.348), particularly in girls. Loss of appetite, which is common during childhood illnesses, is not the same as food refusal, although it may also be caused by anxiety.

Fussy eating habits affect about 1 in 4 children of school age. The fussy child insists on eating only certain foods, but dietary problems rarely occur unless the range of foods is very narrow.

Pica is a craving to eat nonfood substances, such as soil, coal, or chalk. This disorder can sometimes be hazardous. For example, licking or eating certain types of paint can cause severe lead poisoning. Pica usually occurs in children who have other behavioural problems and is possibly associated with a nutritional deficiency, such as a lack of iron.

Overeating commonly leads to obesity. (*see* Obesity in children, below). A child may eat for comfort if he or she feels neglected or insecure.

What might be done?

If your child is reluctant to eat, there are practical ways in which you can help (*see* Encouraging your child to eat, p.551). However, if the child fails to gain weight, loses weight, or has pica, you should consult the doctor, who may refer your child to a child psychologist or psychiatrist.

Obesity in children

A condition in which a child is severely overweight

 Slightly more common with increasing age

 Sometimes runs in families; occasionally associated with certain genetic diseases

 Overeating and a sedentary lifestyle are risk factors

 Gender is not a significant factor

The number of overweight and obese children has increased steadily over the last two decades, and it is now estimated that about 1 in 5 children in the UK is obese. As with adults, obesity in children is assessed using body mass index (BMI) values. An individual's BMI is his or her weight (in kilograms) divided by his or her height (in metres) squared. Unlike in adults, there is no single BMI value that can be used to define overweight or obesity in children. Instead, percentiles are used; this is method of assessment that is based on the percentage of people (in this case, children) that is above or below a particular value (in this case, has a higher or lower BMI). A child is defined as obese if his or her BMI is above the 98th percentile, which means that his or her BMI is higher than that of 98 per cent of children of the same age. A child is con-

sidered overweight if his or her BMI is between the 91st percentile (i.e. 91 per cent of the same-age children have a lower BMI) and the 98th percentile (98 per cent have a lower BMI).

What are the causes?

By far the most common cause of childhood obesity is an unhealthy, high-calorie diet combined with lack of physical activity. Although childhood obesity sometimes runs in families, this is usually because of an unhealthy family lifestyle. However, in very rare cases, there may be a genetic cause for obesity, as in Prader–Willi syndrome, an inherited genetic abnormality that leads to compulsive overeating. Very occasionally, other medical conditions may also cause obesity, such as underactivity of the thyroid gland (*see* Hypothyroidism, p.432) or a brain tumour (p.327).

Are there complications?

During childhood, obesity may lead to a wide variety of health problems, including type 2 diabetes (*see* Diabetes mellitus, p.437); high blood cholesterol levels; high blood pressure (*see* Hypertension, p.242); and digestive system disorders, such as abdominal pain, gallstones (p.412), inflammation of the gallbladder (*see* Cholecystitis, p.413), inflammation of the pancreas (*see* Acute pancreatitis, p.413), and liver disease. The excess weight causes increased stress on the musculoskeletal system, which may lead to bone and joint problems, such as bow legs (*see* Minor leg and foot problems, p.541) or slipped femoral epiphysis (p.541). Accumulation of fat around the airways may cause respiratory problems such as asthma (p.295) and obstructive sleep apnoea (p.292) In some adolescent girls, obesity may also be associated with hormone-related problems, such as early onset of puberty, acne, menstrual irregularities, excessive body hair, and polycystic ovarian syndrome (p.477). As well as physical problems, obesity may also cause emotional and psychological problems, such as depression or eating disorders.

Children who are obese are more likely to be obese as adults and are therefore at increased risk of developing the numerous disorders associated with adult obesity (*see* Obesity in adults, p.400).

What might be done?

The whole family should eat a healthy, balanced diet, with plenty of fruit and vegetables and fresh, home-made food. Fast food, high-calorie snacks, and fizzy drinks should be avoided. You should encourage your child to take plenty of physical exercise, and consider limiting your child's time using a computer or watching television. It is better to reward healthy eating and exercise rather than punishing unhealthy habits. You should aim for a gradual return to a healthy weight, not a dramatic weight loss.

If these measures do not seem to be working or if you are concerned about your child's weight, you should consult your doctor. He or she will calculate your child's BMI, and will carry out a thorough examination to look for any signs of obesity-related disorders. The doctor may also perform tests to check for any underlying disorder that might be a cause of the obesity.

If an underlying causative disorder is found, treatment for the disorder will probably also lead to weight loss. However, in most cases, the cause is simply an unhealthy lifestyle, and the doctor will probably refer you to a dietitian and possibly other specialists, such as a child psychologist and physiotherapist. Occasionally, the doctor may recommend family therapy for all the family members.

Other treatments, such as anti-obesity drugs or surgery (for example, gastric banding) are only recommended in exceptional cases for older children when all other possibilities have failed and the child remains extremely obese and has obesity-related health problems.

Encopresis

Inappropriate defecation after the age at which bowel control is usually attained

 Considered abnormal only after about the age of 4

 More common in boys

 Stress is a risk factor

 Genetics is not a significant factor

Most children have achieved bowel control by the age of 3. If a child is still soiling by the age of 4, there may be a psychological or physical reason. Soiling problems, which are more common in boys, are known as encopresis. Sometimes, the behaviour is simply the result of inadequate toilet training. However, children occasionally begin soiling again after successful training. The most common cause of this recurrence is overflow of liquid faeces from above a hard, constipated stool (*see* Constipation in children, p.560). Some children pass normal faeces in unacceptable places, such as behind furniture. This soiling may be related to emotional stress.

What might be done?

A sympathetic approach to encopresis is vital, because scolding and criticizing a child often makes the problem worse. Usually, patient toilet training is all that is required. If you suspect that your child is constipated, you should change his or her diet to include more fibre.

If simple measures are not effective, you should consult your doctor. In the case of severe constipation, the doctor will probably advise on diet and may prescribe

laxatives (p.597). Causes of emotional distress can often be identified after discussion with the child.

Encopresis usually disappears with unhurried toilet training once constipation has been treated or emotional problems have been addressed.

Autism spectrum disorders

Severely impaired development of normal communication and social skills

 Usually develop before the age of 3

 More common in boys

 Sometimes run in families

 Lifestyle is not a significant factor

Autism was first identified in 1943 and is now estimated to affect about 1 in 100 children in the UK. There are varying forms of autism known as autism spectrum disorders, and affected children have a wide range of symptoms. In general, there is a failure to develop language and communication skills, inability to form social relationships, and a marked need to follow routines. These disorders are more common in boys.

At least 2 in 3 autistic children have generalized learning disabilities (opposite page). Rarely, affected children have normal or above-average intelligence, a form of autism known as Asperger's syndrome. Autism spectrum disorders are possibly caused by abnormalities of the brain. The disorders sometimes run in families, which suggests that genetic factors may be involved. In a very small proportion of autistic children, a specific genetic abnormality is identified as a cause of their condition, such as fragile X syndrome (p.533).

What are the symptoms?

Some autistic children show symptoms from birth, such as arching the back to avoid physical contact. In infancy, a child with autism may bang his or her head against the side of the cot. Other children may appear normal until they are about 12–18 months old, when the following symptoms become apparent:

■ Failure to develop normal speech.
■ Absence of normal facial expression and body language.
■ Lack of eye contact.
■ Tendency to spend time alone.
■ Lack of imaginative play.
■ Repetitive behaviour, such as rocking and hand flapping.
■ Obsession with specific objects or particular routines.
■ Severe learning difficulties.

Rarely, an autistic child has an exceptional skill, such as a particular aptitude for technical drawing, mathematics, or playing a musical instrument. Some affected children develop epilepsy (p.324). Children who have Asperger's syndrome may develop normal speech and language but have difficulty communicating with other people. These children are also rigid in their behaviour and cannot tolerate changes in routine.

Are there complications?

Autism spectrum disorders often have a devastating effect on family life. Bringing up an autistic child can be stressful, especially when the child is unable to show normal responsiveness and affection. Parents may find it difficult to take the child to public places because of his or her unusual or difficult behaviour. Other children in the family may feel neglected because an autistic sibling needs so much attention. A child with autism may also be at risk of self-harm.

What might be done?

Autism spectrum disorders are often first identified by parents who notice that their child's behaviour is different from that of other children in the same age group. The doctor will usually refer the child to a child development specialist or child psychiatrist. There are no specific tests to confirm the diagnosis. However, when a genetic disorder such as fragile X syndrome is suspected, blood tests may be performed to look for the genetic abnormality.

There is no cure for autism spectrum disorders. Treatment normally focuses on education designed to maximize a child's potential. Language and speech therapy (p.621) can improve communication skills. Behaviour therapy (p.622) can help to replace abnormal behaviours with more appropriate ones, and occupational therapy can improve physical skills. A highly structured daily routine is usually recommended.

What is the prognosis?

Most children with autism spectrum disorders cannot lead independent lives and require long-term care. Some people with Asperger's syndrome achieve academic success, although they may always have poor social skills.

Developmental delay

Delay of a child in achieving the abilities expected at a particular age

 Usually apparent by the age of 5

 Lack of stimulation is a risk factor

 Gender and genetics as risk factors depend on the cause

There are significant stages in the first few years of life, known as developmental milestones, when a child is normally expected to have acquired certain basic physical, intellectual, and social skills. Children achieve these milestones at different ages but usually within an established typical age range. Failure to reach the milestones within this range is known as developmental delay.

What are the types?

Delays may be of varying severity and can affect one or more area of development. Children are usually mobile by about 9 months, and most are walking by 15 months. A delay in walking frequently runs in families and often has no obvious cause; most children catch up eventually and continue to develop normally. However, children who have a severe underlying disability, such as cerebral palsy (p.548), will have long-term difficulties with mobility.

Some children are slow to develop movements that involve good hand–eye coordination or fine control, such as catching a ball or using a pencil. These children should be monitored carefully because they are at risk of experiencing specific learning disabilities (right) during their school years.

Delay in acquiring speech and language ranges from minor difficulties in increasing vocabulary (*see* **Speech and language difficulties**, p.554) to the severe communication problems often associated with autism spectrum disorders (opposite page). Sometimes, delay is due to a lack of stimulation in the child's environment. Hearing problems, which can be due to disorders such as chronic secretory otitis media (p.557), may also be a cause of delayed development in speech and language skills.

Certain basic accomplishments, such as learning to use the toilet unaided, are acquired only slowly in some children. Usually, these skills improve with time, but occasionally there may be underlying problems (*see* **Bedwetting**, p.565, and **Encopresis**, opposite page).

Developmental delays that affect all areas of learning and general ability can be caused by underlying disorders, such as Down's syndrome (p.533) or inborn errors of metabolism (p.561), but often the underlying cause cannot be identified. Such delays in development can lead later to a diagnosis of generalized learning disabilities (right).

What might be done?

Developmental delays are usually first noticed by parents who are concerned when a child does not reach the normal milestones for his or her age group. A delay may also be detected at routine developmental checkups during the first 5 years of life. If a problem is suspected, your doctor may arrange for a full developmental assessment, which normally includes hearing tests (*see* **Hearing tests in children**, p.557) and vision tests (*see* **Vision tests in children**, p.555). Tests may be performed on a sample of the child's blood to check for a genetic abnormality.

A child with delay in one area of development may only need encouragement to begin to catch up. Many children with mild delays develop normally over a period of time, especially if the cause is understimulation and the problem is given appropriate treatment. Other children benefit from help, such as speech therapy (p.621), in particular areas of development. A child with more severe delays will need specialized treatment.

Generalized learning disabilities

Difficulties with all areas of learning experienced by children with significantly lower than average intelligence

 Usually becomes apparent in early childhood

 More common in boys

 Genetics as a risk factor depends on the cause

 Lifestyle is not a significant factor

A child with generalized learning disabilities has poor intellectual skills, leading to developmental delay (left). Generalized learning disabilities can affect speech, language, reading, and writing. Physical development may be affected, causing general clumsiness and poor hand–eye cordination. Behavioural problems may also develop.

There is often no obvious cause for mild generalized learning disabilities, which may not be noticeable until an affected child reaches school age. Severe learning disabilities usually have an obvious cause, such as the genetic disorders Down's syndrome (p.533) or fragile X syndrome (p.533).

What might be done?

Mild generalized learning disabilities are usually first suspected by parents or teachers when a child fails to develop skills at the same rate as his or her peers or is experiencing difficulties at school. In more severe cases, delays in development are usually detected at an early stage in childhood, often during routine developmental checkups.

If a child is thought to have generalized learning disabilities, the doctor will probably arrange for a full developmental assessment, including hearing tests (*see* **Hearing tests in children**, p.557) and vision tests (*see* **Vision tests in children**, p.555). Blood tests to check for evidence of genetic abnormalities may also be performed.

Most affected children have special educational needs and will benefit from attending classes or schools where they can have individual attention. Parents will be supported by a team of specialists, who may provide physiotherapy (p.620) and speech therapy (p.621).

Many children with mild generalized learning disabilities can do well if they receive appropriate education and support. Those who are severely affected usually need lifelong supervision.

Specific learning disabilities

Difficulties in one or several areas of learning in a child of average or above average intelligence

 Usually become apparent between the ages of 3 and 7

 More common in boys

 Sometimes run in families

 Lifestyle is not a significant factor

A child whose development is delayed in one or several areas of learning but who has normal intelligence probably has a specific learning disability. Such disabilities are thought to affect up to 15 in 100 otherwise normally developed children and are common cause of poor achievement at school. Specific learning disabilities are more common in boys.

Dyslexia is a common example of a specific learning disability and affects a child's ability to read or write. In dyscalculia, a child has specific problems with mathematics. Dyspraxia is a learning disability that affects coordination, particularly finely controlled movement, often leading to clumsiness.

In most cases, the cause of a particular learning disability is not known. However, such conditions sometimes run in families, suggesting that genetic factors may be involved. In some cases, specific learning disabilities are due to problems with vision or hearing.

What are the symptoms?

The symptoms of specific learning disabilities are usually first recognized in early school years and may include:

- Difficulty coping with reading, writing, and/or mathematics.
- Problems telling left from right.
- Poor coordination and difficulty with sports other physical activities.

A child may also become frustrated and develop behavioural problems, such as extreme shyness or aggression.

What might be done?

If a specific learning disability is suspected, a full assessment of a child's academic and developmental skills will be made. Hearing tests (*see* **Hearing tests in children**, p.557) and vision tests (*see* **Vision tests in children**, p.555) may also be performed to rule out the presence of physical conditions that may cause delays in learning.

Parents and teachers should work together to encourage an affected child. In many cases, specialized teaching is necessary. Disorders causing impaired hearing or vision can often be treated successfully. Many children do well if the appropriate remedial treatment is given, but some children continue to experience difficulties throughout life.

Speech and language difficulties

The slow or abnormal development of understanding and expression of language

 Usually develop in early childhood

 Gender, genetics, and lifestyle as risk factors depend on the type

There is wide variation in the age at which speech and language skills are acquired, but most children are able to communicate verbally well before the age of 3. Many children have some type of speech and language difficulty in their early years, commonly only a minor impediment, such as a lisp, that rapidly improves with increasing maturity.

A common cause of delay in speech and language development is hearing impairment (*see* Chronic secretory otitis media, p.557, and Congenital deafness, p.556). Children who have cerebral palsy (p.558) and those with a cleft lip and palate (p.558) may have difficulty coordinating the movements of their mouth and tongue. Slowness in acquiring speech and language skills may be due to lack of intellectual stimulation or developmental delay (p.553). Severe generalized learning disabilities (p.553) may cause speech and language difficulties.

Difficulties with fluency of speech, for example stuttering, affect about 3 in 100 children, especially boys, and sometimes run in families.

What might be done?
A speech or language difficulty may first be noticed by parents or teachers or at a routine developmental checkup. A full assessment of the child's development and hearing will then be made.

A child with a speech or language difficulty usually catches up with his or her peers when given appropriate guidance. Impaired hearing will be treated when possible. Stuttering can often be improved with speech therapy (p.621).

Once the underlying cause is treated, most speech and language difficulties improve. However, if there is a physical cause, such as cerebral palsy, the speech or language difficulty may persist.

Attention deficit hyperactivity disorder

A behavioural disorder in which a child consistently has a high level of activity and/or difficulty attending to tasks

 Usually develops in early childhood

 More common in boys

 Often runs in families

 Lifestyle is not a significant factor

Attention deficit hyperactivity disorder (ADHD), also sometimes known as hyperkinetic disorder, is a condition that affects an estimated 3–9 per cent of children in the UK. The disorder, which is more common in boys, should not be confused with the normal boisterous conduct of a healthy child. Children with ADHD consistently show abnormal patterns of behaviour over a period of time. An affected child is likely to be restless, unable to sit still for more than a few moments, inattentive, and impulsive.

The causes of ADHD are not fully understood. However, the disorder often runs in families, which suggests that genetic factors may be involved. ADHD is not, as popularly believed, a result of poor parenting or abuse.

What are the symptoms?
The symptoms of ADHD develop in early childhood, usually between the ages of 3 and 7, and may include:
- Inability to finish tasks.
- Short attention span and inability to concentrate in class.
- Difficulty following instructions.
- Tendency to talk excessively and frequently interrupt others.
- Difficulty waiting or taking turns.
- Inability to play quietly alone.
- Physical impulsiveness.

Children with ADHD may have difficulty forming friendships. Self-esteem is often low because an affected child is frequently scolded and criticized.

What might be done?
The doctor will probably refer a child with suspected ADHD to a child psychiatry team. The diagnosis is normally made following discussion with parents and observation of the child. However, ADHD is often difficult to diagnose in preschool children. Parents have a key role in their child's treatment and are usually given training in techniques that help to improve the child's behaviour. These techniques are based on giving praise for good behaviour rather than criticism for inappropriate conduct. An affected child may also benefit from structured teaching in small groups.

For some children, the doctor may prescribe drugs that help to improve concentration and reduce disruptive behaviour (*see* Central nervous system stimulant drugs, p.593).

In most affected children, the disorder continues throughout adolescence, although the behavioural problems may become less severe in older children. A small proportion of those with ADHD later develop conduct disorder (below), in which a child consistently displays antisocial and unruly behaviour.

Conduct disorder

A behavioural disorder in which a child persistently behaves in an antisocial or disruptive manner

 More common in late childhood and adolescence

 More common in boys

 Sometimes runs in families

 An emotionally unstable home environment is a risk factor

Most children are mischievous from time to time, and some may become rebellious, especially as they reach adolescence. Conduct disorder is suspected only if a child or adolescent persists in antisocial or disruptive behaviour.

Many children with conduct disorder have failed to acquire a sense of right and wrong. They may have grown up in an unstable home in which there is family discord or violence and lack of parental supervision. Children with attention deficit hyperactivity disorder (left) are at increased risk of developing conduct disorder in later childhood.

Conduct disorder is more common in boys. The antisocial behaviour usually becomes more obvious towards adolescence, when an affected child may start to become aggressive and play truant from school. In some cases, a child will indulge in substance or alcohol abuse or become involved in criminal activities, such as theft, vandalism, assault, and arson. Children with conduct disorder often have low self-esteem and find it difficult to form relationships.

What might be done?
A diagnosis of conduct disorder is usually based on a psychiatric assessment of the child's behavioural patterns.

The treatment for conduct disorder is always aimed at the whole family. Therapy will be directed at overcoming conflicts or tensions within the family. Parents will be encouraged to reinforce good behaviour, and an aggressive child will be taught how to control his or her anger and to be considerate to others. However, in many children who have conduct disorder, antisocial behaviour persists into adulthood.

Eye and ear disorders

Vision and hearing are important to a child's development because the eyes and ears collect information about the environment and play a key role in the acquisition of speech and language. Eye and ear disorders are often diagnosed during routine examinations in childhood.

The first article covers congenital blindness, in which a child is born with impaired vision. The following articles discuss conditions such as strabismus, in which vision is affected due to misalignment of the gaze of the eyes, and amblyopia, in which a child's vision fails to develop normally. The remaining articles cover ear disorders that affect children, beginning with congenital deafness. A common cause of earache in children is acute otitis media. Chronic secretory otitis media is covered in the following article. Eye and ear disorders that can affect people of any age are covered in other sections of the book (*see* Eyes and vision, pp.351–369, and Ears, hearing, and balance, pp.370–373).

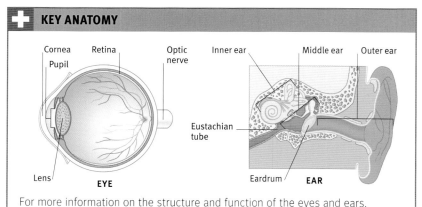

KEY ANATOMY

Cornea · Pupil · Retina · Optic nerve · Lens · EYE

Inner ear · Middle ear · Outer ear · Eustachian tube · Eardrum · EAR

For more information on the structure and function of the eyes and ears, *see* pp.351–369 and pp.370–380.

Congenital blindness

Severely impaired vision that is present from birth

 Present at birth

 Sometimes runs in families

 Gender and lifestyle are not significant factors

Vision plays a very important part in a child's early development. Impaired vision at birth can cause serious delay in certain aspects of development and may lead to learning disabilities, particularly when it is associated with other difficulties, such as congenital deafness (p.556).

Most children considered blind from birth do have some vision, even though it may be as little as recognition of light and dark or shapes.

What are the causes?

In the developed world, many cases of congenital blindness run in families and may be due to a genetic disorder. Other important causes are congenital infections (p.530) such as the protozoal infection toxoplasmosis (p.176) and the viral infection rubella (p.168). These infections are transmitted from the mother to the developing fetus during pregnancy and may lead to impaired vision in a newborn baby. However, congenital rubella is now rare in the developed world due to routine immunization. A baby's eyes may also be affected by cataracts (p.357), in which the eye lenses are opaque, or glaucoma (p.358), in which the optic nerve is damaged due to increased pressure within the eyes. Congenital blindness may also be caused by damage to the brain as a result of lack of oxygen during birth.

What are the symptoms?

Parents usually become aware that their baby has a vision problem within a few weeks of birth. He or she may be less responsive than other babies, lying quietly to make the most of his or her hearing. Parents may also notice that their baby:
- Is unable to fix his or her eyes on a close object.
- Has random eye movements.
- Does not smile by the age of 6 weeks.
- Has abnormally large, cloudy eyes if glaucoma is present.

Parents may find it difficult to bond with a quiet baby who does not smile.

How is it diagnosed?

If congenital blindness is not suspected by the baby's parents, it will probably be picked up during a routine examination in infancy. A child suspected of having impaired vision will be referred to a specialist for an examination and tests (see Vision tests in children, right). His or her hearing will also be tested (see Hearing

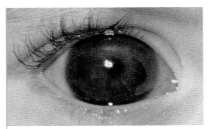

Congenital glaucoma
This child's eye appears enlarged and cloudy due to increased pressure within the eye caused by congenital glaucoma.

tests in children, p.557) because, if the child is severely visually impaired, he or she will rely more on hearing.

What is the treatment?

It is possible to improve vision in only a small number of babies, such as those with cataracts or glaucoma. Early treatment of these conditions is important. Cataracts are usually removed surgically within the first month of life (see Cataract surgery, p.357). Glaucoma may also be treated by surgery to allow fluid to drain from the eye.

If vision cannot be improved, much can be done to help a child to make maximum use of other senses or what little vision he or she has. If your child is diagnosed as blind, a team of specialists, including a teacher for the blind, will be available to give you and your child support and care. You will also be given advice on how to stimulate your child using speech, sounds, and touch and how to

adapt your home so that your child is able to explore it safely and develop self-confidence. Some children require special schooling to learn braille, a system of raised dots that allows blind people to read and write.

Genetic counselling (p.151) is available for parents of an affected child who wish to have more children or for prospective parents who are blind.

What is the prognosis?

Children treated for cataracts or glaucoma will probably still have impaired vision but often have enough sight to perform most activities unaided. Many blind or visually impaired children with no other disabilities go on to have successful personal and professional lives.

Strabismus

Abnormal alignment of the gaze of one of the eyes, also known as crossed eyes or squint

 Often occurs in early childhood

 Sometimes runs in families

 Gender and lifestyle are not significant factors

Strabismus is a common condition in which only one eye points directly at the object being viewed. This abnormal alignment of the eyes causes the brain to receive conflicting

images, which may result in double vision or, in children under the age of 8, suppression of the image from the misaligned eye.

Strabismus can be caused by any disorder of vision, such as longsightedness (see Hypermetropia, p.366) or shortsightedness (see Myopia, p.365), and can run in families, suggesting a genetic factor. The condition may be caused by a structural difference in the muscles that control movement of the eyes. Very rarely, strabismus develops as a result of cancer of the eye (see Retinoblastoma, p.556) or paralysis of the muscles in one eye caused by a serious underlying condition such as a tumour in the brain (see Brain and spinal cord tumours in children, p.550).

Most babies squint occasionally up to the age of about 3 months, and this is normal. However, a squint after the age of about 3 months or a persistent squint at any age is abnormal and parents should consult their doctor.

What are the symptoms?

If the condition is mild, the symptoms occur only when a child is tired, but in severe cases, they are present all the time. The symptoms of strabismus include:
- Misalignment of the gaze of one of the eyes.
- Poor vision in one of the eyes due to lack of use.

A child may cover or close the affected eye to see clearly and hold his or her head at an angle. Left untreated, strabismus

---

▶ **TEST**

Vision tests in children

Vision tests in children are specifically tailored to age and ability and are routinely performed to look for defects that may delay normal development and learning. The need for glasses can be assessed in infants using tests such as retinoscopy, while older children may be asked to match shapes or letters. Once a child can read, a Snellen chart may be used to look for vision defects (see Vision tests, p.367).

Retinoscopy

This test can be performed on infants. Eyedrops are given about 30 minutes beforehand to dilate the pupils and prevent focusing. A beam of light is shone from an instrument called a retinoscope into each eye in turn. The effect of different lenses on the beam of light determines whether glasses are needed.

During the test
The test is performed in a darkened room. Each eye is tested individually.

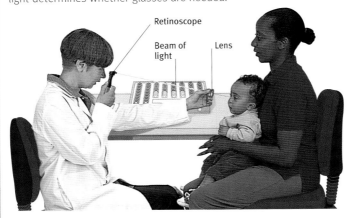

Letter matching test

This test is designed for children of about 3 years of age. A child is given a card with letters printed on it. The doctor then holds up letters of decreasing size at a distance of 3 m (10 ft) and asks the child to identify the same letters on the card. By using an eye patch, each of the eyes can be tested separately.

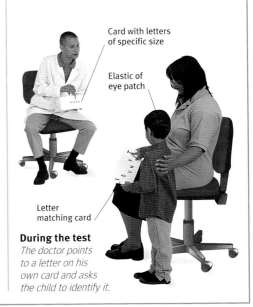

Card with letters of specific size

Elastic of eye patch

Letter matching card

During the test
The doctor points to a letter on his own card and asks the child to identify it.

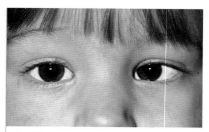

Strabismus
The gaze of this child's eyes is misaligned, a disorder known as strabismus, causing conflicting images to be sent to the brain.

may cause amblyopia (below), in which the vision in the affected eye does not develop normally.

What might be done?

The doctor will arrange for your child to have vision tests (*see* **Vision tests in children**, p.555). If the strabismus has developed suddenly, an imaging test, such as CT scanning (p.132), may be performed to look for a tumour.

The aim of treatment is to correct the strabismus. If your child has a vision disorder such as myopia, he or she may have to wear glasses, which should also correct strabismus. To treat amblyopia, your child may also be given a patch to wear over the unaffected eye for a period of time each day. Wearing the eye patch forces the child to use the weaker eye, which is essential for the normal development of vision. Your child will have regular checkups every 3 or 6 months until the strabismus is corrected. The treatment is usually successful, although the condition can recur. In some cases, surgery on the eye muscles may be necessary. A rare underlying cause, such as a tumour, will be treated if possible.

Amblyopia

Impaired vision in an eye that is usually structurally normal

 Usually develops before the age of 5

 Sometimes runs in families

 Gender and lifestyle are not significant factors

Amblyopia develops in young children if each of the two eyes send a different image to the brain. The development of vision occurs until a child is about 5 years old and depends on the brain learning to combine the images from both eyes. If each eye produces a different image during this period, the brain responds by suppressing images it receives from the more unfocused eye, and vision does not develop normally. If the underlying cause is not treated by the age of 10, later attempts to correct vision will fail.

What are the causes?

Any condition that causes each eye to send a different image to the brain may lead to amblyopia. Misalignment of the gaze of the

eyes (*see* **Strabismus**, p.555) is the most common cause of amblyopia. Other causes include vision disorders in one eye, such as astigmatism (p.366), shortsightedness (*see* **Myopia**, p.365), and longsightedness (*see* **Hypermetropia**, p.366). The condition sometimes runs in families, suggesting that genetic factors are involved.

What might be done?

If you suspect that your child cannot see clearly, you should consult the doctor without delay to minimize the risk of permanent visual impairment. Your child will probably be referred to an ophthalmologist, who will examine your child's eyes and assess vision (*see* **Vision tests in children**, p.555).

Treatment depends on the underlying cause of amblyopia. If your child has a vision disorder such as shortsightedness, this may be corrected by wearing glasses. If vision in one eye is reduced, wearing a patch over the good eye for at least 5 hours each day for several months forces the brain to process visual information from the weaker eye, whatever the underlying cause. If your child has to wear an eye patch to correct amblyopia, he or she will need support and encouragement, especially if vision in the affected eye is poor.

Left untreated, strabismus may lead to amblyopia. In some cases, an operation to correct strabismus is necessary to prevent amblyopia from developing.

What is the prognosis?

The outlook for children with amblyopia depends on when the condition is detected and treatment to correct it begins. Amblyopia is usually at least partially reversible in children under the age of 10. Older children with the condition will probably already have some degree of permanent visual impairment.

Retinoblastoma

A rare cancer of the retina, the lightsensitive membrane at the back of the eye

 Usually develops before the age of 2

 Sometimes runs in families

 Gender and lifestyle are not significant factors

In the UK, about 1 in 20,000 babies is affected with retinoblastoma, a rare cancer of the retina (the light-sensitive membrane at the back of the eye). The condition can develop in one or both of the eyes, usually before a child reaches 2 years of age. About half of all cases are caused by an abnormal gene, which is located on chromosome 13 and is inherited in an autosomal dominant manner (*see* **Gene disorders**, p.151). This inherited form of retinoblastoma often affects both eyes. In the remaining, non-inherited cases, the cause is unknown, and usually only one eye is affected.

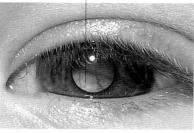
Retinoblastoma

Retinoblastoma
The pale area seen through the pupil of this eye is a retinoblastoma, a rare cancer of the membrane at the back of the eye.

The most common symptom is the development of a whitened area behind the pupil. Impaired vision caused by retinoblastoma may lead to strabismus (p.555). Left untreated, the cancer can spread to other parts of the body.

What might be done?

If the doctor suspects that a child has retinoblastoma, he or she will refer the child to a specialist, who will examine the eyes, possibly under general anaesthesia. The child may also have blood tests to look for the abnormal gene. If retinoblastoma is confirmed, CT scanning (p.132) or MRI (p.133) may be done to see if the cancer has spread.

The aim of treatment is to cure the cancer and, if possible, to retain vision in the affected eyes. It is usually possible to destroy small cancerous tumours in the retina by freezing the tissue. However, surgical removal of the entire eye will probably be necessary to treat large tumours. Treatment with chemotherapy (p.157) and radiotherapy (p.158) may also be required if the cancer has spread.

What is the prognosis?

In most cases, the cancer can be cured, but the child's vision may be severely impaired. Genetic counselling (p.151) is available to relatives of an affected child and to adults treated for retinoblastoma in childhood. The siblings of an affected child should have regular eye tests.

Congenital deafness

Partial or total hearing loss that is present from birth

 Present at birth

 Genetics as a risk factor depends on the cause

 Gender and lifestyle are not significant factors

Normally, a baby reacts to noise from birth, and even a fetus in the uterus is sensitive to sound. Hearing is particularly important for emotional contact between a baby and his or her family and for the development of speech and language skills. Congenital deafness is the rarest form of deafness; only

about 2 in 1,000 babies are born with a hearing impairment that affects both ears. The condition varies from partial hearing loss to profound deafness.

What are the causes?

Congenital deafness is caused by the abnormal development of the inner ear or of the vestibulocochlear nerve, which transmits electrical impulses from the inner ear to the brain. In about half of all cases, the condition runs in families, suggesting that a genetic factor may be involved. Congenital deafness is also associated with the chromosome disorder Down's syndrome (p.533).

Certain infections, such as rubella or cytomegalovirus (CMV), can also cause congenital deafness if they are transmitted from the mother to the fetus during the early stages of development (*see* **Congenital infections**, p.530). The development of hearing may also be affected if the mother takes certain drugs during pregnancy, particularly some types of antibiotic (p.572).

What are the symptoms?

The symptoms of congenital deafness may be noticed in the first few weeks or months after birth and include:

■ Lack of response to loud noise.
■ Failure to make normal baby sounds such as cooing by about 6 weeks of age or babbling by about 3 months.

You should take your baby to the doctor without delay if you suspect that he or she has impaired hearing.

What might be done?

All newborn babies are routinely tested in the first weeks of life for congenital deafness by using otoacoustic emission, and sometimes also by an auditory brainstem response (ABR) test (*see* **Hearing tests in children**, opposite page). Hearing tests are also performed through childhood during routine developmental assessments, as well as whenever a child is suspected of having a hearing impairment.

There is no cure for congenital deafness, but any hearing that a child has can be maximized with a hearing aid (p.376) or, in some children, using a cochlear implant (p.378). In all cases, it is important to ensure that a child can communicate. He or she may be taught sign language and lip-reading. Some children are able to learn to speak.

About half of all children with congenital deafness attend a normal school. Others, such as those with Down's syndrome, need to receive special schooling. Children who have congenital deafness and their families may find it helpful to contact a support group for advice.

Can it be prevented?

Immunization against rubella reduces the risk to the developing fetus. You should not take drugs during pregnancy unless they are known to be safe for the fetus.

▶ **TEST**

Hearing tests in children

Tests to detect impaired hearing are routinely performed in childhood. All newborn babies are given a hearing screening test, usually using the otoacoustic emission test. Sometimes an auditory brainstem response (ABR) test may also be done. In this test, sounds are played to the baby though headphones while electrodes on the baby's head and neck detect the brain's response to the sounds. Further hearing tests are performed as part of the routine developmental assessment and whenever hearing impairment is suspected. Once a child has learned simple language, speech discrimination tests may be performed. By the age of about 4, most children can manage a simple form of audiometry similar to that used to diagnose hearing impairment in adults (*see* **Hearing tests**, p.377).

Otoacoustic emission test

This test detects the echo that is normally emitted by the inner ear in response to sound. An earpiece is placed in the ear canal, and a sound is played through it. The resulting echo is recorded. The test is painless.

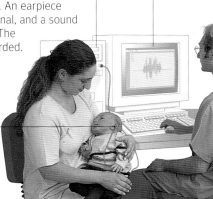

Computer   Monitor

Earpiece

During the test
While the baby is quiet, a sound is played through the earpiece and the response is recorded.

RESULTS

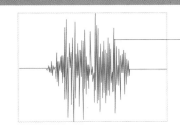

Otoacoustic emission
This normal tracing shows the echo emitted by the inner ear as sound is played through an earpiece. An echo is produced only if the inner ear is healthy and functioning normally.

Sound waves
An echo is produced by the inner ear in response to sounds played

Speech discrimination tests

Speech discrimination tests can be used to detect hearing loss in young children who have a simple vocabulary. For example, the McCormick toy discrimination test is used in children of about 3 years old. The child is shown various toys and is then asked to identify pairs of toys that have similar-sounding names, such as tree and key.

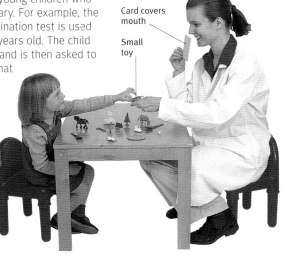

Card covers mouth

Small toy

McCormick test
The doctor prevents the child from lip-reading by covering his or her mouth with a card and then asks the child to identify various toys.

If the condition runs in your family, you may wish to consider genetic counselling (p.151), in which you will be advised about the risks of passing the condition on to your children.

Acute otitis media in children

Infection of the middle ear, which often causes earache

 More common under the age of 5

 Passive smoking is a probable risk factor; more common in children who attend daycare centres

 Gender and genetics are not significant factors

The most common cause of earache in children is acute otitis media, which is caused by infection in the middle ear. Children are at risk because the eustachian tubes, which connect the middle ear to the throat, are small and become obstructed easily. Acute otitis media is often part of an infection of the respiratory system with a virus such as the common cold (p.164). Infection causes inflammation that may block one of the eustachian tubes, causing a build-up of fluid in the middle ear that may then become infected with bacteria.

About 1 in 5 children under the age of 4 has an episode of acute otitis media each year. There is some evidence to suggest that the condition is more common in children whose parents smoke. Children who attend daycare centres are also more susceptible. The condition is less common in children over the age of 5.

What are the symptoms?

The symptoms usually develop rapidly over several hours. A very young child may have difficulty locating the pain, and the only symptoms may be fever, vomiting, and disturbed sleep. In older children, however, the symptoms may be more specific and include:

- Earache.
- Tugging or rubbing the painful ear.
- Temporary impaired hearing in the affected ear.

Left untreated, the eardrum may rupture, relieving the pain but causing a discharge of blood and pus. Recurrent infections in the middle ear may cause chronic secretory otitis media (right).

What might be done?

You should consult your child's doctor if liquid is discharged from the ear or if the earache lasts more than a few hours. He or she will examine your child's ears and may blow air into the affected ear using a special instrument to check that the eardrum is moving normally. Acute otitis media can clear up without treatment; however, the doctor will probably prescribe antibiotics (p.572) if he or she suspects that a bacterial infection is present. Paracetamol or ibupro-

Eardrum

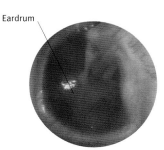

Acute otitis media
The eardrum shown above is bulging and inflamed as a result of the middle-ear infection acute otitis media.

fen (*see* **Painkillers**, p.589) may be given to relieve discomfort. The doctor will re-examine your child after a few days.

The symptoms usually clear up in a few days with appropriate treatment. A ruptured eardrum should heal within a few weeks. In some children, hearing is affected for more than 3 months until the fluid in the ear disappears.

Chronic secretory otitis media

A persistent collection of fluid in the middle ear

 More common under the age of 5

 More common in boys

 Passive smoking is a probable risk factor

 Genetics is not a significant factor

In chronic secretory otitis media, the middle ear becomes filled with a thick, sticky, glue-like fluid. The condition is more common in boys and is the most common cause of impaired hearing in children under the age of 5. Since the disorder can be persistent and usually occurs at a stage of a child's development when good hearing is essential for learning to speak, it may cause a delay in speech development and in the normal acquisition of language skills.

What are the causes?

The middle ear is normally ventilated by the eustachian tube (the narrow tube that connects the middle ear to the back of the throat). However, if this tube becomes blocked, possibly as a result of infection (*see* **Acute otitis media in children**, left), the middle ear may fill with fluid. Often the blockage persists, causing chronic secretory otitis media. In some cases, the cause of the blockage is unknown. However, the disorder is thought to be more common in children whose parents smoke. Children who have asthma (p.544) or allergic rhinitis (p.283) are also more susceptible to chronic secretory otitis media. Children born with Down's syndrome (p.533) or a cleft lip and palate (p.558) are also at an increased risk of developing the disorder.

▶ **TREATMENT**

Grommet insertion

The ear disorder chronic secretory otitis media (p.557) may be treated surgically by inserting a small plastic tube, called a grommet, into the eardrum. This tube ventilates the middle ear and allows fluid to drain away. After insertion of the grommet, hearing in the affected ear usually returns to normal, often within a few days. In most cases, the operation is performed on both ears under general anaesthesia as day surgery.

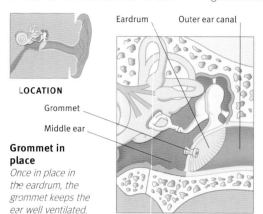

LOCATION

Grommet

Middle ear

Grommet in place
Once in place in the eardrum, the grommet keeps the ear well ventilated.

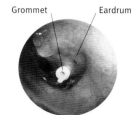

Eardrum | Outer ear canal

Grommet | Eardrum

View of the eardrum
A grommet has been inserted into the eardrum above. Grommets usually fall out 6–12 months after insertion, and the hole in the eardrum closes.

What are the symptoms?
In most cases, symptoms develop gradually and may initially go unnoticed. The symptoms often fluctuate and tend to be worse in winter. They may include:
- Partial hearing loss.
- Immature speech for the child's age.
- Behavioural problems due to frustration at being unable to hear well.

You may notice that your child is sitting close to the television or turning up the volume. His or her school performance may suffer because of difficulty hearing. If you suspect a hearing problem, you should consult the doctor without delay.

How is it diagnosed?
The doctor will examine your child's ears and may then refer him or her to a specialist. Depending on the age of your child, various hearing tests may be performed (*see* **Hearing tests in children**, p.557). The specialist may also perform a test in which air is blown into the affected ear using a special instrument. This test is carried out to measure the amount of movement of the eardrum, which is reduced in chronic secretory otitis media. Since the condition can fluctuate, the specialist will probably wish to examine your child again after about 3 months, when the tests will be repeated. Allergy tests may also be recommended.

What is the treatment?
In most cases, chronic secretory otitis media clears up without treatment. If symptoms persist for several months, an operation may be advised. During the procedure, a small plastic tube called a grommet is inserted in the eardrum (*see* **Grommet insertion**, above). The tube allows air to enter and circulate around the middle ear, drying it out. Some children with chronic secretory otitis media also have enlarged adenoids (p.546), which may be removed in the same operation (*see* **Tonsillectomy and adenoidectomy**, p.546).

What is the prognosis?
As a child grows, the eustachian tubes widen, allowing fluid to drain away from the middle ear more efficiently. As a result, the eustachian tubes are much less likely to become blocked. Chronic secretory otitis media is therefore rare in children over the age of 5.

Protruding ears

Prominent ears, which have no harmful effect on hearing

 Present at birth

 Sometimes runs in families

 Gender and lifestyle are not significant factors

Some children are born with ears that protrude instead of lying almost flat against the head. If the condition is particularly noticeable, a child may be self-conscious and experience psychological distress, usually from the teasing of other children. The condition sometimes runs in families, suggesting that a genetic factor is involved.

What might be done?
Protruding ears can be hidden by a suitable hairstyle. However, in extreme cases, cosmetic surgery may be recommended. During the operation, a thin strip of skin from behind the ear is removed and then the ear is drawn into the desired position. Scarring is hidden behind the ear. This surgery is not usually performed until a child is at least 5 years of age.

Disorders of the digestive system

Throughout early childhood, attacks of diarrhoea and vomiting system are common, and many children have episodes of constipation. Such disorders can often be treated successfully at home with self-help measures. Other rarer disorders may be due to a physical defect present at birth, and these disorders may require surgery.

The first two articles in this section cover problems with the mouth that affect babies: the physical defects of cleft lip and palate, which require surgery, and oral thrush, a common fungal infection. Two other digestive disorders that may affect babies, gastro-oesophageal reflux disease and pyloric stenosis, are covered next. Both can be treated successfully, but pyloric stenosis requires surgery.

A general article follows on vomiting and diarrhoea, including self-help measures for avoiding dehydration. There is also an article on cows' milk protein allergy. The section ends with articles on intussusception, a rare obstruction of the intestines, and constipation. Digestive disorders that affect adults only or affect adults and children are covered in the section on the digestive system (pp.391–423).

For further information on the structure and function of the digestive tract, *see* pp.391–396.

➕ **KEY ANATOMY**

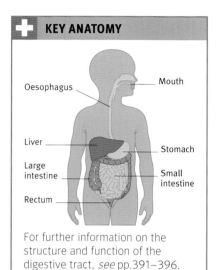

Oesophagus — Mouth

Liver — Stomach

Large intestine — Small intestine

Rectum

Cleft lip and palate

Splits in the upper lip and the roof of the mouth that are present at birth

 Present at birth

 Sometimes runs in families

 Heavy drinking and using some medical drugs in pregnancy are risk factors

 Gender is not a significant factor

A cleft upper lip and palate are among the most common defects in babies and affect about 1 in 700 babies in the UK. These conditions may occur singly or together and are present at birth. These conditions can be upsetting for parents, but plastic surgery (p.614) produces excellent results in most cases.

The defects occur when the upper lip or roof of the mouth does not fuse completely in the fetus. In many cases, the cause is unknown, but the risk is higher if certain anticonvulsant drugs (p.590), such as phenytoin, are taken during pregnancy or if the mother is a heavy drinker. Cleft lip and/or palate sometimes run in families.

If a baby is severely affected, he or she may find it difficult to feed at first, and, if the condition is not treated early, speech may be delayed. Children with a cleft lip and/or palate are also susceptible to persistent build-up of fluid in the middle ear (*see* **Chronic secretory otitis media**, p.557) that impairs hearing and may delay speech.

What might be done?
A cleft lip is usually repaired surgically by the age of 3 months, and a cleft palate is repaired at 6–15 months of age. While waiting for surgery, a plate may be fitted into the roof of the mouth if a baby has feeding problems. Following surgery, a child may have a hearing test (*see* **Hearing tests in children**, p.557) to check for hearing impairment caused by fluid build-up in the ear. A child may also need speech therapy (p.621) when he or she begins to talk. Plastic surgery often produces good results and allows speech to develop normally.

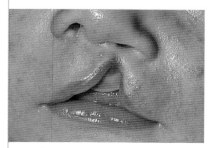

Cleft lip
This child has a split in the upper lip, known as a cleft lip. This can usually be repaired successfully with plastic surgery.

Oral thrush

A fungal mouth infection caused by an overgrowth of a yeast

 Most common under 1 year of age

 Gender, genetics, and lifestyle are not significant factors

Oral thrush is a common fungal infection in the first year of life. It produces white spots inside the mouth and may make a baby reluctant to feed. The infection is caused by an overgrowth of *Candida albicans*, a yeast naturally present in the mouth. The reason for the overgrowth is often unknown.

What are the symptoms?

In most cases, the symptoms of oral thrush include the following:
■ Creamy white spots in the mouth that are difficult to rub off.
■ Sore mouth that may make a baby reluctant to feed.
Oral thrush may be associated with a candida infection in the nappy area (*see* **Nappy rash**, p.538).

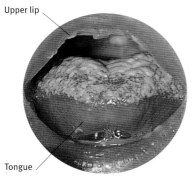

Upper lip

Tongue

Oral thrush
The white patches on the tongue and the lining of this baby's mouth are caused by a common yeast infection, oral thrush.

What might be done?

If you think your baby has oral thrush, you should arrange for him or her to see a doctor within 48 hours. The doctor will examine your baby's mouth and may take a mouth swab to check for *Candida albicans*. He or she may prescribe antifungal drops and, to prevent reinfection if you breast-feed, an antifungal cream for your nipples (*see* **Preparations for skin infections and infestations**, p.577). If you bottle-feed your baby, all the equipment should be thoroughly sterilized. Oral thrush often improves within days of starting treatment and clears up within a week, but the infection may recur.

Gastro-oesophageal reflux disease in infants

Regurgitation of the stomach contents caused by immaturity and weakness of the muscles around the stomach's entrance

 Most common under 1 year of age

 Gender, genetics, and lifestyle are not significant factors

Most babies bring up small amounts of milk after a feed. This regurgitation is normal and does not usually cause distress. However, if an infant regurgitates larger amounts of milk or food regularly, the cause may be gastro-oesophageal reflux disease (GORD). This condition occurs because the muscles at the entrance of a baby's stomach are not fully developed. As a result, the contents of the stomach, including acidic digestive juices, are able to pass back up the oesophagus (the tube between the throat and the stomach). GORD is more common in premature babies and those with cerebral palsy (p.548), who have poor overall muscle tone.

What are the symptoms?

The symptoms of GORD are most noticeable after a feed and may include the following:
■ Regurgitation of milk, usually more pronounced when the baby is lying flat or is crying.
■ Coughing or wheezing if regurgitated milk is inhaled into the lungs.
If GORD is severe, it may prevent the baby gaining weight. Severe reflux may also cause inflammation and bleeding of the lining of the oesophagus, which may make the vomit bloodstained. Sometimes, if milk is inhaled into the lungs, a chest infection, such as pneumonia (p.299), may develop. Rarely, a baby can stop breathing temporarily after inhaling milk.

If your baby regularly regurgitates more than a dribble of milk after feeding or if the vomit is bloodstained, contact a doctor as soon as possible.

How is it diagnosed?

The doctor may be able to diagnose the condition from your baby's symptoms. However, if he or she is unsure of the diagnosis, a test may be carried out to monitor the amount of acid passing up the oesophagus from the stomach over 24 hours. This test involves passing a narrow tube into the baby's nose and down the oesophagus. The doctor may arrange for further tests, including a specialized X-ray (*see* **Barium swallow**, p.404), to check for a structural abnormality in the oesophagus. If a baby has severe reflux with bloodstained vomit, endoscopy (*see* **Upper digestive tract endoscopy**, p.407) may be carried out to look for inflammation of the lining of the oesophagus.

What is the treatment?

In most cases, small, frequent feeds help to prevent GORD. Raising the head end of the cot after giving feeds may also help to prevent regurgitation. The doctor may prescribe a thickener or antacids (p.596) to be added to your baby's milk. In more severe cases, drugs may be given to lower the production of acid in the stomach (*see* **Ulcer-healing drugs**, p.596). With appropriate treatment, symptoms usually improve. Most babies outgrow GORD by the age of about 1 year. In the rare cases that do not clear up by themselves, surgery may be recommended.

Pyloric stenosis in infants

Narrowing of the outlet of the stomach in infancy, causing severe vomiting

 Symptoms usually develop 3–8 weeks after birth

 Five times more common in boys

 Sometimes runs in families

 Lifestyle is not a significant factor

In pyloric stenosis, the ring of muscle that forms the outlet from the stomach to the duodenum (the first part of the small intestine) becomes thickened and narrowed due to excess growth of the muscle tissue. As a result, only a small amount of milk can pass into the duodenum, and the remainder builds up in the stomach until the baby vomits. The condition is five times more common in boys. The cause of pyloric stenosis is unknown, but it may run in families.

What are the symptoms?

The symptoms of pyloric stenosis develop gradually, usually between 3 and 8 weeks after birth, and may include:
■ Persistent vomiting, which is sometimes projectile (ejected forcefully).
■ Immediate hunger after vomiting.
■ Infrequent bowel movements.
If vomiting is persistent or projectile, consult your doctor immediately.

What might be done?

The doctor will examine your baby's abdomen, usually during a feed, to feel for a swelling around the stomach outlet. If pyloric stenosis is suspected, your child will probably be admitted to hospital because affected babies frequently become dehydrated and may need to be given intravenous fluids. To confirm the diagnosis, ultrasound scanning (p.135) and/or specialized X-rays (*see* **Contrast X-rays**, p.132) of the abdomen may be carried out. The treatment for pyloric stenosis is a minor operation to widen the stomach outlet. Feeds can then be increased gradually until the baby's intake is normal. After surgery, babies usually make a full recovery, and the condition does not recur.

Vomiting and diarrhoea

Vomiting and the passage of loose stools caused by allergy, infection of the digestive tract, or an infection elsewhere in the body

 Most common under the age of 5

 Lifestyle as a risk factor depends on the cause

 Gender and genetics are not significant factors

Attacks of vomiting and diarrhoea occur throughout childhood but are more common under the age of 5. There are many causes, some more serious than others, and it may be useful to assess your child (*see* **Symptom chart: Vomiting in children**, p.112, and **Symptom chart: Diarrhoea in children**, p.114). Most cases improve within 24 hours, but prompt treatment with fluids is important because babies and young children become dehydrated rapidly.

What are the causes?

Most episodes of vomiting and diarrhoea develop as a result of a viral or bacterial infection of the digestive tract (*see* **Gastroenteritis**, p.398). Vomiting in young children may also be caused by an infection elsewhere in the body, such as the ear (*see* **Acute otitis media in children**, p.557).

Persistent diarrhoea in children aged between 1 and 3 years is often associated with inability to digest vegetables such as peas and carrots, which may be visible in the stools. This so-called "toddler's diarrhoea" is no cause for concern if your child is otherwise well. However, persistent diarrhoea that is accompanied by failure to gain weight should always be investigated by a doctor.

Persistent vomiting with diarrhoea may be due to conditions such as cows' milk protein allergy (p.560) and sensitivity to gluten, which is found in certain foods, such as wheat, rye, and barley (*see* **Coeliac disease**, p.416).

Are there complications?

If your child has vomiting and diarrhoea that lasts for several hours, he or she may become dehydrated. The symptoms may then also include:
■ Abnormal drowsiness or irritability.
■ Passing of small amounts of concentrated urine.
■ Sunken eyes.
■ In a baby, a sunken fontanelle (the soft spot on the top of a baby's head).
If a child with vomiting and diarrhoea develops symptoms of dehydration, you should seek medical help immediately.

What might be done?

Most cases clear up without treatment. Make sure your child drinks plenty of fluids. Over-the-counter oral rehydration preparations (p.598) that contain the ideal balance of salts and minerals can help to prevent dehydration. If the symptoms persist for over 24 hours or become worse, consult a doctor. He or she will assess the level of hydration and check for infection. If your child is dehydrated, admission to hospital and treatment with intravenous fluids (p.572) may be necessary, and antibiotics (p.572) may be prescribed if the child has a bacterial infection. If the disorder is found to be caused by food sensitivity, a modified diet will be recommended. Treatment is usually successful.

Cows' milk protein allergy

An allergic reaction to the proteins present in cows' milk and cows' milk products

 Usually develops during the first 12 months of life

 Sometimes runs in families

 Gender and lifestyle are not significant factors

An allergy to the proteins in cows' milk occurs in about 1 in 100 babies, usually during the first 12 months of life. Most babies are exposed to these proteins because they are present in formula and, if the mother consumes cows' milk products, in breast milk. If a baby has the allergy, his or her immune system reacts to cows' milk proteins, causing inflammation of the digestive tract. The cause is unknown, but the disorder may run in families, suggesting a genetic factor.

What are the symptoms?
The symptoms of cows' milk protein allergy vary and may include:
- Diarrhoea, with loose stools containing blood and/or mucus.
- Abdominal discomfort, causing the baby to cry and become irritable.
- Vomiting.
- Wheezing and coughing.
- Eczema (p.193) or an itchy, red rash (*see* Urticaria, p.285).
- Failure to gain weight.
If you think that your baby is allergic to proteins in cows' milk, consult a doctor. Rarely, cows' milk protein allergy leads to anaphylaxis (p.285), a potentially life-threatening allergic reaction.

What might be done?
If the doctor suspects cows' milk protein allergy, you may be advised to exclude cows' milk temporarily from your child's diet under a dietitian's supervision. If you are breast-feeding, you will be told to exclude all milk products from your own diet. If symptoms disappear while your child is on the special diet and reappear when cows' milk is reintroduced, the diagnosis is confirmed and the special diet is

continued. Treatment for cows' milk protein allergy is usually successful, and children rapidly put on weight on the modified diet. Your child will be reviewed regularly to check whether the allergy is still present and a special diet is still required. The problem usually disappears between the ages of about 1 and 3 years, but in a minority of affected children it continues in some form into adult life.

Intussusception

A rare condition in which a segment of intestine slides inside the neighbouring part, causing an intestinal obstruction

 Usually develops in early childhood

 More common in boys

 Genetics and lifestyle are not significant factors

Intussusception is a rare condition, but it is the most common cause of intestinal obstruction in children under the age of 2. In intussusception, a section of the intestine "telescopes" into a neighbouring part, forming a tube within a tube. The condition usually affects the last part of the small intestine. If left untreated, the blood supply to the affected "telescoped" part may be cut off and cause tissue death in that section of intestine. The cause of intussusception is usually unknown. However, it may be associated with enlargement of the lymph nodes in the lining of the intestine, possibly due to a viral infection.

What are the symptoms?
The symptoms of intussusception are usually intermittent. Each episode develops suddenly and usually lasts for a few minutes. Symptoms may include:
- Severe abdominal pain, which may cause the child to cry and draw up his or her legs.
- Pale skin.
- Vomiting.
- After a few hours, passage from the rectum of bloodstained mucus that may resemble redcurrant jam.
Between the intermittent episodes of pain and vomiting, your child may feel ill and lethargic. If you suspect intussusception, seek medical attention at once. The disorder progresses rapidly, and prompt treatment is essential.

What might be done?
If your child's doctor suspects intussusception from the symptoms, he or she will arrange for your child to be admitted to hospital immediately.

In hospital, your child will probably be given intravenous fluids to prevent dehydration. In order to confirm the diagnosis, a special X-ray examination that involves

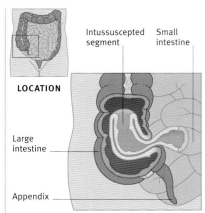

Intussuscepted segment | Small intestine

LOCATION

Large intestine

Appendix

Intussusception
In this example of intussusception, the last part of the small intestine has passed into the adjacent section of large intestine and caused an obstruction.

the use of air or a barium enema may be carried out. In most cases, the gentle pressure exerted by the air or barium forces the displaced intestinal tissue back into the correct position and relieves the obstruction. If this procedure does not correct the problem, surgery is necessary to relieve the obstruction and to remove the damaged part of the intestine. Most affected children recover fully following treatment, and the condition recurs in fewer than 1 in 20 of all cases.

Constipation in children

Difficult, infrequent, and sometimes painful passage of hard faeces

 A low-fibre diet is a risk factor

 Age, gender, and genetics are not significant factors

All children differ in their bowel habits. Some children pass faeces several times a day, and others may do so only once every few days. Both these situations are normal provided that the faeces are not too runny or so hard that they cause discomfort. The presence of hard faeces that are difficult or painful to pass indicates that your child has constipation, a common condition that affects people of all ages. Constipation in children is usually only a temporary problem, and often no cause is found. It is rarely an indication of a serious underlying disorder.

What are the causes?
A common cause of temporary constipation is a change in diet, particularly if there is insufficient fibre or fluid in the diet. Constipation is rare in babies, but the condition may occur during the change from formula or breast milk to cows' milk. Sometimes, temporary constipation occurs during toilet training, when it is common for a toddler to try to avoid defe-

cation. This phase may be associated with a toddler passing faeces in inappropriate places (*see* Encopresis, p.552). Illnesses that cause high fever and vomiting can also cause temporary constipation due to dehydration.

Underlying disorders that may cause persistent constipation include cerebral palsy (p.548), in which there is brain damage that impairs muscular control, and Hirschsprung's disease, a rare disorder in which the nerve supply to the lower bowel fails to develop normally.

What are the symptoms?
If your child has constipation, you may notice the following symptoms:
- Difficult passage of small or bulky hard, dry faeces.
- Infrequent defecation.
- Soiling of clothes due to leakage of faeces associated with constipation.
- Sometimes, loss of appetite.
Your child may be afraid to pass faeces if he or she suffers severe discomfort while defecating, especially if a painful tear develops in the anal tissue (*see* Anal fissure, p.423) caused by straining to pass stools. In these cases, constipation may become a long-term problem.

What can I do?
In most cases, constipation in children does not require medical treatment. You should encourage your child to drink plenty of fluids. If the child is over the age of 6 months, make sure that there is plenty of fibre in the diet. If constipation is linked to problems with toilet training, patience and time will usually solve the problem. Seek medical advice if constipation persists for a week despite self-help measures.

What might the doctor do?
The doctor will probably examine your child's abdomen and may perform a rectal examination, in which a gloved finger is gently inserted into the rectum. He or she may prescribe a short course of drugs to soften the faeces (*see* Laxatives, p.597) and reduce the discomfort of defecation. Softened faeces will also allow an anal tear to heal. Once the pain of defecation is relieved, your child should feel confident to pass faeces normally again. If constipation persists or your doctor suspects a disorder such as Hirschsprung's disease, your child may need an abdominal X-ray (p.131), or a specialized contrast X-ray (p.132) or a biopsy (removal of a tissue sample for examination) of the bowel for a definite diagnosis. Hirschsprung's disease may be treated by surgery to remove the abnormal area of bowel. Severe constipation caused by a condition such as cerebral palsy may require lifelong treatment with laxatives. In other cases, constipation usually clears up within 1–2 weeks of changing the child's diet or of laxative treatment.

Endocrine and metabolic disorders

Some endocrine and most metabolic disorders in children are present from birth and are caused by an abnormal gene that is inherited from one or both parents. Most of these disorders are rare, but, when they do occur, they can adversely affect normal growth and development unless diagnosed and treated early.

Most of the disorders discussed in this section are caused by abnormalities in the production of enzymes that are vital for the metabolic (chemical) processes of the body. The first disorder covered is congenital adrenal hyperplasia, in which deficiency of an enzyme affects production of one or more hormones by the adrenal glands. As a result, important metabolic processes are disrupted and excessive production of male sex hormones may affect the formation of a female baby's genitals. The second article introduces a group of rare inherited metabolic disorders, known as inborn errors of metabolism. The articles that follow cover five of these disorders: phenylketonuria, MCADD, galactosaemia, Tay–Sachs disease, and albinism. The section concludes with a general article on growth disorders. Endocrine and metabolic conditions such as diabetes mellitus that affect adults only or adults in addition to children are discussed in hormones and metabolism (pp.424–441) or in the section that covers the particular body system affected.

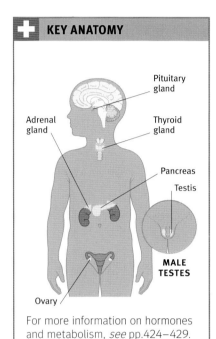

KEY ANATOMY

Pituitary gland

Adrenal gland

Thyroid gland

Pancreas

Testis

MALE TESTES

Ovary

For more information on hormones and metabolism, *see* pp.424–429.

Congenital adrenal hyperplasia

In either sex, abnormally high production of male sex hormones by the adrenal glands

 Present from birth

 Due to an abnormal gene inherited from both parents

 Gender and lifestyle are not significant factors

Congenital adrenal hyperplasia is a rare inherited condition that affects around 1 in 5,000 babies in the UK. In congenital adrenal hyperplasia, the production of one or more hormones in the adrenal glands is abnormal.

In the most common form of congenital adrenal hyperplasia, there is a deficiency of an enzyme that is essential for the production of the adrenal hormones aldosterone, which maintains the salt and water balance in the body, and cortisol, which maintains glucose levels in the blood. As a result, these hormones may be absent or deficient. The condition also leads to excessive production of male sex hormones (androgens).

Congenital adrenal hyperplasia is caused by an abnormal gene that is inherited in an autosomal recessive manner (*see* **Gene disorders**, p.151).

What are the symptoms?

The symptoms of congenital adrenal hyperplasia may be present at birth or may develop later in childhood or adolescence. Raised levels of androgens may lead to the following symptoms:

- In girls, an enlarged clitoris and external genitals that are fused, giving a masculinized appearance.
- In boys, a slight increase in pigmentation of the scrotum, which often goes unnoticed.
- Early puberty in boys.

Lack of aldosterone may cause a "salt-losing crisis" in which there is a sudden loss of salt and fluid. The symptoms of such a crisis may include:

- Lethargy.
- Vomiting.
- Loss of weight.

If it is not treated, the salt-losing crisis may lead to shock (p.248), which may be life-threatening. A lack of cortisol may cause low levels of glucose in the blood (*see* **Hypoglycaemia**, p.440).

What might be done?

Congenital adrenal hyperplasia is usually diagnosed in girls at birth from the appearance of the genitals. The disorder may become apparent in boys due to a salt-losing crisis developing 1–3 weeks after birth.

An affected child will have blood tests to measure the levels of hormones, salt, and glucose. If a baby has a salt-losing crisis, he or she will require emergency treatment in hospital with intravenous salt and glucose solutions. Cortisol and a drug that mimics the actions of aldosterone will also be given. A child who has congenital adrenal hyperplasia will require lifelong treatment to replace the deficient hormones and to normalize the production of androgens. Affected girls may need to have surgery to correct genital abnormalities.

With treatment, most children with congenital adrenal hyperplasia can lead normal lives. If a pregnant woman has already given birth to a child with the disorder or if both partners are known to be carriers, screening tests may be offered, and, if necessary, medication prescribed to minimize the effects of the condition on a female fetus.

Inborn errors of metabolism

Genetic disorders in which chemical processes in the body are disrupted or faulty

 Present from birth

 Due to an abnormal gene usually inherited from both parents

 Gender and lifestyle are not significant factors

Inborn errors of metabolism is a general term used to describe a group of genetic disorders in which the body chemistry (metabolism) is affected by an abnormal gene. In each disorder, this abnormal gene affects the production of a particular enzyme that is essential for specific metabolic processes. The disruption of these processes results in damage to one or more organs of the body, and the severity of a particular disorder depends on the chemical processes affected. Over 200 inborn errors of metabolism have been identified, but each disorder is extremely rare. Most of the abnormal genes that cause these in born metabolic disorders are inherited in an autosomal recessive manner (*see* **Gene disorders**, p.151).

What are the types?

Many inborn errors of metabolism lead to a build-up of harmful chemicals that cause damage to one or more organs in the body. In phenylketonuria (p.562), the accumulation of phenylalanine causes brain damage. In galactosaemia (p.562), the sugar galactose builds up to a dangerously high level and causes damage to the liver and brain. In Tay–Sachs disease (p.562), chemical build-up in the brain results in fatal brain damage.

In MCADD (p.562), lack of an enzyme needed to convert fats into energy can lead to low levels of glucose and a high level of toxins in the blood. In the milder condition albinism (p.563), a deficient enzyme affects the production of the pigment melanin, which gives colour to the skin, eyes, and hair, but there is no harmful chemical build-up.

The symptoms of inborn errors of metabolism are usually present at or soon after birth, although in some cases symptoms may not appear until later in childhood. The symptoms may include unexplained illness and failure to thrive in a newborn, and drowsiness, floppiness, seizures, and developmental delay (p.553) in older babies and children.

What might be done?

Couples planning to have children may be offered screening for the presence of an abnormal gene before beginning a pregnancy if there is a family history of an inborn error of metabolism or if a particular metabolic disorder is common in their ethnic group. A pregnant woman can also be screened for the condition before the baby is born (*see* **Antenatal genetic tests**, p.509).

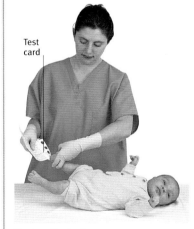

▶ **TEST**

Blood spot screening tests

Shortly after birth, newborn babies are given blood spot screening tests to check for several rare but potentially serious disorders. All babies are offered screening for phenylketonuria (p.562), hypothyroidism (p.432), cystic fibrosis (p.535), sickle cell disease (p.272), and MCADD (p.562). In some areas, babies may also be offered screening for certain other inherited metabolic disorders. The blood sample is obtained by pricking the baby's heel and collecting the blood on a special card for analysis. The results are usually available a few weeks later.

Test card

During the test
After pricking the side of the baby's heel, a few drops of blood are squeezed on to an absorbent test card.

In the UK, all newborn infants are routinely given blood spot screening tests (p.561), which screen for various metabolic disorders as well as certain other conditions, such as cystic fibrosis (p.535).

Some inborn errors of metabolism can be treated easily. For example, the diet of an affected child can be adapted to restrict the intake of substances, such as phenylalanine or galactose, that his or her body cannot process. If the missing enzyme is produced by white blood cells, the condition may sometimes be cured by a stem cell transplant (p.276).

What is the prognosis?
The outlook for inborn errors of metabolism depends on the disorder and how early it is diagnosed. Some disorders, such as albinism, rarely cause serious problems; others, such as galactosaemia, can be treated successfully if diagnosed soon after birth. However, there is no treatment for Tay–Sachs disease, which is usually fatal in early childhood.

Phenylketonuria

An inherited chemical defect that can cause brain damage

 Present from birth

 Due to an abnormal gene inherited from both parents

 Gender and lifestyle are not significant factors

Children with phenylketonuria lack the enzyme that is responsible for breaking down phenylalanine, which occurs naturally in most food containing protein. As a result, phenylalanine is converted into harmful substances that build up in the blood and may damage the developing brain. Although phenylketonuria is rare in the UK, affecting about 1 in 10,000 infants, all newborn babies are screened for the disorder because of the risk of serious brain damage. Like most inborn errors of metabolism, phenylketonuria is due to an abnormal gene that is inherited in an autosomal recessive manner (*see* **Gene disorders**, p.151). If both parents carry the abnormal gene, there is a 1 in 4 chance that their baby will be affected.

What are the symptoms?
At birth, some babies with phenylketonuria have a red, itchy rash similar to eczema, but most affected infants appear healthy. The symptoms of the disorder usually develop gradually over 6–12 months and may include:
- Vomiting.
- Restlessness and sometimes seizures.
- Stale, unpleasant skin odour.
- Delay in development (*see* **Developmental delay**, p.553).

If it is not treated, phenylketonuria may lead to serious brain damage, resulting in severe learning problems (*see* **Generalized learning disabilities**, p.553).

What might be done?
In the UK, a blood test for phenylketonuria is given to all newborn babies (*see* **Blood spot screening tests**, p.561). Early screening is important because prompt diagnosis and treatment are vital. If your baby is diagnosed as having phenylketonuria, he or she will probably be prescribed a special formula or milk substitute that is rich in protein but contains little phenylalanine. Your child should continue with a diet low in phenylalanine, at least throughout his or her childhood until the brain has stopped growing. Most doctors recommend that an affected person should follow a low-phenylalanine diet for life. Women with the condition who are planning a pregnancy are advised to follow a low phenylalanine diet before conception and throughout pregnancy.

With early diagnosis and treatment, children with phenylketonuria develop normally, attend mainstream schools, and do not have reduced life expectancy.

MCADD

A rare inherited condition in which there is lack of an enzyme needed to convert fats to energy

 Present at birth

 Due to an abnormal gene inherited from both parents

 Gender and lifestyle are not significant factors

The abbreviation for medium-chain acyl CoA dehydrogenase deficiency, MCADD is a rare hereditary metabolic disorder in which there is a lack of an enzyme needed to completely convert fats to energy. The body's first source of energy is glucose (a type of sugar), which circulates in the blood. When this glucose is used up – during a long period without food or during an illness, for example – fats from the body's stores are broken down to produce energy. This fat breakdown occurs in several stages, each stage requiring a different enzyme. People with MCADD lack one of these enzymes and so cannot break down fats completely. As a result, there is a build up of partly broken down fats (medium-chain fats), which can accumulate to toxic levels. In addition, because the body's glucose is used up, the blood glucose levels may drop to a dangerously low level.

The underlying cause of MCADD is an abnormal gene on chromosome 1. This gene is carried by about 1 in 80 people in the UK and is inherited in an autosomal recessive manner (*see* **Gene disorders**, p.151), which means that two copies of the abnormal gene, one from each parent, are necessary to develop MCADD. Carriers have only one copy of the abnormal gene and do not have any symptoms. MCADD is rare, affecting about 1 in 10,000 babies.

What are the symptoms?
Typically, symptoms do not appear until between 3 months and 3 years after birth and are often triggered by an infection, a period of poor feeding, or when a baby starts to feed less at night. Initial symptoms may include:
- Irritability and sleepiness.
- Vomiting and diarrhoea.
- Sweating.

Without prompt treatment, breathing problems, seizures, and unconsciousness may develop. In some cases there may be brain damage, heart failure, or even death.

What might be done?
MCADD can be detected shortly after birth as part of the routine blood spot screening tests (p.561). The condition is treated by diet. There is no specific diet but the disorder requires close monitoring of the child to determine "safe" time periods between meals, and a strict feeding schedule to ensure that an affected child does not go for long periods without food. However, during an illness, glucose supplements, as well as a regular diet, may be necessary. If a child is unable to eat or drink normally, it may be necessary to admit him or her to hospital for intravenous feeding. Dietary treatment is usually lifelong but with proper dietary management children with MCADD usually develop normally and lead healthy, active lives.

Galactosaemia

An abnormal build-up of the sugar galactose, due to a deficient enzyme

 Present from birth

 Due to an abnormal gene inherited from both parents

 Gender and lifestyle are not significant factors

Galactosaemia is a rare condition in which harmful amounts of galactose, a sugar that is present in milk, build up in a baby's body tissues. Normally, an enzyme in the liver converts galactose into glucose, but in galactosaemia this enzyme is deficient. If the disorder is not treated, high levels of galactose accumulate, leading to serious damage to the liver, brain, and eyes. In the UK, the disorder affects about 1 in 70,000 infants. Galactosaemia is caused by an abnormal gene inherited in an autosomal recessive manner (*see* **Gene disorders**, p.151).

What are the symptoms?
Symptoms of galactosaemia appear in the first few days of life, often after the baby's first milk feeds, and include:
- Vomiting and diarrhoea.
- Failure to gain weight.
- Yellow coloration of the skin and the whites of the eyes (*see* **Neonatal jaundice**, p.531).

If not treated, cataracts (p.357), chronic liver failure (p.411), and generalized learning disabilities (p.553) may develop.

What might be done?
If a newborn infant develops the above symptoms, the doctor may suspect galactosaemia and arrange for the baby's blood to be tested for the enzyme deficiency. If galactosaemia is confirmed, you will be advised to exclude galactose from your baby's diet and to use milk substitutes in feeds. Usually, a galactose-free diet is recommended throughout childhood and, in some cases, for life. With early treatment, affected children may develop normally, but most have at least mild learning difficulties.

Tay–Sachs disease

An inherited condition in which harmful chemicals accumulate in the brain

 Present from birth

 Due to an abnormal gene inherited from both parents

 Gender and lifestyle are not significant factors

Tay–Sachs disease is a fatal childhood disorder that is most common in the Ashkenazi Jewish population. The condition is caused by the lack of a vital enzyme in the brain. Without the enzyme, abnormal chemicals build up, leading to progressive and fatal brain damage. Tay–Sachs disease is caused by an abnormal gene that is inherited in an autosomal recessive manner (*see* **Gene disorders**, p.151). About 1 in 25 Ashkenazi Jews is a carrier of the abnormal gene, compared with about 1 in 250 in the non-Jewish population.

What are the symptoms?
A baby who has Tay–Sachs disease often appears healthy at birth. The symptoms, which usually start to appear at 3–6 months of age, may include:
- Exaggerated startle response to noise.
- Muscle weakness and floppy limbs.
- Lack of awareness of surroundings.
- Deteriorating vision.

An affected baby may have seizures and gradually become paralysed during the first 6 months of life.

What might be done?
If the doctor suspects that your baby has Tay–Sachs disease, he or she may arrange for a blood test or a test on a sample of skin tissue to confirm that the enzyme is missing. The doctor will also examine the baby's eyes to look for the presence of an abnormal "cherry-red spot" on the retina (the layer of light-sensitive cells at the back of the eye). There is no cure for Tay–Sachs disease, but an affected child will be made as comfortable as possible by treating symptoms as they arise.

People who are at risk of having a child with Tay–Sachs disease can be screened for the abnormal gene before marriage or pregnancy. If both partners are carriers of the gene, there is a 1 in 4 chance of their child being affected. The couple will be offered genetic counselling (p.151) to explain these risks and discuss the options. Affected couples may decide not to have children or to conceive using IVF treatment (*see* **Assisted conception**, p.498), so that the embryo can be tested for the disease before implantation in the uterus.

Tay–Sachs disease is a fatal disorder, and children with the disease do not usually survive beyond the age of 5.

Albinism

An inherited condition in which there is inadequate production of the pigment that gives colour to skin, eyes, and hair

 Present from birth

 Due to an abnormal gene

 Gender as a risk factor depends on the type

 Lifestyle is not a significant factor

Albinism is a rare inherited disorder in which a baby is born with little or no colour in the skin, hair, and eyes or, more rarely, in the eyes only. An inborn error of metabolism (p.428), albinism is caused by a fault in an enzyme that is essential for the production of the pigment melanin. In most cases, albinism is due to an abnormal gene that is inherited in an autosomal recessive manner (*see* **Gene disorders**, p.151) and affects the skin, hair, and eyes. A less common type, in which the abnormal gene is inherited in an X-linked recessive manner from the mother, affects only males. In this type of albinism, only the eyes are affected by lack of melanin. Albinism affects about 1 in 17,000 babies.

What are the symptoms?

The symptoms depend on the amount of melanin that is produced and vary from mild to severe. They may include:
- Unusual eye colour, ranging from pink to pale, watery blue.
- Dislike of bright light.
- Involuntary, jerky eye movements.
- Severe visual impairment.
- White hair and fair skin that does not tan normally.

Children with albinism are at increased risk of developing skin cancer (p.199) in later life from exposure to sunlight.

What might be done?

Albinism is usually diagnosed from the baby's appearance at birth. If albinism is suspected, a blood test is performed to confirm that the enzyme is missing. There is no medical treatment for the condition. However, tinted

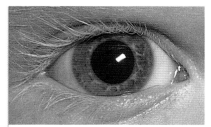

Albinism
The iris of this eye is pink and the eyebrows and eyelashes are white, due to absence of the brown pigment melanin.

lenses can be worn to help with the aversion to bright light, and visual impairment can be corrected with glasses or, when the child is older, with contact lenses. The doctor will also recommend the use of sunscreens and sunblocks (p.577) and a hat to protect your child's skin in bright sunlight. People with albinism have a normal life expectancy.

Growth disorders

Abnormally short or tall stature in babies and children due to a number of causes

 Age, gender, genetics, and lifestyle as risk factors depend on the type

Children of the same age vary greatly in height due to factors such as diet, genetics, and ethnic background. In most cases, tall or short stature is not abnormal and is due to a family tendency to be taller or shorter than average or to reach final height later than usual. Tall or short stature is a cause for concern only if the child's height is well outside the average range for his or her age. Abnormally short or tall stature may be caused by a number of disorders.

What are the types?

Normal growth depends on a nutritionally adequate diet and good general health and is controlled by specific hormones. Disruption of any of these three important factors may lead to a growth disorder that results in a child having abnormally short or tall stature.

Short stature A child may be shorter than normal if his or her diet is inadequate. A long-term illness, such as cystic fibrosis (p.535) or severe asthma (*see* **Asthma in children**, p.544), may also result in poor growth. Crohn's disease (p.417), an inflammatory bowel condition, is another example of a long-term illness that may lead to short stature. Some babies who have severe intrauterine growth retardation (p.514) may be slightly below average height in later life.

Sometimes, short stature is caused by insufficient production of the hormones that are necessary for normal growth. In some children, the pituitary gland does not produce enough growth hormone (*see* **Hypopituitarism**, p.431). Insufficient production of thyroid hormones is another cause of poor growth (*see* **Hypothyroidism**, p.432).

Short stature is also a characteristic feature of Turner's syndrome (p.534), a genetic disorder that only affects girls. In addition, short stature may occur as a result of a skeletal abnormality such as achondroplasia (p.540), an inherited disorder in which the bones of the legs and arms are shorter than normal.

Tall stature Children may be temporarily taller than others of the same age and sex if puberty occurs early (*see* **Abnormal puberty in males**, p.465, and **Abnormal puberty in females**, p.474). However, in these children, final height is usually slightly shorter than normal. In rare cases, exaggerated growth caused by the overproduction of growth hormone results in excessive height, called gigantism. The overproduction may be due to a tumour in the pituitary gland (*see* **Pituitary tumours**, p.430). Boys who have the chromosome disorder known as Klinefelter's syndrome (p.534) may also grow taller than normal.

How is it diagnosed?

Your child's height will be measured during routine checkups. If his or her height is consistently either lower or higher than would be expected, he or she will be measured more frequently. If growth rates continue to be abnormal, tests may be performed to check hormone levels and to look for underlying disorders. In some cases, maturity of a child's bones may be assessed by taking X-rays (p.131) of the hand and wrist.

What is the treatment?

Treatment for growth disorders is most successful if started well before puberty when bones still have the potential for normal growth. Slow growth due to an inadequate diet in infancy usually improves if the diet is modified. Later in childhood, a growth disorder is likely to be the result of long-term illness, and careful control of the illness sometimes results in normal growth. Growth hormone deficiency is usually treated by hormone replacement. Hypothyroidism is treated by replacing thyroid hormone.

Abnormal early puberty is sometimes treated using drugs to halt the advancement of puberty. Gigantism caused by a pituitary gland tumour may be treated by surgical removal of the tumour.

If treated early, most children reach a relatively normal height, but, if treatment is delayed until puberty, normal height is more difficult to achieve. Abnormal stature may cause a child to be self-conscious and unhappy, and he or she may need support such as counselling (p.624).

Disorders of the reproductive and urinary systems

The two main causes of reproductive and urinary disorders in children are abnormal development of the affected systems in the fetus and infection. Prompt treatment of urinary tract infections is important because of the risk of kidney damage.

The first articles in this section cover two disorders of the male reproductive and urinary systems, hypospadias and undescended testis, which are present at birth. In hypospadias, the opening of the urethra (the passage that carries urine from the bladder to the outside of the body) is on the underside of the penis rather than the tip. Undescended testis is a condition in which one testis (or rarely both) fails to descend into the scrotum before birth.

Urinary tract infections, which are more common in girls, are discussed next. All children who have these infections need prompt medical treatment because the kidneys can be damaged if the infection persists. An article follows on bedwetting, a common urinary problem in childhood. The section ends with an article on Wilms' tumour, a rare cancer of the kidney that can often be treated successfully. Circumcision (p.462) is discussed elsewhere.

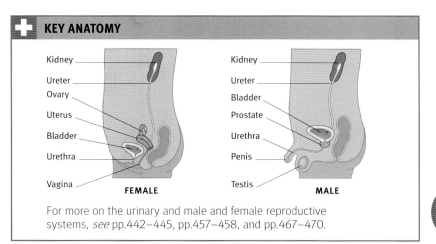

KEY ANATOMY

Kidney, Ureter, Ovary, Uterus, Bladder, Urethra, Vagina — FEMALE

Kidney, Ureter, Bladder, Prostate, Urethra, Penis, Testis — MALE

For more on the urinary and male and female reproductive systems, *see* pp.442–445, pp.457–458, and pp.467–470.

Hypospadias

An abnormality in which the opening of the urethra is on the underside of the penis rather than at the tip

 Present at birth

 Sometimes runs in families

 Lifestyle is not a significant factor

Hypospadias is a common birth defect in which the opening of the urethra (the passage that carries urine from the bladder to outside the body) develops on the underside of the shaft of the penis instead of at the tip. Most commonly, the opening develops near the end of the penis, but in severe cases it can occur far back towards the scrotum. Sometimes, part of the foreskin may be missing and the penis curves downwards, a condition known as chordee. Hypospadias occurs in about 1 in 300 boys and can run in families, which suggests that a genetic factor is involved. If the condition is not treated early, an affected child may need to sit on the toilet to pass urine, unlike other boys, which may make him self-conscious.

What might be done?
Hypospadias is usually detected at birth and treated with surgery before the age of 2. During the operation, the foreskin is used to form an extension to the existing urethra so that it reaches the tip of the penis. It is therefore important that the boy is not circumcised. If chordee is also present, this can be corrected during the same operation. Surgery usually allows the child to pass urine normally. Sexual activity and fertility in later life are usually unaffected.

Undescended testis

A testis that fails to descend into the scrotum before birth

 Present at birth

 Genetics and lifestyle are not significant factors

Normally, the testes descend from the abdomen into the scrotum before birth. In about 4 in 100 boys, one testis (or rarely both) fails to move down. In 2 in 3 affected boys, an undescended testis moves into the scrotum within the first few months of life, but the rest may need surgery to correct the condition. Males who have had an undescended testis are at greater risk of developing cancer of the testis (p.460) in adulthood. They may also be at risk of impaired fertility (*see* **Male infertility**, p.499).

It can be difficult to determine if your son has an undescended testis because the testes of most young boys retract up into the abdomen in response to cold or touch. However, you should consult the doctor if you are concerned.

What might be done?
Examination of the testes is part of the routine check of a newborn boy. If a testis has not descended, regular checks will be carried out. If the testis has not descended by the time the boy is about 6 months old, it is unlikely to do so spontaneously, and treatment is needed.

The condition is usually treated with a small operation called an orchidopexy, in which the testicle is moved down into the scrotum and secured with stitches. This surgery should ideally be carried out before the age of 12 months. After treatment, most boys develop normally, and sexual function is unaffected. However, in some cases, fertility may be reduced, especially if both testes are affected.

Urinary tract infections in children

Infection of the urinary tract, which may lead to kidney damage

 Overall more common in girls

 Sometimes runs in families

 Age and lifestyle are not significant factors

Urinary tract infections develop when bacteria, normally present around the anus, pass up the urethra (the passage from the bladder to outside the body) and infect the bladder (*see* **Cystitis**, p.453) or kidneys (*see* **Pyelonephritis**, p.446). Less commonly, a bacterial infection may be carried to the urinary tract in the bloodstream. Most urinary infections are easily treated, but they may scar the kidneys, increasing the risk of further infection, so treatment must be prompt. Urinary infections tend to be more common in girls, although newborn boys are more susceptible than newborn girls.

The kidney infection pyelonephritis is more common in children who have urinary reflux. In this condition, there is an abnormality of the ureters (the passages from the kidneys to the bladder) where they open into the bladder. This abnormality results in a

---

▶ **TEST**

DMSA scanning

To look for scarring in the kidneys, a type of radionuclide scanning (p.135) called dimercaptosuccinic acid (DMSA) scanning is used. In this procedure, which takes place in hospital, a small amount of radioactive DMSA is injected into a vein in the arm. After 2 hours, the DMSA collects in the kidneys and images of the organs are taken with a gamma camera. The scan takes about 30 minutes and is painless.

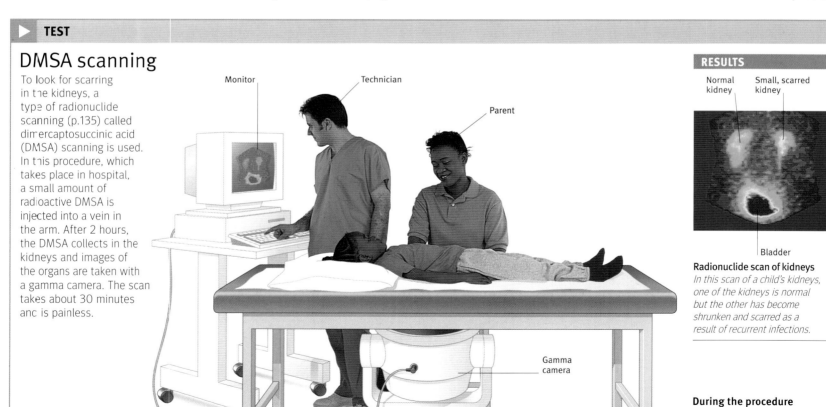

Monitor · Technician · Parent · Gamma camera

RESULTS

Normal kidney · Small, scarred kidney · Bladder

Radionuclide scan of kidneys
In this scan of a child's kidneys, one of the kidneys is normal but the other has become shrunken and scarred as a result of recurrent infections.

During the procedure
Your child will need to lie very still while the radiographer watches the images on the monitor screen. You should be able to stay with your child during the scanning.

Overcoming bedwetting

A child may be helped to overcome persistent bedwetting by using a pad and buzzer system. The pad, which can detect moisture, is placed in the bed and attached to a buzzer. When a child starts to pass urine, the buzzer is activated. The noise wakes the child, who can then get up and go to the bathroom before going back to sleep. After a few weeks, the child will wake automatically without the buzzer if he or she needs to pass urine.

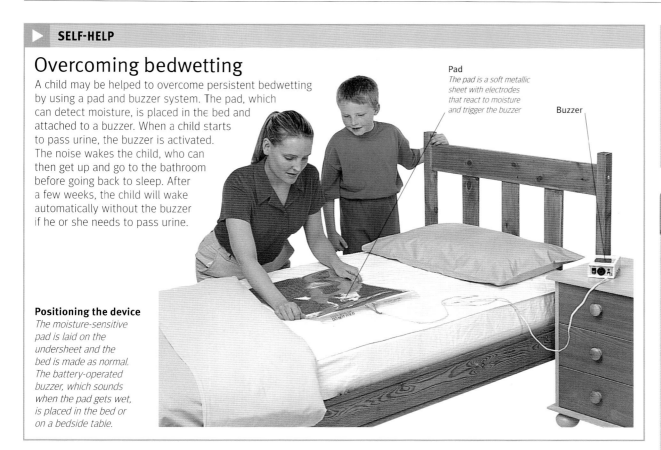

Pad
The pad is a soft metallic sheet with electrodes that react to moisture and trigger the buzzer

Buzzer

Positioning the device
The moisture-sensitive pad is laid on the undersheet and the bed is made as normal. The battery-operated buzzer, which sounds when the pad gets wet, is placed in the bed or on a bedside table.

small amount of urine flowing back up the ureters towards the kidneys when the bladder is emptied. Urinary reflux sometimes runs in families, suggesting a genetic factor.

What are the symptoms?
If your child is under the age of 2, he or she may be unable to describe any specific symptoms, but you may notice:
■ Fever.
■ Vomiting and/or diarrhoea.
■ Irritability or drowsiness.
Older children often have more specific symptoms and can explain how they feel. In addition to the symptoms of young children, an older child may have:
■ Frequent, urgent need to pass urine.
■ Burning sensation on passing urine.
■ Pain in the lower abdomen or side.
■ Bedwetting (right) or daytime wetting after a period of dryness.
If you suspect that your child has developed an infection of the urinary tract, you should consult the doctor at once.

What might be done?
The doctor will test a urine sample for evidence of infection. If the test indicates a possible infection, your child will be treated at once with antibiotics (p.572). The sample will be sent for laboratory testing to identify the bacteria responsible. The antibiotics may be changed when the results are known. If the symptoms suggest pyelonephritis, your child will probably be treated in hospital with intravenous antibiotics and fluids.

Your child may need to have radionuclide scanning (*see* **DMSA scanning**, opposite page) or ultrasound scanning

(p.135) to look for scarring in the kidneys or other abnormalities of the urinary tract. A specialized X-ray to check for urinary reflux may also be carried out. In this procedure, a dye is introduced into the bladder through a narrow tube. X-rays are then taken as the child passes urine. A child with urinary reflux may be given low-dose antibiotics long-term until the kidneys are no longer at risk. In severe cases, surgery may be needed.

With treatment, most children with a urinary tract infection make a complete recovery. However, infections may recur and should always be investigated. If untreated, recurrent infections due to reflux may cause permanent kidney damage.

Bedwetting

Involuntary emptying of the bladder during sleep, also known as enuresis

 Considered abnormal only over the age of 6 years

 Slightly more common in boys

 Sometimes runs in families

 Emotional stress is a risk factor

Children normally stop wetting the bed between the ages of 3 and 6 years. Bedwetting is considered a problem only if it persists after the age of 6 or if it starts again after 6 months or more of dryness. At the age of 5, about 1 in 7 children

wets the bed regularly. At the age of 10, the number is about 1 in 20. The problem is slightly more common in boys. Some children are late staying dry at night because the section of the nervous system that controls bladder function develops slowly. This developmental delay sometimes runs in families. Other children start to bedwet following stressful events such as divorce. Rarely, the condition develops because of an underlying disorder, such as diabetes mellitus (p.437) or a urinary tract infection (*see* **Urinary tract infections in children**, opposite page).

What can I do?
The most important factors in helping your child to stop bedwetting are praise, patience, and encouragement. Talking to your child may reveal worries that could be contributing to the problem. Routine visits to the toilet before bedtime are important, and it may be helpful to wake your child at your own bedtime so he or she can pass urine. It may also help to limit the amount your child drinks in the two hours before bedtime and avoid giving caffeinated drinks such as cola. A chart, on which a star is awarded after each dry night, is a visible reminder of progress. If your child is still wetting the bed after the age of 6 or begins to wet after 6 months or more of being dry at night, consult your doctor.

What might the doctor do?
Your doctor may test a urine sample to exclude diabetes mellitus or a urinary tract infection that may require treatment with antibiotics (p.572).

Children may be helped to overcome persistent bedwetting with a special pad that triggers a buzzer when they start to pass urine (*see* **Overcoming bedwetting**, left). If your child goes away overnight, desmopressin (*see* **Drugs that affect bladder control**, p.606) may be prescribed. If bedwetting persists, your child may be referred to a special clinic for advice. With patience and support, most children eventually stop bedwetting.

Wilms' tumour

A rare cancer of the kidney, also known as a nephroblastoma

 Usually develops before the age of 5

 Sometimes runs in families

 Gender and lifestyle are not significant factors

Wilms' tumour is a rare type of kidney cancer, affecting about 1 in 10,000 children each year. The tumour commonly develops before the age of 5, and it may be present at birth. Usually, one kidney is affected, but in about 1 in 10 children with the disease tumours occur in both kidneys. Wilms' tumour sometimes runs in families, but in most cases the cause is unknown.

What are the symptoms?
A tumour may be large before symptoms appear. Symptoms may include:
■ Obvious swelling in the abdomen.
■ Abdominal pain or discomfort.
■ Occasionally, blood in the urine.
A child with these symptoms should be seen by a doctor immediately.

What might be done?
The doctor will examine your child and test a urine sample for the presence of blood. If the doctor suspects that there is a tumour in the kidney, further tests will be necessary. Ultrasound scanning (p.135) or CT scanning (p.132) of the kidneys may be performed. Other tests, such as a chest X-ray (p.300), may also be carried out to check if the cancer has spread elsewhere in the body.

Surgical removal of the affected kidney is the usual treatment for Wilms' tumour. The remaining healthy kidney can easily perform the work of both. To destroy any remaining cancerous cells, an affected child may have radiotherapy (p.158) and/or chemotherapy (p.157). In rare cases in which both the kidneys need to be removed, dialysis (p.451) or a kidney transplant (p.452) is necessary. Treatment has a high success rate, and about 8 in 10 affected children are free of the cancer after 5 years.

treating disease

MEDICAL AND PHARMACEUTICAL RESEARCH has provided doctors with a broad range of effective treatments, including powerful drugs and precise new forms of surgery. Although there are many treatments that cure a disease or disorder, the majority are designed to relieve symptoms. Some treatments, such as immunizations, are given to prevent diseases developing. Treatments for sick, disabled, and elderly people are provided in hospital and at home by carers ranging from nurses and other professionals to relatives and friends.

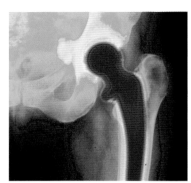

Artificial hip joint
Joints that have been damaged by disease can be replaced by artificial joints to relieve pain and to restore mobility.

When you are ill or injured, the first decision to be made is whether professional medical help is required. This may be obvious in an emergency but less so if the disorder is troublesome but does not appear to be serious. Many minor problems disappear without treatment, and many others can be dealt with using home or over-the-counter remedies.

Most treatments fall into one of three broad categories: drugs, surgery, or some form of supportive therapy or care. In practice, many disorders require a combination of treatments used simultaneously or in sequence, and often supported by nursing care.

Aims of treatment

The purpose of treatment may be to cure a disorder, slow down its progress, relieve symptoms, or prevent an illness developing. Supportive treatments, such as physiotherapy and counselling, focus on speeding up recovery or helping people to come to terms with their illness and live as independently as possible.

The optimal result of treatment is to cure an illness completely with minimum risk and side effects. When no cure is available, the next option is relief of symptoms. Some drugs relieve symptoms common to several conditions. Other drugs relieve symptoms that are specific to particular conditions. For example, bronchodilators are drugs that ease the wheezing that occurs in lung disorders such as asthma. Drugs may also be used to increase the levels of substances in the body, such as hormones and neurotransmitters. Even if a disease is incurable, treatment may still be able to slow its progression and relieve symptoms.

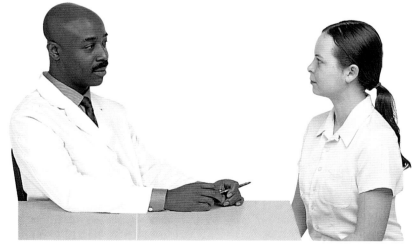

You and your doctor
If you require treatment, your doctor will discuss the benefits and disadvantages of the suggested treatment options and answer any questions so that you can make an informed choice.

Planning treatment

Before starting treatment, your doctor will discuss the available options with you. For minor illnesses or when there is only one suitable treatment, little discussion may be required. However, for a long-term disorder or one that is serious, there may be a choice between treatment with surgery or with drugs, or between different forms of surgery or different drugs. Your doctor will also discuss the risks or possible side effects of your treatment. Your consent will be needed before treatment can begin.

For most disorders, early diagnosis and treatment offer the best chances of a cure. Where there is no prospect of a cure, there may be little benefit in radical treatment. For example, when a person has advanced cancer, chemotherapy and radiotherapy may do little to prolong life and can cause debilitating side effects. The better option may be relief of symptoms in hospital or at home.

Advances and improvements

Advances in medicine have led to new treatments that play a major part in improving life expectancy and reducing long-term illness. New technologies have brought about improvements in surgical techniques that minimize post-operative pain, reduce risks and complications, and allow quicker recovery. However, before a new drug or technique is approved, it must be rigorously tested, and its effectiveness and safety demonstrated in controlled trials.

Development of drugs

Over the past 100 years, medical research has produced safer and more reliably effective synthetic modifications of naturally occurring substances and some completely new drugs. Antibiotics and vaccines have revolutionized the treatment of infections.

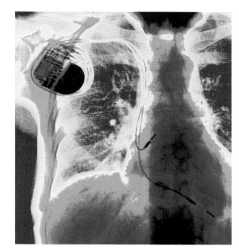

Regulating the heart
Some treatments, such as the fitting of an artificial pacemaker, help to control the effects of a disorder rather than treating the underlying cause.

Genetic engineering is now used to produce human insulin and other hormonal treatments. Research into the underlying mechanisms of disease has produced tailor-made drugs that target a particular part of a disease process. The development of immunosuppressant drugs that reduce the body's rejection of new tissue has enabled transplants to be carried out successfully.

Advances in surgery

Surgery can now often be performed through a natural body opening or a small incision, which is sometimes known as "keyhole surgery", using a viewing tube called an endoscope.

In microsurgery, surgeons use a specialized microscope and tiny instruments to perform operations on minute structures, such as nerves and small blood vessels. For operations on delicate areas, surgeons can wear a headset that displays three-dimensional images. Lasers and electrocautery equipment seal blood vessels as tissue is cut.

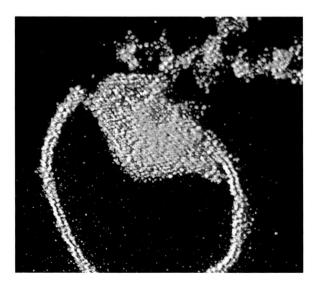

Drug killing a bacterium
A Staphylococcus aureus *bacterium is destroyed by an antibiotic drug.*

Drug treatment

Medicinal drugs are substances that can cure, arrest, or prevent disease, relieve symptoms, or help in the diagnosis of disorders. There are a huge number of drugs available, and new drugs are continually being developed that are more effective at restoring health and saving lives than ever before.

MODERN DRUG THERAPY began when scientists discovered how to isolate the active ingredients in plant sources and how to create synthetic versions of them. This technology, together with a better understanding of how the body functions in health and disease, has enabled the development of drugs that can target specific processes in the body.

Before any new drug is marketed, it is thoroughly tested. The effects that the drug has on people are measured either against the existing standard treatment or against a placebo (an inactive substance that looks and tastes exactly like the drug). In the UK, drugs are approved and licensed by the Medicines and Healthcare products Regulatory Agency (MHRA). A new drug is approved only if it is shown to be safe and effective. The MHRA can withdraw a drug from the market if it later proves to cause unacceptable side effects.

How drugs work

Drugs act in a variety of ways. Some kill or halt the spread of invading organisms, such as bacteria, fungi, and viruses. These drugs include antivirals, antifungals, and antibiotics. Other drugs, known as cytotoxic drugs, kill cells as they divide or prevent their replication. Cytotoxic drugs are mainly used in the treatment of cancer.

Some drugs simply supplement missing or low levels of natural body chemicals such as certain hormones or vitamins. Another group of drugs alters the effectiveness of certain body chemicals. These drugs work either by mimicking the action of natural chemicals to increase their effect or by blocking their action to decrease their effect (see How drugs act on receptors, below). Drugs may also affect the part of the nervous system that controls a particular process, such as the brain's vomiting centre to relieve vomiting.

How drugs are used

There are various different ways in which drugs may be delivered to their intended site of action. Some, such as eyedrops or topical skin preparations, can be applied directly to the target area. These preparations tend to have a very localized effect and do not usually enter the bloodstream in significant quantities. Other preparations are introduced into the bloodstream, which circulates them to their target area in the body. These drugs may be delivered by different routes, depending on which is the most effective way to reach the target area and on how the drugs are metabolized (see Drug metabolism, opposite page).

IN THIS SECTION

✚ **DRUG ACTION**

How drugs act on receptors

Many cells have specialized areas, known as receptors, on their outer surfaces. Natural chemical messengers, such as hormones, bind with these receptors to produce changes in cells and thereby affect body processes. In order to treat some disorders, it may be necessary to increase or decrease the effect of a particular natural chemical. Drugs called agonists bind with specific receptors to produce an effect similar to that of the natural chemical. Antagonist drugs inhibit the effect of the chemical by blocking the receptors.

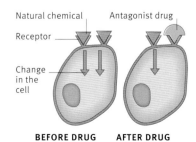

Agonist drugs
An agonist drug mimics the action of body chemicals. It occupies an empty receptor and enhances the natural chemical's effect.

Antagonist drugs
An antagonist drug occupies cell receptors, preventing the body chemicals from binding to them, thereby inhibiting their action.

✚ **PROCESS**

Drugs in your body

Drugs can be introduced into the bloodstream by a number of different routes. Most commonly, they are taken orally in the form of pills, capsules, or liquids. However, if oral treatment is inappropriate, drugs may be given in various other ways. For example, a suppository containing a drug can be inserted into the rectum. If an immediate effect is needed, intravenous injection or infusion ensures rapid delivery of the drug. A long-lasting effect may be achieved by administering a drug in a skin patch or as an implant inserted just under the skin.

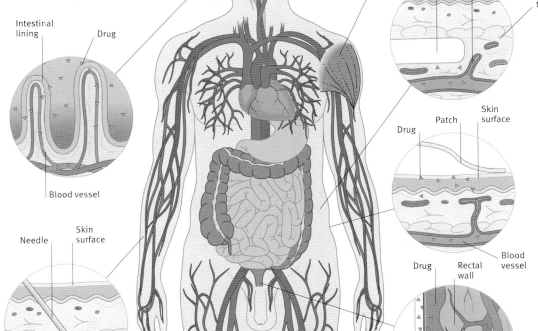

Nasal/sublingual/buccal route
Drugs in a nasal spray, in a sublingual tablet (placed under the tongue), or in a buccal tablet (placed inside the cheek) are absorbed through the thin mucous membrane directly into the bloodstream.

Drug
Blood vessel
Mucus layer
Mucous membrane

Oral route
Drugs in pill, capsule, or liquid form are swallowed and pass into the digestive system. The drugs are then broken down in either the stomach or the intestines and are absorbed in the same way as food.

Intestinal lining
Drug
Blood vessel

Intravenous route
An injection into a blood vessel allows a drug to take effect very quickly. The drug enters the bloodstream directly and is rapidly circulated to the organ or tissues where it is needed.

Needle
Skin surface
Drug
Blood vessel

Intramuscular route
Drugs are injected into a muscle in the upper arm, thigh, or buttock and then disperse into the bloodstream.

Needle
Muscle
Drug in bloodstream

Subcutaneous route
Drugs implanted or injected into fatty tissue just below the skin disperse slowly into the bloodstream.

Implant
Drug
Fatty tissue

Transdermal route
Drugs are released continuously from an adhesive patch or a gel on the skin surface and pass through the skin into blood vessels.

Drug
Patch
Skin surface
Blood vessel

Rectal route
Drugs inserted into the rectum in suppositories, enemas, or foam are quickly absorbed by blood vessels in the rectal wall.

Drug
Rectal wall
Suppository

Drug metabolism

Drugs that are taken orally are absorbed in the intestines and pass through the liver before entering the general circulation. Drugs that are administered by other routes enter the bloodstream before they pass through the liver. Once a drug has entered the bloodstream, it circulates to the site where its action is needed. Most drugs are metabolized (broken down or transformed) each time they pass through the liver. They are eventually excreted by the kidneys in urine and/or by the liver in bile, which is excreted in faeces.

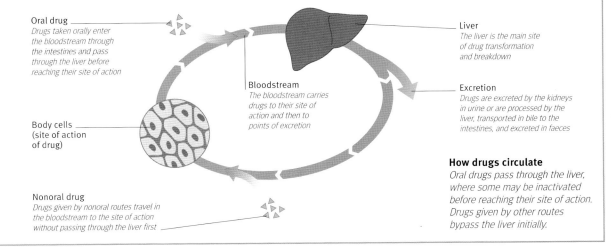

Oral drug
Drugs taken orally enter the bloodstream through the intestines and pass through the liver before reaching their site of action

Body cells (site of action of drug)

Bloodstream
The bloodstream carries drugs to their site of action and then to points of excretion

Nonoral drug
Drugs given by nonoral routes travel in the bloodstream to the site of action without passing through the liver first

Liver
The liver is the main site of drug transformation and breakdown

Excretion
Drugs are excreted by the kidneys in urine or are processed by the liver, transported in bile to the intestines, and excreted in faeces

How drugs circulate
Oral drugs pass through the liver, where some may be inactivated before reaching their site of action. Drugs given by other routes bypass the liver initially.

Understanding drugs

All drugs, even the familiar ones such as aspirin, may have potentially harmful as well as beneficial effects. Whether you are prescribed drug treatment or you choose remedies for yourself, you will gain most benefit from drugs if you understand how they are likely to act and how to use them safely and effectively.

During the last century, advances in drug treatment have enabled doctors to cure many conditions, including a wide range of infectious diseases. Drug treatment can also be used to control symptoms in disorders such as epilepsy and to relieve common symptoms such as itching. Today, there is a vast range of drugs available. Some can be bought over the counter (OTC), but others require a doctor's prescription and are known as prescription-only medicines (POMs).

The first article in this section covers the types of effect that various drugs may have on the body. The second article gives practical advice on how to use medications effectively and how to store drugs safely.

Courses of vaccination
Most drugs are used in the treatment of disease. However, vaccines may be given to prevent certain diseases, such as diphtheria or tetanus, from developing.

▶ **SELF-ADMINISTRATION**

Giving a child medicine

When giving liquid medicines to a baby or a young child, use a syringe or dropper to avoid spillage and ensure that you give the correct dose. If you are unsure how to use the syringe or dropper, ask your pharmacist to show you how to measure and give a dose of medicine. When treating the child, hold him or her securely to give reassurance and keep the child from struggling.

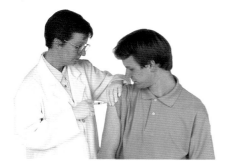

Syringe
Angle the tip of the syringe at the inside of the cheek

Giving medicine with a syringe
Place the tip of the syringe well inside the child's mouth and angle it towards the cheek. Slowly press the plunger, allowing the child time to swallow. Do not aim directly down the child's throat.

How drugs affect you

How drugs act on your body and their possible effects

A drug may have several types of effect on your body as well as the intended action. These include side effects, tolerance, and dependence. Interaction may also occur, in which drugs that are taken together enhance or reduce each other's actions. Some drugs may also interact with certain foods and with complementary remedies. Many drugs can have a powerful psychological benefit called the placebo effect. A number of drugs have unwanted effects, which can be unpleasant or harmful, and your doctor will plan drug treatment to avoid or minimize these effects.

Side effects of drugs

Almost all systemic drugs (drugs that affect the whole body) can cause side effects – undesired reactions resulting from a normal dose. Many side effects occur because drugs act on cells throughout the body, not just in the area to be treated. For example, beta-blocker drugs (p.581) may be used in the treatment of hypertension (p.242). However, they may disrupt sleeping patterns as a side effect of their intended action.

Some side effects, such as the dry mouth caused by some antihistamines (p.585). are predictable because they result from the known chemical effects of a drug. However, drugs may also produce unpredictable reactions such as drug allergy (p.284). Any type of drug, including penicillins (see **Antibiotics**, p.572), can cause allergic reactions that can range in severity from a mild rash to severe

breathing problems. Other unexpected reactions occur in people whose genetic make-up influences their body's ability to process particular drugs. For example, some people of Mediterranean, African, or Southeast Asian origin inherit a condition called G6PD deficiency, which affects the chemistry of red blood cells. If these people take certain types of drug, such as sulphonamides, they may develop haemolytic anaemia (p.273), a condition in which red blood cells are destroyed prematurely. As a result, the blood does not carry enough oxygen to body tissues.

Most side effects are not serious, and they often disappear gradually as your body becomes used to a drug. However, for some drugs used to treat serious disorders, the side effects are severe and potentially fatal. For instance, certain cytotoxic drugs used to treat cancer (see **Anticancer Drugs**, p.586) are toxic to the heart and can cause it to fail. A medical decision to use a drug depends on whether the overall benefit outweighs the risk of harmful effects.

Drug tolerance and dependence

If you take certain drugs for a long time, your body adapts to them in a process known as tolerance. With some drugs, tolerance may be useful, allowing the body to overcome side effects while still responding to the beneficial effects of the drug. However, tolerance may make some drugs less effective so that a higher dose is needed to obtain the same result. The higher dose may increase side effects.

Dependence is a need for a drug. The need can be psychological or physical. If you become dependent on certain drugs, your body may develop tolerance to them. If you then stop taking them, you may suffer unpleasant effects known as withdrawal symptoms.

People at special risk

The effects of a drug may differ from one person to another. This variation occurs because people's bodies absorb and excrete drugs at different rates. In addition, the same dose of a drug may reach different concentrations in the blood depending on factors such as body size and kidney function.

Fetuses Most drugs that are taken during pregnancy pass across the placenta to the fetus. Many can harm the fetus, especially if taken during the first 12 weeks of pregnancy when the fetus's organs are developing. If you know or believe that you are pregnant, check with your doctor or pharmacist before taking any drug, including over-the-counter drugs or complementary remedies. If you take medication for a long-term condition, consult your doctor if you are planning a pregnancy.

Breast-fed babies If a woman takes drugs while breast-feeding, they may pass into her breast milk. Some drugs cause unwanted effects in the baby. For example, antianxiety drugs may make the baby drowsy. If you are breast-feeding, you should check with your doctor or pharmacist before taking any drug, including over-the-counter drugs or complementary remedies.

Babies and children Drugs must be used with care in babies and children. Children's doses are usually smaller than doses for adults and are often calculated on the basis of a child's weight or age. It is very important to give children the correct dose. Never give a child a drug prescribed for an adult.

People with liver or kidney disease Most drugs are broken down by enzymes in the liver. The drugs are then eliminated by the liver or the kidneys and excreted in the urine. If your liver or kidneys are not functioning well, toxic substances may build up in your blood, increasing the risk of side effects. You may need lower doses than normal. Alcohol also affects liver function, so the effect of some drugs may be altered if you drink heavily or regularly.

Older people Older people are at increased risk of side effects. This risk may be due to the decline in the function of organs such as the liver and kidneys as the body ages, which causes toxins to accumulate faster in the body.

Managing your medication

Using prescription and over-the-counter medications safely and effectively

Drugs must always be used with care, and you should be especially careful if you give them to children. It is important to understand how drugs are likely to affect you. Drugs must also be stored safely.

How are drugs obtained?

Some drugs may be bought over the counter, but others require a doctor's prescription. When buying an over-the-counter (OTC) medication, it is wise to consult a pharmacist to make sure you are buying a remedy that is effective and is suitable for you. If you buy on the internet, make sure the website is a registered one. You can check this at www.pharmacyregulation.org/registration/internet-pharmacy

Using drugs safely

Read the instructions carefully and discuss anything you do not understand with your doctor or pharmacist. Find out whether the drug is likely to affect everyday tasks, whether you should take the drug with food, and what you should do if you miss or exceed a dose.

When you discuss your treatment with a doctor or pharmacist, let him or her know if you have recently taken any other medications, including any complementary remedies. If you are planning a pregnancy, consult your doctor before starting treatment.

Taking drugs correctly When taking tablets or capsules, swallow them with plenty of water so that they do not become stuck in your oesophagus. If you are taking liquid medicine, shake the bottle before use to mix the ingredients thoroughly, and measure the doses carefully. Devise a routine for taking the correct doses at the correct time.

Make sure that you complete the full course of any treatment, even if your symptoms seem to have disappeared. **Dealing with side effects** Seek medical help if you develop any unexpected side effects or symptoms that seem unrelated to your illness while taking either prescription or OTC drugs. If you have a severe reaction to a drug, such as difficulty in breathing, call for urgent medical attention. If you have a mild reaction from a prescription drug, see your doctor as soon as possible. If you have a mild reaction from an OTC drug, stop taking it and consult your doctor.

Taking long-term medication If you need drug treatment that continues for a long time, you may be given a prescription that can be renewed without visiting your doctor each time. Never stop taking your medication suddenly without consulting your doctor. Talk to your doctor or pharmacist before using any additional drugs, including OTC drugs and complementary remedies. If you need hospital treatment, tell the staff which drugs (prescription, OTC, and complementary remedies) you are taking.

Giving drugs to children
It is normally simpler to administer liquid medicine by syringe or dropper (*see* **Giving a child medicine**, opposite page). Older children may be given tablets, but if you need to crush them first, check with the pharmacist that this will not affect absorption. A child who dislikes medicine can have a pleasant drink afterwards.

How should drugs be kept?
Follow storage directions to prevent drugs from deteriorating. Always keep medicines out of reach of children, preferably in a locked cabinet.

Do not keep medicines beyond their expiry dates and make sure that you always dispose of drugs carefully.

Drugs for infections and infestations

As recently as 50 years ago, infectious diseases were a leading cause of death in children and young adults. That picture has changed with the introduction of immunization against the major childhood diseases, antibiotics to kill bacteria, and a wide range of other anti-infective drugs.

This section describes the drugs that are used to protect the body against infectious disease as well as to control or cure infections and infestations once they have developed.

The first article discusses vaccines and immunoglobulins, which are given to provide immunity against certain infections and to prevent the spread of diseases. The next article describes antibiotics, a large group of drugs used widely to treat bacterial infections. In the UK, millions of prescriptions are written for these drugs each year.

The following articles in this section explain how drugs are used to treat infections caused by viruses, protozoa, and fungi. The information includes discussion of the prevention and cure of malaria and of recent advances made in the treatment of HIV infection and AIDS. The final article deals with drugs to eradicate parasitic worm infestations.

✚ KEY ELEMENTS

FUNGI

BACTERIA

1 mm

WORMS

PROTOZOA

VIRUSES

For more information on the structure and function of infectious organisms, *see* pp.161–163.

Vaccines and immunoglobulins

Preparations that immunize the body against certain infectious diseases

COMMON PREPARATIONS

Vaccines
- BCG (tuberculosis) ■ Cholera ■ Diphtheria ■ Hepatitis A ■ Hepatitis B ■ Hib (Haemophilus influenzae type b) ■ HPV (human papillomavirus) ■ Influenza ■ Meningitis A, C, W & Y ■ Meningitis B ■ Meningitis C ■ MMR (measles/mumps/rubella) ■ Pertussis ■ Pneumococcus ■ Polio ■ Rabies ■ Rotavirus ■ Shingles ■ Tetanus ■ Typhoid ■ Varicella zoster ■ Yellow fever

Immunoglobulins
- Anti-D ■ Hepatitis B ■ Normal immunoglobulin ■ Rabies ■ Tetanus

A variety of vaccines and immunoglobulins is available to provide protection against particular infectious diseases. The use of these preparations is known as immunization (p.12). Vaccines contain infectious organisms that have been modified or killed. Immunoglobulins contain antibodies (proteins made by white blood cells that neutralize or destroy infectious organisms) extracted from the blood of a person who has already had a specific disease. The body's own defence mechanism, the immune system, is able to combat many infections, but it cannot protect people against all infectious diseases. Immunization with vaccines or immunoglobulins is therefore used to give added protection. The incidence of a number of highly infectious diseases has declined dramatically worldwide since the introduction of immunization programmes. One disease, smallpox, has been eradicated worldwide.

How do they work?
There are two forms of immunization, which are known as active immunization and passive immunization (*see* **How immunization works**, p.572). In active immunization, vaccines are given to stimulate the immune system to produce its own antibodies. A different vaccine must be given for each disease because each type of infectious organism triggers the production of a specific type of antibody. Some vaccines contain live organisms that have been altered and made harmless. Others contain killed organisms, part of an organism, or a toxin (poison) made by bacteria. All forms of vaccine have the same effect of priming the body's immune system to produce appropriate antibodies so that the body is ready to fight off particular invading organisms. Passive immunization uses immunoglobulins and works by introducing donated antibodies into the blood. These antibodies destroy infectious organisms that are present or that enter the body shortly afterwards.

Why are they used?
Some highly infectious diseases cannot be treated effectively or can be so serious that prevention, in the form of active or passive immunization, is recommended. Active immunization with vaccines is used mainly to prevent diseases from spreading within a community. If most people are vaccinated, some diseases may eventually disappear. In developed countries, children are routinely given active immunization against a range of diseases from the age of 2 months, including diphtheria (p.172), measles (p.167), tetanus (p.173), poliomyelitis (p.168), and pertussis (whooping cough) (p.301) (*see* **Routine immunizations**, p.13).

Other vaccines are used for specific groups of people. For example, immunization against seasonal influenza (p.164) is recommended for people who are at high risk of becoming seriously ill if they develop the disease. Those at high risk include elderly people, those who have reduced immunity because of diseases such as diabetes mellitus (p.437), and people with long-term heart or lung disease. There are many different types (strains) of influenza, and a specific vaccine is required for each one. New influenza vaccines are usually created each year to match the viral strains of seasonal influenza predicted to be most widespread. Specific vaccines may also be created for unexpected outbreaks of new strains of nonseasonal influenza, such as H1N1 influenza (swine flu).

Vaccines are also used for people at increased risk of catching certain infections. For example, travellers to a developing country are advised to receive immunization against diseases common in that region (*see* **Travel immunizations**, p.35).

The main use of passive immunization with immunoglobulins is in cases where rapid protection against disease is necessary, for example after exposure to infection. This process is also used to provide antibodies against particular infections in people whose immune systems are suppressed due to disorders such as HIV infection and AIDS (p.169) or as a result of certain drug treatments (*see* **Immunosuppressants**, p.585).

How are they used?
Most vaccines are given by injection (although cholera vaccine is given orally and typhoid may be given orally or by injection). Many vaccines provide lifelong immunity with one dose or a course of several doses, but some may not give full protection or may be effective for only a few months or years. The degree of protection depends largely on the strength of the immune reaction a vaccine provokes. Additional doses (booster doses) may be needed at regular intervals to reinforce the effect of the original course of a vaccine and to maintain immunity.

Often, vaccines against more than one infection are given in a combined preparation, limiting the number of injections that are needed. For example, vaccines against measles, mumps, and rubella (MMR) are given together.

Immunoglobulins are given by injection into a muscle or intravenously. They are effective for a short period only, and protection diminishes over several weeks, partly depending on the dose. If continued protection is needed, the treatment must be repeated.

What are the side effects?

Some vaccines, such as the polio vaccine, cause few side effects. Others, such as the measles, mumps, and rubella (MMR) vaccine, may produce mild forms of the diseases. Many vaccines may cause a red, tender area at the injection site and a mild fever or flu-like illness that lasts a few days. Severe side effects, including the allergic reaction anaphylaxis (p.285), are rare. For most people, the risks are far outweighed by the protection given. In some cases, vaccines should not be given. If you or your child has a fever, vaccination should be postponed until the fever has subsided. Vaccines containing live organisms should not be given during pregnancy or to those who have some types of cancer or whose immune systems are suppressed (although HIV-positive people can have MMR unless they are severely immunosuppressed).

Side effects of immunoglobulins are uncommon but may include tenderness at the injection site and fever. Repeated immunoglobulin treatment may result in an allergic reaction, such as a rash.

Antibiotics

A group of drugs used primarily to treat infections caused by bacteria

COMMON DRUGS

Penicillins
- Amoxicillin - Ampicillin - Co-amoxiclav
- Flucloxacillin - Phenoxymethylpenicillin

Cephalosporins
- Cefaclor - Cefalexin - Cefixime
- Cefradine - Ceftazidime - Cefuroxime

Macrolides
- Azithromycin - Clarithromycin
- Erythromycin

Tetracyclines
- Doxycycline - Lymecycline - Minocycline
- Oxytetracycline - Tetracycline

Aminoglycosides
- Amikacin - Gentamicin - Neomycin
- Streptomycin - Tobramycin

Sulphonamides
- Co-trimoxazole - Sulfadiazine

Quinolones
- Ciprofloxacin - Levofloxacin - Norfloxacin
- Ofloxacin

Other antibiotics
- Chloramphenicol - Clindamycin
- Fusidic acid - Metronidazole
- Trimethoprim - Vancomycin

Antibiotics are among the most commonly prescribed drugs in the world. They are used to treat and prevent bacterial infections. The drugs work either by killing bacteria directly or by halting their multiplication so that the body's immune system is able to overcome the remaining infection.

Antibiotics are classified in groups, such as penicillins, cephalosporins, and tetra-

---

How immunization works

The most commonly used method of immunization is known as active immunization or vaccination. This involves the introduction into the body of a harmless form of an infectious organism that stimulates the body to produce antibodies against that organism. To provide immediate protection, a method called passive immunization is used. This introduces into the body "ready-made" antibodies extracted from people or animals who already have immunity to the infection.

Active immunization

Many vaccines are made from weakened forms of a disease-causing organism; these are known as live vaccines. Others use an inactive form or just a part of the organism, such as a protein. Protection may be lifelong, or booster shots may be needed.

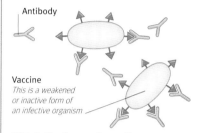

Vaccine
This is a weakened or inactive form of an infective organism

[1] *Antibodies are formed in response to the organisms in the vaccine. A "memory" of these antibodies is retained by the immune system.*

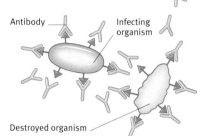

[2] *If the same organism invades the body at a later date, the immune system will recognize it and will rapidly produce antibodies to destroy it.*

Passive immunization

Immunity to an infectious organism can be achieved by the introduction of donated antibodies. This is needed if no active immunization is available or if rapid protection against an organism is vital, especially for people with weakened immune systems.

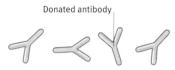

Donated antibody

[1] *Antibodies taken from humans or animals with immunity to the infection are introduced into the body.*

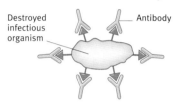

[2] *When exposed to the infectious organism, the antibodies immediately destroy it. They also provide short-term protection against future infection.*

---

cyclines, according to their chemical composition and the way in which they work. One of the most commonly used groups of antibiotics is penicillins (*see* **How penicillins work**, below). Some antibiotics work against a wide range of bacteria and are called broad-spectrum antibiotics. Other antibiotics work against only one or two types of bacteria and are known as narrow-spectrum antibiotics. Some also work against other types of infection, such as those caused by certain protozoa (*see* **Antiprotozal drugs**, p.574).

Why are they used?

Antibiotics are most commonly used for the short-term treatment of minor infections, such as infections of the ear, throat, or urinary tract. The drugs may also be used in the treatment of serious infections, such as septicaemia (p.171) and bacterial meningitis (p.325).

On occasion, long-term treatment with low-dose antibiotics may be given to prevent infection in people whose immunity is reduced, such as those with HIV infection or AIDS (p.169) and people who are taking immunosuppressants (p.585). Long-term use of antibiotics may also be prescribed for other conditions, such as acne (p.197).

How are they used?

Most bacterial infections are treated with oral antibiotics. Eye and ear infections are often treated using antibiotic drops (*see* **Drugs for eye and ear disorders**, pp.593–595). To treat severe infections, when high doses of antibiotics are needed

---

immediately, the drugs may be given by intramuscular injection or by intravenous injection or infusion.

If you have a bacterial infection, your doctor will probably prescribe a specific antibiotic that is effective against the bacterium which is most likely to be causing that infection. For certain conditions, such as pneumonia (p.299) or a wound infection, your doctor may carry out tests to identify the specific infecting organism before prescribing a narrow-spectrum antibiotic. In the meantime, you will probably be treated with

---

a broad-spectrum antibiotic. More than one antibiotic may be prescribed to reduce the risk of antibiotic resistance developing.

When you are taking antibiotics, you should continue treatment even after your symptoms improve. Finish the entire course prescribed by your doctor in order to eradicate the infection. Bacterial resistance to antibiotics is increasing, due in part to incorrect use.

Antibiotics are available by prescription only. The choice of antibiotic may be restricted if you are pregnant, have a

---

How penicillins work

Penicillin antibiotics are used to treat many bacterial infections. Penicillins are bactericidal, which means that they actually destroy the bacteria causing infection. Most other types of antibiotic work by altering chemical activity in the bacteria, thereby preventing them from reproducing. The immune system is then able to overcome the remaining infection.

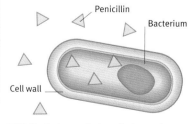

Penicillin
Bacterium
Cell wall

[1] *Bacteria are single-celled organisms that have protective cell walls. The penicillin enters the bacterium, beginning a process that will destroy it.*

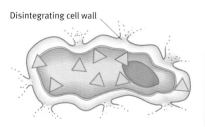

Disintegrating cell wall

[2] *The drug interferes with chemicals needed by the bacterium to form its cell walls. This causes the cell walls to disintegrate, and the bacterium dies.*

history of drug allergy, have impaired kidney or liver function, or if you are taking other drugs that might interact with a particular antibiotic.

What are the side effects?

Antibiotics do not usually cause serious side effects. The most common is diarrhoea, although it is not usually severe. Antibiotics can alter the balance between normal bacteria and the yeast *Candida albicans* that occurs naturally in or on the body; this imbalance may lead to an overgrowth of the yeast (*see* **Candidiasis**, p.177). In some cases, antibiotics destroy harmless bacteria in the bowel that prevent the growth of disease-causing organisms. Rarely, this results in the potentially serious condition pseudomembranous colitis, which can cause diarrhoea and severe dehydration.

Penicillins may cause rashes and in some people a rare, life-threatening allergic reaction known as anaphylaxis (p.285). This is more common when the drugs are given by injection and occurs mainly in people who have previously had a mild allergic reaction to a penicillin. If you are allergic to one type of penicillin, you will be allergic to others in the same group. About 1 in 10 people who is allergic to penicillin is also allergic to cephalosporins. If you have an adverse reaction, such as a rash, stop taking the drug and see your doctor promptly. If you have previously had a reaction, tell your doctor.

Tetracyclines can cause changes to growing bones and teeth and are therefore not prescribed for young children or pregnant women. In some rare cases, aminoglycosides can damage the kidneys, cause severe skin rashes, and affect the sense of hearing and balance.

Quinolones occasionally cause convulsions and should not be taken by people with epilepsy. They may rarely cause tendon damage and, in children, damage to joints.

Sulphonamides sometimes cause serious side effects, such as rashes and kidney damage.

Antituberculous drugs

Drugs used in the treatment of the bacterial infection tuberculosis

COMMON DRUGS

- Capreomycin ■ Cycloserine ■ Ethambutol
- Isoniazid ■ Pyrazinamide ■ Rifabutin
- Rifampicin ■ Streptomycin

Antituberculous drugs are antibiotics (p.572) used mainly or exclusively to treat tuberculosis, or TB (p.300). The initial infection usually develops in the lungs, but may spread to other parts of the body, such as the kidneys, lymph nodes, and sometimes the membranes covering the brain and spinal cord (*see* **Meningitis**, p.325). Usually, several antituberculous drugs are given together to prevent drug resistance from developing.

How are they used?

If you are diagnosed with TB, the strain of bacteria causing the infection will be tested to determine its sensitivity to specific antituberculous drugs. While you are waiting for the results, which can take up to 2 months, your doctor will prescribe an initial combination of four drugs to be taken orally. The main drugs used are isoniazid, pyrazinamide, ethambutol, and rifampicin. After the initial 2 months, isoniazid and rifampicin are used. Treatment with these drugs is usually continued for 4 months to ensure that the infection is eradicated. In some cases, this treatment may need to be continued for a longer period, depending on the organs affected. For example, treatment may need to continue for 12 months if the infection has led to meningitis.

It is important that you complete the course of drugs as instructed by your doctor. If you fail to do so, the bacteria may not be eradicated and drug-resistant strains may develop, which can then be transmitted to other people.

What are the side effects?

Antituberculous drugs may cause side effects, such as nausea, vomiting, rashes, and abdominal pain. Isoniazid, pyrazinamide, and rifampicin may damage the liver, so you will have liver function tests before treatment. If your liver function is found to be impaired, you will have regular liver function monitoring during treatment. Kidney function will also be checked before treatment; if your kidney function is impaired, a reduced drug dosage will be given. Rifampicin may turn urine and other body secretions red, but this effect is harmless. However, it can also reduce the effectiveness of some types of contraception, such as the combined contraceptive pill. Isoniazid may affect the nerves, causing numbness or tingling in the hands or feet. Ethambutol may rarely damage the nerves in the eyes, causing vision problems. People taking it are usually advised to have regular vision tests. If you are taking it and develop blurred vision or cannot distinguish colours, see your doctor promptly.

Antiviral drugs

Drugs that are used to treat certain infections caused by viruses

COMMON DRUGS

- Aciclovir ■ Boceprevir ■ Famciclovir
- Foscarnet ■ Ganciclovir ■ Inferferon alfa
- Lamivudine ■ Oseltamivir ■ Ribavirin
- Telaprevir ■ Valaciclovir ■ Zanamivir

Drugs for HIV infection and AIDS (right)

Various drugs are available to treat viral infections. Although these drugs may not eliminate an infection, they are often effective in reducing its severity. Many viral illnesses are mild and clear up without

treatment because healthy people can usually fight off infection quickly. Sometimes, antiviral drugs help to relieve symptoms and hasten recovery. However, because viruses invade body cells in order to multiply, antiviral drugs can damage body cells as well as the targeted viruses. Their use is therefore usually limited to treating severe or recurrent infections. Some antiviral drugs are more effective against certain viruses than others. A particular range of antivirals is used to treat HIV infection (*see* **Drugs for HIV infection and AIDS**, right).

Why are they used?

The main use for antivirals is in the treatment of infections that recur or persist over a prolonged period, such as herpes, HIV, and chronic hepatitis B and C. Some drugs are also effective in treating or preventing infections in people with impaired immune systems who are at increased risk of severe illness and complications.

Antivirals such as aciclovir, valaciclovir, and famciclovir are most commonly used to treat herpes simplex infections (p.166) in people who have severe or recurrent genital herpes or cold sores. These drugs are also effective against the varicella–zoster virus, which causes chickenpox (p.165) as well as shingles (*see* **Herpes zoster**, p.166).

Some antivirals are used for specific infections, especially in at-risk people such as those whose immunity is impaired by disease or by drug treatment (such as chemotherapy) and those with certain conditions such as diabetes, chronic kidney disease, and significant cardiovascular disease. For example, oseltamivir and zanamivir may be used to treat severe cases of influenza, and to treat otherwise healthy people in certain situations, such as pandemics. Ganciclovir is used for preventing or treating cytomegalovirus infection (p.167), especially in people with reduced immunity. Ribavirin may be used to treat babies with a severe form of bronchiolitis (p.545). It may also be used to treat Lassa fever (*see* **Viral haemorrhagic fevers**, p.169). In addition, ribavirin in combination with interferon alfa and/or boceprevir or telaprevir, may be used to treat chronic hepatitis C. Lamivudine and interferon alfa are used in the treatment of chronic hepatitis B.

How do they work?

Viruses invade body cells, where they use human genetic material (DNA) to reproduce. Antiviral drugs block this process, either by causing changes within body cells to prevent the virus from replicating or by preventing the virus from entering cells. If treatment is started early, the drugs usually work rapidly and relieve symptoms within a few days. However, some viruses develop resistance to the effects of drugs, which can make particular infections difficult to treat.

How are they used?

The drugs used to treat herpes infections, such as aciclovir, can be applied as a topical preparation or taken orally, depending on

the site and severity of the infection, or given by injection for urgent treatment of a serious infection. For mild infections, topical antivirals can be bought over the counter.

Ganciclovir and interferon are given by injection in hospital. Ribavirin can be given by inhaler to babies with bronchiolitis, by injection for Lassa fever, and orally for hepatitis C. For influenza, zanamivir is given by inhaler, and oseltamivir is given orally.

What are the side effects?

Aciclovir, valaciclovir, and famciclovir do not usually produce side effects, although when taken orally they may cause nausea. Rarely, when aciclovir is given by injection, the drug can cause kidney damage and may produce symptoms such as confusion and seizures. Ganciclovir may cause skin rashes and nausea. This drug can reduce red blood cell production, causing anaemia (p.271), and white blood cell production, increasing susceptibility to further infections. Ganciclovir may also lead to impairment of kidney function. The side effects of oseltamivir include nausea, vomiting, and other intestinal disturbances, and sometimes headache, insomnia, and dizziness. Zanamivir rarely produces side effects, although it may cause breathlessness and wheezing in some people, so it is used with caution in those with existing respiratory problems such as asthma. Ribavirin can cause anaemia and fetal abnormalities.

Interferon alfa commonly produces side effects, including nausea and flu-like symptoms such as tiredness, fever, and aching muscles. These effects are usually mild and may diminish with continued treatment. However, prolonged treatment can lead to decreased production of red and white blood cells and also depression.

Drugs for HIV infection and AIDS

A range of drugs that are used to treat HIV infection and its complications

COMMON DRUGS

Reverse transcriptase inhibitors
- Abacavir ■ Didanosine ■ Efavirenz
- Emtricitabine ■ Etravirine ■ Lamivudine
- Nevirapine ■ Stavudine ■ Tenofovir
- Zidovudine

Protease inhibitors
- Atazanavir ■ Darunavir ■ Fosamprenavir
- Indinavir ■ Ritonavir ■ Saquinavir
- Tipranavir

Fusion inhibitors
- Enfuvirtide

Other anti-HIV/AIDS drugs
- Maraviroc ■ Raltegravir

For people with HIV infection and AIDS (p.169) continued advances in drug treatments that slow or halt the progression of the disease have enabled most people to stay healthier for longer and to live comparatively normal lives.

However, drug treatments cannot cure the disease and a vaccine to protect against infection has not been developed.

The human immunodeficiency virus (HIV) infects and gradually destroys white blood cells of the body's immune system, known as CD4 lymphocytes, which normally help to fight infections. People with HIV infection may remain symptom-free for many years, or they may experience frequent or prolonged mild infections. If a specific infection or tumour occurs, a person is said to have AIDS (acquired immunodeficiency syndrome). These conditions, called AIDS-defining illnesses, include a number of severe infections, such as pneumocystis infection (p.177), toxoplasmosis (p.176), and certain cancers, such as Kaposi's sarcoma (p.201) and non-Hodgkin's lymphoma (p.279).

Why are they used?

The drugs currently in use to treat HIV infection have made it possible to suppress the level of the virus in the blood, with the aim of reducing it so that the virus becomes undetectable. If this aim is achieved, the immune system can recover sufficiently to deal with infections. The drugs may also be able to prevent the progression of HIV infection to AIDS. Evidence to support this is very encouraging, and many people have shown a dramatic improvement in their condition and also in their life expectancy.

Treatment of HIV infection involves combinations of antiretroviral drugs, which act against the virus itself, and anti-infective drugs such as antibiotics (p.572), which are used to treat the diseases that develop as a result of reduced immunity.

Treatment with antiretroviral drugs is believed to be beneficial for anybody with HIV infection or AIDS. In general, it is usually recommended that treatment begins when a patient's CD4 cell count falls below a certain level, although in some cases starting treatment at a higher CD4 count may be advised.

People who have been in contact with blood or other body fluids from a person with HIV are given immediate treatment with antiretroviral drugs for 1 month. This treatment is known as post-exposure prophylaxis or PEP. Antiretrovirals are also recommended for HIV-positive mothers during pregnancy to reduce the risk of the baby being born with the virus.

How do they work?

There are two main groups of antiretroviral drugs used in the treatment of HIV infection and AIDS: reverse transcriptase inhibitors and protease inhibitors. The drugs work by blocking the processes necessary for viral replication without significantly damaging the body cells that the virus has invaded. Reverse transcriptase inhibitors, such as zidovudine, inhibit viral enzymes involved in replication. Protease inhibitors, such as atazanavir, prevent the production of viral proteins necessary for replication. Fusion inhibitors and maraviroc inhibit the entry of HIV into body cells. Raltegravir works by

preventing HIV from integrating its genetic material into the chromosomes of human cells, thereby preventing viral replication inside cells.

How are they used?

Treatment of HIV infection and AIDS is subject to rapid change as knowledge about the virus increases. Currently, antiretroviral drugs are generally used in combination to destroy the virus more effectively and help to prevent the development of drug-resistant strains of HIV. Most people are treated with a combination of three or more antiviral drugs, and the development of combined preparations with multiple drugs in a single pill has simplified treatment for many people.

What are the side effects?

If you have HIV infection, your doctor will discuss your treatment options with you at length because the drugs have side effects that should be weighed against the benefits of treatment.

Antiretroviral drugs can cause nausea, vomiting, and diarrhoea, which may be very severe. Other serious side effects include inflammation of the pancreas (see Acute pancreatitis, p.413) and damage to the nerves, liver, or kidneys. There may also be redistribution of body fat, and anaemia (p.271) may develop. You need regular checkups and blood tests to look for warning signs of side effects. Pregnant women need expert advice on having treatment with antiretrovirals; these drugs may prevent transmission of HIV to the fetus but the effects of most antiretrovirals on fetal development are not known.

Antiprotozoal drugs

A group of drugs that is used to treat infections caused by protozoa

COMMON DRUGS

- Atovaquone ■ Co-trimoxazole ■ Diloxanide furoate ■ Mepracrine hydrochloride ■ Metronidazole ■ Pentamidine ■ Pyrimethamine with sulfadiazine ■ Sodium stibogluconate ■ Sulfadiazine ■ Tinidazole

A range of drugs is used to treat infections caused by single-celled organisms called protozoa. Some antiprotozoals, such as metronidazole and sulfadiazine, are also used for bacterial infections. A specific group of these drugs is used to treat malaria, a serious disease caused by protozoa that affects millions of people worldwide (see Antimalarial drugs, right).

Antiprotozoals act in various ways; some of the drugs work by preventing protozoa from multiplying.

Why are they used?

Antiprotozoals are commonly used to treat infections such as trichomoniasis (p.492) and giardiasis (p.176). Metronidazole or tinidazole is often taken for these disorders. Another use for antiprotozoals, particularly

pyrimethamine with sulfadazine, is to treat toxoplasmosis (p.176), an infection that can cause severe illness in fetuses and people with reduced immunity. Co-trimoxazole and pentamidine may be used for pneumocystis infection (p.177), a form of pneumonia that is potentially fatal in people whose immunity is reduced.

How are they used?

For minor infections, antiprotozoals are usually taken for about a week. Severe infections may need treatment for several months, especially in people with reduced immunity, such as those who have HIV infection or AIDS (p.169).

Most antiprotozoals are taken orally, but some may be injected to treat severe infections. Pentamidine is administered by injection or taken through an inhaler. This drug is given only under the supervision of a specialist.

What are the side effects?

Antiprotozoal drugs often cause side effects, including nausea, diarrhoea, and abdominal cramps. If you are taking metronidazole, you should avoid alcohol because it can cause vomiting. Another side effect of the drug is darkening of the urine. Pentamidine may cause a severe drop in blood pressure, either when it is administered or directly afterwards. In rare cases, pyrimethamine reduces red blood cell production, causing anaemia (p.271). If you have unusual bruising or bleeding while taking this drug, notify your doctor because these may be signs of a blood disorder.

Antimalarial drugs

A group of drugs that is used for the prevention and treatment of malaria

COMMON DRUGS

- Artemether with lumefantrine ■ Chloroquine ■ Doxycycline ■ Mefloquine ■ Primaquine ■ Proguanil ■ Proguanil with atovaquone ■ Pyrimethamine with sulfadoxine ■ Quinine

Antimalarial drugs are prescribed as a preventive measure against infection with malaria (p.175) and also as treatment if the disease develops. There are various types of antimalarial drug. Some are suitable only for treatment of the infection, while others are used for both prevention and treatment.

Malaria is a serious infectious disease caused by protozoa that are transmitted to humans by the bites of infected mosquitoes. The protozoa travel through the blood to the liver, where they multiply before re-entering the blood and circulating throughout the body. At this stage, the symptoms of malaria appear.

No antimalarial provides complete protection against the disease because malarial protozoa continually develop drug resistance. For this reason, you should protect yourself from mosquito bites if you

visit an area where malaria occurs. It is important to keep your body well covered and to use insect repellents and netting (see Travel health, p.35).

How do they work?

Antimalarial drugs are effective at different stages in the life cycle of the malarial protozoa. When taken to prevent malaria, the drugs act by killing the protozoa when they enter the liver or the red blood cells. To treat malaria once symptoms have appeared, higher doses of drugs are given to destroy the protozoa when they are released from the liver into the blood. In some cases, the protozoa lie dormant in the liver and reactivate to cause recurrent episodes of malaria. These protozoa are difficult to eradicate and are treated with primaquine.

How are they used?

The choice of drug usually depends on the part of the world you plan to visit or where you contracted the disease.

If you plan to visit a malarial risk area, you need to start preventive treatment up to 3 weeks before departure, continuing for 1–4 weeks after your return (the exact timings depend on the drugs taken). Antimalarials are usually taken orally, either once a day or once a week. To increase protection against the most drug-resistant strains, combinations of drugs may be given. For example, proguanil may be taken with chloroquine.

If you develop malaria, the drugs used for treatment may be taken orally or, in serious cases, given by intravenous drip. If you have recurrent bouts of malaria, your doctor will prescribe an oral antimalarial such as primaquine for 2–3 weeks or more to eradicate the protozoa.

What are the side effects?

Antimalarial drugs can cause a number of side effects, including nausea, diarrhoea, headaches, rashes, and blood disorders. Quinine can cause ringing in the ears (see Tinnitus, p.378), blurred vision, and hot flushes. Mefloquine can cause some people to experience panic attacks, dizziness, hallucinations, and depression.

If you are, or think you might be, pregnant, you should consult your doctor or pharmacist before taking antimalarial drugs. Mefloquine and chloroquine should not be taken by people with epilepsy.

Antifungal drugs

A group of drugs that is used to treat infections caused by fungi

COMMON DRUGS

- Amphotericin ■ Clotrimazole ■ Econazole ■ Fluconazole ■ Flucytosine ■ Griseofulvin ■ Itraconazole ■ Ketoconazole ■ Miconazole ■ Nystatin ■ Sulconazole ■ Terbinafine

Various drugs are available to treat fungal infections. These antifungal drugs have a wide range of uses because disorders resulting from fungal infections can occur on or in many different parts of the body. For example, treatment may be needed for infections of superficial areas such as the skin, nails, or genitals; rarely, internal organs, such as the heart or lungs, may also be infected.

Most antifungals work by damaging the walls of fungal cells. This causes vital substances within the cell to leak out, destroying the fungus.

Why are they used?

Antifungal preparations are frequently used to treat minor fungal infections of the skin, such as athlete's foot (p.205) and ringworm (p.205), or of the nails (see **Nail abnormalities**, p.209). These types of drug are also effective against candidiasis (p.177), a common fungal infection that can affect moist areas of the body, in particular the mucous membranes that line the mouth (see **Oral thrush**, p.559) and the vagina (see **Vaginal thrush**, p.482).

Antifungal drugs may also be used for the long-term treatment of potentially serious fungal infections such as aspergillosis (p.177), which may affect the lungs and spread to other organs. People with reduced immunity, such as those who have HIV infection or AIDS (p.169), are at high risk from severe fungal infections, and in such cases antifungal drugs may be life-saving.

How are they used?

If you have a fungal infection of the skin, your doctor may prescribe a cream containing an antifungal such as ketoconazole. Symptoms normally start to improve within about a week. However, you should continue the treatment for the full period recommended by your doctor to ensure that the infection has been eradicated. If topical treatment is ineffective, an oral antifungal drug may be prescribed. Nail infections are treated with a drug such as terbinafine, taken orally for several months. It may take much longer than this for the infected part of the nail to grow out. Dandruff may be treated with shampoo containing ketoconazole.

Drugs used to treat vaginal thrush are available over the counter. Commonly used drugs include fluconazole and clotrimazole. Fluconazole is taken orally; clotrimazole is inserted into the vagina, either as a cream using a special applicator or in the form of a pessary. Some preparations are available as a single dose; others need a 3-day course of treatment. Oral thrush is treated by antifungal drugs given as lozenges, which are dissolved slowly in the mouth, or as gels or solutions applied directly to the affected area.

Serious infections of internal organs need to be treated with potent antifungal drugs, such as amphotericin, which are initially given intravenously. Further treatment with oral drugs may then be continued for months.

What are the side effects?

Antifungal drugs used topically on the skin, scalp, or mucous membranes do not often cause side effects, but some irritation may occur. Nystatin used as a cream may stain clothing yellow.

Potent oral antifungal drugs may cause nausea and vomiting. Less frequently, serious side effects may occur, such as kidney damage and blood disorders. Oral treatment with the drug ketoconazole may cause liver damage.

Anthelmintic drugs

A group of drugs that is used to eradicate parasitic worm infestations

COMMON DRUGS

- Albendazole
- Ivermectin
- Mebendazole
- Praziquantel
- Tiabendazole

Anthelmintic drugs are used to eradicate worm (helminth) infestations of the intestine or of the tissues of other organs, such as the lungs. The most common intestinal worm infestation occurring in the UK is threadworm (see **Threadworm infestation**, p.178).

Infestations affecting the intestines are treated with anthelmintics that kill or paralyse the worms, which then pass out of the body in the faeces. Worm infestations of other body tissues are treated with anthelmintic drugs that circulate in the bloodstream and are absorbed by the tissues, where they kill the worms by preventing them from obtaining essential nutrients.

How are they used?

Many anthelmintic drugs are appropriate only for certain types of infestation. Your doctor will therefore need to identify the worm before prescribing the drug to be taken. In most cases, infestations are treated easily with a short course of oral drugs.

The most commonly used drug for intestinal infestations is mebendazole. Threadworms can often be eradicated with a single dose of mebendazole, provided that treatment is combined with good hygiene measures, such as careful handwashing, to prevent reinfestation. Your doctor may suggest that the whole family be treated with the drug at the same time, because threadworms can spread very rapidly to other people.

Worm infestations of the tissues, such as hydatid disease (p.180), which can affect the lungs, liver, or bones, may be treated with albendazole. Tissue infestations are difficult to eradicate, and it may be necessary to continue taking the drug for several weeks.

Anthelmintics usually do not cause side effects. However, sometimes the drugs produce diarrhoea, headaches, and dizziness. Albendazole may impair liver function; this may necessitate regular monitoring during treatment.

Drugs acting on the skin

Drugs acting on the skin are commonly used to relieve dryness and itching, to reduce inflammation, or to treat skin infections and infestations. Most treatments are applied directly to the skin as ointments, creams, or gels. Treatment with oral drugs may be necessary if a skin condition is severe or widespread.

The first article in this section covers emollients and barrier preparations, which are widely used to moisturize the skin and to protect it against the effects of irritant substances. Retinoid drugs, discussed next, are used to treat specific disorders, such as severe acne.

The following two articles in this section cover antipruritic drugs, which are used to relieve itching, and topical corticosteroids, which may be given to reduce inflammation of the skin. Preparations that are applied to the skin to treat infections and infestations are discussed next. Oral anti-infective drugs to treat the skin are described elsewhere (see **Drugs for infections and infestations**, pp.571–572).

The final article covers sunscreens and sunblocks, which protect the skin against the damaging effects of the sun. Drug treatments for other specific disorders are discussed elsewhere (see **Skin, hair, and nails**, pp.281–286).

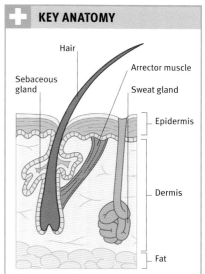

✚ KEY ANATOMY

Hair · Arrector muscle · Sebaceous gland · Sweat gland · Epidermis · Dermis · Fat

For more information about the structure and function of the skin, see pp.191.

Emollients and barrier preparations

Preparations that moisturize and protect the skin against water and other irritants

COMMON DRUGS

Emollients
- Aqueous cream
- Petroleum jelly

Barrier preparations
- Dimeticone
- Zinc ointment

Emollients are commonly used to treat dry, scaly, or itchy skin that results from skin disorders such as eczema (p.193), contact dermatitis (p.193), seborrhoeic dermatitis (p.194), and psoriasis (p.192). Emollients increase the moisture content of the skin by forming an oily film that stops water from evaporating from the skin's surface, thereby soothing and softening the skin. Emollient preparations are available over the counter in the form of creams, ointments, lotions, bath additives, and washes.

Barrier preparations often contain water-repellent substances and are used to protect the skin from water and irritants. They are useful for protecting the skin around pressure sores (p.203) and leg ulcers (p.203). They can also be applied to the nappy area in babies to help to prevent nappy rash (p.538).

How are they used?

Emollients and barrier preparations are available without a prescription. They should be rubbed gently on to clean, dry skin. However, the effects of the preparations are short-lived, and they may need to be applied frequently, especially after washing. Emollient bath additives and washes are used in place of normal soap. Occasionally, ingredients that are commonly added to emollient preparations, such as lanolin, irritate the skin. If sensitivity occurs, you should discontinue using the product. In some cases, emollients may need to be used for an extended period of time, such as in the treatment of severe psoriasis.

Retinoid drugs

A group of drugs used for skin conditions such as acne, psoriasis, and sun damage

COMMON DRUGS

- Acitretin
- Isotretinoin
- Tretinoin

Retinoid drugs are used to treat a number of skin conditions, including acne, psoriasis, and sun damage. These drugs are related chemically to vitamin A, which is needed to maintain healthy skin. Tretinoin and isotretinoin are used mainly in the treatment of severe acne (p.197). In addition, tretinoin may be used to treat mottling, fine wrinkles, and roughness in sun-damaged skin. However, the effects are only temporary, and the drug is not effective on deep wrinkles. Acitretin is used mainly to treat some types of severe psoriasis (p.192), a condition in which the skin becomes red, thickened, and scaly.

How do they work?
Retinoid drugs act on cells in the outer layers of the skin. The precise way in which tretinoin and isotretinoin work is unknown, but both drugs increase the rate at which the outer layers of skin are shed. This action helps to prevent acne by unblocking hair follicles clogged by sebum (oil) that might develop into blackheads or whiteheads. Isotretinoin also reduces the production of sebum by sebaceous glands in the skin.

Acitretin reduces the rate of production of keratin, a protein found in the outer layer of the skin. Keratin is produced in excessive amounts in the skin of people with psoriasis. Acitretin also has anti-inflammatory properties and may help to relieve the inflammation of the joints that is sometimes experienced by people who have severe psoriasis.

 WARNING

Retinoid drugs can damage a developing fetus. You should discuss your contraception needs with your doctor before starting treatment.

How are they used?
Topical tretinoin preparations should be applied as a liquid, gel, or cream once or twice daily in a thin layer over the affected area. Skin affected by acne will probably improve after 2–3 weeks, although the maximum effect may not be apparent for 8–12 weeks. Skin that has been damaged by exposure to strong sunlight is treated with a cream preparation. You will probably notice an improvement in your skin's condition after 2–4 weeks, but treatment may last up to 6 months.

Isotretinoin is available in capsule form and is prescribed by a specialist only when acne is very severe. It should be taken daily with food. After 4 weeks, your doctor may adjust the dose, depending on how your skin has responded to the treatment. A 12–16 week course of the drug often clears up acne entirely. A repeat course is not usually recommended.

Acitretin, which is used to treat psoriasis, is only taken orally. If your doctor prescribes acitretin, it will have to be taken daily, and you will usually see an improvement in your skin after about 2–4 weeks. The full benefit is usually seen after 4–6 weeks. Your doctor will pre-

scribe acitretin for no longer than 6 months, but treatment may resume after a 3–4 month break. If you take acitretin, you should not get pregnant for 3 years after you stop taking the drug or give blood for 1 year afterwards.

What are the side effects?
Using topical preparations that contain tretinoin may cause your skin to peel and become red and inflamed.

If you are taking isotretinoin or acitretin, your skin may become dry, flaky, and itchy, and you may experience sore lips and eyes, nosebleeds, and hair loss. Acitretin and isotretinoin can also affect the liver, and your blood will be tested regularly during treatment to monitor liver function. Women who are taking these drugs may find that their periods become irregular.

All retinoid drugs can cause severe birth defects, and this effect persists for some time after stopping treatment. For this reason, any woman who is pregnant (or thinks she might be) or who is planning a pregnancy should tell her doctor, who will be able to advise about suitable contraception. Long-term treatment with retinoid drugs may lead to pain in the joints and bones. In very rare cases, the treatment may also result in thinning or thickening of the bones in the spine, knees, and ankles.

Antipruritic drugs

Drugs used to control itching, a condition also known as pruritus

COMMON DRUGS

Topical corticosteroids
- Hydrocortisone

Antihistamines
- Antazoline ■ Diphenhydramine
- Mepyramine

Local anaesthetics
- Benzocaine ■ Lidocaine ■ Tetracaine

Soothing preparations
- Calamine lotion ■ Emollients

Antipruritic drugs are used to relieve itching, a symptom with a variety of possible causes, including inflammation or dryness of the skin, allergy, hormone deficiency in older women, exposure to irritant substances, and skin infections and infestations. Scratching the skin may cause further inflammation and itching, which may continue after the initial cause of the itching has disappeared.

This cycle may be broken by the use of antipruritics, which can be applied to the skin or taken orally. Most antipruritic drugs are available over the counter. However, itching should be investigated by your doctor in case there is an underlying cause that needs specific treatment. If you have an infection or infestation, you may be prescribed an alternative treatment (*see* **Preparations for skin infections and infestations**, opposite page).

▶ **SELF-ADMINISTRATION**

Applying ointments, creams, and gels

When applying medication in the form of ointments, creams, or gels, it is important to use the correct amount. Too much may increase the chance of side effects, whereas too little may not achieve the desired effect. The fingertip unit is a simple measure that can help you to work out how much medication you need to apply over an area of skin.

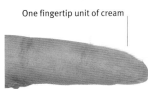

One fingertip unit of cream

A fingertip unit
One unit is the amount of the preparation that can be squeezed in a line onto the tip of the index finger as far as the first joint.

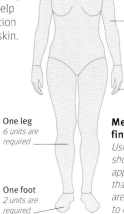

Face and neck
2.5 units are required

Trunk
7 units are required for front or back

One arm
3 units are required

One hand
(both sides)
1 unit is required

One leg
6 units are required

One foot
2 units are required

Measuring with fingertip units
Using the measures shown here as a guide, apply an amount of cream that is proportional to the area of skin that you need to cover.

What are the types?
The main types of antipruritic drug include topical corticosteroids (opposite page), antihistamines (p.585), local anaesthetics, and soothing preparations, such as emollients (*see* **Emollients and barrier preparations**, p.575). A topical corticosteroid can help to relieve itching caused by skin inflammation; antihistamines may be used to relieve itching caused by an allergic reaction; local anaesthetics numb small areas of skin, reducing itchiness caused by insect bites or stings; and soothing preparations ease itching caused by a variety of disorders, including eczema (p.193).

Topical corticosteroids A corticosteroid preparation may be applied to the skin to reduce inflammation and thereby relieve itching caused by skin conditions such as psoriasis (p.192), contact dermatitis (p.193), or eczema. Corticosteroids affect a wide range of body processes, including virtually all aspects of the inflammatory process. Their exact mechanism of action is still unclear, but one of their effects is to reduce the production of substances called prostaglandins, which play a key role in triggering inflammation.

Antihistamines Topical ointments or creams that contain antihistamine are commonly used for localized itching, such as that caused by an insect bite or sting. Widespread itching that is caused by a disorder such as chickenpox (p.165) can often be treated more effectively with an oral antihistamine.

 WARNING

Do not apply an antipruritic drug to broken or infected skin except on the advice of a doctor.

Antihistamines relieve itching by inhibiting the action of histamine, which is produced by body tissues in response to tissue damage or the presence of an allergen (a substance that triggers an allergic reaction, such as wasp venom). Histamine causes itching, swelling, and other symptoms of allergic reaction.

Topical antihistamines may themselves cause an allergic skin reaction, and you should stop using the product if additional irritation occurs. Certain oral antihistamines may make you feel drowsy, which can be useful if itching has prevented you from sleeping.

Local anaesthetics Small regions of skin irritation, such as those caused by insect stings or bites, may be soothed using a local anaesthetic cream or spray. These products stop itching by blocking the transmission of impulses along the nerves in the affected area. Local anaesthetics are inappropriate for widespread itching and can worsen symptoms by causing an allergic reaction in the skin.

Soothing preparations Itching, such as that caused by insect bites, sunburn (p.207), or an allergic rash such as urticaria (p.285), can often be soothed using calamine lotion or cream or an emollient. Emollient preparations reduce moisture loss from the skin, preventing dryness and easing itching, and can be used to relieve the symptoms of eczema, psoriasis, and other dry skin conditions.

Topical corticosteroids

Drugs related to natural hormones that are applied directly to the skin to reduce inflammation

COMMON DRUGS

Very potent corticosteroids
- Clobetasol ▪ Fluocinonide ▪ Halcinonide

Potent corticosteroids
- Beclometasone ▪ Betamethasone
- Fluocinolone ▪ Fluticasone
- Hydrocortisone butyrate ▪ Mometasone
- Triamcinolone

Moderately potent corticosteroids
- Alclometasone

Mild corticosteroids
- Hydrocortisone

Corticosteroids (p.600) are chemically similar to the natural hormones produced by the adrenal glands. They are used topically as cream or ointment preparations to relieve skin inflammation and itching caused by conditions such as eczema (p.193), contact dermatitis (p.193), seborrhoeic dermatitis (p.194), and, less commonly, for psoriasis (p.192). If inflammation is caused by a bacterial or fungal infection of the skin, topical corticosteroids may be used in conjunction with an anti-infective preparation (*see* **Preparations for skin infections and infestations**, right).

When applied directly to the skin, corticosteroids are absorbed into the underlying layers of tissue, where they reduce inflammation and relieve itching. These drugs have complex effects on many body processes, including almost all aspects of the inflammatory process, and one of their effects is to reduce the production of prostaglandins, substances that play a key role in triggering inflammation.

How are they used?

Your doctor will prescribe a corticosteroid cream or ointment that is potent enough to relieve your symptoms while at the same time minimizing the risk of side effects. You should follow your doctor's instructions on how often to apply the cream or ointment (usually once or twice a day) and use the correct amount (*see* **Applying ointments, creams, and gels**, opposite page). Some mild topical corticosteroid preparations are available over the counter.

What are the side effects?

Mild topical corticosteroid preparations used sparingly and for a short time do not usually cause side effects. However, prolonged use of these preparations can cause permanent changes to the skin. Most commonly, the treated skin becomes thin and easily damaged. If corticosteroids are applied to infected skin, the condition may worsen.

More potent topical corticosteroids used long-term may rarely cause more severe side effects, such as an increased blood pressure and a susceptibility to bruising. If you are using potent topical corticosteroids,

your doctor will review your condition regularly. Do not stop using corticosteroids without first consulting your doctor.

> ❌ **WARNING**
>
> Do not use a topical corticosteroid on your face or on a baby's skin except on the advice of a doctor.

Preparations for skin infections and infestations

Preparations applied directly to the skin to treat skin infections and infestations

COMMON DRUGS

Antiseptic preparations
- Chlorhexidine ▪ Triclosan

Antibiotics
- Fusidic acid ▪ Mupirocin ▪ Neomycin

Antiviral drugs
- Aciclovir ▪ Penciclovir

Antifungal drugs
- Clotrimazole ▪ Econazole ▪ Ketoconazole
- Miconazole ▪ Nystatin ▪ Terbinafine
- Tioconazole

Antiparasitic drugs
- Benzyl benzoate ▪ Malathion ▪ Permethrin

Topical anti-infective or antiparasitic skin preparations are used to prevent or treat a number of skin infections and infestations. These preparations contain an active ingredient, which is mixed with a cream, ointment, lotion, or detergent base. The preparations are easy to apply and are formulated so that the drug remains on the surface of the skin, where its effect is needed. Some preparations that are used to treat skin infections and infestations may themselves irritate or inflame the skin or result in an allergic reaction, and, if this occurs, treatment should be discontinued.

What are the types?

Topical treatments for skin infections include antiseptic preparations, which are effective against a wide range of microorganisms; antibiotics (p.572), used to prevent or treat infection with bacteria; and antiviral drugs (p.573) and antifungal drugs (p.574), used to treat viral and fungal infections respectively. Antiparasitic drugs are commonly used to treat skin infestations.

Antiseptic preparations These preparations contain chemicals that kill or prevent the growth of microorganisms that can cause infection in damaged skin. Antiseptic solutions and creams can be bought over the counter. Antiseptic solutions are added to water and used to clean broken skin; creams should be applied to wounds after they have been thoroughly cleansed. Antiseptics are also included in some shampoos and soaps to prevent minor scalp and skin problems, but they are of doubtful benefit.

Antibiotics These drugs are used in topical preparations to treat bacterial infections of

the skin, such as infected eczema (p.193) or impetigo (p.204). Severe burns may also be treated with a topical antibiotic in order to prevent infection. In some cases, a preparation containing two or more antibiotics is used to make sure that all bacteria are eradicated. You should always follow your doctor's instructions on how long to continue using a topical antibiotic preparation. Stopping early may allow a skin infection to recur.

Antiviral drugs Some topical antivirals used to treat conditions such as cold sores (p.205), which are caused by herpes viruses, can be bought over the counter. These drugs are most effective used early in an attack. Most common viral infections that cause a rash, such as rubella (p.168), do not need treatment, and many infections in the skin, such as warts (p.206), do not respond to topical antiviral drugs. However, herpes zoster (p.166) and genital herpes (p.493) are treated effectively with oral antivirals.

Antifungal drugs These drugs are used to treat fungal infections, including athlete's foot (p.205), ringworm (p.205), thrush (*see* **Vaginal thrush**, p.482, and **Oral thrush**, p.559), and fungal nail infections (*see* **Nail abnormalities**, p.209). Treatment of nail infections may need to be continued for several months to allow healthy nail to grow. Some topical antifungals can be bought over the counter. However, some fungal infections do not respond to topical preparations and require treatment with oral drugs.

Antiparasitic drugs Topical antiparasitic drugs are used to destroy adult parasites and their eggs and to treat infestations, including head lice (p.539), pubic lice (p.493), and scabies (p.207).

Infestations of head lice are treated with an antiparasitic lotion or cream rinse that is washed off later. For pubic lice, your doctor will prescribe a lotion or cream to apply to the pubic area. Scabies is treated with a lotion or cream applied all over the body and washed off after 8–24 hours. All members of a household affected by head lice or scabies should be treated at the same time to avoid reinfestation. In the case of infestation with pubic lice, sexual partners should be checked for lice and treated simultaneously if necessary.

Sunscreens and sunblocks

Preparations containing chemicals that help to protect the skin from the damaging effects of the sun's ultraviolet radiation

COMMON DRUGS

- Aminobenzoic acid ▪ Avobenzone
- Bemotrizinol ▪ Bisoctrizole ▪ Dioxybenzone
- Ethylhexyl methoxycinnamate
- Methylbenzylidene camphor ▪ Octinoxate
- Octocrilene ▪ Oxybenzone ▪ Padimate-O
- Para-aminobenzoic acid ▪ Titanium dioxide
- Zinc oxide

Sunscreens and sunblocks contain a variety of chemicals that help to protect the skin from the damaging effects of ultra-

> ❌ **WARNING**
>
> Reapply sunscreens regularly, particularly after swimming or if you are sweating.

violet (UV) radiation present in sunlight. UV radiation is composed of UVA and UVB rays, both of which age the skin. In addition, UVA rays cause tanning, and UVB rays cause burning (*see* **Sunburn**, p.207). Excessive exposure to sunlight also increases the risk of skin cancer (p.199). The sun's rays can cause cancerous changes to occur in the skin because they progressively damage the genes that control important functions in the skin, such as cell division.

Using sunscreens or sunblocks protects against these harmful effects and is advisable for anyone spending time in the sun. The use of these preparations is particularly important for people with fair skin and young children, whose skin is more vulnerable to sun damage (*see* **Safety in the sun**, p.34).

If your skin becomes sensitive to the sun (*see* **Photosensitivity**, p.195), you may need to use sunscreen or sunblock even when you are not exposed to strong sunlight. UV sensitivity may develop in people who are taking certain types of drug, such as antibiotics (p.572), thiazide diuretics (*see* **Diuretic drugs**, p.583), and rarely some oral contraceptives (*see* **Contraception**, p.28).

How do they work?

Sunscreens protect the skin by absorbing UVB rays, thereby reducing the amount that enters the skin; sunblocks provide a physical barrier that reflects or scatters UVA and UVB rays. Substances in sunscreens that absorb UVB rays include para-aminobenzoic acid (PABA) and padimate-O. Sunblocks contain chemicals such as zinc oxide and titanium dioxide, which are opaque and therefore reflect and scatter both UVB and UVA rays. Sunscreens are graded using a sun protection factor (SPF), which is a measure of the level of protection they provide against UVB rays. The higher the rating, the greater the protection against this type of radiation. However, even sunscreens with a high SPF do not provide complete UVB protection.

How are they used?

Sunscreens and sunblocks are available as creams, lotions, gels, and sprays. All products need to be applied frequently and generously to maintain protection, especially after swimming. You may experience irritation or an allergic rash when using certain sun protection products, particularly those containing PABA.

Drugs for musculoskeletal disorders

Pain in the bones, muscles, or joints is a common problem. In many cases, it is due to a minor muscular injury, and drugs are used to relieve the pain while the problem gets better. More serious disorders may cause persistent pain or disability, and long-term medication is needed to control the symptoms.

The first two articles in this section cover nonsteroidal anti-inflammatory drugs and locally acting corticosteroids. These drugs can relieve symptoms of musculoskeletal disorders, such as inflammation and pain, but have no effect on the underlying causes.

Drugs used to treat specific joint and bone disorders are discussed in the next two articles. Antirheumatic drugs are commonly used to treat rheumatoid arthritis. They can slow or halt joint damage, thereby preventing the disability that may be the long-term result of this disorder. The next article covers drugs for bone disorders. These drugs prevent or halt the abnormal growth or breakdown of bone that occurs in bone disorders such as Paget's disease and osteoporosis.

The final article in this section covers muscle relaxants, drugs that are used to relieve muscle spasms resulting from a variety of disorders.

✚ KEY ANATOMY

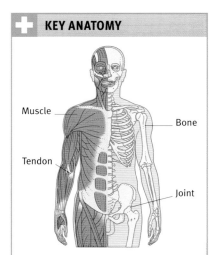

Muscle

Bone

Tendon

Joint

For information on the structure and function of the musculoskeletal system, *see* pp.211–216.

Nonsteroidal anti-inflammatory drugs

A group of drugs that are used to relieve pain and inflammation, particularly in muscles, ligaments, and joints

COMMON DRUGS

- Acemetacin ■ Aspirin ■ Diclofenac
- Etocolac ■ Fenbufen ■ Fenoprofen
- Flurbiprofen ■ Ibuprofen ■ Indometacin
- Ketoprofen ■ Mefenamic acid ■ Meloxicam
- Nabumetone ■ Naproxen ■ Piroxicam
- Sulindac ■ Tenoxicam ■ Tiaprofenic acid

COX-2 inhibitors
- Celecoxib ■ Etoricoxib

Nonsteroidal anti-inflammatory drugs (NSAIDs) are nonopioid painkillers (p.589) that are used to relieve the discomfort and inflammation caused by a variety of musculoskeletal disorders. These drugs are also commonly used to treat other types of pain and inflammation, such as headache (p.320).

Although it is technically an NSAID, aspirin is not usually classed with other types of NSAID because it has only a limited anti-inflammatory effect at normal doses. For this reason, NSAIDs with a more powerful anti-inflammatory action are normally prescribed to treat inflammatory conditions.

NSAIDs may be used for conditions that develop suddenly, such as ligament damage and muscle strains and tears (p.234). They usually reduce symptoms within a few hours. NSAIDs are also used to relieve pain and inflammation caused by long-term musculoskeletal disorders such as osteoarthritis (p.221) and rheumatoid arthritis (p.222). When used to treat these conditions, NSAIDs can rapidly relieve pain, but they may take about 2 weeks to reduce inflammation. Although NSAIDs are effective in alleviating symptoms, they do not cure the underlying condition.

NSAIDs reduce pain and inflammation by blocking the action of the enzyme cyclo-oxygenase (COX), which is involved in the production of prostaglandins, substances that trigger inflammation and the transmission of pain signals to the brain but which also protect the stomach lining. There are two types of COX, COX-1 and COX-2, which act at different sites in the body. Most NSAIDs block both COX-1 (leading to stomach irritation) and COX-2 (providing the anti-inflammatory effect). COX-2 inhibitors block COX-2 alone, thereby reducing the risk of stomach irritation.

How are they used?

NSAIDs are most commonly taken orally, although occasionally they may be applied as a gel or given by injection.

▶ **DRUG ACTION**

How NSAIDs work

Nonsteroidal anti-inflammatory drugs (NSAIDs) are used to treat a variety of conditions, including inflammatory disorders such as rheumatoid arthritis (p.222). The inflammatory response is triggered by substances called prostaglandins, which are released when tissue is damaged. NSAIDs reduce inflammation by blocking the production of prostaglandins.

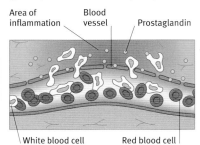

Area of inflammation | Blood vessel | Prostaglandin

White blood cell | Red blood cell

Before drug
Prostaglandins are released in damaged tissue, causing the blood vessels to widen and leak fluid. White cells move into the tissue. The area becomes red and swollen.

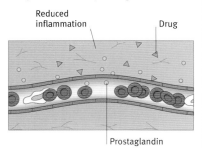

Reduced inflammation | Drug

Prostaglandin

After drug
NSAIDs limit the release of prostaglandins, thereby reducing the inflammation. The leaky blood vessels return to normal, and swelling and redness subside.

Certain NSAIDs are available in a slow-release form, which may be effective for up to 24 hours. This reduces the need to take pills frequently when long-term conditions are being treated. Slow-release NSAIDs also provide a more constant level of pain relief. For many conditions, these drugs are used in combination with other treatments, such as physiotherapy (p.620). Some NSAIDs, such as ibuprofen, can be bought over the counter.

What are the side effects?

NSAIDs have varying potential to irritate the stomach lining, which may cause nausea, indigestion, bleeding from the stomach, and occasionally peptic ulcer (p.406). If you are given certain NSAIDs, such as ibuprofen, for long-term use, you may also be given an anti-ulcer drug (*see* **Ulcer-healing drugs**, p.596) to protect the stomach lining. COX-2 inhibitors cause less stomach irritation than other NSAIDs but, because they are associated with an increased risk of heart disease and stroke, they are not generally recommended for people who have had, or who are at risk of having these conditions. Some other NSAIDs, such as diclofenac and ibuprofen, may also increase the risk of heart attack and stroke, especially when used at high doses for long periods. Consequently, NSAIDs should be used at the lowest dose for the shortest period.

NSAIDs may also cause allergic reactions (*see* **Drug allergy**, p.284), including rashes and a condition called angioedema (p.285), in which temporary, painless swellings develop in the skin and mucous membranes. People who have had a reaction to any NSAID should avoid all NSAIDs. Some people may develop photosensitivity (p.195), in which the skin becomes abnormally sensitive to sunlight. People who have asthma (p.295) or a kidney disorder may be advised not to take NSAIDs because the drugs can make these conditions worse.

Locally acting corticosteroids

Drugs that are injected directly into body tissues to reduce inflammation

COMMON DRUGS

- Betamethasone ■ Dexamethasone
- Hydrocortisone ■ Methylprednisolone
- Prednisolone ■ Triamcinolone

Locally acting corticosteroids are anti-inflammatory drugs that are injected into a specific area of the body to reduce inflammation in that area. The drugs block the body's response that triggers production of natural chemicals that cause inflammation and pain. Corticosteroids can be injected into joints to relieve inflammation due to conditions such as rheumatoid arthritis (p.222). Injections can also be given around ligaments and tendons to relieve conditions such as tennis elbow (p.230). A local anaesthetic may be injected with a corticosteroid to relieve pain quickly.

Side effects do not often occur with injected corticosteroids; if they do, they are usually limited to the site of injection. These local side effects can include thinning of the skin or fat at the injection site, which may produce a dimple. There may be a temporary increase in pain; rarely, the area becomes infected.

Antirheumatic drugs

Drugs used in the treatment of rheumatoid arthritis and certain other conditions caused by autoimmune disease

COMMON DRUGS

Disease-modifying antirheumatic drugs (DMARDS)
- Auranofin ■ Azathioprine ■ Chloroquine
- Ciclosporin ■ Cyclophosphamide
- Hydroxychloroquine ■ Leflunomide
- Methotrexate ■ Penicillamine ■ Sodium aurothiomalate ■ Sulfasalazine

Biological DMARDS
- Abatacept ■ Adalimumab ■ Anakinra
- Etanercept ■ Infliximab ■ Rituximab

Painkillers (p.589)

Nonsteroidal anti-inflammatory drugs (p.578)

Corticosteroids (opposite page, and p.600)

Antirheumatic drugs are used to treat rheumatoid arthritis (p.222), an autoimmune disease in which the immune system attacks the body's own tissues, primarily the joints. Some antirheumatic drugs may also be used to treat other autoimmune disorders, such as systemic lupus erythematosus (p.281). Various types of drugs may be used in the treatment of rheumatoid arthritis, usually in combination with other treatments, such as physiotherapy.

What are the types?
The main drugs used to treat rheumatoid arthritis are known as disease-modifying antirheumatic drugs (DMARDs). These drugs modify the disease process itself by altering the activity of the body's immune system, which leads to a reduction in symptoms such as pain and inflammation and can also limit further joint damage. Many of the DMARDs are immunosuppressants; the newer ones, often known simply as "biologicals", reduce the level of a natural chemical called tumour necrosis factor-alpha (TNF-alpha), which plays a key role in causing inflammation in joints.

In addition to DMARDs, painkillers, nonsteroidal anti-inflammatory drugs (NSAIDs), and corticosteroids may also be used during the initial treatment of rheumatoid arthritis or to control flare-ups of symptoms.

How are they used?
In most cases, treatment with DMARDs is started as soon as possible after rheumatoid arthritis has been diagnosed. Treatment with these drugs is started under specialist supervision, and before DMARDs are prescribed you will be given various tests to check whether you have any condition that might preclude the use of any particular drug. When DMARD treatment is started, you will probably be given a combination of drugs. Because it can take weeks, or even months, before DMARDs produce any noticeable effect, you may also be prescribed painkillers, NSAIDs, and/or corticosteroids to relieve symptoms in the interim.

It may be necessary to try various DMARDs to find the most suitable for you.

If none of the standard DMARDs is found to be suitable, you may be prescribed one of the newer biological DMARDs. Once a suitable DMARD has been found, you will then probably need to take it indefinitely.

What are the side effects?
DMARDs are a diverse group of drugs and may therefore produce a wide range of side effects. Rarely, they may cause serious side effects, such as kidney, liver, blood, or eye problems, and for this reason people taking DMARDs are monitored regularly. Because DMARDs affect the immune system, they may not be suitable for some people with impaired immunity. Some DMARDs should not be used by women who are breast-feeding, and some may cause fetal abnormalities and should not be used during pregnancy.

> ### ✖ WARNING
> If you are taking an antirheumatic drug, you should report any sign of infection, unusual bleeding, rash, sore throat, cough, or breathlessness to your doctor immediately.

Drugs for bone disorders

Drugs used to treat disorders affecting bone formation, replacement, and repair

COMMON DRUGS

Bisphosphonates
- Alendronic acid ■ Etidronate
- Ibandronic acid ■ Risedronate
- Zoledronic Acid

Calcium and vitamin D
- Calcitriol ■ Calcium carbonate
- Ergocalciferol ■ Vitamin D

Oestrogen and compounds with oestrogen-like effects
- Conjugated oestrogens ■ Estradiol
- Raloxifene ■ Tibolone

Other drugs for bone disorders
- Calcitonin ■ Parathyroid hormone
- Teriparatide ■ Strontium ranelate

The body constantly breaks down and rebuilds bone. Disorders can develop if the balance between breakdown and renewal is upset. Drugs that affect bone turnover are used to treat disorders in which either too much bone is broken down or bone grows abnormally. For example, in osteoporosis (p.217), bone is broken down faster than it is replaced; in Paget's disease of the bone (p.218), there is abnormal bone formation.

What are the types?
Drugs used to treat bone disorders include bisphosphonates; calcium and vitamin D; oestrogens and compounds with oestrogen-like effects; certain hormones involved in bone breakdown and rebuilding, such as calcitonin and parathyroid hormone, and synthetic variants of such hormones, such as teriparatide; and strontium ranelate.

Bisphosphonates These drugs have replaced hormone replacement therapy (p.605) as the first-line treatment for osteoporosis; they are also used to treat Paget's disease. The drugs work by reducing abnormally high rates of bone breakdown and renewal and are usually taken orally. Side effects may include nausea, diarrhoea, and indigestion.

Calcium and vitamin D These substances are essential for maintaining healthy bone. Supplements may be used to treat bone disorders. Postmenopausal women require a daily calcium intake of about 1,200–1,500 mg, much of which can be obtained in the diet. Calcium supplements may cause constipation. Vitamin D helps the body to absorb calcium from food. Deficiency is rare but can cause rickets in children and osteomalacia in adults (p.217). Taken at the recommended dose, vitamin D supplements usually cause no side effects.

Oestrogen and compounds with oestrogen-like effects The sex hormone oestrogen and compounds with oestrogen-like effects slow the breakdown of bone and may be used to prevent osteoporosis or to slow its progress. However, oestrogens, either alone or with progestogens, and tibolone are no longer usually recommended as the first-line treatment for the prevention or treatment of osteoporosis. Raloxifene is used for the prevention and treatment of osteoporosis after the menopause. Side effects include hot flushes, leg cramps, rashes, and breast discomfort. There is also a risk of thromboembolism (p.259).

Other drugs Calcitonin and parathyroid hormone help regulate bone turnover in the body. As medication, calcitonin may be used to treat Paget's disease and to reduce the risk of osteoporotic fractures in some postmenopausal women. It may be given as a nasal spray or by injection. Side effects may include irritation at the injection site, gastrointestinal disturbances, and hot flushes.

Parathyroid hormone and teriparatide are given by injection and may be used to treat osteoporosis in some women at a high risk of fractures; teriparatide may also be used to treat some men at risk of osteoporotic fractures. Possible side effects of both drugs include gastrointestinal disturbances, palpitations, and irritation at the site of injection.

Strontium ranelate stimulates bone formation and reduces bone breakdown. It may be used to treat osteoporosis in some women for whom other treatments are not suitable. Possible side effects include gastrointestinal disturbances, headache, and venous thromboembolism. Very rarely, it may cause a life-threatening allergic reaction; if you

> ### ✖ WARNING
> If you are taking strontium ranelate and develop a rash, particularly if it is accompanied by fever and swollen glands, you should stop taking the drug and consult your doctor immediately.

develop a rash while taking strontium ranelate, you should stop using the drug and consult your doctor immediately.

Muscle relaxants

A group of drugs that are used to treat muscular stiffness and cramps

COMMON DRUGS

- Baclofen ■ Botulinum toxin ■ Dantrolene
- Diazepam ■ Quinine ■ Tizanidine

Muscle relaxants are used for the relief of muscle spasm. They are also used to ease the movement of limbs that are stiff because of nervous system disorders such as multiple sclerosis (p.334) and cerebral palsy (p.548). Muscle relaxants are sometimes prescribed to treat conditions such as night-time muscle cramps (p.230) and torticollis (p.230). Certain muscle relaxants are used to paralyse muscles during surgery under general anaesthesia.

How do they work?
Muscle relaxant drugs work in a variety of ways. Some muscle relaxants, such as tizanidine, baclofen, and the antianxiety drug diazepam, work by reducing transmission of nerve signals from the brain and spinal cord to the muscles, causing the muscles to relax.

Dantrolene relieves spasm by acting directly on muscles and making them less sensitive to nerve signals from the brain and spinal cord. Botulinum toxin relaxes muscles by blocking transmission of signals from nerve endings to muscle cells. The way in which quinine works is not fully understood.

How are they used?
Doses of muscle relaxants need careful adjustment. Too little has no effect, and too much may lead to muscle weakness. For long-standing conditions such as multiple sclerosis, doses begin at a low level and are increased gradually to reach a balance between symptom control and muscle strength.

Involuntary contractions of the neck and facial muscles can be relieved by injecting tiny amounts of botulinum toxin directly into the affected area. A single injection is usually effective for about 3 months. Quinine taken at bedtime, also in tiny amounts, helps to prevent cramp developing in the night.

What are the side effects?
A common side effect of many muscle relaxants is drowsiness, which usually decreases as treatment progresses. With long-term use, the body may become dependent on a muscle relaxant; if the drug is withdrawn suddenly, muscle spasms may become worse than they were before treatment began. Dantrolene can cause diarrhoea. This drug may also cause severe liver problems, as may tizanidine. If you are taking either of these drugs, your doctor will carry out regular blood tests to check your liver function.

Drugs for cardiovascular disorders

Disorders of the cardiovascular system are a major cause of poor health and early death in the developed world. In some cases, cardiovascular disorders can be improved by changes in lifestyle, such as improving diet or giving up smoking. In other cases, cardiovascular disorders require treatment with drugs that act on the blood vessels, the heart, or the kidneys.

The opening article in this section discusses the drugs used to treat high blood pressure, a disorder that affects a large number of people in developed countries. A number of these drugs are effective not only in lowering blood pressure, but also in the treatment of heart failure, angina, and coronary artery disease.

The next article gives an overview of the types of drug that may be used in the treatment of arrhythmias, a group of disorders in which the heart beats extremely rapidly or with an abnormal rhythm.

Specific classes of drugs are discussed in separate articles. Beta-blockers and calcium channel blockers are used to treat certain arrhythmias; these drugs and nitrates also treat coronary artery disease; diuretics, ACE inhibitors, and beta-blockers are helpful in treating congestive heart failure; and most are useful in lowering high blood pressure.

Lipid-lowering drugs, which are used to reduce the risk of heart attack by lowering levels of fats in the blood, are discussed elsewhere (*see* **Drugs acting on the endocrine system and metabolism**, pp.600–604).

KEY ANATOMY

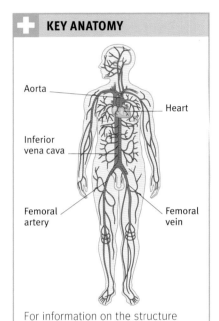

Aorta

Heart

Inferior vena cava

Femoral artery

Femoral vein

For information on the structure and function of the cardiovascular system, *see* pp.235–240.

Antihypertensive drugs

Drugs used to treat high blood pressure, a condition also known as hypertension

COMMON DRUGS

ACE inhibitor drugs (p.532)

Alpha-blocker drugs
- Doxazosin   Prazosin   Terazosin

Angiotensin II blocker drugs (p.582)

Beta-blocker drugs (p.581)

Calcium channel blocker drugs (p.582)

Centrally acting drugs
- Methyldopa   Moxonidine

Diuretic drugs (p.583)

Other antihypertensive drugs
- Diazoxide   Hydralazine   Minoxidil
- Nitroprusside

High blood pressure (*see* **Hypertension**, p.242) requires treatment mainly because it increases the risk of both coronary artery disease (p.243) and stroke (p.329). Antihypertensive drugs are most often used when changes in your lifestyle, such as improving your diet, doing more exercise, and giving up smoking, fail to produce an adequate fall in blood pressure over a short period of time. Antihypertensives may also be used to treat hypertension in pregnancy (*see* **Pre-eclampsia and eclampsia**, p.513).

What are the types?

There are many different types of antihypertensive drugs. The types that are most commonly used are beta-blocker drugs (p.581), ACE inhibitor drugs (p.582), angiotensin II blocker drugs (p.582), calcium channel blocker drugs (p.582), and diuretic drugs (p.583). Less commonly, alpha-blocker drugs, centrally acting drugs, and other drugs, including diazoxide, hydralazine, and minoxidil, are used.

Most types of antihypertensive drug reduce high blood pressure by increasing the diameter of the blood vessels (a process known as vasodilation) or by reducing the force with which the heart pumps the blood. ACE inhibitors, alpha-blockers, angiotensin II blockers, calcium channel blockers, and centrally acting drugs act in a variety of ways to cause vasodilation. Beta-blockers lower blood pressure by reducing the force with which the heart pumps. This effect is achieved by blocking the action of substances produced naturally by the body that increase heart rate and blood pressure. Diuretics cause the kidneys to excrete more water and salts than usual, which reduces the volume of blood that is present in the circulation and thereby lowers blood pressure.

How are they used?

Antihypertensives are normally taken orally over long periods of time and usually for life. However, in some cases it is possible to reduce the dose gradually and eventually stop the drugs if blood pressure returns to normal following long-term changes in weight or lifestyle. The choice of drug depends on several factors, including age, other medical conditions that might be present, and severity of the high blood pressure. Certain drugs are especially likely to cause side effects in elderly people.

At the beginning of treatment for mild or moderate hypertension, a single drug is usually used. For some people this may be an ACE inhibitor or angiotensin II blocker, whereas for others the initial treatment may be with a calcium channel blocker or diuretic. If a single drug does not reduce your blood pressure sufficiently, a combination of these drugs may be used. Some people who have moderate hypertension also require an additional drug, in which case an alpha-blocker or beta-blocker may also be prescribed.

If you have mild or moderate hypertension, your doctor will usually start you on a low dose of a drug. The dose is then gradually increased until your blood pressure is normal or until you experience side effects.

People with severe hypertension are usually treated with a combination of several drugs, which may need to be given in high doses. Your doctor may need to try a number of drugs before finding a combination that controls your blood pressure without producing unacceptable side effects.

Everybody receiving treatment for hypertension will have their blood pressure monitored regularly.

❌ WARNING

Do not suddenly stop taking an antihypertensive drug without first consulting your doctor. Abrupt withdrawal of the drug could cause a rapid increase in blood pressure.

What are the side effects?

All antihypertensive drugs, in particular ACE inhibitors and alpha-blockers, can cause a sudden drop in blood pressure (*see* **Hypotension**, p.248) when you first take them. This drop in blood pressure can cause light-headedness. Some drugs may also cause drowsiness. If you experience these side effects, your doctor may reduce the dose or may give you a different drug. You should not stop taking an antihypertensive without first consulting your doctor.

Other side effects are associated with specific types of antihypertensive drugs. Several types of these drugs, especially beta-blockers and some diuretics, may cause erectile dysfunction; ACE inhibitors sometimes cause a dry cough and calcium channel blockers may cause swollen ankles, flushing, and headaches. Long-term use of diuretics may increase the risk of gout (p.224). Minoxidil may result in excessive hair (p.209) and hydralazine may cause palpitations.

Antiarrhythmic drugs

Drugs used to treat abnormal heart rates and rhythms (arrhythmias)

COMMON DRUGS

Beta-blocker drugs (opposite page)

Calcium channel blocker drugs (p.582)
- Diltiazem   Verapamil

Digitalis drugs (p.582)
- Digoxin

Other antiarrhythmic drugs
- Adenosine   Amiodarone   Disopyramide
- Flecainide   Lidocaine   Mexiletine
- Moracizine   Procainamide   Propafenone

Abnormalities in heart rhythm and rate, known as arrhythmias (p.249), are caused by a disturbance in the electrical signals that control heart action. Often, minor disturbances do not need treatment. However, some arrhythmias do require treatment to restore normal heart rhythm, thereby reducing symptoms such as palpitations, shortness of breath, light-headedness, and chest pain.

Antiarrhythmics are commonly prescribed to treat the arrhythmias atrial fibrillation (p.250) and supraventricular tachycardia (p.250), both of which cause the heart to beat very rapidly. They are also used to treat ventricular arrhythmia, which may develop after a heart attack (*see* **Myocardial infarction**, p.245) and, if left untreated, may lead to cardiac arrest (p.252).

Commonly used antiarrhythmics include beta-blockers (opposite), the calcium channel blockers verapamil and diltiazem, and the digitalis drug digoxin. There are various other types of antiarrhythmics, some of which are mostly used to treat ventricular arrhythmias.

How are they used?

Once an antiarrhythmic is required, you may have to take the drug indefinitely. For long-term treatment, the drugs are given orally, and initially you may need to take several doses a day. When your heartbeat has been stabilized, your doctor may test the drug levels in your blood in order to correct the dose.

The type of drug your doctor selects depends on which form of arrhythmia you have. For example, a beta-blocker, calcium channel blocker, or the digitalis drug digoxin may be useful in reducing a rapid heart rate in atrial fibrillation; flecainide or amiodarone may be used to restore a regular rhythm in atrial fibrillation; and amiodarone or propafenone may be used to treat ventricular arrhythmia.

If you have developed arrhythmia suddenly and the condition is severe, you may be given a drug such as adenosine intravenously as an emergency measure to restore normal heart activity. When the initial symptoms have been brought under control, your doctor may prescribe drugs for long-term treatment to prevent future attacks.

What are the side effects?
Many types of these drugs reduce blood pressure. This may cause light-headedness when you stand up. You may also experience nausea and blurred vision.

Other side effects are specific to certain drugs. For example, amiodarone causes skin sensitivity to sunlight and may also affect the function of the thyroid gland and lungs. If you are taking the digitalis drug digoxin, contact your doctor immediately if you experience nausea, diarrhoea, vomiting, or visual disturbances. These symptoms may indicate that the dose is too high.

You should tell your doctor if you are taking other drugs because of the risk of an adverse interaction with an antiarrhythmic. You should not stop taking an antiarrhythmic without consulting your doctor, as abrupt withdrawal of the drug may make your condition worse.

Beta-blocker drugs

Drugs that block the transmission of certain nerve impulses and are used to treat disorders of the heart and circulation

COMMON DRUGS

Cardioselective beta-blockers
■ Acebutolol ■ Atenolol ■ Bisoprolol
■ Esmolol ■ Metoprolol

Noncardioselective beta-blockers
■ Carvedilol ■ Labetolol ■ Nadolol
■ Oxprenolol ■ Pindolol ■ Propanolol
■ Sotalol ■ Timolol

Beta-blocker drugs, or beta-adrenergic blocking agents, are widely prescribed to treat disorders of the heart and circulation and also to treat other conditions. Cardioselective beta-blockers act mainly on the heart. Other beta-blockers act on blood vessels throughout the body and on other target tissues such as the cells that secrete fluid in the eye.

Why are they used?
Beta-blockers are prescribed principally to treat heart and circulatory disorders such as angina (p.244), a disabling chest pain caused by too little oxygenated blood reaching the heart muscle, some irregularities of heart rhythm (*see* **Arrhythmias**, p.249), and high blood pressure (*see* **Hypertension**, p.242). They are also sometimes given after a heart attack (*see* **Myocardial infarction**, p.245) to reduce the likelihood of further damage to the heart muscle.

Beta-blockers are also used to treat other conditions, such as migraine (p.320) and glaucoma (p.358), in which the pressure in the eye is increased by a build-up of excess

fluid. Some beta-blockers are used to reduce the physical symptoms of anxiety, such as tremor. The drugs also help in the treatment of an overactive thyroid gland (*see* **Hyperthyrodism**, p.432) by controlling the symptoms caused by excess production of thyroid hormone, such as sweating, tremor, and rapid heart rate.

How do they work?
Beta-blockers work by blocking the action of epinephrine (adrenaline) and norepinephrine (noradrenaline), two chemicals produced by the body that increase heart rate and raise the blood pressure. Cardioselective beta-blockers are especially effective at slowing heart rate and reducing the force of the heartbeat, thereby reducing the workload of the heart. These actions make beta-blockers effective in the treatment of angina, hypertension, and some types of arrhythmia. Other beta-blockers have a more widespread action and block many of the effects that norepinephrine has throughout the body, such as narrowing blood vessels and causing tremor and sweating. As a result, they may be effective in treating some physical symptoms caused by this chemical, such as tremor. Beta-blockers do not treat the underlying causes of these conditions.

Beta-blockers are used for migraine because they block the effects of norepinephrine on blood vessels in the head. They also reduce fluid formation, and thus pressure, in the eyeball, and so are used to treat glaucoma.

How are they used?
If you have angina, high blood pressure, or recurrent migraine, you may be given long-term treatment with oral beta-blockers. Your doctor may initially prescribe a low dose and increase it until the desired effect is reached. If you have glaucoma, you may be prescribed eyedrops that contain the beta-blocker timolol. A beta-blocker may be given intravenously in hospital if you experience sudden severe angina or if you have a heart attack.

Beta-blockers are also used along with other types of drug, especially in the treatment of angina, high blood pressure, and some types of heart failure.

What are the side effects?
Beta-blockers may precipitate asthma (p.295), which can be life-threatening. They should therefore not be used by anybody who has, or has ever had, asthma or similar breathing problems, except in exceptional circumstances and under specialist supervision, when a cardioselective beta-blocker may be given.

Beta-blockers can also mask some of the symptoms of hypoglycaemia (low blood glucose), which is a serious condition that must be recognized and treated immediately, and the drugs may therefore not be suitable for some people who need to take insulin for diabetes mellitus (p.437).

If you are taking a beta-blocker, your sleeping pattern may be disrupted, and your hands and feet may feel cold because the blood circulation in the extremities is reduced. Men sometimes experience erectile dysfunction, but normal sexual function usually returns when the drug is stopped. Rarely, beta-blockers cause rashes and dry eyes. All these side effects tend to be more common and more severe in elderly people.

If you need to stop taking a beta-blocker, your doctor will advise you on how to reduce the dose gradually to avoid rebound high blood pressure, a recurrence of angina, or a heart attack.

Nitrate drugs

A group of drugs used to prevent and treat angina (chest pain) caused by coronary artery disease

COMMON DRUGS
■ Glyceryl trinitrate ■ Isosorbide dinitrate
■ Isosorbide mononitrate

Nitrate drugs are often used in conjunction with various other drugs in the treatment of angina (p.244), a disabling chest pain that occurs when too little oxygen reaches the heart muscle.

Nitrates may be prescribed to prevent angina attacks or to relieve the symptoms of an attack when it happens. However, nitrates do not treat the underlying cause of angina, which is usually narrowing of the coronary arteries due to build-up of fatty deposits (*see* **Coronary artery disease**, p.243).

How do they work?
Nitrates cause blood vessels in the body to dilate (widen), making it easier for the heart to pump blood around the body. This reduces the oxygen requirement of the heart muscle. Nitrates also make the coronary arteries dilate, which improves the blood supply to the heart muscle.

How are they used?
Nitrates may be used either to provide rapid relief from an angina attack or to prevent an attack occurring. "Reliever" nitrates provide fast relief from chest pain in the event of an angina attack, but are effective for only 20–30 minutes. These drugs are available as tablets that you place under your tongue or between your upper lip and gum, and as an aerosol spray that is sprayed under the tongue (*see* **Using sublingual sprays**, below). Your doctor may advise you to use a fast-acting nitrate just before exerting yourself.

A long-acting nitrate takes more time to become effective than a fast-acting nitrate but it may continue to have an effect for several hours. Long-acting nitrates may be prescribed as skin patches or tablets, usually taken once or twice a day. Skin patches, which may be applied to the chest, arm, back, abdomen, or thigh, are useful if you have angina at night. Skin patches should be applied to a different part of the skin each day. Nitrate drugs may also be administered intravenously in hospital as an emergency treatment to relieve an angina attack.

What are the side effects?
Nitrates commonly cause a throbbing headache and flushing. They can also cause a fall in blood pressure, resulting in light-headedness when you stand up.

If you are using a long-acting nitrate, you may develop tolerance, resulting in a reduction of the drug's effectiveness. Tolerance can be avoided by interrupting use of a skin patch or an ointment for 4–8 hours each day. Usually, long-acting nitrate pills allow levels of the drug in the blood to fall overnight.

▶ SELF-ADMINISTRATION
Using sublingual sprays
Sublingual sprays are used when immediate drug action is needed. For example, they are used to relieve the symptoms of an angina attack. The drugs are absorbed into the blood through the tongue's rich supply of blood vessels. This is a much faster route than absorption from the digestive tract, which occurs when drugs are taken orally.

Using the spray
With an open mouth, touch the roof of your mouth with your tongue and spray on to the underside of your tongue. Avoid inhaling through your mouth at the same time as you spray the drug.

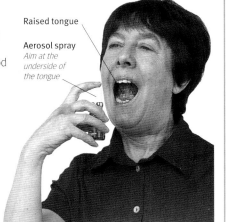

Raised tongue

Aerosol spray
Aim at the underside of the tongue

Calcium channel blocker drugs

A group of drugs used to treat several disorders of the heart and circulation

COMMON DRUGS

- Amlodipine ▪ Diltiazem ▪ Felodipine
- Isradipine ▪ Lacidipine ▪ Nicardipine
- Nifedipine ▪ Verapamil

Calcium channel blocker drugs may be prescribed to treat angina (p.244), a disabling chest pain that occurs when too little oxygen reaches the heart muscle. These drugs may also be used in the treatment of high blood pressure (*see* **Hypertension**, p.242). The calcium channel blockers verapamil and diltiazem are used to treat some abnormal heart rhythms (*see* **Arrhythmias**, p.249). Nifedipine may be used to treat Raynaud's phenomenon (p.262), a disorder in which spasm of arteries in the hands or feet restricts the blood supply to the fingers or toes. Verapamil may be taken regularly to reduce the frequency of cluster headaches (p.320), in which blood vessels in the head may constrict and then widen, causing severe headache.

How do they work?

Muscle cells need calcium to contract. Calcium channel blockers reduce the amount of calcium entering the muscle cells in blood vessel walls. This action causes the muscle cells to relax and the blood vessels to widen, thereby reducing blood pressure. This widening of blood vessels is thought to be the reason why calcium channel blockers work in the treatment of Raynaud's phenomenon and in the prevention of cluster headaches. Since the drugs reduce the amount of calcium that enters heart muscle cells, they reduce both the force and the rate of the heartbeat and therefore help to relieve angina.

Verapamil and diltiazem also slow down the flow of electrical impulses through the heart and thus slow the heartbeat. They may be used in treating some arrhythmias in which the heart beats excessively fast.

How are they used?

Calcium channel blockers may be used alone or in combination with other drugs that are used in the treatment of angina, hypertension, or certain types of arrhythmia. Usually, the drugs are initially prescribed at a low dose, and the dose is gradually increased to an effective level. The ideal dose for you will be one that is high enough to allow the drug to be effective without causing troublesome side effects.

What are the side effects?

The most common side effects of calcium channel blockers are headache, light-headedness, flushing, and swollen ankles. Constipation can sometimes be a problem, particularly if you are taking verapamil. Grapefruit may increase the effects of some of these drugs and should be avoided. Occasionally, taking calcium channel blockers can cause nausea, palpitations, excessive tiredness, and rashes. Some calcium channel blockers may not be suitable for people with heart failure because they may make the symptoms worse.

✖ WARNING

Do not suddenly stop taking a calcium channel blocker drug without first consulting your doctor. Abrupt withdrawal could cause worsening of your angina.

ACE inhibitor drugs

A group of drugs used to treat heart failure and high blood pressure

COMMON DRUGS

- Captopril ▪ Enalapril ▪ Fosinopril
- Lisinopril ▪ Moexipril ▪ Perindopril
- Quinapril ▪ Ramipril ▪ Trandolapril

Angiotensin converting enzyme (ACE) inhibitor drugs are commonly used in the treatment of chronic heart failure (p.247), in which the efficiency of the heart in pumping blood around the body is reduced. ACE inhibitors are also used to treat high blood pressure (*see* **Hypertension**, p.242), and may also be used to treat diabetic kidney disease (p.450). In this disorder, small blood vessels in the filtering units of the kidneys are damaged and, as a result, protein leaks into the urine.

How do they work?

ACE inhibitors prevent the normal formation in the body of angiotensin II, a hormone that causes constriction (narrowing) of blood vessels. By reducing the amount of angiotensin II present in the blood, ACE inhibitors allow blood vessels to dilate (widen). This widening of blood vessels throughout the body reduces blood pressure, which makes it easier for the heart to pump blood and therefore alleviates heart failure.

The mechanism by which ACE inhibitor drugs are effective in relieving diabetic kidney disease is not entirely understood. ACE inhibitors are not given to people with certain other types of kidney damage because they may make the condition worse.

How are they used?

ACE inhibitors may also be used alone or in combination with diuretic drugs (opposite page) or calcium channel blockers (left) to reduce blood pressure when a single drug is not sufficiently effective.

You will probably need to take these drugs for several months at least, and sometimes years. Before you are given an ACE inhibitor to treat heart failure or high blood pressure, you may have a blood test to check that your kidney function is normal. Your doctor is likely to prescribe a low oral dose of the drug initially. The dose is gradually increased over several weeks until an effective level is reached. You may be advised to take the first dose at bedtime because it may cause your blood pressure to fall rapidly, making you feel light-headed. If you are elderly or taking another drug for high blood pressure, such as a diuretic, your doctor may suggest that you try a small dose while still in the doctor's surgery so that you can be monitored in case you have a sudden drop in blood pressure.

✖ WARNING

If you are taking an ACE inhibitor drug, do not take a nonsteroidal anti-inflammatory drug (p.578) without first consulting your doctor because the combination may increase the risk of kidney damage.

What are the side effects?

Light-headedness can occur if there is a temporary fall in blood pressure and not enough blood reaches the brain. If light-headedness persists, you should consult your doctor. He or she may wish to adjust your dose. You should not drive or undertake hazardous tasks until you know how you are affected by the drug.

Other common side effects that ACE inhibitors may cause include a persistent dry cough, muscle cramps, diarrhoea, and occasionally the skin condition urticaria (p.285). A rare but serious side effect is kidney damage.

Angiotensin II blocker drugs

A group of drugs used to treat high blood pressure and heart failure

COMMON DRUGS

- Candesartan ▪ Irbesartan ▪ Losartan
- Olmesartan ▪ Telmisartan ▪ Valsartan

Angiotensin II blocker drugs, a group of drugs also known as angiotensin II receptor blockers (ARBs), are used to treat high blood pressure (*see* **Hypertension**, p.242) and chronic heart failure (p.247). The drugs may be used to treat people with high blood pressure who also have thickening of the heart muscle or diabetes mellitus (p.437). ARBs are also commonly prescribed for people with high blood pressure who have unacceptable side effects from other antihypertensives, particularly ACE inhibitors. Occasionally, an ARB may be used in combination with an ACE inhibitor to treat some cases of heart failure.

ARBs work by blocking the action of the substance known as angiotensin II, which is produced naturally by the body and causes blood vessels to constrict. As a result, the blood vessels are able to dilate and blood pressure is reduced.

How are they used?

ARBs, available as oral preparations, are usually prescribed at a low dose initially. The dose is then gradually increased over several weeks until the lowest effective dose is found.

The most common side effects that ARBs cause are light-headedness and dizziness but they are usually mild. ARBs are much less likely than ACE inhibitors to cause a persistent dry cough and are therefore a possible alternative for people who have to discontinue ACE inhibitors because of the side effects.

Digitalis drugs

A group of plant-derived drugs used to treat certain heart disorders

COMMON DRUGS

- Digitoxin ▪ Digoxin

Digitalis drugs belong to a group of drugs called cardiac glycosides, the most commonly used of which is digoxin. Digitalis drugs may be used to treat chronic heart failure (p.247), in which the heart fails to pump blood effectively. These drugs increase the strength of the heart's contraction. They also slow an abnormally rapid heart rate and allow the heart to pump more blood with each beat. This results in improved blood flow.

Digitalis drugs may also be used to treat a very rapid, irregular heartbeat, such as atrial fibrillation (p.250). However, in this condition, digitalis drugs may slow the heart rate without correcting the irregularity.

✖ WARNING

Contact your doctor immediately if you experience nausea, vomiting, diarrhoea, or visual disturbances while you are taking the digitalis drug digoxin.

How are they used?

You will normally be prescribed oral digitalis drugs. You may be given a large initial dose so that the drug becomes effective quickly. If your heart failure is life-threatening, very rapid treatment will be needed immediately, and the drug may be administered by infusion into a vein.

While you are taking a digitalis drug, your doctor will monitor your heart rate regularly. He or she may also arrange for you to have blood tests to check the levels of the drug in your blood. You may need to take a digitalis drug for a prolonged period.

What are the side effects?

You are most likely to experience side effects from taking the drug if the dose you are taking is too high. These side effects often develop slowly and may include nausea, vomiting, diarrhoea, abdominal pain, and headache. You may also experience other side effects such as loss of appetite and fatigue. Visual disturbances, such as seeing coloured haloes around lights, may occur, and, in rare cases, drowsiness, confusion, hallucinations, and delirium may also be experienced. You should report any of these side effects to your doctor without delay.

Diuretic drugs

Drugs that increase the volume of urine and that are used to remove excess fluid from the body

COMMON DRUGS

Thiazide drugs
- Bendroflumethazide (bendrofluazide)
- Chlortalidone   ■ Cyclopenthiazide
- Indapamide   ■ Metolazone

Loop diuretic drugs
- Bumetanide   ■ Furosemide (frusemide)
- Torasemide

Potassium-sparing diuretic drugs
- Amiloride   ■ Spironolactone   ■ Triamterene

Other diuretic drugs
- Acetazolamide   ■ Brinzolamide
- Dorzolamide   ■ Mannitol

Diuretic drugs are commonly used in the treatment of high blood pressure (*see* **Hypertension**, p.242) and chronic heart failure (p.247). Diuretics are also used to treat other conditions in which excess fluid accumulates in the body, such as liver or kidney disorders and glaucoma (p.358). Acetazolamide may be used to prevent altitude sickness (p.186) and to treat the inner ear condition Ménière's disease (p.380).

How do they work?
Diuretics act on the kidneys to increase the volume of water that is excreted from the body as urine. Water, salts (such as sodium and potassium), and waste products are removed from the blood as it passes through small tubules in the kidneys. Most of the water and salts are reabsorbed into the bloodstream. What is not reabsorbed is then excreted, along with waste products, as urine. Diuretics reduce the reabsorption of water and salts into the blood, thereby increasing the volume of urine that is produced. This action of diuretics relieves the accumulation of fluid that occurs in the body due to heart failure, and the reduced blood volume helps to reduce blood pressure. Some diuretics also dilate (widen) blood vessels in the body, which also has the effect of lowering blood pressure.

What are the types?
The diuretic drugs that are most frequently prescribed are thiazide drugs, loop diuretic drugs, and potassium-sparing diuretic drugs, which vary in their potency. Different types of diuretic affect reabsorption at different sites along the kidney tubules. The type of diuretic that your doctor prescribes is likely to depend on the condition being treated, your age, and any other existing medical conditions that you may have.

Thiazides These are the most commonly used diuretics for the treatment of high blood pressure. Thiazides lower blood pres-

sure by reducing blood volume as well as by dilating (widening) blood vessels. These types of diuretic are usually taken orally once a day and have an effect at low doses.

Thiazides generally cause few side effects. However, the increased frequency with which you need to pass urine may be inconvenient. This effect is most noticeable at the start of treatment. You may find it convenient to take the diuretic early in the morning so that your sleep is not interrupted at night.

Occasionally, thiazide diuretics cause light-headedness due to a drop in blood pressure. Thiazides can cause excessive loss of potassium from the body, which can result in confusion, weakness, and, in rare cases, an abnormal heart rhythm. Blood tests are used to monitor the levels of potassium in the body. To correct low levels, you may be given a potassium supplement or a potassium-sparing diuretic either in place of or in combination with a thiazide.

Thiazides may also cause increased levels of uric acid in the blood. When the level of uric acid becomes too high, crystals may be deposited in the joints, which may cause the painful condition gout (p.224). Thiazides are sometimes avoided in people with diabetes mellitus (p.437) because they may make control of the condition more difficult. In addition, these drugs can cause the skin to become sensitized to sunlight.

Loop diuretics These diuretics have a more powerful effect than thiazides and are used to treat the accumulation of fluid due to heart failure, some kidney disorders, and some liver disorders. They may also be given as an injection for the emergency treatment of acute heart failure.

Loop diuretics cause the production of urine to increase dramatically. In men with an enlarged prostate gland (p.463), this problem may lead to urinary retention (p.455). The drugs may also cause nausea. In addition, loop diuretics can deplete the body's supply of potassium. If you are affected by potassium loss, your doctor may prescribe a potassium supplement or a potassium-sparing diuretic to be taken in combination with a loop diuretic.

Potassium-sparing diuretics Most of these drugs are mild diuretics and are used either alone or in combination with a thiazide or loop diuretic if potassium depletion has occurred. The side effects of potassium-sparing diuretics may include digestive disturbances, such as flatulence and nausea, a dry mouth, and rashes. One drug, spironolactone, may cause breast enlargement in men (*see* **Gynaecomastia**, p.466).

Other diuretic drugs Acetazolamide is occasionally used to prevent altitude sickness and attacks of dizziness associated with the inner ear condition Ménière's disease. It may also be used to relieve the excessive pressure in the eye that occurs in glaucoma. Glaucoma may also be treated with brinzolamide or dorzolamide. Mannitol may be used to treat cerebral oedema (a build-up of fluid in the brain).

Drugs for blood and immune system disorders and cancer

Improved understanding of blood and immune system disorders has led to advances in certain drug treatments. For example, there are now drugs that reduce the risk of heart attacks caused by blood clots. Recently developed drugs that act on the immune system also allow some forms of cancer to be controlled.

There are a number of potentially serious disorders that alter the clotting mechanism of the blood, resulting in either abnormal bleeding or the formation of unwanted clots. The first articles in this section describe the drugs that help to keep the clotting factors of the blood at normal levels.

The body's immune system combats disease by activating white blood cells and proteins in the blood against infections and cancers. Sometimes, this system malfunctions and needs to be treated with drugs. Types of drug used to treat immune system malfunction include antiallergy drugs, which counter overreaction of the immune system; immunosuppressants, which prevent the immune system attacking the body's own tissues; and interferon drugs, which boost immunity. Drugs for the immune deficiency disease AIDS are discussed elsewhere (*see* **Drugs for HIV infection and AIDS**, p.573). The final article in this section describes anticancer drugs, which can destroy cancerous cells or prevent them from spreading elsewhere in the body. The use of anticancer drugs is known as chemotherapy (p.157).

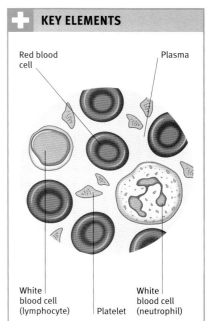
Drugs that promote blood clotting

Drugs used to treat disorders in which blood fails to clot normally

COMMON DRUGS

Blood products
- Dried prothombin complex
- Factor VIII   ■ Factor IX   ■ Fresh frozen plasma

Vitamin K
- Phytomenadione

Antifibrinolytic drugs
- Tranexamic acid

Several types of disorder cause spontaneous internal bleeding or excessive bleeding after even minor injuries (*see* **Bleeding disorders**, p.274). These disorders are usually treated with drugs that promote blood clotting or slow the breakdown of existing clots.

What are the types?
The three main types of drug that are used to promote the formation of blood clots and to prevent or reduce abnormal bleeding are blood products, vitamin K, and antifibrinolytic drugs.

Blood products Normal blood clotting depends on the presence in the blood of certain proteins called clotting factors. People who lack one of these clotting factors (often due to an inherited disorder) may be given specific blood products, which are concentrated supplements of the missing protein. For example, a blood product called Factor VIII is needed for the treatment of the inherited bleeding disorder haemophilia A (*see* **Haemophilia**, p.274), in which a defective gene causes a deficiency of natural Factor VIII in the blood. Other blood products (fresh frozen plasma or dried prothrombin complex) are given to counteract abnormally prolonged or severe bleeding due to causes such as an excessive dose of anticoagulants (*see* **Drugs that prevent blood clotting**, p.584).

All blood products are administered intravenously, either in hospital or at home, and may be used regularly as a preventive treatment or given when abnormal bleeding occurs.

Some people experience side effects, including chills and fever, when being given blood products. These side effects may result from an allergic reaction.

Vitamin K This vitamin is essential for the production of several vital blood-clotting factors. Newborn babies (who are born with no stores of vitamin K) and people who are deficient in vitamin K may need a supplement, which is either given by injection or taken orally. Vitamin K is also used to reverse the effect of an excessive dose of oral anticoagulants. No side effects are known to be associated with its use.

Antifibrinolytic drugs These drugs may be used when bleeding is difficult to control, as may occur after surgery, or to reduce menstrual bleeding that is excessively heavy (see **Menorrhagia**, p.471). Antifibrinolytic drugs affect the clotting process of blood by slowing the breakdown of existing clots. The drugs may be injected or given by infusion into a vein if bleeding must be stopped urgently or may be taken orally for the treatment of menorrhagia. Side effects such as headaches, diarrhoea, nausea, and vomiting are sometimes experienced by people who are taking these drugs.

Drugs that prevent blood clotting

Drugs used to prevent unwanted blood clots developing or to stabilize existing blood clots

COMMON DRUGS

Antiplatelet drugs
■ Aspirin ■ Clopidogrel ■ Dipyridamole ■ Prasugrel ■ Ticagrelor

Oral anticoagulants
■ Apixaban ■ Dabigatran ■ Rivaroxaban ■ Warfarin

Injected anticoagulants
■ Dalteparin ■ Enoxaparin ■ Heparin ■ Tinzaparin

Drugs may be prescribed to prevent unwanted blood clots (thrombi) from developing in blood vessels. They may also be used to prevent existing blood clots from enlarging and to reduce the risk of an embolism, in which a piece of an existing clot in a vein breaks off and travels to a vital organ. Thrombolytic drugs (right) are used when a blood clot needs to be dissolved rapidly.

What are the types?

Antiplatelet drugs and anticoagulants are used to prevent blood clots from forming. In general, antiplatelet drugs are used to prevent clots from forming in arteries and anticoagulants are prescribed to prevent clots from forming or enlarging in veins or within the heart.

Antiplatelet drugs These drugs are used to help prevent blood clots from forming in the arteries. The drugs work by reducing the tendency of platelets, a type of blood cell that plays a vital role in the clotting process, to stick together. If you have symptoms of coronary artery disease, such as angina (p.244), or have had a heart attack (see **Myocardial infarction**, p.245), a stroke

(p.329), or a transient ischaemic attack (p.328), you may need to take an antiplatelet drug for the rest of your life.

Aspirin is the most commonly prescribed antiplatelet drug. However, you should not take aspirin if you are pregnant, breast-feeding, or have a peptic ulcer. Clopidogrel works by reducing the "stickiness" of platelets in a similar way to aspirin and is often recommended as an alternative for people who cannot take aspirin. Combination treatment with clopidogrel and aspirin may be recommended for people who have had a heart attack, a severe attack of angina (p.244), or who have undergone a coronary angioplasty and stenting (p.246). When used together with aspirin in this way, clopidogrel further reduces the likelihood of another heart attack or a stroke during such periods of high risk. The drug should not be taken if you are breast-feeding.

Oral anticoagulants These drugs are given as a long-term treatment to prevent deep vein thrombosis (p.263) and pulmonary embolism (p.302). Oral anticoagulants may also be given to people with the heart rhythm disorder atrial fibrillation (p.250). There are two types of oral anticoagulant: warfarin, and the newer drugs apixaban, dabigatran, and rivaroxaban, which are known as novel oral anticoagulants (NOACs).

Warfarin acts by preventing the formation of clotting factors, the proteins that are essential for normal blood clotting. NOACs work by blocking the action of clotting factors. Warfarin and NOACs usually take about 48–72 hours to become effective.

While you are taking warfarin, you will need frequent blood tests for the first few days and then regular tests during your treatment so that the dose can be adjusted to your needs. If the dose is too high, these drugs may cause abnormal bleeding. For this reason, you should consult your doctor immediately if you develop symptoms such as nosebleeds or blood in your urine. To treat abnormal bleeding, your doctor may prescribe drugs that reverse the effect of anticoagulants (see **Drugs that promote blood clotting**, p.583). If you are taking NOACs, you will not need regular blood tests. Unlike with warfarin, if abnormal bleeding occurs while you are taking a NOAC, the effects cannot easily be reversed.

Warfarin may cause other side effects, including rashes, diarrhoea, easy bruising, hair loss, and impaired liver function. You should avoid drinking alcohol and making any sudden changes to your diet, both of which may affect the action of the drug. Since many drugs interact with anticoagulants, you should not take other medications, particularly aspirin, without first consulting your doctor. It is very important that you inform your doctor if you plan to become pregnant because certain anticoagulants can cause abnormalities in a developing fetus. You should not discontinue anticoagulant drug treat-

ment suddenly. You will be given an anticoagulant treatment card or a medical alert bracelet or pendant, which you should always carry with you to inform health professionals in case of an emergency.

Injected anticoagulants If blood clotting must be controlled quickly, an anticoagulant, such as heparin, may be given by injection or infusion so that it has immediate effect. These fast-acting injected anticoagulants are used to treat disorders such as pulmonary embolism before oral anticoagulants take effect. Injected anticoagulants are given as a preventive measure before orthopaedic surgery. They may also be given before surgery to people who are at particular risk of blood clotting and are often prescribed for people who are immobilized during treatment in hospital.

Some longer-acting drugs, such as tinzaparin, which need be given only once a day, can be self-administered for the treatment of deep vein thrombosis. Injected anticoagulants may cause side effects such as skin rashes.

Thrombolytic drugs

A group of drugs, also known as fibrinolytics, used to dissolve blood clots

COMMON DRUGS

■ Alteplase ■ Reteplase ■ Streptokinase ■ Tenecteplase

Thrombolytic drugs act rapidly to dissolve unwanted blood clots (thrombi) in blood vessels. In some cases they may be given as an emergency treatment for heart attacks (see **Myocardial infarction**, p.245). They may also be used to treat ischaemic strokes (p.329).

A heart attack is usually caused by a blood clot blocking one of the coronary arteries, which supply blood to the heart muscle. Left untreated, such a clot can cause irreversible damage to the heart, which can be fatal. Ischaemic strokes are caused by a blood clot blocking the supply of blood to an area of the brain.

Thrombolytics may be used to dissolve a blood clot in a vein deep within the body, often in the legs (see **Deep vein thrombosis**, p.263). These fast-acting drugs may also be used to treat pulmonary embolism (p.302), where the flow of blood to the lungs becomes blocked.

Thrombolytic drugs work by dissolving the mesh of fibrin, a stringy protein that

How thrombolytic drugs work

Thrombolytic drugs are used to dissolve unwanted blood clots, known as thrombi. A blood clot consists of blood cells and platelets that are held together by a mesh of fibrin strands. Thrombolytics dissolve the fibrin strands, thereby breaking up the blood clot.

Red blood cell　　Fibrin　　Blood clot　　Platelet

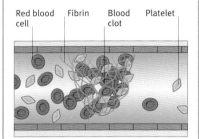

Before drug
A clot, made up of red and white blood cells and platelets bound together by strands of fibrin, has formed in a blood vessel, restricting blood flow.

Drug　　Blood clot dissolving

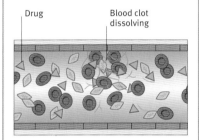

After drug
The thrombolytic drug dissolves the fibrin strands that bind the blood clot together. The clot is broken down and normal blood flow resumes.

binds a blood clot together (see **How thrombolytic drugs work**, right). When the blood clot has been dissolved by the drugs, normal blood flow to the affected area is restored.

How are they used?

Thrombolytics are given by injection or by infusion. In the treatment of a heart attack, the drugs must be given within 6–12 hours (ideally, within 1 hour) of the start of the attack to be effective. In the case of a stroke, the drugs must be given within 3 hours (ideally, within 1 hour) of the onset of symptoms.

These drugs may cause side effects such as nausea and vomiting, as well as an increased susceptibility to bruising and bleeding. Streptokinase, which is one of the most frequently used thrombolytics, can cause allergic reactions, often in the form of a rash. Occasionally, a life-threatening allergic reaction called anaphylaxis (p.285) occurs.

Antiallergy drugs

Drugs used to prevent and treat allergic conditions and allergic reactions

COMMON DRUGS

Antihistamines (right)

Mast cell stabilizers
■ Nedocromil sodium ■ Sodium cromoglicate

Corticosteroids (p.600)

Leukotriene antagonists
■ Montelukast ■ Zafirlukast

Allergen extracts

Other antiallergy drugs
■ Epinephrine (adrenaline)

Antiallergy drugs are used in the treatment of a variety of allergic disorders, such as allergic conjunctivitis (p.355), hay fever (*see* **Allergic rhinitis**, p.283), and atopic eczema (p.193). Antiallergy drugs can be used to prevent an allergic response from occurring or to relieve the symptoms of allergy, such as sneezing.

What are the types?

Several groups of drugs are used to treat allergic reactions. The most commonly used are antihistamines (right), mast cell stabilizers, corticosteroids (p.600), leukotriene antagonists, allergen extracts, and the drug epinephrine (adrenaline).

Antihistamines These drugs are most commonly used to relieve the symptoms of hay fever, to treat allergic rashes such as urticaria (p.285), and to relieve itching due to insect bites. They block the action of histamine, a chemical that is released by the body in an allergic reaction.

Mast cell stabilizers These may be prescribed to prevent allergic reactions. The drugs block the release of histamine, a chemical that is stored in mast cells (a type of white blood cell present in blood and most body tissues). Histamine is released from these cells in allergic reactions. The most commonly used mast cell stabilizer is sodium cromoglicate, which is given for allergic conjunctivitis, hay fever, asthma in children (p.544), and exercise-induced asthma (p.295) in adults. Since these drugs cannot be absorbed when taken orally, they are used topically as eyedrops, nasal sprays, or inhalers. The drugs are taken as preventive treatment; they do not relieve symptoms.

Corticosteroids These drugs reduce inflammation caused by allergic reactions. They may be included in skin creams used to treat atopic eczema (*see* **Topical corticosteroids**, p.577) and in nasal sprays to relieve the symptoms of hay fever (*see* **Corticosteroids for respiratory disease**, p.588). For severe or persistent allergies, corticosteroids may be given orally or intravenously.

Leukotriene antagonists When used with corticosteroids, these drugs help to prevent asthma attacks. They block the action of leukotrienes, chemicals that cause airway inflammation in asthma.

Allergen extracts Substances that can cause allergic reactions, such as bee venom or grass pollen, are called allergens. Tiny amounts of an allergen may be used to desensitize a person who has a severe allergy to that substance. The treatment is usually given as a series of weekly injections containing gradually increasing doses. Treatment may last for several months. Allergen extracts can themselves cause life-threatening allergic reactions and are given only where emergency treatment is available.

Epinephrine (adrenaline) This drug is used to treat anaphylaxis (p.285), a life-threatening allergic reaction. The drug reverses the swelling of the throat, narrowing of the airways, and drop in blood pressure that occurs in anaphylaxis. Epinephrine is injected in repeated doses until the condition improves. If you are at risk of anaphylaxis because of a severe allergy, you should carry a syringe prefilled with epinephrine for emergency treatment (*see* **Emergency aid for anaphylaxis**, p.285).

Antihistamines

Drugs that block the effects of histamine, a chemical released during allergic reactions

COMMON DRUGS

Nonsedating antihistamines
■ Acrivastine ■ Cetirizide ■ Desloratadine
■ Fexofenadine ■ Loratadine ■ Mizolastine

Sedating antihistamines
■ Alimemazine (trimeprazine)
■ Chlorphenamine ■ Clemastine
■ Promethazine

Antihistamines are used mainly to prevent or relieve symptoms of allergies, such as hay fever (*see* **Allergic rhinitis**, p.283), and to treat allergic rashes, such as urticaria (p.285). These drugs are also effective in relieving itching and irritation due to insect bites or stings. Antihistamines are sometimes included in cold and flu remedies (p.588) because they dry up mucus. Since some types of antihistamine also depress the vomiting reflex in the brain, these drugs may also be taken to relieve nausea, vomiting, vertigo, and motion sickness (*see* **Antiemetic drugs**, p.595). Certain antihistamines have a sedative effect and are recommended if you have regular nighttime itching.

Antihistamines are normally taken orally, but some types are available for topical use as nasal sprays, eyedrops, or skin lotions. Antihistamines may also be given by injection as emergency treatment for the life-threatening allergic reaction anaphylaxis (p.285).

How do they work?

Antihistamines prevent or relieve the symptoms of an allergic reaction by blocking the action of histamine, a chemical

▶ DRUG ACTION

How antihistamines work

Antihistamine drugs are used to prevent or relieve the symptoms of allergic reactions, such as a rash. Allergens, such as grass pollen, can trigger the release of the chemical histamine from body cells. This chemical acts on small blood vessels, glands, and other tissues, causing the symptoms of allergy. The drugs work by blocking the action of histamine.

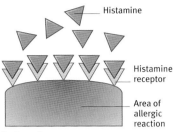

Before drug
Histamine is released in response to an allergen and attaches to sites on tissue cells known as histamine receptors. This causes an allergic reaction in the tissue.

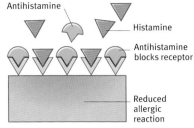

After drug
The antihistamine drug occupies some of the histamine receptors, thereby preventing histamine from attaching to them. This reduces the severity of allergic symptoms.

that is released from certain cells in the blood and body tissues when they are exposed to an allergen (*see* **How antihistamines work**, above). The effects of histamine include widening of the small blood vessels in the affected area, often the skin, nose, and eyes, leading to redness and swelling and increased production of mucus. By blocking the action of histamine, antihistamine drugs can reduce some of the symptoms of allergies, such as swelling, rash, itching, runny nose, and sneezing.

What are the side effects?

Generally, topical antihistamines do not usually cause side effects, although occasionally there may be local irritation. With oral antihistamines, the older, sedating types may cause difficulty in passing urine and therefore may not be suitable for men with prostate problems. These drugs also may not be suitable for some people with glaucoma. If you have either of these conditions, you should check with your pharmacist or doctor before taking an older type of antihistamine.

Oral antihistamines may also cause varying degrees of drowsiness, problems with coordination, dry mouth, constipation, and blurred vision. These problems are more likely with sedating antihistamines but may also occur with the nonsedating ones. If an antihistamine causes drowsiness, coordination problems, and/or blurred vision, you should not drink alcohol, drive, or operate machinery. In some children, antihistamines may cause hyperactive behaviour.

Oral antihistamines may interact with a variety of other medications, including some antidepressants, beta-blockers, and antibacterial drugs. If you are taking any medications, you should check with your pharmacist or doctor before taking an antihistamine.

Immunosuppressants

Drugs used to reduce the activity of the body's immune system

COMMON DRUGS

Corticosteroids (p.600)

Cytotoxic anticancer drugs
■ Azathioprine ■ Chlorambucil
■ Cyclophosphamide ■ Methotrexate

Disease-modifying antirheumatic drugs (p.579)

Other immunosuppressants
■ Alemtuzumab ■ Antithymocyte
immunoglobulin ■ Basiliximab
■ Glatiramer acetate ■ Natalizumab
■ Sirolimus ■ Tacrolimus

Immunosuppressants reduce the activity of the body's immune system. The immune system protects the body against infection and helps to destroy diseased cells. However, in certain conditions, known as autoimmune disorders (p.280), the immune system acts against the body's healthy tissues, and immunosuppressant drugs may be required to protect them from damage. Immunosuppressants are also used to prevent rejection of donor tissue and organs after transplant surgery (p.614). Some immunosuppressants are also used to treat certain cancers.

People who are taking immunosuppressant drugs are at increased risk of infection because the drugs reduce the body's ability to fight disease.

What are the types?

There are various types of drugs that suppress the activity of the immune system. The most commonly used ones are corticosteroids (p.600), disease-modifying antirheumatic drugs (p.579), and some cytotoxic anticancer drugs (p.586).

Corticosteroids Oral corticosteroids are widely used in the treatment of autoimmune disorders, such as systemic lupus erythematosus (p.281) and rheumatoid arthritis (p.222). They are also used to prevent transplant rejection and some, such as prednisolone, are used to treat some types of cancer, such as certain leukaemias (p.276) and lymphomas (p.279). They inhibit the activity of white blood cells, which are an essential component of the immune response, and also reduce inflammation.

Prolonged used of oral corticosteroids may cause acne, the development of a moon-shaped face, and weight gain. They also increase the risk of developing osteoporosis (p.217), high blood pressure (see **Hypertension**, p.242), and diabetes mellitus (p.437), and may make some otherwise minor infections, such as chickenpox (p.165), life-threatening. You should not stop taking oral corticosteroids suddenly. Your doctor or pharmacist will issue a card giving details of your treatment, which you should carry at all times in case of a medical emergency.

❌ **WARNING**

When taking immunosuppressant drugs, it is important to report any signs of infection, such as a sore throat or fever, or any unusual bruising or bleeding to your doctor immediately. If you are taking oral corticosteroids, you should not stop them suddenly.

Disease-modifying antirheumatic drugs
Often known as DMARDs, these drugs are used to treat rheumatoid arthritis and certain other autoimmune disorders, such as systemic lupus erythematosus. Some of these drugs, such as ciclosporin, are also used to prevent transplant rejection, and others, such as rituximab, are used to treat certain cancers.

DMARDs are a diverse group of drugs and affect the immune system in a variety of different ways, although in general they reduce its activity. They may cause potentially serious side effects, such as kidney, liver, blood, or eye problems, and therefore people taking them are monitored regularly.

Cytotoxic anticancer drugs
These drugs are used primarily to treat cancers such as leukaemia and lymphoma but some, such as methotrexate and cyclophosphamide, have an immunosuppressant effect and are also used to treat noncancerous autoimmune disorders such as rheumatoid arthritis. Cytotoxic immunosuppressants suppress the immune system by inhibiting the growth of new white blood cells in the bone marrow.

Cytotoxic immunosuppressants can cause side effects including nausea, vomiting, diarrhoea, hair loss, and abnormal bleeding. People taking such drugs need regular blood tests to monitor the drug's effects.

Other immunosuppressants
In addition to the drugs already discussed, various other drugs also have an immunosuppressant effect. Some of these drugs are used to prevent transplant rejection, for example,

antithymocyte immunoglobulin, basiliximab, and tacrolimus, which work by suppressing lymphocytes (types of white blood cells), and sirolimus, which works by inhibiting the production of antibodies (substances made by white blood cells to neutralize foreign proteins in the body). Alemtuzumab, which suppresses lymphocytes, is used to treat some cases of leukaemia. Glatiramer acetate, whose method of action is unknown, and natalizumab, which inhibits the movement of white blood cells, are used to treat multiple sclerosis (p.334).

These drugs may cause a wide range of side effects, most commonly gastrointestinal disturbances, such as nausea and vomiting, fever, and chills. They may also cause various potentially more serious side effects, such as hypersensitivity reactions, high or low blood pressure, and heart, kidney, liver, nervous system, or blood disorders. For this reason, people taking these drugs are monitored regularly.

Interferon drugs

A group of drugs that inhibit the multiplication of viruses and also act against certain tumours

COMMON DRUGS

- Interferon alfa   ■ Interferon beta   ■ Interferon gamma   ■ Peginterferon alfa

---

Interferons are a group of proteins produced naturally by the body's immune system in response to viral infections and certain other challenges, such as tumours. Synthetic versions that mimic the action of these natural interferons are used as drugs to treat a number of disorders. There are three main types of synthetic interferon: alfa, beta, and gamma. Peginterferon alfa is a modified form of interferon alfa that remains in the blood for longer.

Interferon alfa is used in the treatment of some types of cancer, such as certain lymphomas (p.279) and leukaemias (p.276), malignant melanoma (p.201), multiple myeloma (p.277), carcinoid tumours (a type of tumour that affects the intestines or bronchus), AIDS-related Kaposi's sarcoma (p.201), and some kidney tumours (p.456). Interferon alfa or peginterferon alfa may be used in the treatment of chronic hepatitis B and C (see **Chronic hepatitis**, p.409).

Interferon beta is used to treat some patients with multiple sclerosis (p.334), although not all respond to the drug. Interferon gamma is used in the treatment of chronic granulomatous disease (an inherited condition in which certain cells of the immune system do not work properly) and some cases of severe osteopetrosis (abnormally dense, brittle bones), both of which are rare.

How do they work?
Interferons work in several ways. They bind to body cells and cause them to produce antiviral proteins; they stimulate certain types of white blood cell (which form part

of the body's immune system) to resist viral infection and to destroy virus-infected cells; and they slow down the multiplication of cancerous cells.

Interferon drugs are given only by injection, and in most cases the drugs can be self-administered. Your doctor or nurse will teach you how to inject yourself.

What are the side effects?
The most common side effects of interferon drugs are loss of appetite; nausea; a flu-like syndrome in which you may have a fever, aches, and a headache; tiredness; and lethargy. Less commonly, there may be redness and swelling at the injection site; tingling in the hands and feet; and depression. Interferons may also produce other adverse effects, including liver, kidney, and heart and circulatory problems. If you are taking an interferon drug, your doctor will arrange for regular tests to monitor changes in your body functions.

Anticancer drugs

A group of drugs used to destroy or slow the growth of cancerous cells

COMMON DRUGS

Cytotoxic drugs
- Bleomycin   ■ Busulfan   ■ Carboplatin
- Chlorambucil   ■ Cisplatin
- Cyclophosphamide   ■ Cytarabine
- Dacarbazine   ■ Doxorubicin
- Etoposide   ■ Fluorouracil   ■ Gemcitabine
- Hydroxycarbamide (hydroxyurea)
- Irinotecan   ■ Melphalan   ■ Methotrexate
- Paclitaxel   ■ Pemetrexed   ■ Procarbazine
- Temozolomide   ■ Trastuzumab   ■ Vincristine

Hormones and hormone antagonists
- Aminoglutethimide   ■ Anastrozole
- Diethylstilbestrol   ■ Flutamide
- Goserelin   ■ Leuprorelin
- Medroxyprogesterone   ■ Megestrol
- Octreotide   ■ Tamoxifen

Other drugs
- Aldesleukin   ■ Bevacizumab   ■ Cetuximab
- Erlotinib   ■ Imatinib   ■ Interferon alfa
- Lapatinib   ■ Rituximab   ■ Sorafenib
- Sunitinib

Cancers are a broad group of diseases in which abnormal body cells form and multiply, interfering with the function of surrounding tissues. Cancerous cells may affect vital organs and can spread to other parts of the body through the bloodstream. Anticancer drugs either destroy the cancer cells or prevent them from spreading. Treatment with these drugs, known as chemotherapy (p.157), is normally managed by an oncologist, a doctor who specializes in the medical treatment of cancer.

Anticancer drugs may be given with the aim of curing the cancer, prolonging life, or relieving symptoms. In some cases, chemotherapy is used in combination with surgery and/or radiotherapy (p.158). Anticancer drugs may be used to shrink the tumour before the other treatments, or they may be used after surgery or radiotherapy to prevent the growth of cancer cells that may have spread around the body.

What are the types?
The group of drugs most commonly used to treat cancer are cytotoxic drugs, which damage or destroy both cancerous and healthy body cells. Some hormonal drugs, such as the synthetic female sex hormones medroxyprogesterone and megestrol, are also used to treat certain forms of cancer, as are hormone antagonist drugs, which work by blocking the effects of hormones that stimulate cancer growth. Other anticancer drugs include drugs that stimulate the immune system and drugs that disrupt specific biological processes of cancer cells.

Cytotoxic drugs There are several types of cytotoxic drug, which kill cells or prevent cancer cells from increasing in number. The drugs either act directly on the cells' genetic material, DNA, or prevent the cells from using the nutrients they need to divide normally. The effect of the drugs is concentrated on areas of tissue where cells are rapidly dividing, and they are therefore effective in treating rapidly growing cancers, such as those of the lymphatic system (see **Lymphoma**, p.279), various forms of leukaemia (p.276), many childhood cancers, and some types of cancer of the testis (p.460). Some cytotoxic anticancer drugs, such as methotrexate, are also used to treat noncancerous conditions such as severe psoriasis (p.192) and rheumatoid arthritis (p.222). Cytotoxic drugs are usually administered in hospital. Several short courses of the drugs are given over a number of weeks, with drug-free periods in between to allow time for the normal body cells to recover.

Cytotoxic drugs can cause severe side effects because they affect any area of the body where there is rapid cell division, including the bone marrow, the hair follicles, and the lining of the mouth and the intestines. Damage to the bone marrow may reduce the numbers of red and white blood cells and platelets in the blood. Some anticancer drugs may also cause folic acid deficiency. These problems can lead to anaemia (p.271), an increased susceptibility to infection, and reduced ability of the blood to clot. Nausea and vomiting are particularly common side effects of cytotoxic drugs and may be severe. Certain drugs may cause mouth ulcers and hair loss.

The severity of many side effects can be reduced by additional treatment with other drugs. For example, antiemetic drugs (p.595) are commonly given and are usually effective in preventing vomiting. Most side effects are temporary and do not result in long-term damage. However, some types of cytotoxic drug can cause irreversible damage to the ovaries, which leads to premature menopause, or to the testes, resulting in abnormal or reduced sperm production. Men who wish to have children in the future can arrange to have their sperm frozen and stored before treatment. For women, the harvesting of ovarian tissue or eggs for future use is a possibility.

How chemotherapy treatment works

Anticancer drugs (chemotherapy) may be given in a series of treatments. The drugs kill cancer cells, but they also destroy some normal cells. For this reason, there are recovery periods between treatments during which the number of normal cells is allowed to rise again. Treatment is stopped when no cancer cells are detectable.

CHEMOTHERAPY TREATMENT

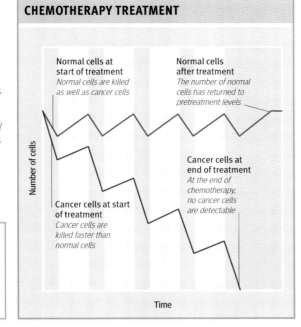

Normal cells at start of treatment
Normal cells are killed as well as cancer cells

Normal cells after treatment
The number of normal cells has returned to pretreatment levels

Cancer cells at end of treatment
At the end of chemotherapy, no cancer cells are detectable

Cancer cells at start of treatment
Cancer cells are killed faster than normal cells

Number of cells

Time

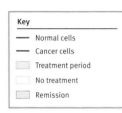

Key

— Normal cells
— Cancer cells
▢ Treatment period
▢ No treatment
▢ Remission

If you are taking cytotoxic drugs, you will have regular blood tests, including a blood count, before each course of treatment to measure the levels of different types of blood cell. See your doctor at once if you develop new symptoms, such as a sore throat, because they may indicate a low number of white blood cells.

Hormones and hormone antagonists Treatment with hormones may be suitable for certain types of cancer whose growth is influenced by hormones. This type of treatment may be used following surgery or radiotherapy to prevent any remaining cancer cells from growing and spreading. The treatment may involve the use a hormone that halts the progression of the cancer. For example, megestrol is used to slow the progression of cancer of the uterus (p.479).

Alternatively, a hormone antagonist drug may be used. Drugs of this type oppose the effects of the hormone that stimulates the growth of the cancer. For example, hormone antagonists such as tamoxifen are often effective in halting the progression of certain types of breast cancer (p.486) that are stimulated by the female sex hormone oestrogen. The drug blocks the action of oestrogen on breast cells. The growth of cancerous cells that have spread from a cancer in the prostate gland may be slowed by using the drug goserelin, which blocks the secretion of the male sex hormone testosterone.

Hormonal drugs are usually taken orally or injected, and sometimes treatment is continued for several years. Most of these hormonal drugs have milder side effects than cytotoxic drugs. However, treatment with tamoxifen slightly increases the risk of developing cancer of the uterus; you should report abnormal vaginal bleeding to your doctor immediately.

Other anticancer drugs These drugs include biological agents (sometimes called simply "biologicals"), which are being used increasingly in the treatment of cancer. Some biologicals work by stimulating the immune system against cancer, whereas other work by disrupting specific biological processes of cancer cells, thereby inhibiting their growth or destroying them.

Biologicals that are thought to work primarily by stimulating the immune system include aldesleukin, used to treat some advanced kidney cancers; and interferon alfa (*see* **Interferon drugs**, p.586), which may be used to treat several types of cancer, including certain lymphomas (p.279), leukaemias (p.276), malignant melanomas (p.201), kidney tumours (p.450), and AIDS-related Kaposi's sarcoma (p.201). Biologicals that work primarily by disrupting cancer cells' biological processes include bevacizumab, used to treat some breast cancers; cetuximab (some bowel cancers); erlotinib (some lung cancers); imatinib (some leukaemias); lapatinib (some breast cancers); sorafenib (some kidney and liver cancers); and sunitinib (some kidney cancers). Rituximab is a monoclonal antibody that may be used to treat some lymphomas and leukaemias. It is not known exactly how it works.

Side effects vary according to the specific drug. Generally, however, common side effects include fever, muscle aches, vomiting, fatigue, rash, and diarrhoea. More serious side effects, such as heart, liver, or blood disorders, may also occur and therefore these drugs are given under specialist supervision.

✖ WARNING

Many anticancer drugs are potentially harmful to a developing fetus. You should consult your doctor about your contraception needs before starting treatment.

Drugs for respiratory disorders

Conditions affecting the airways and lungs range from minor illnesses, such as the common cold, to long-term disorders, such asthma. The discomfort of coughs and colds may be eased with over-the-counter remedies. However, the symptoms of long-term disorders, such as shortness of breath, can be severe and require specific medical treatment.

This section describes some of the drugs used to treat both common illnesses, such as coughs and colds, and more serious conditions that affect the airways and lungs.

The first three articles in this section discuss drugs used to treat common symptoms of upper respiratory tract infections, such as nasal congestion, cough, and fever. The next article discusses bronchodilator drugs, which widen the airways of the lungs and are used to treat respiratory conditions in which breathing becomes difficult, such as asthma (p.295) and chronic obstructive pulmonary disease (p.297). The final article in this section covers the use of corticosteroids in the treatment of respiratory conditions, including their use in preventing attacks of asthma. Drugs used for hay fever and other allergic disorders that affect the respiratory system are described elsewhere (*see* **Antiallergy drugs**, p.585), as are antibiotics used in the treatment of respiratory infections (*see* **Drugs for infections and infestations**, pp.571–572).

➕ KEY ANATOMY

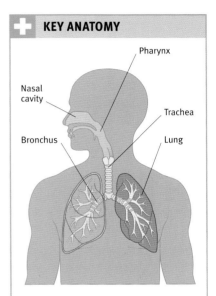

Pharynx

Nasal cavity

Trachea

Bronchus

Lung

For further information on the structure and function of the respiratory system, *see* pp.286–289.

Decongestants

Drugs that are used to reduce swelling of the membranes lining the nose and sinuses

COMMON DRUGS

- Ephedrine
- Phenylephrine
- Xylometazoline
- Oxymetazoline
- Pseudoephedrine

Decongestants act to relieve congestion in the nose and sinuses. A blocked nose or sinuses (*see* **Sinusitis**, p.290) may be caused by a viral infection, such as the common cold (p.164), or by an allergic condition, such as hay fever (*see* **Allergic rhinitis**, p.283).

Infections and allergic reactions can cause inflammation of the delicate lining of the nose or sinuses. The blood vessels in the lining enlarge, and increased volumes of fluid pass into the mucous membranes, which swell and produce excessive amounts of mucus. Decongestants act directly on the blood vessels to constrict them and reduce the swelling and mucus secretion.

Decongestants are available as sprays or drops that are used in the nose or as oral pills or capsules. Some cold and flu remedies (p.588) that are available over the counter also contain a small amount of decongestant. You can spray or insert decongestant drops directly into your nose to provide rapid relief. When taken orally, decongestants work more slowly, but the effects last longer.

Decongestant sprays or drops should be used in moderation and for no longer than a week. After that time, they may lose their capacity to constrict blood vessels. When the last effective dose wears off, the blood vessels widen again, and congestion may become worse.

Used sparingly, decongestant sprays or drops have few side effects. If you have heart disease or high blood pressure, you should check with your doctor or pharmacist before using decongestants because they sometimes cause a rapid, irregular heartbeat and raise blood pressure. Decongestants must be avoided by people taking MAOIs (monoamine oxidase inhibitors, a group of antidepressant drugs) because the drugs may interact to cause a dangerous rise in blood pressure. Decongestants may also cause a slight tremor in the hands.

✖ CAUTION

Avoid using decongestants for longer than a week because the drugs may become ineffective or worsen your condition.

Cough remedies

Preparations containing various drugs used to treat coughing

COMMON DRUGS

- Codeine ■ Dextromethorphan
- Guaifenesin ■ Pholcodine

Coughing is a natural reflex that helps to clear the lungs of sputum produced by infections. The effectiveness of cough medicines is doubtful, which is why doctors rarely prescribe them for minor respiratory disorders. However, there are many cough remedies available over the counter. Almost all of these are syrups to which a variety of drugs and flavourings have been added. Most are of little medicinal value, although some may have soothing properties.

The main groups of drugs used to treat coughs are expectorants, mucolytics, and suppressants. Expectorants are supposed to encourage productive coughs (which produce sputum), but their benefit is not proven.

Mucolytic preparations make sputum less sticky and easier to cough up, but they are of little benefit to most people. However, mucolytic drugs are used in the treatment of cystic fibrosis (p.535), in which abnormally thick, sticky sputum is produced.

Cough suppressants which often contain drugs such as codeine or pholcodine, are usually effective in relieving a troublesome cough. They can cause drowsiness, which may be helpful if a cough interrupts sleep. However, if you feel drowsy after taking the drugs, you should not drive or operate machinery. They should be taken according to your doctor's or the manufacturer's instructions. They are not advised for a cough that is producing large amounts of sputum because preventing the expulsion of sputum can delay recovery from an infection.

Cold and flu remedies

Preparations containing drugs that ease the symptoms of colds and flu

COMMON DRUGS

Painkillers
■ Aspirin ■ Ibuprofen ■ Paracetamol

Decongestants
■ Ephedrine ■ Oxymetazoline
■ Phenylephrine ■ Pseudoephedrine
■ Xylometazoline

There are no cures for the common cold (p.164) or influenza (p.164), but there are various remedies that may suppress the symptoms and ease discomfort. Most of these remedies are combinations of drugs, which may include a painkiller (p.589), such as paracetamol or ibuprofen, to lower fever and relieve muscle aches, sore throat, and headache; decongestants (p.587) to relieve congestion; caffeine, which acts as a mild stimulant; and vitamin C. Generally, doctors

advise taking single drugs to treat individual symptoms rather than medicines that contain several different types of drug, some of which are not necessary. Antiviral drugs (p.573) may occasionally be used to treat influenza.

✖ WARNING

Do not give aspirin to children under 16 years, except on the advice of a doctor, because it increases the risk of Reye's syndrome.

How are they used?

Dosages for cold and flu remedies tend to vary. It is important to follow the instructions given with the product and not to exceed the recommended daily dose of paracetamol, because high doses can cause liver damage. Children under the age of 16 should not be given aspirin, except on the advice of a doctor, because this drug is linked with Reye's syndrome (p.550). You should avoid taking cold and flu remedies containing aspirin or ibuprofen if you have asthma (p.295), a peptic ulcer (p.406), indigestion (p.397), or gout (p.224).

Bronchodilator drugs

Drugs that widen the airways to ease breathing difficulties

COMMON DRUGS

Sympathomimetics
■ Bambuterol ■ Formoterol ■ Salbutamol
■ Salmeterol ■ Terbutaline

Anticholinergics
■ Aclidinium bromide ■ Glycopyrronium
■ Ipratropium bromide ■ Tiotropium
■ Umeclidinium

Xanthines
■ Aminophylline ■ Theophylline

Bronchodilator drugs are used to dilate (widen) the bronchi (airways) inside the lungs (*see* **How bronchodilator drugs work**, right). Widening the airways prevents or relieves the wheezing, tightness of the chest, and shortness of breath that can result from conditions such as asthma (p.295) and chronic obstructive pulmonary disease (p.297), a progressive disease of the lungs.

Many bronchodilator drugs are inhaled through a metered-dose inhaler, a small aerosol pump that delivers a controlled amount of the drug to be inhaled into the lungs. Spacers, which are plastic chambers into which a dose of the drug is released before it is inhaled, and breath-activated inhalers are also available. You may prefer to use a spacer if you have difficulty using an inhaler on its own (*see* **Taking inhaled asthma drugs**, p.297). If you have severe shortness of breath, you may need to take bronchodilator drugs by means of a nebulizer, a device that delivers the drug in aerosol form through a mask or a mouthpiece. Certain bronchodilators are taken orally on a regular basis to prevent asthma attacks.

▶ DRUG ACTION

How bronchodilator drugs work

Bronchodilator drugs are often used to prevent or relieve wheezing and shortness of breath caused by disorders such as asthma. In these conditions, the bronchi (airways in the lungs) become abnormally narrowed because muscles in their walls contract. Bronchodilators work by widening the airways and thereby increasing the air flow.

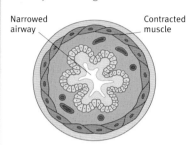

Narrowed airway
Contracted muscle

Before drug
The airway narrows as the muscle layer in its walls contracts. The flow of air to the lungs becomes reduced.

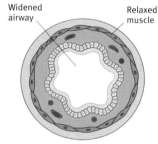

Widened airway
Relaxed muscle

After drug
The drugs act on the muscle cells of the airway. The muscles relax, and the airway widens, increasing air flow.

During any discussion about your bronchodilator treatment, you should let your doctor know if you are pregnant or breast-feeding.

What are the types?

Bronchodilator drugs are divided into three main groups: sympathomimetics, anticholinergics, and xanthines. When inhaled, some sympathomimetics take effect within 10 minutes and are often used for rapid relief from shortness of breath; anticholinergics and xanthines are slower acting. Two or more types of drug may be used simultaneously.

Sympathomimetics These are the most commonly used bronchodilators. They relax muscles in the wall of the airways, causing the airways to widen.

These drugs are usually inhaled and are of two main types: short-acting and longer-acting. Short-acting types, such as salbutamol, act within minutes and remain effective for 4–6 hours. Other types, such as salmeterol, are slower acting and longer

lasting, taking up to 4 hours to act and lasting for about 12 hours. Formoterol acts rapidly and also lasts for about 12 hours.

Usually, inhaled sympathomimetics are used at the first sign of symptoms or to prevent symptoms developing, for instance before physical activity. These drugs may cause slight tremor, agitation, insomnia, and, rarely, a rapid heartbeat.

Anticholinergics The drugs in this group are often used in combination with sympathomimetics to treat chronic obstructive pulmonary disease. Anticholinergics work in a similar way to sympathomimetics. They may cause some side effects, including a dry mouth, difficulty in passing urine, and blurred vision. In rare cases, they may trigger an attack of acute glaucoma (p.358), an eye disorder that can permanently damage vision and needs immediate treatment.

Xanthines These bronchodilator drugs have a prolonged action, which makes them useful in preventing night-time asthma attacks. Xanthines act on the muscle cells of the airway walls, causing the airways to widen.

Oral xanthines may be taken daily as a preventive measure. If you have a severe attack of shortness of breath, you may be given aminophylline intravenously through a drip. These drugs sometimes cause nausea and headache and, taken in high doses, occasionally produce a rapid and irregular heartbeat. For this reason, xanthines are used less commonly than other bronchodilators.

Corticosteroids for respiratory disease

A group of anti-inflammatory drugs used to treat several respiratory disorders

COMMON DRUGS

- Beclometasone ■ Budesonide
- Ciclesonide ■ Fluticasone ■ Hydrocortisone
- Mometasone ■ Prednisolone

Corticosteroids (p.600) are drugs that are related to natural hormones. When used to treat respiratory disorders, these drugs reduce or prevent inflammation of the airways. Corticosteroids are frequently prescribed to prevent attacks of asthma (p.295). They are also occasionally prescribed for people with chronic obstructive pulmonary disease (p.297). In addition, corticosteroids are sometimes helpful in preventing or treating inflammation of the nasal passages in allergic conditions such as hay fever (*see* **Allergic rhinitis**, p.283).

Less commonly, corticosteroids are used to treat people with sarcoidosis (p.304), a disorder in which the lung tissue becomes inflamed.

How do they work?

The lining of the airways in the lungs becomes inflamed in asthma. This reaction causes the airways to narrow and restricts air flow. Corticosteroids reduce inflammation by inhibiting the release of natural chemicals, called prostaglandins, that play a key role in triggering the inflammatory response. Reducing inflammation widens the airways and thereby relieves or prevents asthma attacks. When they are used in treating hay fever, corticosteroids act on the lining of the nose to reduce inflammation. In people with sarcoidosis, the reduction in inflammation slows down and minimizes damage to lung tissues.

How are they used?

Your doctor may prescribe an inhaled corticosteroid if you are experiencing attacks of asthma or if you find that you need to use bronchodilator drugs (p.588) more than a few times a week. Regular use of inhaled corticosteroid drugs can prevent asthma attacks occurring, and, over time, it may be possible to reduce the dose. If you have a severe asthma attack, you may need to take an oral corticosteroid drug for a few days. Long-term use of low-dose oral corticosteroids is usually necessary only if you have severe asthma that cannot be controlled by inhaled drugs. If you are admitted to hospital with a severe attack, you may be given an intravenous corticosteroid. To treat hay fever, corticosteroids are taken as a nasal spray. People who have sarcoidosis will probably be prescribed long-term treatment with oral corticosteroids.

If you have been taking oral corticosteroids for more than a few weeks, do not stop taking them suddenly. If the drugs are taken for a prolonged period, they can suppress the body's own production of corticosteroids, which are needed to fight infection. The dose should be reduced gradually to allow natural corticosteroid production to resume.

If you are prescribed an oral corticosteroid for longer than a few weeks, your doctor or pharmacist will give you a treatment card to carry with you at all times.

What are the side effects?

The side effects from inhaled corticosteroids are usually minimal because the drugs act directly on the airways with little effect elsewhere in the body. The most common side effect is oral thrush (*see* **Candidiasis**, p.177), a fungal infection more commonly associated with other areas of the body. To avoid this infection, rinse your mouth with cold water after using your inhaler.

Your doctor will prescribe the lowest dose for your condition to reduce the risk of side effects. However, if oral corticosteroids are taken on a long-term basis, there is a risk of side effects, including an increased susceptibility to infections, osteoporosis (p.217), cataracts (p.357), bruising, glaucoma (p.358), and slowed growth in children.

✖ WARNING

Do not suddenly stop taking oral corticosteroids without first consulting your doctor.

Drugs acting on the brain and nervous system

Many of the drugs that act on the brain and nervous system relieve symptoms such as pain, insomnia, and anxiety. Others treat the disorders that cause the symptoms. As understanding of the chemical changes that occur in disorders such as depression improves, treatment is becoming more effective.

The opening article in this section describes groups of drugs known as painkillers. Most of these drugs work by preventing pain signals from being produced or altering the way in which the brain perceives pain. Drugs for migraine are covered next, followed by general anaesthetic drugs, which induce unconsciousness so that no pain can be felt during surgery. Local anaesthetic drugs, which block the transmission of pain signals in a specific body part, are then discussed.

The next articles in this section cover anticonvulsant drugs, sleeping drugs, and antianxiety drugs. Most work by reducing electrical activity in the brain to relieve symptoms but do not treat the underlying disorder.

Antidepressant drugs, which are described next, work by increasing levels of chemicals in the brain that regulate mood. Reduced levels of these chemicals can usually be found in people who are depressed.

In the final articles, antipsychotic drugs, mood-stabilizing drugs, and central nervous system stimulants are described. All of these drugs work by altering chemical activity in the brain.

✚ KEY ANATOMY

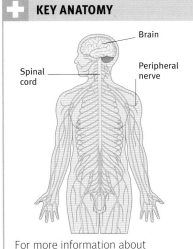

For more information about the structure and function of the brain and nervous system, *see* pp.311–318.

Painkillers

Drugs of varying potency that are used to relieve pain

COMMON DRUGS

Opioid painkillers
- Buprenorphine
- Codeine
- Diamorphine
- Fentanyl
- Methadone
- Morphine
- Pethidine
- Tramadol

Nonopioid painkillers
- Aspirin
- Celecoxib
- Diclofenac
- Etodolac
- Etoricoxib
- Fenoprofen
- Ibuprofen
- Indometacin
- Ketoprofen
- Mefenamic acid
- Naproxen
- Paracetamol
- Piroxicam

Combination painkillers
- Aspirin with codeine
- Dihydrocodeine with paracetamol
- Ibuprofen with codeine
- Paracetamol with codeine

Painkillers work in different ways, depending on the type of preparation. Some drugs block the nerve pathways that transmit pain signals from a part of the body to the brain. Other painkillers reduce the perception of pain by preventing further transmission of pain signals once they reach the brain. However, pain relief for most long-term disorders depends on treatment of the underlying cause.

What are the types?

The two main types of painkiller are opioid (narcotic) and nonopioid (non-narcotic). A number of commonly used painkillers are combinations of more than one drug. Opioid painkillers are mainly used to relieve severe pain. Nonopioid painkillers, most of which are nonsteroidal anti-inflammatory drugs (p.578), may be used to ease mild to moderate pain. Combinations of two or more painkillers and, in some cases, another drug may provide greater pain relief than a single drug.

Opioid painkillers These drugs are the strongest painkillers available. They may be given for pain during a heart attack (*see* **Myocardial infarction**, p.245) or following surgery or serious injury. They are also widely used in pain relief for cancer (p.159). Opioids act on the brain, altering the perception of pain. These drugs work in a similar way to natural substances called endorphins, which are released in the brain in response to pain. Opioids bind to the same receptors in the brain as endorphins and stop the transmission of pain signals from cell to cell (*see* **How opioid painkillers work**, right).

Prolonged use of opioids may lead to dependence. However, you are very unlikely to become dependent if you take the drugs for a few days to relieve severe pain. Dependence is also not usually a cause for concern in the treatment of pain in a terminally ill person. However, prolonged use leads to tolerance, which means that progressively higher doses are needed to achieve the same level of pain relief.

Opioids may be taken orally or, if the pain is extremely severe or accompanied by vomiting, may be given by injection. They are also available as patches. Side effects include constipation, nausea, vomiting, and drowsiness. Larger doses can depress breathing and may also cause confusion and impaired consciousness. Overdose may be fatal.

Nonopioid painkillers These types of drug are less potent than opioids, and a number are available over the counter. They include paracetamol and non-steroidal anti-inflammatory drugs (NSAIDs)

▶ DRUG ACTION

How opioid painkillers work

Opioid drugs are often used to relieve severe pain. Pain signals are transmitted along nerves from the source of pain to the brain. Opioids block the transmission of pain signals in the brain, and thus reduce the sensation of pain.

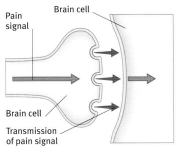

Before the drug
On reaching the brain, the pain signal is transmitted from one brain cell to the next until it reaches the part of the brain that interprets the signal as pain.

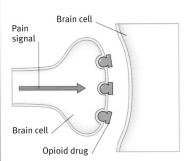

After the drug
Opioid painkillers block transmission of the pain signal in the brain, thereby reducing the sensation of pain.

❌ WARNING

Do not give aspirin to children under 16 years, except on the advice of a doctor, because it increases the risk of Reye's syndrome.

such as aspirin and ibuprofen. Nonopioids are used mainly for pain such as headache or menstrual pain and also lower fever and reduce inflammation in conditions such as arthritis.

Side effects are rarely a problem if you take nonopioid painkillers occasionally and at the doses recommended for pain relief. However, when used repeatedly, aspirin and other NSAIDs may damage the lining of the stomach and intestines. NSAIDs may also cause various other adverse effects; for a fuller discussion of these effects, and warning about use of NSAIDs, see p.578.

Paracetamol relieves pain and lowers fever, but, unlike NSAIDs, it does not reduce inflammation. The drug works by blocking pain impulses in the brain. Paracetamol is dangerous if taken in doses above the recommended maximum daily intake. Overdose can cause severe liver and kidney damage.

Combination painkillers Combination painkillers, which may contain other, non-painkiller types of drug, are available as over-the-counter remedies for headaches, backache, menstrual pain, and other minor disorders. However, caffeine, an ingredient included in some remedies, may itself cause headaches.

Antimigraine drugs

Drugs that are used in the prevention and treatment of migraine

COMMON DRUGS

Drugs to prevent migraine
- Amitriptyline ■ Clonidine ■ Cyproheptadine ■ Methysergide ■ Propranolol ■ Pizotifen ■ Sodium valproate

Drugs to relieve migraine
- Ergotamine ■ Naratriptan ■ Rizatriptan ■ Sumatriptan ■ Zolmitriptan

Painkillers (previous page)
- Aspirin ■ Codeine ■ Ibuprofen ■ Paracetamol

Migraine attacks (see **Migraine**, p.320) produce severe headaches and are often accompanied by nausea and vomiting. These symptoms may be preceded by visual disturbances. Some drugs used to treat migraine are taken regularly to prevent attacks, while others are taken during an attack to alleviate the symptoms. Painkillers (previous page) may help to relieve headaches.

How do they work?

During a migraine attack, blood flow inside the brain changes. Initially, the blood vessels narrow, reducing blood flow. After this initial phase, the vessels rapidly widen, and a severe headache develops. Drugs that are used to prevent migraine, such as propranolol (see **Beta-blocker drugs**, p.581), prevent these changes in blood vessel size. However, the exact mechanism by which they work is not understood.

Triptan drugs, such as sumatriptan, and ergotamine relieve the symptoms of an attack by returning widened blood vessels to their normal size. Painkillers can provide some relief if taken early in an attack.

How are they used?

Most people who experience migraines have attacks infrequently and can control the pain by taking drugs such as paracetamol, aspirin, ibuprofen, or codeine. If you experience frequent, severe migraine attacks, your doctor may recommend that you use a preventive drug, such as the beta-blocker propranolol, to be taken daily for a few months.

Severe migraine that is not relieved by painkillers may respond to triptans. You should take these antimigraine drugs as soon as you notice symptoms developing. Triptans can be taken orally, but if you regularly experience episodes of very severe migraine, especially if they are accompanied by nausea and vomiting, your doctor may prescribe triptans in a form that can be given by injection or nasal spray. Ergotamine may occasionally be prescribed instead of a triptan, but is rarely used because of its adverse side effects.

There are various over-the-counter preparations for migraine. These may contain one or more painkillers and an antiemetic drug (p.595) to help to relieve nausea and vomiting.

What are the side effects?

You may experience side effects when taking drugs to treat migraine. Taking propranolol may cause cold hands and feet and tiredness. Triptans can make you feel drowsy and can sometimes cause flushing, dizziness, tingling sensations, and chest pain. Ergotamine may cause nausea, vomiting, abdominal pain, diarrhoea, and muscle cramps. Excessive use of triptans or ergotamine may reduce their effectiveness. You should not exceed the recommended dose of any antimigraine drug.

General anaesthetics

Drugs that act on the brain to induce unconsciousness for surgery

COMMON DRUGS

Injected anaesthetics
- Etomidate ■ Ketamine ■ Propofol ■ Thiopental

Inhaled anaesthetics
- Isoflurane ■ Nitrous oxide ■ Sevoflurane

General anaesthetics produce reversible loss of consciousness and sensation and are therefore used in people undergoing surgery (see **Having a general anaesthetic**, p.609). The drugs are rapidly absorbed by the brain and produce unconsciousness by reducing the flow of nerve impulses in the brain.

How are they used?

Initially, a short-acting drug such as etomidate or propofol is injected to induce anaesthesia. The effect of these drugs wears off quite quickly so to maintain anaesthesia, inhaled anaesthetics are administered, either via a face mask or an endotracheal tube (a flexible tube passed into the windpipe through the nose or mouth). Often, a muscle relaxant drug is given in addition to the general anaesthetics. This relaxes all the muscles in the body, including those of the throat and respiratory system. Consequently, breathing has to be assisted artificially and vital body functions, such as heart rate and blood pressure, are monitored continuously during a general anaesthetic.

Various general anaesthetics are often combined so that only a minimum dose of each drug is needed to maintain unconsciousness. This method reduces the potential for side effects from any of the drugs. For minor surgical procedures, an injected general anaesthetic is sometimes used without inhaled anaesthetics.

When the surgical procedure is completed, the anaesthetics are stopped and, if necessary, drugs are administered to reverse muscle relaxation.

What are the side effects?

Modern general anaesthetics have few side effects and recovery is usually prompt. The most common side effects on regaining consciousness are nausea and vomiting, which can be controlled with antiemetic drugs (p.595) if necessary, and tiredness. Rarely, some inhaled anaesthetics may cause liver damage if given repeatedly. Your doctor or anaesthetist will ask if you have had a general anaesthetic within the last 3 months and whether you have had any adverse reactions to an anaesthetic.

Certain other drugs, such as those used to treat high blood pressure, may interact with anaesthetics. You should inform your anaesthetist about any drugs you have been taking, whether prescription, over-the-counter, recreational, or complementary remedies.

Local anaesthetics

Drugs that block pain sensations in a limited region of the body

COMMON DRUGS

- Benzocaine ■ Bupivacaine ■ Lidocaine ■ Mepivacaine ■ Procaine ■ Tetracaine

Local anaesthetics produce reversible loss of sensation in a specific area of the body. They have a wide range of uses, including the prevention of pain during minor surgical procedures or diagnostic tests. The drugs are also used to produce regional anaesthesia, sometimes called a nerve block, in which a large area of the body is anaesthetized. Local anaesthetics vary in potency and in the duration of their effect. They work by temporarily preventing the conduction of pain signals along nerve fibres.

How are they used?

A local anaesthetic may be injected directly into the site at which sensation needs to be blocked (see **Having a local anaesthetic**, p.608). For example, local anaesthesia may be used to numb a small area of skin before the removal of a mole. Local anaesthetics may also be applied to the skin or the mucous membranes as a cream, gel, or spray. Some products that contain a local anaesthetic are available over the counter; these include throat lozenges and suppositories or ointments used to relieve painful haemorrhoids (p.422).

Regional anaesthesia is used to anaesthetize a large area of the body. The drug is usually injected at a site close to a nerve or bundle of nerves that supplies a specific area of the body (see **Having a regional anaesthetic**, p.610). The anaesthetic then numbs the entire area supplied by that nerve or nerve bundle. One example of this type of anaesthesia is epidural anaesthesia, in which a local anaesthetic is injected into the space around the spinal cord. This procedure anaesthetizes the whole of the lower body and is sometimes used as a form of pain relief during labour (see **Epidural anaesthesia in labour**, p.518).

What are the side effects?

Some local anaesthetics applied to the skin can cause an allergic reaction if they are used repeatedly. If a large dose of local anaesthetic becomes absorbed into the bloodstream, it may lead to symptoms such as dizziness.

Following an epidural anaesthetic, you may have a headache or backache that can last for several days.

Anticonvulsant drugs

Drugs used to prevent and treat epileptic seizures and other types of seizures

COMMON DRUGS

Benzodiazepines
- Clonazepam ■ Diazepam ■ Lorazepam

Other anticonvulsant drugs
- Carbamazepine ■ Ethosuximide ■ Gabapentin ■ Lamotrigine ■ Phenobarbital ■ Phenytoin ■ Primidone ■ Sodium valproate ■ Topiramate

Anticonvulsant drugs are mainly used to prevent recurrent seizures caused by epilepsy (p.324) and as an emergency treatment for prolonged seizures. Left untreated, prolonged seizures may cause brain damage. Rarely, an anticonvulsant drug is used for seizures not due to epilepsy, such as febrile convulsions (p.550), which can occur in children. Some anticonvulsant drugs are used to treat pain due to nerve damage, such as trigeminal neuralgia (p.338), which causes severe pain on one side of the face.

How do they work?

Anticonvulsants have a direct effect on electrical activity in the brain. A seizure occurs when excessive electrical activity spreads from one part of the brain to other areas, causing uncontrolled stimulation of nerves supplying many parts of the body. Anticonvulsants reduce these abnormally high levels of electrical activity and thereby prevent or reduce the muscle spasms that are characteristic of a seizure. The mechanism by which anticonvulsants relieve nerve pain in disorders such as trigeminal neuralgia is not clearly understood.

How are they used?

If you have recurrent seizures, you are likely to need anticonvulsants for a prolonged period to reduce the frequency and severity of your seizures or, if possible, to prevent them altogether. Your doctor will initially prescribe a single drug that is appropriate for the type of seizure that you have. For example, if you experience absence seizures, in which brief periods of detachment from reality occur, your doctor will usually give you either ethosuximide or sodium valproate. If seizures are tonic-clonic (characterized by uncontrolled movement of the limbs and trunk) or partial (involving minor twitching movements), your treatment may be with sodium valproate, lamotrigine, or carbamazepine. Drugs such as gabapentin may be used if other anticonvulsants do not control seizures or cause severe side effects.

If a seizure is prolonged, diazepam may be given by intravenous injection, or as a liquid that is administered into the rectum. Once the seizure has been brought under control, intravenous infusions of phenytoin or another drug may be given for a few hours afterwards to prevent seizures from recurring.

The dose of an anticonvulsant is adjusted so that the drug is effective without causing unwanted side effects. You may find that you have occasional seizures while taking anticonvulsants. If this is the case, your doctor may try another drug, either as an alternative or as an additional treatment.

If you have epilepsy you will probably be given a card, bracelet, or pendant giving the details of your condition and treatment. It is advisable to carry this identification with you at all times for others to refer to if you have a seizure.

If you have an isolated seizure that is not due to epilepsy, liquid midazolam may be given for buccal absorption (absorption through the inside of the cheek into the

WARNING

- If you are taking anticonvulsants, you should consult your doctor immediately if you develop a rash, fever, mouth ulcers, swollen glands, sore throat, bruising, or bleeding.
- Do not stop taking or alter the dose of an anticonvulsant without first consulting your doctor. Stopping the drug abruptly could cause withdrawal symptoms and a recurrence of the original problem.
- Anticonvulsants can harm a developing fetus. If you are planning a pregnancy, you should discuss this with your doctor.

bloodstream). Alternatively, diazepam may be given rectally. If you have trigeminal neuralgia (sudden, short attacks of severe facial pain), you may need long-term treatment with an oral anticonvulsant.

What are the side effects?

Anticonvulsants can affect memory and coordination and may induce lethargy and impair concentration. You should consult your doctor immediately if you develop signs of a hypersensitivity reaction, such as rash, fever, mouth ulcers, and swollen glands, or develop an infection, because some anticonvulsants reduce the effectiveness of the immune system. If you are planning to become pregnant, you should also arrange to see your doctor to discuss your treatment needs during pregnancy.

Sleeping drugs

Drugs that reduce nerve cell activity in the brain and are used to treat insomnia

COMMON DRUGS

Benzodiazepines
- Flurazepam - Nitrazepam - Temazepam

Antihistamines (p.585)

Other sleeping drugs
- Chloral hydrate - Zaleplon - Zolpidem
- Zopiclone

Sleeping drugs may be prescribed to reestablish sleep patterns after a period of insomnia (p.343) or when insomnia is the result of a stressful event, such as a death in the family. They may also be used if you need to adjust your sleep patterns to suit your work. However, sleeping drugs do not treat the cause of insomnia, which may be depression (p.343) or anxiety (*see* Anxiety disorders, p.341). You should not drink alcohol when taking sleeping drugs because the sedative effect is enhanced.

WARNING

Sleeping drugs can affect your ability to drive or to operate machinery; these effects may persist the following day.

Sleeping drugs should always be taken in the smallest effective dose for the shortest period of time. In general, they should be used for no longer than 3 weeks, and preferably for no longer than 1 week and not every night.

What are the types?

There are a variety of sleeping drugs available. One type of these is benzodiazepines, which are also used to treat anxiety disorders. Over-the-counter remedies containing an antihistamine (p.585) are also available to treat insomnia. If insomnia is caused by depression, your doctor may prescribe antidepressant drugs (p.592) to relieve the symptoms of depression, including insomnia. Barbiturates are no longer recommended for treating sleeping problems as they may cause serious side effects and dependence.

Benzodiazepines These drugs reduce the level of activity in the brain, causing drowsiness. They are usually used only to treat insomnia that is severe or disabling and, if your doctor does prescribe a benzodiazepine, you will usually have only a limited supply and be advised not to take the drug every night. This is because prolonged use may result in dependence and tolerance, in which progressively larger doses of the drug are needed to produce the same effect. When you take the drug, side effects such as confusion, dizziness, and poor coordination may develop even between doses. If you are elderly, you should take particular care because these drugs can increase the risk of falling. You may also experience withdrawal symptoms when you stop taking benzodiazepines, including a recurrence of insomnia and increased dreaming, restlessness, and anxiety. Reducing the dose gradually can minimize withdrawal symptoms.

Antihistamines Some sleep preparations containing an antihistamine may be purchased over the counter. They do not cause dependence and have only a few minor side effects, but you should not take any of them for longer than a few days without first consulting your doctor. Antihistamines sometimes cause a dry mouth and blurred vision.

Other sleeping drugs Zaleplon, zolpidem, and zopiclone reduce electrical activity in the brain, so that falling asleep is easier. Their effects are brief and they are less likely to cause dependence, but they are not recommended for long-term use.

Chloral hydrate is now used only if other sleeping drugs prove unsuccessful. Side effects include stomach upsets and nausea.

Antianxiety drugs

Drugs that are used to reduce and control the symptoms of stress and anxiety

COMMON DRUGS

Benzodiazepines
- Chlordiazepoxide - Diazepam - Lorazepam
- Oxazepam

Beta-blocker drugs
- Oxprenolol - Propranolol

Antidepressant drugs (p.592)

Other antianxiety drugs
- Buspirone

Antianxiety drugs, sometimes known as anxiolytics or minor tranquillizers, are used to treat anxiety disorders (p.341), in which feelings of foreboding and fear may be accompanied by physical symptoms such as palpitations and tremor. The underlying cause of the anxiety may also need to be treated at the same time, possibly using one or more psychological therapies (pp.622–624). Some drugs are used specifically to relieve the physical symptoms of anxiety.

What are the types?

Several types of drug are used in the treatment of anxiety. Benzodiazepines are the drugs most commonly prescribed for the short-term treatment of psychological symptoms of anxiety.

Where physical symptoms, such as muscle tremor, are the main problem, beta-blocker drugs (p.581) may be used instead. Buspirone is sometimes prescribed to treat anxiety because it is less sedating than benzodiazepines. Some antidepressants, such as selective serotonin reuptake inhibitors, may also be used to treat anxiety, as well as post-traumatic stress, phobias, and certain other psychological problems.

WARNING

Benzodiazepine drugs often cause drowsiness and may affect your ability to drive vehicles or operate machinery.

Benzodiazepines These drugs may be used for the treatment of severe anxiety. They reduce agitation and make you feel relaxed.

Benzodiazepines slow mental activity by reducing the signals between brain cells. They are also used as sleeping drugs (left) because they often cause drowsiness. You should not drink alcohol while taking the drugs because it increases the sedative effect. These drugs can also cause confusion, dizziness, lethargy, and poor coordination.

Tolerance to benzodiazepines (in which progressively larger doses are needed to produce the same effect) can develop after as little as 3 days and there is a high risk of users becoming physically and psychologically dependent on the drugs, even after only a few weeks' use. For these reasons, most doctors are reluctant to prescribe benzodiazepines unless they are absolutely necessary, and then usually only for a maximum period of 4 weeks. Stopping the drugs may also cause withdrawal symptoms, such as excessive anxiety and insomnia. Reducing the dose gradually can minimize such symptoms.

Beta-blocker drugs Physical symptoms that can occur together with anxiety may be reduced with beta-blockers. These drugs should only be used occasionally and are not suitable for long-term treatment.

The drugs block the actions of two hormones, epinephrine (adrenaline) and norepinephrine (noradrenaline), that produce the physical symptoms of anxiety. Beta-blockers reduce heart rate, may prevent palpitations, and can also help to reduce muscle tremor. If you take a beta-blocker, you may find that your sleep is disturbed and that your hands and feet feel cold.

Beta-blockers may precipitate asthma (p.295), which can be life-threatening. They should therefore not be used by anybody who has, or has ever had, asthma or similar breathing problems, except in exceptional circumstances and under specialist supervision. Beta-blockers can also mask some of the symptoms of hypoglycaemia (low blood glucose), and the drugs may therefore not be suitable for some people who need to take insulin for diabetes mellitus (p.437).

Other antianxiety drugs The most common of the other drugs used to reduce anxiety is buspirone, which is less addictive than the benzodiazepines and has a less sedative effect. Buspirone can take up to 2 weeks to become fully effective and is therefore not used when immediate relief from stress or anxiety is needed. The drug may cause side effects, such as nervousness, headache, and dizziness. It may also affect your ability to drive or operate machinery.

Antidepressant drugs

Drugs that are used to treat the symptoms of depression

COMMON DRUGS

Selective serotonin reuptake inhibitors (SSRIs)
- Citalopram ■ Escitalopram
- Fluoxetine ■ Fluvoxamine
- Paroxetine ■ Sertraline

Tricyclics (TCAs)
- Amotriptyline ■ Clomipramine ■ Dosulepin
- Imipramine ■ Lofepramine ■ Nortriptyline
- Trimipramine

Monoamine oxidase inhibitors (MAOIs)
- Isocarboxazid ■ Moclobemide ■ Phenelzine
- Tranylcypromine

Other antidepressant drugs
- Flupentixol ■ Mianserin ■ Mirtazapine
- Reboxetine ■ Maprotiline ■ Trazodone
- Venlafaxine

Antidepressant drugs help to relieve many symptoms of depression (p.343), such as despair, lethargy, poor appetite, insomnia,

▶ **DRUG ACTION**

How SSRIs work

SSRI drugs are often used to treat depression. Depression is associated with low levels of serotonin, a chemical that acts on certain brain cells involved in thoughts and mood.

Nerve cells in the brain constantly release and reabsorb the chemical serotonin. SSRIs reduce the rate of reabsorption, resulting in higher levels of serotonin in the brain.

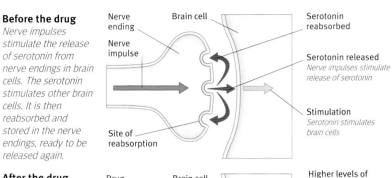

Before the drug
Nerve impulses stimulate the release of serotonin from nerve endings in brain cells. The serotonin stimulates other brain cells. It is then reabsorbed and stored in the nerve endings, ready to be released again.

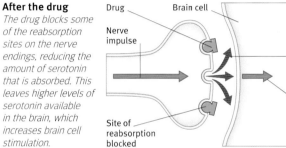

After the drug
The drug blocks some of the reabsorption sites on the nerve endings, reducing the amount of serotonin that is absorbed. This leaves higher levels of serotonin available in the brain, which increases brain cell stimulation.

and thoughts of suicide. Some types of antidepressants, such as selective serotonin reuptake inhibitors (SSRIs), are also effective in treating certain other psychological problems, such as anxiety and post-traumatic stress.

People who are depressed have been shown to have reduced levels of certain chemicals called neurotransmitters in the brain. Serotonin and norepinephrine (noradrenaline) are two neurotransmitters that are thought to increase brain activity and improve mood. They are usually reabsorbed by brain cells and inactivated by an enzyme called monoamine oxidase. In a depressed person, levels of serotonin or norepinephrine are frequently lower than normal. Antidepressants work by helping to restore these chemicals to normal levels.

Antidepressants are taken orally and usually take 2–3 weeks to have an effect on depression. Side effects may develop immediately but gradually lessen. Your doctor will usually advise you to take an antidepressant for at least 4–6 months after your depression has lifted to prevent symptoms recurring and then to reduce the dose gradually. You should avoid alcohol while you are taking these drugs because it enhances the sedative effect.

What are the types?

Most of the drugs used to treat depression belong to one of three main groups: selective serotonin reuptake inhibitors (SSRIs), tricyclics, and monoamine oxidase inhibi-

tors (MAOIs). There are also several other types of antidepressant. All of these drugs treat depression by increasing levels of the neurotransmitters in the brain that lift mood.

SSRIs These drugs are the most commonly used type of antidepressant. They may also be used to treat anxiety disorders (p.341) and post-traumatic stress disorder (p.342). SSRIs cause fewer side effects than other types of antidepressant and are less toxic if more than the prescribed amount is taken. The drugs work by blocking the reabsorption of the neurotransmitter serotonin, leaving more of the chemical to stimulate brain cells (*see* **How SSRIs work**, above). SSRIs may cause side effects, including diarrhoea, nausea and vomiting, reduced sex drive, and headache. They may also cause restlessness and anxiety. Most SSRIs are not recommended for treating depression in those under 18 years old.

Tricyclics Tricyclics are often used to treat depression. They interfere with the reabsorption of serotonin and norepinephrine in the brain; as a result, levels of these mood-lifting chemicals increase. They are also sometimes used to treat pain from damaged nerves in conditions such as trigeminal neuralgia (p.338).

Tricyclics cause a number of side effects, including a dry mouth, blurred vision, constipation, and difficulty in passing urine. The side effects are usually worse when the drug is first started and become less of a problem as you get used to the drug. Tricyclics are dangerous if you

 WARNING

Antidepressant drugs can cause drowsiness and may affect your ability to drive vehicles or operate machinery.

exceed the usual dose. They may cause seizures and heart rhythm irregularities, which can be fatal.

MAOIs These drugs are usually only used when other types of antidepressant drug are ineffective. They work by blocking the activity of monoamine oxidase (the enzyme that makes serotonin and norepinephrine inactive) in brain cells. The side effects may include light-headedness, drowsiness, insomnia, headache, a dry mouth, constipation, and other digestive problems. MAOIs interact with a wide range of other drugs and with food and drink containing tyramine (for example, cheese, meat and yeast extracts, pickled herring, fermented soya bean extract, red wine, and some other alcoholic and low-alcohol drinks). These interactions can cause a dangerous rise in blood pressure and it is therefore important that you follow your doctor's instructions about taking MAOIs and consult your doctor or pharmacist before taking any over-the-counter medications or complementary remedies. When planning to stop taking an MAOI, the dose should be reduced gradually to minimize the risk of dangerous changes in blood pressure.

Other antidepressant drugs Mianserin and trazodone are related to tricyclic antidepressants. They are used to treat depression when sedation is required. Trazodone is less likely to cause heart rhythm problems than other tricyclics. Mirtazepine increases serotonin and norepinephrine levels in the brain. It initially causes sedation and may sometimes cause potentially serious blood disorders. Flupentixol may cause restlessness and agitation and is therefore not suitable for people who are easily excitable and overactive. Reboxetine inhibits the reuptake of norepinephrine in the brain, and venlafaxine inhibits the reuptake in the brain of both serotonin and norepinephrine. Venlafaxine tends to produce fewer side effects than many antidepressants, but you should consult your doctor if you develop a rash while taking it.

Antipsychotic drugs

Drugs used to treat schizophrenia and other severe psychiatric disorders

COMMON DRUGS

- Amisulpride ■ Chlorpromazine ■ Clozapine
- Fluphenazine ■ Haloperidol ■ Olanzapine
- Pimozide ■ Promazine ■ Quetiapine
- Risperidone ■ Trifluoperazine ■ Zotepine

Antipsychotic drugs are used to control symptoms such as hallucinations and disturbed patterns of thought in schizophrenia (p.346) and other psychotic disorders. Some of these drugs are also used to stabilize mood in people with bipolar affective disorder (p.344), where episodes of mania tend to alternate with episodes of depression, although people with this condition are also likely to be treated with a mood-stabilizing drug (right) such as lithium. Occasionally, an antipsychotic drug is used to control vomiting or uncontrollable hiccups where other treatments have failed. Antipsychotic drugs may also be prescribed to treat severe anxiety and agitation.

How do they work?
Many antipsychotic drugs block the action of the neurotransmitter (brain chemical) dopamine. This chemical is released in the brain at higher than normal levels in people with psychotic disorders and is believed to play a part in producing symptoms. Some antipsychotic drugs also block the action of serotonin and other chemicals involved in regulating mood.

How are they used?
The type of antipsychotic drug prescribed will depend on factors such as how much sedation is needed and your susceptibility to side effects.

The drugs are usually taken orally, although they may be injected if a person is very agitated. A low dose of the drug is prescribed initially, and the dose is then increased gradually until the symptoms are under control. A depot injection, which is an injection deep into a muscle from which the drug is slowly released, may be used so that you do not have to take the drug every day. Depot injections provide enough of the drug to last up to 4 weeks.

If you have bipolar affective disorder, your doctor may prescribe lithium or another mood-stabilizing drug. These drugs take time before they become fully effective. For this reason, you may initially be given a short course of an antipsychotic drug that acts rapidly to make you feel calmer until the mood-stabilizing drug reaches its full effect.

What are the side effects?
Antipsychotics may cause a dry mouth, blurred vision, and dizziness due to lowering of blood pressure, and some may make you feel drowsy. They may also cause restlessness and, rarely, movement disorders such as parkinsonism (p.333) and tardive dyskinesia (involuntary, rhythmic movements of the face, jaw, and tongue). These side effects tend to disappear when you stop taking the drug although, after a long period of use, some antipsychotic drugs may cause permanent tardive dyskinesia.

You should never suddenly stop taking any antipsychotic drug without first consulting your doctor. If you need to stop taking the drug, the dose will be reduced gradually by your doctor.

Mood-stabilizing drugs

Drugs used to treat severe psychiatric disorders involving excessive mood swings

COMMON DRUGS

- Carbamazepine ■ Lithium ■ Valproic acid

Mood-stabilizing drugs are used for the treatment of bipolar affective disorder (p.344), which is also known as manic-depressive disorder, and less commonly for severe depression (p.343). In bipolar affective disorder, cycles of mania (elation) and severe depression may occur. Lithium is the drug most commonly used to treat this disorder and can control or reduce the intensity of mania. It may also prevent or reduce the frequency of attacks and lift depression. Two other drugs, carbamazepine and valproic acid, may be used as mood stabilizers if lithium is ineffective in treating bipolar affective disorder or if it causes unacceptable side effects.

How are they used?
Lithium is taken orally. It may take at least 3 weeks before the drug's effects are noticeable and several weeks more for it to take full effect. For this reason, a rapidly acting antipsychotic drug (p.592) is often prescribed at the same time for initial control of mania. Lithium will then be continued to prevent further episodes.

Treatment with lithium can cause nausea, diarrhoea, tremor, and excessive thirst. These side effects usually reduce in severity if treatment is continued. High levels of lithium may cause blurred vision, increased gastrointestinal disturbances, drowsiness, rash, and possibly hypothyroidism (underactivity of the thyroid gland) and kidney damage. For this reason, your doctor will carry out regular tests to monitor lithium levels in the blood, and you should report any side effects promptly to your doctor. Carbamazepine or valproic acid may be given if lithium is unsuitable, but may cause memory and coordination problems. If you are taking either of these drugs, your doctor may also carry out regular blood tests to monitor blood levels of the drugs.

If you are taking lithium, you will be given a treatment card, bracelet, or pendant, which you should carry with you at all times. You should be careful not to make changes in your diet that might alter the amount of salt you take in because this may affect lithium levels in your body. It is also important to avoid dehydration, which may occur if you develop diarrhoea or vomiting or travel to a region with a particularly hot climate.

Central nervous system stimulant drugs

Drugs that are used to increase mental alertness and wakefulness

COMMON DRUGS

- Atomoxetine ■ Caffeine ■ Dexamfetamine
- Methylphenidate ■ Modafinil

Central nervous system (CNS) stimulant drugs act by increasing activity in the brain, which increases wakefulness and mental alertness. Their main use is in the treatment of narcolepsy (p.325), a disorder in which a person experiences recurrent episodes of involuntary sleep during the day. Some CNS stimulants, including atomoxetine and methylphenidate, are used to improve the attention span of children who have attention deficit hyperactivity disorder (p.544).

How do they work?
CNS stimulants improve concentration and increase wakefulness by acting on a part of the brain that regulates mental alertness. These stimulants promote the release of certain chemicals in the brain (neurotransmitters) that increase nerve activity in this part of the brain.

How are they used?
CNS stimulants are given orally long-term for the treatment of narcolepsy and as part of a treatment programme for children with severe, persistent attention deficit hyperactivity disorder. If CNS stimulants are prescribed for a prolonged period of use in a child, the child's growth may be monitored because of possible slowing of growth with long-term treatment with some of these drugs.

What are the side effects?
While you are taking CNS stimulants, you may experience reduced appetite, tremor, and palpitations. These drugs can also cause restlessness, sleeplessness, anxiety, shaking, and sweating. Some CNS stimulants produce symptoms similar to those of schizophrenia (p.346), such as hallucinations. Other side effects include rashes and allergies. If you take a CNS stimulant long-term, stopping treatment may cause withdrawal symptoms, including lethargy, depression, and increased appetite.

Drugs for eye and ear disorders

Eye and ear problems need prompt attention because they affect our most important senses. Many infections and chronic (long-term) conditions can be treated effectively with drugs. Medication for eye and ear disorders can often be administered easily as drops or ointments.

Most eye and ear disorders are minor and clear up rapidly with appropriate treatment. More serious and persistent problems may need medical attention and long-term use of drugs.

The first article in this section discusses drugs used to treat infections and inflammation of the eye. It also covers artificial tears, which relieve dry eyes, and mydriatics, a group of drugs that are used in the treatment of the inflammatory disorder uveitis.

Drugs that are used for glaucoma, a potentially serious condition if left untreated, are described in the next article. These drugs work in a variety of ways to relieve excess accumulation of fluid in the eye. As a result, the pressure that can damage the optic nerve is relieved, thereby diminishing the likelihood of partial or complete loss of vision.

The final article in this section discusses drugs used to treat disorders of the ear. These drugs range from treatments for bacterial infections and excess earwax to treatments for nausea and vomiting, symptoms that are commonly seen in inner ear disorders and can affect the balance mechanism. Drugs that relieve nausea and vomiting are discussed further elsewhere (*see* **Antiemetic drugs**, p.595).

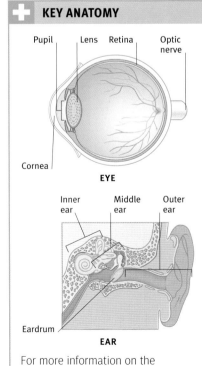

✚ KEY ANATOMY

Pupil   Lens   Retina   Optic nerve

Cornea

EYE

Inner ear   Middle ear   Outer ear

Eardrum

EAR

For more information on the structure and function of the eyes and ears, *see* pp.351–354 and pp.370–373.

Drugs acting on the eye

Drugs that are used to treat a variety of disorders affecting the eye

COMMON DRUGS

Anti-infective drugs
- Aciclovir - Chloramphenicol - Ciprofloxacin
- Gentamicin - Neomycin - Polymyxin B

Anti-inflammatory drugs
- Betamethasone - Dexamethasone
- Emedastine - Nedocromil sodium
- Prednisolone - Sodium cromoglicate

Artificial tears
- Carmellose - Hydroxyethylcellulose
- Hypromellose - Polyvinyl alcohol

Mydriatics
- Atropine - Cyclopentolate - Phenylephrine

Many eye disorders can be treated by applying drugs directly to the eye in the form of eyedrops (*see* **Using eyedrops**, right) or ointments. Minor eye problems, such as dryness or irritation due to allergy, can often be relieved with over-the-counter remedies. Drugs for eye infections and for other serious conditions, such as uveitis (p.357) or scleritis (p.357), in which the eye is inflamed, are available only on prescription.

What are the types?
The main types of drug used to treat eye disorders are anti-infective drugs and anti-inflammatory drugs. Anti-infective drugs are commonly used to treat bacterial, viral, and, less commonly, fungal infections of the eye. Anti-inflammatory drugs are used to relieve the redness and swelling that may develop as a result of infection, allergic reactions, or autoimmune disorders (in which the immune system attacks the body's own tissues). Artificial tears are used to relieve dryness of the eyes (*see* **Keratoconjunctivitis sicca**, p.365). Mydriatics dilate (widen) the pupil and are commonly used to treat uveitis.

Anti-infective drugs There are two main groups of drugs used to treat eye infections. Antibiotics (p.572), such as chloramphenicol, may be used to treat bacterial infections such as conjunctivitis (p.355) and blepharitis (p.364).

Antiviral drugs (p.573), such as aciclovir, are used to treat corneal ulcers (p.356) that occur as a result of infection with herpes viruses.

Antibiotics are usually applied as eyedrops or ointment directly on to the site of infection in the eye. However, if a bacterial infection is severe, it may be necessary to take oral antibiotics as well as using eyedrops. Viral infections of the eye may be treated with both antiviral eyedrops and oral antiviral drugs.

When using antibiotic eyedrops or ointment you may experience temporary stinging or itching. You may also notice a bitter taste as the eyedrops run down inside the tear ducts and into your nose and mouth. Medication in the form of eye ointment may have a longer-lasting effect than if applied as

---

Using eyedrops

Eyedrops deliver a drug directly to the area where its effect is needed. Always wash your hands before using the drops and do not touch the eye or the skin around it with the dropper. If you wear contact lenses, check with your doctor or pharmacist before using eyedrops because some preparations may be unsuitable.

Instilling the drops
Tilt your head backwards and draw the lower lid away from the affected eye. Drop the eyedrops on to the inside of your lower lid. Try to avoid blinking immediately.

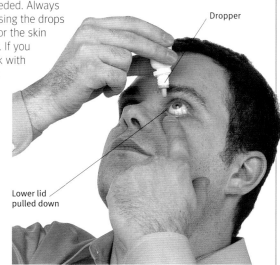

Dropper

Lower lid pulled down

---

eyedrops. To reduce the risk of contaminating the eye, always wash your hands before applying the ointment and do not touch the affected eye with your fingers or the tube.

Anti-inflammatory drugs The drugs most commonly prescribed to treat the inflammation that accompanies many eye disorders are corticosteroids (*see* **Topical corticosteroids**, p.577) and antiallergy drugs (p.585).

Corticosteroids are applied as eyedrops or as ointment squeezed just inside the eyelids. If you are predisposed to develop chronic glaucoma (p.359), in which the pressure of fluid in the eye becomes abnormally high, the use of corticosteroids may slightly increase your risk of developing drug-induced glaucoma (p.358). Corticosteroids are available on prescription and must be used under the supervision of a doctor.

Short-term inflammation caused by allergy is often treated with antihistamine or sodium cromoglicate eyedrops. Some antiallergy eyedrops, such as those used to treat eye irritation associated with hay fever (*see* **Allergic rhinitis**, p.283), are available over the counter. Some antiallergy drugs may cause side effects such as blurred vision and headache.

Artificial tears Eyedrops containing chemicals to relieve dryness are available for people whose eyes do not produce enough natural tear fluid. Artificial tears form a moist film on the cornea (the transparent front part of the eye), soothing and rehydrating the surface of the eyes. You can buy artificial tear preparations over the counter. They may be applied as often as necessary.

Mydriatics These drugs are used to treat uveitis, an inflammatory condition affecting the iris (the coloured part of the eye) and the muscles that control focusing. If the iris becomes inflamed, there is a danger that it may stick to the lens of the eye. Most mydriatics, such as atropine and cyclopentolate, relax the ring of muscles in the iris, causing

---

dilation of the pupil. Mydriatics may also be used to dilate the pupil during eye examinations and eye surgery.

Mydriatics are usually prescribed as eyedrops or eye ointment. While using a mydriatic drug, you may find that bright lights cause discomfort, and you may also have difficulty in focusing. These drugs can cause contact dermatitis (p.193) and various other side effects, including dry mouth, constipation, and difficulty in passing urine. Certain mydriatics, such as phenylephrine, can also raise blood pressure and are therefore unsuitable for people who have high blood pressure (*see* **Hypertension**, p.242).

Drugs for glaucoma

Drugs that are used to reduce abnormally high pressure inside the eye

COMMON DRUGS

Beta-blocker drugs
- Betaxolol - Carteolol - Levobunolol
- Metipranolol - Timolol

Prostaglandin analogues
- Bimatoprost - Latanoprost - Travoprost

Carbonic anhydrase inhibitors
- Acetazolamide - Brinzolamide
- Dorzolamide

Miotics
- Pilocarpine

Other drugs
- Apraclonidine - Brimonidine - Mannitol

Fluid is produced in the front part of the eye to maintain its shape and to nourish the tissues. To achieve a steady pressure, the fluid drains from the eye at the same rate at which it is produced. In glaucoma, abnormally high pressure develops in the eye because of an excessive build-up of fluid. This build-up is due to a defect in the internal

---

drainage system between the iris (the coloured part of the eye) and the cornea (the transparent outer part of the front of the eye). There are two common types of glaucoma (acute and chronic) and two rarer types (secondary and congenital).

High pressure in the eye can be relieved by surgery, which usually eliminates the symptoms and limits any sight loss, or by using drugs that either increase fluid drainage from the eye or reduce the production of fluid.

Prompt treatment is necessary when glaucoma occurs suddenly (*see* **Acute glaucoma**, p.358) to avoid permanent damage to the eye. Once the condition is detected, immediate drug treatment will be given by intravenous injection, as eyedrops, or by mouth in order to reduce the pressure in the eye. If glaucoma develops gradually (*see* **Chronic glaucoma**, p.359), and is diagnosed early, eyedrops may be prescribed to reduce pressure in the eyes. The condition may be treated by long-term use of these drugs to reduce and maintain normal pressure in the eye.

What are the types?
The types of drugs that are most commonly used in the treatment of glaucoma include beta-blockers, prostaglandin analogues, carbonic anhydrase inhibitors, and miotics. These drugs act in various ways to lower pressure inside the eye.

Beta-blocker drugs In chronic glaucoma, a beta-blocker such as timolol may be used to decrease the amount of fluid produced inside the eye. The drug works by blocking the transmission of nerve signals that stimulate the production of fluid by certain cells in the eye.

Rarely, beta-blockers may slow your heart rate and lower blood pressure. Beta-blocker eyedrops are not usually prescribed for people who have asthma or chronic obstructive pulmonary disease (p.297).

Prostaglandin analogues These drugs are used to treat some cases of chronic glaucoma. Available as eyedrops, prostaglandin analogues work by increasing the outflow of fluid from the eye, thereby lowering the pressure inside the eye.

Side effects of prostaglandin analogues tend to be minimal; they include changes in the colour of the iris and increased thickness and length of the eyelashes. Rarely, the drugs may cause headaches and may worsen asthma.

Carbonic anhydrase inhibitors This type of drug is often used in cases of acute glaucoma. The drugs may also be used to treat chronic glaucoma if other drugs are not effective. Carbonic anhydrase inhibitors rapidly reduce fluid pressure inside the eye by blocking an enzyme necessary for fluid production. Some carbonic anhydrase inhibitors may be given as eyedrops, while others, such as acetazolamide, are given by intravenous or intramuscular injection or are taken orally.

Carbonic anhydrase inhibitors used as eyedrops may cause stinging, itching, and inflammation of the eye. If you are having carbonic anhydrase inhibitors by injection or taking the drugs orally, you may experience loss of appetite, drowsiness, and painful tingling in the hands and feet. You may also experience mood changes. In rare cases, carbonic anhydrase inhibitors may cause the formation of kidney stones (p.447).

Miotics Both acute and chronic glaucoma can be treated using a miotic, such as pilocarpine. Miotic drugs cause the pupil to constrict, thereby moving the iris away from the cornea. This increases the size of the opening (the drainage angle) through which fluid flows out of the eye. Miotics are usually administered as eyedrops.

While taking miotics, you may find it harder to see in dim light because the drugs constrict the pupil. You may also experience irritation of the eye, blurred vision, and headache.

Other drugs Various other drugs are used to treat glaucoma. For example, brimonidine reduces pressure in the eye by both decreasing the production of fluid and increasing the outflow of fluid from the eye. Mannitol encourages excess fluid to be absorbed from the eye into surrounding blood vessels. It may be given by intravenous infusion as emergency treatment for acute glaucoma or to relieve pressure within the eye just before surgery.

Drugs acting on the ear

Drugs that are used to treat disorders of the outer, middle, or inner ear

COMMON DRUGS

Antibiotics and antifungals
■ Chloramphenicol ■ Clioquinol ■ Clotrimazole ■ Gentamicin ■ Neomycin

Anti-inflammatory drugs
■ Aluminium acetate ■ Betamethasone ■ Dexamethasone ■ Hydrocortisone ■ Prednisolone ■ Triamcinolone

Earwax softeners
■ Docusate ■ Olive oil ■ Sodium bicarbonate ■ Urea–hydrogen peroxide

Other drugs
■ Betahistine ■ Hyoscine ■ Prochlorperazine

Drugs can be used to treat conditions affecting the outer, middle, or inner ear. They may also be used to relieve the symptoms that accompany these conditions, such as pain, inflammation, and nausea. The drugs can be applied topically in the form of drops (*see* **Using eardrops**, right) or sprays or they can be taken orally.

What are the types?
Several types of drug are used to treat ear disorders, including antibiotics (p.572), antifungals (p.574), anti-inflammatory drugs, and earwax softeners. Antibiotics are prescribed for bacterial infections, sometimes in combination with anti-inflammatory drugs, such as aluminium acetate, or mild corticosteroid drugs (*see* **Topical corticosteroids**, p.577). Earwax softeners loosen excess earwax so that it can be removed easily. Various other drugs are used to treat symptoms that accompany disorders of the balance mechanism in the inner ear.

Antibiotics and antifungals If you have a bacterial or fungal infection of your outer ear, such as otitis externa (p.374), your doctor will probably prescribe antibiotic or antifungal eardrops, which act directly on the infected area of the ear. Infections of the middle ear, such as otitis media (p.374), may be treated with oral antibiotics.

Anti-inflammatory drugs The anti-inflammatory drugs most commonly prescribed are corticosteroid eardrops. Eardrops containing aluminium acetate are sometimes used to treat mild inflammation of the outer ear. You may notice a slight stinging sensation as the eardrops are applied.

Earwax softeners If excess wax builds up in your ear canal (*see* **Wax blockage**, p.374), your doctor will probably recommend olive oil drops or sodium bicarbonate drops, available over the counter, to soften the wax. Over-the-counter products containing docusate or urea–hydrogen peroxide are also available but can cause mild irritation of the skin inside the ear. The earwax may come out with these treatments alone but if it does not, your doctor or a nurse may syringe your ears to remove it.

Other drugs Nausea, vomiting, and vertigo are common symptoms of inner-ear disorders such as Ménière's disease (p.380) and labyrinthitis (p.380). Mild symptoms may be relieved by treatment with antihistamines (p.585). However, if these drugs are ineffective, you may be prescribed the antiemetic drug prochlorperazine. Betahistine is used specifically to treat the nausea, dizziness, and ringing in the ears (*see* **Tinnitus**, p.378) that occur in Ménière's disease. Antiemetic drugs are usually taken orally, but if you are vomiting repeatedly, the drugs may be administered as an injection or by suppository or skin patch.

▶ SELF-ADMINISTRATION

Using eardrops

It is usually easier to have someone else apply eardrops for you than to do it yourself. If the eardrops are being kept in the fridge, allow them to warm to room temperature before they are applied.

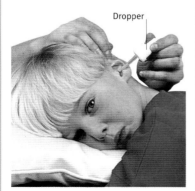
Dropper

Instilling eardrops
Tilt the head and squeeze the eardrops into the ear canal. Keep the head tilted for a minute to let the eardrops settle.

Drugs for digestive disorders

Minor digestive problems, such as indigestion, constipation, or bouts of vomiting or diarrhoea, are common and short-lived, and most do not require treatment. However, drugs may sometimes be used to relieve digestive symptoms and treat specific disorders. Many of these drugs are available over the counter.

The first articles in this section discuss drugs that act on the upper digestive tract. These include antiemetics, which relieve nausea and vomiting; antacids, which relieve indigestion; and ulcer-healing drugs, which are used to treat peptic ulcers. Drugs that act on the lower digestive tract are described next. These include aminosalicylate drugs, which are used to treat long-term inflammation of the intestines; antidiarrhoeal drugs, which relieve diarrhoea; and laxatives, which are used to relieve constipation or to clear the intestine before a medical procedure. Antispasmodic drugs and motility stimulants, used to treat disorders caused by abnormal muscle action in the digestive tract, are discussed in the following article. The final article covers oral rehydration preparations, which replace water and other essential substances that are lost in vomiting and diarrhoea.

✚ KEY ANATOMY

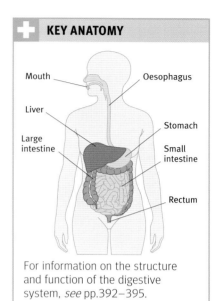

Mouth, Oesophagus, Liver, Stomach, Large intestine, Small intestine, Rectum

For information on the structure and function of the digestive system, *see* pp.392–395.

Antiemetic drugs

A group of drugs used to prevent or relieve nausea and vomiting

COMMON DRUGS

Anticholinergics
■ Hyoscine hydrobromide

Antihistamines
■ Cinnarizine ■ Cyclizine ■ Promethazine

Motility stimulants
■ Domperidone ■ Metoclopramide

Phenothiazines
■ Chlorpromazine ■ Perphenazine ■ Prochlorperazine

Serotonin antagonists
■ Dolasetron ■ Granisetron ■ Ondansetron

Others
■ Betahistine ■ Nabilone

Antiemetic drugs are used to prevent or relieve nausea and vomiting due to a variety of conditions, including motion sickness (p.379), vertigo (p.379), migraine (p.320), Ménière's disease (p.380), and labyrinthitis (p.380). They may also be used to relieve the nausea and vomiting that may occur during chemotherapy (p.157), radiotherapy (p.158), or after a general anaesthetic (p.590), and, more rarely, to treat severe vomiting in pregnancy (*see* **Hyperemesis**, p.510). Antiemetics are not normally used to alleviate vomiting due to food poisoning because the body needs to rid itself of harmful substances.

Antiemetic drugs work in various ways. For example, antihistamines and anticholinergics (also known as antimuscarinics) suppress the vomiting reflex; motility stimulants work by increasing movement through the gastrointestinal tract; and serotonin antagonists suppress signals to and from the vomiting centre in the brain.

What are the types?
There are many different types of antiemetics. They are normally taken orally but may be given by injection or as a suppository if vomiting is severe. Some are also available as skin patches.

Anticholinergics Hyoscine hydrobromide may be prescribed as a skin patch to relieve motion sickness; it is also available over the counter as tablets. Side effects may include dry mouth, drowsiness, difficulty passing urine, and dizziness.

Antihistamines These drugs may be taken to ease nausea due to Ménière's disease and labyrinthitis and to prevent motion sickness. Some types for motion sickness can be bought over the counter. Possible side effects include drowsiness, blurred vision, dry mouth, difficulty passing urine, and problems with coordination. They may also affect driving ability.

Motility stimulants Domperidone may be prescribed for the relief of nausea and vomiting, particularly that due to chemotherapy or radiotherapy. Side effects are uncommon but may include gastrointestinal disturbances, breast enlargement, reduced sex drive, and a rash. Domperidone is also associated with a small increased risk of serious effects on the heart. Metoclopramide is used to relieve nausea and vomiting due to gastrointestinal disorders such as gastro-oesophageal reflux disease (p.403), migraine, chemotherapy, or radiotherapy. Side effects of metoclopramide include muscle spasms, especially of the face. This side effect is particularly likely to occur in young people and the drug is therefore not usually given to those under 20 years old.

Phenothiazines These drugs may be used to treat nausea and vomiting due to radiotherapy, chemotherapy, general anaesthetics, vertigo, or labyrinthitis. They may also sometimes be used to treat severe vomiting in pregnancy. Prochlorperazine is available over the counter to treat nausea and vomiting due to previously diagnosed migraine in people over 18 years old. Side effects of phenothiazines include dizziness, restlessness, muscle spasms, and tremor.

Serotonin antagonists These drugs are used mainly to prevent or relieve severe vomiting caused by chemotherapy or radiotherapy. They are usually started shortly before chemotherapy or radiotherapy begins and continued for up to a few days after the final dose of chemotherapy drugs or radiotherapy is given. Serotonin antagonists may also be used to prevent vomiting after surgery under general anaesthesia. They cause very few side effects.

Other drugs Betahistine is used specifically to treat Ménière's disease. It is taken orally and generally produces few side effects, the main one being gastrointestinal disturbance. Nabilone is mainly used to treat nausea and vomiting caused by chemotherapy when other antiemetic drugs have been ineffective. It commonly causes drowsiness and dizziness. It may also cause mood changes and various nervous system side effects, such as incoordination, visual disturbances, difficulty concentrating, sleeping problems, confusion, and disorientation.

Antacids

Drugs that neutralize excess acid to relieve indigestion or help peptic ulcers to heal

COMMON DRUGS

■ Alginates ■ Aluminium hydroxide
■ Calcium carbonate ■ Magnesium hydroxide
■ Simeticone ■ Sodium bicarbonate

Antacids are used to relieve upper abdominal discomfort caused by irritation of the stomach or duodenum (*see* Indigestion, p.397). Antacids can also relieve the discomfort caused by gastro-oesophageal reflux disease (p.403), in which stomach acid is regurgitated into the oesophagus. They may help to ease symptoms due to peptic ulcers (p.406).

▶ **DRUG ACTION**

How antacids work

Antacids are used to treat symptoms caused by acid in the digestive juices. This acid may inflame eroded areas in the layer of mucus that lines the stomach, irritating the stomach walls.

Antacids are mild alkaline substances that are taken orally. They work by neutralizing acidity in the digestive juices, thereby allowing eroded areas in the mucus layer to recover.

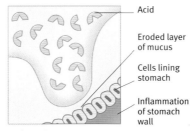

Before drug
The digestive juices contain acid, which may inflame eroded areas in the mucus layer and irritate the stomach lining.

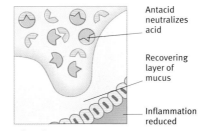

After drug
The antacid combines with some of the stomach acid and neutralizes it, reducing irritation of the stomach lining.

Antacid preparations may contain aluminium and/or magnesium salts, both of which neutralize stomach acid (*see* **How antacids work**, above). Some contain additional ingredients such as simeticone, which disperses bubbles of gas to reduce bloating, or alginates, which provide a protective coating for the oesophagus if regurgitation of the stomach contents occurs. If indigestion persists for more than a week, see your doctor.

What are the side effects?
Most antacid preparations have very few side effects. However, antacids containing aluminium can occasionally cause constipation, while those that contain magnesium may cause diarrhoea. The antacid sodium bicarbonate may produce excess gas in the stomach, which can cause abdominal bloating. Sodium bicarbonate may cause fluid retention in people who have kidney disease or chronic heart failure (p.247) and should therefore be avoided by anyone with these conditions.

Consult your doctor before using antacids if you are already taking other medication; antacids can interfere with the body's absorption of certain drugs.

✖ WARNING

You should not take antacids regularly, unless advised to do so by your doctor, because they may suppress the symptoms of a potentially serious disorder or provoke serious complications.

Ulcer-healing drugs

Drugs that reduce the secretion of acid by the stomach, helping peptic ulcers to heal

COMMON DRUGS

Proton pump inhibitors
■ Lansoprazole ■ Omeprazole ■ Pantoprazole
■ Rabeprazole

H$_2$-receptor antagonists
■ Cimetidine ■ Famotidine ■ Nizatidine
■ Ranitidine

Other drugs
■ Bismuth ■ Misoprostol ■ Sucralfate

Ulcer-healing drugs are used to treat peptic ulcers (p.406), which are eroded areas in the lining of the stomach or duodenum. One group of these drugs, called proton pump inhibitors, is used in combination with two antibiotics (p.572) to heal ulcers that are caused by the bacterium *Helicobacter pylori* (*see* **Helicobacter pylori infection**, p.405). Ulcer-healing drugs may also be given without antibiotics to treat peptic ulcers and other digestive disorders that are not due to *H. pylori*, such as nonulcer dyspepsia (p.397) and gastro-oesophageal reflux disease (p.403).

What are the types?
The two main groups of ulcer-healing drugs are proton pump inhibitors and H$_2$-receptor antagonists. Both of these types of drugs work by reducing production of acid in the stomach, although proton pump inhibitors do so more effectively than H$_2$-receptor antagonists. Other drugs used to treat ulcers include misoprostol, sucralfate, and bismuth, which work by protecting the stomach lining from stomach acids. Ulcer-healing drugs are usually taken orally.

Proton pump inhibitors Drugs in this group may be given as a 4–8 week course, although some people may need to take them for longer periods. Proton pump inhibitors are usually used to reduce stomach acid. Omeprazole is available over the counter for the short-term relief of heartburn. Proton pump inhibitors may also be given with a 1- or 2-week course of antibiotics as part of the treatment for ulcers caused by *H. pylori*. The drugs do not usually cause serious side effects, but you may have headaches, constipation, diarrhoea, or other side effects such as dizziness, blurred vision, rashes, and muscle aches.

H$_2$-receptor antagonists These drugs are usually given as an initial course of 4–6 weeks to reduce stomach acid. You may then have to continue taking a lower dose to prevent ulcers from recurring. Some of these drugs can be bought over the counter for the short-term relief of heartburn and indigestion. Side effects are rare, but you may experience dizziness, tiredness, and rashes. In elderly people, the drugs can cause confusion.

Other drugs Your doctor may prescribe misoprostol if you need to take nonsteroidal anti-inflammatory drugs (p.578), such as ibuprofen, long term. These drugs may cause peptic ulcers if taken for a long time, and misoprostol can help prevent ulceration by protecting the stomach lining. It can cause diarrhoea, which may be severe; other side effects may include abdominal pain, nausea and vomiting, and flatulence. Do not take misoprostol if you are or may be pregnant; it can cause uterine contractions and may cause fetal abnormalities. Sucralfate coats the ulcer, providing a barrier against stomach acid. This drug can cause side effects such as constipation, indigestion, diarrhoea, nausea, and dizziness.

Bismuth seems to combat bacteria and protect ulcers from stomach acids. Side effects include a darkened tongue, black faeces, nausea, and vomiting.

Aminosalicylate drugs

A group of drugs used to reduce persistent inflammation of the intestines

COMMON DRUGS

■ Balsalazide ■ Mesalazine ■ Olsalazine
■ Sulfasalazine

Aminosalicylates are a group of anti-inflammatory drugs, chemically related to aspirin, that are used to treat persistent inflammation of the digestive tract. They work by suppressing the body's production of prostaglandins, which are naturally occurring chemicals that trigger tissue inflammation. Aminosalicylates are often used to treat Crohn's disease (p.417), in which there is inflammation of parts of the digestive tract. They are also given to treat ulcerative colitis (p.417), in which only the large intestine is inflamed. The drugs can also be used to help to prevent attacks of these conditions.

Aminosalicylates are usually taken orally but may be given as enemas or suppositories if inflammation mainly affects the lower part of the large intestine. Treatment is started with a high dose. Dosage is then reduced to a lower level for long-term use.

What are the side effects?
Aminosalicylates can cause side effects such as nausea, vomiting, abdominal pain, headache, rashes, and diarrhoea. Taking these drugs can also sometimes cause increased susceptibility to infections or abnormal bleeding.

Antidiarrhoeal drugs

Drugs that stop diarrhoea by slowing the passage of the intestinal contents or regulating the action of the intestine

COMMON DRUGS

Opioids
- Codeine phosphate ■ Diphenoxylate
- Loperamide

Bulk-forming agents
- Bran ■ Ispaghula ■ Methylcellulose
- Sterculia

Adsorbents
- Kaolin

Antidiarrhoeal drugs are used to relieve diarrhoea (p.397), which is the frequent passing of loose, watery faeces. They may be used as a short-term measure to control a sudden attack of diarrhoea or long term for diarrhoea that persists due to disorders such as diverticular disease (p.420) or irritable bowel syndrome (p.415). Some drugs also relieve abdominal pain associated with diarrhoea.

In most cases, an attack of diarrhoea clears up in about 48 hours and drug treatment is not normally required. Drinking plenty of fluids, but not milk, to compensate for the water that the body loses in diarrhoea is usually all that is needed. However, infants and young children are at higher risk of dehydration and may need to be given oral rehydration preparations (p.598). If an attack of diarrhoea lasts longer than 48 hours, consult your doctor. Do not give antidiarrhoeal drugs to children.

What are the types?
The main types of antidiarrhoeal drug are opioids, bulk-forming agents, and adsorbents. All types of antidiarrhoeal drug should be taken with plenty of water to prevent constipation.

Opioids These drugs reduce the muscle contractions of the intestine. As a result, the intestine moves faeces more slowly and therefore has more time to absorb water from food residue. Opioid drugs may also help to relieve pain in the lower abdomen associated with frequent contractions of the intestinal muscle. Loperamide, although chemically similar to opioids, does not have opioid-like effects on the brain. Some opioid antidiarrhoeal drugs are available over the counter.

Bulk-forming agents These preparations absorb water, resulting in larger and firmer stools produced at less frequent intervals. Bulk-forming agents are often given to regulate intestinal action over a long period if you have had an operation on your intestine, such as a colectomy (p.421), or if you have persistent diarrhoea due to a disorder such as diverticular disease. Since they help to regulate intestinal action, bulk-forming agents are sometimes also used as laxatives (below). Some types are available over the counter, others only on prescription. All types are usually supplied as granules, powder, or tablets. Do not take a bulk-forming agent when taking opioids; the combination could cause faeces to obstruct the intestine. Drink plenty of water when taking a bulk-forming agent.

Adsorbents These substances attract and bind to irritants and other substances in the intestine, such as harmful microorganisms. As the adsorbents are moved through the intestine and excreted, the irritants are carried with them. Like bulk-forming agents, adsorbents are used to control the consistency of the faeces and to regulate intestinal action. They are usually used to treat mild diarrhoea. The adsorbent kaolin can be bought over the counter.

Laxatives

Drugs used to relieve constipation or clear the intestine before a medical procedure

COMMON DRUGS

Bulk-forming agents
- Bran ■ Ispaghula ■ Methylcellulose
- Sterculia

Osmotic laxatives
- Lactulose ■ Magnesium salts ■ Phosphates
- Sodium citrate

Faecal softeners/lubricants
- Arachis oil ■ Liquid paraffin

Stimulant laxatives
- Bisacodyl ■ Dantron ■ Docusate sodium
- Glycerol ■ Senna ■ Sodium picosulfate

Laxatives make faeces pass more easily through the intestines. They are most commonly used to treat constipation (p.398), the difficult, infrequent passing of stools that are hard and dry. However, laxatives may be prescribed for other reasons. For example, they may be given to clear the intestine before a colonoscopy (p.418), in which an instrument for viewing the colon is passed through the anus. Laxatives may also be prescribed to counteract the constipating effect of other drugs such as morphine or codeine.

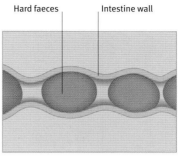
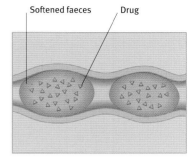
Laxatives can be bought over the counter. If you are taking laxatives for constipation, use them only until your bowel movements have returned to normal. If the constipation continues for more than a few days, you should see your doctor. Do not take more than the recommended dose because some laxatives can cause severe abdominal pain. Never give laxatives to children without first consulting your doctor.

What are the types?
Laxatives can be classified into different types, depending on how they work. Bulk-forming agents, osmotic laxatives, and faecal softeners all make stools softer and easier to pass. Stimulant laxatives make the intestinal muscles move faeces more rapidly. Most laxatives are taken orally, but some osmotic and stimulant laxatives may be administered as enemas or suppositories.

Bulk-forming agents These preparations cause the faeces to retain water, keeping them soft and increasing their volume, and thereby stimulating intestinal muscle action. They are mainly available as granules or powders that are taken orally. It may take several days for these agents to have their full effect.

Bulk-forming agents are mostly prescribed to treat long-term constipation. For example, they may be used in the treatment of irritable bowel syndrome (p.415) or diverticular disease (p.420). You may also be given bulk-forming agents to make passing stools easier after childbirth or abdominal surgery.

Bulk-forming laxatives are the safest type of preparation for the long-term treatment of constipation because their action is similar to the natural action of fibre in food. You should drink plenty of water when taking these laxatives because the bulky stools may otherwise eventually block the intestine. Side effects of bulk-forming laxatives may include excess intestinal gas and abdominal pain and bloating.

Osmotic laxatives These drugs work by preventing the body from removing water from faeces. As a result, the faeces stay soft and increase in bulk. Osmotic laxatives are available on prescription and over the counter. The most commonly prescribed osmotic laxative is lactulose, a synthetic form of sugar that the body does not absorb. Lactulose can cause side effects such as intestinal gas and abdominal cramps, which may gradually lessen with continued use. In elderly people, long-term use of lactulose can eventually cause dehydration and lead to a chemical imbalance in the blood.

Other drugs that retain water in the intestines, including magnesium salts, phosphates, and sodium citrate, may be used to achieve rapid bowel evacuation, particularly before procedures such as colonoscopy, radiological investigation, or surgery on the lower digestive tract. Some of these laxatives are taken orally, others are given by enema. They work by drawing water into the gut from the body and therefore may cause dehydration. You should be sure to drink plenty of water when taking these laxatives. Side effects may include intestinal gas and abdominal bloating.

Faecal softeners These laxatives act by softening faeces. They also lubricate faecal matter, enabling it to pass more easily through the intestine. Arachis oil is available over the counter and is administered as an enema. Because the oil is derived from peanuts, you should not use it if you have a nut allergy. Liquid paraffin is also available over the counter and is taken orally. You should not take this laxative over a long period because it can cause anal irritation. Liquid paraffin can also prevent your body from absorbing certain vitamins, which may lead to nutritional deficiencies (p.399) in the long term.

Stimulant laxatives These laxatives stimulate the intestinal muscles to contract more strongly, resulting in more frequent bowel movements. Stimulant laxatives are sometimes used to clear the intestines quickly if other drugs have failed to work. Some of these drugs can be bought over the counter. You should not take stimulant laxatives regularly because your body may come to depend on them to stimulate bowel movements. Side effects commonly include abdominal cramps and diarrhoea. Dantron may colour the urine red.

 CAUTION

When taking a bulk-forming laxative such as bran, be sure to drink plenty of water; otherwise, the bulky faeces that are produced may cause an intestinal blockage.

Antispasmodic drugs and motility stimulants

Drugs used to relieve muscle spasms in the intestine or to stimulate the passage of food through the digestive tract

COMMON DRUGS

Direct smooth-muscle relaxants
■ Alverine ■ Mebeverine ■ Peppermint oil

Anticholinergics
■ Atropine ■ Dicycloverine (Dicyclomine)
■ Hyoscine ■ Propantheline

Motility stimulants
■ Metoclopramide

Antispasmodics and motility stimulants regulate the waves of muscular contraction that propel food through the digestive tract. Both these types of drug are used to treat conditions caused by abnormal muscle action in the digestive tract, including irritable bowel syndrome (p.415) and diverticular disease (p.420). In some cases, these drugs may be used to relieve the symptoms of nonulcer dyspepsia (p.397). Motility stimulants are also used to treat gastro-oesophageal reflux disease (p.403), in which acidic stomach contents are regurgitated into the oesophagus.

Changes in diet, such as altering the amount of fibre eaten, may help to regulate intestinal contractions in people with conditions such as irritable bowel syndrome. Other changes in lifestyle, such as decreasing your alcohol intake and learning how to reduce stress, may also help. Your doctor may initially suggest that you make such changes to see whether they bring about an improvement. However, if self-help measures are not effective, your doctor may recommend that you take antispasmodic drugs or motility stimulants.

What are the types?
Antispasmodic drugs can be classified into two groups: direct smooth-muscle relaxants and anticholinergic drugs. Both types may be used to relieve the abdominal pain

that occurs in gastrointestinal conditions such as irritable bowel syndrome and diverticular disease. Motility stimulants are sometimes given to relieve some of the symptoms caused by nonulcer dyspepsia and gastro-oesophageal reflux disease.

Direct smooth-muscle relaxants These drugs have a direct action on the intestinal wall, which contains smooth muscle. Direct smooth-muscle relaxants work by causing the muscle to relax, thereby relieving painful intestinal cramps. The drugs are taken orally. Some preparations containing low doses of direct smooth-muscle relaxants are available over the counter. Some preparations contain a direct smooth-muscle relaxant combined with a bulk-forming agent (see p.597). It is important to drink plenty of water if you are taking a direct smooth-muscle relaxant combined with a bulk-forming agent because otherwise an intestinal blockage may occur. In addition, you should not take these drugs before going to bed.

Direct smooth-muscle relaxants occasionally cause headache or nausea. Peppermint oil capsules can irritate the mouth or oesophagus; for this reason, they should always be swallowed whole with plenty of water.

Anticholinergics These drugs help to reduce muscle spasm by lessening the transmission of nerve signals to the intestinal wall. They are usually taken orally and are available by prescription and also over the counter.

Side effects of anticholinergic drugs may include headache, constipation, a dry mouth, flushed skin, and blurred vision. These drugs may also cause difficulty in passing urine. Children and elderly people in particular are at risk of developing side effects.

Motility stimulants Motility stimulants work primarily by causing the contents of the stomach to empty into the small intestine more rapidly than would otherwise happen. In this way, they help to prevent the occurrence of gastro-oesophageal reflux disease and relieve attacks of nonulcer dyspepsia. Motility stimulants also cause the muscular valve between the stomach and the oesophagus to close with more force. This also helps to prevent gastro-oesophageal reflux disease from occurring.

Motility stimulants are usually taken orally. They are available by prescription only. Metoclopramide may cause a number of different side effects, including diarrhoea and drowsiness. Occasionally, it may cause uncontrollable muscle spasms, particularly of the face, tongue, mouth, and neck. These muscle spasms are more likely to occur in children and young adults. For this reason, metoclopramide is not recommended for those under 20 years old. Metoclopramide may be also used to relieve nausea and vomiting (*see* **Antiemetic drugs**, p.595).

Oral rehydration preparations

Preparations used to treat dehydration resulting from diarrhoea and vomiting

Oral rehydration preparations are made up of water and essential minerals, such as sodium and potassium, that are lost during severe attacks of diarrhoea (p.397) or vomiting. Usually, drinking plenty of fluids to replace the water that the body loses in diarrhoea or vomiting is the only treatment needed for adults. However, it may be necessary to give oral rehydration preparations to treat fluid loss that occurs in infants and young children. These groups are at a higher risk of dehydration because any water lost accounts for a higher proportion of the total water content in their bodies.

Rehydration preparations contain the minerals sodium, which is necessary for the body to retain water, and potassium, which is vital for the functioning of nerves and muscles. Both these minerals may be lost very quickly and in large amounts as a result of diarrhoea and vomiting. Rehydration preparations also contain glucose, a sugar that improves the absorption of sodium and water through the wall of the intestine and into the bloodstream.

Rehydration preparations can be purchased over the counter as soluble tablets or as powder for reconstitution with water. Some are flavoured to make them more palatable. Once you have made up a batch of rehydration solution, it should be used within an hour unless it is stored in a refrigerator, when it can be kept for up to 24 hours. When used according to instructions, oral rehydration preparations do not cause side effects.

Vitamin and mineral supplements

A well-balanced diet should contain adequate amounts of all vitamins and minerals required for health. For most people, supplements are unnecessary, and high doses may even be harmful. However, certain groups of people are vulnerable to vitamin or mineral deficiencies. Doctors may prescribe vitamin or mineral supplements for people in these groups to prevent a deficiency or to treat a deficiency that has already developed.

Groups who are particularly prone to developing vitamin and mineral deficiencies include young children, pregnant women, and elderly people, especially those who live alone. Those who are seriously ill due to injury or long-term illness, or those who have disorders that impair their ability to absorb nutrients from the digestive tract (*see* **Malabsorption**, p.415), are also at increased risk of deficiencies, not only of vitamins and minerals but also of other nutrients (*see* **Nutritional deficiencies**, p.399). These people may require dietary supplementation with extra proteins, carbohydrates, and fats as well as vitamins and minerals. In the case of individuals who are unable to eat and drink normally

because of illness, such as a stroke, which prevents them from swallowing, nutrients sometimes have to be given in a liquid form by tube, either through the nose down to the stomach or directly into the stomach. More rarely, for example in people who have very severe intestinal disorders, nutrients may be administered directly into the bloodstream through a vein.

The body needs some nutrients, such as carbohydrates, proteins, and fats, in relatively large quantities but requires vitamins and minerals in only small amounts. The articles in this section describe the vitamins and minerals that doctors most commonly prescribe as dietary supplements. The first article deals with vitamins and the second with minerals.

Vitamins

Chemical compounds that enable the body to carry out essential functions

Vitamins are complex chemicals that are essential for the normal growth, development, and functioning of the body. The principal source of most vitamins is a bal-

anced diet (*see* **Good sources of vitamins and minerals**, p.18). Most healthy people do not need vitamin supplements because a healthy, balanced diet provides enough of all the vitamins needed. However, supplements may be prescribed for people with conditions such as alcohol dependence (p.350) that deplete the body's supply of certain vitamins. They may also be prescribed for people who need larger than normal quantities of certain vitamins because they are recovering from serious injuries or they are taking medications that affect the action or absorption of particular vitamins.

What are the types?

Many types of vitamin are necessary for the maintenance of good health. They are broadly categorized into two main groups: fat-soluble and water-soluble. Fat-soluble vitamins, such as A, D, E, and K, are not readily excreted in urine. They are stored in fatty body tissues, such as the liver, for long periods and do not normally need to be supplemented by a daily intake. Water-soluble vitamins, which include B, C, and folic acid, are rapidly excreted in urine. The body cannot hold long-term reserves of these vitamins, and they must be replaced on a daily basis through food sources to prevent deficiencies.

Vitamin A This vitamin is required for growth, healthy skin and surface tissues, and good eyesight and night vision. Vitamin A is also necessary for fertility in both sexes. Supplements may be prescribed for people with conditions that can cause deficiency, such as certain intestinal disorders. Supplements of vitamin A are also recommended for children between 6 months and 5 years old. Diets that are too low in fat may also lead to vitamin A deficiency.

Taking excessive doses of vitamin A, however, can cause dry skin, nose-bleeds, and hair loss. Excess vitamin A, especially in the form of retinol, has also been associated with a higher risk of bone fractures. You should not take vitamin A supplements if you are either pregnant or planning to become pregnant because taking too much of this vitamin may cause fetal abnormalities; you should also avoid eating liver and liver products because they contain high levels of vitamin A.

> ### ❌ WARNING
>
> Vitamin A may harm a developing fetus. Do not take supplements if you are pregnant or planning to conceive, except on medical advice.

Vitamin B₁ (thiamine) This vitamin is necessary for the normal functioning of the brain and peripheral nerves, the heart, and the muscles. Thiamine is present in unprocessed food, and most people should be able to obtain enough by eating a balanced diet. A severe lack of thiamine can cause certain deficiency diseases, such as beriberi, which affects the nervous system. Your doctor may prescribe supplements for conditions in which severe thiamine deficiency can occur, such as alcohol dependence (p.350) or alcohol-related liver disease (p.409).

The risk of developing side effects from thiamine supplements is very low. However, when given intravenously, this vitamin may sometimes cause serious allergic reactions.

Vitamin B₃ (niacin) This vitamin, also known as nicotinic acid, plays a vital role in the activities of many enzymes involved in energy metabolism. Severe niacin deficiency can result in the skin disorder pellagra, which primarily occurs in rural areas of poor countries. You may be prescribed niacin supplements if you have alcohol-related liver disease, in which niacin deficiency can occur, or a bowel disorder that results in poor absorption of food, a condition known as malabsorption (p.415).

Large doses of niacin inhibit the body's synthesis of some fats and are used to treat high levels of cholesterol and triglycerides (*see* **Lipid-lowering drugs**, p.603). Niacin may cause some side effects, including itching, flushing, and headaches. If excessive amounts of niacin are taken, liver damage and gout (p.224) can occur as a result.

Vitamin B₆ (pyridoxine) Vitamin B₆ aids the activities of enzymes and hormones involved in the body's processing of carbohydrates, proteins, and fats, the manufacture of red blood cells and antibodies, the functioning of the digestive and nervous systems, and the maintenance of healthy skin. Supplements may be required by people with malabsorption or severe alcohol dependence, those taking certain drugs (such as penicillamine and isoniazid), and elderly people who have a poor diet. Low-dose vitamin B₆ may also sometimes be given to help relieve the symptoms of premenstrual syndrome (p.472). Long-term use of high-dose pyridoxine supplements has been associated with nerve damage, which may result in symptoms such as numbness and impaired physical coordination.

Vitamin B₁₂ (cobalamin) This vitamin plays a vital role in the activities of various enzymes in the body and is important in the production of genetic material (and therefore in growth and development) and red blood cells, in the utilization of dietary folic acid, and in the functioning of the nervous system. The most common cause of B₁₂ deficiency is pernicious anaemia (*see* **Megaloblastic anaemia**, p.272), in which a substance necessary for the absorption of the vitamin is not produced by the body. Less commonly, deficiency may also result from a gastrectomy (the removal of all or part of the stomach), malabsorption, or a vegan diet (because B₁₂ occurs naturally only in animal products). The effects of B₁₂ deficiency include megaloblastic anaemia, sore mouth and tongue, and symptoms resulting from damage to the spinal cord, such as numbness and tingling in the limbs; there may also be depression and memory problems.

Treatment for pernicious anaemia and B₁₂ deficiency due to a gastrectomy involves regular injections of the vitamin. Side effects are very uncommon but can include itching, flushing, and nausea. If deficiency results from a vegan diet or malabsorption, oral supplements may be required.

Folic acid This vitamin is needed for nervous system function and for the formation of red blood cells. Dietary sources include green leafy vegetables, liver, and nuts. Supplements may be advised if you are taking certain drugs, including some antimalarials (p.574) or anticonvulsant drugs (p.590), which deplete folic acid. Folic acid also lowers levels of the amino acid homo-cysteine, high levels of which may increase the risk of coronary artery disease (p.243).

Women are advised to take the recommended dose of folic acid supplements before conception and during the first 12 weeks of pregnancy to reduce the risk of neural tube defects (p.547), such as spina bifida, in the fetus; a higher dose may be recommended if a woman is at high risk of having a child with a neural tube defect.

Vitamin C This vitamin is needed for the formation of bones, teeth, ligaments, and blood vessels. It is found in fresh fruit and vegetables, and severe deficiency is uncommon. Severe deficiency causes a disorder called scurvy, which is rare in developed countries. However, mild deficiency is common among people who eat a poor diet, and particularly among elderly people living alone.

Supplements of vitamin C are rarely necessary except to treat scurvy. In some people who are prescribed iron supplements, supplementary vitamin C may also be prescribed because the vitamin improves the efficiency of iron absorption by the body. Supplements of vitamin C are also recommended for children between 6 months and 5 years old. There is no evidence that vitamin C supplements can protect against or alleviate the symptoms of colds, or promote wound healing.

Vitamin D This vitamin helps to regulate the amount of calcium in the body. The body's requirements for the vitamin are usually met by normal diet and exposure to sunlight, which the body needs to make vitamin D. However, some people may not receive sufficient sun exposure, especially in winter, to make enough vitamin D and are therefore at risk of deficiency. Those most at risk are people with dark skin who live in northern latitudes. Vitamin D deficiency can cause a disorder in which the bones become weak and soft (*see* **Osteomalacia and rickets**, p.217).

Vitamin D supplements may be given to increase calcium levels in people with hypoparathyroidism (p.434). Supplements are sometimes given to elderly people and to premature infants, who may not obtain enough dietary vitamin D or sun exposure. They may also be recommended for some dark-skinned people at risk of deficiency. Supplements are recommended for children between 6 months and 5 years old. In some cases, babies under 6 months old may also need supplements; consult your health visitor or midwife for advice. Supplements may also be given in combination with calcium to prevent or treat osteoporosis (p.217). Women who are pregnant or breast-feeding are also advised to take supplementary vitamin D.

> ### ❌ WARNING
>
> Do not exceed the prescribed dose of vitamin D. Excessive intake can cause a dangerous rise in the level of calcium in the blood.

Taking high doses of vitamin D may increase levels of calcium in the body, which may lead to calcium deposits in soft tissues, impaired kidney function, or impaired growth in children.

Vitamin E Vitamin E is the collective term for a group of substances that are essential for normal cell structure, for maintenance of the activities of certain enzymes, and for the formation of red blood cells. Vitamin E also protects the lungs and other tissues from damage by pollutants and is believed to slow cell aging. Dietary deficiency of vitamin E is rare; it is most common in people with malabsorption or certain liver disorders, and in premature infants. Deficiency leads to destruction of red blood cells, which eventually results in anaemia. In infants, it causes irritability and oedema (accumulation of fluid in tissues). Supplementary vitamin E is prescribed only to treat established deficiency. Prolonged excessive intake of the vitamin may cause abdominal pain, nausea, and diarrhoea. It may also reduce intestinal absorption of vitamins A, D, and K.

Vitamin K This vitamin is essential for the formation of blood clotting factors, substances that are necessary for blood to clot. Most of the required amount of vitamin K is produced by bacteria in the intestines, but the body also obtains some from dietary sources, such as green leafy vegetables, eggs, and liver.

Newborn babies lack the intestinal bacteria that produce vitamin K and, as a result, are at risk of developing a condition called haemorrhagic disease of the newborn, which results in easy bruising and internal bleeding. For this reason, newborn babies are given vitamin K routinely. Supplements may be given to older children and adults taking antibiotics for long periods because these drugs destroy the intestinal bacteria that produce vitamin K. In addition, people who are unable to absorb nutrients, or those who experience abnormal bleeding as a side effect of oral anticoagulant drugs (*see* **Drugs that prevent blood clotting**, p.584), may be given supplements of this vitamin.

Multivitamins Preparations containing a combination of vitamins are used to treat people who have nutritional deficiencies, alcoholism, and other conditions in which dietary vitamin intake is insufficient. Some of these multivitamin preparations contain iron and other minerals. Multivitamins can be purchased over the counter.

Minerals

Chemical elements that enable the body to perform essential functions

Minerals are chemical elements that are necessary to maintain health. The body does not manufacture minerals and therefore it must obtain them from dietary sources (*see* **Good sources of vitamins and minerals**, p.18).

Your doctor may prescribe mineral supplements if you have a medical condition that interferes with the ability of your body to absorb minerals (see **Malabsorption**, p.415) or if you need extra amounts of certain minerals, as may happen in pregnancy. Most people should not need mineral supplements because a balanced diet usually provides sufficient amounts. You should not take mineral supplements unless you need them because excessive doses of some minerals can be toxic.

What are the types?

Many minerals are necessary to maintain good health. The most important minerals prescribed to treat deficiencies include iron, calcium, magnesium, zinc, fluoride, iodine, and phosphorus.

Iron This mineral is a vital component of haemoglobin, the oxygen-carrying pigment in blood. A correctly balanced diet usually provides sufficient supplies of iron but deficiency sometimes occurs in women with heavy menstrual periods (see **Menorrhagia**, p.471), pregnant women, and women who have recently given birth. Vegans, and people who have persistent blood loss due to conditions such as a peptic ulcer (p.406), may also be deficient in iron.

Iron is usually taken orally as a liquid or tablets and can be purchased over the counter. Side effects of taking iron supplements may include darker stools, constipation or diarrhoea, nausea, and abdominal pain. In certain cases when the body cannot absorb sufficient iron from the digestive tract, for example following extensive bowel surgery, injections of iron may be needed. Although these injections are given deep into muscle, staining of the skin at the injection site may result.

Calcium This is essential for formation and maintenance of bones and teeth, as well as for muscle contraction and transmission of nerve impulses. Dairy products usually provide sufficient calcium.

An increased dietary intake is recommended for women who are pregnant or breast-feeding because both fetal bone formation and maternal milk production require large amounts of calcium. Elderly people may need supplements because the body absorbs calcium less efficiently with age. Calcium supplements may also be prescribed to prevent bone disorders such as osteoporosis (p.217) and to increase blood levels of calcium in people who have hypoparathyroidism (p.434) or kidney failure (p.450). In addition, calcium may be given by intravenous injection to treat cardiac arrest

(p.252). Severe calcium deficiency leads to cramps and muscle spasms and may be treated with calcium injections. Side effects of calcium include constipation and nausea.

Magnesium This mineral is needed for healthy teeth and bones, muscle action, and transmission of nerve impulses. Magnesium supplements may be prescribed for certain conditions that can interfere with the absorption of magnesium from food, including alcohol dependence (p.350), repeated vomiting, or long-term diarrhoea. Excessive doses of magnesium may cause nausea, vomiting, diarrhoea, and dizziness.

Zinc This mineral is used for growth and to help wounds to heal. Deficiency is rare; it usually occurs only in malnourished elderly people, and may also occur in people with severe burns or other traumatic injury because zinc is used up rapidly in the healing process. In these cases, zinc supplements are sometimes prescribed. Zinc is usually taken orally but may also be given as a topical treatment for skin disorders, such as nappy rash. Taking overly large doses of oral zinc may cause side effects such as fever, nausea, vomiting, headaches, and abdominal pain.

Fluoride The mineral fluoride helps to prevent tooth decay and makes bones stronger. Water is very often the main dietary source because fluoride occurs naturally in some water supplies or is added to the drinking water in some areas. Fluoride is also an ingredient in most toothpastes. If you have an excessive fluoride intake, you may develop fluorosis, in which the teeth become discoloured (see **Discoloured teeth**, p.386).

Iodine This mineral is essential for the formation of thyroid hormones, which control the rate at which the body uses energy and which are vital for normal growth in childhood. Supplements are rarely needed because sufficient iodine is usually present in the diet. Important sources of iodine include seafood, bread, and dairy products. Radioactive iodine may be given to people with a goitre (p.433) or hyperthyroidism (p.432) in order to shrink the thyroid gland. Excessive amounts of iodine can suppress the activity of the thyroid gland, leading to hypothyroidism (p.432).

Phosphorus The mineral phosphorus is an essential part of the diet. It is present in many foods, including cereals, dairy products, eggs, and meat. Much of the phosphorus contained in the body is combined with calcium to form the structure of the bones and teeth. Hypophosphataemia, in which the body contains an abnormally low level of phosphorus, may occur in some forms of kidney disease, hyperparathyroidism (p.434), and malabsorption.

Deficiencies of this mineral can be treated with phosphate supplements. In addition, hypercalcaemia, in which blood levels of calcium are abnormally high, may be treated using phosphates. Diarrhoea is a potential side effect of phosphate supplements.

Drugs acting on the endocrine system and metabolism

Disorders of the endocrine system and metabolism, such as diabetes mellitus and hypothyroidism, may have wide-ranging, serious effects, and in some cases may be fatal if left untreated. Drug treatments can control the symptoms of these disorders and in many cases restore normal health to affected people.

The first article in this section covers corticosteroids, which are synthetic hormones that are chiefly used to treat inflammation in a variety of disorders and may also be used as hormone replacement therapy. The next four articles discuss drugs that control levels of insulin, thyroid hormones, and sex hormones in the body. Drugs that replace, inhibit, or stimulate some of the many hormones produced by the pituitary gland, which is the major hormone-secreting gland in the body, are covered next. The final article looks at lipid-lowering drugs, which control disorders in which the blood contains excessive levels of lipids (fats and related substances).

Topical corticosteroids (p.577), which are used to treat certain skin disorders, are covered elsewhere, as are locally acting corticosteroids (p.600), which are used in the treatment of inflamed joints or muscles.

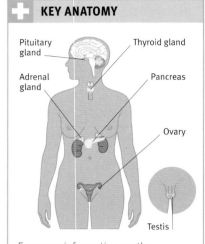

➕ KEY ANATOMY

Pituitary gland
Thyroid gland
Adrenal gland
Pancreas
Ovary
Testis

For more information on the endocrine system and metabolic disorders, see pp.437–441.

Corticosteroids

Drugs similar to the natural corticosteroid hormones produced by the adrenal gland

COMMON DRUGS

- Beclometasone ■ Betamethasone
- Cortisone ■ Dexamethasone
- Fludrocortisone ■ Fluocinolone
- Fluticasone ■ Hydrocortisone
- Methylprednisolone ■ Prednisolone
- Triamcinolone

Corticosteroids are related to corticosteroid hormones produced by the body. The production of corticosteroid hormones by the adrenal glands is regulated by corticotropin, a pituitary hormone.

The main use for corticosteroid drugs is in the treatment of inflammatory conditions that may affect the joints, skin, digestive tract, respiratory system, eyes, and ears. These drugs are also prescribed as replacement therapy if the body is unable to produce sufficient natural corticosteroid hormones on its own (see **Addison's disease**, p.436, and **Hypopituitarism**, p.431).

In addition, corticosteroids may be given as long-term treatment following transplant surgery because their action suppresses the body's immune system. This action helps to prevent rejection of the transplanted organs or tissue.

How do they work?

Corticosteroids affect many body processes, including virtually all aspects of the inflammatory process. Their exact mechanism of action is unknown, but one of their effects is to reduce the production of prostaglandins, substances that play a key role in triggering inflammation. Corticosteroids also suppress the immune system by reducing the production and effectiveness of certain white blood cells that are an important part of the body's immune response.

How are they used?

Corticosteroids can be given in a variety of ways. The drugs may be injected directly into body tissues near inflamed areas such as tendons and joints (see **Locally acting corticosteroids**, p.578). Used in this way, they may improve symptoms in joint disorders such as osteoarthritis (p.221) and rheumatoid arthritis (p.222). Frequent injections are avoided because of the risk of side effects.

Topical corticosteroids (p.577) in the form of creams and ointments are used to reduce inflammation and itching in some skin conditions. Corticosteroids may be used topically as suppositories, orally, or by injection to treat the gastrointestinal disorders ulcerative colitis (p.417) and Crohn's disease (p.417). Oral corticosteroids are used for severe rheumatoid arthritis and for respiratory disorders such as asthma (p.295) and sarcoidosis (p.304). They are also used after transplant surgery (*see* **Immunosuppressants**, p.585) and to treat Addison's disease and hypopituitarism. Corticosteroids may be injected to treat severe Addison's disease or anaphylaxis (p.285) and can be administered by inhaler to prevent asthma attacks (*see* **Corticosteroids for respiratory disease**, p.588).

What are the side effects?
Short-term use of corticosteroids rarely produces side effects. Such effects are also rare in long-term replacement therapy for Addison's disease and hypopituitarism because the drugs replace the body's natural hormones. Doctors use these drugs sparingly for other conditions because of side effects.

Prolonged use of strong topical corticosteroid drugs can damage the skin in the affected areas, causing thinning, wrinkling, and loss of pigmentation. Particular care is needed when using these drugs on the face or on a baby's skin. Locally injected or inhaled corticosteroids are unlikely to cause serious side effects, but may cause local problems such as minor throat infections. Inhaled corticosteroids may also cause oral thrush (p.559).

Long-term treatment with oral corticosteroids may cause easy bruising, acne, a moon-shaped face, and weight gain (*see* **Cushing's syndrome**, p.435). Prolonged use can also cause raised blood pressure and osteoporosis (p.217). Children taking corticosteroids will have their height monitored during treatment, as the drugs can slow growth. The risk of infections, especially viral infections, is increased by the drugs because they suppress the immune system.

Corticosteroids suppress the body's own production of corticosteroid hormones. As a result, the body may not be able to produce sufficient corticosteroid hormones if treatment is stopped suddenly. An abrupt withdrawal from long-term, high-dose corticosteroids can lead to a rapid fall in blood pressure and, sometimes, shock (p.248), which can be fatal. If your doctor prescribes corticosteroid drugs for you for more than 3 weeks, you will be given a medical alert card that gives details of your medication to inform any health professional who treats you. You should avoid coming into contact with anyone with chickenpox or shingles because of the risk of a severe infection. If you develop an infection or if you sustain injuries, a higher dose of corticosteroids may be needed. If you are prescribed systemic corticosteroids (that is, when the drugs reach all parts of the body, rather than just a localized area), your doctor will give you a leaflet detailing precautions, side effects, and warnings about the drugs.

Drugs for diabetes mellitus

Drugs used to treat diabetes mellitus that control blood glucose (sugar) levels

COMMON DRUGS

Insulin

Biguanides
- Metformin

Sulphonylurea drugs
- Glibenclamide
- Gliclazide
- Glimepiride
- Glipizide
- Tolbutamide

Gliptins
- Saxagliptin
- Sitagliptin
- Vildagliptin

Other drugs for diabetes
- Acarbose
- Dapagliflozin
- Exenatide
- Glucagon
- Liraglutide
- Nateglinide
- Pioglitazone
- Repaglinide

In diabetes mellitus (p.437), levels of blood glucose are too high because the body produces too little or is resistant to the action of the hormone insulin, which is secreted by the pancreas and regulates blood glucose. Drugs for diabetes mellitus keep blood glucose at normal levels.

There are two types of diabetes mellitus. In type 1 diabetes, the body does not produce sufficient insulin, and synthetic insulin is needed. In type 2 diabetes, the body tissues have reduced sensitivity to the action of insulin. Mild forms of type 2 diabetes may be controlled by making changes to the diet and without having to use drugs.

What are the types?
The main drugs for diabetes mellitus are insulin, which is always given for type 1, and antidiabetic drugs, which are used to treat type 2. The most common antidiabetic drugs are metformin and the sulphonylureas, although the drugs acarbose, repaglinide, nateglinide, and pioglitazone may also be prescribed. If antidiabetic drugs are ineffective, insulin may be used to treat type 2 diabetes.

Insulin Injections of insulin are given to replace missing natural insulin. This replacement mimics the body's normal patterns of insulin production, maintaining low background levels with peaks at meal times when glucose enters the blood. Most insulin is genetically engineered to be identical to human insulin.

There are several types of insulin preparation whose durations of action differ. Short-acting insulins are taken 15–30 minutes before meal times, giving high levels of insulin in the blood to coincide with high levels of glucose. Longer-acting insulins are taken once or twice a day. Many people take a combination of both types. The dose will be tailored to your individual needs.

Since insulin is destroyed by stomach acids it cannot be taken orally and is always injected. Your doctor or nurse will teach you how to inject insulin (*see*

Injecting insulin, p.439), and you will be shown how to measure your blood glucose levels (*see* **Monitoring your blood glucose**, p.439). You should measure your glucose levels at regular intervals during the day to see whether your insulin dose is at the correct level. For type 1 diabetes that is hard to control, newer types of long-acting insulin may be appropriate. Alternatively, if these long-acting insulins do not provide adequate control, continuous and timed doses of insulin can be given by a pump.

Taking excess insulin or too little food may cause hypoglycaemia (p.440), in which blood glucose levels are abnormally low. You will be taught how to recognize the symptoms, which include sweating, hunger, faintness, and anxiety. If you have an attack, you should eat or drink something sweet immediately. An injection of glucagon, which increases blood glucose levels, may be given for severe hypoglycaemia. Common injection sites for insulin include the abdomen and thighs. Some of the preparations used contain an additive that can cause soreness and inflammation at the injection site when you start using insulin, but this is usually temporary and will disappear after a short while.

▶ **DRUG ACTION**

How sulphonylurea drugs work
Sulphonylurea drugs are used to treat type 2 diabetes. In this type of diabetes, body tissues have reduced sensitivity to insulin. Sulphonylurea drugs stimulate cells in the pancreas to secrete more insulin to compensate for the reduced sensitivity.

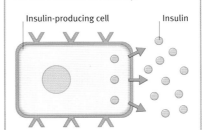

Before drug
The amount of insulin made by the insulin-secreting cells in the pancreas is not sufficient for the body's needs.

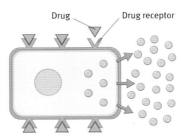

After drug
The sulphonylurea drug acts on the insulin-producing cells, stimulating them to increase production of insulin.

Biguanides Metformin is the drug of first choice for most people with type 2 diabetes and is particularly useful for those who are overweight or those of normal weight whose diabetes cannot be controlled by dietary changes alone. It can be used together with sulphonylureas or another drug such as pioglitazone to increase the sensitivity of body tissues to insulin. Metformin also increases the utilization of glucose by the tissues.

Metformin is unlikely to cause weight gain and is less likely to cause an attack of hypoglycaemia than sulphonylureas, but it may initially cause nausea, diarrhoea, abdominal bloating, low appetite, and facial flushing. These side effects often disappear after a few weeks of use.

Sulphonylurea drugs These drugs stimulate the insulin-producing cells in the pancreas to increase insulin production (*see* **How sulphonylurea drugs work**, below left). This helps to compensate for the low sensitivity of body tissues to insulin that occurs in type 2 diabetes. Sulphonylurea drugs are usually taken orally once or twice a day, and treatment is combined with dietary restrictions. However, in many people, increased appetite and weight gain are side effects.

Gliptins These drugs block the breakdown of a hormone called GLP-1 that stimulates insulin release from the pancreas; as a result, more insulin is released. They are taken once daily and may be combined with sulphonylureas or metformin. Gliptins are usually well tolerated but may increase the likelihood of urinary infections or infections of the nose and throat.

Other drugs for diabetes In addition to other treatments for type 2 diabetes, your doctor may prescribe drugs such as acarbose, exenatide, liraglutide, dapagliflozin, repaglinide, nateglinide, or pioglitazone. These drugs work in a variety of different ways. Acarbose slows the absorption of glucose from the intestines and prevents a rapid rise in blood glucose levels after meals. Exenatide and liraglutide are synthetic forms of the hormone GLP-1. They may cause gastrointestinal side effects such as abdominal distention, nausea, vomiting, and increased weight loss. Dapagliflozin reduces high blood glucose levels by increasing the amount of glucose lost in the urine. It may increase the risk of urinary tract infections and vaginal thrush (p.482). Repaglinide and nateglinide stimulate the release of insulin from the pancreas. These drugs may cause side effects in some people, including flatulence, abdominal discomfort, diarrhoea, and rarely, rashes. Pioglitazone increases the uptake of insulin by body tissues, leading to a reduction in blood glucose levels. It may cause side effects including intestinal disturbances, weight gain, headache, and anaemia. Pioglitazone should not be used by people with heart failure (p.247) or a history of heart failure, and may not be suitable for those with other heart problems or peripheral vascular disorders (p.260).

Drugs for hypothyroidism

Synthetic thyroid hormones used to treat underactivity of the thyroid gland

COMMON DRUGS
- Levothyroxine (thyroxine) ▪ Liothyronine

In hypothyroidism (p.432), the thyroid gland produces insufficient amounts of thyroid hormones, particularly thyroxine, causing symptoms such as tiredness and weight gain. This disorder can be caused by inflammation of the thyroid gland, known as thyroiditis (p.433), which may be either a short-term or long-term condition. Hypothyroidism may also be the result of previous radioiodine treatment for overactivity of the thyroid gland (*see* **Drugs for hyperthyroidism**, below), or it may be present from birth (*see* **Inborn errors of metabolism**, p.561). Hypothyroidism usually needs lifelong treatment with synthetic thyroid hormones.

How are they used?
Newborn babies who have hypothyroidism may initially need injections of the hormones. In adults, synthetic thyroid hormones are taken orally every day. Drugs are started at a low dose and the dose is increased gradually until an effective level is reached without causing side effects. The drugs take a few weeks to become effective, and it may take up to 6 months for symptoms to disappear completely.

What are the side effects?
Given at the correct dose, synthetic thyroid hormones cause no side effects. To ensure that the correct dose is maintained, you will have regular blood tests. If the dose that you are given initially is too high, you may develop symptoms of hyperthyroidism (p.432), which may include tremor, weight loss, and rapid, sometimes irregular heartbeat. These symptoms will disappear once the correct dose for you has been established.

Drugs for hyperthyroidism

Drugs that are used to treat overactivity of the thyroid gland

COMMON DRUGS

Antithyroid drugs
- Carbimazole ▪ Propylthiouracil

Radioiodine

Hyperthyroidism (p.432) is a disorder in which the thyroid gland is overactive and secretes excessive amounts of thyroid hormones. The symptoms of hyperthyroidism may include weight loss, per-

---

How antithyroid drugs work

Antithyroid drugs are used to treat hyperthyroidism, in which the thyroid gland produces excessive quantities of hormones. Active hormones are formed when iodine combines with precursor (inactive) hormone. Antithyroid drugs block this combination, reducing the formation of thyroid hormones.

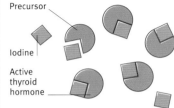

Before drug
Active thyroid hormone is formed when iodine binds to precursor (inactive) hormones in the thyroid gland.

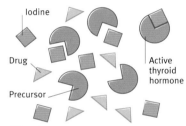

After drug
The drug prevents iodine binding to precursors, reducing the amount of active thyroid hormone produced.

---

sistent tremor, and rapid, sometimes an irregular heartbeat. Drugs for hyperthyroidism are given to reduce the activity of the thyroid gland.

What are the types?
An overactive thyroid gland may be treated using antithyroid drugs, radioiodine, or surgery. The drugs take several weeks to become effective, and a beta-blocker drug (p.581) may be prescribed in the interim to control symptoms such as rapid heartbeat.

Antithyroid drugs These drugs are used for long-term treatment of hyperthyroidism. They may also be used in preparation for surgery to remove all or part of an overactive thyroid gland. The drugs decrease the production of thyroid hormones (*see* **How antithyroid drugs work**, above).

Carbimazole is the antithyroid drug that is most commonly used. Antithyroid drugs are taken on a daily basis. Levels of hormones are usually reduced to normal, and symptoms of hyperthyroidism should begin to improve over a period of 1–2 months. In the interim, beta-blockers may be given to alleviate symptoms. Treatment with antithyroid drugs usually continues for 12–18 months, in which time the underlying disorder that is responsible for the hyperthyroidism may have cleared up.

During the treatment of hyperthyroidism, blood tests are performed on a regular basis to monitor levels of thyroid hormones in the blood so that the dose of antithyroid drugs can be adjusted if necessary. These tests are necessary to ensure that thyroxine levels do not become too high or too low.

The side effects of antithyroid drugs are usually minor and include nausea, headache, rashes, itching, and joint pains. Reduced production of white blood cells is a rare but potentially serious side effect that can occur during treatment with carbimazole. Decreased levels of these cells reduce the body's ability to fight infection. If you develop symptoms of an infection or a severe sore throat while taking carbimazole, inform your doctor immediately.

Radioiodine A radioactive form of iodine, called radioiodine, may be used to treat an overactive thyroid gland. Normally, the thyroid gland uses iodine from the diet to produce thyroid hormones. If radioiodine is given, it is taken up by the thyroid gland instead of normal iodine. The radioiodine then destroys part of the thyroid tissue, thereby reducing hormone production.

After treatment for an overactive thyroid gland, levels of thyroid hormone should return to normal within 2–3 months. Sometimes, levels of thyroid hormone increase for a short period after radioactive treatment before decreasing. If the levels are still high after 4 months, you will probably be given a second dose of radioiodine.

Following treatment, you may develop symptoms of hypothyroidism (p.432), such as dry, thickened skin, hair thinning, weight gain, and tiredness, because your thyroid gland has become underactive. Your doctor will regularly monitor the levels of thyroid hormones in your blood. If the levels become too low, you will need to take synthetic thyroid hormones to compensate (*see* **Drugs for hypothyroidism**, left); you will need to continue this treatment for the rest of your life. When given in correct doses, the drugs cause no side effects.

Radioiodine treatment is not given during pregnancy because there is a risk of damage to the developing fetus.

Radioactive iodine may also be used after surgery to treat thyroid cancer (p.434) but at a much higher dose in order to destroy any remaining thyroid tissue that may be cancerous. After treatment, you will need to take synthetic thyroid hormones for life.

Sex hormones and related drugs

Drugs that are used to increase levels of female and male sex hormones or block their release or action

COMMON DRUGS

Female sex hormones
- Desogestrel ▪ Estradiol ▪ Ethinylestradiol
- Levonorgestrel ▪ Medroxyprogesterone
- Tibolone

Anti-oestrogens
- Clomifene ▪ Tamoxifen

Gonadotrophins (*see* Drugs for infertility, p.604)

Danazol

Male sex hormones
- Mesterolone ▪ Testosterone

Antiandrogens
- Abiraterone ▪ Bicalutamide ▪ Cyproterone
- Dutasteride ▪ Finasteride ▪ Flutamide

Gonadorelin and gonadorelin analogues
- Buserelin ▪ Gonadorelin ▪ Goserelin
- Leuprorelin ▪ Nafarelin ▪ Triptorelin

Various forms of sex hormones and sex hormone antagonists (chemicals that block the release or action of hormones) are used to treat disorders in which there are abnormally high or low levels of sex hormones in the body.

A brain area called the hypothalamus produces gonadotrophin-releasing hormone. This hormone then stimulates the further production of follicle-stimulating hormone (FSH) and luteinizing hormone (LH) by the pituitary gland, a pea-sized gland at the base of the brain. FSH and LH, in turn, regulate sexual development by stimulating the release of the sex hormones: testosterone by the testes in males, and oestrogen and progesterone by the ovaries in females.

What are the types?
The hormones and drugs used to treat hormonal disorders in women include forms of the female hormones oestrogen and progesterone. Anti-oestrogens are sex hormone antagonists and may be used to block the action of oestrogen. The male hormone testosterone is used to treat certain hormonal disorders in boys and men; male sex hormone antagonists called antiandrogens may also be necessary to block the action of testosterone. Gonadorelin, a synthetic form of gonadotrophin-releasing hormone, and gonadorelin analogues, which block the release of gonadotrophin, are also used to treat hormonal disorders.

Female sex hormones Synthetic forms of the hormones oestrogen and progesterone have several uses. By far the most widespread use is as oral contraceptives (*see* **Contraception**, p.28), in which the two hormones are taken together, or progesterone is taken alone, to prevent pregnancy. Oestrogen and progesterone are used in lower doses in hormone replacement therapy (p.605) to relieve the symptoms of the menopause.

The drugs may be administered by injection, taken orally, or used as skin patches, depending on the type of drug and the reason for its use. Side effects are most likely to occur at the higher doses and may include fluid retention, headache, nausea, weight gain, and depression. In addition, premenopausal women may experience some bleeding between periods while taking synthetic sex hormone drugs.

Anti-oestrogens Clomifene is often used to treat infertility in women (see **Female infertility**, p.497). Because clomifene stimulates egg production, there is a risk of multiple pregnancy. Possible side effects of clomifene include visual disturbances, hot flushes, abdominal discomfort, nausea, and vomiting. Tamoxifen is used to treat breast cancer (p.486) and some forms of female infertility. Prolonged use of tamoxifen may be associated with a slightly increased risk of uterine cancer. Tamoxifen may cause menstrual irregularities, abnormal vaginal bleeding, and pelvic pain; if you experience any of these symptoms, you should see your doctor promptly. Other side effects include hot flushes, genital irritation, headache, and light-headedness. There may be an increased risk of thromboembolism (see **Thrombosis and embolism**, p.259).

Male sex hormones Synthetic forms of male sex hormones are used to treat certain conditions caused by low levels of testosterone, including delayed puberty in boys (see **Abnormal puberty in males**, p.465) and decreased libido in men (see **Decreased sex drive**, p.494). Given in low doses, synthetic testosterone mimics the action of the natural hormone, and side effects are rare.

Antiandrogens Some antiandrogens, such as finasteride, are used to treat an enlarged prostate gland (p.463); others, such as flutamide and abiraterone, are used in the treatment of prostate cancer (p.464). In addition, virilization (p.474), in which women develop a number of masculine characteristics such as excessive facial and body hair, may also be treated using one of these drugs, usually cyproterone. Antiandrogens act by blocking the action or synthesis of the natural male sex hormones. A common side effect of treatment with antiandrogens is tiredness. The drugs can also affect liver function and are not normally given to anyone with a history of liver problems.

Danazol This drug is used to treat endometriosis (p.475). Side effects of danazol include hirsutism (excessive hair growth), acne, and voice changes, as well as changes in libido and disturbances to the menstrual cycle.

Gonadorelin and gonadorelin analogues Gonadorelin is a synthesized version of a natural hormone called gonadotrophin-releasing hormone. This drug is used to assess whether the pituitary gland is producing the right levels of LH and FSH.

Gonadorelin analogues are prescribed for certain female reproductive disorders,

such as endometriosis and female infertility. These drugs may also be used to treat prostate cancer and breast cancer. Their initial effect is to stimulate the release of LH and FSH from the pituitary gland. When given over a long period of time, gonadorelin analogues reduce production of these hormones. This, in turn, inhibits the release of oestrogen, progesterone, and testosterone.

Gonadorelin analogues are given by injection or as a nasal spray. Side effects of the drugs may include acne, nausea and vomiting, and headache. In premenopausal women, these drugs may cause bleeding between periods, hot flushes, and increased sweating.

Pituitary drugs

Drugs that replace, stimulate, or inhibit some of the hormones produced by the pituitary gland

COMMON DRUGS

Growth hormone
- Somatropin

Growth hormone antagonists
- Bromocriptine ■ Lanreotide ■ Octreotide

Prolactin inhibitors
- Bromocriptine ■ Cabergoline

Drugs for diabetes insipidus
- Desmopressin ■ Vasopressin

The pituitary gland, located at the base of the brain, produces a number of hormones. These hormones include growth hormone, prolactin, which controls the production of breast milk in women, and vasopressin, which regulates the function of the kidneys.

Drugs for pituitary disorders work in various ways. Some drugs are synthetic hormones that replace missing natural hormones, and others, known as antagonists, reduce the production or action of pituitary hormones.

Drugs that act on the hormones produced directly by the pituitary gland are discussed below. Other drugs whose action on the pituitary gland affects the production of hormones in other parts of the body are discussed elsewhere. These drugs include sex hormones and related drugs (p.602), drugs for infertility (p.604), corticosteroids (p.600), and drugs for labour (p.605).

What are the types?
A number of drugs are used to treat pituitary disorders. Growth hormone and growth hormone antagonists are given to adjust levels of growth hormone that are either too low or too high. Prolactin inhibitors are given to reduce levels of prolactin in the treatment of disorders in which there is excessive production of prolactin by the pituitary gland. The pituitary disorder diabetes insipidus (p.431), which results from insufficient vasopressin, is treated by replacement of the hormone with a synthetic equivalent.

Growth hormone If the pituitary gland does not secrete sufficient growth hormone during childhood, a synthetic form of the growth hormone can be prescribed to replace it. Low levels of growth hormone in childhood can cause impaired growth (see **Growth disorders**, p.563). If a child begins the treatment at an early age, well before puberty, normal growth usually takes place. The drug is usually administered daily by injection. This treatment normally continues for several years until the child reaches adult height. Side effects may include aching muscles and joints and headaches.

Growth hormone antagonists If too much growth hormone is produced by the pituitary gland, adults may be given growth hormone antagonists such as octreotide. Excess growth hormone can cause abnormal enlargement of certain parts of the body, particularly facial features, hands, and feet, a condition that is known as acromegaly (p.430). In adults, overproduction of growth hormone is most commonly caused by a pituitary tumour (p.430). Drugs that block the production of growth hormone may be prescribed as a temporary measure prior to surgery or radiotherapy. However, where surgery is not possible, these drugs may be given long term.

The drugs octreotide and lanreotide are given by injection. Bromocriptine is taken orally. Possible side effects of octreotide and lanreotide include diarrhoea and cramping abdominal pain. Bromocriptine may cause nausea, vomiting, constipation, headache, drowsiness, confusion, nasal congestion, and hallucinations. It has also been associated with abdominal, heart, and lung problems, and your doctor may therefore monitor you regularly.

Prolactin inhibitors These drugs are used to suppress production by the pituitary gland of the hormone prolactin, to treat conditions such as noncancerous pituitary tumours (see **Prolactinoma**, p.430). The drugs may also be used to suppress milk production after childbirth and to treat Parkinson's disease (p.333). Prolactin inhibitors are most commonly taken orally. The drugs may cause a wide range of side effects, including nausea, vomiting, constipation, headache, drowsiness, confusion, nasal congestion, and hallucinations. They have also been associated with certain abdominal, lung, and heart problems, and people taking these drugs may therefore be monitored regularly by their doctor.

Drugs for diabetes insipidus You may be given vasopressin or a synthetic form of this hormone (desmopressin) if you have cranial diabetes insipidus (p.431). In this disorder, the pituitary gland produces insufficient vasopressin to regulate kidney function, which controls the amount of water retained in the body. It may be given orally, as a nasal spray, or by injection.

Vasopressin or desmopressin may cause some side effects, including nausea, belching, and abdominal cramps.

Lipid-lowering drugs

Drugs used to reduce the level of lipids (fats and related substances) in the blood

COMMON DRUGS

Statins
- Atorvastatin ■ Fluvastatin ■ Pravastatin
- Rosuvastatin ■ Simvastatin

Fibrates
- Bezafibrate ■ Ciprofibrate ■ Fenofibrate
- Gemfibrozil

Nicotinic acid and derivatives
- Acipimox ■ Nicotinic acid

Drugs that bind to bile salts
- Colestipol ■ Colestyramine

Other lipid-lowering drugs
- Ezetimibe ■ Omega-3 compounds

Lipid-lowering drugs reduce excessive levels of lipids, particularly cholesterol and triglycerides, in the blood. They are used to treat, or provide protection against, hyperlipidaemia (p.440). They also help to prevent or slow the progression of atherosclerosis (p.241), which in turn reduces the risk for cardiovascular disorders such as coronary artery disease (p.243), myocardial infarction (p.245), and stroke (p.329).

For maximum cardiovascular risk reduction, lipid-lowering drugs should be used together with other measures, such as stopping smoking, a lipid-lowering diet (see **Diet and health**, pp.16–20), regular exercise, and control of raised blood pressure.

What are the types?
The main types of lipid-lowering drug are statins, fibrates, nicotinic acid and its derivatives, and drugs that bind to bile salts. Other lipid-lowering drugs include ezetimibe and omega-3 compounds.

Your doctor's choice of drug treatment will depend on which type of lipid is causing your condition. In some instances, your doctor may prescribe a combination of drugs. Lipid-lowering drugs are taken orally on a daily basis, and most need to be taken long term.

Statins These drugs reduce the formation of cholesterol and triglycerides in the body. Side effects may include nausea, headaches, abdominal pain, and diarrhoea or constipation. Statins may also cause muscle inflammation; you should inform your doctor if you develop any unexplained muscle pain, tenderness, or weakness. Long-term use of statins may affect liver function, so you may need regular liver function tests. You should also tell your doctor if you are planning a pregnancy, are pregnant, or are breast-feeding because statins can harm a fetus or baby.

Fibrates These drugs are effective in lowering levels of both cholesterol and triglycerides in the blood. Fibrates are unsuitable if you have a disorder of the kidneys, liver, or gallbladder. The drugs occasionally cause side effects, including muscle pain, nausea, headache, and erectile dysfunction. Muscle pain may be more common if you have a disorder of the kidneys or are also receiving a statin. Fibrates can harm a fetus or baby, and it is important to tell your doctor if you are planning a pregnancy, are pregnant, or are breast-feeding.

Nicotinic acid and derivatives Excessively high levels of cholesterol or triglycerides in the blood may be reduced by treatment with nicotinic acid or its derivative. However, these drugs often cause side effects and are generally used only when other drugs have proved ineffective. The side effects may include facial flushing, unsteadiness, headache, nausea and vomiting, and itching. Muscle pain may develop if these drugs are used together with a statin. Women who are planning a pregnancy or who are pregnant or breast-feeding should avoid these drugs because they may harm a fetus or baby.

Drugs that bind to bile salts These drugs lower blood cholesterol levels by reducing fat absorption from the intestines. They may be used in combination with other lipid-

lowering drugs, such as fibrates and statins. You should take any other lipid-lowering drugs at least 1 hour before or 4–6 hours after taking a drug that binds to bile salts because they can interfere with the absorption of the other lipid-lowering drugs.

Drugs that bind to bile salts have few side effects, although they sometimes cause nausea, abdominal discomfort, and constipation. Supplements of vitamin K may be necessary in long-term treatment with drugs that bind to bile salts because the drugs reduce the body's absorption of these vitamins.

Other lipid-lowering products Ezetimibe and omega-3 compounds are used to reduce blood levels of cholesterol and triglycerides respectively. Each is usually used in combination with a statin and/or dietary measures. Possible side effects of ezetimibe include gastrointestinal disturbances, headache, tiredness, and muscle pain. Omega-3 compounds may cause gastrointestinal disturbances; other side effects are rare.

Drugs acting on the reproductive and urinary systems

Advances in our understanding of how the reproductive and urinary systems function have led to improved drug treatments for conditions such as infertility and prostate disorders. Drugs can also prevent problems of the menopause or labour.

Drugs are used to increase the likelihood of conception f infertility is due to hormonal imbalances. These drugs are discussed in the first article of this section. The second article covers hormone replacement therapy, which helps to reduce the symptoms of the menopause, which occurs when levels of sex hormones decline.

The next article covers drugs for labour, which are most often used to prevent premature labour or to induce or hasten labour. They may also be used to prevent bleeding after delivery. In the following article, the various drug treatments for

prostate disorders, including prostate cancer, are covered. The final article deals with drugs that affect bladder control. These drugs are used to treat urinary incontinence and retention.

Further information on drugs for the male and female reproductive and urinary systems, including articles on contraception (p.28) and on the use of sex hormones and related drugs (p.602), can be found elsewhere. In addition, antibiotics (p.572) are widely used to treat infections of the reproductive and urinary systems.

KEY ANATOMY

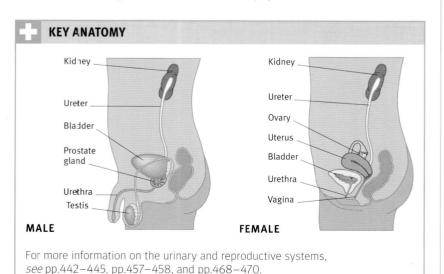

MALE

Kidney
Ureter
Bladder
Prostate gland
Urethra
Testis

FEMALE

Kidney
Ureter
Ovary
Uterus
Bladder
Urethra
Vagina

For more information on the urinary and reproductive systems, *see* pp.442–445, pp.457–458, and pp.468–470.

Drugs for infertility

Drugs that are used to treat couples who are unable to conceive

COMMON DRUGS

Anti-oestrogens
■ Clomifene ■ Tamoxifen

Gonadotrophins
■ Follitropin ■ Human chorionic gonadotrophin
■ Menotrophin

Gonadorelin analogues
■ Buserelin ■ Goserelin ■ Nafarelin

Drugs can be used to help a woman to become pregnant when a couple's inability to conceive is caused by a hormonal imbalance in either the male or the female (*see* **Infertility**, pp.497–499). For conception to occur, all the following steps must take place: ovulation (the release of a mature egg by an ovary), fertilization of the egg by a sperm, transport of the fertilized egg along the fallopian tube to the uterus, and implantation of the egg in the uterus lining.

Fertility is influenced by hormones produced in the brain by the hypothalamus and the pituitary gland. The hypothalamus secretes gonadotrophin-releasing hormone, which regulates the release of gonadotrophin hormones from the pituitary gland. The main gonadotrophin hormones are known as follicle-stimulating hormone (FSH) and luteinizing hormone (LH). These hormones control fertility. In females, FSH stimulates the ripening of eggs, and LH triggers ovulation (release of the egg). In males, FSH and LH regulate sperm production. An imbalance or deficiency of these hormones may lead to infertility. In such cases, drugs may be used to stimulate the ovaries to produce eggs, or less commonly, to stimulate a man to produce more sperm.

In women, drugs may also be used to stimulate the ovaries to produce more eggs than normal as part of techniques called assisted conception (p.498), such as in-vitro fertilization (IVF), gamete intrafallopian transfer (GIFT), and zygote intrafallopian transfer (ZIFT). These techniques are infertility treatments that involve mixing eggs and sperm outside the body.

Women who are having treatment with fertility drugs are monitored using blood tests and ultrasound scanning (p.135) because there is a small risk that the ovaries may become overstimulated, which can be a life-threatening condition. Symptoms of overstimulation can include nausea, vomiting, and abdominal pain and swelling. Infertility treatment also increases the likelihood of multiple pregnancy.

Treatments for infertility may not be effective immediately. These treatments often need to be continued for several months to increase the likelihood of conception.

What are the types?

In females, low levels of FSH and LH can be boosted by using an anti-oestrogen (also known as an oestrogen antagonist). Synthetic gonadotrophin hormones may also be given to influence fertility directly in both males and females. A gonadorelin analogue may sometimes be given in conjunction with gonadotrophin drugs in the treatment of female infertility.

Anti-oestrogens The naturally occurring hormone oestrogen suppresses the production of FSH and LH. Treatment with an oral anti-oestrogen, such as clomifene or tamoxifen, blocks this effect and stimulates the pituitary gland to produce more FSH and LH, thereby encouraging ovulation.

Clomifene may cause side effects such as visual disturbances, headache, nausea, hot flushes, breast tenderness, and abdominal pain. Ovarian cysts occasionally develop, but may shrink when the dose is reduced. If you take the drug for longer than 6 months, there may be an increased risk of developing cancer of the ovary (p.477). The drug may also cause multiple pregnancies.

Tamoxifen may cause side effects such as menstrual irregularities, and may increase the risk of thromboembolism and uterine cancer (*see* **Sex hormones and related drugs**, p.602).

Gonadotrophins Men and women who produce very low levels of FSH or LH may be given injections of synthetic FSH, such as follitropin, or human chorionic gonadotrophin (HCG), a hormone that mimics the action of LH. Gonadotrophins may also be used if treatment with the anti-oestrogen drug clomifene is unsuccessful. These synthetic hormones can be used to stimulate the production of several eggs in women undergoing assisted conception. In men, they can be used to increase sperm production. Several monthly courses may be needed. Possible side effects include headaches, tiredness, and mood changes. In men, the breasts may enlarge.

Gonadorelin analogues These drugs are sometimes given to women undergoing assisted conception who are also being given synthetic gonadotrophins. When given intermittently, gonadorelin analogues stimulate the release of FSH and LH. However, when taken continuously, they block the effects of natural gonadotrophin-releasing hormone, thus reducing the production of FSH and LH. Blocking the production of natural gonadotrophins makes it easier for doctors to control the action of synthetic gonadotrophins. Gonadorelin analogues are given by injection or as a nasal spray. Side effects include hot flushes, itching, loss of libido, nausea, and vomiting.

Hormone replacement therapy

Drugs that act in a similar way to female sex hormones and that are used to reduce symptoms associated with the menopause

COMMON DRUGS

Oestrogens
- Conjugated oestrogens ▪ Estradiol
- Estrone ▪ Estropipate ▪ Ethinylestradiol

Progestogens
- Levonorgestrel ▪ Medroxyprogesterone
- Norethisterone ▪ Norgestrel

Other drugs
- Tibolone

At the menopause, there is a decline in the levels of the sex hormone oestrogen. Hormone replacement therapy (HRT) can be used to restore oestrogen to pre-menopausal levels. Reduced oestrogen levels may lead to symptoms such as hot flushes and vaginal dryness. In the long term, low levels of oestrogen may increase the risk of osteoporosis (p.217) and heart disease. Menopausal symptoms may be particularly severe after surgical removal of the ovaries or following radiotherapy of the pelvic area in the treatment of cancer. Whether they occur naturally or after surgery or radiotherapy, the symptoms of the menopause are usually relieved by HRT.

HRT usually consists of a combination of oestrogen and a progestogen (a synthetic form of the hormone progesterone). Oestrogen that is taken alone is associated with a higher than normal risk of cancer of the uterus (p.479). For this reason, most women are also prescribed a progestogen, which gives protection against uterine cancer. In the case of women who have had a hysterectomy (p.479), usually oestrogen alone is prescribed. Tibolone combines the action of both oestrogen and progestogen in a single preparation.

How is it used?

HRT is usually given in the form of tablets, skin patches, or as a combination of the two. Tablets are taken daily; patches are usually changed twice a week and should be placed on a different area of skin each time. Other forms of HRT include a gel that is rubbed into the skin daily and a vaginal ring impregnated with oestrogen. Oestrogen creams, applied to the vagina for several weeks to treat vaginal dryness, may also be used. Courses of treatment with creams can be repeated if necessary, but the smallest effective dose should be used to minimize possible effects on other parts of the body.

In women with a uterus, HRT involves taking a continuous dose of an oestrogen, which is combined with a progesterone for 10 to 13 days of the 28-day cycle. The progesterone causes bleeding similar to that of menstruation, which is necessary to prevent excessive thickening of the lining of the uterus and the risk of it becoming cancerous. Alternatively, when more than a year has passed since the last menstrual period, continuous, bleed-free HRT or a single drug with both oestrogenic and progestogenic effects (such as tibolone) may be used. Women who have had a hysterectomy need only take oestrogen drugs.

HRT does not provide contraception, and you should consult your doctor about how long contraception should be used and the type most suitable for you.

Whether or not treatment with HRT is appropriate is a complicated issue and varies according to the particular woman concerned. For this reason, it is important to discuss with your doctor the risks and benefits of HRT that may apply in your specific case. However, in general, HRT is usually only advised for short-term use around the menopause to treat symptoms such as hot flushes and vaginal dryness. In addition, it is advised that the minimum effective dose of HRT is used for the shortest duration. HRT is no longer recommended for long-term use for the relief of menopausal symptoms nor for the treatment of osteoporosis because of the increased risk of disorders such as breast cancer, stroke, and thromboembolism (*see* **Thrombosis and embolism**, p.259). There may also be an increased risk of coronary artery disease (p.243) in women who start HRT more than 10 years after the menopause. The increased risk of breast cancer is related to duration of HRT use; the risk reduces to its previous level within about 5 years of stopping HRT.

What are the side effects?

If you are taking oestrogen, you may experience some side effects. These include nausea, headaches, and mood swings. Oestrogen may also cause breast tenderness, fluid retention, fluctuating weight, and

---

▶ **SELF-ADMINISTRATION**

Using skin patches

Adhesive skin patches are a simple and effective way to deliver drugs, such as HRT, gradually into the body. Drugs that are administered in this way are released slowly and steadily and are absorbed directly into the bloodstream.

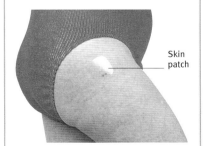

Skin patch

Using skin patches
Patches should be placed on dry, unbroken skin. Patches for HRT are usually placed on the lower abdomen, lower back, buttocks, or thigh.

---

eye irritation when wearing contact lenses. Progestogens can produce similar side effects to oestrogen, and occasionally cause acne and skin rashes. Such side effects are usually temporary and disappear after 1–2 months of treatment.

Drugs for labour

Drugs that are used to prevent or start labour or for associated problems

COMMON DRUGS

Uterine stimulant drugs
- Carboprost ▪ Dinoprostone
- Ergometrine ▪ Gemeprost
- Oxytocin

Uterine muscle relaxant drugs
- Atosiban ▪ Ritodrine
- Salbutamol ▪ Terbutaline

Magnesium

Drugs may be used during labour, either as a routine part of medical care or to treat specific problems. Among the most commonly used drugs during childbirth are epidural anaesthetics (*see* **Epidural anaesthesia in labour**, p.518).

It may be necessary to use drugs to induce labour (start labour artificially) if the health of the mother or the fetus is at risk. The most common reasons for the induction of labour (p.515) include continuation of pregnancy beyond the due delivery date or complications, such as poor growth of the baby. Drugs may also be given to speed up labour if it does not progress as quickly as it should or to prevent bleeding after delivery.

If labour starts early (before the 34th week of pregnancy), drugs are often used to stop or delay delivery.

What are the types?

Drugs are used during labour either to stimulate contractions of the uterus or to relax the uterus. The most commonly used drugs are known as uterine stimulants. These drugs induce labour by starting contractions or speed up labour by strengthening contractions. Uterine stimulants may also be used for the termination of pregnancy (p.510). Drugs that relax the uterus to delay premature labour are called uterine muscle relaxants. Magnesium may be used to prevent seizures during labour in women with the condition pre-eclampsia (*see* **Pre-eclampsia and eclampsia**, p.513).

Uterine stimulant drugs If labour is going to be induced or if it is necessary to terminate pregnancy, a pessary that contains a prostaglandin uterine stimulant may be inserted into the vagina. Prostaglandins not only stimulate contractions but also soften and widen the cervix. Prostaglandins may also be administered in the form of gel. During treatment with a prostaglandin, you may occasionally experience some side effects, such as nausea, vomiting, diarrhoea, and hot flushes.

Oxytocin, another uterine stimulant, is given by infusion into a vein to induce labour or to speed up prolonged labour by increasing the strength, duration, and frequency of contractions. The dose will be adjusted carefully, as excess oxytocin may result in painful, continuous contractions, nausea, vomiting, and fluid retention.

A combination of oxytocin and ergometrine, another uterine stimulant drug, is given by intramuscular injection to most women just as the baby is delivered. The drugs cause strong uterine contractions that hasten delivery of the placenta and also constrict the blood vessels in the uterus to reduce bleeding after delivery. A common side effect of ergometrine is nausea. In rare cases, headache, light-headedness, and ringing in the ears may occur.

Uterine muscle relaxant drugs If labour begins prematurely, the doctor may give you drugs to relax the muscles of your uterus, thereby preventing further contractions. Uterine muscle relaxants are given continuously by infusion into a vein. These drugs may have side effects such as nausea, hot flushes, and rapid heartbeat; your blood pressure may drop, causing light-headedness.

Magnesium This mineral may be used to prevent seizures that can occur during labour in women with pre-eclampsia. It may also be used to try to stop premature labour, especially in multiple pregnancy (p.512). Side effects may include flushing, sweating, and low blood pressure.

Drugs for prostate disorders

Drugs that are used to treat disorders affecting the prostate gland

COMMON DRUGS

Alpha-blocker drugs
- Alfuzosin ▪ Doxazosin
- Tamsulosin ▪ Terazosin

Antiandrogen drugs
- Abiraterone ▪ Bicalutamide ▪ Cyproterone
- Dutasteride ▪ Finasteride ▪ Flutamide

Gonadorelin analogues
- Goserelin ▪ Leuprorelin

The main disorders that affect the prostate are noncancerous enlargement of the prostate (*see* **Enlarged prostate gland**, p.563), prostate cancer (p.564), and infection (*see* **Prostatitis**, p.563). Drugs may be used to treat all of these conditions, sometimes in conjunction with surgery or other treatments. An enlarged prostate gland constricts the urethra, the tube along which urine flows from the bladder. There may also be obstruction if the muscle at the outlet of the bladder fails to relax. This can cause problems, such as a frequent urge to pass urine but difficulty in doing so. Prostate cancer can cause similar difficulties in passing urine, and may also spread to other parts of the body.

Infection of the prostate may cause symptoms including fever and pain in the lower back, around the anus, or around the base of the penis. You may also have other symptoms, including frequent, painful passing of urine and discoloured semen that contains blood.

What are the types?

The main types of drug used to treat prostate disorders are alpha-blockers and antiandrogens. Alpha-blockers are used to improve the flow of urine from the bladder. Antiandrogens are used to treat both noncancerous and cancerous enlargement of the prostate. Gonadorelin analogues may also be used to treat prostate cancer.

Prostate infections are usually treated with a course of antibiotics (p.572). The course of treatment may need to be continued for several weeks before the infection clears up completely.

Alpha-blocker drugs Drugs of this type, such as doxazosin and alfuzosin, relax the ring of muscle at the outlet of the bladder, thereby improving urine flow. Alpha-blockers are taken orally and may need to be used indefinitely because symptoms often recur when the drugs are stopped. Alpha-blockers may lower blood pressure, leading to light-headedness. The drugs may also cause drowsiness, tiredness, mood changes, a dry mouth, headache, and nausea.

Antiandrogen drugs Androgens are male sex hormones (testosterone, for example) that play an important but incompletely understood role in the development of noncancerous enlargement of the prostate gland and of prostate cancer. Antiandrogens work by counteracting the effects of androgens.

The main antiandrogens used for cancerous enlargement of the prostate gland are cyproterone, flutamide, and bicalutamide. They work by preventing the nuclei of prostate cells from being stimulated by testosterone, thereby inhibiting or stopping tumour growth. Certain other antiandrogens (called 5-alpha-reductase inhibitors), such as finasteride, are used to treat noncancerous enlargement of the prostate. These drugs work by inhibiting the metabolism of testosterone, which leads to a reduction in the size of the prostate. The 5-alpha-reductase inhibitors can be used as an alternative to alpha-blockers but may take several months to have a beneficial effect.

Antiandrogens are taken orally. They produce some side effects, which include reduced libido, erectile dysfunction, and breast tenderness.

Gonadorelin analogues These drugs are commonly used to treat prostate cancer that has spread beyond the prostate gland. The drugs affect the release of gonadotrophin hormones from the pituitary gland in the brain, thereby reducing the production of testosterone, the hormone that promotes the growth of prostate tumours. Gonadorelin analogues are either given by injection or are given as an implant under the skin. They may initially make symptoms worse. However, this effect may be treated with an antiandrogen, such as flutamide. Gonadorelin analogues may cause side effects such as hot flushes, itching, loss of libido, nausea, and vomiting.

Drugs that affect bladder control

Drugs for disorders that affect the ability of the bladder to store or expel urine

COMMON DRUGS

Anticholinergic drugs
- Flavoxate
- Imipramine
- Oxybutynin
- Propantheline
- Solifenacin
- Tolterodine

Desmopressin

Alpha-blocker drugs
- Alfuzosin
- Doxazosin
- Tamsulosin
- Terazosin

Other drugs for bladder disorders
- Dutasteride
- Finasteride
- Imipramine

Drugs may be used to treat disorders that affect the normal functioning of the bladder. These disorders fall into two main groups: urinary incontinence (p.454), in which there is involuntary leakage of urine; and urinary retention (p.455), in which there is difficulty emptying the bladder.

Urinary incontinence may occur for many reasons, including involuntary contractions of the muscle of the bladder wall, loss of nerve control due to a disorder such as stroke (p.329), or poor muscle tone at the bladder outlet, which is common in postmenopausal women. Bedwetting (p.565) is a common form of incontinence in young children. Normally, bedwetting stops by the age of 6, but some children do not gain full bladder control until they are older.

Urinary retention can also occur for a variety of reasons, including damage to nerves supplying the muscle of the bladder wall or an obstruction that prevents the outflow of urine from the bladder, which is commonly caused by an enlarged prostate gland (p.463).

What are the types?

Anticholinergic drugs (also called antimuscarinics) are used to treat incontinence. Desmopressin may occasionally be used to treat bedwetting in children. Urinary retention may be treated with alpha-blocker drugs.

Drugs for incontinence You may be prescribed an anticholinergic drug if you have frequent, sudden urges to pass urine and cannot control your bladder. These drugs work by relaxing the muscle in the bladder wall. This increases the bladder's capacity and reduces the urge to pass urine. If you are taking these drugs, you may have side effects such as a dry mouth, blurred vision, constipation, and nausea; they may also worsen glaucoma (p.358).

Bedwetting in children is sometimes treated with desmopressin, which is a synthetic version of a natural hormone produced by the pituitary gland that reduces urine production. Desmopressin may be given either orally or as a nasal spray. Side effects of the drug may include fluid retention, salt imbalance, nausea, and headache. Rarely, desmopressin can cause seizures.

Other drugs that may be helpful for overcoming bedwetting in children are tricyclic antidepressants (p.592) such as imipramine. This type of drug is given in small doses and is rarely used for longer than 3 months.

Drugs for urinary retention Alpha-blockers, such as doxazosin, may be used to treat urinary retention that develops gradually due to noncancerous enlargement of the prostate gland. The drugs work by relaxing the muscles at the bladder outlet, allowing urine to flow out more easily. Alpha-blockers sometimes cause drowsiness, headache, dry mouth, nausea, and mood changes. They may also lower blood pressure, resulting in light-headedness.

In some cases, finasteride or dutasteride (*see* Drugs for prostate disorders, p.605) may be used to shrink the prostate gland and allow urine to flow more easily. However, these drugs may take several months to become effective.

Surgery

Advances in technology have changed surgery from a risky procedure, often used only as a last resort, to a safe and effective treatment with many applications. New surgical techniques and improved anaesthetic drugs have reduced risks, increased success rates, and shortened recovery times. Many new types of surgery are far less invasive than techniques used previously, and a stay in hospital is now often unnecessary. These improvements have done much to reduce most people's anxiety about having an operation.

SURGERY NOW HAS such a wide range of applications that it has become the first choice treatment for many disorders, often bringing about immediate relief or even a complete cure.

Surgical procedures can be used to remove, repair, or replace damaged tissue anywhere in the body. A surgeon can take out a diseased body part, such as an inflamed appendix, or remove a tumour. Broken bones and torn tendons can be repaired following an accident. Diseased body organs, such as the kidneys, heart, and liver, can now be replaced with healthy donor organs, and artificial body parts, such as heart valves, can be implanted. Artificial joint replacement is now a routine operation.

Surgery can also be used to improve the efficiency of body functions. For example, blood flow to the heart muscle can be substantially improved by an operation to bypass blocked blood vessels using grafted lengths of veins taken from another part of the body.

known as an endoscope is used. The endoscope is inserted through a small incision made in the body or through a natural body opening. It is now possible to use an endoscope to perform many operations that would previously have needed open surgery, such as coronary artery bypass and stenting, and gallbladder removal. Recovery time in hospital from endoscopic surgery is much shorter than after open surgery, in which larger incisions are made in the skin. Endoscopes can also be used to take samples of diseased tissue, which are sent for laboratory examination.

Surgeons also use microscopes and tiny instruments to carry out detailed work on minute structures, such as blood vessels and nerves. Lasers are used for delicate operations on the eye, to remove skin blemishes, and to destroy tumours without damaging surrounding tissue. High-intensity,

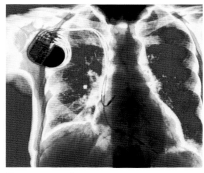

Heart pacemaker
Surgery sometimes involves implanting semi-permanent artificial devices, such as the pacemaker that can be seen in the upper chest in this X-ray.

focused ultrasound and surgical techniques using high or low temperatures are increasingly being used to destroy tumours, and robotic surgery is starting to be used for certain operations, such as hernia repair and prostate cancer surgery.

Today, a wide range of body organs can be transplanted, largely due to the development of immunosuppressant drugs, which help the body to accept new organs by reducing the likelihood of rejection after transplant surgery.

There have also been improvements in care and monitoring before, during, and after surgical operations, as well as new anaesthetic drugs that have fewer side effects. Many operations can now

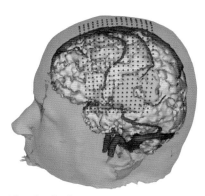

Planning brain surgery
Sophisticated imaging may be used to plan complex surgery, such as removal of a brain tumour (the large green area in this 3D MRI scan).

be performed under local or regional anaesthesia. As a result of these developments, many people who might once have been considered too ill for surgery can be operated on successfully.

Choices in surgery

Advances in surgery mean that any operation now involves decisions that the patient and doctor need to make together. Many minor procedures can now be done in the doctor's surgery rather than in hospital, and operations such as cataract removal, which used to require general anaesthesia, are now offered under local anaesthesia. Where the operation takes place and the type of anaesthesia used largely depend on the condition being treated, and on the patient's age, general state of health, personal preference, and whether care can be provided at home following surgery.

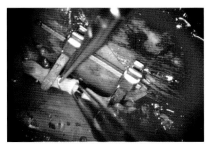

Microsurgical repair
Microsurgery involves a surgeon using a microscope to perform delicate procedures, such as repairing a severed blood vessel, as shown here.

Surgical advances

In recent years, advances in surgical techniques have changed the way in which operations are performed. The most dramatic change has been the development of endoscopic surgery, in which a tube-like viewing instrument

---

➕ PROCEDURE

Undergoing surgery

All types of surgery follow set procedures before, during, and after the operation. Before anaesthesia and surgery, you are given a preoperative assessment. Afterwards, your condition is assessed by your doctor before you are allowed to go home. Major surgery is always carried out in hospital, but minor operations may be performed in the doctor's surgery or in an outpatient clinic.

A surgical procedure
Before surgery, a physical assessment will check your fitness for anaesthesia and surgery. Your recovery time depends on your general state of health and the type of surgery you have.

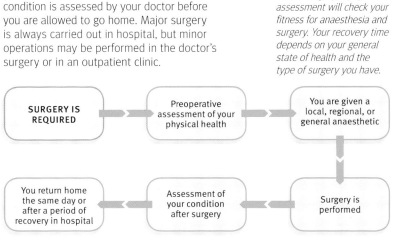

Having an operation

Many people face having an operation at some point in their lives. While some operations require a stay in hospital as an inpatient, an increasing number of procedures can be performed as day surgery. Advances in surgical procedures and anaesthesia have made having an operation safer than ever, with shorter recovery times and fewer side effects.

The first article covers minor surgical procedures that may be carried out in your doctor's surgery or in hospital on an outpatient basis. The second article outlines what you can expect to take place when you have major surgery, including your recovery afterwards. Major surgery is always performed in hospital. All hospitals and surgical procedures vary, but there are certain routines that are common to all, such as a thorough physical assessment before an operation to check your overall fitness for anaesthesia and surgery. This assessment may take place weeks or days before you are admitted to hospital. The final article discusses convalescence once you have returned home after major surgery. Different types of surgery are described in a separate section (*see* **Types of surgery**, pp.611–615).

Having minor surgery

Minor surgical procedures that take a short time to perform and usually require only local anaesthesia

Minor surgical procedures are those that can be done quickly, usually with only a local anaesthetic (*see* **Having a local anaesthetic**, right). Examples of these procedures include removal of moles, drainage of cysts or abscesses, and vasectomy (p.461). Most minor surgical procedures involve instruments. However, in some situations no instruments are needed, such as in the manipulation of a simple fracture (p.232).

Minor surgery is usually carried out in hospital as a day case or on an outpatient basis, or your doctor may carry out the procedure in his or her surgery.

What does it involve?
A minor operation that involves little blood loss requires only minimal preparation when performed on a healthy individual. The doctor will usually discuss the procedure with you, carry out a brief physical examination, and ask you to sign a consent form.

You may be given a local anaesthetic, usually by injection. Anaesthetic creams, gels, and sprays can also be used, but these are much less effective than injected anaesthetics. However, they may sometimes be used to numb the skin before giving a local anaesthetic injection.

The doctor then scrubs up and puts on a sterile gown and gloves; he or she may or may not wear a mask. An antiseptic liquid is used to clean the area that will be operated on (which will previously have been shaved, if necessary), and sterile drapes will be put around the area to prevent bacteria on the surrounding skin from entering the wound.

Once the skin around the affected area is clean and anaesthetized, the doctor carries out the procedure. Some procedures involve cutting through the skin and leave a wound, which is closed after surgery using stitches (sutures), tape, staples, clips, or glue (*see* **Rejoining tissue**, p.611). Other procedures, such as draining abscesses, leave an open wound, which is covered with a dressing.

What happens after surgery?
Your doctor or a nurse will give you instructions on how to look after the wound until it has healed, and arrangements may be made to have dressings changed regularly. Most wounds are watertight after about 24 hours and do not need to be specially protected to prevent infection. However, the tissue at the site remains delicate for about 5–10 days and usually needs protection against physical injury.

You may need to take painkillers (p.589) to relieve any discomfort when the local anaesthetic wears off. You may also need a course of antibiotics (p.572) to prevent infection. Your doctor will prescribe these drugs for you if necessary.

After some minor procedures, you may feel uncomfortable or a little faint, and you may need someone to take you home. You may be given a follow-up appointment so that the doctor can check that the procedure has been successful and that the wound is healing. If you have clips or staples, they will need to be removed. If you have stitches, they will also need to be removed unless the type of stitch that dissolves on its own was used.

▶ PROCEDURE

Having a local anaesthetic

A local anaesthetic is used to prevent pain during minor procedures such as removing moles or stitching cuts. The anaesthetic drug numbs the nerve endings around the site where it is administered. A local anaesthetic is usually given by injection, although it may also be applied as a cream, gel, or spray.

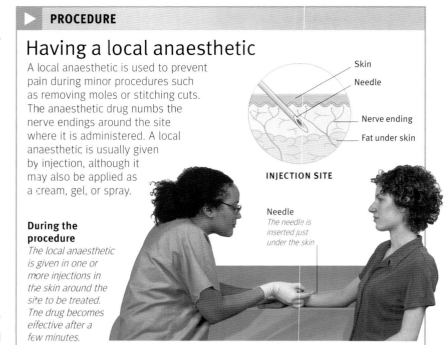

Skin
Needle
Nerve ending
Fat under skin

INJECTION SITE

Needle
The needle is inserted just under the skin

During the procedure
The local anaesthetic is given in one or more injections in the skin around the site to be treated. The drug becomes effective after a few minutes.

Having major surgery

Major surgical procedures carried out under general or regional anaesthesia

Major surgery always takes place in hospital and usually involves a procedure performed on tissue deep inside the body. For example, surgery to remove a section of intestine or implant an artificial hip would be considered major surgery (*see* **Types of surgery**, pp.611–615).

Before you undergo a major surgical procedure, your doctor will discuss with you why surgery is necessary, exactly what the procedure involves, where the operation will take place, and how long it will take. You will be fully informed about possible risks associated with the operation, and you will be asked to sign a consent form to say that you understand the risks and agree to surgery.

Before the procedure is performed, your general health and fitness for surgery will be assessed. On the day of the operation, you will be prepared for surgery and given an anaesthetic. Usually, major surgery is performed under general anaesthesia (*see* **Having a general anaesthetic**, opposite page). However, an increasing number of procedures are now carried out under regional anaesthesia (*see* **Having a regional anaesthetic**, p.610), in which you remain fully conscious but free of pain. A sedative may be given along with regional anaesthesia to help to keep you calm and reduce anxiety. The type of anaesthesia you have depends largely on the nature of the procedure, but your general health and age may also play a part.

After the operation has been completed there is a recovery period. An increasing number of operations now need only a short recovery period in hospital – often only 24 hours – although it may sometimes be necessary to stay in hospital for several days or longer. Your doctor will be able to advise you on how long it will take for you to recover from your operation. There may be particular practical issues that you wish to clarify with the doctor. For example, you may want to check whether further treatment will be needed after the operation and how long it is likely to be before you are able to carry out your normal day-to-day activities.

Preoperative assessment
Before you undergo a major surgical procedure, you will be given a preoperative assessment. The main purpose of this assessment is to find out whether you have an underlying medical condition, such as heart disease, that may require special precautions during the operation in order to minimize the risk of complications developing.

During the preoperative assessment, a doctor reviews your medical history and carries out a physical examination. Routine tests, such as blood tests and an ECG (p.243) to assess the condition of your heart, will also be carried out, together with any other investigations that may be needed because of your age, general health, or an underlying condition.

You may also be seen by an anaesthetist, who checks your suitability for anaesthesia, discusses how the anaesthetic will be administered, and answers any questions you may have.

Medical history and examination
You will be asked about your current condition and about other serious illnesses or allergies you have experienced in the past (*see* **Medical history**, p.127). It is important to tell the doctor about any allergies,

and also about any medications (including complementary remedies) you are taking because they may affect the safety of the surgery. It is helpful if you bring any medications and/or complementary remedies with you to show the doctor.

You will then be given a full medical examination (*see* **Physical examination**, p.127) to help identify any underlying medical conditions that may increase the risk of complications developing either during or after the operation.

Routine tests You may have a number of routine tests, many of which require a sample of blood or urine to be taken. Blood tests usually require no more than two or three small tubes of blood to be withdrawn through a single needle. A full blood count of your red and white blood cells and the level of haemoglobin (the oxygen-carrying molecule in red blood cells) will usually be checked. The levels of certain chemicals, such as urea and salts, in your blood may be measured because they reflect the function of organs such as the kidneys. Your blood group may be checked and a sample of blood may be saved for cross-matching against blood from the blood bank if you need to have a blood transfusion (p.272) during surgery.

In addition to these tests, you may also be given an ECG (electrocardiogram) to check the condition of your heart, particularly if your medical history suggests that you may have a heart condition.

Other presurgical investigations Depending on the outcome of your initial physical examination, your doctor may decide that other investigations are needed before you undergo surgery. For example, if there is a possibility that you have a heart or lung disorder, a chest X-ray (p.300) may also be performed. The results of these tests may influence how the surgery is carried out and the level of monitoring that is required during the operation. In some cases, these initial test results indicate the need for further investigations, such as exercise testing (p.244), which evaluates the flow of blood to the heart while a person is at rest and during the physical stress of exercise.

Preparations for surgery

On the day of your surgery, you will be prepared for the operation. After arriving in the operating theatre, you will then be given the anaesthetic.

You should not eat or drink non-clear fluids for about 6 hours before an operation under general anaesthesia. If you have food in your stomach there is an increased risk of vomiting while you are unconscious. If the acidic contents of the stomach are inhaled, serious damage to your lungs may result. You may drink clear fluids up to about 2 hours before the operation. You may also need to fast if you are having a regional anaesthetic, in case it becomes necessary to give you a general anaesthetic during surgery.

General preparations An hour or two before your operation, you will be asked to remove all jewellery and to change into a surgical gown. You will be asked to remove dentures, if you have them, or to point out loose teeth or crowns, which could be damaged when the breathing tube for anaesthetic gases is inserted. If a surgical incision is to be made in an area of skin that is covered with hair, the area may be shaved to make the skin easier to clean. The surgeon will mark your skin on the side of the operation or around the operation site. To reduce the risk of blood clots forming in the legs (*see* **Deep vein thrombosis**, p.363), you will probably be asked to wear special calf compression stockings, and you may also be given an injection of heparin (*see* **Drugs that prevent blood clotting**, p.583). Just before your operation, a nurse will take you to the operating theatre.

Anaesthesia When you arrive in the operating theatre, theatre staff will go through a checklist to make sure you are having the right operation, then you will be given an anaesthetic. For longer operations carried out under general anaesthesia, the anaesthetic is given in two parts. First, an anaesthetic is injected into a vein on the back of your hand. Although this injection induces anaesthesia rapidly, it is not long-lasting. Second, inhaled gases are given to maintain unconsciousness. For shorter operations, a single injected or inhaled anaesthetic may be used.

The initial anaesthetic drug is injected into a thin plastic tube called a catheter. This tube is inserted into a vein either in the back of your hand or in your arm, and the anaesthetic drug causes almost immediate loss of consciousness.

The anaesthetist then inserts a breathing tube, called an endotracheal tube, through your mouth and down into your trachea (windpipe). The tube is connected to a ventilator, which regulates the speed and depth of breathing throughout surgery. You will be given a mixture of gases to breathe, including oxygen and an inhaled anaesthetic. You will also be given a drug through the catheter that relaxes your muscles and enables the surgeon to cut and move muscles easily. By doing this, the surgeon can obtain a clear view of the operating area.

If you are having a regional anaesthetic, the anaesthetic drug is given by injection. The injection site varies according to the procedure to be performed. For some types of regional anaesthesia, such as epidural or spinal anaesthesia, the skin around the injection site is first numbed with a local anaesthetic.

In the operating theatre

As soon as you are anaesthetized, the surgeon or assistant surgeon uses an antiseptic solution to clean the appropriate area of your skin. The solution used may leave pink or brown stains on the skin for a short time after the operation. The remaining nonsterile parts of your skin are covered with sterile drapes, and the procedure is then carried out. During the operation, further precautions will be taken to prevent deep vein thrombosis, such as supporting your calves and/or fitting calf vein pumps around your legs.

▶ **PROCEDURE**

Having a general anaesthetic

General anaesthesia is used in surgery to induce unconsciousness and thereby to prevent pain. First, a rapidly acting drug is injected through a catheter into a vein in the back of your hand or in your arm. A drug given at the same time relaxes the muscles. Once unconscious, you are given a mixture of gases, including oxygen, through a tube inserted into your trachea (windpipe).

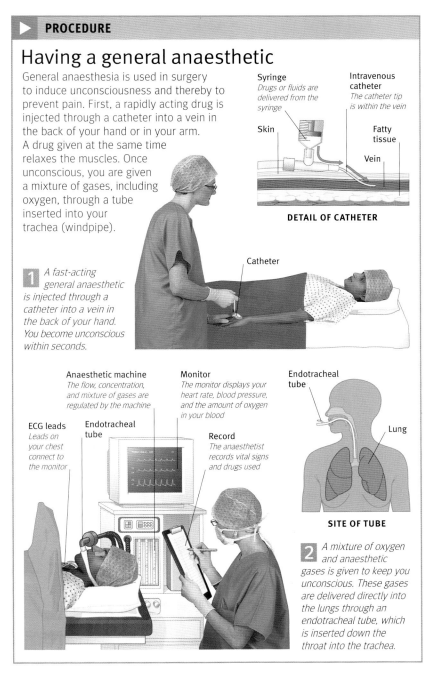

DETAIL OF CATHETER

Syringe
Drugs or fluids are delivered from the syringe

Intravenous catheter
The catheter tip is within the vein

Skin

Fatty tissue

Vein

Catheter

1 *A fast-acting general anaesthetic is injected through a catheter into a vein in the back of your hand. You become unconscious within seconds.*

Anaesthetic machine
The flow, concentration, and mixture of gases are regulated by the machine

Monitor
The monitor displays your heart rate, blood pressure, and the amount of oxygen in your blood

Endotracheal tube

ECG leads
Leads on your chest connect to the monitor

Endotracheal tube

Record
The anaesthetist records vital signs and drugs used

Lung

SITE OF TUBE

2 *A mixture of oxygen and anaesthetic gases is given to keep you unconscious. These gases are delivered directly into the lungs through an endotracheal tube, which is inserted down the throat into the trachea.*

When the procedure is completed, the wound is closed up (*see* **Rejoining tissue**, p.611) by the surgeon. For some types of wound, you may have internal stitches as well as those that are visible on your skin. Usually, a local anaesthetic is injected around the wound to reduce any pain and the amount of painkilling drugs needed when you wake up. If you have been given a general anaesthetic, the proportion of anaesthetic gases you are breathing will be reduced and the proportion of oxygen you are given will be increased to allow you to wake up.

In the recovery room

As soon as you show signs of breathing on your own, the anaesthetist will remove the endotracheal tube. You may hear someone telling you the operation is over, but you will probably wake up only briefly. You will then be moved to the recovery room. If you have had a general anaesthetic, the recovery room is probably the first place that you will remember after the operation. When you wake up, you may have an intravenous drip in your arm, drainage tubes near the operation site, and a catheter in your bladder. For the first hours after a major operation, your temperature, blood pressure, and pulse are checked frequently. When you are taken back to the ward, usually when you are fully awake, these checks are repeated, but less frequently.

Some major surgery requires intensive nursing care afterwards and you may be transferred to an intensive therapy unit (p.618) or a high-dependency unit (which provides more specialist nursing care and monitoring than is available on an ordinary ward but less than in an intensive therapy unit) rather than being taken directly back to an ordinary ward. You will be transferred to an ordinary ward when you are no longer dependent on specialized equipment and medical personnel.

▶ **PROCEDURE**

Having a regional anaesthetic

A regional anaesthetic blocks the transmission of pain along a nerve or group of nerves. The anaesthetic is injected around targeted nerves, and you remain awake throughout the procedure. Regional anaesthesia can be used in many parts of the body. A spinal nerve block, shown here, anaesthetizes the whole of the lower body below the site of injection.

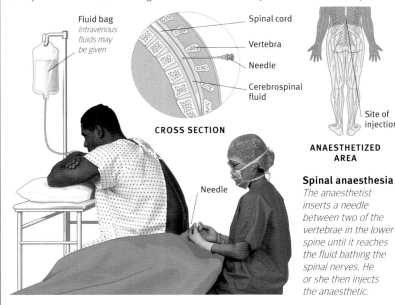

Fluid bag
Intravenous fluids may be given

Spinal cord

Vertebra

Needle

Cerebrospinal fluid

CROSS SECTION

Needle

Site of injection

ANAESTHETIZED AREA

Spinal anaesthesia
The anaesthetist inserts a needle between two of the vertebrae in the lower spine until it reaches the fluid bathing the spinal nerves. He or she then injects the anaesthetic.

Back to the ward

After major surgery, you will be transferred to the ward so that you can be monitored and given any further treatment that you may need. Postoperative monitoring is carried out in order to identify any complications as early as possible. If necessary, you will be given pain relief. Generally, the more extensive the operation, the longer it will take for you to recover. Usually, your recovery is faster and complications, such as deep vein thrombosis, are less likely to occur if you start moving around as soon as possible after the effects of the anaesthetic have worn off.

If you have had a general anaesthetic, you are likely to remain drowsy for a few hours. After regional anaesthesia, you will not experience the drowsiness that normally follows general anaesthesia. The numbing effects of a regional anaesthetic usually wear off after about an hour.

Treatment and monitoring You may be attached to tubes and equipment that monitor your condition or help you to perform particular bodily processes. For example, you may be attached to an ECG machine that monitors your heart function. You may have a urinary catheter if surgery has involved the bladder or nearby organs, such as the prostate gland. The catheter makes it possible to monitor the amount of urine that you produce. An intravenous drip may be placed in your arm or the back of your hand to deliver fluids and medication if necessary. Fluids help to prevent you becoming dehydrated until you are able to eat and drink normally. After certain procedures, there may be a tube called a drain coming from a small hole in the skin near the surgical wound. This tube is often attached to a vacuum bottle and allows excess tissue fluid or blood to drain away from the operation site. It is usually removed after a few days. You may also have a tube called a central line coming from the side of your neck or just below your collarbone. This tube is held in place by stitches and is used to monitor your fluid balance and blood pressure and to give you extra fluids or drugs if these are needed. This tube will be removed as soon as continuous monitoring and fluids are no longer necessary.

Pain relief You may not feel much pain when you wake up because of the effects of the drugs you have received during anaesthesia, and because the surgeon may have injected a local anaesthetic into the edges of the surgical wound. After a few hours, you may become more uncomfortable and require painkillers (p.589). These drugs may be administered by suppository, orally, or by injection, depending on the drug, the severity of your pain, and your ability to absorb the medication. You may be able to administer your own painkillers in small, safe doses as often as you need using a patient-controlled analgesic pump attached to a tube that is inserted into a blood vessel in your arm. This type of pump has a built-in device to prevent you from receiving too much medication.

Other treatments Some major surgery may necessitate other treatments to prevent complications. For example, deep vein thrombosis (blood clots in the legs) may develop if you are immobile for long periods of time. These clots may break off and travel to the heart or lungs, which may be life-threatening. If clots are likely to form after surgery, your doctor will prescribe injections of a drug that reduces blood clotting. You may also need to wear support stockings for a few days until you are fully mobile.

If you have had an operation on an infected area such as an abscess, you may be given antibiotics. Depending on the type of operation you have had, you may be offered physiotherapy (p.320) or other treatment while in hospital to help you to return to full mobility.

Leaving the hospital

You will be discharged from hospital when you no longer need close monitoring or special treatment. You usually need to be eating and drinking normally without the aid of tubes and to be able to pass urine without a catheter. The medical staff need to be satisfied that you have someone to accompany you home and that you will be adequately looked after if you are unable take care of yourself. Home nursing (*see* **Home care**, p.618) may need to be organized in advance. If you require special aids, such as a bath lift, you may be assessed by an occupational therapist (*see* **Occupational therapy**, p.621) before you are discharged from hospital.

Before you leave hospital, you will be provided with any medication that you need, and a follow-up appointment will be made to check on your progress and, if necessary, to remove stitches.

Convalescence after major surgery

The period of adjustment and recovery following a major operation

After surgery, there may be a period of time before you are able to return to work and resume your normal activities. This period of convalescence often involves some bed rest, and you may need help with day-to-day tasks. In addition to physical recovery, convalescence following major surgery may also involve a period of psychological adjustment. It is not unusual to feel emotional or depressed after surgery, and many people find counselling (p.624) helpful.

Developments in surgical techniques, for example endoscopic surgery (p.612), and improvements in the control and relief of pain have shortened the time needed for convalescence. In general, the older you are, the more extensive the surgery, and the poorer your general health, the more time you will need to convalesce.

You are likely to need a period of rest after surgery and may be in enough discomfort to restrict movement. However, this must be balanced with the need for you to gradually increase your level of activity in order to regain your strength and reduce the risk of deep vein thrombosis (p.263). If your muscles are weak from lack of use, such as after surgery on bones or joints, you may be offered regular physiotherapy (p.620) to regain mobility and muscle strength. You may also need help from a specialist nurse to make lifestyle changes, such as learning how to manage a colostomy (p.422).

Resuming activity

To help you recover as quickly as possible after surgery, it is important to try to be as physically active as you can. Make sure that you have appropriate medication to allow you to move around without excessive pain. After some types of surgery, particularly operations on the abdomen, it may hurt to cough, and secretions may remain in the lungs. In this case, you will be shown breathing exercises and how to reduce discomfort when you cough before you leave hospital, and you should continue to use these techniques during convalescence. As you recover from surgery, you should gradually be able to resume many of your day-to-day activities. With time, you will be able to return to your normal lifestyle, resume sexual activity, and drive again.

Work You should follow your doctor's advice on when to return to work, taking into account the progress of your recovery and the nature of your occupation. Manual work naturally requires a higher level of physical fitness than office work. You may be able to arrange to resume your work duties gradually. You may find that travelling to and from work is more tiring than usual, and even working from home may be more demanding than you anticipate.

Sex Few surgical operations require you to abstain from sexual activity afterwards for physical reasons, but your surgeon will tell you if there is a particular risk. However, sometimes you may wish to avoid sex for reasons of comfort as well as from medical necessity, such as after surgery on a hernia (p.419) in the groin. You may also need time for your sexual feelings to return to normal, since it is very common for sex drive to disappear during a period of illness. If you have sexual problems that continue for some time after surgery, consult your doctor.

Driving You may be advised not to drive if your operation or medical condition could affect your concentration or your ability to drive safely, for example if you are unable to wear a seat belt or stop quickly in an emergency. It may be unsafe for you to drive while you are taking certain painkillers or other drugs. Your doctor will advise you when you can start driving again.

Identifying complications

Something may be seriously wrong if you suddenly feel ill or if a symptom that was improving begins to get worse. Symptoms such as fever, shortness of breath, coughing, bleeding or a new discharge from the surgical wound, or pain in the legs, chest, or operation site that becomes worse may indicate a problem. If you develop any of these symptoms, you should seek advice promptly from your doctor or a contact at the hospital, who can distinguish between normal postoperative symptoms and serious complications.

Types of surgery

Surgery at its most basic level consists of cutting through body tissues, treating a problem, and sewing up the wound. However, the development of surgical techniques using new technology, such as microsurgery and laser treatment, has enabled more complex operations to be performed with increasing precision.

Open surgery, in which internal body structures are accessed through large incisions, is still a very common type of surgery and is discussed in the opening article. However, an increasing number of operations are now performed using endoscopic surgery, which is discussed next. Endoscopic surgery requires only a small incision or none at all.

Further articles cover other specialized surgical techniques, including microsurgery and laser treatment, both of which are used in plastic surgery to reconstruct or repair tissues. Microsurgery can be performed on tiny structures, such as the nerves. Laser treatment has many uses, such as removing birthmarks and repairing delicate structures of the eye. The final article discusses transplant surgery, which enables diseased and failing body parts to be replaced with healthy ones.

What happens before, during, and after surgery is covered elsewhere (*see* **Having an operation**, pp.608–610).

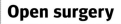

A surgical procedure
Almost all surgical procedures involve cutting through tissues and then securing the tissue edges together to promote healing, reduce bleeding, and prevent infection.

Open surgery

Surgical procedures in which internal body structures are accessed by large incisions made in the skin

Many operations are still carried out using open surgery. In this type of surgery, an incision is made in the skin large enough to allow the surgeon to see clearly the internal body parts that require treatment and the surrounding tissues. A large incision provides easy access, but it may leave an obvious scar.

Open surgery is used for all internal organ transplant operations and for caesarean sections (p.518). Open surgery may also be necessary for the removal of certain types of tumour or in cases in which the extent of the problem is not known. Sometimes, open surgery may need to be performed urgently in order to deal promptly with an emergency such as internal bleeding.

What happens during the operation?
There are a number of open surgery procedures, such as a caesarean section, that may be performed under regional anaes-

thesia (*see* **Having a regional anaesthetic**, opposite page). However, most open surgery is carried out under general anaesthesia (*see* **Having a general anaesthetic**, p.609). Once you are fully anaesthetized, the surgeon makes an incision through the skin and the layers of fat and muscle below it. The skin and muscles may be held back by clamps, and organs and tissues that are not being operated on are pulled out of the way by retractors. When the area to be treated is clearly visible, the surgeon is able to carry out the procedure.

Blood vessels that have to be severed during surgery are sealed in order to prevent serious loss of blood. This is done using electrocautery, a process in which blood vessels are sealed by an electric current applied through a pen-like instrument, or by tying off the severed ends of the vessels with synthetic thread. Lasers are also sometimes used during open surgery to seal blood vessels (*see* **Laser treatment**, p.613).

The operation site is kept free of blood and other fluids to ensure that the surgeon can see clearly what he or she is doing. Sponges and suction tubes are positioned around the area to remove fluids. The number of sponges used is counted carefully and is checked after the operation to make sure that they have all been removed. The surgeon checks that there is no internal bleeding before

---

▶ **TECHNIQUE**

Rejoining tissue

Tissues are rejoined after surgery to promote healing, stop bleeding, and prevent infection. There are various rejoining techniques and materials that can be used depending on the site and the type of tissue. Some materials are designed to dissolve as the tissues heal, and these are particularly useful for internal use. Materials that do not dissolve are used if healing is likely to take a long time or needs assessment before the stitches are removed.

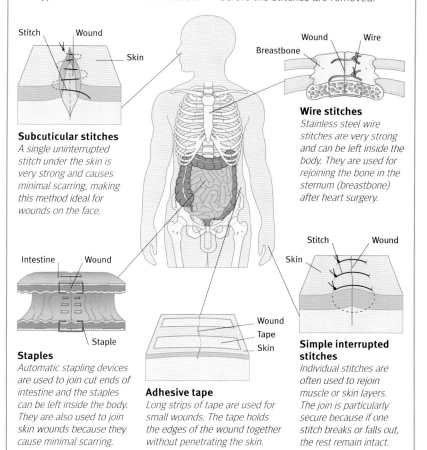

Subcuticular stitches
A single uninterrupted stitch under the skin is very strong and causes minimal scarring, making this method ideal for wounds on the face.

Staples
Automatic stapling devices are used to join cut ends of intestine and the staples can be left inside the body. They are also used to join skin wounds because they cause minimal scarring.

Adhesive tape
Long strips of tape are used for small wounds. The tape holds the edges of the wound together without penetrating the skin.

Wire stitches
Stainless steel wire stitches are very strong and can be left inside the body. They are used for rejoining the bone in the sternum (breastbone) after heart surgery.

Simple interrupted stitches
Individual stitches are often used to rejoin muscle or skin layers. The join is particularly secure because if one stitch breaks or falls out, the rest remain intact.

---

he or she sews up the wound (*see* **Rejoining tissue**, above). The wound may be covered with a sterile dressing.

What are the risks?
All surgical procedures, whether major or minor, involve some risk. For example, there may be an adverse reaction to the anaesthetic, excessive bleeding, formation of blood clots, or infection.

A general anaesthetic can provoke changes in heart rhythm during or after surgery. The risk of this is higher if you are elderly, have a heart problem, or are overweight. In rare cases, an allergic reaction to the anaesthetic may occur.

Rarely, if blood vessels are not fully sealed, excessive bleeding may occur during the operation, or there may be persistent bleeding afterwards. In either case, a blood transfusion (p.272) may be required. A supply of cross-matched (compatible) blood is made available for each person having major surgery.

After surgery, blood has an increased tendency to clot, which may lead to the formation of blood clots in the deep veins of the legs (*see* **Deep vein thrombosis**, p.263). These blood clots may cause pain and swelling in the leg, and they can sometimes travel to the lungs. If a blood clot becomes lodged in an artery that supplies a lung, it can cause chest pain and shortness of breath and may be life-threatening (*see* **Pulmonary embolism**, p.302). To reduce the risk of blood clots developing, you will be encouraged to move around as soon as you can after the operation. Treatment with drugs such as heparin (*see* **Drugs that prevent blood clotting**, p.584) may be given during and after surgery to thin the blood. Painkillers (p.589) may also help to prevent the formation of blood clots by allowing you to move around more easily without pain.

Infection may occur if bacteria or other microorganisms enter a wound during or after surgery, preventing or delaying the healing process and causing tissue damage and fever. The risk of infection is minimized by performing the operation in a highly sterile environment with instruments that have been carefully sterilized. Antibiotics (p.572) may be given before, during, or after surgery to help to prevent infection.

Endoscopic surgery

Surgical procedures that use a viewing instrument inserted through a natural body opening or through skin incisions

Endoscopic surgery is a technique that enables various procedures to be performed without making large incisions in the skin. An endoscope is a tube-like viewing instrument with a light source. Some endoscopes have a built-in miniature camera.

Endoscopes are inserted either through a natural body opening, such as the anus, or through a small incision, depending on the site to be accessed. Endoscopic surgery performed through skin incisions is often referred to as minimally invasive surgery (*see* Having minimally invasive surgery, below). Endoscopes may be flexible or rigid (*see* Flexible endoscopy, p.138, and Rigid endoscopy, p.139) and are used to provide a view of the inside of body cavities, either directly through the endoscope or on a screen.

Endoscopes may be used to carry out treatment, to examine a particular area, or to take tissue samples. Tiny instruments, such as forceps and scissors, are passed through small incisions in the skin or through side channels in the endoscope to reach the operating site. These instruments are operated by the surgeon, who is guided by the view through the endoscope or on the screen.

Since endoscopic surgery may not involve any incisions or only require small ones, the length of stay in hospital and recovery time are shorter than for open surgery. Bleeding from any small incisions that have been made is minimal. Therefore, the wounds heal more quickly and are less likely to become infected than the large incisions that are needed in open surgery.

When is it used?

Endoscopic surgery may be used to operate inside any part of the body that is large enough for the instruments to be inserted into and moved around. Suitable sites include the chest, abdominal cavity, pelvic cavity, digestive tract, large joints, such as the knee and hip, and the nasal sinuses. Endoscopes have different names according to the part of the body in which they are used. For example, laparoscopes are

▶ **PROCEDURE**

Having minimally invasive surgery

Minimally invasive surgery allows the surgeon to examine and treat disorders in body cavities, such as the abdomen, through small incisions. An endoscope (a tube-like viewing instrument with a light source and a camera) is inserted through one incision to provide a view of the cavity.

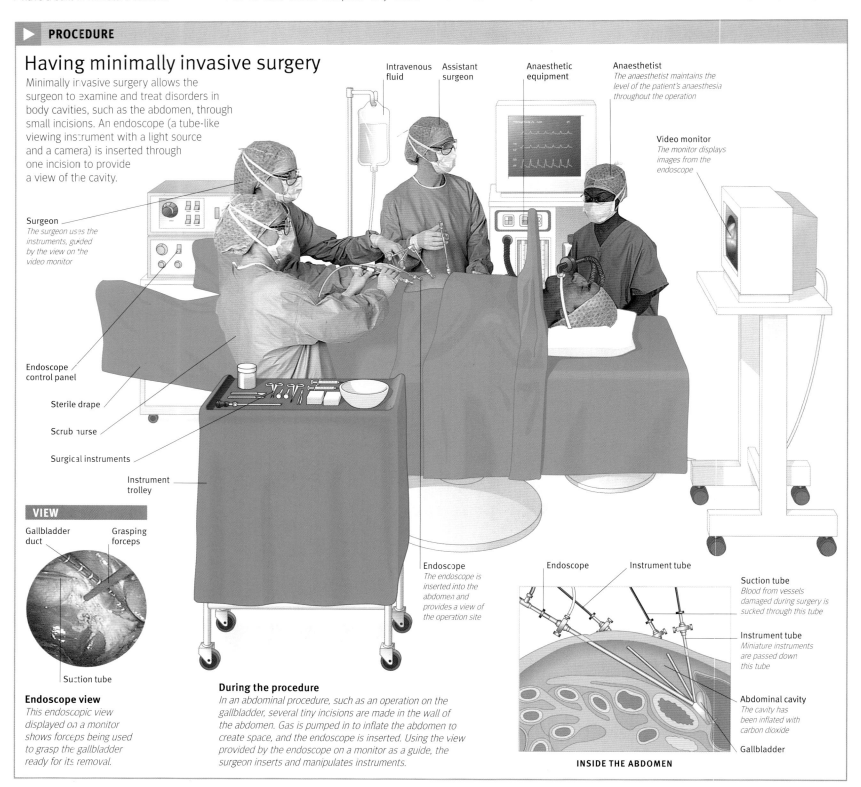

Intravenous fluid

Assistant surgeon

Anaesthetic equipment

Anaesthetist
The anaesthetist maintains the level of the patient's anaesthesia throughout the operation

Video monitor
The monitor displays images from the endoscope

Surgeon
The surgeon uses the instruments, guided by the view on the video monitor

Endoscope control panel

Sterile drape

Scrub nurse

Surgical instruments

Instrument trolley

Endoscope
The endoscope is inserted into the abdomen and provides a view of the operation site

Endoscope

Instrument tube

Suction tube
Blood from vessels damaged during surgery is sucked through this tube

Instrument tube
Miniature instruments are passed down this tube

Abdominal cavity
The cavity has been inflated with carbon dioxide

Gallbladder

INSIDE THE ABDOMEN

VIEW

Gallbladder duct

Grasping forceps

Suction tube

Endoscope view
This endoscopic view displayed on a monitor shows forceps being used to grasp the gallbladder ready for its removal.

During the procedure
In an abdominal procedure, such as an operation on the gallbladder, several tiny incisions are made in the wall of the abdomen. Gas is pumped in to inflate the abdomen to create space, and the endoscope is inserted. Using the view provided by the endoscope on a monitor as a guide, the surgeon inserts and manipulates instruments.

used in the abdominal cavity, broncho-scopes are used to look in the lungs, and colonoscopes are used inside the colon.

If you have symptoms that suggest a disorder of the reproductive system, diges-tive tract, lungs, sinuses, or bladder, an endoscope may be inserted through the vagina, anus, mouth, nose, or urethra in order to investigate the affected area. Endoscopy through natural openings may be repeated safely many times and can be used to monitor a condition such as a peptic ulcer (p.406).

When the area under investigation can-not be accessed through a natural body opening, small incisions need to be made for the endoscope and other instruments. For example, if you have a disorder of the gallbladder, appendix, or some parts of the female reproductive system, such as the fallopian tubes, a laparoscope may be inserted through an incision in the abdomen to carry out investigations or treatment (*see* **Laparoscopy**, p.476). Laparascopes are also used in female sterilization (p.476). If you have a dis-order of the joints, such as arthritis, or a damaged cartilage or ligament, an arthroscope inserted through a small incision may be used to view and possibly to operate on the affected joint (*see* **Arthroscopy**, p.228).

What happens during the operation?

Endoscopic surgery through natural open-ings in the body, such as the throat or anus, may not need an anaesthetic or may take place under sedation or local anaes-thesia. This means that you remain conscious, but the area being operated on is numb (*see* **Having a local anaesthetic**, p.608, and **Having a regional anaesthetic**, p.610). After the endoscope has been inserted into the body opening, surgical instruments may be introduced through specific channels in the endoscope.

The majority of endoscopic surgical procedures through incisions are per-formed under general anaesthesia (*see* **Having a general anaesthetic**, p.609). An incision about 13 mm (½ in) long is made for the endoscope, and then further tiny incisions are made so that instruments, such as lasers (*see* **Laser treatment**, p.614) and scissors, can be inserted if needed. In a laparoscopic operation on the abdomen, a tube is inserted through an incision, and gas is pumped through it to inflate the abdominal cavity, giving the surgeon a better view and more operating space.

The surgeon looks at the procedure through an eyepiece on the endoscope and also observes a magnified image of the operating site transmitted to a video monitor. The surgeon's colleagues can also watch the procedure on the screen.

When the operation is complete, the endoscope and all the instruments are removed. The incisions are then closed, often with a single stitch.

▶ PROCEDURE

Having microsurgery

Microsurgery is a technique that allows delicate operations to be performed on very small structures in the body. The technique is used for a number of procedures, such as repairing damaged blood vessels and nerves. Microsurgery is also frequently used to remove the eye lens of someone with a cataract and to operate on the tiny bones in the middle ear.

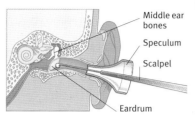

INSIDE THE EAR
During the procedure
The surgeon views the operating site through a powerful microscope and uses extremely small instruments. Here an operation is being carried out on delicate structures inside the ear.

Middle ear bones
Speculum
Scalpel
Eardrum

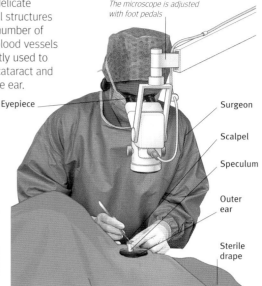

Operating microscope
The microscope is adjusted with foot pedals

Eyepiece
Surgeon
Scalpel
Speculum
Outer ear
Sterile drape

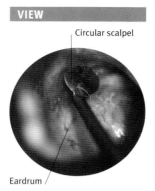

VIEW
Circular scalpel
Eardrum

The operation site
This view through the operating microscope shows a tiny circular scalpel being used to make a small incision in the eardrum to give the surgeon access to the bones of the middle ear.

What are the risks?

The risk of damage to a body organ or blood vessel is slightly greater with endoscopic surgery than it is with open surgery (p.611) because the surgeon has to work in a more restricted area. As with all types of surgery, there is a risk of an adverse reaction to the anaes-thetic. During the operation, the surgeon may need to access a larger area and per-form open surgery. For this reason, before an endoscopic operation you will also be asked for your consent to open surgery.

Microsurgery

Surgical procedures that use magnifying equipment and tiny surgical instruments to operate on small or delicate structures

Microsurgery makes it possible to perform operations on extremely small or delicate tissues in the body. In this form of surgery, a surgeon uses a binocular microscope to view the operating site and specially adapted small operating instruments. Using microsurgery, delicate surgical procedures can be carried out that would be difficult or impossible with other surgical techniques.

When is it used?

Microsurgery is most commonly used to operate on tissues such as nerves and blood vessels and on small structures in the eye, middle ear, and reproductive sys-tem. For example, microsurgery can be used to repair a detached retina (*see* **Retinal detachment**, p.360). It can also be used to remove the diseased eye lens of someone with a cataract and replace it with

an artificially made lens (*see* **Cataract sur-gery**, p.357). In the disorder otosclerosis (p.375), deafness may occur when a bone in the middle ear becomes diseased and is unable to transmit sound. Hearing can be restored using microsurgery to replace the diseased bone with an artificial substitute.

During an operation to reattach a sev-ered limb or digit, microsurgery is used to reconnect severed nerves and blood vessels. Microsurgery is also used to try to reverse two sterilization procedures: tubal ligation in women (*see* **Female steriliza-tion**, p.476) and vasectomy (p.461) in men. Sterilization in women involves cutting or sealing the fallopian tubes. In a vasectomy, the narrow tubes that carry sperm from the testes to the penis are severed, preventing the release of sperm. In both cases, micro-surgery procedures can be used to rejoin the sealed or severed tubes accurately, and, in many cases, a person's reproductive function can be restored.

What happens during the operation?

Microsurgery is normally carried out under general anaesthesia (*see* **Having a general anaesthetic**, p.609). However, regional or local anaesthesia (*see* **Having a regional anaesthetic**, p.610, and **Having a local anaesthetic**, p.608) may be used for some minor surgical procedures, such as cataract operations.

During the operation, the surgeon views the operating site through a binocu-lar microscope, which is operated using foot pedals. This leaves his or her hands free to use small precision instru-ments, including scissors, forceps, and clamps (*see* **Having microsurgery**, above). To repair nerves and blood vessels, small needles and fine thread are used to make tiny stitches.

What are the risks?

Any type of surgery involves some risk, whether from a reaction to the anaesthetic, excessive bleeding, formation of blood clots, or infection. Some microsurgical operations take longer to carry out than other similar surgical procedures, which means that the time under anaesthesia is longer. This increases the risk of adverse reaction to the anaesthetic and may extend the recovery time from anaesthe-sia. The risk of infection may be greater with microsurgery since the operating site is exposed for a relatively long time com-pared with other procedures.

There is a high success rate for many of the most routine microsurgical procedures, such as cataract removal and repair of reti-nal detachment. However, some procedures, such as reattachment of severed limbs or reversal of female sterilization, have lower success rates, which are partly determined by the extent of the tissue damage. Nevertheless, without microsurgery, opera-tions such as these could not be attempted.

Laser treatment

Procedures using intense beams of light to cut, join, or destroy tissue

Light from a laser can cut or destroy tissue or repair damaged tissue by fusing together torn edges. This ability allows lasers to be used in a number of surgical procedures in place of scalpels, scissors, and stitches.

A wide range of lasers is used for various purposes, including treatment of skin problems, operations on the eye, and internal operations that are carried out in conjunction with endoscopes (*see* **Endoscopic surgery**, opposite page).

Since laser beams can be focused precisely, small sections of tissue can be treated without causing damage to the surrounding tissues. Lasers produce differing wavelengths of light that are absorbed by different types of tissue. For example, a wavelength of light that is absorbed by melanin (the dark pigment that gives skin its colour) may be effective in removing a mole caused by the overproduction of melanin. A wavelength that is absorbed by blood causes clotting to occur and prevents bleeding from tissues cut during treatment.

Lasers generate intense heat, and laser treatment is therefore given in short bursts to avoid burning.

When is it used?

Laser treatment is used in gynaecological procedures. A laser beam can be directed into the body through an endoscope to remove scar tissue inside the fallopian tubes, which may cause infertility. Lasers are also used to remove cysts that form in the pelvic area due to endometriosis (p.475) and to destroy abnormal cells on the cervix that, if left untreated, may develop into cancer (see **Cervical intraepithelial neoplasia**, p.480).

Small tumours or precancerous cells in other internal body areas, such as the larynx or inside the digestive tract, can be destroyed by laser beams directed through an endoscope. The technique can also be used to open arteries that have become narrowed by fatty deposits (see **Atherosclerosis**, p.241). In ophthalmic surgery, laser beams can be used to seal small tears in the retina, the light-sensitive layer at the back of the eye (see **Retinal detachment**, p.360).

Laser treatment is often used on the skin, especially on the face, for reducing scar tissue and birthmarks (p.537), noncancerous moles (p.199), wrinkles, or tattoos (see **Laser treatment on the skin**, below). The results depend on the extent of the problem but in most cases scarring is minimal, and the appearance of the skin is much improved.

External laser treatment can also be used to treat conditions such as spider veins and to remove warts (p.206) on the skin and genital warts (p.493).

What happens during the treatment?

Most forms of laser treatment are performed under either local or general anaesthesia, depending on the type of surgery and the area to be treated. However, for minor skin conditions, laser treatment causes little discomfort and may be performed without anaesthesia. There may be some swelling, redness, and blistering, which usually disappear within a week. Large areas of skin may need to be treated over several sessions.

What are the risks?

Occasionally, laser treatment may cause scarring, or there may be incomplete removal of damaged tissue. Skin treated by laser may also be vulnerable to infection until it has healed completely. The intense heat of the laser can sometimes lead to coarsening of the skin.

▶ **PROCEDURE**

Laser treatment on the skin

Lasers can be used to remove tattoos and birthmarks from the skin by destroying cells with a particular colour, such as cells in red birthmarks. A laser beam can also be used to reduce the severity of scars and the effects of aging, such as wrinkles, by removing the top layer of cells to smooth the skin. The beam of high-intensity light is precise and does not cause damage to surrounding cells.

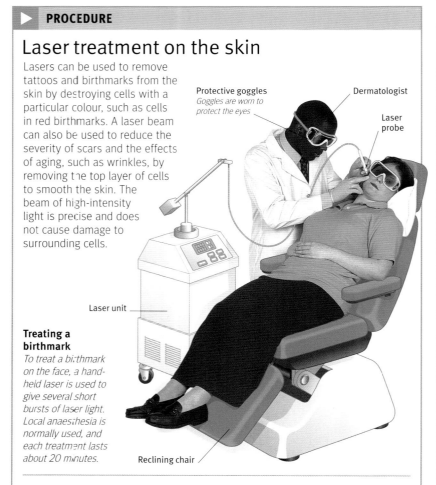

Protective goggles
Goggles are worn to protect the eyes

Dermatologist

Laser probe

Laser unit

Treating a birthmark
To treat a birthmark on the face, a handheld laser is used to give several short bursts of laser light. Local anaesthesia is normally used, and each treatment lasts about 20 minutes.

Reclining chair

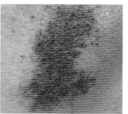

BEFORE TREATMENT

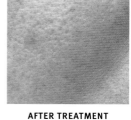

AFTER TREATMENT

Effect of treatment
Laser treatment destroys the cluster of blood vessels under the skin that make up the birthmark. In some cases, a course of several treatments is needed before noticeable improvement is seen and the birthmark disappears completely.

Plastic surgery

Procedures used to repair and reconstruct skin and underlying tissue or alter its appearance

Skin or tissue that has been damaged or destroyed as a result of disease or injury or that has been malformed since birth can often be repaired or reconstructed using plastic surgery. The aim of plastic surgery is to restore the appearance and function of the affected area as much as possible with minimal visible scarring. A form of plastic surgery known as cosmetic surgery may be used in healthy people to disguise the signs of aging or to change the shape of part of the body. Cosmetic surgery may also be used following disease or injury. For example, skin grafting (p.183) can improve the appearance of burned skin, and breast reconstruction is often carried out after a mastectomy has been performed (see **Surgery for breast cancer**, p.488).

Some congenital conditions, such as a cleft lip and palate (p.558), can be corrected by plastic surgery. Plastic surgery can also be used in sex change operations to create or remove breasts and male and female genitals.

Before you have plastic surgery, it is important to obtain as much information as possible about the risks of the procedure and the likelihood of a good outcome. You should also check that the surgeon is well qualified and experienced in the techniques to be used.

What happens during the operation?

In most plastic surgery, general anaesthesia is needed (see **Having a general anaesthetic**, p.609). However, minor procedures, such as removing a mole, may be performed under local anaesthesia (see **Having a local anaesthetic**, p.608). Various surgical techniques may be used, depending on the nature of the operation. A technique that is commonly used in plastic surgery is skin grafting, in which a piece of healthy skin is detached from one part of the body and is placed over a damaged area in another part. Another commonly used technique is the skin and muscle flap, in which a section of skin and underlying muscle is moved from one area of the body to replace damaged tissue in another area. This technique may be used together with an implant to reconstruct a breast following a mastectomy.

Cosmetic surgery uses a range of techniques that are either the same or similar to those used in plastic surgery to alter a person's appearance. For example, in cosmetic surgery the techniques used to alter breast size are similar to those used to reconstruct a breast following a mastectomy.

What are the risks?

Plastic surgery carries the risks of infection and bleeding that all other types of surgery share. Swelling and bruising after the operation are also common. When skin is grafted, the graft sometimes fails to attach properly to the new area, and the procedure needs to be repeated.

There is also the risk that plastic surgery may not produce as satisfactory an effect as initially expected, and any operation in which the skin is cut will leave visible scars, although the surgeon will ensure that scarring is as minimal and unobtrusive as possible.

Transplant surgery

Operations carried out to replace failing body organs or tissues with healthy ones

Diseases can occasionally cause major organs, such as the heart, kidneys, or liver, to fail irreversibly. Dialysis (p.451) can take over the functions of the kidneys but may lead to a deterioration in health. Dialysis also has to be carried out frequently and is time-consuming. Replacing the diseased organ with a transplanted one is usually the best longterm treatment. In the case of a failing heart or liver, a transplant may be the only chance of survival if the organ has deteriorated significantly.

Many body organs and tissues can be transplanted. Kidney transplants are now common, and liver, heart, lung, and cornea transplants are performed routinely. Transplants of the intestines and pancreas are carried out less often. More than one organ may be transplanted at the same time, as in the case of heart and lung transplants. Stem cell transplants (which have largely replaced bone marrow transplants) are also performed.

▶ **TECHNIQUE**

Surgery using a heart–lung machine

A heart–lung machine takes over the function of the heart and the lungs. This allows the surgeon to operate on the heart during certain major chest operations, such as coronary artery bypass grafts, a heart transplant, or heart valve replacements. The heart is cooled and paralysed to stop it beating during surgery, and blood is diverted to the heart–lung machine, which oxygenates the blood, removes carbon dioxide, and then returns the blood to the body. Afterwards, the heart is restarted with an electric shock and the circulation is restored.

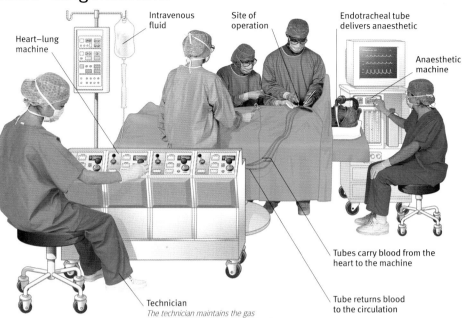

Heart–lung machine

Intravenous fluid

Site of operation

Endotracheal tube delivers anaesthetic

Anaesthetic machine

Tubes carry blood from the heart to the machine

Tube returns blood to the circulation

Technician
The technician maintains the gas content and temperature of the blood

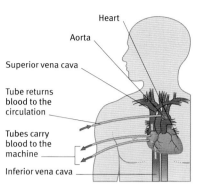

Heart

Aorta

Superior vena cava

Tube returns blood to the circulation

Tubes carry blood to the machine

Inferior vena cava

SITE OF THE CONNECTIONS

During the operation
Tubes from the heart–lung machine are inserted into the blood vessels entering and leaving the heart to divert blood through the machine. The heart is then stopped and the operation performed. Afterwards, the heart is restarted and disconnected from the machine.

Transplants are carried out not only to treat life-threatening conditions but also to improve quality of life when a condition is not potentially fatal. For example, a damaged cornea that causes loss of vision can be repaired by a corneal graft to restore sight.

Organ and tissue transplants can be carried out only if a suitable donor organ can be found at the right time and if the person receiving the transplant has no other medical problems that could hinder his or her recovery.

Who are the donors?
Transplants are usually performed only when the tissue type and blood group of the donor and recipient are similar. This is necessary because the recipient's immune system will attack any organ it identifies as "foreign", a process known as rejection. Most transplant organs are removed from donors who have very recently been declared dead and who are unrelated to the recipient. However, stem cells and single kidneys can be taken from living donors without damaging their health. Part of the liver can also be donated by a living donor, because the remaining liver

tissue regenerates and liver function returns to normal within about 6–12 weeks of donation. When stem cells, a kidney, or part of the liver are donated by a close, living, genetic relative, often a brother or sister, the transplants are far less likely to be rejected by the recipient's body because the tissue types are likely to match more closely.

In the case of organ transplants from a donor who has recently died, most come from people in whom brain function has ceased irreversibly but whose other organs have been kept functioning by a life-support machine.

What happens during the operation?
Most transplant surgery requires general anaesthesia (*see* **Having a general anaesthetic**, p.609).

In an organ transplant, the organ to be transplanted is removed from the donor and chilled in a salt-containing solution until it reaches the operating room. This prolongs the time the organ can safely be deprived of its normal blood supply by a few hours. In most cases, the diseased organ is replaced by the donor organ.

However, in kidney transplants (p.452) the defective organ may be left in place and the new kidney placed in the pelvis, where it is connected to the appropriate blood vessels. During a heart transplant (p.257), the major blood vessels are connected to a heart–lung machine to oxygenate the blood and remove the carbon dioxide from it while the heart transplant is being carried out (*see* **Surgery using a heart–lung machine**, above).

In a stem cell transplant (p.276), cancerous or otherwise abnormal blood-producing cells are replaced by healthy cells from a related or unrelated donor, or from the recipient's own blood before the start of treatment. They are taken directly from the blood in a procedure similar to that of a blood donation. Before the transplant, the recipient is given chemotherapy and radiotherapy to eliminate abnormal stem cells. The healthy cells are then introduced directly into the bloodstream using a catheter.

After a transplant, you will probably spend several days in a critical care unit. With all transplants except the cornea, you will need to take immunosuppressant drugs (p.585) indefinitely to prevent your immune

system from rejecting the new organ or tissue. You should be able to leave hospital after a few weeks if the transplant has been successful. Recovery time for a corneal graft is shorter, and it is usually possible to go home after a few days.

What are the risks?
Transplant surgery, like other forms of major surgery, involves a risk of excessive bleeding and an adverse reaction to the anaesthetic. Transplant surgery carries a higher risk of infection than other types of surgery because immunosuppressant drugs interfere with the body's natural defences. However, the greatest risk of this type of surgery is that the transplanted organ will be rejected by the immune system and that this will cause the organ to fail.

Following a major transplant operation, the chances of long-term survival improve significantly once the first year after the operation has passed. However, survival depends on the transplanted organ not being rejected and on the recipient remaining free of a serious infection. The best outcomes are usually in people who were otherwise healthy when the original organ failed.

Care and therapies

In spite of advances in the prevention and early detection of disease, most of us need treatment from time to time to relieve symptoms or cure an illness. Major surgery and treatment for serious short-term illness still take place on an inpatient basis in hospital, although people are now discharged as soon as possible. However, many long-term treatments and procedures now take place in the home or in an outpatient department without the need for admission to hospital.

THE RANGE OF care and therapies that is available today to treat illness and injury is extensive. The first choice for most people is treatment recommended by their doctor, which is usually with drugs, surgery, or, in some cases, with therapies such as physiotherapy or occupational therapy. Your doctor recommends such treatments because their effectiveness is supported by evidence from properly conducted trials. There is also a wide range of complementary therapies available, such as acupuncture, homeopathy, and hypnotherapy. However, in most cases there is little or no scientifically sound evidence to support their effectiveness. Consequently, your doctor will not usually recommend complementary therapies, although he or she may sometimes suggest a complementary therapy if there is evidence that it is effective and if he or she feels it might be useful in your particular case.

Location of care
The current emphasis is on providing care and therapies either in the home or in outpatient departments rather than in hospital. There are two reasons for this trend. The first is that the cost of hospital care is far greater than the cost of care as an outpatient. Secondly, visiting an outpatient department or receiving care in familiar surroundings is, for most people, preferable to being in hospital. However, there are times when hospital facilities and a skilled medical team are essential, as in the case of severe illness or injury or when a person who has a long-term illness cannot be cared for at home.

Choice of therapies
The type of care or therapy that is most appropriate for an individual depends on the severity of the illness or injury. Choice is an important element, and

health-care professionals always try to consider the wishes of the individual. At one extreme, a person with an acute illness or a serious injury may require emergency admission to hospital and treatment in an intensive therapy unit. At the other extreme, a person who has strained a muscle may only need to have a short course of physiotherapy in a local outpatient department.

Therapies such as physiotherapy and occupational therapy are used to rehabilitate a person, usually following an acute illness or injury. They also help a person to remain independent during a long-term illness. Of equal importance are psychological therapies that are used to treat mental health problems, such as depression.

Complementary therapies have been used for centuries and many have seen a surge in popularity in recent years. However, doctors tend to restrict their recommendation of complementary

therapies to the ones that, like all conventional medical treatments, are backed by sound evidence from controlled trials, and few complementary therapies meet this criterion.

Care of the dying
Over the last few decades, there has been an increasing awareness that a person who is dying has unique needs. As a result, caring for people with a terminal illness has become a medical

speciality. The medical and nursing care that addresses the needs of people who are dying is known as palliative care, and its main focus is on relieving distressing symptoms, such as pain and shortness of breath, with drugs and other techniques. The overall aim of palliative care is to provide a comfortable and dignified death while giving support to the partner and/or family of the dying person.

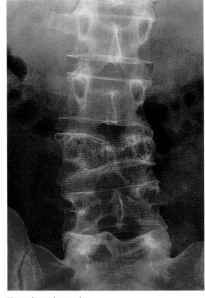

Treating the spine
Either conventional or complementary therapies may be used to relieve back pain.

✚ PROCEDURE

Care at home

If you have an illness or disability that does not require admission to hospital, you will probably be cared for at home by a partner, close friend, or relative. Helping you with daily tasks, such as washing and dressing, does not necessarily require particular nursing skills. However, if you are very disabled, these tasks may require extra time and patience.

Dressing and undressing
If you have a disability, such as a weak limb following a stroke, you may require help from your carer to dress and undress.

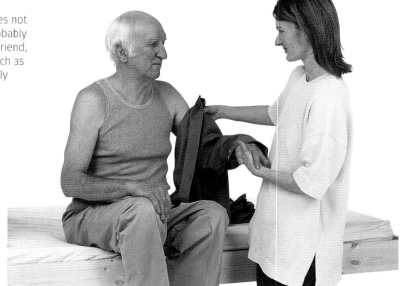

Care of the sick

Many people are referred for treatment or need nursing care at some time in their lives, but increasingly this takes place without a stay in hospital. The high cost of care in hospital and advances in medical techniques have created a trend for treatment on a day care basis, either in hospital or another medical facility, such as an outpatient clinic, and for nursing care at home.

The first article in this section looks at ways of accessing hospital care, either through accident and emergency services or when you are referred to a specialist for treatment.

Day care (care that does not need an overnight stay in hospital), also known as ambulatory care, is provided in a number of settings. The development of less invasive surgical techniques has enabled many treatments that would once have required a hospital stay of several days to be carried out on a day care basis.

The article on hospital care looks at the various reasons why you might be admitted to hospital and provides an overview of hospital routines. The different levels of care, from routine care on a general hospital ward to intensive care for people who are critically ill, are also described here.

Finally, the advantages of nursing care in the home are discussed, including the need for support for carers.

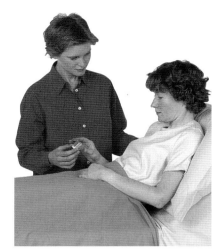

Care in the home
Drugs and other treatments, including some that require specialized equipment or medical expertise, can often be delivered just as effectively at home as in hospital.

Accessing hospital care

Being referred to hospital for secondary care or going straight to hospital in an emergency

Most health problems can be diagnosed and treated at primary health care level by general practitioners (GPs) or other primary care medical personnel. However, if you have an injury or illness that requires special tests and/or expertise, you may need to go to hospital or another secondary care unit.

The usual way of accessing hospital or secondary care is by referral, either from a GP or from another medical professional at a primary care centre (a walk-in centre, for example). People also have direct access to hospital treatment when they go to an accident and emergency department. Some hospital clinics are also run on the basis of self-referral, such as clinics for sexually transmitted infections (called STI clinics or genito-urinary medicine clinics).

Referral to hospital
If your GP or another medical practitioner at a primary care centre thinks that your condition may be serious and requires urgent attention, he or she will refer you to hospital for immediate assessment and treatment or will arrange for an urgent appointment with an appropriate specialist. For less urgent conditions, you may have to wait longer after referral for an appointment with a specialist.

Going straight to hospital
People with urgent medical problems may be treated in the accident and emergency department of a hospital, and are sometimes admitted to hospital for further care if it is needed.

You may be taken to hospital by ambulance after an accident, or emergency admission may be arranged by your GP or another medical practitioner. For example, if you have severe chest pain that suggests a heart attack, you may be taken straight to hospital by ambulance. If your condition is serious, paramedics may stabilize your condition or begin treatment on the way.

Many people go to the accident and emergency department themselves after an accident or because they have severe symptoms, such as bleeding. However, every year thousands of people arrive at hospital with minor health problems that could have been dealt with by their GP or another health practitioner at a primary care centre. If your injuries or symptoms are not severe, you should consider seeing your GP, going to a walk-in centre or minor injury unit, or calling the NHS 111 service (dial 111) for advice.

Day care treatment

Secondary care that does not require an overnight stay in hospital

Many secondary-care treatments are now carried out without the need for an overnight stay in hospital. For example, you may be treated in an outpatient clinic or attend hospital or another medical centre and return home on the same day as your treatment. This form of care is also known as ambulatory care. Most first consultations with a specialist take place in an outpatient clinic or day care unit. You may also need to go to an outpatient clinic, diagnostic and treatment centre, or go to hospital on a day care basis for more complex tests, such as coronary angiography (p.245).

What treatment can be provided?
Many elements of hospital care, including giving specialist advice, prescribing drugs, and monitoring a person's condition, can be provided on a day care basis. In addition, a wide range of tests and treatments, including some surgical procedures, can be carried out successfully in outpatient clinics or day care units. For example, cataract surgery (p.357) on the eye is usually performed on a day care basis. Even some types of surgery performed under a general anaesthetic can now be done without needing an overnight hospital stay.

Hospital care

Medical and nursing care that require a stay in hospital

Day care treatment (above) is the preferred option for many procedures, but complicated treatments and severe illness may require hospital admission. Hospitals provide specialized medical and nursing care as well as expertise, treatments, and technology not available elsewhere. A stay in hospital is always necessary for major surgery. You may also need to be kept in hospital after minor surgery if you have a long-term disorder, such as a heart or lung disease, that increases the risk of complications.

You may need to be treated in hospital if you develop a serious illness or sustain a severe injury, or if you have a flare-up of an existing disorder, such as asthma (p.295). An elderly person may need time in hospital if his or her general health is poor. Children may be admitted to hospital for all of the above reasons or in particular circumstances, for example if a non-accidental injury is suspected. If a doctor is unsure about the cause of a child's symptoms, such as a high temperature or abdominal pain, the child may be need to be admitted to hospital for observation and investigations.

You may need to be cared for in hospital if you are living alone and become too ill to look after yourself adequately.

What are the types of care?
Many routine operations and procedures can be arranged in a hospital near your home, but some conditions may need treatment in a specialist centre. For example, some types of cancer, and rare metabolic disorders are sometimes treated in hospitals that have particular expertise in these disorders. In addition, there are specialist hospitals for people who have long-standing mental health problems, although, whenever possible, care is arranged in the community.

Routine admissions are to a general ward, but, if you are severely ill, you may need to be treated in an intensive therapy unit (p.618). Usually, children are cared for on children's wards in general hospitals, although there are some hospitals specifically for children.

General wards Most people are admitted to a general ward, which provides a wide range of routine care, or to a general surgical ward if they are to have surgery. There may also be wards that are designated for a particular branch of medicine or type of disease, such as oncology wards for cancer and coronary wards for heart disease.

You are usually allocated to a team of nurses who will be responsible for your care. Any medication that is needed will be given on a regular schedule, although drugs such as painkillers (p.589) will be given as and when they are needed. Your temperature, pulse, and blood pressure will be measured at regular intervals and recorded on charts so that your doctor can monitor your progress.

A particular consultant, with a team of doctors, is in charge of your treatment in hospital. Decisions about your care are made on medical rounds, when this team of professionals will examine you and discuss your condition. This is usually the best opportunity for you to ask questions about the results of tests, your treatments, and progress.

Most wards allow visiting for most of the day, but visitors may be advised to avoid early morning visits when staff are busiest. Visiting may be restricted immediately after a general anaesthetic.

Intensive therapy units People who are critically ill are usually admitted to an intensive therapy unit. These units differ from general wards in that they have a higher ratio of nurses to patients. They are also fully equipped with specialized equipment for treating and monitoring people who are seriously ill.

Admission to an intensive therapy unit is often necessary for monitoring after major surgery, such as transplant surgery (p.614) or heart surgery, or during a serious acute illness, such as a severe attack of asthma (p.295) or septicaemia (p.171). Intensive therapy may also be required after a person sustains a head injury (p.322) or other major injury.

Intensive therapy unit

Many hospitals have an intensive therapy unit, sometimes called an intensive care or critical care unit, that is devoted to caring for people in a critical or unstable condition who need continuous monitoring. Frequently, patients in these units require mechanical ventilation to assist or take over their breathing.

Blood pressure is checked continuously and heart rate and rhythm are monitored on an ECG machine. Fluids are given intravenously. If nutrients are required, they are supplied to the stomach through a tube or intravenously.

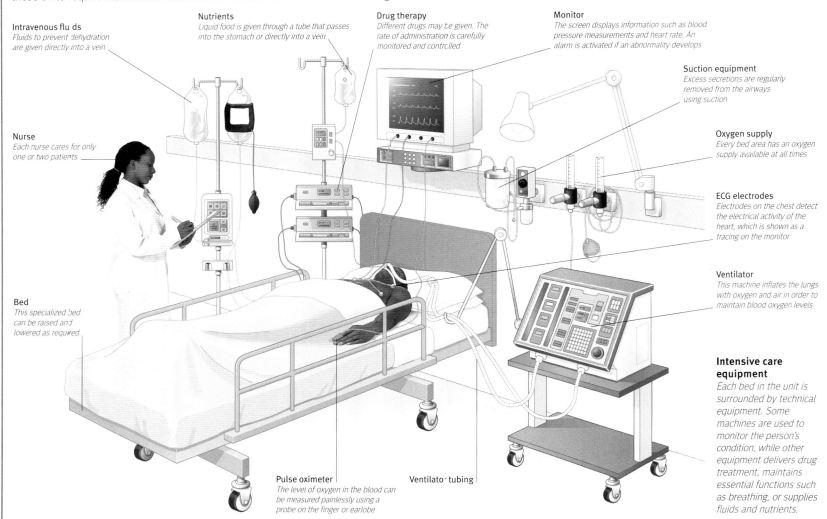

Intravenous fluids
Fluids to prevent dehydration are given directly into a vein

Nutrients
Liquid food is given through a tube that passes into the stomach or directly into a vein

Drug therapy
Different drugs may be given. The rate of administration is carefully monitored and controlled

Monitor
The screen displays information such as blood pressure measurements and heart rate. An alarm is activated if an abnormality develops

Suction equipment
Excess secretions are regularly removed from the airways using suction

Nurse
Each nurse cares for only one or two patients

Oxygen supply
Every bed area has an oxygen supply available at all times

ECG electrodes
Electrodes on the chest detect the electrical activity of the heart, which is shown as a tracing on the monitor

Bed
This specialized bed can be raised and lowered as required

Ventilator
This machine inflates the lungs with oxygen and air in order to maintain blood oxygen levels

Intensive care equipment
Each bed in the unit is surrounded by technical equipment. Some machines are used to monitor the person's condition, while other equipment delivers drug treatment, maintains essential functions such as breathing, or supplies fluids and nutrients.

Pulse oximeter
The level of oxygen in the blood can be measured painlessly using a probe on the finger or earlobe

Ventilator tubing

Some intensive therapy units specialize in treating particular conditions. For example, if you have had a heart attack (*see* **Myocardial infarction**, p.245), you will be treated in a coronary care unit where your treatment can be monitored continuously. Some hospitals have separate intensive therapy units for people who have serious kidney, liver, or nervous system disorders. Some hospitals also have a separate high-dependency unit, which provides more specialist nursing care and monitoring than is available on a general ward but less than in an intensive therapy unit. Newborn babies who are premature or unwell are usually monitored and treated in a special care baby unit (opposite page) or, if they are seriously ill, in a neonatal intensive therapy unit.

Children's wards Children are almost always admitted to children's wards, staffed by doctors and nurses who specialize in the treatment of children. There is often a playroom attached to the unit to allow sick children the stimulation and company of other children. Play therapists and teachers may visit to provide educational support. Usually, a child's main concern is being separated from the family, and parents are encouraged to spend as much time as possible with their child. There are usually facilities for parents to stay overnight.

Leaving hospital

The decision to discharge you from hospital will be made by your consultant after discussion with other members of the medical team and with you and your family. Ideally, your discharge will be planned in advance to allow time for any drugs that are needed to be prescribed and issued and any necessary follow-up care to be arranged.

After discharge from hospital, most people need no further care apart from follow-up appointments at an outpatient clinic or in a GP's surgery to check on their recovery. However, if you have a long-term disease or a disability as a result of illness, you may need rehabilitation, such as physiotherapy (p.620) or occupational therapy (p.621), at an outpatient clinic or in your own home.

Home care

Nursing care and medical treatment delivered in a person's own home

As part of the trend away from hospital admission, many people are now treated at home. Even when hospital treatment is unavoidable, time spent in hospital is kept to the minimum, and care is often transferred to the home. Depending on your circumstances, you may be cared for by visiting health-care professionals working with family carers or friends.

Apart from the comfort and convenience of familiar surroundings, one of the main advantages of home care is that it reduces the risk of infections that are sometimes acquired in hospital.

Home care may be required for only a short period of time, such as after minor surgery, or may need to be established on a long-term basis for a person who has a long-standing illness, such as multiple sclerosis (p.334) or Alzheimer's disease (p.331). Some people in the end stages of terminal illness choose to be at home for the final weeks of their lives.

Preparing the home

Depending on the severity of your illness and the extent of your disability, you may be advised to make practical adaptations to your home. Usually, an occupational therapist (*see* **Occupational therapy**, p.621) suggests which changes need to be made.

▶ **SETTING**

Special care baby unit

Premature or ill babies need treatment and monitoring in a special care baby unit. The normal mechanisms that regulate breathing and body temperature may not be fully developed in a premature baby. A heater keeps the baby's body at a constant temperature, and the baby may be attached to a ventilator if he or she needs assistance to breathe.

Intravenous fluids
Fluids given to avoid dehydration are carefully controlled

Wall panel
Electricity and oxygen supplies are delivered from a wall panel

Drug control unit
This unit regulates delivery of an intravenous drug

Parent
A baby's parents are encouraged to spend as much time as possible with their child

Heater
An overhead heater radiates constant heat to keep the baby's temperature at the correct level

Monitor
The baby's heart rate, blood pressure, and blood oxygen levels are continuously displayed on the screen

Ventilator
This machine takes over the baby's breathing by blowing oxygen-rich air into the baby's lungs

Cot
The baby may be placed in an open cot or in an incubator

Baby care equipment
A sophisticated machine monitors each baby and closely controls his or her environment. Other equipment assists body functions or supplies drugs, fluids, and nutrients.

If you are only temporarily immobilized following an injury such as a leg fracture, you may need to have wheelchair ramps placed over steps. If you are likely to be permanently immobile, doorways can be widened and equipment, such as a lift to manoeuvre you from a chair to the bed or into the bath, can be installed to minimize the physical strain on your carer.

What care can be provided?

A growing number of treatments can now be carried out at home, including drug treatments, basic and specialist nursing care, and rehabilitation. You or your carer can be shown how to manage many simple and some more complex procedures yourselves on a day-to-day basis, while remaining under the overall supervision of visiting professionals.

Drug treatment Drugs are usually given orally, but some are given as injections or using a nebulizer that delivers drugs in aerosol form through a mask. Some painkillers, anticancer drugs, and anti-nausea drugs may be given by continuous infusion using a syringe pump. Injected, nebulized, and infusion drugs are usually first given by a nurse, but you or your carer may be shown how to administer them.

Nursing care Nursing help at home may include changing wound dressings, monitoring healing, and helping to prevent pressure sores (p.203) in a person who

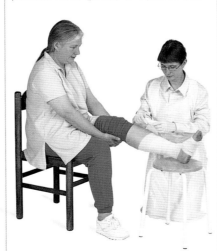

Changing a dressing
If necessary, a nurse can visit you regularly in your own home to change dressings and monitor the healing of a wound.

is confined to bed. Specialized support may be needed. For example, a person with a stoma, an opening from the bowel that has been surgically created in the wall of the abdomen (*see* **Colostomy**, p.422), will be shown how to manage it by a visiting stoma nurse.

Rehabilitation After major surgery or a disabling illness such as a stroke, you may need intensive rehabilitation to restore as much function as possible. A physiotherapist will arrange a programme of physical treatments, including massage and exercise (*see* **Physiotherapy**, p.620). You may also have occupational therapy (p.621) or speech therapy (p.621), depending on which skills you have lost.

Technical treatments Advances in technology have made some kinds of medical equipment much easier to use. As a result, treatments such as kidney dialysis (p.451) can sometimes be carried out at home. If you have difficulty eating or swallowing, nasogastric feeding, in which liquid nutrients are pumped through a nasal tube to the stomach, may also be performed in your own home. If the eating or swallowing difficulty is long term, you

may be given a PEG tube instead. This is a tube inserted through the abdominal wall and into the stomach, enabling nutrients to be delivered directly to the stomach. Like a nasogastric tube, a PEG tube enables feeding to be performed at home; unlike a nasogastric tube, a PEG tube cannot be seen while wearing clothes.

You as carer

As the partner, relative, or friend of a person who is ill, you may have made a conscious decision to become a carer. However, sometimes the role is taken on gradually as an ill, disabled, or elderly person becomes less able to cope. The role of carer can be physically and emotionally demanding, and you may find yourself neglecting your own health because of your other responsibilities. It is important that you do not ignore your own need for support. Joining a local support group to share experiences with people in a similar situation can make a difference. It may be possible to organize a period of respite care for the person you care for in a residential home, nursing home, or hospital.

Moving into long-term care

Eventually, long-term care may be needed for people with severe mental health problems, physical and/or learning difficulties, a degenerative disease such as multiple sclerosis, or a terminal illness. Elderly people who are physically frail or mentally impaired may also need to move into a long-term care facility, such as a residential home or a hospice.

Rehabilitation therapies

Rehabilitation therapies aim to allow people to live independent lives, either after an illness or injury or because of a problem present since birth. Some therapies are used to treat children with developmental problems. Although some of these therapies may be started in hospital, treatment frequently continues at home.

This section describes three major types of therapy used in rehabilitation: physiotherapy, occupational therapy, and speech and language therapy. Rehabilitation may involve more than one type of therapy, and usually a programme is developed to meet an individual's needs and circumstances, for example, cardiac rehabilitation following a heart attack or pulmonary rehabilitation for people with chronic obstructive pulmonary disease.

The goal of physiotherapy is to improve mobility and maintain the normal function of the body using physical techniques, such as exercise and massage. Occupational therapy helps people who have physical or mental illnesses to cope with everyday living and to remain as independent as possible. Speech therapy may be used to help people with communication problems or who have swallowing difficulties after a stroke.

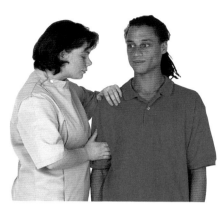

Assisting recovery
A variety of rehabilitation therapies can be used to relieve pain, speed the process of recovery, and help an individual to regain independence after an injury or illness.

▶ TECHNIQUE

Chest physiotherapy

Several techniques, including chest clapping and breathing exercises, are used in chest physiotherapy to prevent the accumulation of mucus in the lungs, which may otherwise lead to a chest infection. Chest physiotherapy is often used to help people with chronic obstructive pulmonary disease, elderly people after major surgery, and children with the inherited disorder cystic fibrosis.

Chest clapping
Parents of children with cystic fibrosis can be taught how to clap the child's chest to loosen mucus in the lungs. The child lies over pillows with the head low, and the chest is tapped with cupped hands. Mucus can then be coughed up easily.

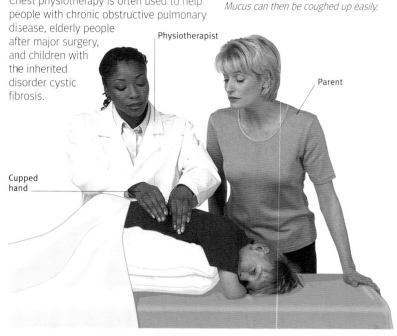

Physiotherapist

Parent

Cupped hand

Physiotherapy

The use of physical techniques, such as exercise and massage, to restore or maintain mobility and function

Physiotherapy is used to restore muscle strength and flexibility and to improve physical mobility after surgery, injury, or illness. It may also be used to help a person with a long-term disorder, such as arthritis (p.220), to maintain normal use of the body. In addition, physiotherapy can help to relieve pain and prevent complications from developing following an operation or an illness.

Physiotherapy may be combined with other types of treatment, such as drugs and occupational therapy (opposite page).

What does it involve?

The physiotherapist starts by taking a detailed medical history and evaluating your condition. Assessment may involve determining the strength and flexibility of your muscles, how well you are able to get in and out of bed, and whether you are able to walk unaided or need to use a walking aid or wheelchair. The physiotherapist draws up a treatment plan using one or more physiotherapy techniques. These may include exercise, heat and cold treatments, massage, hydrotherapy, electrical stimulation, ultrasound, and gait training. A form of therapy called chest physio-

therapy (right) may be used to prevent chest infections in people who are vulnerable because of illness or surgery.

Exercise Usually, the aim of exercise therapy is to strengthen weak muscles and increase flexibility. Exercise therapy is useful for anyone who has reduced movement in a limb. For example, this may occur after a person is confined to bed following knee surgery, after the limb has been immobilized to treat a fracture, or after a stroke. Anyone who has been confined to bed with a serious or long-term illness is likely to have lost muscle bulk and will also benefit from exercise. Your physiotherapist may show you exercises that you can do on your own, or, if you are unable to move a joint or limb, the physiotherapist may manipulate it to extend your range of movement. Equipment such as weights, treadmills, and exercise bicycles may be used in an exercise programme.

Heat and cold treatments A physiotherapist often uses heat to treat muscle injuries and joint stiffness caused by excessive exercise or arthritis. The application of hot packs to the affected area stimulates blood flow, relaxes tense muscles, and relieves pain. Cold treatments using ice or cold packs may be used to reduce pain and swelling.

Massage A physiotherapist uses his or her hands or specialized massage tools to knead muscles and stroke the body using circular or long, sweeping movements. Massage stimulates blood flow, which helps to reduce inflammation and relieve

fluid retention. Massage techniques are also used by physiotherapists to promote relaxation, which in turn helps to relieve localized pain and muscle spasm.

Hydrotherapy This form of therapy usually takes place in a heated pool and uses water to support the body, making movements easier or providing resistance to motion during exercise. Gentle exercise can help to improve muscle strength, flexibility, and general fitness. Hydrotherapy is helpful if you are unable to bear weight on a limb because of injury or a disorder such as arthritis.

Electrical stimulation In this type of therapy, a mild electric current is passed through pads applied to the surface of the skin to generate heat, which relieves stiffness and improves mobility in joints affected by injury or illness.

Ultrasound This form of therapy uses high-energy sound waves to create heat in the tissues, which helps to relieve pain and inflammation. This technique is often used to treat soft tissue injuries involving a ligament, tendon, or muscle and may be given in several sessions. A gel is applied to the skin, and an ultrasound probe is then placed on the skin and moved over the area being treated. After each session of ultrasound therapy, you may experience a slight tingling sensation in the affected area.

Gait training This training is used to help a person to walk again after an injury or an illness such as a stroke (p.329) or if

the person has a long-term disability. Various techniques may be used, including strength training, electrical stimulation, biofeedback, and treadmill training.

Chest physiotherapy This form of physiotherapy is used to manage breathlessness in people with chronic obstructive pulmonary disease (p.297), and to help prevent chest infections in people who have had major surgery or who have an illness that prevents them from clearing their lungs. In particular, elderly people who have had a major operation and children with the inherited disorder cystic fibrosis (p.535) may accumulate mucus in their lungs, which may cause infections. You may be shown breathing and coughing exercises that help to expand the chest and fill the lungs with air. Some techniques involve lying in a position that allows mucus to drain from the lungs while the chest is tapped with cupped hands (*see* **Chest physiotherapy**, above). If your child needs regular chest physiotherapy, you may be taught to use these techniques at home.

What can I expect?

You may need only a brief course of physiotherapy after a minor injury, but long-term therapy may be required after a major injury or illness. Physiotherapy helps to slow the progression of long-term disorders, such as cystic fibrosis, and reduce complications.

Occupational therapy

Treatment to encourage independence following a physical illness or injury or in people with a mental health disorder

The purpose of occupational therapy is to help a person with a physical or mental health problem to be as independent as possible. The therapy is tailored to each individual's needs and may include help with daily tasks, such as dressing, bathing, driving, food preparation, and going to the toilet. It can also help a person who is returning to work after a long illness or severe injury and help children with a disability to develop their full potential. Usually, referral for occupational therapy comes from your own doctor or a hospital doctor. Occupational therapy is incorporated in a comprehensive treatment plan, which may also include drugs and physiotherapy (opposite page).

When is it used?

Occupational therapy is used to help people cope with everyday living if simple tasks have become difficult because of a long-term disorder, such as multiple sclerosis (p.334) or arthritis (p.220). It is also used to aid recovery following hand or upper arm injuries or after a major illness, such as a stroke (p.329). An occupational therapist teaches a person how to conserve energy by using specialized techniques for daily tasks. A person may be shown how to use different muscles to carry out actions or to work with a variety of specialized aids.

Children who have learning difficulties or problems with coordination can benefit from occupational therapy. This therapy also helps elderly people to remain independent and active and may make enough difference to allow a person to stay in his or her own home.

Walking aid

If you need a walking aid, your occupational therapist will make sure that it is suitable for your needs at home as well as for outdoor use.

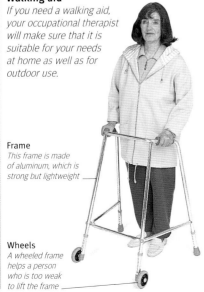

Frame
This frame is made of aluminum, which is strong but lightweight

Wheels
A wheeled frame helps a person who is too weak to lift the frame

In addition, occupational therapy is useful for people with a mental health problem such as schizophrenia (p.346). Once the main symptoms of the illness are under control, occupational therapy can help a person to adjust to living in the community by gradually increasing his or her independence, providing support, and preventing a relapse.

What does it involve?

At your first consultation, the occupational therapist starts by assessing your current health problems and past medical history. The therapist may arrange to visit you at home to observe how you manage with routine activities, such as dressing and bathing. The therapist may also ask you to perform specific tasks, such as making a hot drink. If your child needs to have occupational therapy, he or she is likely to be assessed by an occupational therapist who specializes in treating children.

Your occupational therapist will plan a therapy programme based on his or her initial assessment. The programme may include therapeutic activities and practical exercises to improve your performance of daily tasks. Your therapist may suggest or provide you with specialized equipment to make tasks easier.

Practical work If you need to build muscle strength, stamina, and concentration, your occupational therapist may recommend an activity such as a handicraft or cooking. For example, you may initially find it difficult to write following a stroke. Practical activities such as woodwork can help to improve your strength and fine muscle control, which may help you to regain near-normal dexterity and coordination. Fine muscle control of the hands and hand–eye coordination may also be improved by computer games.

Help with aids and equipment Your occupational therapist can provide a wide range of equipment to help you to increase your independence. For example, items such as slings or splints can help provide support for a weakened part of the upper body. If you have a long-term disorder that restricts mobility, you may need to use a walking aid. Some adaptations to your home, such as raised chairs, handrails, or a stairlift, may be necessary. You may be offered specially adapted devices that can help to make everyday tasks, such as opening jars, dressing, and eating, easier.

What can I expect?

Your occupational therapist may see you several times to check your progress and to ensure that your treatment is effective. You will be helped to regain as much of your independence as possible, although the extent to which this is achieved will depend on the severity of your disability and your mental attitude.

Speech therapy

Treatment to help people develop, improve, or recover their ability to speak

Speech therapy is used to help children and adults who have verbal communication problems. Speech therapy can benefit children whose speech is delayed by impaired hearing or learning difficulties or by physical problems, such as a cleft lip and palate (p.558).

People with a fluency problem, such as stuttering, may be given speech therapy, as may people who forget words or who have problems with comprehension or swallowing after a stroke (p.329). A speech problem with a physical cause, such as cancer of the larynx (p.294), may be helped by exercises or artificial aids.

What does it involve?

At your first appointment, your speech therapist will assess the extent of your speech problem and evaluate the effect that it has on your daily life. For children, the assessment is usually through observation of play. Adults are assessed on their ability to carry on a conversation and to perform tasks such as describing a picture. Part of the assessment conversation may be recorded on a computer and analysed later. This recording is used to determine whether your speech patterns, vocabulary, and the pitch, range, and volume of your voice are within normal ranges. If you find swallowing difficult as a result of a stroke, your speech therapist will advise you on eating and drinking safely.

The approach used in speech therapy depends on the problem, its cause, and the age of the person affected. Play therapy is often used to help children to improve their speech and is likely to be combined with other approaches, such as voice exercises. Parents or carers are taught useful games and exercises so that the child's speech improvement can continue at home.

Adults may be taught voice exercises or how to use artificial devices to aid communication. Speech difficulties that have been caused by a neurological problem such as a stroke may be helped by learning other ways of communicating. For example, you may be given a chart to indicate your basic needs until you are able to speak again.

Play therapy Children are frequently treated for speech problems using play therapy and games and by encouraging them to use both verbal and nonverbal communication. The speech therapist may also teach parents or carers how to encourage speech development at home by playing games that incorporate verbal description or naming.

Exercises If you have a condition that affects your mouth, tongue, or larynx (voice box), you may be given exercises that help to improve your articulation. For disorders that affect your fluency, you may be shown exercises to help you to control your speech and make you feel less anxious. If you have speech difficulties as a result of brain damage, such as a stroke, you may need to do exercises, such as describing pictures, to improve your word-retrieval abilities. In cases in which the larynx has been damaged or removed to treat cancer, a person can be taught to produce speech sounds by trapping air in the oesophagus and gradually releasing it.

Use of artificial devices There are a number of different electronic voice-synthesizers and artificial voice aids that may be used if speech difficulties are the result of a major physical problem. For example, if the larynx has been removed as part of treatment for cancer, a device called a tracheoesophageal voice prosthesis may be fitted. This device is inserted between the windpipe and oesophagus and uses inhaled air to produce sound. The sounds produced by the device can be converted into speech sounds using the lips, tongue, and teeth. Alternatively, a person may be taught to speak using a hand-held electromechanical device that generates sounds when it is pressed against the neck.

What can I expect?

Some problems, such as mild articulation problems, may improve with only a few weekly sessions of speech therapy. For other, more serious problems, regular speech therapy sessions over several months or years may be needed. Early treatment for children is particularly important because delayed speech affects the ability to relate to other people and may interfere with learning.

Psychological therapies

Many mental health problems, including depression, personality disorders, addictions, and eating disorders, may be helped by psychological therapies. There is a variety of therapies available, some of which explore a person's past while others focus on current behaviour or thought processes. The person in therapy is often encouraged to take an active role in the treatment.

The treatment of mental health problems with psychological therapy, or psychotherapy, was developed by Sigmund Freud at the end of the 19th century. Since that time, a number of different forms of psychological therapy have evolved. Some of the major types of therapy are described in this section, beginning with forms of psychoanalytic-based psychotherapy, in which the therapist tries to give a person insight into the effect of past experiences. The next two articles look at behaviour therapy and cognitive–behavioural therapy, which are based on changing the way people act or think. Both person-centred therapy and group therapy emphasize supporting the individual and helping people to achieve self-awareness and understanding. In the last article in this section, counselling is discussed. Counselling can help people who need to learn how to cope with personal problems and crises.

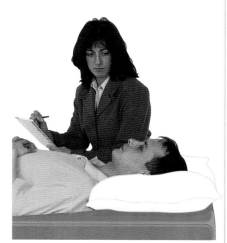

Psychoanalysis
In psychoanalytic-based psychotherapy, your therapist encourages you to talk freely about your past experiences. You work together to resolve your problems.

Psychoanalytic-based psychotherapy

Treatment that may help a person to overcome psychological problems by uncovering suppressed feelings

Psychoanalytic-based therapy tries to help people to identify, confront, and eventually work through their psychological problems. The therapy, which is also called psychoanalysis, is based on the theory that some painful feelings and memories are suppressed and confined to an unconscious part of the mind, and that these feelings may resurface as psychological problems.

In psychoanalytic-based psychotherapy, you are encouraged to talk freely about your past experiences and express openly the emotions that these recollections cause. Your therapist interprets the information you give to help you to gain insight into your psychological history and problems.

Classical psychoanalysis, as developed by Sigmund Freud, is the most intensive form and involves seeing a therapist several times a week for years. Today, other forms of psychoanalytic therapy that are less time-intensive than classical psychoanalysis are available.

When is it used?
Various forms of psychoanalytic-based psychotherapy may be helpful for people in whom the cause of their psychological problems is not immediately apparent. The aim of the therapy is to increase a person's awareness of the way in which past experiences may have shaped his or her present feelings and behaviour. For this reason, psychoanalytic-based therapy may be used to help people with long-term problems, such as chronic anxiety, panic attacks, depression, and relationship difficulties.

What does it involve?
During classical psychoanalysis, you will probably lie on a couch, with your therapist sitting nearby. The therapist will encourage you to talk freely about whatever comes to mind. This technique, known as free association, helps to uncover painful feelings or memories that you may have repressed. You may have 3–5 sessions per week, each session lasting for up to 1 hour, for 3–5 years.

In newer, less intensive psychotherapies based on psychoanalytical principles, you may sit with your therapist for sessions that typically take place once or twice a week. Therapy usually continues for 6 months to 2 years. All forms of psychoanalytic-based psychotherapy use similar basic techniques and methods. The therapist interprets your memories and dreams, and the feelings you express, and uses the interpretation as a basis for discussion.

The principal difference between the classical and the newer forms lies in the role of the therapist. In the newer forms, the therapist is more active in helping you to reveal information about your past.

A good relationship between you and your therapist is vital to successful treatment because you work together to resolve your problems over a relatively long period of time.

What can I expect?
Classical psychoanalysis is a time-consuming process, which you may find emotionally distressing at times. During the course of treatment, you may experience periods of vulnerability and despair when unwelcome feelings resurface before you feel able to deal with them. Supporters of psychoanalysis feel that the self-understanding that results from such distress leads to a resolution of psychological problems that outweighs the level of distress itself.

You might find the newer, briefer forms of therapy more acceptable than classical psychoanalysis because therapy with a time limit may motivate you to tackle specific issues by identifying and working through the underlying cause. You may find that your psychological problems are more likely to recur with shorter-term therapy, but you may be able to avoid this problem by obtaining support from group therapy (p.624) when your psychoanalytic-based therapy has come to an end.

Behaviour therapy

Techniques for changing inappropriate behaviour by substituting new behaviour

The aim of behaviour therapy is to alter abnormal or maladjusted behaviour associated with certain psychological conditions. The therapist works to modify a person's current behaviour but does not explore the underlying reasons, as would occur in psychoanalytic-based therapy (left).

Treatment is based on two ideas: desirable behaviour can be encouraged by using a system of rewards, and exposure to a feared experience or object under conditions where you feel safe will make it less threatening. Behaviour therapy is often used in combination with cognitive–behavioural therapy (opposite page), which explores and can change the thought processes and actions that lead to abnormal behaviour.

When is it used?
Behaviour therapy is useful in the treatment of a person with a phobia (p.341), which is an irrational fear that occurs in response to a particular object, creature, or circumstance. For example, a person may have an overwhelming fear of insects or air travel. Some people have a complex phobia, such as agoraphobia, which typically involves multiple fears about being trapped in crowds or being alone in open spaces.

People who have habitual behaviour, such as frequent, repeated handwashing (*see* **Obsessive–compulsive disorder**, p.342), or who lack assertiveness can also benefit from this therapy.

Behaviour therapy can also be used to treat certain eating disorders, such as anorexia nervosa (p.348) and bulimia (p.349), and it may help people with an anxiety-related problem such as panic attacks (*see* **Anxiety disorders**, p.341).

What does it involve?
Behaviour therapy begins with the therapist making a detailed analysis of your behaviour by interviewing you at length. You may be asked to rate the severity of your symptoms on a scale of 1 (mild) to 10 (extremely severe). Improvement may also be measured in this way. The therapist will discuss with you the best approach to overcoming your problem. The techniques that might be used include desensitization, and flooding, assertiveness training, and response prevention. Since changing ingrained behaviour often causes anxiety, you will probably be taught to use techniques such as controlled breathing and muscle relaxation to help you cope.

Desensitization and flooding Both desensitization and flooding are used to treat phobias. Desensitization involves gradually increasing exposure to the object or circumstance of the phobia (*see* **Desensitization therapy**, opposite page) and uses relaxation techniques to help you deal with the anxiety. For example, if you have agoraphobia, in early sessions you might walk just outside your house with the therapist. As sessions continue, you may try walking from the house to the end of the street with your therapist until, over time, you can travel alone without anxiety.

Flooding forces you to confront the focus of your fear directly for prolonged periods. You will be supported throughout by your therapist. After you have confronted the object or circumstance of your phobia, either gradually or in one step, the distress associated with it is reduced and may eventually disappear completely.

Assertiveness training This therapy uses role-play to demonstrate the appropriate responses to different situations, for example someone acting aggressively towards you. Your therapist shows you an appropriate response and, by copying it, you become more confident in your ability to deal with real situations.

Response prevention This technique is used in the treatment of compulsive rituals, such as repeated handwashing. You are encouraged to resist the urge to carry out the action, even though resistance results in intense anxiety. The therapist gives you support and suggests relaxation techniques. If you continue to successfully resist the compulsion, eventually the anxiety will lessen.

What can I expect?
You may find that improvement is slow at first and that it is difficult to avoid returning to your unwanted behaviour when your

▶ **TECHNIQUE**

Desensitization therapy

Desensitization therapy may help you to overcome a phobia. With the help of relaxation exercises in weekly sessions for several months, you will face the object or circumstance that you fear. You learn to overcome your phobia by facing the focus of it in its least distressing form and gradually working towards more direct contact.

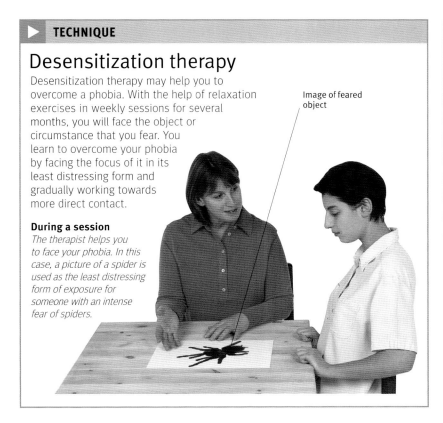

Image of feared object

During a session
The therapist helps you to face your phobia. In this case, a picture of a spider is used as the least distressing form of exposure for someone with an intense fear of spiders.

therapist is not there to support you. Group therapy (right) may be recommended to provide extra support when individual therapy ends.

Improvements in your behaviour can be maintained after your therapy has finished by carrying on with the techniques that you have learned.

Cognitive–behavioural therapy

An approach to overcoming psychological problems that aims to change unhelpful thoughts, beliefs, and behaviour

Often known simply as CBT, cognitive–behavioural therapy is based on the idea that some psychological problems arise from a person's erroneous or unhelpful cognitions (ways of perceiving and thinking about the world and/or oneself). These faulty cognitions can, in turn, result in unhelpful behaviour. CBT helps people to recognize and understand their current thought patterns and behaviour and shows them ways to consciously adopt more helpful thinking styles and behaviour. CBT does not always look at past events, although it incorporates methods of doing so when necessary.

When is it used?
People who suffer from depression (p.343) or those who lack confidence often benefit from CBT because it helps them to identify and change the thoughts and behaviour that contribute to their low mood or poor self-esteem. Such thoughts

may include "I am a failure", and "no one likes me because I am ugly"; such behaviour may include withdrawal from other people and avoiding situations that are perceived as being threatening.

By pointing out inconsistencies in thinking, cognitive–behavioural therapists can help people who have extreme concerns about their body shape, such as those with anorexia nervosa (p.348). Similarly, CBT can help people to break habitual patterns of thought and behaviour in, for example, obsessive–compulsive disorder (p.342).

In conjunction with drug treatment, CBT has been found to help some people with schizophrenia (p.346) to cope better with some of their symptoms, such as hearing voices.

What does it involve?
At the initial session your therapist assesses your problem, and together you decide on an approach to solve it.

People undergoing CBT are often asked to keep a diary of their thoughts, feelings, and behaviour. For example, someone suffering from anxiety might be asked to record the thoughts and feelings that precede and accompany an anxiety attack as well as what they did to cope.

During a therapy session, the therapist helps you to analyse the thoughts, feelings, and behaviour you have recorded and asks if you now feel they were appropriate to the circumstances. Once you identify the ones that are inappropriate, your therapist will then help you develop techniques for changing them.

In some people, attempts to change ingrained ways of thinking may produce anxiety. To help people cope with this

anxiety, the therapist may teach techniques such as breathing exercises and muscle relaxation.

You will probably see your therapist weekly for sessions lasting about 45 minutes to 1 hour. If you have a specific problem, such as stopping an unwanted habit, your therapy may last only for a few weeks. For more complex problems, such as low self-esteem, you may see your therapist for months.

What can I expect?
Once therapy is finished, you will probably need to make a conscious effort to analyse and challenge your thoughts, feelings, and behaviour for a while. However, many people find that their new, more appropriate patterns eventually become incorporated unconsciously.

Person-centred therapy

A process that aims to increase a person's self-esteem and encourages self-reliance

Person-centred therapy is based on the concept that an individual's behaviour arises from their inner feelings and self-image rather than from their responses to people or past experiences. Person-centred therapists avoid interpreting or explaining the information a person gives them, in contrast to therapists in psychoanalytic-based therapies (opposite page). Instead, the therapist gives a person support as he or she develops greater self-esteem and self-reliance.

The person-centred therapist is nondirective and helps to clarify a person's feelings and thoughts rather than telling him or her what to do or think.

When is it used?
Person-centred therapy may be used to treat long-term depression (p.343) and low self-esteem. This therapy is also used in crisis intervention to help people who are becoming increasingly overwhelmed by multiple stressful events. These events may be a combination of stresses such as problems at work, the failure of a marriage, or a physical or sexual assault. Person-centred therapy can be helpful in providing support, especially to individuals who need to work through their difficulties in an environment that feels safe.

Person-centred therapy is not often recommended for people with severe disorders, such as schizophrenia (p.346), in which the individual has no insight into his or her behaviour. Nor is this therapy considered appropriate for a person with severe mood swings (*see* **Bipolar affective disorder**, p.344) or obsessive–compulsive disorder (p.342).

What does it involve?
You and your therapist sit face to face while you speak about yourself, your relation-

ships, and your environment. From time to time, your therapist summarizes what you have said but does not judge or interpret it.

You will probably see your therapist for a weekly session of about 1 hour. The duration of the treatment depends on the time it takes you to feel more confident and in control of your life. It may take months if you are trying to overcome a specific crisis, such as the loss of a loved one. However, if you have a less specific problem, such as long-term depression, it may take more than a year.

Group therapy

Interaction with a small group of people to share experiences and feelings and gain insight or support

Group therapy is thought to be helpful in improving a person's ability to cope with and solve problems by discussing his or her experiences and emotions with a small group of people.

Each group session has one or more therapists who primarily help to guide the interaction that takes place. You may join a group directly or be referred to one in the course of individual therapy. Group therapy may use techniques from other forms of psychotherapy, such as psychoanalytic-based therapy (opposite page), behaviour therapy (opposite page), cognitive–behavioural therapy (left), and person-centred therapy (left).

When is it used?
Group therapy is used to treat a wide range of problems. For instance, it is helpful for people with irrational fears, those who have suffered serious physical or sexual assault, and those with addictions or habits that they are trying to break. It is also used to support and continue the therapy of people who have finished individual therapy.

Group therapy is not suitable for people who particularly need personal attention and privacy in which to examine their own experiences and feelings. It is also unsuitable for people who are shy or extremely introverted, or for those with severe disorders, such as schizophrenia (p.346) or bipolar affective disorder (p.344).

What does it involve?
There are two main types of group therapy. One is supportive therapy, in which people with similar problems share their experiences and learn how to cope from each other. In the other type of group therapy, people with diverse problems are brought together. The therapist conducts the sessions so that the interactions among the group members can be explored, with the aim of enabling individual members to develop increased self-understanding. The group setting also allows an individual to test out opinions or newly learned ways of thinking in the group before applying them to everyday life.

Supportive groups are usually run as open groups. The number of meetings is unlimited and members may join and leave when they choose. By contrast, mixed groups are usually run as closed groups. The therapist selects the members, who meet for a limited number of sessions, sometimes as few as six.

Groups usually meet weekly for sessions of 1–2 hours (see **Having group therapy**, below).

What can I expect?

It may take several sessions before you feel completely at ease in the group. You may also find that it will take some time before what you have learned in the group becomes part of your usual behaviour and thoughts. Some people find group therapy more useful than individual therapy, particularly if their problems relate to difficulties in interacting with other people.

Counselling

Support in identifying and addressing personal problems

People who are having trouble coping with their problems may use counselling to provide support and relieve distress. Counsellors act as a sounding board and encourage people to express their feelings, allowing them to take the lead in dealing with their problems.

Counselling can help support people who are sad, worried, or facing a crisis. You may find it helpful if you are having difficulty dealing with bereavement or if you are facing a terminal illness. However, if you have more deep-seated psychological problems, you may need a form of therapy in which the therapist plays a stronger and more active role, such as behaviour therapy (p.622) or cognitive–behavioural therapy (p.623).

For some problems, you may need a specific form of support. For example, you may require relationship counselling if you are in a troubled relationship or debt counselling if you are continually in financial difficulty.

What does it involve?

At the first session, which may take one hour or longer, the counsellor asks you about yourself and your background to build up a clear picture of you and your problem. You may also discuss what you want counselling to achieve.

At counselling sessions, which are usually held once a week, you decide, with the counsellor's guidance, what you discuss and the pace at which you discuss it. Your counsellor may suggest problem-solving exercises to help you deal with your problems one by one.

Counselling may be short-term if you are dealing with a situation such as a bereavement, or long-term to help with a more complex problem.

What can I expect?

You may find that talking about your problems is enough to help you to find a solution. With your counsellor's support, you should be able to develop ways to solve your problems. In counselling, it is often easier than in some other therapies to see whether specific goals have been achieved.

▶ **TECHNIQUE**

Having group therapy

Group therapy encourages people to share problems and feelings with others, and some people find that it provides better motivation for change than individual therapy. Supportive group therapy may help you to overcome lack of self-esteem or confidence or an addiction. Therapy in groups of people with diverse problems may be useful because the relationships within the group raise issues and help to solve problems.

During a session
A therapist and up to 12 group members sit informally in a circle. The therapist directs group discussions and encourages one member at a time to talk in front of the group about their problems or feelings. The group may also be coached through role-play sessions.

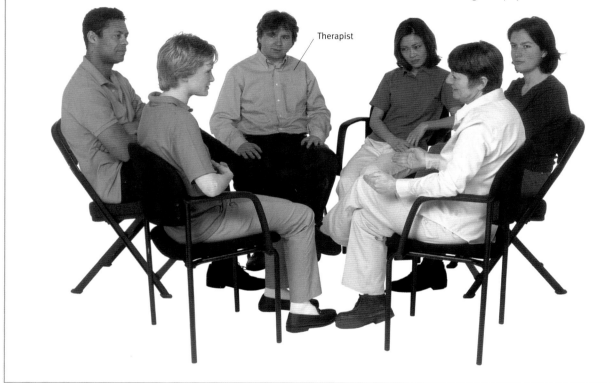

Therapist

Index

A page number in *italic typeface* indicates a separate illustration, an illustrated box, or a table.

Acknowledgments

The publisher would like to thank the following for their help in previous editions:

LOAN OF EQUIPMENT A.K (UK); Heather Auty, Cochlear Implant Ltd.; Roseanne Aitken, Oxford Instruments Medical Systems Division; Robert Bosch Ltd.; Central Medical Equipment Ltd.; Department of Clinical Neurophysiology, University College London Hospital NHS Trust; Dukes Avenue Practice; Peter Edwards, Birmingham Optical; Keep Able Ltd.; London Laser Clinic; Mothercare UK Ltd.; PC Worth Ltd.; Porter Nash Medical Showroom; data for the graph on page 25 was derived from *The Health Benefits of Smoking Cessation*, US Department of Health and Human Services, Centers for Disease Control, DHHS Publication No. (CDC) 90-8416, 1990.

EXPERT MEDICAL ADVICE Sue Bateman MB ChB FRCOG DObst, Obstetrics and Ultrasound Department, St. Peter's Hospital, Chertsey; Valerie Dawe; Department of Clinical Neurophysiology, The Royal Free Hospital NHS Trust, London; Department of Clinical Neurophysiology, University College London Hospital NHS Trust; Anthony C. de Souza FRCS, Cardiology Department, Royal Brompton Hospital, London; Karen Ferguson, Department of Surgery, The Royal Free Hospital NHS Trust, London; Penelope Hooper; Ken Lang; Alan Lawford and Malcolm Nudd, Benenden Hospital, Benenden; Elizabeth Liebson MD; Janet Page BSC MB BS MRCP FRCR, Radiology Department, Redhill Hospital, Redhill; John Perry; Paul Pracy MB BS FRCPS; Ann Shaw CNM FMP MSN; Susan Whichello, Radiography Department, King's College Hospital, London; Mary H. Windels MD

ADDITIONAL ILLUSTRATORS Paul Banville, Joanna Cameron, Gary Cross, John Egan, Simone End, Mick Gillah, Mark Iley, Jason Little, Brian Pearce, Peter Ruane, Les Smith, Philip Wilson, Deborah Woodward

PHOTOGRAPHERS Andy Crawford, Steve Gorton, Gary Ombler, Tim Ridley

OTHER PHOTOGRAPHY Steve Bartholomew, Jo Foord, Dave King, Susanna Price, Jules Selmes, Debi Treloar

MODELS Peter Adams, C. Adebusuti, Francesca Agati, Zamir Akram, Danielle Allan, Richard Allen, Susan Alston, Evi Antoniou, Rebecca Ashford, Bert Audubert, Simone Aughterlony, Andrew Baguley, Bridget Bakokodie, Tricia Banham, Austin Barlow, John C. Barrett, Maria Bergman, Lisa Bissell, Acam Blaug, Clare Borg, Lucy Bottomley, Tirzah Bottomley, Laurence Bouvard, Natasha Bowden, Jacqui Boydon, Catherine Brennan, Alison Briegal, Lisa Brighten, Ashley Brown, Garfield Brown, Dominica Buckton, Tom Busch, Bibi Campbell, Steve Capon, Alesandra Caporale, Nefertiti Carnegie, Daniel Carter, Jane Cartwright, Julie Clarke, Sean Clarke, Adam Cockerton, Sam Cocking, Ciro Coleman, Declan Collins, Madeline Collins, Siobhan Contreras, Jonah Coombes, Kevin Cooper, Lilly Cooper, Alan Copeland, Carol Copeland, Barbara Cordell, Caitlin Cordell, Catherine Cordell, Liam Cordell, Ryan Cordell, Sam Cosking, Will Cox, Julia Crane, Andy Crawford, Grace Crawford, Sarah Crean, Mark Cronin, Jessica Currie, Nigel Currie, Laverne Daley, Tariq Daley, Jeff Daniel, Undra Dashdavaa, Katherine Davidson, Lucy de Kinder, Nora Dennis, Terence Dennis, N. J. Deschamps, Flavio Dias, R. S. Dudoo, Maree Duffy, Barbara Egervary, Tony Elgie, Belinda Ellington, Fred English, Mehmet Ergan, Michael Esswood, Steve Etienne, Carole Evans, Julian Evans, Nadia Faris, Jane Farrell, Eric Ferretti, Mary Ferretti, Yvonne Fisher, Larry Francis, Ephraim Frank Otigbah, Annie Fraser, Jane Garioni, Laura Gartry, Hilda Gilbert, Timor Golan-Weyl, Anthony Grant, Sharon Green, Daniel Greendale, Culver Greenidge, Robin Grey, John Gunnery, Maudie Gunzi, Hainsley Guthrie, Charlotte Halfhide, Sarah Halfhide, Carmen Hanlan, Alfie Harrison, Christine Henry, B. M. Hewson, A.W. Hewson, Nigel Hill, Richard Hill, Kit Hillier, Lorraine Hilton, Jignesh Hirani, Manjula Hirani, Chris Hirst, Michael Hoey, Alfred Hoffman, Leila Hoffman, Anthony Howes, Tracey Hughes, Isaac Hughes-Batley, Lewis Hughes-Batley, Richard Hurdle, Faron Isaac, Robert Isaacs, Nora J. Dennis, Ouseynou Jagne, Beverly James, Kaye James, James Jeanes, Jane Jeanes, Thomas Jeanes, Cornell John, Christine Lloyd Jones, Marcia McKoy Jones, Andy Jones-Leopoldie, Cheryl Johnson, Fiona Johnson, John Johnson, Andy Jones, Mahesh Kanani, Hayley Kay, Taryn Kay, L. Keller, Cameron Kelleher, Peter Kelleher, Susan Kelleher, Mark Kennell, Alison Kerl, Amanda Kernot, Claudia Keston, Aline Kleinubing, Deborah Kright, Mahan Krinde, Krishna Kunari, Jane Law, Lisa Law, Roland John Leopoldie, Sarah Layesh-Melamed, Simon Lewandowski, William Liam, Kate Liasis, Leon Liasis, Nina Loving, Doreen Llm, Joanna Lyn Thompson, Denise Mack, Janey Madlani, Lee Mannion, Bryan Marsh, Maija Marsh, Jason Martin, Bobby Maru, David Mathison, Mary Matson, Nicole McClean, Maria McKerzie, Suzanne McLean, Phyllis McMahon, Karen McSween, Jeremy Melling, Hannah Mellows, Paul Mellows, Fiona Mentzel, Hilary Michel, Tony Mills, Olive Mitchell, Catherine Mobley, Alan Montgomery, Lee Moone, Robert Morrison, Teresa Munoz, Nicki Mylonas, Faron Naai, Terry Nelson, Charlotte Nettey, Julie Nettey, Nicole Nnonah, Eva Nowojenska, James O'Connor, Scarlett O'Hara, Akudo Okereafor, Roli Okorodudu, Simon Oon, Chris Orr, E. F. Otilbah, Lucinda Page, Gemma Papineau, Katie Paine, Ann Parkes, Derek Parkes, Nella Passarella, Josephine Peer, Sarah Peers, Flora Pereira, Cecilia Peries, Anthony Perry, Daniela Pettena, Joyce-lyn Phillips, Carol Pieters, Hamilton Pieters, Marcus Pieters, Sheila Power, Erick Rainey, Rebecca Rainsford, Alan Rawlings, Giles Rees, Valerie Renay, John Robey, Erroline Rose, Stuart Rose, Dawn Rowley, Rosie Ruddock, Sam Russell, Sol Rymer, H. Sajjan, Ruth Samuel, Paul Samuels, Rita Sanyaolu, Titi Sanyaolu, Mai Sasaki, Callum Savage, Angela Seaton, Tony de Sergio, Isaac Shaahu, Marianne Sharp, Hannah Vidal-Simon, Phyllis Slegg, Anthony Smalling, Ronella Smalling, Edwin So, Sally Somers, Susan Stowers, Itsuko Sugawara, Cara Sweeney, Sheila Tait, Kaz Takabatake, Flavia Taylor, Peter Taylor, Ann Theato, Graeme Thomas, Jack Thomas, Joanna Thomas, Ian Tilley, Jenny-Ann Topham, C. Turnbull, Andrew Turvill, D. Venerdiano, Richard Vidal, Ahmani Vidal-Simon, Philippe Von Lanthen, Teo-nu Vuong, Alison Waines, Aidan Walls, Rosie Walls, Tim Webster, Chris Wells, Alexander Williams, Henderson Williams, John Williams, Miranda Wilson, Seretta Wilson, Stefan Wilson, Syanice Wilson, Harsha Yogasundram, Matt Yoxall, Dominic Zwemmer

PICTURE CREDITS

The publisher would like to thank the following for permission to reproduce images:

123RF: Tomwang 438 bl; **Alamy Images:** BSIP SA 127 ca; **Courtesy of Dr. R. N. Allan, Q.E.H., University Hospital, Birmingham:** 417 bl; **Courtesy of Miss Sue Bateman, Obstetric Ultrasound Department, St. Peter's Hospital, Chertsey:** 512 b; **Baxter, USA, Carpentier-Edwards, ® S. A. V. ®, Bioprosthesis:** 253 bl; **Biophoto Associates:** 8 t, 149 b, 157 cl, 269 t, 269 ctr, 278 t, 409 b, 442 t, 449 bc, 464 cr; **Courtesy of Dr. D. A. Burns, Leicester Royal Infirmary:** 192 t, b, 193 t, 194 t, 194 br, 203 bl, br, 206 c; **Courtesy of Professor Keith Cartwright, Public Health Laboratory, Gloucester Royal Hospital:** 326 c; **Corbis:** Peter Andrews 29 fcl, 29 tl; Michael Keller 29 fcr; Pascal Parrot/Sygma 8br; **Courtesy of Dr. Erika Denton:** 130 tl, 135 br, 302 t, c, 328, 403 cla, 404 r, 414 r, 418 t, b, 420 r, 474, 487 br; **Courtesy of Mr J. M. Dixon, Edinburgh Breast Unit, Western General Hospital:** 484 t, 486 t; **Courtesy of Professor Peter Ell, Institute of Nuclear Medicine, University College London Medical School:** 137 tl; **Courtesy ESL Healthcare, FLA:** 221 bc; **Courtesy of Dr. A. G. Fraser & Dr. A. Ionescu, University of Wales, College of Medicine, Cardiff:** 255 t, b; **Courtesy of Professor Gleeson, Guy's Hospital, London:** 370; **iStockphoto:** Jaroslaw Wojcik 379 l; **Courtesy of Donald R. Kauder, MD FACS:** 181 bl; **Courtesy of Dr. Gordon, Anatomic Pathology Division of Department of Pathology and Laboratory Medicine, University of Pennsylvania Medical Center:** 433 br; **Great Ormond Street Hospital for Sick Children, Department of Medical Illustration:** 422, 543 b, 548 b, 551, 563; **Courtesy of Dr. C. Dyer & Dr. Owens:** 525 tr, 540 br; **Courtesy of Professor Terry Hamblin, The Royal Bournemouth Hospital Medical Illustration Department:** 278 b; **Robert Harding Picture Library:** Ansell Horn/Phototake NYC 530 b; GJLP/CNRI/Phototake, NY 245 tr, 616 t; **Courtesy of Mr T.Hillard, Poole Hospital, Dorset:** 470 b; **Courtesy of Mr Howard, Institute of Laryngoscopy, National Ear, Nose and Throat Hospital:** 293 t, 294 r; © **Photographic Unit, The Institute of Psychiatry, London:** 349 t; **Courtesy of KeyMed (Medical & Industrial Equipment) Ltd., Southend-on-Sea:** 456 r; **Dr. Alex Leff, MRC Cyclotron Unit, Hammersmith Hospital, London:** 318; **The Leprosy Mission, Peterborough, England:** 173 t, b; **Professor Valerie Lund, Institute of Laryngology & Otology, University College London Medical School:** 129 bl, 291 br; **Professor William Wei, Queen Mary Hospital, Hong Kong:** 294 l; **Courtesy of Dr. N. K. I.McIver, North Sea Medical Centre, Great Yarmouth:** 187; **Mediscan:** 181 br; **Shout Pictures** 181 l; **Moorfields Eye Hospital, London, Department of Medical Illustration:** 361 b; **Courtesy of Dr. Keith Morris, Nottingham City Hospital:** 258; **Oxford Medical Illustration OMI, John Radcliffe Hospital:** 174 r, 262 tl, 549; **Courtesy of Dr. Janet Page, East Surrey Hospital & Community Healthcare Trust:** 131 bl, 157 tc, 288 tl, tr; **Dr. N. R. Patel:** 220 t, 231, 466; **K. R. Patel, Queen Mary's University Hospital, Roehampton:** 473; © **Philips Medical:** 134 br; **Dr. Porter, University College London Hospital:** 273; **PowerStock Photolibrary/Zefa:** 221 cl; **Professor R. H. Rezneck, St. Bartholomew's Hospital, London:** 436; **Courtesy of Mr R. C. G. Russell:** 612 b; **Science Photo Library:** 9 br, 15 b, 130 cbl, 131 tl, br, 132 t, 199 t, 205 t, 214 b, 216 b, 232 bl, bc, 238 br, 254, 264 l, 349 br, 364 t, b, 402 c, 480 t, 481 t, 492 tl, 493 tl, 497, 501; Michael Abbey 171, 211 cl; Department of Clinical Cytogenetics, Addenbrookes Hospital 150 b; Jonathan Ashton 484 br; AJ Photo 489 bl; Dr. Lewis Baxter 345 t; Robert Becker/Custom Medical Stock Photo 265 b; Dr. Beer-Gabel/CNRI 137 br, 407 t; Z. Binor/Custom Medical Stock Photo 476, 477 l; Francis Leroy, Biocosmos 268 b; Biology Media 269 br; Chris Bjornberg 161 b, 330; Simon Brown 214 tr; BSIP Dr. T. Prichard 135 bl; BSIP Estiot 399; BSIP VEM 9 cr, 260 t, 381 t, 386 b, 413, 545; Dr. Jeremy Burgess 189; Dr. Monty Buchsbaum, Peter Arnold Inc. 347; Scott Camazine 251 cr, 567 t, 607; Dr. L. Caro 162 t; CDC 326 t; Department of Nuclear Medicine, Charing Cross Hospital 130 tr, 564; CNRI/Clinique Ste Catherine: 130 ctl; CNRI 4 tr, 124 t, 129 tr, 130 ctr, br, 136 br, 143 t, 144 b, 145 b, 147 b, 158 cl, 175 c, 176 t, 214 ctl, 245, 269, 290, 307 l, 311 t, b, 320, 329 t, c, 352 bl, 381 b, 391 t, 405, 417, 527, 567 b; Custom Medical Stock Photo 352 tr; Mike Devlin 223 tl; Martin Dohrn 351 t; John Durham 269 bl, 566 b; Ralph Eagle 351 cr, 352 br; Ken Eward 265 c, 383 br; Don Fawcett 424 b; Professor C. Ferlaud/CNRI 289 cl, cr; Sue Ford 126 bl, 210 b, 357 bl; Cecil H. Fox153 t, 391 b; Simon Fraser/Medical Physics, RVI, Newcastle-upon-Tyne 465; Simon Fraser/Neuroradiology Department/Newcastle General Hospital 214 cb, 327 b, 329 b; Dr. Freiburger, Peter Arnold Inc. 219 cl; GCa, CNRI 130 cbl, 133 t, 214 ctr, 220 c, 411 tr, 412 tr, 548 t; GJLP-CNRI 227, 477 r; Dr. Peter Gordon 387 bl, br; Eric Grave 126 cr, 180, 272 crb, 316; E. Gueho, CNRI 163 bl; Innersrace Imaging 216 c; Manfred Kage 216 t, 269 bcr, 312, 382, 467 b; Keith/Custom Medical Stock Photo 9 cl, 525 bl; James King-Holmes 499 ca; Mehau Kulyk 4 tl, 5 t, 6 t, 9 bl, 130 bl, 155, 214 cbr, 217, 314, 380, 430 b, 481 b, 500tl, 566 t; David Leah 525 cr, br; Dr. Andrejs Liepins 142 t, 152 b; Lunagrafix 15 t, 132 bl, 236 tr; David McCarthy 152 clb; Dr. P. Marazzi 165, 166 br, 167 t, 168 b, 182, 194 cr, 200 t, 207, 222, 223 tc, 229, 256, 263, 274 br, 279 b, 284 bl, br, 293 b, 339, 363 l, 386 t, 401 bl, 403 t, 493 t, 523 b, 537 c, 538, 546, 556 tl, 558 b, 559; Matt Meadows 133 cr, 503; Astrid & Hanns-Frieder Michler 190 bl, 305 b, 410, 424 t, 460 bl, 491; MIT AI Lab, Surgical Planning Lab, Brigham & Women's Hospital 607 c; Moredun Animal Health Ltd. 163 tr; Professor P. M. Motta & E. Vizza 467 t, 469 tr; Professor P. M.Motta, G. Macchiarelli, & S. A. Nottola 469 tl; Professor P. Motta & A. Caggiati, University "La Sapienza," Rome 395 tl; Professor P. Motta, Correr, & Nottola, University "La Sapienza," Rome 286; Professor P. Motta, Department of Anatomy, University "La Sapienza," Rome 211 cr, 212, 265 t, 267, 269 ctl, 289 bl, 373, 374 bl, 394, 429 tr, 442 b, 470 tl, tr; Professors P. Motta & T. Naguro 395 tr, 429 tl; Professors P. Motta, K. R. Porter, & P. M. Andrews 269 cr; Professors P. M. Motta & J. Van Blerkom 529 cra; Sidney Moulds 396; Larry Mulvehill 174 bc; Dr. Gopal Murti 125 b, 237 cl; National Cancer Institute 179 tr; National Institute of Health 137 c, 332; NIBSC 8 bl, 143 b, 170; Dr. Yorgos Nikas 500 tr; Ohio Nuclear Corporation 132 br; Dr. G. Oran 372 bl; David Parker 205 b, 206 t, 208; Paul Parker 360 cr, 361 t, c, 362 b; Alfred Pasieka 27 b, 129 br, 130 tc, 393, 408; Petit Format/CSI 490; Petit Format/E. M. de Monasterio 354 cr; Petit Format/Nestle 502 t, b; Petit Format/Nestle/Steiner 313 t; Petit Format/CSI 147 t; Dr. M. Phelps & Dr. J. Mazziotta et al/Neurology 354 cl, 372 br; D. Phillips 9 tl, 190 tr, 238 t, 489 t; Philippe Plailly 157 c, 237 br; Parviz M. Pour 457 t; Chris Priest 136 t; Princess Margaret Rose Orthopaedic Hospital 223 cr, 232 cl, 245 cb, 529 crb; Quest 9 tr, 154 t, 429 b, 445; John Radcliffe Hospital 283 r, 326 b, 402 b, 475; Ed Reschke, Peter Arnold Inc. 268 bl; J. C. Revy 4 br, 140, 218 t; Dr. H. C. Robinson 168 t; Salisbury District Hospital 406; Department of Clinical Radiology, Salisbury District Hospital 259 t, b, 307 r, 309, 322, 334 r, 450, 478 b, 512 t; Francoise Sauze 176 br, 530 t; David Scharf 179 bl; Dr. K. F. R. Schiller 392; Science Source 457 b; Secchi, Lecaque, Roussel, UCLAF, CNRI 315, 317, 444, 458, 529 bc; Dr Gary Settles 164, 289 br; St. Bartholomew's Hospital 342, 512 c; Josh Sher 29 tr; St. Stephen's Hospital 183 t, 184; Sinclair Stammers 163 br, 178 b, 214 cl; Dr Linda Stannard, UCT 160 t; Volker Steger/Siemens 152 t; James Stevenson 25 cl, cr, 282 607 b; Andrew Syred 460 br, 529 t; Alexander Tsiaras 139 c; Dr. E. Walker 125 t, 448; M. I. Walker 213; Garry Watson 407 b; Richard Wehr/ Custom Medical Stock Photo 4 bl, 36 t; Wellcome Department of Cognitive Neurology 343 t; Western Opthalmic Hospital 356, 362 t, 363 t; **Dr. D. Singh, Institute of Orthopaedics, Royal National Orthpaedic Hospital, London:** 223 tr; **St. John's Institute of Dermatology, London:** 195 b, 198 cra, 201 t, 204, 210 t; **Courtesy of Dr. Peter Stradling c/o Dr. John Stradling, Osler Chest Unit, Churchill Hospital, Oxford:** 308 b; **Viewing Medicine:** 135 t, 202 t, 300 br, 305 t, 484 bl; **M. I. Walker, Microworld Services:** 190 br, 480 b; **Dr. Jean Watkins:** 167 b, 486 cl; **Philip Watson:** 6 b, 498; **The Wellcome Trust MPL:** 137 tr, 166 t, 172 bl, 188, 195 cr, 196, 200 b, 201 b, 202 cb, 219 t, 223 cl, 224, 230, 246, 251 cl, 253 br, 260 b, 261, 262 r, 264 t, 274 b, 279 t, 281 l, r, 283 t, 285 t, bl, 301, 302 b, 304 l, 327 t, 340, 345 b, 348, 355 t, 364 c, 371, 374 bc, 389, 390, 401 br, 404 l, 411 tl, 412 tl, 420 l, 431, 433 bl, 435, 456 l, 492 tr, 525 tl, 534, 537 b, 539 b, 540 bl, 541, 542, 543 t, 555, 556 tr, 557 tr, 558 t, 614 bl, br; **Dr David Williams & Dr Paula Hannant:** 195 t, & V. Ankrett 198 clb, 199 b, 202 cl, 232 cr, 355 b; **Courtesy of Professor A. Wright, Institute of Laryngology and Otology, Royal Free and University College Medical School, London:** 613 t.

All other images © Dorling Kindersley
For further information see: www.dkimages.com